Infectious
Diseases
in Primary Care

Infectious Diseases in Primary Care

CHARLES S. BRYAN, MD, FACP, FRCP (Edin)

Heyward Gibbes Distinguished Professor of Internal Medicine
Director, Center for Bioethics and Medical Humanities
Assistant Dean for Medical Humanities
Formerly Chair, Department of Medicine
University of South Carolina School of Medicine
Columbia, South Carolina

W.B. SAUNDERS COMPANY
An Imprint of Elsevier Science
Philadelphia   London   New York   St. Louis   Sydney   Toronto

W.B. Saunders Company
An Imprint of Elsevier Science

The Curtis Center
Independence Square West
Philadelphia, Pennsylvania 19106

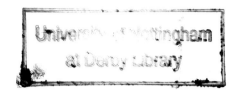

Library of Congress Cataloging-in-Publication Data

Bryan, Charles S.
    Infectious diseases in primary care / Charles S. Bryan.
        p. ; cm.
    Includes bibliographical references and index.
    ISBN 0-7216-9056-4
    1. Communicable diseases. 2. Primary care (Medicine) I. Title.
    [DNLM: 1. Bacterial Infections. 2. Primary Health Care. 3. Virus Diseases. WC 200
B915i 2002]
    RC111 .B745 2002
    616.9—dc21
                                                                        2001044752

Acquisitions Editor: Elizabeth Fathman
Publishing Services Manager: Patricia Tannian
Book Design Manager: Gail Morey Hudson
Cover Designer: Diane Beasley

INFECTIOUS DISEASES IN PRIMARY CARE   ISBN 0-7216-9056-4

Printed in United States of America
GW/MVY

Last digit is the print number   9   8   7   6   5   4   3   2   1

For

Donna, and Chandlee and Emily, and Anna and Amelia

Contributors

ROBERT T. BALL, M.D., M.P.H.
Director, HIV/AIDS Services,
South Carolina Department of Health and Environmental Control,
Columbia, South Carolina

WILLIAM H. BARKER, M.D.
Professor of Preventive Medicine and Gerontology,
University of Rochester School of Medicine and Dentistry,
Rochester, Minnesota

ERIC R. BRENNER, M.D.
Clinical Professor of Medicine,
University of South Carolina School of Medicine,
Columbia, South Carolina;
Chargé de Coeurs, University of Geneva School of Medicine,
Geneva, Switzerland

EDWIN A. BROWN, M.D.
Associate Professor of Medicine,
Medical University of South Carolina,
Charleston, South Carolina

CHARLES S. BRYAN, M.D.
Heyward Gibbes Distinguished Professor of Internal Medicine,
Director, Center for Bioethics and Medical Humanities,
Assistant Dean for Medical Humanities,
University of South Carolina School of Medicine,
Columbia, South Carolina

CHARLES CAMISA, M.D.
Professor and Vice-Chairman,
Department of Dermatology, The Cleveland Clinic,
Cleveland, Ohio

J. ROBERT CANTEY, M.D.
Professor of Medicine,
Director, Division of Infectious Diseases,
Medical University of South Carolina,
Charleston, South Carolina

VALDA CHIJIDE, M.D.
Fellow, Division of Infectious Diseases,
Medical College of Georgia,
Augusta, Georgia

RADU CLINCEA, M.D.
Fellow, Division of Infectious Diseases,
Medical University of South Carolina,
Charleston, South Carolina

MYRON S. COHEN, M.D.
Professor of Medicine, Microbiology, and Immunology,
Chief, Division of Infectious Diseases,
University of North Carolina School of Medicine,
Chapel Hill, North Carolina

SUSAN M. COX, M.D.
Professor of Obstetrics and Gynecology,
Assistant Dean for Professional Education,
University of Texas Southwestern Medical Center,
Dallas, Texas

C. WARREN DERRICK, Jr., M.D.
William Weston Professor and Chair,
Department of Pediatrics,
University of South Carolina School of Medicine,
Columbia, South Carolina

SRI EDUPAGANTI, M.D.
Clinical Assistant Professor of Medicine,
University of North Carolina School of Medicine,
Chapel Hill, North Carolina

DAVID O. FREEDMAN, M.D.
Associate Professor of Medicine,
Director, UAB Travelers Health Clinic,
Division of Geographic Medicine,
University of Alabama School of Medicine,
Birmingham, Alabama

R. BROOKS GAINER II, M.D.
Clinical Associate Professor of Medicine,
University of West Virginia School of Medicine,
Morgantown, West Virginia

JOHN R. GRAYBILL, M.D.
Professor of Medicine,
Director, Division of Infectious Diseases,
University of Texas Health Sciences Center,
San Antonio, Texas

STEPHEN B. GREENBERG, M.D.
Herman Brown Teaching Professor and Associate Chairman,
Baylor College of Medicine;
Chief, Medicine Service, Ben Taub General Hospital,
Houston, Texas

DAVID GREENHOUSE, M.D.
Assistant Professor of Family and Preventive Medicine,
University of South Carolina School of Medicine,
Columbia, South Carolina

SANJEEV GREWAL, M.D.
Assistant Professor of Ophthalmology,
University of South Carolina School of Medicine,
Columbia, South Carolina

NILI GUJADHUR, M.D.
Fellow, Division of Allergy, Immunology, and Infectious Diseases,
University of Medicine and Dentistry of New Jersey—
    Robert Wood Johnson Medical School,
New Brunswick, New Jersey

DAVID R. HABURCHAK, M.D.
Professor of Medicine and Director,
Internal Medicine Residency Program,
Medical College of Georgia,
Augusta, Georgia

SALLY A. HARDING, M.D.
Clinical Professor of Pathology,
University of South Carolina School of Medicine;
Medical Director,
Microbiology and Molecular Pathology Laboratories,
Palmetto Richland Memorial Hospital,
Columbia, South Carolina

STEPHEN J. HAWES, M.D.
Clinical Professor of Medicine,
University of South Carolina School of Medicine,
Columbia, South Carolina

TONYA JAGNEAUX, M.D.
Chief Resident, Louisiana State University
    Internal Medicine Residency in Baton Rouge,
Baton Rouge, Louisiana

JOSEPH F. JOHN, Jr., M.D.
Professor of Medicine,
University of Medicine and Dentistry of New Jersey—
    Robert Wood Johnson Medical School,
New Brunswick, New Jersey

GEORGE H. KARAM, M.D.
Professor of Medicine,
Louisiana State University School of Medicine in New Orleans;
Head, Department of Medicine, Earl K. Long Medical Center,
Baton Rouge, Louisiana

JOSEPH E. KOHN, Pharm.D.
Assistant Professor of Pharmacy,
University of South Carolina,
Columbia, South Carolina

GEORGE S. KOTCHMAR, Jr., M.D.
Associate Professor of Clinical Pediatrics,
Director, Division of Infectious Diseases,
University of South Carolina School of Medicine,
Columbia, South Carolina

JULIE Y. LO, M.D.
Fellow, Maternal-Fetal Medicine,
University of Texas Southwestern Medical Center,
Dallas, Texas

SHARON J. LONGSHORE, R.Ph., M.D.
Fellow, Department of Dermatology,
The Cleveland Clinic,
Cleveland, Ohio

J. DAVID OSGUTHORPE, M.D.
Professor of Otolaryngology–Head and Neck Surgery,
Medical University of South Carolina,
Charleston, South Carolina

BOSKO POSTIC, M.D.
Professor of Medicine,
Director, Division of Infectious Diseases,
University of South Carolina School of Medicine,
Columbia, South Carolina

AMAR SAFDAR, M.D.
Associate Professor of Medicine,
University of South Carolina School of Medicine,
Columbia, South Carolina

ARLENE C. SEÑA, M.D.
Clinical Assistant Professor of Medicine,
University of North Carolina School of Medicine,
Chapel Hill, North Carolina

JEANNE S. SHEFFIELD, M.D.
Assistant Professor, Department of Obstetrics and Gynecology,
University of Texas Southwestern Medical Center,
Dallas, Texas

JAMES R. STALLWORTH, M.D.
Associate Professor of Pediatrics,
Director, Division of General Pediatrics,
University of South Carolina,
Columbia, South Carolina

ROBERT L. SWORDS, M.D.
Fellow, Division of Infectious Diseases,
Medical University of South Carolina,
Charleston, South Carolina

ROHIT TALWANI, M.D.
Assistant Professor of Medicine,
University of South Carolina School of Medicine,
Columbia, South Carolina

NATHAN M. THIELMAN, M.D., M.P.H.
Assistant Professor of Medicine,
Duke University Medical Center,
Durham, North Carolina

Preface

Infectious Diseases in Primary Care began in 1967 with the following case:

> A 24-year-old man was admitted to the medical service of a major teaching hospital with fever and anterior neck pain of recent onset. Examination revealed a tender, symmetric swelling anterior to the trachea just above the sternal notch. He was treated with aspirin for acute thyroiditis. Corticosteroids were added when fever, tachycardia, and anorexia progressed. On the fifth hospital day, concern for his increasing systemic toxicity prompted surgical exploration, which revealed an abscess that contained thin, watery, foul-smelling pus. Cardiac arrest occurred on the operating table, and resuscitation was unsuccessful.

As an intern in pathology that year, I performed the autopsy. I was fascinated by the disease and its bacteriology, but deeply troubled by the human dimension. The patient was an employee in the hospital where he died. His wife was expecting their first child. This case and others prompted me to do an internship in internal medicine the next year, and I came to realize that my greatest joys and sorrows usually involved infectious diseases. In 1974 I returned to my hometown as the first fully trained adult infectious diseases specialist in central South Carolina, and since then I have kept up four career identities: infectious diseases consultant, hospital epidemiologist, medical school faculty member, and editor of a state medical journal. In each of these roles I have treasured especially my relationships with primary care physicians. The purpose of this book is to present information about infectious diseases that is relevant and up to date for primary care.

The goals of *Infectious Diseases in Primary Care* are to help primary care clinicians, in order of priority, to (1) prevent tragedy, (2) practice cost-effective medicine, (3) promote conservative use of antimicrobials, and (4) appreciate the limitations of our knowledge, perhaps prompting questions that will add to the knowledge base. These goals are discussed more fully in Chapter 1. Special emphasis is given to emergencies (Chapter 6) because of the recognition that primary care clinicians, compared with their hospital-based counterparts, are at a huge disadvantage. Primary care clinicians often see patients who harbor life-threatening infections, but before the telltale symptoms and signs have appeared. Yet primary care clinicians are under increasing pressure to maintain crammed schedules and to be "cost effective," with parsimonious use of laboratory tests and imaging studies. To determine specific problems that need highlighting, a survey was conducted among fellows of the Infectious Diseases Society of America. The findings (see Chapter 6) were somewhat surprising and, it is hoped, will be helpful.

The book is written mainly for the primary care clinician working in the ambulatory care setting. He or she may also make rounds in a nursing home, follow up on patients being treated with parenteral antimicrobial therapy at home, and write (or call in) the initial orders for patients being admitted to the hospital. However, the primary care physician will nearly always seek assistance for difficult diagnostic or therapeutic problems, including the care of the seriously ill patient. The definition of primary care and its delineation from specialty and subspecialty care are, of course, arbitrary and controversial. However, clinicians who follow their patients in the hospital, and especially in the intensive care unit, will want access to one or more of the superb comprehensive textbooks of infectious diseases. I welcome suggestions for improving the book and can be reached at cbryan@richmed.medpark.sc.edu.

Acknowledgments

My debts to colleagues in infectious diseases and in the various primary care disciplines are too numerous to mention. I am especially indebted to Sanchia Mitchell for her secretarial assistance, Patricia Stoud for reviewing literature citations, and Field Branham, Rebecca A. Wilson, Shirley Frick, and Peter A. Zvejnieks for help with the illustrations.

Charles S. Bryan
Columbia, South Carolina
December 2001

Contents

Infectious
Diseases
in Primary Care

1 Approach to Infectious Diseases in Office Practice

CHARLES S. BRYAN

Mankind has three great enemies, fever, famine, and war. And of these by far the greatest, by far the most terrible, is fever.

William Osler, 1897

Infectious disease is one of the few genuine adventures left in the world . . . however secure and well regulated civilized life may become, bacteria, protozoa, viruses, infected fleas, lice, ticks, mosquitoes and bedbugs will always lurk in the shadows ready to pounce when neglect, poverty, famine or war lets down the defenses.

Hans Zinsser, 1935

This book is designed to help primary care clinicians recognize life-threatening emergencies, practice cost-effective medicine, promote rational use of antimicrobials, and contribute to the knowledge base of clinical medicine, in that order of priority.

Recognition of life-threatening emergencies receives top priority because of the serious consequences of improperly managed infections, whether measured as death, disability, or staggering health care costs. Primary care clinicians see countless patients with such nonspecific complaints as fever, headache, and myalgias. These illnesses are usually self-limited and go undiagnosed; hence the common term "viral syndrome." Occasional patients with nonspecific complaints have life-threatening disease such as staphylococcal septicemia or Rocky Mountain spotted fever. In preparing this book, we conducted a survey among fellows of the Infectious Diseases Society of America (IDSA) concerning mistakes they had encountered over the years that led to death, disability, or litigation (see Chapter 6). We hope the findings will help primary care clinicians keep such errors to an irreducible minimum.

Practice of cost-effective medicine receives second priority because infectious diseases include many of the more common problems encountered in primary care practice. Which patients can be self-diagnosed and treated over the telephone? Which can be managed in the office by standard protocols, without being seen by a physician? Which require attempts to make a precise etiologic diagnosis by cultures, serologic tests, and other methods? Which require imaging studies to delineate the extent of disease? Which require antimicrobials and, if so, which drugs? What should be the frequency of scheduled follow-up visits? When can patients return to school or work? Billions of dollars of direct and indirect health care costs hang in the balance. We hope that the information in this book will help primary care clinicians design and implement cost-effective strategies, and to that end we have made liberal use of guidelines and algorithms.

Promotion of rational antimicrobial use receives third priority because of the mounting problem of drug resistance. Some authorities believe that the success of antibiotics will prove to be a short-lived phenomenon and that we are entering a postantibiotic era. Yet primary care clinicians face enormous pressures from patients to prescribe. Social historians observe that the introduction of penicillin in civilian medical practice during the 1940s changed forever the nature of the doctor-patient relationship. From that time patients have increasingly expected and insisted on technical solutions, not wise counsel. We hope that the information in this book will help primary care clinicians devise strategies for rational use of antimicrobials through optimal prescribing practices and patient education.

Contribution to the knowledge base of clinical medicine receives priority because we believe that primary care clinicians have much to add. Computer-based technologies should enable clinicians, working together, to provide meaningful data regarding the optimal management of commonly encountered problems. DNA-based technologies should enable primary care clinicians, working in concert with diagnostic laboratories, to obtain data regarding the epidemiology and pathogenesis of infectious diseases. Primary care clinicians are often the first to bring previously undescribed diseases to the attention of public health officials (legionnaire's disease is a recent example). We hope that the information in this book will stimulate primary care clinicians to ask questions and design research protocols that will modify or change many of the conclusions reached herein.

This book is designed for the primary care clinician who practices mainly in the office setting. The clinician who undertakes the diagnosis and management of more complicated infectious disease problems in the hospital setting will want access to the excellent encyclopedic textbooks in this field. We hope that the information in the book will not always satisfy the primary care clinician's desire for up-to-date information, and to that end Appendix 5 discusses ways to keep up with breaking information. This chapter provides an overview of the diagnosis, management, and prevention of infectious diseases in the office setting.

SUGGESTED READING

Armstrong D, Cohen J, eds. Infectious Diseases. London: Mosby; 1999.

Gantz NM, Brown RB, Berk SL, et al., eds. Manual of Clinical Problems in Infectious Diseases. 4th ed., Philadelphia: Lippincott Williams & Wilkins; 1999.

Gorbach SL, Bartlett JG, Blacklow NR, eds. Infectious Diseases. 2nd ed., Philadelphia: W.B. Saunders; 1998.

Mandell GL, Bennett JE, Dolin R, eds. Mandell, Douglas, and Bennett's Principles and Practice of Infectious Diseases. 5th ed., Philadelphia: Churchill Livingstone; 2000.

Root RK, Waldvogel F, Corey L, Stamm WE, eds. Clinical Infectious Diseases: A Practical Approach. New York: Oxford University Press; 1999.

Rose BD, ed. UpToDate. Wellesley, MA: UpToDate, Inc.; 2000 (www.uptodate.com).

Shulman ST, Phair JP, Peterson LR, Warren JR, eds. The Biologic and Clinical Basis of Infectious Diseases. 5th ed., Philadelphia: W.B. Saunders; 1997.

Epidemiology

Infections still cause about one third of deaths worldwide and are the leading cause of death, mainly because of disease in developing countries. In developed countries, including the United States, improvements in sanitation and hygiene during the 19th century lowered the death rates from infectious diseases even before the dramatic impact of antimicrobial agents and new vaccines. However, recent data suggest that mortality from infectious diseases in the United States is actually increasing. Between 1980 and 1992, mortality from infections increased by 58% and age-adjusted death rates increased by 39%, so that taken as a group infectious diseases were the third leading cause of death (up from fifth in 1980). The epidemiology and pathogenesis of infection can be discussed in several complementary ways.

First, consider the formula for infection:

$$\text{Likelihood of infection} = \frac{\text{Virulence of microorganism} \times \text{Number of microorganisms}}{\text{Likelihood of infection host resistance}}$$

Microorganisms are virulent to the extent that they cause disease in previously healthy individuals—that is, when host resistance is high. Virulent microorganisms are capable of eluding host defenses, invading tissues, and elaborating toxins. Highly virulent pathogens, such as *Mycobacterium tuberculosis, Francisella tularensis* (tularemia), and *Yersinia pestis* (plague), require only a few microorganisms to cause infection in a normal host. Most of the pathogens encountered in daily clinical practice, such as *Streptococcus pneumoniae*

and *Staphylococcus aureus,* require many thousands of microorganisms to cause disease. Infection is therefore preceded by colonization, the multiplication of microorganisms on epithelial surfaces without evidence of disease. Low host resistance allows less virulent or opportunistic pathogens to cause infection. Examples are *Staphylococcus epidermidis* infection in patients with surgically implanted foreign bodies, anaerobic bacterial infection in patients whose tissues have been disrupted or deprived of adequate blood supply, and *Cryptococcus neoformans* infection in patients taking immunosuppressive drugs. The many factors that lower host resistance are discussed in Chapter 3. Virulence is sometimes defined in terms of the percentage of infected persons in whom serious disease develops or in some instances as the case-fatality rate.

A second framework for understanding infections is the epidemiologic triad, or chain of infection:

Reservoir → Means of transmission → Susceptible host

All pathogens must have a reservoir or sanctuary in which they survive and multiply before causing disease. For some the reservoir consists of the animate or inanimate environment; for others the only reservoir is *Homo sapiens sapiens.* The reservoir is often but not always the source from which the infection is acquired. For example, a food handler colonized with *Salmonella enteritidis* might be the reservoir, whereas custard prepared by the same food handler might be the source of an outbreak of salmonellosis. Infections transmitted from other vertebrates are known as zoonoses. Some human pathogens actively multiply in water, soil, or plants. Others, such as *Legionella pneumophila* (legionnaires' disease), *Bacillus anthracis,* and the spores of *Clostridium tetani* (tetanus), can survive for long periods without multiplying in hostile environments. The means of transmission from the reservoir or source to a susceptible host can be direct or indirect. Direct transmission includes physical contact and droplets (produced, for example, by coughing or sneezing). Three types of indirect transmission are recognized: (1) transmission by vehicles (contaminated water, food, biologic products, including blood products and transplanted organs, or physical objects); (2) transmission by vectors (usually insects, such as mosquitoes or ticks); and (3) transmission by aerosols, that is, airborne suspensions of tiny particles (1 to 5 μm in diameter and thus much smaller than particles such as droplets, in which is direct transmission).

A third framework for understanding infections concerns exogenous versus endogenous microorganisms. Exogenous infections arise from the animate or inanimate environment, whereas endogenous infections arise from the patient's flora. Clinicians often witness a dynamic interplay between exogenous and endogenous infection, as illustrated by the following case:

PATIENT 1

In a 70-year-old man in previously good health but with a history of frequent respiratory infections, an upper respiratory tract infection developed, followed by pneumonia. *Streptococcus pneumoniae, Moraxella catarrhalis,* and *Haemophilus influenzae* were isolated from sputum cultures. The pneumonia did not resolve, and an empyema containing foul-smelling pus developed. The patient died of hemorrhage into the empyema cavity 3 months after the onset of illness.

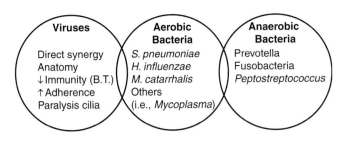

Time

FIG. 1-1   In respiratory disease a progression often occurs from viral infection (exogenously acquired) to infection by virulent bacteria (endogenously acquired, through colonization) to infection by opportunistic bacteria (such as anaerobic bacteria that are part of the normal bacterial flora). This model also applies to certain other types of infection. (From Brook I. Oropharyngeal anaerobes. In: Johnson JT, Yu VL, eds. Infectious Diseases and Antimicrobial Therapy of the Ears, Nose, and Throat. Philadelphia: W.B. Saunders Company; 1997: 193-200.)

This case from the preantibiotic era—the year was 1919 and the patient was Sir William Osler—illustrates how viral upper respiratory tract infection, acquired exogenously from other humans, predisposes to infection from virulent bacterial pathogens, which in turn predisposes to infection by opportunistic pathogens such as anaerobes (as evidenced by the foul-smelling pus). This sequence of events is well recognized in the case of respiratory infections (Figure 1-1). Another example is pelvic inflammatory disease; an exogenous pathogen (*Neisseria gonorrhoeae* or *Chlamydia pneumoniae*) predisposes to pelvic inflammatory disease in which numerous opportunistic pathogens, mainly anaerobic bacteria, are present.

We should remember that infectious disease is usually an accidental event in a world in which each of us lives intimately with billions of microorganisms. In many cases we depend on them, as they on us, for survival. Death is undesirable from the microbe's perspective as well as ours. It is sometimes better to tolerate colonization or even infection with potential pathogens than to stamp it out at all costs.

 KEY POINTS

EPIDEMIOLOGY

⊃ Morbidity and mortality from infectious diseases in the United States are increasing because of the combined impact of the acquired immunodeficiency syndrome/human immunodeficiency virus (AIDS/HIV) epidemic, an aging population, diseases of medical progress, immigration, and emergence of new pathogens.

⊃ Human factors promoting the emergence and spread of infectious diseases include suburbanization, outdoor activities, centralized food processing and distribution, ventilation systems, and international travel.

⊃ Often a dynamic interplay occurs between exogenous infections (arising from the animate or inanimate environment) and endogenous infections (arising from a person's own resident flora).

SUGGESTED READING

Cohen ML. Changing patterns of infectious diseases. Nature 2000; 406: 762-767.

Nelson KE, Williams CM, Graham NMH. Infectious Diseases Epidemiology: Theory and Practice. Gaithersburg, Maryland: Aspen Publishers, Inc.; 2001.

Pinner R, Teutsch SM, Simonsen L, et al. Trends in infectious diseases mortality in the United States. JAMA 1996; 275: 189-193.

Rothman KJ, Greenland S, eds. Modern Epidemiology: 2nd ed., Lippincott Williams & Wilkins; 1998.

Swartz MN. Impact of antimicrobial agents and chemotherapy from 1972 to 1998. Antimicrob Agents Chemother 2000; 44: 2009-2016.

Host Defenses

Infectious diseases are often discussed with military metaphors; hence we speak of host defenses and invaders. Host defenses include intact epithelial barriers, the B-lymphocyte system (responsible for antibody synthesis or humoral immunity), the T-lymphocyte system (responsible for cell-mediated immunity), the complement system (which facilitates the inflammatory response and assumes responsibility for humoral immunity in the absence of specific antibodies), and polymorphonuclear neutrophils (responsible for phagocytosis and killing of virulent bacteria). These specific components act selectively against specific pathogens. In recent years the knowledge of host defenses has been enhanced by the discovery of cytokines, small molecules released by cells that help to orchestrate the immune response by communicating with other cells. This section briefly reviews these components.

Epithelial Barriers to Infection

A psalmist observed, "My wounds stink and are corrupt because of my foolishness" (Psalms 38:5). In providing perhaps the first account of an anaerobic bacterial infection (the foul odor of his wounds is diagnostic thereof), the psalmist bore witness to the importance of intact epithelial barriers. Few organisms can penetrate intact skin. Mucosal surfaces, being moist, support microbial colonization more readily but are equipped with physical barriers (e.g., mucus and cilia, peristalsis) and secretions having antimicrobial properties. These include lysozyme and secretory immunoglobulin A. Potential pathogens that successfully breach the epithelial barriers encounter two defense systems: the acute inflammatory response, which can be activated within minutes to hours and is nonspecific (i.e., it needs no prior experience with the pathogen in question), and the specific immune response, which depends on B and T lymphocytes and, in the absence of prior experience with the pathogen in question, requires days to weeks to become fully operative.

Acute Inflammatory Response

The familiar signs of local inflammation, known in Latin as *calor, rubor, dolor,* and *tumor* and in English as warmth, erythema (redness), pain, and swelling, reflect a process designed to contain invading microorganisms and to initiate the development of specific immunity. The key elements are polymorphonuclear neutrophils (PMNs), monocytes and macrophages, the complement system, and various small molecules known as cytokines and chemokines. Eosinophils are important when the invading microorganisms are parasites.

The earliest event seems to be the secretion of cytokines and chemokines by various cells—monocytes, macrophages, fibroblasts, stromal cells, and others—that sense the presence of invaders. One chemokine, interleukin-8, changes the shape of circulating PMNs so that they can migrate through the vascular endothelium (diapedesis) and move toward the invading pathogens (chemotaxis). Other cytokines prompt the bone marrow to release stored PMNs and to increase its production of new ones, causing the familiar leukocytosis of acute bacterial infection. PMNs are able on their own to trap microorganisms against surfaces and ingest them (phagocytosis), but this process works more efficiently when the microorganisms have been coated with antibodies or complement factors (opsonization, from the Greek "to prepare for a meal"). The complement system consists of more than 30 serum proteins that are activated in an orderly fashion (called the complement cascade) by either of two pathways: the classical pathway (which requires specific antibody or C-reactive protein, an acute-phase reactant) or the alternative pathway (a more primitive system that does not require specific antibody). Activated complement proteins enhance the acute inflammatory response, neutralize viruses, opsonize bacteria and other microorganisms, kill certain gram-negative bacteria, and promote the development of specific immunity. Although PMNs, aided by complement, provide the most dramatic and visible aspects of the acute inflammatory response, monocytes and macrophages (collectively known as mononuclear phagocytes) also have at least two key roles: they elaborate important cytokines, and they digest and process the invading microorganisms in a way that initiates the development of specific immunity.

The events that make up the acute inflammatory response are often designated the acute-phase response to infection. Clinically detectable features of the acute-phase response include leukocytosis; fever; changes in the levels of numerous serum proteins, including C-reactive protein; mobilization of energy sources from muscle, fat, and albumin; and increased production of several key hormones, including both insulin and glucagon from the pancreas. Leukemoid reactions (extremely high white blood cell counts), marked hypoalbuminemia, hypoglycemia, and, in patients with diabetes mellitus, hyperosmolar coma or ketoacidosis occasionally result.

Humoral Immunity (B-Cell Immunity)

Specific immunity is broadly divided into B-cell (humoral) and T-cell (cell-mediated) immunity on the basis of the lymphocytes and other cells involved.

Antibodies (immunoglobulins) are complex glycoprotein molecules that bind with high affinity to molecules recognized as foreign, such as peptides, proteins, polysaccharides, and glycolipids. Such molecules are known as antigens; an antigen that elicits a specific immune response is also called an immunogen. The antibody-producing limb of the immune system is called humoral immunity because its products, antibodies with antigen-binding specificity, are present throughout the circulation, ready to act almost anywhere on short notice. The functions of antibodies include opsonization of particles, permitting more efficient ingestion by phagocytic cells (PMNs and monocyte-macrophages); activation of complement through the classical pathway; neutralization of microbial toxins and viruses (hence the basis for most vaccines); and facilitation of contact-dependent killing by cytotoxic natural killer cells.

Antibodies are of five types:

- Immunoglobulin M (IgM). This is the first antibody to be synthesized in response to a new antigen. It is a large molecule, and its size prevents it from leaving the bloodstream or from crossing the placenta. One of its primary functions is to activate complement, which facilitates the inflammatory response by causing vasodilatation, attracting PMNs to the site of infection, and promoting phagocytosis. IgM normally makes up about 10% of serum immunoglobulin and has a half-life in serum of only 2 to 3 days.

- Immunoglobulin G (IgG). This antibody appears after IgM following the first contact with a new antigen. Compared with IgM it has more antigen-binding specificity. Unlike IgM, it enters extravascular compartments (tissues and body fluids) and crosses the placenta. IgG is by far the most abundant serum antibody, making up about 75% of serum immunoglobulin, and has a half-life of 23 to 70 days. For these reasons, IgG represents the major specific defense against numerous microorganisms. Four subclasses of IgG, designated IgG_1 through IgG_4, are recognized. IgG_1, which activates complement and binds especially to protein antigens, is the most abundant. IgG_2 binds especially to polysaccharide antigens and is therefore an essential defense against encapsulated bacteria such as *H. influenzae* and *S. pneumoniae*. IgG_3 is important for neutralization of viruses. IgG_4, although representing only about 4% of the total IgG, may be especially important for protection of the respiratory tract, since selective IgG_4 deficiency is associated with respiratory infections such as sinusitis and bronchiectasis.

- Immunoglobulin A (IgA). This antibody consists of two subclasses, IgA_1 and IgA_2, which tend to differ in structure and function. IgA_1 is produced mainly in the bone marrow, is the predominant form of IgA found in serum, and is usually monomeric (i.e., consisting of a single antibody molecule). IgA_2 provides important local immunity on mucosal surfaces, since it is the major antibody in tears, saliva, nasal secretions, and gastrointestinal secretions. IgA does not bind complement. Some of the newer strategies for vaccination take advantage of the protective role of IgA on mucosal surfaces. In some bacteria, however, specific enzymes known as IgA proteases destroy IgA.

- Immunoglobulin E (IgE). This antibody is present in serum in only small amounts but is present on receptors on mast cells and basophils. In clinical medicine it is known mainly for the unwanted effects associated with immediate hypersensitivity reactions (type I reactions, characterized by anaphylaxis, bronchospasm, angioedema, or urticaria). Its original purpose may have been to protect against parasitic infections, and it possibly plays a gatekeeper role in regulating humoral immunity.

- Immunoglobulin D (IgD). IgD represents less than 0.2% of serum antibody and has no known major function.

Most infectious diseases evoke an antibody response, and measurement of IgM and IgG antibodies is the traditional basis for serologic diagnosis. High levels of antibodies (hypergammaglobulinemia) characterize many infections. Undesirable aspects of antibodies include the formation of circulating immune complexes (which can cause glomerulonephritis and other localized pathology), cryoglobulins (which can cause vasculitis associated with purpura, arthralgia, and glomerulonephritis), and autoantibodies (which can cause rheumatic heart disease and also various types of connective tissue disease).

Cell-Mediated Immunity (T-Cell Immunity)

The term "cell-mediated immunity" encompasses specific immune responses that are mediated not by antibodies but rather by lymphocytes, macrophages, and cytokines. The lymphocytes involved in cell-mediated immunity, called T cells because their instructions come from the thymus gland, are recruited to sites of foreign invasion by various signals. T cells maintain a constant surveillance system against antigens they have encountered in past experience. For example, the patient with a positive tuberculin skin test possesses T lymphocytes that devote their lives to searching for the antigens of *M. tuberculosis*. The functions of cell-mediated immunity include discrimination of "self" from "nonself" or "foreign" to keep one's immune system from turning against one's own body; destruction of cells infected with certain viruses; destruction of intracellular bacteria such as *M. tuberculosis, Listeria monocytogenes,* and *Salmonella* species; defense against many fungal and parasitic infections; and destruction of cells that show evidence of neoplasia (cancer).

T cells require that antigen-presenting cells present antigens to them in an orderly fashion. All cells except red blood cells can present antigens, but certain cells, sometimes called professional antigen-presenting cells, are crucial to the development of specific immunity. These include monocytes, macrophages, dendritic cells (which are modified macrophages), and B lymphocytes. In response to a foreign antigen, antigen-presenting cells take up the antigen by phagocytosis, break it down into small peptide molecules, assemble major histocompatibility (MHC) antigens on the cell's outer surface, and present on the surface a package that includes the processed foreign antigen, the T-cell receptor, and the MHC molecule. In this way the lymphocyte simultaneously "sees" both the foreign antigen (properly dressed for presentation) and also the "self" nature of the antigen-presenting cell (represented by the MHC molecule, since histocompatibility antigens enable the immune system to distinguish between "self" and "nonself"). CD4 lymphocytes respond to antigen-presenting cells that exhibit MHC class II antigens, whereas CD8 lymphocytes respond to antigen-presenting cells that exhibit MHC class I antigens. CD4 cells are essential to initiating an immune response, since the antigen presented is invariably foreign (nonself). The term "cell-mediated immunity" denotes an intricate system that patrols against foreign antigens in the context of distinguishing "self" from "nonself."

Further mention should be made of cytokines, the small molecules that serve as biologic response modifiers (or modulators) of the immune system. Initially, cytokines were given names that seemed to describe their functions, such as interferon, colony-stimulating factor, and tumor necrosis factor. When it later became apparent that cytokines can have several functions and often work at cross-purposes, newly discovered or renamed cytokines were called interleukins and assigned a number (e.g., interleukin-1, interleukin-6, interleukin-18). Cytokines are produced by cells of many types, but especially by macrophages and dendritic cells. Interleukin-1 causes fever and induces the acute-phase response, the production of other cytokines, B- and T-cell activation, and bone marrow cell proliferation. Tumor necrosis factor-α also causes fever, activates macrophages and neutrophils, induces the production of other cytokines, and mediates shock caused by gram-negative bacteria. Efforts to determine whether cytokines or their antagonists will be useful therapeutically are well under way.

 ## KEY POINTS

HOST DEFENSES

⊃ Epithelial barriers to infection—intact skin and mucosal surfaces—are formidable obstacles to most microorganisms under most circumstances.

⊃ The nonspecific acute inflammatory response, mobilized within minutes to hours of tissue invasion by a microorganism, depends on polymorphonuclear neutrophils (PMNs), monocytes and macrophages, the complement system, and small molecules known as cytokines and chemokines.

⊃ Specific immunity, which develops days to weeks after invasion by a microorganism, is of two types: humoral (or B-cell) immunity and cell-mediated (or T-cell) immunity.

⊃ Humoral immunity is concerned with the production of antibodies (immunoglobulins), which opsonize foreign particles for phagocytosis, activate complement, neutralize microbial toxins and viruses, and facilitate contact-dependent killing by cytotoxic natural killer cells.

⊃ Cell-mediated immunity is concerned with discrimination between "self" and "nonself" or "foreign" and in this context destroys cells infected with certain viruses; destroys intracellular bacteria such as *M. tuberculosis, L. monocytogenes,* and *Salmonella* species; defends against many fungal and parasitic infections; and helps prevent neoplasia (cancer).

SUGGESTED READING

Cunningham MW, Fujinami RS, eds. Effects of Microbes on the Immune System. Philadelphia: Lippincott Williams & Wilkins; 2000.

Delves PJ, Roitt IM. The immune system. N Engl J Med 2000; 343: 37-49, 108-117.

Gallin JI, Snyderman R. Inflammation: Basic Principles and Clinical Correlates. 3rd ed., Philadelphia: Lippincott Williams & Wilkins; 1999.

Medzhitov R, Janeway C Jr. Innate immunity. N Engl J Med 2000; 343: 338-344.

Nielsen CH, Fischer EM, Leslie RG. The role of complement in the acquired immune response. Immunology 2000; 100: 4-12.

Parkin J, Cohen B. An overview of the immune system. Lancet 2001; 357: 1777-1789.

Normal and Colonizing Bacterial Flora

We have already discussed the difference between exogenous pathogens (acquired from the animate or inanimate environment) and endogenous pathogens (acquired from a person's own normal or colonizing body flora). Viral, chlamydial, rickettsial, spirochetal, and parasitic infections are nearly always exogenous, since little or no "normal flora" is in these categories. Fungal infections are usually exogenous with the exception of candidiasis. Bacterial infections are often endogenous, since many of the body's epithelial surfaces are heavily colonized with bacteria at all times (Table 1-1). Colonization begins at birth and is of two

TABLE 1-1
Normal and Colonizing Bacterial Flora

Microorganism	Skin	Conjunctiva	Upper respiratory tract	Mouth	Lower intestine	External genitalia	Anterior urethra	Vagina
AEROBIC AND FACULTATIVELY ANAEROBIC BACTERIA								
Staphylococci	+	+	+	+	±	+	+ +	+
Streptococci								
Viridans	±	±	+	+ +	+	+	±	+
Group A			±	±				
S. pneumoniae		±	+	+				
Enterococci			±	+	+ +	+	+	+
Neisseria species		±	±	+			+	±
Corynebacteria	+	+	+	+	+	+	+	+
Haemophilus species		±	+	+				
Enterobacteriaceae*			±	±	+ +	+	+	±
ANAEROBIC BACTERIA								
Clostridia				±	+ +		±	±
Propionibacteria	+ +		+	±	±		±	
Actinomyces			+	+	±			
Lactobacilli				+	+		±	+ +
Bifidobacteria				+	+ +			+ +
Bacteroides species†			+	+ +	+ +	+	+	+
Fusobacterium species			+	+ +	+	+	+	±
Anaerobic gram-positive cocci	+		+	+ +	+ +	+	±	+
Anaerobic gram-negative cocci			+	+ +	+		±	+

From Eisenberg HD. Clinical microbiology. In: Gorbach SL, Bartlett JG, Blacklow NR. Infectious Diseases. 2nd ed., Philadelphia: W.B. Saunders Company; 1998: 123-145.
Scale: ±, irregular; +, common; + +, prominent.
Escherichia coli is the usual species of Enterobacteriaceae found in normal flora, but others such as *Klebsiella, Enterobacter, Proteus,* and *Serratia* species can be found, especially in patients who have received antibiotics.
†Includes *Prevotella melaninogenicus* (formerly *Bacteroides melaninogenicus*).

types: permanent colonization by bacteria that are generally part of the normal flora, and transient colonization by potential pathogens. Examples of the former are "diphtheroid" bacteria (*Propionibacterium* and *Corynebacterium* species) on the skin, viridans streptococci in the oral cavity, and *Escherichia coli,* enterococci, and *Bacteroides* species in the colon. Examples of the latter are *Streptococcus pneumoniae, Haemophilus influenzae,* and *Neisseria meningitidis* in the upper respiratory tract. Colonization is not a haphazard event. Microorganisms have on their surfaces specialized molecules, called adhesins, that bind with specific receptors on host epithelial cells or with extracellular matrix materials. An appreciation of the major components of the body's normal and colonizing bacterial flora promotes understanding of many of the common infections encountered in primary care.

Staphylococcus Aureus

Potential sites of colonization by *S. aureus* include the skin, perineal area, and gastrointestinal tract, but by far the most important site is the nasal mucosa (anterior nares). *S. aureus* nasal carriage is extremely common. At a given time, 20% to 40% of adults would have positive nasal swab cultures for *S. aureus*. Many persons (up to 25% of the population) are permanent nasal carriers of *S. aureus.* Most people (about 60% of the population) exhibit intermittent colonization with *S. aureus,* while about 20% of persons never show colonization. Because most of us (whether we admit it or not) put our fingers in our noses on a regular basis, person-to-person transmission of *S. aureus* by hand contact is a universal phenomenon. Viral upper respiratory tract infection in patients with nasal colonization by *S. aureus* sometimes results in wide dispersal of the organism in the immediate environment; this phenomenon has long been recognized in pediatrics as "cloud babies," but recently "cloud adults" have also been reported. Some persons with staphylococcal nasal colonization are prone to styes, folliculitis, or furunculosis (boils). Most, however, remain asymptomatic until the organism is given the opportunity to invade the skin through a wound, abrasion, vascular access line, or surgical incision. *S. aureus* pneumonia develops in some persons, especially during influenza epidemics because influenza A increases the density of staphylococcal colonization. Staphylococcal bacteremia can arise from colonization, local infection, trauma, foreign bodies, or pneumonia. Complications of staphylococcal bacteremia, which often manifests itself as a nonspecific flulike illness, include septic shock, endocarditis, and metastatic infection (Figure 1-2).

Viridans Streptococci

Most of the α-hemolytic streptococci present in the normal flora are loosely known as "viridans" (Latin *viridis,* "green") because they cause green hemolysis on blood agar plates, but 13 individual species are now recognized on the basis of physiologic, biochemical, and molecular typing methods. Under normal circumstances these bacteria constitute the major aerobic component of the flora of the human mouth (Table 1-1), making up nearly 50% of all bacteria that can be cultured from saliva. Individual species of viridans streptococci occupy distinct ecologic niches. *Streptococcus sanguis* and *S. mitis* adhere preferentially to the buccal mucosa, and *S. salivarius* and *S. mitis* to the dorsal surface of the tongue; *S. sanguis, S. mitis, S. oralis, S. gordonii,* and *S. anginosus* are frequently found in dental plaques. *S. mutans,* which adheres to teeth in large numbers and ferments dietary sugars into acids, is strongly associated with dental caries, no doubt the world's most prevalent bacterial infection. One group of viridans streptococci, variably known as the *S. milleri* group or *S. anginosus,* is associated with purulent infections, including brain abscess. Nearly all of the viridans streptococci occasionally cause endocarditis, usually in persons with diseased heart valves. With these

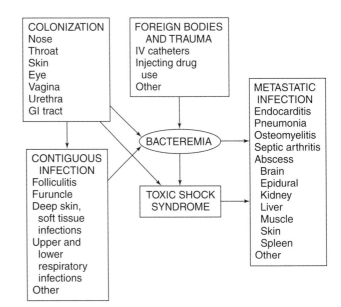

FIG. 1-2 Dynamics of colonization and infection by *Staphylococcus aureus.* Nasal colonization is especially important. Staphylococcal bacteremia carries the potential for metastatic infection in numerous organs and tissues. Toxin-producing strains can cause the staphylococcal toxic shock syndrome.

three exceptions, colonization by viridans streptococci is nearly always harmless; indeed, it is highly beneficial because it provides resistance to colonization by more virulent microorganisms.

Streptococcus Pyogenes (Group A Streptococcus)

S. pyogenes is a major pathogen in primary care not only because of the frequency of streptococcal pharyngitis and impetigo, but also because of the potential for life-threatening complications. Complacency engendered by the declining incidence of acute rheumatic fever has given way to renewed concern because of the streptococcal toxic shock syndrome and necrotizing fasciitis. *S. pyogenes* is a frequent colonizer of the human pharynx, especially in children, who have carriage rates reported to be as high as 20%. Asymptomatic colonization is less common in adults. Streptococcal M protein enables the organism to resist phagocytosis and multiply in blood. The development of antibodies against M protein confers lasting immunity, but unfortunately, the immunity is type specific and more than 90 types of M protein have been identified. The diverse manifestations of *S. pyogenes* infection are summarized in Figure 1-3 and discussed further in Chapters 6, 10, and 15.

Streptococcus Pneumoniae

Increasing resistance to β-lactam antibiotics and other drugs, including the fluoroquinolones, makes the pneumococcus—a common cause of otitis media, sinusitis, pneumonia, meningitis, and other serious infections—more dangerous today than at any time since the preantibiotic era. Most humans are intermittently colonized in the nasopharynx by this organism, especially during midwinter. Prevalence studies indicate that 20% to 40% of children and 5% to 10% of adults are col-

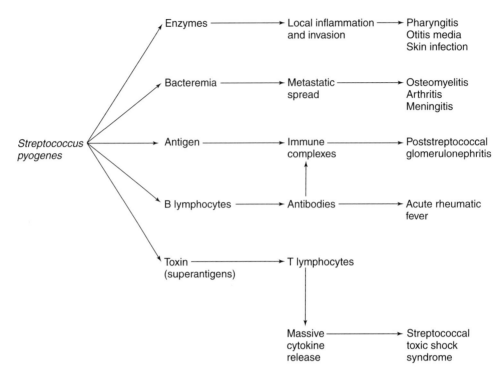

FIG. 1-3   The diverse clinical manifestations of infection by *Streptococcus pyogenes* as currently understood in terms of pathogenesis. In recent years, toxin-producing strains have been associated with necrotizing fasciitis and the streptococcal toxic shock syndrome.

onized at a given time. From the nasopharynx, pneumococci have access to the eustachian tubes, the ostia to the paranasal sinuses, and the tracheobronchial tree (see Figure 10-1).

Enterococci, Streptococcus Bovis, and Group B Streptococci

Group D streptococci formerly included the enterococci, *S. bovis,* and *S. equinus.* Newer classifications give enterococci their own genus with at least 12 species, of which *Enterococcus faecalis* (80% to 90%) and *E. faecium* are the major isolates from humans. Enterococci form a major part of the normal flora of the lower gastrointestinal tract and are the predominant aerobic gram-positive bacteria in stools. In primary care, enterococci occasionally cause urinary tract infection and endocarditis. However, the ability of enterococci to cause disease by themselves (i.e., as sole pathogens) is limited. Enterococci are commonly involved in hospital-acquired infections and are frequently isolated from urine of patients with obstructive uropathy and from wounds, including decubitus ulcers. Resistance to numerous antibiotics complicates treatment of enterococcal infection.

S. bovis is occasionally found in the human gastrointestinal tract, especially in patients with cancer or precancerous lesions of the bowel; documented *S. bovis* bacteremia is an indication for colonoscopy. Group B streptococci *(S. agalactiae),* found in the genital tract or colon in 5% to 40% of women, are of concern primarily because of neonatal and puerperal sepsis but also cause disease in adults with impaired host defenses.

Neisseria Meningitidis

Although rarely encountered in most primary care practices, the meningococcus is one of the few microorganisms capable of killing a previously healthy person within a few hours. However, asymptomatic colonization is relatively common, having been found in 18% of "normal" family members over a 32-month period. Asymptomatic carriage of meningococci leads to the development of protective antibodies directed against the organism's polysaccharide capsule. Most cases of invasive meningococcal disease (see Chapter 6) occur among the newly colonized. Studies suggest that men often bring the organism into a household; respiratory transmission leads to colonization of other family members, with children the most likely victims of invasive disease.

Haemophilus Influenzae and Moraxella Catarrhalis

Haemophilus influenzae is a small, pleomorphic, aerobic, gram-negative coccobacillus found mainly in the upper respiratory tract. Some strains contain a polysaccharide capsule, the major virulence factor, and are typed (a through f) according to the nature of the capsule. Most instances of life-threatening disease such as meningitis are caused by type b strains. Wide deployment of the conjugate vaccine against *H. influenzae* type b has greatly diminished the importance of this scourge of early childhood. Nonencapsulated strains are frequently associated with sinusitis, otitis media, exacerbations of chronic bronchitis in patients with chronic obstructive pulmonary disease (COPD), and conjunctivitis. About 30% to 80% of healthy persons have nasopharyngeal colonization by nonencapsulated strains of *H. influenzae.* About 2% to 4% of children were colonized by type B strains prior to the vaccine. *H. influenzae,* like *N. meningitidis,* preferentially colonizes nonciliated epithelial cells in the nasopharynx.

Moraxella catarrhalis, previously known as *Neisseria catarrhalis* and then *Branhamella catarrhalis,* is a gram-negative diplococcus associated with upper and lower respiratory tract infections in children and adults. Up to two thirds of infants, but only 1% to 5% of healthy adults, are colonized by this microorganism, which causes a spectrum of disease similar to that caused by *H. influenzae.*

Escherichia Coli and Other Aerobic Gram-Negative Rods

E. coli, the major aerobic gram-negative rod (bacillus) found in the lower gastrointestinal tract, is of enormous importance in primary care because of its role in the great majority of cases of community-acquired urinary tract infection (UTI), in occasional deep tissue infections such as vertebral osteomyelitis in patients with underlying medical problems, in rare cases of colitis caused by enteropathogenic or enterohemorrhagic strains (see Chapter 12), and in the well-publicized problem of hemorrhagic colitis and hemolytic syndrome caused by strains of the O157:H7 serotype. Probably all humans (except those who have received broad-spectrum antimicrobial therapy) are colonized with *E. coli,* but asymptomatic colonization with enteropathogenic or enterohemorrhagic strains is rare if it occurs at all. UTI in otherwise healthy women, the syndrome caused by *E. coli* most frequently seen in office practice, is nearly always preceded by colonization of the vaginal introitus. *E. coli* strains with a notable propensity to cause UTI are called "uropathogenic" strains and typically possess unique pili associated with pyelonephritis ("Pap pili") or *P. fimbriae.* Women who are especially prone to UTI are likely to be nonsecretors of P group blood substance, and studies also indicate that these women possess a unique receptor for Pap pili on their uroepithelial cells. These findings raise the possibility that a large portion of UTIs may someday be preventable by vaccination.

Proteus mirabilis causes up to 10% of community-acquired UTIs and presumably colonizes the normal human gastrointestinal tract. Other aerobic gram-negative rods cause infections in patients with underlying diseases who have received broad-spectrum antimicrobial therapy. *Klebsiella, Enterobacter,* and *Serratia* species are often found in the stool flora of patients who have received broad-spectrum antibiotics. *Enterobacter cloacae* is a frequent nosocomial or nosohusial (home-acquired) pathogen, since it is resistant to most of the β-lactam antibiotics. *Pseudomonas aeruginosa* can be part of the normal fecal flora but, unlike *E. coli* or *P. mirabilis,* is rarely associated with community-acquired UTI in the absence of a predisposing factor such as urologic instrumentation. *Acinetobacter* species, which often resist the action of soap, can be found in the skin flora in up to 25% of persons but rarely cause community-acquired disease. *Salmonella* and *Shigella* species are not considered part of the normal intestinal flora.

Anaerobic Bacteria

Anaerobic bacteria are operationally defined by their failure to grow on solid media in the presence of 10% carbon dioxide (or 18% oxygen). Most of the common aerobic bacteria encountered in medicine can grow under anaerobic conditions as well and are therefore sometimes called "facultative" (i.e., they can grow either aerobically or anaerobically). The term "anaerobic" is usually reserved for *strict* anaerobes. Quantitatively, these bacteria are the most important component of the normal human flora. Saliva contains anaerobic bacteria in numbers of 10^7 to 10^8/mL, the terminal ileum 10^4 to 10^6/mL, and the colon, where anaerobes outnumber aerobes by a ratio of about 1000:1, 10^{11} or more per gram of stool (dry weight). Anaerobes are also highly prevalent in the normal flora of the skin, vagina, and periurethral tissues. Anaerobic bacteria are commonly found in odontogenic infections, including infected root canals; chronic sinusitis; chronic otitis media; and pelvic inflammatory disease. Otherwise, anaerobic bacteria rarely assume importance in primary care unless the patient has serious underlying disease or the infection is so severe that hospitalization is clearly indicated. This is the case because anaerobic bacteria cause serious infection only when a major disruption of tissue has occurred (e.g., a wound or perforated bowel) or when the oxidation-reduction potential has been lowered (e.g., by ischemia, necrotic tumors, or foreign bodies). To the contrary, anaerobic bacteria have major importance for human well-being because they protect against colonization by more pathogenic organisms.

When anaerobic bacteria cause disease, they generally arise from the indigenous body flora. The primary exception is the clostridial syndromes such as tetanus *(Clostridium tetani)* and botulism *(C. botulinum)* (see Chapter 6). The species most commonly isolated from deep tissue infections include peptostreptococci ("anaerobic streptococci"), which are normally present in all of the sites mentioned previously; *Prevotella, Porphyromonas,* and *Fusobacterium* species, which are normally present in the oral cavity; and the *Bacteroides fragilis* group of bacteria, which make up the bulk of the normal fecal flora. The most important clue to an anaerobic infection is its foul odor. This sign is diagnostic although present in only about one half of cases. Other clues include tissue gas (observed as bullae or as crepitation on physical examination, or found on x-ray examination), tissue necrosis, the presence of multiple bacterial morphologies on Gram stain of a specimen, and the failure of bacteria to grow on a routine aerobic culture ("sterile pus"). Settings in which anaerobic bacteria should be suspected include bite wounds, aspiration pneumonia, lung abscess, pleural empyema, brain abscess, necrotizing fasciitis, myonecrosis (gas gangrene), diabetic foot ulcers, decubitus ulcers, and septic thrombophlebitis.

 KEY POINTS

NORMAL AND COLONIZING BACTERIAL FLORA

⊃ Colonization by bacteria is of two types: permanent colonization by bacteria that are generally part of the normal flora at all times, and transient colonization by potential pathogens.

⊃ Anaerobic bacteria are quantitatively the most important component of the normal bacterial flora. These bacteria cause disease under special circumstances but also serve to prevent colonization by more virulent bacteria.

SUGGESTED READING

Brook I. Microbial factors leading to recurrent upper respiratory tract infections. Pediatr Infect Dis J 1998; 17 (Suppl 8): S62-S67.

Kluytmans J, van Belkum A, Verbrugh H. Nasal carriage of *Staphylococcus aureus:* epidemiology, underlying mechanisms, and associated risks. Clin Microbiol Rev 1997; 10: 505-520.

Schaechter M, Engleberg NC, Eisenstein BI, Medoff G. Mechanisms of Microbial Disease. 3rd ed., Philadelphia: Lippincott Williams & Wilkins; 1999.

von Eiff C, Becker K, Machka K, et al. Nasal carriage as a source of *Staphylococcus aureus* bacteremia. N Engl J Med 2001; 34: 11-16.

Cost-Effectiveness: Prevention

Primary care is considered to be more cost effective than specialty and subspecialty care, especially when the focus is on prevention. However, decisions made by primary care physicians regarding the management of infectious diseases have huge cost implications. When and to what extent should expensive, sophisticated laboratory tests and imaging procedures be obtained? Which patients should be hospitalized? When is parenteral antimicrobial therapy (as opposed to oral therapy) indicated, and for how long? It behooves practitioners to examine the cost implications of their practice styles in relation to the styles of their peers. Clinicians with stable office practices, who know their patients through and through, are well positioned to practice cost-effective diagnosis and treatment, since they can usually be assured of close follow-up and compliance with recommendations. Clinicians working in walk-in clinics and emergency rooms tend toward a more expensive style of practice because they suspect they have only one chance at diagnosis and treatment. By far the most cost-effective measure used by primary care physicians is prevention.

Preventive measures are usually classified as primary, secondary, or tertiary. Primary prevention includes active immunization with vaccines, passive immunization with preformed antibiotics, and administration of antimicrobial agents before exposure. Primary prevention should be systematic:

- The database for each patient should reflect immunization status with regard to universally indicated vaccines (see Chapters 4 and 25).
- The patient's problem list should indicate conditions for which special immunizations are indicated and the date of the most recent immunization (e.g., "Asplenia secondary to splenectomy for trauma [10/15/89], last pneumococcal vaccine booster 11/27/00"), or even better, a computer-generated reminder should be issued to the patient when the next immunization is due.
- A system should be in place to administer the yearly "flu shot" to patients in high-risk categories for influenza, including everyone over age 65.
- Patients with cardiac lesions requiring prophylaxis against endocarditis should be given thorough instructions about what to do before dental and other procedures (see Chapter 26).
- A system should be in place to advise travelers about immunizations, malaria prophylaxis, and other measures before their departure dates (see Chapter 24).

Secondary prevention involves early detection of infection and aggressive therapy before the appearance of disease. The most common example in infectious diseases consists of screening programs for detection of sexually transmitted disease (STD). Tertiary prevention aims to control complications of established disease; an example would be aggressive management of AIDS/HIV disease. Most primary care clinicians consider prevention to be extremely rewarding.

 KEY POINTS

COST-EFFECTIVENESS: PREVENTION

⊃ Primary prevention (active and passive immunization and use of prophylactic antibiotics) should be systematic and displayed prominently in the medical record.

⊃ Patients with conditions that predispose to specific infections should receive specific instructions, to be shared with other health care providers.

⊃ Secondary prevention involves early detection of disease followed by aggressive therapy (e.g., screening for sexually transmitted disease).

SUGGESTED READING

Jenson HB. Pocket Guide to Vaccination and Prophylaxis. Philadelphia: W.B. Saunders Company; 1999.

Cost-Effectiveness: Diagnosis

Diagnosis is of two types: presumptive and definitive. Presumptive diagnosis is usually based on the history and physical examination, sometimes supported by laboratory and radiographic findings. Definitive etiologic diagnosis usually requires cultures and serologic methods. In primary care, most diagnoses of infectious diseases are presumptive. This is understandable, since the conditions most commonly encountered tend to be self-limited and often involve the upper respiratory tract (Table 1-2). This section reviews some principles of diagnosis of infectious diseases in the ambulatory setting.

Principle 1: Assume the Worst-Case Scenario

Skilled clinicians assume that the patient's symptoms might reflect the worst possible disease process. Mention of such possibilities in the medical record is frequently appropriate even when the probability seems low and the clinician believes that specific testing is not indicated. This is conveniently done in the assessment portion of the familiar problem-oriented format (subjective/objective/assessment/plan). Thus an office note for a patient with vague flulike complaints and low back pain might read in part, "*Assessment:* Probable self-limited viral syndrome. I have considered the possibility of a more serious condition such as endocarditis or spinal epidural abscess as an explanation for the patient's subjective feverishness and low back pain, but I really think the probabilities are low, especially since the WBC and sedimentation rate are normal. I have urged return visit should symptoms worsen or fail to resolve."

Principle 2: Search for a Syndrome

Confronted with a patient whose symptoms suggest infectious disease, the clinician should begin at once to search for a syndrome. In most instances the seasoned clinician

TABLE 1-2
Frequency of Some Common Syndromes in Primary Care, and Recommendations for Cost-Effective Diagnosis and Therapy

Syndrome	Estimated annual number of office visits, United States*	Physical examination usually necessary?	Recommendations for cost-effective diagnosis and therapy
Common cold	27 million	No	Treatment by telephone is acceptable practice, but antibiotic prescribing is to be discouraged (see Chapter 10).
Otitis media	24.5 million	Yes	Otoscopic examination provides a basis for decision-making (see Chapter 10).
Urinary tract infection	10 million	No	Treatment by telephone is acceptable practice for acute uncomplicated UTI in many situations, and empiric treatment based on the dipstick methods in others. Care must be taken, however, to exclude sexually transmitted disease (see Chapters 5, 14, and 16). Physical examination and culture are indicated for patients with systemic symptoms (e.g., fever, flank pain, nausea) and those with complicated UTI.
Vaginitis	10 million	Yes	Etiologic diagnosis can usually be made by physical examination supplemented by microscopy (see Chapter 16).
Acute sinusitis	2 million	Yes	Unfortunately, physical examination has limited value. Strategies for evaluation and treatment are summarized in Chapter 10 (see text and also algorithms for management of children and adults).
Infectious diarrhea	1.5 million	No	Small-volume diarrhea with blood and pain on defecation suggests colitis, which should be evaluated. The extent to which other cases of diarrhea need extensive evaluation depends on the patient's age and underlying medical condition and the severity of the diarrhea (see Chapter 12).
Bite wounds	800,000	Yes	Bite wounds should receive aggressive local care and preventive antimicrobial therapy (see Chapter 26).

UTI, Urinary tract infection.
*Data from various sources, especially Mandell GL, Bennett JE, Dolin R, eds. Mandell, Douglas, and Bennett's Principles and Practice of Infectious Diseases. Philadelphia: Churchill Livingstone; 2000.

quickly narrows the diagnostic possibilities and suggests the likely diagnosis based on a targeted history and physical examination in the context of the patient's basic health profile. Often a "virus" of one sort or another is suggested by the stereotyped complaints of many persons in the community. Associations often point the differential diagnosis in one direction or another; examples are fever and headache (e.g., meningitis, sinusitis, brain abscess, Rocky Mountain spotted fever), fever and productive cough (pneumonia), fever and heart murmur (endocarditis), fever with flank pain and dysuria (urinary tract infection), fever and diarrhea (enterocolitis), fever and lymphadenopathy (see Chapter 8), and fever and arthritis (see Chapter 15). Seemingly bizarre questions may yield huge dividends. Has the patient skinned rabbits, explored caves, or been around parakeets or other pet birds? To save time, the clinician may ask the patient to sit in a quiet place for 10 to 15 minutes and reflect on (and write

down) any possible unusual exposures. Sometimes the correct diagnosis is made only after multiple attempts to elicit the essential clue.

PATIENT 2
A 24-year-old resident physician had fever, generalized aching, and headache that largely resolved after several days but recurred the following week along with a stiff neck. Lumbar puncture revealed clear cerebrospinal fluid (CSF) with cell count, differential white cell count, glucose, and protein consistent with aseptic meningitis. A skilled consultant obtained the clue after multiple workups had failed. In response to specific questioning, the resident remembered that, while swimming in a freshwater lake, she had approached an object in the water and found it to be a dead animal. Leptospirosis was later confirmed by serology.

Principle 3: Recognize the Sepsis Syndrome

Often there is little or nothing to suggest a specific disease apart from self-limited "viral syndrome." This diagnosis usually proves correct, but the clinician should consider whether the patient might have the sepsis syndrome. Among the many life-threatening causes of sepsis syndrome encountered in primary care are *S. aureus* bacteremia, endocarditis, Rocky Mountain spotted fever, unusually severe ehrlichiosis, meningococcemia, and acute appendicitis. The clinician should pay close attention to the vital signs. Increased rate or depth of breathing, best assessed by placing a hand on the patient's abdomen and timing the excursions, is a subtle clue to respiratory compensation for metabolic acidosis. Hypotension, considered in relation to the patient's baseline blood pressure, should always be taken seriously. The clinician should appreciate the sepsis syndrome as currently understood: progression of local inflammation to a generalized inflammatory response that if unchecked can progress inexorably to multiorgan failure and death (Figure 1-4; see also Chapter 6).

Principle 4: Look for Atypical Features

A famous story tells of a family physician who, having been asked to see a family with six children, all of whom had fever, nausea, and "stomachache," concluded, "These five have gastroenteritis. Little Sally has a ruptured appendix." Is there a clinical finding from the history, examination, or laboratory testing that does not fit the diagnosis of self-limited viral illness? This question assumes great importance when influenza is prevalent in a community.

> **PATIENT 3**
> During an influenza epidemic a 64-year-old woman had a fever and aches all over, which began to resolve after several days but were followed by localized pain over the thoracic spine. Evaluation revealed epidural abscess caused by *S. aureus.* With surgery and antimicrobial therapy the woman made a complete recovery.

Principle 5: Pay Attention to the Peripheral Blood Smear

The physician should "listen to the leukocytes" for at least three kinds of valuable clues: (1) shift to the left (bandemia) with toxic changes (toxic granulations, vacuolization of the cytoplasm, and Döhle bodies), suggesting acute bacterial disease or other life-threatening disease such as rickettsial infection; (2) predominance of lymphocytes with atypical lymphocytosis, suggesting viral infection, including mononucleosis caused by the Epstein-Barr virus or cytomegalovirus; and (3) in rare instances a specific pathogen, such as malaria parasites, histoplasmosis, or bacteria (asplenic patients are especially likely to have bacteremia of such intensity that microorganisms can be seen on routine peripheral blood smears). Unfortunately, several factors now make it difficult for clinicians to examine their patients' peripheral blood smears: lack of time, lack of adequate facilities, and regulations resulting from the Clinical Laboratory Improvement Amendments of 1988 (CLIA).

Principle 6: Perform Diagnostic Testing Only When Results Will Alter Patient Management, but Arrange for Close Follow-Up

Experts suggest that between 75% and 85% of information necessary for diagnosis of a syndrome can be obtained from the medical history. Unfortunately, harried clinicians may find it more expedient to order tests than to take a meticulous history. Furthermore, patients often seem to obtain greater reassurance from a negative test result than from a clinician's well-reasoned opinion. Diagnostic testing is crucial mainly when an acute, life-threatening disease enters the differential diagnosis (see above). *The clinician should consider the more serious diagnostic possibilities and then decide whether elaborate testing is appropriate.* When lumbar puncture is performed, an extra tube of cerebrospinal fluid (CSF) should be saved to spare the patient another puncture if further tests are desired.

Principle 7: Arrange for Follow-Up

Seasoned clinicians appreciate that "tincture of time" is often the best strategy. When the clinician has determined with reasonable certainty that the problem is benign and self-limited, but cannot entirely exclude the possibility of more serious disease, close follow-up should be arranged. A further office visit or at least a telephone call should be scheduled. The clinician should make clear his or her availability for further diagnostic consideration. The clinician might also enlist the collaboration of the patient's spouse, a family member, or a roommate by prescribing a "buddy check" (see Appendix 3).

Principle 8: Document the Level of Diagnostic Certainty

The level of diagnostic certainty should be conveyed in the medical record. Such phrases as "suspected but not proven" reflect intellectual honesty and attention to detail. For example, a final diagnosis of "Pneumonia, right lower lobe, cause undetermined (suspected pneumococcal)" would be accurate in a case of gram-positive diplococci on sputum Gram stain, *S. pneumoniae* on sputum culture, and a therapeutic response to β-lactam antibiotic therapy, but sterile blood cultures (since

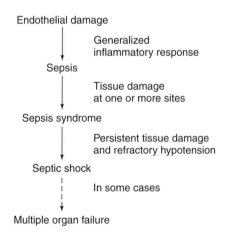

FIG. 1-4   Sepsis, if unchecked, leads to the sepsis syndrome, which can then progress to septic shock and in some cases to multiple organ failure.

positive blood or body fluid cultures are the only definitive means of diagnosis). By indicating in writing the level of diagnostic certainty, the clinician guards against the habit of taking intellectual shortcuts, which sooner or later leads to serious error.

Principle 9: Think of Tuberculosis and Endocarditis

Tuberculosis (see Chapter 22) is now uncommon and is usually encountered in persons who are disadvantaged for one reason or another: the frail elderly, the socioeconomically deprived, patients with HIV disease, immigrants from developing countries, and prisoners. However, it can occur in anyone and often presents unexpectedly and in unfamiliar guises. Most primary care clinicians have limited experience with this disease, and studies indicate that tuberculosis is often poorly managed in primary care practice. Endocarditis (see Chapter 6) is an uncommon disease with symptoms that often direct attention away from the heart. If a patient has fever and a significant heart murmur, even when the source of the fever seems obvious, endocarditis should be considered and blood cultures should be obtained. Many patients with acute endocarditis (which is usually caused by *S. aureus*) do not have a murmur.

PATIENT 4

A 52-year-old schoolteacher with learning disabilities was struck in the mouth by a pupil who refused to take part in a fire drill, resulting in dislodgment of two teeth. One week later a persistent fever developed. Over the course of several weeks she was given four different antibiotics, and a penicillin allergy developed. Although she was known to have a grade 3/6 systolic murmur owing to mitral valve prolapse, the diagnosis of endocarditis was not considered until the sixth week of illness. The causative microorganism, *Streptococcus sanguis,* was determined to be penicillin resistant (probably as a result of the ineffective oral antibiotic therapy). Three courses of intensive antimicrobial therapy were necessary to obtain an eventual cure.

Principle 10: Understand the Principles of Clinical Reasoning and the Elements of Probability Theory as Applied to Diagnostic Testing

The major categories of clinical reasoning are, in ascending order of importance, pattern recognition, probabilistic thinking, and pathophysiology. For example, an 18-year-old woman has a chief complaint of burning on urination. Pattern recognition and probabilistic thinking suggest uncomplicated UTI and hence a quick prescription for a 3-day course of antimicrobial therapy. The pathophysiologic approach, however, would be to ask further questions to determine whether the dysuria is external rather than internal and whether risk factors for STD are present. The physician then decides whether to perform a pelvic examination and obtain studies for STD and a urine culture before beginning therapy.

What diagnostic tests should be obtained, and when? Generations of medical students have learned such gems as Sutton's law ("Go where the money is," after Willie Sutton, the bank robber), Occam's razor ("Seek the one, simplest explanation," after William of Occam, the philosopher), and Anselm's ass ("Do something; don't just stand there in the middle," referring to an animal tethered between two bales of hay, both just out of reach). A better and more sophisticated approach is to consider the properties of tests within the context of probability theory.

All clinicians must be familiar with "sensitivity," "specificity," and related terms (Figure 1-5). Sensitivity basically means "positive in disease"; we say a test is 99% sensitive if positive test results are obtained in 99% of persons judged to have the disease on the basis of a "gold standard" test, such as biopsy or autopsy. Specificity basically means "negative in health"; we say that a test is 99% specific if positive test results are obtained in only 1% of persons who clearly do not have the disease.

It is extremely important to consider "sensitivity," "specificity," and related concepts in the context of pretest probability—the likelihood that the patient has the disease. This concept is best captured by Bayes' theorem, which holds that the likelihood that a positive test result is actually false positive rather than true positive varies inversely with the prevalence of the disease in the population. (Careful study of Figure 1-6 will clarify Bayes' theorem.) The likelihood that a positive test result is false positive rather than true positive is 100% if nobody in the population represented by the patient has the disease, but zero if everybody has the disease. Between these extremes the relationship is described not by a straight line, but rather by a hyperbolic curve. In sum, *if the pretest probability is extremely low, the*

$$
\begin{array}{cc}
 & \text{DISEASE} \\
 & \begin{array}{cc} \text{Present} & \text{Absent} \end{array} \\
\text{TEST RESULT} \begin{cases} \text{Positive} \\ \text{Negative} \end{cases} & \begin{array}{|c|c|} \hline a & b \\ \hline c & d \\ \hline \end{array}
\end{array}
$$

$$\text{Sensitivity} = \frac{a}{a+c}$$

$$\text{Likelihood ratio for a positive test result} = \frac{\text{Sensitivity}}{1-\text{Sensitivity}}$$

$$\text{Specificity} = \frac{d}{b+d}$$

$$\text{Likelihood ratio for a negative test result} = \frac{1-\text{Sensitivity}}{\text{Sensitivity}}$$

$$\text{Pretest probability (prevalence)} = \frac{a+c}{a+b+c+d}$$

$$\text{Pretest odds} = \frac{\text{Prevalence}}{1-\text{Prevalence}}$$

$$\text{Positive predictive value} = \frac{a}{a+b}$$

$$\text{Posttest odds} = \text{Pretest odds} \times \text{Likelihood ratio}$$

$$\text{Negative predictive value} = \frac{d}{c+d}$$

$$\text{Posttest probability} = \frac{\text{Posttest odds}}{\text{Posttest odds}+1}$$

FIG. 1-5 Data pertaining to test results (positive or negative) in the presence or absence of disease are used to define at least 10 concepts useful to clinical reasoning. Sensitivity means that a test is "positive in disease," whereas specificity means that a test is "negative in health." Test results must, however, be interpreted within the context of the pretest odds that the disease is present.

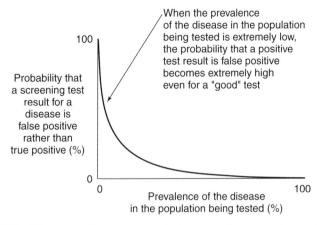

When the prevalence of the disease in the population being tested is extremely low, the probability that a positive test result is false positive becomes extremely high even for a "good" test

FIG. 1-6 Bayes' theorem as applied to a positive screening test result for a given disease (see text).

chances are overwhelming that a positive screening test result is actually a false-positive result even if the sensitivity and specificity of the test are superb.

Increasingly, the concept of pretest probability is being expressed as the likelihood ratio, and nomograms are available for evaluating of the usefulness of a test. An example is the testing for HIV antibodies. The enzyme-linked immunosorbent assay (ELISA) is extremely sensitive, and the Western blot test is extremely specific. However, in populations with low prevalence of the disease (i.e., no recognized risk factors for HIV infection), the odds become extremely high that a positive test result is false positive, which causes numerous problems for the patient, including psychological trauma. Screening makes sense in populations with high pretest probability (e.g., male prisoners with history of injecting drug use). Similarly, using specific treponemal tests (such as the fluorescent treponemal antibody absorption [FTA-ABS] and *Treponema pallidum* microhemagglutination [MHA-TP]) as screening tests for syphilis in persons with low pretest probability is associated with a high rate of false-positive tests despite the reputation of these tests for specificity. Unfortunately, these concepts have been rigorously applied to the diagnosis of infectious diseases in only a few instances. (See Chapter 14 for a discussion of applying this concept to interpretation of urine cultures.)

 KEY POINTS

COST-EFFECTIVENESS: DIAGNOSIS

⊃ Most infectious diseases encountered in primary care are self-limited; most diagnoses are presumptive rather than definitive and etiologic.
⊃ When patients have fever or other symptoms possibly caused by infectious disease, the clinician should ask, "What is the worst-case scenario?" Ideally, the medical record reflects this thought process.
⊃ "Probable viral syndrome" should be stated as the diagnosis only after careful consideration of the possibility that the patient has the sepsis syndrome. This includes close attention to vital signs and search for clinical findings that are atypical of nonspecific viral illness.

⊃ Examination of the peripheral blood smear for bandemia and toxic changes in the PMNs helps differentiate patients with sepsis syndrome from those with nonspecific viral illness and occasionally provides a specific diagnosis.
⊃ Elaborate diagnostic testing (beyond such basic tests as complete blood count and urinalysis) should be obtained only when the results will alter patient management.
⊃ When the likely diagnosis seems to be nonspecific viral syndrome but the remote possibility of life-threatening infection cannot be excluded on clinical grounds, the clinician should arrange for close follow-up and prescribe a "buddy check" (see Appendix 3).
⊃ The level of diagnostic certainty should be conveyed in the medical record, with use of such words as "probable" and "suspected," to avoid the habit of taking intellectual shortcuts, which leads inevitably to serious error.
⊃ The concepts of sensitivity and specificity must be interpreted in the context of the pretest probability of disease, or likelihood ratio.

SUGGESTED READING

Ioannidis JP, Lau J. State of the evidence: current status and prospects of meta-analysis in infectious diseases. Clin Infect Dis 1999; 29: 1178-1185.

Cost-Effectiveness: Treatment

The aphorism that the three most important principles of treatment are diagnosis, diagnosis, and diagnosis has merit, since surety of diagnosis usually allows the clinician to prescribe a standard, cost-effective drug regimen. The major determinants of cost of therapy are acquisition cost, administration cost, monitoring cost, and cost of complications. The least expensive antimicrobial regimen would consist of a drug that is available generically, provides excellent bioavailability when given by the oral route, requires no special monitoring, and has few serious complications. Parenteral therapy (see Chapter 27), even when given at home, is much more expensive than oral therapy because of the cost of administration and the need in many instances to monitor such parameters as serum drug levels and renal function.

Primary care clinicians should "think generically" about antibiotics. When a new drug is introduced, the clinician should make a conscious effort to memorize the generic name as well as the trade name. Primary care clinicians receive new information from pharmaceutical representatives on a regular basis. Pharmaceutical representatives provide a useful societal function, but their *raison d'être* in part is to publicize the subtle advantages of their drugs over those of competitors and thereby encourage the clinician to prescribe a particular brand. The habit of thinking generically promotes cost-effective prescribing and helps the busy clinician keep abreast of current knowledge, since articles in the major peer-reviewed journals emphasize generic rather than brand names.

Ideally, antimicrobial therapy is based on the results of culture and sensitivity tests. In practice this is usually not the case. The severity of the clinical situation often mandates presumptive therapy before the availability of laboratory results. In many of the syndromes commonly seen in primary care, such as upper and lower respiratory tract infections, "clean" specimens for bacteriologic tests are difficult to obtain without putting the patient at some risk. Presumptive therapy poses a delicate trade-off. On the one hand, death or disability can result from withholding therapy for what later proves to be (for example) staphylococcal septicemia or Rocky Mountain spotted fever. On the other hand, presumptive therapy complicates the diagnostic process, causes unwanted side effects, adds to the cost of medical care, and promotes the emergence of drug-resistant microorganisms.

Presumptive therapy should be based on three questions: What infectious syndrome might be present? How severe is the illness? How serious is the patient's underlying medical condition (Figure 1-7)?

■ What infectious syndrome might be present? The syndrome should be defined as accurately as possible by history, physical examination, appropriate radiographic studies, and simple laboratory tests such as examination of peripheral blood smears, Gram stains, and urinalyses. This definition should include the anatomy of the infection: for example, is it tracheobronchitis or pneumonia? Cystitis or pyelonephritis? Fever without localizing symptoms or signs poses a special situation in which the history must be carefully explored and reexplored.

■ How severe is the illness? Do subjective and objective data suggest that it may be life threatening? Or do all of the parameters point to a self-limited disorder or one in which a 24- to 72-hour delay before institution of therapy is unlikely to have adverse consequences?

■ How serious is the patient's underlying medical condition? Many researchers have shown that patients with "ultimately fatal disease," defined as a process that if untreated would probably cause death within 5 years, are much more likely to die of an acute infection than patients with "nonfatal" underlying conditions. In doubtful situations the physician should err toward giving presumptive therapy to such patients.

In many situations presumptive therapy is more cost effective than expensive laboratory tests. However, the potential for disaster should be kept in mind. Presumptive therapy can, for example, precipitate Stevens-Johnson syndrome or obscure the diagnosis of endocarditis.

When the clinician has determined that presumptive therapy is indicated, three additional questions should be asked:

■ What are the most likely pathogens, and to what extent is it necessary to cover all or most of the possible pathogens? Narrow-spectrum, relatively inexpensive therapy may be chosen if the etiology seems reasonably certain and the likelihood of serious consequences from missing the target seems small (e.g., suspected community-acquired *E. coli* urinary tract infection in an otherwise healthy young woman). Broad-spectrum therapy, even if quite expensive, should be chosen if the infection is life threatening (e.g., fever and petechiae suggesting either meningococcemia or Rocky Mountain spotted fever) or the patient is severely compromised (e.g., the patient is elderly, is receiving corticosteroids, or has an "ultimately fatal" underlying disease as defined previously). The physician should keep in mind potential pathogens that might be poorly covered by the chosen regimen.

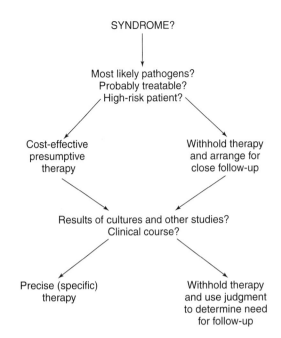

FIG. 1-7 Accurate definition of the syndrome being treated provides the starting point for an algorithmic approach to presumptive antimicrobial therapy (see text).

■ What is the response to initial therapy, and what do laboratory studies (including the results of culture and sensitivity tests) show? All aspects of the illness should be reviewed within 48 to 72 hours after treatment is begun. Within 48 to 72 hours the patient usually shows a favorable response to treatment unless the chosen regimen is ineffective or complicating factors are present, such as an obstructed tube (e.g., an obstructed duct or ureter) or an undrained abscess. Within 48 to 72 hours cultures usually reveal the causative pathogen unless the pathogen will never "grow out," the pathogen is a slow-growing or fastidious microorganism, or antimicrobial therapy was given before specimens were obtained for culture.

■ What should be the duration of therapy? The optimal duration of antimicrobial therapy is well defined for only a few infections, such as endocarditis and pulmonary tuberculosis. According to one quip, the duration of therapy should resemble a plausible football score: 3, 7, 10, 24, 28, or 42 days. However, as discussed elsewhere in this book, a growing number of studies are addressing the optimal duration of uncomplicated lower UTI (3 days versus 7 days), acute pharyngitis, and other syndromes. When in doubt, the physician should usually err toward a slightly longer duration of therapy.

Some regimens for presumptive therapy are summarized in Appendixes 1 and 2.

Treatment usually becomes straightforward when cultures or other studies identify a specific pathogen as the cause of the patient's illness. The clinician should, however, be wary when cultures show a single pathogen in a clinical setting where polymicrobial infection is the rule rather than the exception. Examples of this phenomenon are bite wounds, infected decubitus ulcers, aspiration pneumonia from "mouth flora," deep intraabdominal or pelvic infections, and gas-forming subcutaneous infection in a patient with diabetes mellitus. Such polymicrobial infections often involve anaerobic pathogens even when no foul odor is obvious. Some drugs of choice against specific pathogens are summarized in Table 19-5.

 KEY POINTS

COST-EFFECTIVENESS: TREATMENT
- ⊃ The major determinants of cost of antimicrobial therapy are acquisition cost, administration cost, monitoring cost, and cost of complications.
- ⊃ The clinician should "think generically."

Problem of Drug Resistance

Overuse of antimicrobials is attracting the attention of governments and regulatory agencies as a major public health problem. In most studies the relationship between antibiotic usage and resistance has been shown to be roughly linear. Bacteria develop resistance by four basic mechanisms: altered target sites, decreased accumulation into the cell (by decreased permeability or by efflux), enzymatic inactivation or modification, and bypass of the metabolic system affected by the drug. Such resistance can be transferred either by chromosomal DNA or by plasmids (bits of extrachromosomal DNA that can be spread by bacterial viruses or by conjugation). Of greatest concern in the United States at this time are the following:

- Penicillin-resistant *Streptococcus pneumoniae* (PRSP). Although "penicillin resistance" is a misnomer—most strains have reduced susceptibility to penicillin but remain susceptible to high doses of penicillin—this problem threatens to limit the continued usefulness of β-lactam agents against a common pathogen (see Chapter 11). In many communities 30% or more of pneumococcal blood and CSF isolates now show reduced susceptibility to penicillin. Overuse of amoxicillin in small children is thought to be a major risk factor.
- Methicillin-resistant *Staphylococcus aureus* (MRSA). These strains are actually "broadly β-lactam resistant" in that other β-lactam antibiotics are ineffective even if they appear to be active by in vitro susceptibility testing. The mechanism of resistance, like that of PRSP, involves reduced affinity of the target site (known as a penicillin-binding protein) for the drug.
- Vancomycin-intermediate *Staphylococcus aureus* (VISA [or GIPA]) and vancomycin-resistant *Staphylococcus aureus* (VRSA). Although only a few such strains of *S. aureus* have been identified to date, this problem causes alarm because of the specter of *S. aureus* infections that are essentially untreatable.
- Vancomycin-resistant enterococci (VRE). As discussed previously, enterococci are important mainly as nosocomial pathogens. One concern raised by the rapid spread of VRE is that resistance to vancomycin will be transmitted to pneumococci and staphylococci.
- Gram-negative rods that produce extended-spectrum β-lactamases (ESBLs). Strains of *Enterobacter* and other species have evolved β-lactamases that render them resistant to nearly all of the β-lactam antibiotics, including the newer third- and fourth-generation cephalosporins.

Although bacteria receive most of the publicity, drug resistance among viruses, fungi, and parasites is also increasing at an alarming relate. To what extent are primary care clinicians responsible, and what can be done?

Studies suggest that about 50% of antibiotic prescriptions in primary care are not indicated on the basis of evidence-based guidelines. Moreover, between 18% and 60% of patients with colds receive antibiotics. Primary care clinicians are under enormous pressure to prescribe: patients insist on drugs to "knock out" infection; industry promotes new drugs with hyperbole and free samples; employers (such as those in health maintenance organizations) insist on "efficiency" (writing a prescription is usually more efficient than explaining why one is not needed); and clinicians fervently want to *do something* for their patients. Although the overprescription of antibiotics, especially for upper respiratory tract infection (URI), is widely acknowledged, the reduction in major suppurative complications of URI, such as peritonsillar abscess, retropharyngeal abscess, and the Lemierre syndrome (see Chapter 6), cannot be denied. Unfortunately, we have little or no idea how many patients must be treated to prevent a single severe suppurative complication.

Systematic reduction in antimicrobial prescribing will almost surely require a nationwide effort with national policies and guidelines. In Finland, nationwide reduction in macrolide usage led to a decline in frequency of erythromycin resistance among group A streptococci. The achievement of such a nationwide reduction in use of any antibiotic in a pluralistic society such as the United States is problematic. The best clinical strategies for individual physicians include keeping up with national guidelines for antibiotic use issued by major organizations (e.g., the American Academy of Pediatrics) and setting up systems for patient education.

 KEY POINTS

PROBLEM OF DRUG RESISTANCE
- ⊃ Overuse of antimicrobial agents causes selection of drug-resistant strains of bacteria, viruses, fungi, and parasites.
- ⊃ Major problems in the United States today include penicillin-resistant pneumococci (MRSA), methicillin-resistant staphylococci (MRSA and MRSE), vancomycin-resistant enterococci (VRE), and gram-negative rods that produce extended-spectrum β-lactamases (ESBLs).
- ⊃ In the ambulatory care setting, national policies may be necessary to effect meaningful changes in prescribing that will reduce the incidence of drug resistance.
- ⊃ In the absence of national policies the best clinical strategies for limiting antibiotic use may be to follow guidelines issued by national organizations and to set up systems for patient education.

SUGGESTED READING

Carrie AG, Zhanel GG. Antibacterial use in community practice: assessing quantity, indications and appropriateness, and relationship to the development of antibacterial resistance. Drugs 1999; 57: 871-881.

Fridkin SK. Vancomycin-intermediate and -resistant *Staphylococcus aureus:* what the infectious disease specialist needs to know. Clin Infect Dis 2001; 32: 108-115.

Hayden MK. Insights into the epidemiology and control of infection with vancomycin-resistant enterococci. Clin Infect Dis 2000; 31: 1058-1065.

Hellinger WC. Confronting the problem of increasing antibiotic resistance. South Med J 2000; 93: 842-848.

Jones RN, ed. Global aspects of antimicrobial resistance among key bacterial pathogens: results from the 1997-1999 SENTRY antimicrobial program. Clin Infect Dis 2001; 32: S81-S167.

Kaye KS, Framow HS, Abrutyn E. Pathogens resistant to antimicrobial agents: epidemiology, molecular mechanisms, and clinical management. Infect Dis Clin North Am 2000; 14: 293-319.

McCaig LF, Hughes JM. Trends in antimicrobial drug prescribing among office-based physicians in the United States. JAMA 1995; 273: 214-219.

Seppälä H, Klaukka T, Vuopio-Varkila J et al. The effect of changes in the consumption of macrolide antibiotics on erythromycin resistance in group A streptococci in Finland. N Engl J Med 1997; 337: 441-456.

Swartz MN. Use of antimicrobial agents and drug resistance. N Engl J Med 1997; 337: 491-492.

Fever: Friend or Foe?

Although we no longer attribute fever to yellow bile or demonic influences, the subject remains enshrouded in superstition and dogma. The definition of fever and the desirability of suppressing it with antipyretic drugs merit brief comment.

Fever can be defined as elevation of the thermoregulatory set point in response to a stimulus, resulting in a substantial increase in core body temperature above its baseline value. The normal baseline value is a subject of some dispute. "Normal" temperature is an abstract concept. When a patient says, "My usual temperature is below normal," the patient is referring to 98.6° F (37° C), established as the normal body temperature in 1868 by Carl Reinhold August Wunderlich. Recent studies suggest that the mean normal oral temperature of healthy adults is between 98.1° and 98.2° F (or between 36.7° and 36.8° C). The 99th percentile for temperature measured at 4 PM in healthy adults is 99.9° F (37.7° C). Some authorities, while recognizing the arbitrariness of any cutoff value, suggest that fever consists of a temperature of 100° F (37.8° C) at any time during the day or 99° F (37.2° C) in the early morning. Rectal temperatures are usually 0.8° F (0.4° C) higher than oral temperatures, and oral temperatures can vary as much as 1.7° F (0.95° C) depending on whether the thermometer is placed in the anterior floor of the mouth or in the rear sublingual pocket. Axillary temperatures are often useful in neonates but are unreliable in older children and adults.

Intactness of thermoregulation (the body's ability to balance heat gain with heat loss) distinguishes fever from hyperthermia caused by such conditions as heatstroke. Stated differently, the body is out of control during hyperthermia but remains in control during fever. Hyperthermia is a medical emergency that, since it does not respond to antipyretic drugs, requires cooling of the body by physical means. Little or no evidence has shown that fever per se is harmful. In fever, in contrast to hyperthermia, the temperature never goes above a "glass ceiling." Thus fever rarely causes core temperature to exceed 105.8° F (41° C), the level at which adverse consequences begin to appear. Substantial evidence suggests that fever is an adaptive response. The cytokines largely responsible for fever—interleukin-1, tumor necrosis factor-α, interleukin-6, and interferon-γ—also participate in the immune response to infection. Clinical data indicate that patients who mount a febrile response to bacteremic illness are more likely to survive the illness than patients with normal or subnormal temperature. Antipyretic drugs (such as aspirin, other nonsteroidal antiinflammatory drugs, and acetaminophen) have not been shown to improve the outcome of infection or prevent febrile convulsions in children. Some evidence suggests that antipyretic drugs may actually be harmful.

Body temperature and fever are subject to many interpretations. The following points are worth emphasizing:

- Temperatures above 101° F (38.3° C) are usually of diagnostic usefulness in that the patient probably has a definite abnormality that, if rigorously pursued, could be identified. Lower temperatures in healthy adults often lack diagnostic utility, and some patients (especially women) habitually run higher than normal temperatures (in the range of 100° to 100.9° F [37.8° to 38.3° C]).

- Withholding antipyretics is often advisable if the clinician is uncertain about the diagnosis and concerned about the remote possibility that a serious disease such as meningitis or Rocky Mountain spotted fever might be present.

- The main indication for antipyretics is to make the patient more comfortable. Some of the benefits are due to analgesia, which might also be achieved with analgesics that do not have antipyretic properties. Putative indications for antipyretics include reducing metabolic demands in patients with serious underlying disease such as heart failure or chronic obstructive pulmonary disease and minimizing confusion in the elderly.

- Some patients paradoxically become more uncomfortable when given antipyretics. Antipyretics can also predispose to adverse effects from other medications.

- Antipyretics, if given, should be administered at regular intervals rather than on an as-needed basis. The latter approach often results in extreme fluctuations that make the patient even more uncomfortable.

- Aspirin should not be given to young children with fever because of the risk of Reye's syndrome.

 KEY POINTS

FEVER: FRIEND OR FOE?

⊃ The mean normal body temperature of healthy adults is between 98.1° and 98.2° F (or 36.7° and 36.8° C), rather than 98.6° F (37° C). Any cut-off value for "fever" is arbitrary, but a reasonable definition of fever seems to be an oral temperature of 100° F (37.8° C) at any time during the day or 99° F (37.2° C) in the early morning.

⊃ In fever the body's thermoregulatory mechanisms remain intact and the core temperature rarely exceeds 105.8° F (41° C), the level at which adverse consequences begin to appear. This distinguishes fever from hyperthermia caused by such conditions as heatstroke, in which the body has lost control of thermoregulation.

⊃ Temperatures above 101° F (38.3° C) in healthy adults usually point to a definite disorder. Lower temperatures are of much less diagnostic utility.

⊃ Fever seems to be an adaptive response, and little or no evidence has shown that suppressing it improves the clinical outcome.

⊃ It is often wise to withhold antipyretics if the patient might have a serious, undiagnosed disease, to avoid masking the clinical symptoms.

⊃ If used, antipyretics should be administered on a regular rather than an as-needed basis.

⊃ Aspirin should not be given to young children with fever because of the risk of Reye's syndrome.

SUGGESTED READING

Aranoff DM, Neilson EG. Antipyretics: mechanisms of action and clinical use in fever suppression. Am J Med 2001; 111: 304-315.

Cunha BA, ed. Fever. Infect Dis Clin North Am 1996; 10: 1-222.

Mackowiak PA, ed. Fever. Basic Mechanisms and Management. 2nd ed., Philadelphia: Lippincott-Raven; 1997.

Mackowiak PA. Concepts of fever. Arch Intern Med 1998; 158: 1870-1881.

Mackowiak PA, Wasserman SS, Levine MM. A critical appraisal of 98.6° F, the upper limit of the normal body temperature, and other legacies of Carl Reinhold August Wunderlich. JAMA 1992; 268: 1578-1580.

Rabinowitz RP, Cookson ST, Wasserman SS, et al. Effects of anatomic site, oral stimulation and body position on estimates of body temperature. Arch Intern Med 1996; 156: 777-780.

Prolonged Perplexing Fever

The term "fever of unknown origin" (FUO) should be reserved for a specific clinical situation: prolonged fever that is undiagnosed despite a substantial, conscientious effort to establish the cause. The classic definition, known as the Petersdorf-Beeson criteria, consists of (1) an illness of at least 3 weeks' duration, (2) measured temperature greater than 101° F (38.3° C) on several occasions, and (3) no diagnosis after a week of intensive diagnostic efforts in the hospital. Today's emphasis on carrying out procedures in

TABLE 1-3
Major Causes of Fever of Unknown Origin (FUO)*

Category (frequency)†	Disease‡	Clues
Infections (23% to 36%; relatively more common as a cause of FUO in persons >65 years than in younger persons)	Tuberculosis	Miliary tuberculosis and various syndromes of extrapulmonary tuberculosis can be difficult to diagnosis. Repeat tuberculin tests and physical examinations are often useful (Chapter 22).
	Intraabdominal abscess and other occult abscesses	Newer imaging techniques (ultrasound, CT scans, MRI scans) have revolutionized the diagnostic approach to occult abscess, but some cases remain difficult to diagnose and scans are occasionally false negative.
	Hepatobiliary disease	Elevation of the serum alkaline phosphatase is usually a valuable clue. Recurrent bouts of ascending cholangitis (Charcot's intermittent fever) are often associated with sepsis due to gram-negative bacteria.
	Endocarditis	Improved methods for processing blood cultures and echocardiography make endocarditis a less common cause of FUO than was formerly the case (Chapter 6). Subtle skin and mucous membrane findings often assume great diagnostic importance.
	Pyelonephritis	Atypical urinary tract infections including renal carbuncle and perinephric abscess sometimes cause FUO; symptoms combined with appropriate imaging procedures often provide the clue.
	Cytomegalovirus infection	Cytomegalovirus infection is an important cause of FUO in younger persons, who usually do not appear ill and have a paucity of physical findings (Chapter 8).
	Miscellaneous infections	Other relatively common causes include sinusitis, catheter-related infections, osteomyelitis, malaria, brucellosis, psittacosis, and disseminated fungal disease.
Tumors (7% to 31% of cases, relatively more common in persons >65 years of age compared to younger persons)	Leukemias, lymphomas, and multiple myeloma	Hodgkin's disease is a classic cause of FUO, although the hectic "Pel-Ebstein" fever pattern is relatively uncommon. Severe itching at night (obligate nocturnal pruritus) is sometimes an important clue.
	Solid tumors	Carcinoma of the kidney sometimes presents as FUO without other manifestations. Many tumors cause fever when liver metastases are present.

the ambulatory setting removes the latter criterion; we might substitute "no diagnosis after running the gamut of consultations, blood tests, imaging procedures, and biopsies that might reasonably be performed." In primary care practice, most unexplained fevers resolve well within the 3-week time limit required for the diagnosis of "FUO." Keeping the strict definition of FUO is useful because it frames the patient's problem in a way that directs further investigation (Table 1-3).

True FUO is an uncommon problem in primary care. Most infectious disease specialists see relatively few patients who fulfill the classic criteria, and those patients often have known major underlying problems, including HIV/AIDS, cancer, or diseases requiring immunosuppressive drug therapy. A general familiarity with the causes of FUO is useful for primary care clinicians, however, because these disorders will also be encountered in other ways. The three main categories of FUO are infections, tumors, and connective tissue diseases. Infections are especially likely to include granulo-matous diseases (tuberculosis, histoplasmosis, and others), endocarditis, and atypical intraabdominal infections. Tumors that commonly cause FUO include lymphoma (especially Hodgkin's disease and diffuse histiocytic lymphoma) and renal cell carcinoma. Connective tissue diseases include systemic lupus erythematosus and Still's disease in younger persons and temporal arteritis or polyarteritis nodosa in older persons. Numerous diseases are occasionally manifested as FUO. Diagnosis of FUO can be extremely difficult, and in many patients (especially younger ones) the condition remains undiagnosed. Patients whose FUO remains undiagnosed after intense evaluation often do extremely well on long-term follow-up.

Another uncommon problem in primary care is periodic fever—episodes of fever that often occur with remarkable periodicity, with intervening good health. Familial Mediterranean fever, an autosomal dominant syndrome often associated with amyloidosis, is a classic cause but is uncommon in the United States. Some patients with periodic fever have

TABLE 1-3—cont'd
Major Causes of Fever of Unknown Origin (FUO)*

Category (frequency)†	Disease‡	Clues
Connective tissue diseases (9% to 20%, more common in persons >65 years of age than in younger persons)	Adult Still's disease	An important cause of FUO for which there are no specific diagnostic tests. Features include high fever sometimes with a double quotidian pattern (two spikes per day), arthritis or arthralgia, lymphadenopathy, sore throat, leukocytosis, and an evanescent, salmon-pink rash.
	Temporal arteritis	An important cause of FUO especially in elderly white women. Key symptoms include diplopia (or other visual symptoms) and pain on chewing (intermittent masticatory claudication). The sedimentation rate is usually elevated (>100 mm/hour). Temporal artery biopsy is the diagnostic procedure of choice.
	Polyarteritis nodosa and other forms of vasculitis	Clues to classic polyarteritis nodosa include isolated peripheral neuropathies (mononeuritis multiplex), renal involvement with active urine sediment, and occasionally eosinophilia. Other forms of vasculitis causing fever include hypersensitivity angiitis, Wegener's granulomatosis, and vasculitis accompanying rheumatoid arthritis.
Miscellaneous causes (17% to 24%, more common in persons <65 years of age than in older persons)	Granulomatous diseases including sarcoidosis	Granulomatous diseases are commonly due to infection (see above), but sarcoidosis, Crohn's disease, and granulomatous hepatitis of unknown origin can cause FUO. Diagnosis nearly always requires biopsy and rigorous exclusion of infection.
No diagnosis (7% to 26%; more common in persons <65 years of age than in older persons)	No diagnosis made despite extensive studies	Patients without a definite diagnosis despite extensive studies over a prolonged period of time and whose general health remains good (i.e., no weight loss, anemia, or other evidence of systemic disease) generally have a favorable prognosis.

*FUO as defined by the Petersdorf-Beeson criteria, modified to take into account the current trend of carrying out procedures on an outpatient basis (see text).
†Percentage of cases in various major series.
‡Factitious fever (1% to 4% of cases in older series) is probably less common today because of the advent of the digital thermometer. Occasional causes of FUO include thromboembolic disease (e.g., recurrent pulmonary embolism and pelvic thrombophlebitis), liver disease (alcoholic hepatitis, cirrhosis), hematologic and related conditions (myeloproliferative syndromes, hemoglobinopathies, paroxysmal hemoglobinuria, hemolytic anemias, thrombotic thrombocytopenic purpura, immunoblastic lymphadenopathy, histiocytosis X, Castleman's disease, lymphomatoid granulomatosis, subacute necrotizing lymphadenitis), cardiovascular diseases (dissecting hematoma of the aorta, atrial myxoma, aortitis, pericarditis, venoocclusive disease), subtle diseases of other organ systems (allergic alveolitis, pheochromocytoma, thyroiditis, thyrotoxicosis, pancreatitis), and hypersensitivity reactions (drug fever, erythema multiforme, serum sickness).

cyclic neutropenia, the diagnosis of which is established by documenting leukopenia during febrile episodes. Young children with periodic fever and aphthous stomatitis may have PFADA (periodic fever, aphthous stomatitis, pharyngitis, and cervical adenitis; also known as Marshall's syndrome) (see "Mouth Ulcers," Chapter 10). Many patients with periodic fever have an entirely benign course, remaining well over years of observation despite the puzzling febrile episodes.

Drug fever is much more relevant than FUO and periodic fever to primary care practice. Fever sometimes develops within 10 days after a new drug is started, but it can develop after months or even years of uneventful therapy. Fever is frequently the only manifestation of drug reaction. Eosinophilia is helpful if present but is usually absent. The best diagnostic approach is to discontinue all nonessential drugs while maintaining a temperature diary. Usually a definite downward trend in the temperature pattern is seen within 72 hours. Exceptions to this generalization are patients receiving rifampin or phenytoin (Dilantin) and those with an unusually severe rash.

Night sweats without fever can be associated with drugs and with many conditions, including neoplasms, neurologic disorders, and endocrine disorders. There is no standardized approach to this problem.

 KEY POINTS

PROLONGED PERPLEXING FEVER

⊃ The term "fever of unknown origin" (FUO) should be reserved for patients who have (1) an illness of at least 3 weeks' duration, (2) measured temperature greater than 101° F (38.3° C) on several occasions, and (3) no diagnosis after running the gamut of blood tests, imaging procedures, and biopsies that might reasonably be performed.

⊃ True FUO, an uncommon problem in primary care, is usually caused by disease in one of three categories: infection, neoplasm, or connective tissue disease.

⊃ Drug fever should always be considered as a cause of FUO and periodic fever in the ambulatory setting. The best approach to diagnosis is to discontinue all nonessential drugs. In most instances a definite improvement in the temperature pattern occurs within 72 hours.

SUGGESTED READING

Chambliss ML. What is the appropriate diagnostic approach for patients who complain of night sweats? Arch Fam Med 1999; 8: 168-169.

de Kleijn EMHA, Vandenbroucke JP, van der Meer JWM. Fever of unknown origin (FUO). I. A prospective multicenter study of 167 patients with FUO, using fixed epidemiologic entry criteria. The Netherlands FUO Study Group. Medicine (Baltimore) 1997; 76: 392-400.

Iikuni Y, Okada J, Kondo H, et al. Current fever of unknown origin 1992-1992. Intern Med 1994; 33: 67-73.

Knockaert DC, Vanneste LJ, Bobbaers HJ. Recurrent or episodic fever of unknown origin: review of 45 cases and survey of the literature. Medicine (Baltimore) 1993; 72: 184-196.

Knockaert DC, Vanneste LJ, Bobbaers HJ. Fever of unknown origin in elderly patients. J Am Geriatr Soc 1993; 41:1187-1192.

Reimann HA, McCloskey RV. Periodic fever: diagnostic and therapeutic problems. JAMA 1974; 228: 1662-1664.

Psychiatric Disorders in Infectious Diseases

Infectious diseases mingle with psychiatric disorders and vice versa. Patients with chronic infections, most notably those with HIV/AIDS, need monitoring for symptoms and signs of depression, anxiety, and other psychiatric problems. Patients with psychiatric problems sometimes show symptoms of infectious disease and are frequently convinced that they suffer from a chronic infection.

Somatization disorder is probably the psychiatric condition most likely to be associated with symptoms suggesting infectious disease. This disorder begins before age 30, seems to affect women disproportionately, persists at least several years, causes functional disability, and is defined basically by a "positive review of systems" with complaints in numerous areas. It has been suggested that the functional somatic syndromes are a single disorder with different names conferred by different specialists. Patients often seek specific diagnoses to validate their symptoms. Moreover, the *idea* of a specific disease entity, transmitted by the lay press or through the Internet, sometimes acts as an infectious agent. Examples familiar to infectious disease specialists are Lyme disease, chronic Epstein-Barr virus infection, and chronic "fever" in which the daily temperature seldom if ever exceeds 101° F (38.3° C). Management of patients with somatization disorder is difficult, since they are often dissatisfied with the clinician's failure to propose a medical diagnosis and specific treatment. My approach includes the following elements:

■ Consider the diagnosis of somatization disorder only if the results of a complete physical examination and carefully selected laboratory tests (e.g., complete blood cell count with sedimentation rate, thyroid-stimulating hormone level, and HIV antibody test) are normal.

■ Acknowledge that it is entirely possible that the symptoms have an organic basis, but state that you are reasonably certain that an "organic" diagnosis cannot be made on the basis of currently available medical knowledge and science.

■ Counsel the patient that he or she is probably vulnerable to overuse of medical services, including increased likelihood of major surgery (e.g., hysterectomy, appendectomy, or cholecystectomy) and exposure to unscrupulous persons who offer extremely expensive testing and treatment services.

■ Schedule follow-up visits during which the history will be reviewed and the physical examination repeated, with a careful survey for evidence of organic disease.

■ Consider formal psychological testing, which can form the basis for recommending counseling or support groups and also for determining which patients should be treated with drugs for anxiety or depression.

The primary care physician may encounter some less common disorders. Factitious disorder can present as unexplained fever, bizarre skin infections, and rarely the Munchausen syndrome (feigned medical disorder, often quite complicated and with "textbook" symptoms). Digital thermometers have probably made factitious fever less common than was formerly the case. Bizarre skin infections can present as cellulitis or abscess, aspirates of which may reveal "mouth flora" bacteria by Gram stain and culture. Patients with disease caused by factitious injections of microorganisms often have a medical background. Persons with delusional disorder often have a firm conviction that infection is present; the most common example is probably delusions of parasitosis (see Chapter 23). A related problem is veneroneurosis (also known as syphilophobia or "genitally focused hypochondriasis"), in which patients are convinced that they have an STD (e.g., syphilis or HIV), often as a result of a sexual transgression in the remote past. Such patients sometimes become extremely knowledgeable about the nuances and pitfalls of serologic testing for syphilis. Patients with obsessive-compulsive disorder commonly fear that they will be contaminated, and about half of them manifest compulsive handwashing. Malingering, conversion disorders, and phobias are other less common disorders.

 KEY POINTS

PSYCHIATRIC DISORDERS IN INFECTIOUS DISEASES
⊃ Patients with somatization disorder frequently have symptoms suggestive of infectious diseases and seek medical validation of their complaints.
⊃ Factitious disorders include unexplained fever and bizarre skin infections (cellulitis and abscesses), often caused by "mouth flora" microorganisms.
⊃ Delusional disorders include delusions of parasitosis. In veneroneurosis, patients are convinced that they have an STD.

SUGGESTED READING
Barsky AJ. The patient with hypochondriasis. N Engl J Med 2001; 345: 1395-1399.
Ross SE. "Memes" as infectious agents in psychosomatic illness. Ann Intern Med 1999; 131: 867-871.
Wessely S, Nimnuan C, Sharpe M. Functional somatic syndromes: one or many. Lancet 1999; 354: 936-939.
Wurtz R. Psychiatric diseases presenting as infectious diseases. Clin Infect Dis 1998; 26: 924-932.

Infection Control in Office Practice

Rigorous infection control is a moral imperative and legal requirement. All medical personnel should know the basic principles of disease transmission and control. Each clinic or practice should have an infection control officer (who is often the head nurse) responsible for designing and implementing a comprehensive infection control plan (Table 1-4). The elements of the plan will vary according to the intensity of procedures performed in the office and, to a lesser extent, the nature of the patient population.

The terminology of precautions (or "isolation") can be confusing and tends to change. During the mid-1980s, regulatory agencies such as the Centers for Disease Control and Prevention (CDC) and the Occupational Safety and Health Administration (OSHA) popularized "universal precautions" for prevention of spread of bloodborne pathogens, notably HIV and hepatitis viruses. Barrier-type devices (gloves and in many cases goggles or face shields) were recommended for all potential exposures to blood and certain body fluids, such as vaginal secretions and semen. The term was later changed to "body substance isolation," by which was meant "all body substances." More recently the CDC has combined these two concepts into "standard precautions." Through the changing terminology runs a common thread: all patients should be treated alike, and all body substances should be regarded as potentially infectious. Good infection control requires rigorous attention to detail, including disinfection practices and the keeping of logs to document such matters as refrigerator temperatures, glutaraldehyde efficacy, autoclave functioning, and hepatitis B immunization (Table 1-5).

The following is a brief review of disease transmission as it applies to preventing infection in the office setting:

- Contact transmission involves person-to-person or object-to-person touching of mucous membranes or open skin. This is an important means of transmission of staphylococci, *C. difficile,* and some respiratory viruses, including respiratory syncytial virus. Frequent handwashing is the major defense against contact transmission, but attention should also be paid to routine disinfection of stethoscopes, toys, bathroom fixtures, and other objects in patient care areas.
- Droplet transmission involves coughing, sneezing, or suctioning procedures (as in bronchoscopy), resulting in a spray of secretions capable of contacting conjunctiva, nasal mucosa, and lips within a 3-foot radius. This is an important means of transmission of meningococci, influenza viruses, and pertussis. The use of eye protection, including goggles and shields, during certain procedures is a defense against droplet transmission.
- Airborne transmission involves inhalation of particles much smaller than droplets, often referred to as "droplet nuclei." This is an important means of transmission when organisms remain suspended in the air after coughing in the form of "droplet nuclei," as in tuberculosis (pulmonary and laryngeal), chickenpox, and measles (rubeola). Masks, ultraviolet lights, and immunization constitute some of the defenses. The infection control plan should pay particular attention to tuberculosis.
- Vehicle transmission by contaminated items, although now uncommon in health care settings as a result of tight regulations, still occurs and can cause outbreaks or even epidemics. Causes include use of expired medications or antiseptics, irrigation fluids that have been left in open containers, and diluted bleach solution that is over 24 hours old. Disease frequently involves organisms that survive well in water, such as *Pseudomonas* species. Defenses include monitoring refrigerator temperatures, checking for expired medications, discarding irrigation solutions without preservatives at the end of the day of opening, and selecting disinfectants that do not require dilution.
- Vector transmission by insects or animals is extremely rare in today's health care facilities.

The infection control officer, working in concert with the office manager, should ascertain that all employees know their tuberculin skin status and their immunization status against measles (rubeola), mumps, rubella, hepatitis B, and varicella-zoster virus. A common situation is the exposure of a nonimmune employee to the varicella-zoster virus through a case of chickenpox or shingles. Extending a furlough from the 10th day after the first exposure through the 21st day after the last exposure is expensive and inconvenient. Therefore

TABLE 1-4
Elements of an Infection Control Program for Primary Care Clinicians' Offices

Element	Comment
Handwashing	A mild lotion-type soap is recommended for general use in clinicians' offices. Disposable containers are desirable, since refilling of soap containers without proper care of the container has been shown to promote bacterial growth. Soaps containing antimicrobial products (chlorhexidine, iodophors, triclosan, or alcohol) can be used before invasive procedures such as minor surgery.
Standard precautions	Barrier devices (gloves and other devices) should be donned before anticipated or planned contact with blood, secretions, nonintact skin, or mucous membranes. Gloves should be changed between patients, and hands should be washed immediately after removal of gloves. Additional barriers such as gowns, plastic aprons, masks, goggles, full face shields, or glasses with eye shields should be worn when secretions, blood, or other body fluids are likely to soil the clothing and skin or splash into the face. Use of both eye protection *and* mask/face shield protects both eyes and mucous membranes. Soiled reusable articles, grossly contaminated laundry, and contaminated trash should be placed in a bag bearing the biohazard symbol. Disposable needles and sharp instruments should be placed in puncture-resistant containers. These containers should be checked daily to prevent overfilling, and when three-quarters full they should be closed and disposed of for incineration by the vendor. Recapping of needles, if indicated, should be done *only* by using the one-handed "scoop" method or a recapping device. Patients with illnesses transmitted via the airborne route (e.g., tuberculosis, measles, and chickenpox [varicella]) should be placed in examining rooms as soon as possible. They should be encouraged to cough into tissues and to wear surgical masks. Workers in the office should wear gloves and gowns when cleaning up blood or body fluid spills.
Infectious waste disposal	Solid waste that is grossly contaminated with blood or body fluids is considered to be infectious waste and should be disposed of in a manner consistent with state law. Sanitary napkins, adult diapers, and baby diapers are not considered infectious waste and can be disposed of as regular trash unless supersaturated (saturated to the point of dripping spontaneously with light pressure) with blood or other body fluids.
Cleaning and disinfection of reusable instruments and equipment	Medical devices, equipment, and surgical supplies are divided into three general categories based on the potential risk of infection involved with their use: noncritical, semicritical, and critical. *Noncritical items*—for example, blood pressure cuffs, percussion hammers, bandage scissors, scales, examination tables, canisters for supplies, all work surfaces, and carpets, can be cleaned with a detergent or detergent-disinfectant solution. *Semicritical items*—for example, thermometers, ear specula, ear curettes, endoscopes, tonometers, ear wash equipment, diaphragm-fitting rings, vaginal specula, and nasal specula—should be cleaned and then disinfected or sterilized. *Critical items*—for example, surgical instruments, needle electrodes, cautery tips, and biopsy forceps used with endoscopes—should be cleaned and then sterilized. Sterilization should follow the manufacturer's recommendations. Each sterilizer should be monitored and a written record kept.
Environmental cleaning	Examination tables and horizontal surfaces in examination rooms should be wiped down at the end of each day with dilute disinfectants. Special attention should be paid to stirrups, stools, and lighted instrument handles. All examination tables and baby scales should be covered with a sheet or table paper, which should be changed between patients. Instruments that have been soaking should be rinsed and positioned for drying overnight. Sharps containers should be checked and replaced if three-quarters full. Blood or body fluid spills should be cleaned with an EPA-approved disinfectant or a fresh 1:10 bleach/water solution, paper towels, absorbent material or kitty litter, dustpan and scraper, and infectious waste bag.

TABLE 1-4—cont'd
Elements of an Infection Control Program for Primary Care Clinicians' Offices

Element	Comment
Storage of sterilized supplies	Storage areas should not accommodate cross traffic. In very small areas, sterile supplies should be stored on the upper shelves and clean supplies on the lower shelves. Items used for direct patient contact (and also chemicals) should not be stored under sinks because of the possibility of plumbing leaks. Patient supplies and medications should never be stored on the floor. Like goods should be stored together to prevent puncturing of packages with unlike goods. All supplies and medications should be monitored for expiration dates on a monthly basis. Attention should be paid to stock rotation (*Stocking:* on the bottom—-on the left—in the back; *Dispensing:* from the top—from the right—from the front).
Refrigerators	Contents of refrigerators should be separated into medication, biohazard, and food. Storage of medications in the door of the refrigerator is undesirable, since frequent opening and closing make this the warmest area. Temperature readings on operational days of the clinic or office should be documented in a log. All refrigerators should be defrosted and cleaned monthly.
Cleaning and disinfection of endoscopes	Efficacy of the 2% glutaraldehyde solution should be tested before each use and the results recorded in a log maintained for this purpose. The entire scope and also endoscopic accessories should be cleaned and rinsed according to the manufacturer's recommendations.
OSHA bloodborne pathogen exposure control plan	An exposure control officer, designated from among the office personnel, should review the exposure control plan annually, train employees, identify and recommend engineering controls that will increase worker safety, and assist with implementation of infection control policies. Positions within the office are classified according to whether employees have potential exposure to bloodborne pathogens. Eligible employees are offered the hepatitis B vaccine, and documentation of their acceptance or refusal of the vaccine is maintained in a log. All employees are made aware of a postexposure plan for management of actual or potential exposures to bloodborne pathogens.
Tuberculosis control plan	A written tuberculosis control plan should be based on risk assessment, which takes into account the number of patients with active tuberculosis seen in the office during the prior year. The plan should be reviewed and updated annually. Baseline tuberculin skin test status should be established for all employees. When it has been recognized that a patient with unsuspected, untreated active pulmonary tuberculosis was in the office, contact investigation should be carried out among employees.

Modified from Rapp D. Infection Control Policy and Reference Manual for Medical Offices. Columbia, SC: Privately published; 2000. Copies of the complete manual can be obtained from the author (AVHmouse@aol.com).
EPA, Environmental Protection Agency; *OSHA,* Occupational Safety and Health Administration.

TABLE 1-5
Suggested Work Restrictions for Medical Personnel Exposed to or Infected with Various Conditions

Condition	Recommendations*
Conjunctivitis	Restrict from patient contact (category II) or require the use of disposable gloves for all patient contact† (category II).
Diarrheal disease, acute stage	Restrict from patient contact (category II).
Enteroviral infections	Restrict from care of infants, neonates, and immunocompromised patients (category II).
Hepatitis A	Restrict from patient contact until 7 days after onset of jaundice (category IB).
Hepatitis B	Restrict persons with acute hepatitis B and those with chronic hepatitis B who are positive for the 'e' antigen from performing exposure-prone invasive procedures† (category II).
Hepatitis C	No recommendation.
Herpes simplex on fingers or hands (herpes whitlow)	Restrict from patient contact and from contact with patient's environment (category II).
Herpes zoster	*Localized zoster in a healthy person:* Cover the lesions and restrict from care of high-risk patients until all lesions are dry and crusted (category II). *Generalized zoster or localized zoster in an immunosuppressed person:* Restrict from patient contact until all lesions are dry and crusted (category IB).
Chickenpox, postexposure, susceptible personnel	Restrict from active duty from the 8th day after the first exposure through the 21st day (28th day if VZIG is given) after the last exposure or, if varicella occurs, until all lesions are dry and crusted (see text).
HIV	Restrict from exposure-prone invasive procedures† (category II).
Measles, postexposure, susceptible personnel	Exclude from duty from the 5th day after the first exposure through the 21st day after the last exposure and/or 4 days after the rash appears (category IB).

all employees lacking a clear history of chickenpox should receive the varicella-zoster vaccine (see Chapter 25). A controversial issue concerns what to do when an employee has conjunctivitis (pink eye). Adenoviral conjunctivitis is highly contagious, but the disease is usually mild and serious consequences are extremely rare even in immunocompromised persons. Although the CDC suggests restricting a person with conjunctivitis from patient contact as a category II recommendation (Table 1-5), in most instances such persons can reasonably be allowed to work provided they receive counseling about transmission, wear a new pair of disposable gloves before each patient contact, and wash their hands between patients. The issue of employees with chronic hepatitis B or HIV disease is less urgent in the clinic setting than in the hospital setting, since clinic employees are rarely if ever involved in "exposure-prone invasive procedures" (i.e., manipulating sharp objects by feel in blind cavities). Medical personnel who have transmitted the hepatitis B virus to patients have invariably tested positive for the hepatitis B "e"

antigen and negative for the hepatitis B "e" antibody. Transmission of HIV in the health care setting is extremely rare; theoretically, effective transmitters would be patients with HIV who have high viral loads (see Chapter 17). When doubt exists about an employee's ability to work because of these or any other infectious disease, convening an expert review panel is appropriate.

Primary care clinicians and their staffs will find employees at the local health department to be valuable allies in the effort to diagnose, treat, and prevent infectious diseases. Clinicians should be aware of reportable diseases as required by state law. A strategy that has been successful in the United Kingdom—where every citizen is registered with a primary care physician—and that should be used more widely in the United States is the use of "sentinel physicians" to report diseases seen in their practices as an index to infectious disease epidemiology. Those with particular interest in infectious diseases will find the CDC's *Morbidity and Mortality Weekly Report* to be a lively and pertinent source of breaking information.

TABLE 1-5—cont'd
Suggested Work Restrictions for Medical Personnel Exposed to or Infected with Various Conditions

Condition	Recommendations*
Mumps, postexposure, susceptible personnel	Exclude from duty from the 12th day after the first exposure through the 26th day after the last exposure or until 9 days after the onset of parotitis (category II).
Rubella, postexposure, susceptible personnel	Exclude from duty from the 7th day after the first exposure through the 21st day after the last exposure (category IB).
Scabies	Restrict from patient contact until cleared by medical evaluation (category IB).
Staphylococcus aureus infection with active, draining skin lesions	Restrict from patient contact and from contact with patient's environment until the lesions have resolved (category IB). The *S. aureus* carrier state is not a basis for restriction unless personnel have been linked epidemiologically to transmission of the organism (category IB).
Streptococcus pyogenes (group A streptococcal) infection	Restrict from patient care, contact with patient's environment, or food handling until 24 hours after adequate treatment has been started (category IB).
Varicella, postexposure, susceptible personnel	Exclude from active duty from the 10th day after the first exposure through the 21st day (or 28th day if VZIG is given) after the last exposure (category IA).
Viral respiratory infection, acute febrile	Consider excluding from the care of high-risk patients or contact with their environments during community outbreaks of influenza or respiratory syncytial virus infection (category IB).

Modified from Hospital Infection Control Practices Advisory Committee Membership, Centers for Disease Control and Prevention: Guideline for infection control in healthcare personnel, 1998. Infect Control Hosp Epidemiol 1998; 19: 407-463.
VZIG, Varicella-zoster immune globulin.
*Category IA: strongly recommended and supported by rigorous studies; category IB: strongly recommended and considered to be effective by experts on the basis of strong rationale and suggestive evidence; category II: suggested for implementation on the basis of suggestive clinical or epidemiologic studies, a strong rationale, or studies that are applicable to some settings.
†See text for further comment.

 KEY POINTS

INFECTION CONTROL IN OFFICE PRACTICE

⊃ Medical offices should have an infection control plan coordinated, enforced, and updated by a single infection control officer, who will often be the head nurse.

⊃ All employees should know the basic ways by which pathogens are transmitted, the desirability of handwashing between patients, and the need to maintain a clean environment with regular disinfection of objects in patient care areas.

⊃ All medical personnel with patient contact should know their tuberculin skin test status and their immunization status concerning measles (rubeola), mumps, rubella, hepatitis B, and varicella-zoster virus.

⊃ Primary care clinicians and their office staffs should establish relationships with the local health department, where they will find valuable allies in their efforts to diagnose, treat, and prevent infections.

SUGGESTED READING

Bennett JV, Brachman PS, eds. Hospital Infections. 4th ed., Philadelphia: Lippincott-Raven; 1998.

Hospital Infection Control Practices Advisory Committee Membership, Centers for Disease Control and Prevention: Guideline for infection control in healthcare personnel, 1998. Infect Control Hosp Epidemiol 1998; 19: 407-463.

Mayhall CG, ed. Hospital Epidemiology and Infection Control. 2nd ed., Philadelphia: Lippincott Williams & Wilkins; 1999.

McDonnell G, Russell AD. Antiseptics and disinfectants: activity, action, and resistance. Clin Microbiol Rev 1999; 12: 147-179.

Wenzel RP, ed. Prevention and Control of Nosocomial Infections. 3rd ed., Baltimore: Williams & Wilkins; 1997.

2 Use of Laboratories

CHARLES S. BRYAN, SALLY A. HARDING

Advances in general microbiology, immunology, and molecular biology continue to simplify the diagnosis of infectious diseases. However, cost constraints and regulations of the Clinical Laboratory Improvement Amendments of 1988 (CLIA) limit the extent of on-site testing in all but the largest primary care practices. The purpose of this chapter is to provide a brief overview of clinical microbiology from the perspective of primary care. Discussions of appropriate tests for specific syndromes and pathogens are included in later chapters. No attempt has been made to catalog all the laboratory tests now available. (A useful, comprehensive book can be obtained from Specialty Laboratories in Santa Monica, Calif., phone 1-800-421-4449.)

SUGGESTED READING

Cockerill FR III, ed. The role of the clinical mirobiology laboratory in the diagnosis and therapy of infectious diseases. Infect Dis Clin North Am 2001; 15: 1009-1311.

Koneman EW, Allen SD, Janda WM, et al. Color Atlas and Textbook of Diagnostic Microbiology. 5th ed., Philadelphia: Lippincott; 1997.

Peters JB. Use and Interpretation of Laboratory Tests in Infectious Disease. 6th ed., Santa Monica, Calif.: Specialty Laboratories; 2000.

Robinson A, Marcon M, Mortensen JE, et al. Controversies affecting the future practice of clinical microbiology. J Clin Microbiol 1999; 37: 883-889.

Shanson DC. Microbiology in Clinical Practice. 3rd ed., Oxford: Butterworth-Heinemann; 1999.

CLIA Regulations and Their Implications

Concerns about the accuracy of laboratory test results prompted the U.S. Congress to pass the CLIA regulations in 1988 (issued in 1992 as a final rule). CLIA regulations cover all laboratory tests except those performed for research or forensic purposes. All physician office laboratories must register with CLIA through the U.S. Department of Health and Human Services (DHHS). Only offices that collect specimens and perform no testing are exempt. CLIA is funded by user fees, which means that facilities must pay an annual fee for an updated certificate.

The U.S. Food and Drug Administration (FDA) categorizes tests on an ongoing basis, as follows:

- Waived tests. These procedures are simple to perform, are virtually foolproof, and in the event of an erroneous result are unlikely to have a negative impact on the patient. However, the laboratory must have personnel standards, documented training and competency (initially, at 6 months, and then annually), strict adherence to manufacturers' guidelines for individual tests, quality controls, and appropriate compliance and billing procedures.

- Provider-performed microscopy. Any physician with a CLIA license can perform microscopic examination of urine sediment, vaginal secretions for *Trichomonas vaginalis* and *Candida* species, and stool for cellular constituents and pinworm. Proficiency testing is desirable.

- Moderate-complexity tests. Tests of this type must meet all the criteria for waived tests, but the standards for personnel and competency are higher. Proficiency testing must be carried out. Validation of the method must include sensitivity, specificity, precision, and accuracy. The testing site is inspected at least every 2 years.

- High-complexity tests. These tests must meet all of the above criteria and also have higher personnel standards and specific training requirements for the licensed CLIA laboratory director.

Complete blood cell (CBC) count, differential blood counts, and examination of specimens stained with Gram's method are considered to be moderate-complexity tests. Many primary care clinicians no longer perform these essential tests in the office because of the expense and inconvenience of complying with CLIA regulations.

Most primary care clinicians deal with laboratories at three levels:

- An in-house laboratory, typically for waived tests and provider-performed microscopy and usually offering phlebotomy service for send-out specimens

- A laboratory at a local hospital or other facility for most types of routine cultures, fungal cultures, mycobacterial (acid-fast bacillus [AFB]) cultures, and various serologic tests

- One or more reference laboratories for specialized tests that are beyond the scope of local laboratories; when needed, local laboratories can make recommendations or referrals

Adequate microbiology services require prompt specimen transport and close communication with the laboratory. For this reason, local hospital laboratories usually provide better service than large, remotely situated commercial laboratories.

Systems must be in place for collection and transport of specimens and for ensuring that results affect the patient's management. The following vignettes illustrate the importance of a systematic and carefully documented approach to laboratory test result communication:

- Surgeons performing a lobectomy for presumed bronchogenic carcinoma never received the results of a positive AFB culture, which had been reported to a pulmonary specialist. The entire operating room staff was exposed to *Mycobacterium tuberculosis.*
- A pediatrician treating a patient with fever and arthralgia never received the results of blood cultures positive for viridans streptococci, which had been reported to a partner. The patient sustained a myocardial infarction resulting from septic embolism and, later, subarachnoid hemorrhage caused by a ruptured mycotic aneurysm.
- A family physician who had treated a patient for presumed gastroenteritis received the results of white blood cell (WBC) and differential counts (marked leukocytosis and bandemia) too late to be helpful to the patient, who died of meningococcemia the next morning.

Laboratories are now required to document the initial reporting, usually by telephone, of potentially critical results such as AFB cultures and blood cultures. Ideally, the primary care clinician keeps a running list of pending laboratory tests that might critically affect patient outcomes and has procedures in place for ensuring that the clinician receives all laboratory results in a timely fashion.

 KEY POINTS

CLIA REGULATIONS AND THEIR IMPLICATIONS
- All clinical laboratories must register with CLIA.
- Waived tests and provider-performed microscopy fall well within the scope of primary care.
- Tests of moderate complexity can be performed in the primary care setting but require more resources and are subject to a higher degree of regulation.
- Tests of high complexity are generally referred to a hospital or reference laboratory.
- Systems for specimen collection, prompt specimen transport, and appropriate responses to test results should be in place.

SUGGESTED READING
Health Care Financing Administration. Medicare, Medicaid and CLIA programs. Regulations implementing the Clinical Laboratory Improvement Amendments of 1888 (CLIA). Fed Register 1992; 57: 7002-7186 (http://www.fda.gov/cdrh/clia).

St John TM, Lipman HB, Krolak JM, et al. Improvement in physician's office laboratory practices, 1989-1994. Arch Pathol Lab Med 2000; 124: 1066-1073.

Waived Tests and Provider-Performed Microscopy

An updated list of waived tests, including a list of manufacturers and brand names, can be obtained at http://www.fda.gov/cdrh/clia/testswaived.html. A computer-assisted course is available at http://www.vh.org/Providers/CME/CLIA/CLIAHP. Laboratories with certificates of waiver are not inspected routinely. However, they may be inspected to investigate complaints or inspected on a random basis to determine whether only waived tests are being performed. The following tests were waived at the time of this writing:

- Dipstick urinalysis
- Rapid tests for group A streptococcus
- Rapid tests for mononucleosis antibodies (mono spot test)
- Rapid test for influenza A and B antibodies
- Rapid tests for *Helicobacter pylori* antibodies

Clinicians performing such tests must obtain a CLIA license and designate a CLIA laboratory director.

Clinicians supervising waived tests can also carry out provider-performed microscopy, which means that the primary care clinician must personally examine the specimen. The following are examples:

- Spun urine sediment (see Chapter 14), useful in the diagnosis of cystitis and pyelonephritis
- Unspun urine (the presence of one bacterium per high-power field usually correlates with a bacterial concentration of $>10^5$ colony-forming units [CFUs]/mL on urine culture)
- Wet mount preparation of vaginal secretions. A drop of secretion is mixed with a drop of physiologic saline on a glass slide, and a coverslip is applied. With use of a dim substage light, the slide is examined under the $10\times$ or $45\times$ objective of the microscope for *T. vaginalis* (see Chapter 16).
- Potassium hydroxide (KOH) preparation of vaginal secretions. The technique is similar to the wet mount preparation except that 10% to 20% KOH is added instead of physiologic saline. The slide is examined for yeast elements (notably *Candida* species; see Chapter 16).
- Potassium hydroxide preparation of other specimens, such as skin scrapings. After KOH is added, the specimen is allowed to stand for 10 to 15 minutes or, alternatively, the slide is gently heated from below. KOH lyses background material and debris, allowing the fungal elements to be identified.
- Methylene blue examination for fecal leukocytes. A drop of methylene blue (or reticulocyte stain) is added to a drop of diarrheal stool on a glass slide, and a coverslip is applied. The specimen is examined for polymorphonuclear leukocytes (see Chapter 12).

Microscopy can be an extremely rewarding aspect of office practice, and the interested clinician will find other applications, such as examination of unstained expectorated sputum for eosinophils in cases of suspected asthma.

White Blood Cell Count, Differential Count, and Acute-Phase Reactants

The WBC count, differential count, and acute-phase reactants (erythrocyte sedimentation rate and C-reactive protein level) are commonly used as nonspecific indicators of infection. Abnormal results suggest disease, but normal results are less helpful in excluding disease. These tests are moderately complex and require proficiency testing.

Complete Blood Cell and Differential Counts

The range for normal WBC count varies with age (higher in children and adolescents), with time of day (higher in the afternoon), and with race (higher in whites than in African-Americans). "Leukocytosis" can be arbitrarily defined for adults as >11,000 WBCs per microliter of blood (in various studies, the 95% confidence limit for the upper limit of the WBC count has been 9206 to 10,900 WBCs per microliter). Leukocytosis represents a nonspecific response to illness or stress. Marked leukocytosis (>25,000 WBCs per microliter) often indicates severe illness. Lesser degrees of leukocytosis support the clinician's suspicion that something is wrong but are less helpful in suggesting a bacterial, viral, or noninfectious etiology. *A normal WBC count should not be used as grounds for rejecting the possibility of acute, potentially serious illness.* Leukocytosis is absent in up to 40% of bacteremic infections in adults. "Leukopenia," which can be arbitrarily defined for adults as <4000 WBCs per microliter, is often present in severe infection, especially in persons who are elderly, debilitated, or suffering from alcoholism.

Information obtained from examining the peripheral blood smear is more helpful than the total WBC count. Bandemia, defined as an elevated percentage of immature polymorphonuclear neutrophils (PMNs) in proportion to segmented PMNs, is often used as a laboratory sign of significant infection. The definition of band forms is subject to observer bias. Moreover, the differential blood count is subject to chance variation (up to 15%) in the percentages of various cell types based on counting 100 cells. Vacuolization of the cytoplasm of PMNs is found in up to 90% of patients with serious bacteremic infection. Lymphocytopenia is commonly present during acute bacterial infection. Lymphocytosis, and especially atypical lymphocytosis, suggests the possibility of mononucleosis (see Chapter 8). Occasionally, bacterial, fungal, or parasitic organisms are observed in the peripheral blood smear. Examination of the peripheral blood smear can be pivotal to early diagnosis of certain infections, including malaria, babesiosis, disseminated histoplasmosis, and sepsis in asplenic persons (see Chapter 1).

Acute-Phase Reactants: Erythrocyte Sedimentation Rate and C-Reactive Protein

The erythrocyte sedimentation rate (ESR) and C-reactive protein (CRP) are commonly used to suggest the presence or absence of significant disease, although rigorous validation for this purpose is lacking. With the notable exception of trichinosis, most infectious diseases tend to elevate the ESR. The ESR is usually elevated in endocarditis, tuberculosis, and osteomyelitis. However, the ESR can be elevated in >10% of persons without disease, especially the elderly. The greatest value of the ESR in primary care may be to reassure the "worried well" who have nonspecific complaints, do not appear ill, and have unrevealing results on physical examination. Many such patients require a "laboratory test" for adequate reassurance, and the relatively inexpensive ESR can be useful in this regard. Many clinicians use the ESR to monitor response to therapy of certain infections, notably osteomyelitis. An ESR >100 mm/hr has diagnostic utility in temporal arteritis but can also indicate infection, malignancy, and other systemic diseases.

Bacterial infections usually cause an abrupt, dramatic rise in the C-reactive protein level. Many authorities believe the

CRP to be a better test than the ESR as an indicator of acute infection. However, neither test should be used as a basis for decision making in acute situations.

 KEY POINTS

WHITE BLOOD CELL COUNT, DIFFERENTIAL COUNT, AND ACUTE-PHASE REACTANTS

⊃ Leukocytosis is a nonspecific response to illness or stress. A high WBC count supports the diagnosis of infection, but a normal WBC count should not be used to exclude the possibility of serious infection.

⊃ Examination of the peripheral blood smear provides more useful information than does the total WBC count.

⊃ The erythrocyte sedimentation rate and C-reactive protein level are often used as indicators of the presence of disease but are nonspecific.

SUGGESTED READING

Brigden ML, Heathcote JC. Problems in interpreting laboratory tests: what do unexpected results mean? Postgrad Med 2000; 107: 145-146, 151-152, 155-158.

Callahan M. Inaccuracy and expense of the leukocyte count in making urgent clinical decisions. Ann Emerg Med 1986; 15: 774-781.

Carragee EJ, Kim D, van der Vlugt T, et al. The clinical use of erythrocyte sedimentation rate in pyogenic vertebral osteomyelitis. Spine 1997; 22: 2089-2093.

Shapiro MF, Greenfield S. The complete blood count and leukocyte differential count: an approach to their rational application. Ann Intern Med 1987; 106: 65-74.

Sox HC, Liang MH. The erythrocyte sedimentation rate: guidelines for rational use. Ann Intern Med 1986; 104: 515-523.

General Microbiology

Cultures continue to be the "gold standard" for diagnosis of many infectious diseases and are especially important for diseases requiring prolonged therapy, such as tuberculosis, endocarditis, and osteomyelitis. Microscopic examination of specimens submitted for culture often suggests the final diagnosis.

Specimen Collection and Transport

Proper choice, collection, and transport of clinical specimens are essential.

The specimen must be from an appropriate source. Specimens from inappropriate sources can be dangerously misleading, suggesting the need to use potent and potentially toxic drugs against microorganisms that in reality are only surface colonizers (see Chapter 1).

Inappropriate sources for specimens are, in general, heavily colonized body surfaces, substances, and fluids. The following are examples:

- Surface material from diabetic foot ulcers, decubitus ulcers, and other open wounds, including the margins of nonviable amputations
- Sinus tract drainage from patients with chronic osteomyelitis (see discussion in Chapter 15)

- Nasal swab specimens from patients with sinusitis
- Nasopharyngeal cultures from patients with otitis media

Specimens from heavily colonized body surfaces, substances, and fluids are appropriate only if the physician seeks to identify one or several specific pathogens. The following are examples:

- Throat cultures for *Streptococcus pyogenes* (see Chapter 10)
- Stool cultures for enteric pathogens (see Chapter 12)
- Cultures of urethra, cervix, or rectum for *N. gonorrhoeae* and other sexually transmitted pathogens (see Chapter 16)
- Vaginal cultures for *Candida* species (see Chapter 16)
- Nasal cultures for *Staphylococcus aureus* colonization (see Chapters 1 and 15)
- Cultures of decubitus ulcers or other wounds in a search for drug-resistant organisms such as methicillin-resistant *S. aureus* or vancomycin-resistant enterococci

In these instances the clinician should specify the sought-after pathogen(s).

Appropriate sources for specimens include especially body fluids and tissues that are normally sterile:

- Blood
- Other body fluids: cerebrospinal fluid (CSF), pleural fluid, ascitic fluid, synovial fluid
- Voided urine (with adequate decontamination of periurethral tissue)
- Biopsy specimens (obtained with aseptic technique)
- Aspirates of subcutaneous tissue or soft tissue lesions (obtained with aseptic technique, described below)

Cultures for anaerobic bacteria are seldom necessary in primary care practice. Clinical clues to anaerobic infection include foul odor, infection contiguous to a heavily colonized mucosal surface, tissue gas, and the presence of numerous bacterial morphologies on Gram stain.

For cultures requiring aseptic technique, such as blood cultures, aspirates, and biopsy specimens, the site must be carefully prepared. The site should be cleaned with 70% to 95% isopropyl or ethyl alcohol and then disinfected with an iodophor (Betadine and others) or 2% tincture of iodine. Some data suggest that tincture of iodine is superior to the iodophors, but the latter is more commonly used because it is less likely to cause skin sensitization. The iodophor must be allowed to dry completely before the specimen is obtained, since these compounds require contact for 1 to 2 minutes to exert their antimicrobial effect.

Swabs are commonly used to obtain cultures in office practice. *It is a mistake to send a swab specimen when a generous amount of purulent material is available.* When an abscess has been aspirated, for example, it is best to submit the syringe, capped after removal of the needle. Currently available swabs are tipped with cotton, calcium alginate, rayon, or polyester. Cotton-tipped swabs are acceptable for throat cultures but generally are less preferred because cotton is more toxic to microorganisms than the alternatives. Calcium alginate inactivates herpes simplex virus and can interfere with tests based on the polymerase chain reaction (PCR), and therefore swabs tipped with calcium alginate should not be used for most viral studies. Swabs should be placed immediately in transport media to prevent drying.

Specimens should be correctly identified, including the date and time of collection and the precise source. Specifying the suspected pathogen(s) is often useful. Ideally, the microbiology laboratory receives the specimen within 1 hour after collection. Primary care clinicians who must rely on remote laboratories are therefore at a disadvantage. Blood cultures and cultures for *Neisseria gonorrhoeae,* anaerobic bacteria, fungi, and *T. vaginalis* should be kept at room temperature. Other specimens should usually be kept at refrigerator temperature (36° to 47° F [2° to 8° C]) if prompt transportation to the microbiology laboratory is not possible. Transport systems to preserve specimen integrity for up to 24 hours are available and are often provided by the reference laboratory. Accrediting agencies require laboratories to reject such specimens as the following:

- Specimens inappropriate for a particular test
- Specimens that are unlabeled or improperly labeled
- Specimens that are obviously contaminated
- Specimens that are received in broken, cracked, or leaking containers
- Unpreserved specimens that are received more than 12 hours after collection

Sputum cultures are a special case. Specimens should be rejected if they show heavy contamination by saliva (see later discussion).

Microscopic Examination of Stained Specimens

Microscopic examination of stained specimens for microorganisms, classified by CLIA as a moderate-complexity test, requires adequate specimen collection, preparation, and quality control.

Gram staining is used to sort bacteria into two groups based on the composition of their cell walls. The slide containing the dried specimen is flooded in turn with four reagents: crystal violet or gentian violet, Gram's iodine, a decolorizing agent (95% ethanol or acetone-ethanol), and a red counterstain (safranin). Bacteria that resist decolorization appear purple and are called gram positive. Bacteria that are decolorized appear red with the counterstain and are called gram negative. Precipitates of crystal violet can be mistaken for gram-positive bacteria. Excessive decolorization causes gram-positive bacteria to appear red, whereas incomplete decolorization causes gram-negative bacteria to appear purple. Gram staining, although simple, requires adequate controls and a measure of skill. The sensitivity of the stain varies according to the density of bacteria in the specimen, ranging from about 25% for $<10^3$ CFUs/mL to 95% for $\geq 10^5$ CFUs/mL. Appearances of common bacteria on Gram stain of sputum are shown in Chapter 11.

AFB stains are used to identify mycobacteria and *Nocardia* species. Acid-fast organisms are so called because they resist decolorization with acid-alcohol. Fluorochrome stains (such as the auramine-rhodamine or Truant stain) are more sensitive than the conventional basic fuchsin stains (Kinyoun and Ziehl-Neelsen stains) and are therefore used for screening by many laboratories. Because sensitivity of a single AFB smear for tuberculosis ranges from 20% to 80%, three specimens are customarily collected (see Chapter 22). The predictive value of a positive AFB smear is critically dependent on the pretest probability of tuberculosis.

Other stains for microorganisms that are useful in primary care practice are Wright and Giemsa stains of peripheral blood (see earlier discussion), methylene blue stain for fecal leukocytes (see Chapter 12), calcofluor white and periodic acid–Schiff stains for fungi, and cytologic stains (Papanicolaou [Pap] and Tzanck preparations) for multinucleated giant cells caused by herpes simplex virus infection.

Cultures

Cultures should be obtained before therapy whenever possible.

Blood Cultures

Patients with clear evidence of sepsis are usually referred to a hospital for blood cultures and management. Some patients who do not appear to be acutely ill also have positive blood cultures. This phenomenon is familiar to pediatricians as "walk-in bacteremia" but also occurs in adults. The most important indication for blood cultures for patients who are not acutely ill is the suspicion of endocarditis (see Chapter 6). When blood cultures are obtained, the skin should be decontaminated as thoroughly as possible (see earlier discussion). Gloves should be worn during the venipuncture. With rare exception, notably AFB blood culture for patients with human immunodeficiency virus (HIV) disease (see Chapter 17), a single blood culture is insufficient. For adults, two blood cultures obtained by separate venipunctures, with a total volume of 30 to 40 mL of blood, will detect about 99% of bacteremias that can be detected by multiple cultures. Three blood cultures are recommended when endocarditis is strongly suspected. Recent data largely dispel the time-honored notions that blood for cultures should be drawn at intervals at least 60 minutes apart, that six blood cultures should be obtained in cases of endocarditis, and that the needle should be changed before the bottle is inoculated. The laboratory should be notified and special media used when the practitioner has reason to suspect a fastidious microorganism, a fungus, or an unusual pathogen such as *Brucella* species.

Cerebrospinal Fluid Cultures (see also Chapter 6)

CSF cultures for bacteria should be of adequate volume (5 mL or more) and hand delivered to the laboratory as soon as possible. *Neisseria meningitidis* is temperature sensitive. Usually an extra tube (5 to 10 mL) of CSF should be saved in the event that the CSF findings (WBC and differential counts and glucose and protein levels) suggest the need for special studies, including AFB and fungal cultures.

Cultures of the Upper Respiratory Tract (see also Chapter 10)

Throat cultures are generally performed only for *S. pyogenes* (group A streptococci). Specimens are obtained by the swabbing of areas of exudate in the pharynx and often the tonsillar pillars. When the presence of *N. gonorrhoeae* is suspected, the specimen should be plated directly onto selective agar (e.g., modified Thayer-Martin agar, Martin-Lewis agar, New York City agar) as for genital cultures (see later discussion). When unusual pathogens such as *Corynebacterium diphtheriae* or *Bordetella pertussis* are suspected, special arrangements should be made with the microbiology laboratory, since immediate direct plating on selective media is required.

Sputum Cultures (see also Chapter 11)

Although their value has been debated for many years, sputum Gram stain and culture are still advisable for patients with severe pneumonia who are producing purulent sputum.

More than 10 squamous epithelial cells per low-power field (10× objective) indicates heavy contamination with saliva, which is grounds for rejection of the culture.

Urine Cultures (see also Chapter 14)

Since bacteria in urine double about every 20 minutes at room temperature, specimens of voided urine must be promptly refrigerated if they cannot be plated out in the physician's laboratory. Many transport systems for office-based and even home-based urine culture have been introduced over the years.

Genital Cultures (see also Chapter 16)

Sources of specimens for patients with suspected sexually transmitted disease include the urethra, cervical os, rectum, and throat. Calcium alginate swabs are commonly used, since swabs tipped with cotton or rayon are toxic to *N. gonorrhoeae*. Specimens obtained for *N. gonorrhoeae* should be inoculated directly onto selective media (such as modified Thayer-Martin agar) or placed in modified Stuart's medium and transported promptly to the laboratory. Cell culture for *Chlamydia trachomatis* has been largely replaced by DNA amplification techniques. When culture for *C. trachomatis* is desired, the specimen for *N. gonorrhoeae* should be obtained first, since vigorous swabbing for epithelial cells is recommended for chlamydial isolation. Methods of viral culture for herpes simplex are discussed below.

Stool Cultures (see also Chapter 12)

Although some authorities endorse rectal swab specimens, most recommend fresh, unformed stools. "Routine" stool culture is usually limited to *Salmonella, Shigella,* and *Campylobacter* species. The laboratory should be notified when there is strong reason to suspect other pathogens such as Shiga toxin–producing strains of *E. coli.*

The presence of fecal leukocytes suggests inflammatory diarrhea. As a screen for *Salmonella, Shigella,* or *Campylobacter,* fecal leukocytes were found to have a sensitivity of 29%, specificity of 93%, positive predictive value of 20%, and negative predictive value of 96%. The sensitivity of fecal leukocytes is 30% or less for colitis caused by *C. difficile,* for which the preferred test is the assay for toxin.

Cultures of Skin, Subcutaneous Tissue, Abscesses, and Wounds (see also Chapter 15)

The transient skin flora includes potential pathogens such as *S. aureus* and viridans streptococci, and therefore swab cultures are seldom if ever indicated. Culture of skin biopsy specimens for mycobacteria, fungi, and other pathogens is occasionally worthwhile.

Aspiration of subcutaneous tissue is sometimes indicated in the presence of inflammatory lesions such as nodules, abscesses, and cellulitis, possibly because of atypical microorganisms. One technique is as follows. The skin is thoroughly cleansed and then swabbed with an iodophor (see earlier discussion). Anesthesia is obtained by the intracutaneous injection of lidocaine, performed with a tuberculin syringe. A small amount (2 to 5 mL) of sterile saline *without preservative* is drawn up into a 20-mL syringe attached to a large-bore needle (e.g., 19 gauge). The needle is then inserted into the lesion, and an attempt is made to aspirate fluid. If no fluid is obtained, saline solution is injected into the lesion and a second aspiration is performed. The needle is then removed, the syringe capped, and the specimen transported promptly to the laboratory with specific instructions.

Cultures of surgical wounds often require special microbiologic techniques and are not generally carried out in primary care.

 KEY POINTS

GENERAL MICROBIOLOGY

⊃ Body sites that normally contain a resident flora are, in general, appropriate for culture only if one is seeking to identify one or several specific pathogens.

⊃ Swab specimens should not be submitted to the laboratory when abundant purulent material is available.

⊃ Strict aseptic technique is especially important when obtaining blood cultures, since contamination can lead to unnecessary treatment.

SUGGESTED READING

Bowler PG, Duerden BI, Armstrong DG. Wound microbiology and associated approaches to wound management. Clin Microbiol Rev 2001; 14: 244-269.

Bryan CS. Clinical implications of positive blood cultures. Clin Microbiol Rev 1989; 2: 329-353.

Epstein D, Raveh D, Schlesinger Y, et al. Adult patients with occult bacteremia discharged from the emergency department: epidemiological and clinical characteristics. Clin Infect Dis 2001; 32: 559-565.

Forbes BA, Sahm DF, Weissfeld AS. Bailey & Scott's Diagnostic Microbiology. 10th ed., St. Louis: Mosby; 1998.

Murray PR, Baron EJ, Pfaller MA, et al., eds. Manual of Clinical Microbiology. 7th ed., Washington, D.C.: ASM Press; 1999.

Wilson ML. General principles of specimen collection and transport. Clin Infect Dis 1996; 22: 766-777.

Diagnostic Immunology

Many infectious diseases are detected by serology or by antigen detection techniques that use serologic or molecular methods.

Diagnosis of an infectious disease by serologic testing for antibodies generally requires a diagnostic titer or demonstration of seroconversion by a four-fold increase in titer from "acute" to "convalescent" specimens. The acute and convalescent specimens should be tested under identical conditions. Therefore it is often appropriate to obtain an "acute serology" specimen, which is frozen until the convalescent sample is obtained a minimum of 7 to 10 days later. Determination of IgM antibody titers is replacing reliance on acute and convalescent specimens in many instances, but the clinician should recognize that IgM titers are sometimes nonspecifically elevated during the immune response, resulting in a false-positive test.

Serologic methods to detect antibodies or antigens include the following:

■ Precipitation, in which the reaction between antigen and antibody forms an insoluble complex. Tests based on precipitation have been largely replaced by newer methods.

■ Agglutination, in which antigen-containing particles on a slide or in a tube clump together in the presence of antibody. This method is used by laboratories to identify the presence of antibodies and is also used to serotype infectious agents. In a variant known as coagglutination, latex particles (or killed staphylococci) that have been coated with antibodies agglutinate in the presence of antigens. This principle is used to detect antigens, including *S. pyogenes* (group A streptococci) in throat swabs, *Cryptococcus neoformans* in CSF, and bacterial polysaccharide antigens (*Streptococcus pneumoniae, Haemophilus influenzae* type b, and *N. meningitidis*) in CSF.

■ Complement fixation, in which antigen is added to the patient's heated serum to which is then added guinea-pig complement. This time-honored test is technically difficult and has been largely replaced by newer methods.

■ Indirect fluorescent antibody tests, in which the patient's serum is added to slides containing specific antigen, which are then incubated and washed. Fluorescein-labeled antihuman immunoglobulin is added to slides, causing apple-green fluorescence if antigen-binding antibodies were present in the patient's serum. This test is sensitive and specific, but labor intensive.

■ Direct fluorescent antibody tests, in which fluorescein-labeled antibody against a specific pathogen is added to a slide containing the specimen. This test, which takes only 30 minutes to 3 hours to perform, is used to identify such pathogens as *C. trachomatis, Legionella* species, *S. pyogenes, Pneumocystis carinii, B. pertussis, Giardia* species, and *Cryptosporidium* species.

■ Enzyme-linked immunosorbent assay (ELISA), in which antigen or antibody in a specimen is allowed to a bind to a solid phase (such as the walls of microtiter wells). Enzyme-labeled antihuman immunoglobulin or antigen is added, causing a color to appear when antigen-antibody complexes have formed. ELISA tests can be used to detect either antigen or antibody. Relatively low cost, long shelf life of reagents, lack of radioactivity, and adaptability to many variations make ELISA tests increasingly popular for diagnosis of a wide range of infectious diseases. Many kits allow testing for both IgG and IgM antibodies.

■ Immunoblotting (Western blot tests), which test for antibodies to a range of microbial proteins that have been separated by exposure to a detergent solution and polyacrylamide gel electrophoresis. This method is used for confirmatory testing in the serologic diagnosis of Lyme disease and HIV disease.

These and other innovations make serology an increasingly important aspect of the primary care clinician's armamentarium.

At present, serologic testing for antibodies is especially useful in the diagnosis of pneumonia caused by "atypical" pathogens such as *Mycoplasma pneumoniae, Chlamydia pneumoniae, Chlamydia psittaci, Legionella pneumophila,* and *Francisella tularensis* (see Chapter 11), mononucleosis caused by Epstein-Barr virus or cytomegalovirus (see Chapter 8), causes of fever and rash such as Rocky Mountain spotted fever, ehrlichiosis, and leptospirosis (see Chapter 8), viral hepatitis (see Chapter 13), toxoplasmosis (see Chapters 8 and 17), HIV infection (see Chapters 4 and 17), and childhood exanthems (see Chapters 4 and 8). Serologic testing for antigens in clinical specimens is especially useful in the diagnosis of streptococcal pharyngitis (rapid strep test; see Chapter 10), *C. difficile* colitis (see Chapter 12), and three sexually transmitted pathogens: herpes simplex virus, *C. trachomatis,* and *N. gonorrhoeae* (see Chapter 16). Serologic techniques can also be applied to biopsy specimens for specific diagnosis.

In the past, testing for "febrile agglutinins" was often requested for patients with unexplained fever. The practice is now discouraged unless a reason exists to suspect a specific disease entity such as brucellosis or tularemia.

 KEY POINTS

DIAGNOSTIC IMMUNOLOGY

⊃ Serologic methods now offer a wide array of tests for both antibodies and antigens.

⊃ Serologic diagnosis can be based on a diagnostic antibody titer, a four-fold increase in titer between acute and convalescent specimens, or an IgM antibody test.

⊃ For patients with undiagnosed problems, obtaining and storing a serum sample in the acute stage of the illness for later use is often appropriate.

⊃ Serologic tests should generally be used to answer specific questions. The practice of requesting tests for "febrile agglutinins" should be discouraged.

SUGGESTED READING

Rose NR, de Macario ED, Folds JD, et al. Manual of Clinical Laboratory Immunology. 5th ed., Washington, D.C.: ASM Press; 1997.

Storch GA. Diagnostic virology. Clin Infect Dis 2000; 31: 739-751.

Turgeon ML. Immunology and Serology in Laboratory Medicine. 2nd ed., St. Louis: Mosby; 1996.

Molecular Diagnostics

Breakthroughs in molecular biology may in the foreseeable future revolutionize the diagnosis of infectious diseases. The PCR and other nucleic acid amplification techniques already have important clinical applications. Molecular amplification methods are also being used to facilitate genotyping in order to detect mutations associated with drug-resistant pathogens, including HIV (see Chapter 17).

The PCR is based on the ability of an enzyme, DNA polymerase, to make large quantities of new double-stranded DNA fragments out of three basic ingredients. These are a generous supply of nucleosides (adenine, cytosine, guanine, and thymidine, the four building blocks of DNA), a pair of primers (short sequences of nucleotides that are specific for the nucleic acid sequence of a given pathogen), and the DNA contained in the clinical specimen (usually added to the mixture as an unknown). The specimen is heated to separate the DNA strands, which then bind to the primers. Taq polymerase adds nucleosides to form new double-stranded DNA fragments. The specimen is heated again, and the process is repeated. In this way billions of DNA copies can be generated from a few DNA strands present in the specimen.

PCR testing is exceedingly sensitive and also specific, if carefully controlled. The extreme sensitivity is its Achilles' heel, since low-level contamination can cause false-positive results. Various body substances, including blood, sputum, urine, and other fluids, may contain inhibitors of PCR that can cause false-negative results, necessitating controls for the presence of inhibitors.

PCR is proving useful in the diagnosis of herpes simplex encephalitis (see Chapter 6), tuberculous meningitis (see Chapter 22), HIV, hepatitis C, and infections caused by *C. trachomatis* and *N. gonorrhoeae.* The detection of human papillomavirus (HPV) serotypes in liquid-based cytology preparations by molecular methods has recently shown value in the evaluation of patients with low-grade abnormalities on Pap smear (atypical squamous cells of uncertain significance [ASCUS]). The detection of high-risk serotypes of HPV identifies a woman who is at significantly increased risk for progression to high-grade dysplasia and will therefore need colposcopy and biopsies (see Chapter 16). If only low-risk HPV or no HPV nucleic acid is detected, routine follow-up can be used. Primary care clinicians also find PCR to be especially useful for resolving questions that arise when blood donors receive the information that their serum tested positive or equivocal for antibodies to various pathogens such as HIV and hepatitis C. Quantitation of RNA or DNA using PCR is known as the "viral load test" and is used for follow-up of patients with HIV and hepatitis C and also in other situations, such as cytomegalovirus infection.

Other molecular diagnostic technologies are in various stages of development and clinical use. Examples include the ligase chain reaction (LCR) and Qβ replicase system (probe amplification technologies), self-sustaining sequence replication reaction (3SR), nucleic acid sequence—based amplification (NASBA), transcription-mediated amplification (TMA) and strand-displacement amplification (SDA) (target amplification technologies), and branched DNA (bDNA) assay (a signal amplification technology). Molecular techniques are also being applied to biopsy specimens and cytologic preparations to establish infectious etiologies. We have seen only the beginning.

 KEY POINTS

MOLECULAR DIAGNOSTICS

⊃ Molecular diagnostic methods in current use include nucleic acid amplification and signal amplification technologies.

⊃ The PCR is especially useful in the diagnosis of herpes simplex encephalitis, HIV, hepatitis C, and HPV infection.

SUGGESTED READING

Fredricks DN, Relman DA. Application of polymerase chain reaction to the diagnosis of infectious diseases. Clin Infect Dis 1999; 29: 475-488.

Procop GW, Wilson M. Infectious disease pathology. Clin Infect Dis 2001; 32: 1589-1601.

Tang Y-W, Hibbs JR, Tau KR, et al. Effective use of polymerase chain reaction for diagnosis of central nervous system infections. Clin Infect Dis 1999; 29: 803-806.

3

Host Considerations

ROHIT TALWANI, CHARLES S. BRYAN

The Elderly
Patients with Diabetes Mellitus
Patients Receiving Corticosteroids
Patients with Prosthetic Devices
Patients with Alcoholism or Liver Disease
Injecting Drug Users
Patients with Lymphoma, Leukemia, or Other
    Malignancies
Patients with Spinal Cord Injuries
Organ Transplant Recipients
Primary Immunodeficiency Syndrome Manifested in
    Adulthood
Special Populations

Care more particularly for the individual patient than for the special features of the disease.

William Osler

The careful clinician keeps in mind the predispositions of specific patients to specific diseases. Important examples are the predisposition of asplenic persons to overwhelming sepsis caused by *Streptococcus pneumoniae* and other pathogens (see Chapter 6), of persons with sickle cell disease to pneumococcal infections and osteomyelitis caused by *Salmonella* species (see Chapter 15), and of persons with cystic fibrosis to bronchiectasis (see Chapter 11). Infections associated with childhood (see Chapter 4) and pregnancy (see Chapter 5) are also discussed elsewhere. In this chapter we review some of the host factors predisposing to infection and likely to be encountered in primary care.

SUGGESTED READING

Cunha BA, ed. Infections in the compromised host. Infect Dis Clin North Am 2001; 15: 335-708.
Glauser MP, Pizzo PA, eds. Management of Infections in Immunocompromised Patients. Philadelphia: W.B. Saunders Company; 2000.

The Elderly

Primary care clinicians must be conversant with the susceptibility of elderly persons to certain types of infections. The importance of the pneumococcal and influenza vaccines cannot be overemphasized.

Problems in Host Defenses

Progressive dysregulation of the immune system occurs throughout life and affects cell-mediated immunity to a greater extent than humoral immunity. Immunization is often less effective in older persons. Physiologic problems that predispose to infection include impairments of cough reflex, blood circulation, micturition, and wound healing. Blunting of the febrile and pain responses often renders the symptoms and signs of infection more subtle in older persons than in younger ones. A suggested criterion for fever in an older person residing in a long-term care facility is 100° F (37.8° C) rather than the standard 101° F (38.3° C) used for younger persons (Table 3-1). The possibility of infection must be kept in mind, especially as a cause of clinical deterioration in an older person living in a long-term care facility.

Pneumonia

Pneumonia (see Chapter 11) is the most important cause of infectious disease mortality in older persons. Community-acquired pneumonia is 50 times more common in persons in their seventies than in teenagers. Pneumonia is often a subtle disease in older persons. Confusion, delirium, and impaired level of consciousness may be the presenting features. The temperature is commonly normal. Sputum may be absent because of impairment of the cough reflex. The chest x-ray film may be normal or difficult to interpret because of heart failure, chronic obstructive lung disease, or pulmonary scars from previous infections. Recent data indicate that an increase in the respiratory rate to more than 25 breaths per minute may be the most useful bedside sign of the presence of pneumonia in an older person (90% sensitive and 95% specific in one study). An increase in the respiratory rate should prompt further evaluation that may include pulse oximetry, complete blood cell count (CBC), chest x-ray examination, and sputum collection for Gram stain and culture. When life-threatening pneumonia is suspected, the patient should be hospitalized unless the preferences of the patient or the family (as indicated by advance directives or health care power of attorney) dictate otherwise.

Urinary Tract Infection

Urinary tract infection (UTI; see Chapter 14) occurs frequently in older men and women. In women, common predisposing causes are incontinence, atrophic changes in the bladder neck and the urethra, and impaired neuromuscular function. In men, prostatism is the usual predisposing cause. About 20% of elderly women and 10% of elderly men have asymptomatic bacteriuria, and the prevalence can be as high as 50% in nursing homes. The etiology varies depending on the circumstances. *Escherichia coli* is likely to be the cause in persons who have not received prior genitourinary instrumentation or antimicrobial therapy for UTI. In persons who have received prior treatment, which is common in the institutionalized elderly population, common pathogens include gram-negative rods (other than *E. coli*), enterococci, *Staphylococcus aureus,* and yeasts.

Asymptomatic bacteriuria in elderly patients should usually be left untreated, since therapy predisposes to UTI caused by microorganisms that are more difficult to treat. These include *Pseudomonas aeruginosa,* yeasts, and, increasingly, vancomycin-resistant enterococci. Treatment is indicated when clinical symptoms and signs of sepsis such as fever and flank pain are present. The diagnosis of urosepsis should be made with care even when pyuria and bacteriuria are present. UTI is the cause of only about two thirds of febrile episodes

in nursing home residents with pyuria and bacteriuria. UTI is the most common cause of documented bacteremia in elderly patients in nursing homes, but the case-fatality rate for these episodes is low compared with the case-fatality rate for bacteremia pneumonia. Nevertheless, older persons with urosepsis should be evaluated carefully for the possibility of obstructive uropathy. Ultrasound and computed tomography (CT) are now preferred for this purpose (see Chapter 14).

Tuberculosis

Tuberculosis (TB; see Chapter 22) is the most common reportable disease in elderly patients. Nearly 25% of cases of TB in the United States occur in persons over 65 years of age. Data obtained primarily by Dr. William Stead in

TABLE 3-1
Evaluation of Fever and Infection in Patients in Long-Term Care Facilities*

Aspect	Comments
Temperature	The definition of "fever" should be liberal, using a criterion of 100° F (37.8° C) rather than 101° F (38.3° C). In one study 101° F had only a 40% sensitivity for infection, while lowering the criterion to 100° F raised the sensitivity to 70%, with 90% specificity. In another study a single temperature reading of 100° F or greater had a positive predictive value of 55% for infection.
Respiratory rate	The respiratory rate should be measured carefully as a guide to serious infection and specifically pneumonia. In one study, a respiratory rate >25 beats/min was 90% sensitive and 95% specific for pneumonia, with positive and negative predictive values of 95%.
Complete blood count	A complete blood count should be obtained for all persons with suspected infection. Total white blood cell count $\geq$14,000/mm³ or >6% band forms (or total band count $\geq$1500/mm³) suggests the need for further evaluation.
Blood cultures	*Blood cultures are not recommended in the nursing home setting,* since (1) patients with suspected bacteremia should be admitted to a hospital (pending the patient's and family's preferences) and (2) the 24-hour mortality rate for patients with bacteremia is high.
Evaluation for pneumonia	Pulse oximetry should be performed on patients with respiratory rates >25/min. An oxygen saturation <90% is consistent with pneumonia. Chest x-ray examination should be performed if hypoxemia is present. In patients producing sputum, a sputum Gram stain should be obtained and a sputum culture performed if the specimen is acceptable (<25 squamous epithelial cells per low power field). When an outbreak of respiratory infection is suspected, throat and nasopharyngeal swab specimens should be obtained from several residents for virus diagnostic studies (see Chapter 20).
Evaluation for UTI	Urinalysis and urine culture should be performed when urosepsis is suspected. The clinician should keep in mind that asymptomatic UTI is common in this population and that fever may not be due to UTI even when UTI is present. Treatment of asymptomatic UTI is not recommended (see Chapter 14).
Evaluation for infectious diarrhea	If antibiotics have been given within the past 30 days, stool should be submitted for *Clostridium difficile* toxin assay. If the patient has no history of antibiotic therapy, appropriate workup includes evaluation for fecal leukocytes and stool culture for relatively frequent pathogens *(Salmonella* and *Shigella* species, *Campylobacter jejuni, Escherichia coli* O157:H7). In an outbreak situation, a stool test for rotavirus may also be appropriate.
Evaluation of skin and soft tissue infections	In patients with suspected cellulitis, fine-needle aspiration (after injection of a small amount of sterile saline without preservative) is appropriate in selected circumstances (especially in patients with diabetes mellitus or with cellulitis that is not typical of erysipelas; see Chapter 15). Patients with decubitus ulcers should usually receive surgical attention.

UTI, Urinary tract infection.
*For further discussion and citations of data summarized here, see Bentley DW, Bradley S, High K, et al. Practice guideline for evaluation of fever and infection in long-term care facilities. Clin Infect Dis 2000; 31: 640-653.

Arkansas reshaped the understanding of TB in several ways that are important to the care of elderly persons, especially in nursing homes:

- Many persons outlive their tubercle bacilli and are therefore vulnerable to reinfection. This observation refutes the notion that tubercle bacilli remain viable within macrophages in the lung apices for the remainder of the person's life.
- TB can occur as a major epidemic in nursing homes. The symptoms and signs of TB in older persons are often subtle and may be misattributed to another process, such as presumed carcinoma of the lung. Thus many persons may be exposed.
- Preventive therapy with isoniazid (INH) can be given safely to older persons provided procedures for monitoring toxicity are in place.
- Baseline tuberculin skin testing followed by annual testing is cost effective in the nursing home setting. Use of INH for latent TB infection has been shown to extend life, including years with a good quality of life.
- TB should be suspected as a cause of deterioration in an older person's general health or of failure to thrive. Unexplained fever, cough, night sweats, or lymphadenopathy should also raise the possibility of this diagnosis.

Meningitis

Bacterial meningitis (see Chapter 6) is an uncommon but preventable cause of mortality in older persons, in whom the mortality level is increased (50% versus 10% for younger patients in one study) and complications are more frequent. *S. pneumoniae* is the most common cause, followed by *Listeria monocytogenes* and *H. influenzae*. The signs of acute bacterial meningitis are often muted. Nuchal rigidity in older patients is commonly attributed to arthritis or neurologic disease. Chronic meningitis, most commonly caused by *Mycobacterium tuberculosis* or *Cryptococcus neoformans*, must be kept in mind as a treatable cause of mental deterioration. The key to diagnosis of meningitis is a low threshold for performing lumbar puncture, which is often done most easily with use of fluoroscopy because of the presence of degenerative disease of the lower spine.

Endocarditis

Infective endocarditis (see Chapter 6) is increasingly a disease of the elderly. An older person with degenerative valvular heart disease (e.g., calcific aortic stenosis or calcification of the mitral valve annulus) has replaced a younger person with rheumatic heart disease as the usual patient. More than 50% of cases of endocarditis now occur in persons over 60 years of age. Symptoms and signs of endocarditis in older persons can be subtle and include anorexia, malaise, confusion, weakness, and weight loss. Studies indicate that fever and heart murmur are as common in the elderly as in younger patients but that the significance of these findings is often misinterpreted in older persons. However, complications of endocarditis are often more dramatic in older adults. These include heart failure, stroke, embolic occlusion of large arteries, myocardial infarction, cardiac conduction abnormalities, arrhythmias, myocarditis, and myocardial abscess. Any of these symptoms and signs should prompt three sets of blood cultures. As in younger persons, gram-positive bacteria are the usual cause of endocarditis in older adults.

Gastroenteritis and Intraabdominal Infection

Gastroenteritis and intraabdominal infections (see Chapter 12) are more common, often more subtle, and associated with higher mortality in older persons than in younger ones. About half of U.S. deaths from gastroenteritis occur in persons over 74 years of age. Epidemics of diarrhea caused by rotaviruses and other agents sometimes occur in nursing homes and can cause death in the frail elderly. Intraabdominal infections, including perforated bowel caused by appendicitis and diverticulitis, frequently have subtle presentations in older persons and can be life threatening. Older persons with acute appendicitis usually have some combination of fever, right lower quadrant pain, and leukocytosis, but the significance of these findings is often misinterpreted. Biliary tract disease is more common in older persons, who die disproportionately from acute cholecystitis or cholangitis.

> ### PATIENT 1
> A 75-year-old man with a history of four strokes was admitted to the hospital with complaints of abdominal pain and "falling down." Examination revealed slurred speech and right upper quadrant abdominal tenderness. One family member gave a history of cholecystectomy. White blood cell (WBC) count was 27,000/mm³ with 5% band forms; serum bilirubin level was 5.2 mg/dL (direct 3.8 mg/dL), and alkaline phosphatase level was 236 units/dL (normal up to 115) with aspartate aminotransferase (AST) level 123 mg/dL and alanine aminotransferase (ALT) level 252 mg/dL. Ultrasound of the abdomen revealed a dilated gallbladder with a thickened wall (Figure 3-1). A necrotic gallbladder was removed at surgery (the history of cholecystectomy thus proving to have been erroneous).

Septic Arthritis and Osteomyelitis

Septic arthritis (see Chapter 15) occurs disproportionately in elderly persons (about 25% of cases) and is often associated with impaired host defenses. A painful, swollen joint can be misinterpreted as gout or rheumatoid arthritis. *S. aureus* is the usual cause of septic arthritis, but aerobic gram-negative rods

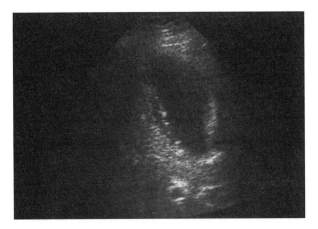

FIG. 3-1 Ultrasound examination of the abdomen, showing dilated gallbladder with thickened wall in a 75-year-old man who was admitted with abdominal pain and was unable to give a history because of four previous strokes. A gangrenous gallbladder was removed at surgery.

are a relatively common cause. Acute septic arthritis should be viewed as a medical emergency because of the high risk of joint destruction. Hematogenous osteomyelitis in older persons has special predilection for the vertebrae and can be misinterpreted as nonspecific low back pain. Spinal epidural abscess (see Chapter 6) is a potential complication. Patients with decubitus ulcers are vulnerable to osteomyelitis of the sacrum, and patients with diabetes mellitus are vulnerable to polymicrobial osteomyelitis of the small bones of the feet (see Chapter 15).

Fever of Undetermined Origin

Fever of undetermined origin (FUO), as defined by the modified Petersdorf-Beeson criteria (see Chapter 1), is an uncommon problem in the elderly but has important implications. Various studies indicate that a precise diagnosis of FUO is made in 87% to 95% of elderly patients with this problem, which is a much higher rate than in younger persons. Moreover, about half of cases of FUO in older persons are due to a curable disease such as temporal arteritis, endocarditis, tuberculosis, or intraabdominal abscess. Neoplasms, especially diffuse histiocytic lymphoma and Hodgkin's disease, are also relatively important causes of FUO in older persons.

Special Problems in Long-Term Care Facilities

Primary care clinicians whose practice includes patients in long-term care facilities should have a general familiarity with guidelines for infection control. Urinary catheters should be used only when necessary. If patients have impaired neurologic function, close attention must be paid to feeding (to prevent aspiration pneumonia) and to frequent turning (to prevent decubitus ulcers). Drug-resistant bacteria, especially methicillin-resistant *S. aureus* (MRSA) and vancomycin-resistant *Enterococcus faecium,* are becoming a problem at most long-term facilities in the United States. The heavy use of fluoroquinolone antibiotics for presumptive treatment of pneumonia and other infections is a possible risk factor. Outbreaks of viral or bacterial infection are relatively common in long-term facilities and sometimes involve more than one pathogen. Outbreaks of scabies (see Chapter 23) can be frustrating for both patients and staff and are often caused by failure to diagnose the initial case properly. Recent guidelines for evaluation of fever in residents of long-term care facilities take into account the need to pay close attention to the patient's mental status and vital signs, to use laboratory tests selectively, and to consider preferences expressed by the patient and family concerning the desirability of hospitalization (Table 3-1).

 KEY POINTS

INFECTIONS IN THE ELDERLY

⊃ The increased incidence of infections is due in part to waning T- and B-cell immunity, impairment of physiologic processes, and comorbid conditions.

⊃ Clinical presentations of infection are often subtle. Fever may be blunted or absent, pain vague or atypical, and laboratory evidence of infection less dramatic.

⊃ Persons over 65 years of age should receive the pneumococcal vaccine and yearly immunization against influenza.

⊃ Indwelling urinary catheters should be avoided when possible.

⊃ Pneumonia is the major infectious cause of death in elderly persons and can be difficult to diagnose.

⊃ UTI is common in the elderly, but death from urosepsis is confined mainly to the severely debilitated.

⊃ Tuberculosis is the most common reportable infectious disease in the elderly and often has subtle presentations such as tuberculous meningitis or "cryptic" miliary tuberculosis. Two-step tuberculin testing and chemoprophylaxis are important in nursing home patients.

⊃ Meningitis carries a greater than 50% mortality in the elderly. *S. pneumoniae* is the most common cause, but others are *L. monocytogenes,* aerobic gram-negative rods, and *M. tuberculosis.*

⊃ Endocarditis is now primarily a disease of the elderly, often occurring in patients with "degenerative" lesions such as aortic sclerosis and calcification of the mitral valve annulus.

⊃ True fever of unknown origin (FUO) in the elderly, compared with younger persons, is more likely to be caused by a diagnosable disease, and about half of the diagnosed causative conditions are potentially curable.

SUGGESTED READING

Bentley DW, Bradley S, High K, et al. Practice guidelines for evaluation of fever and infection in long-term care facilities. Clin Infect Dis 2000; 31: 640-653.

Bonomo RA. Multiple antibiotic-resistant bacteria in long-term-care facilities: an emerging problem in the practice of infectious diseases. Clin Infect Dis 2000; 31: 1414-1422.

Butler JC, Cetron MS. Pneumococcal drug resistance: the new "special enemy of old age." Clin Infect Dis 1999; 28: 730-735.

Castle SC. Clinical relevance of age-related immune dysfunction. Clin Infect Dis 2000; 31: 578-585.

Marrie TJ. Community-acquired pneumonia in the elderly. Clin Infect Dis 2000; 31: 1066-1078.

Mouton CP, Bazaldua OV, Pierce B, et al. Common infections in older adults. Am Fam Physician 2001; 63: 257-268.

Nicolle LE. Infection control in long-term care facilities. Clin Infect Dis 2000; 31: 752-756.

Nicolle LE, The SHEA Long-Term Care Committee. Urinary tract infections in long-term-care facilities. Infect Control Hosp Epidemiol 2001; 22: 167-175.

Norman DC. Fever in the elderly. Clin Infect Dis 2000; 31: 148-151.

Smith PW, Black JM, Black SB. Infected pressure ulcers in the long-term-care facility. Infect Control Hosp Epidemiol 1999; 20: 358-361.

Turnheim K. Drug dosage in the elderly: is it rational? Drugs Aging 1998; 13: 357-379.

Yeh SS, Schuster MW. Geriatric cachexia: the role of cytokines. Am J Clin Nutr 1999; 70: 183-197.

Yoshikawa TT, Norman DC, eds. Infectious Disease in the Aging. Totowa, NJ: Humana Press; 2001.

Patients with Diabetes Mellitus

The assertion is often made that patients with diabetes mellitus have increased susceptibility to infection. Some authorities counter that statistical evidence for such an association remains scanty. However, several infections, although uncommon, are more likely to occur in patients with diabetes mellitus: malignant otitis externa, rhinocerebral mucormycosis, osteomyelitis of the small bones of the feet, and gas-forming infections such as emphysematous cholecystitis, emphysematous pyelonephritis, and soft tissue infections including cellulitis and fasciitis.

Problems in Host Defenses

Patients with uncontrolled diabetes mellitus, and especially during ketoacidosis, have impaired function of polymorphonuclear leukocytes. Chemotaxis, phagocytosis, and intracellular killing by these "professional phagocytes" may all be deficient. Control of hyperglycemia improves neutrophil function and may be important during high-risk surgical procedures. Studies on the effects of diabetes mellitus on lymphocyte function have borne inconsistent results.

Clinical Infections

Pneumonia in patients with diabetes mellitus is more likely to be caused by *S. aureus,* gram-negative rods, and *M. tuberculosis* than is pneumonia in nondiabetic patients. Bacteremic pneumococcal pneumonia in patients with diabetes mellitus is associated with increased mortality. Patients with diabetes mellitus are at increased risk of mortality during influenza epidemics and pandemics. Diabetic persons should receive the pneumococcal vaccine and an annual immunization against influenza.

UTI is more common in patients with diabetes mellitus. Women with diabetes mellitus have a two- to four-fold greater incidence of asymptomatic bacteriuria and are more likely to have pyelonephritis. Complications of UTI in patients with diabetes mellitus include papillary necrosis and perinephric abscess. Complicated UTI should be suspected when fever fails to resolve within 4 days of beginning antimicrobial therapy. Patients with diabetes mellitus are also vulnerable to fungal UTI, which occasionally causes ureteral obstruction because of a fungus ball.

Emphysematous pyelonephritis is a rare form of UTI that occurs mainly in persons with diabetes mellitus (90% of cases). Clues to this diagnosis include systemic toxicity, severe pain, and occasionally an abdominal mass. Gas in the kidneys is apparent on plain x-ray examination in about one third of patients. The left kidney tends to be involved more often than the right, but the disease is bilateral in about 5% of cases. When this diagnosis is suspected, CT scanning is currently the imaging procedure of choice. Patients with suspected emphysematous pyelonephritis should be admitted to the hospital and referred for surgical consultation. A serum creatinine level >1.4 mg/dL or platelet count <60,000/mm³ is associated with an especially high risk of death, but all cases of emphysematous cystitis should be viewed as medical emergencies. Emergency nephrectomy is the standard treatment, although CT-guided percutaneous drainage is being studied as an alternative.

Cholecystitis is possibly more common in patients with diabetes mellitus and may carry an increased mortality rate. The question is sometimes raised whether diabetic patients with asymptomatic gallstones should undergo cholecystectomy. The current consensus is no. Gallstones are present in only about one half of patients with emphysematous cholecystitis, a form of cholecystitis that occurs disproportionately in patients with diabetes mellitus (about 35% of cases). This infection is frequently polymicrobial, involving both aerobic and anaerobic bacteria, and often progresses rapidly to gangrene and perforation of the gallbladder wall. The overall mortality is 15%. The possibility of emphysematous cholecystitis should be raised when a patient with diabetes mellitus presents with fever, nausea, vomiting, and pain in the right upper quadrant of the abdomen. Gas is sometimes apparent on palpation of the abdomen (crepitance, which is an ominous sign) or on plain x-ray or ultrasound examination, but it is more readily demonstrated by CT scanning. Emergency cholecystectomy is generally required in addition to broad-spectrum antibiotics.

Soft tissue infections are possibly more common in patients with diabetes mellitus than in other patients, and they tend to be more severe. Infections of the foot include cellulitis and ulcer, which often progresses to osteomyelitis (see Chapter 15). Serious infections of the upper extremity also occur and may require amputation. There is a general impression that necrotizing fasciitis is more common in patients with diabetes mellitus. In about 90% of cases necrotizing fasciitis associated with diabetes mellitus is polymicrobial, typically involving aerobic gram-negative rods and various anaerobic pathogens such as *Clostridium* species and *Bacteroides fragilis* (type I necrotizing fasciitis). Streptococci cause the remaining 10% of cases (type II necrotizing fasciitis). Pain and systemic toxicity disproportionate to the findings on physical examination are frequent clues to the diagnosis of necrotizing fasciitis. When necrotizing fasciitis is a possibility, nonsteroidal antiinflammatory drugs should probably not be used (see Chapter 6). Nonclostridial gas gangrene (another polymicrobial infection) may also be more common in patients with diabetes mellitus.

Necrotizing fasciitis involving the male genitalia (Fournier's gangrene) occurs disproportionately in patients with diabetes mellitus. This infection usually involves the scrotum but can also involve the perirectal tissues (where it often originates), perineum, penis, and abdominal wall. The same process also affects women and children. In all forms of necrotizing fasciitis, prompt surgery and broad-spectrum antibiotics (usually including clindamycin in addition to penicillin and gentamicin) are mandatory. Recent data suggest that Fournier's gangrene is often a more insidious process than in the classic description, that a source is usually apparent, and that the overall mortality is about 16% to 38%.

Invasive otitis externa (also called malignant otitis externa) is an uncommon infection that usually affects patients with diabetes mellitus. Initial symptoms and signs suggest uncomplicated otitis externa. Multiple attempts at topical therapy with various ear drops usually ensue. Eventually, the epithelium of the ear canal becomes macerated with cellulitis and formation of polypoid granulation tissue. Affected patients have pain, continued drainage from the ear (otorrhea), and hearing loss. The usual organism is *P. aeruginosa,* but other bacteria, including anaerobic pathogens, can be involved. Small vessel disease is thought to be a predisposing factor. The causative bacteria pass through gaps between the ear cartilages (fissures of Santorini) and gain access to the temporal bone, resulting in osteomyelitis. Further extension to the base of the brain can lead to involvement of the meninges, sigmoid sinus, jugular bulb, and several cranial nerves (VII, IX, X, and XII) (Figure 3-2). Magnetic resonance imaging (MRI) with gadolinium enhancement is probably the best imaging procedure to confirm the diagnosis. Appropriate management includes referral to an otolaryngologist for aggressive débridement of the ear and systemic antimicrobial therapy directed against *P. aeruginosa.*

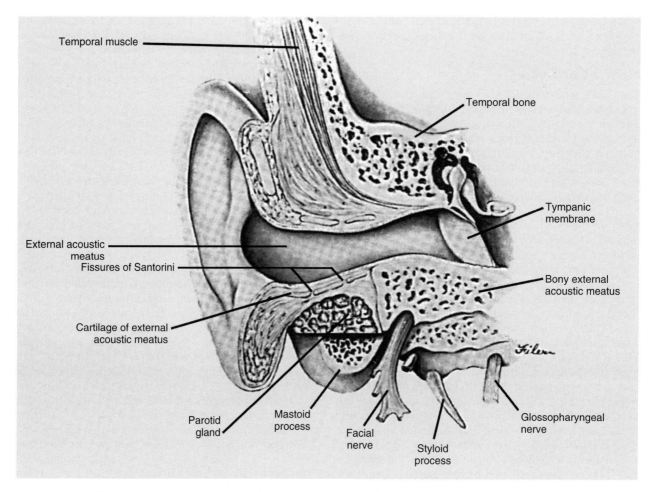

FIG. 3-2   Anatomy of the external ear. In necrotizing (malignant) otitis externa, microorganisms (usually *Pseudomonas aeruginosa*) pass through the fissures of Santorini into the deeper soft tissue, from which they spread to the temporal bone and the base of the skull. This life-threatening infection is seen mainly in patients with diabetes mellitus. (From Grandis JL, Yu VL. Necrotizing [malignant] external otitis. In: Johnson JT, Yu VL. Infectious Diseases and Antimicrobial Therapy of the Ears, Nose and Throat. Philadelphia: W.B. Saunders Company; 1997: 314-320.)

Rhinocerebral mucormycosis is an uncommon infection that tends to affect patients with diabetes mellitus (about one half of patients). Many patients have a prior history of ketoacidosis. Nasal stuffiness and facial pain are often early signs. Early symptoms sometimes suggest sinusitis; indeed, the paranasal sinuses have been called "way stations on the way to the brain" in the pathogenesis of this infection. The presence of a black eschar on the nasal mucosa or on the palate provides a clue to early diagnosis. On this basis, it has been suggested that follow-up examination of the nasal mucosa and of the palate be routine after treatment of diabetic ketoacidosis. The fungi that cause mucormycosis notoriously invade the walls of blood vessels, causing tissue infarction. When it extends to the brain, the infection can cause cavernous sinus thrombosis, ophthalmoplegia, and vision loss. MRI scanning may help to define the extent of brain involvement, but the diagnosis is best made by demonstrating the broad, nonseptate, irregularly branching hyphae typical of

the agents of mucormycosis (see Chapter 21). Patients with rhinocerebral mucormycosis should be admitted to the hospital for aggressive surgery and amphotericin B.

Foot infections including polymicrobial osteomyelitis are common in patients with diabetes mellitus and are discussed more fully in Chapter 15.

 KEY POINTS

INFECTIONS IN PATIENTS WITH DIABETES MELLITUS

⊃ Whether the overall incidence of infections is increased in patients with diabetes mellitus is unclear. However, poor glycemic control and ketoacidosis impair polymorphonuclear leukocyte function.

⊃ In patients with diabetes mellitus undergoing major surgery, the serum glucose level should be kept at <200 mg/dL.

- Four syndromes occur mainly in patients with diabetes mellitus: malignant otitis externa, rhinocerebral mucormycosis, polymicrobial osteomyelitis of the small bones of the feet, and gas-forming infections in general.
- The mortality from influenza and bacteremic pneumococcal pneumonia is increased in patients with diabetes mellitus. Influenza and pneumococcal vaccines should be used liberally in this population.
- Persons with diabetes mellitus, especially women, have an increased frequency of UTI and are more likely to experience pyelonephritis and such complications as perinephric abscess and papillary necrosis.
- Emphysematous pyelonephritis should be suspected when UTI with severe toxicity and abdominal pain develops in a person with diabetes mellitus. Gas in the kidney is seen on plain x-ray films in about one third of cases. CT scanning is the imaging procedure of choice. Emergency nephrectomy is often required for cure of this life-threatening infection.
- Emphysematous cholecystitis is a life-threatening infection that, although uncommon, occurs disproportionately in patients with diabetes mellitus (about 35% of cases). It is characterized by significant toxicity with gas in the gallbladder. Prompt cholecystectomy is necessary.
- Necrotizing fasciitis may be more common in diabetic patients and is usually (90% of cases) polymicrobial. Clues include severe pain and systemic toxicity. Crepitance is present in about one half of cases, and gas can be demonstrated more commonly by radiographic studies.
- Invasive otitis externa (malignant otitis externa) should be suspected in diabetic patients when persistent external otitis with otorrhea, pain, and hearing loss develops.
- Rhinocerebral mucormycosis often follows ketoacidosis and is characterized by facial and ocular pain, proptosis, ophthalmoplegia, and vision loss. Morbidity and mortality result from brain involvement, which includes cavernous sinus thrombosis and thrombosis of the carotid artery or jugular vein. Finding a black eschar on the nasal mucosa or palate facilitates early diagnosis.
- Foot infections in diabetes mellitus include ulcers and polymicrobial osteomyelitis.

SUGGESTED READING

Bryan CS, Reynolds KM, Metzger WT. Bacteremia in diabetic patients: comparison of incidence and mortality with nondiabetic patients. Diabetes Care 1985; 8: 244-249.

Eke N. Fournier's gangrene: a review of 1726 cases. Br J Surg 2000; 87: 718-728.

Eliopoulos GM, ed. Infections in diabetes mellitus. Infect Dis Clin North Am 1995; 9: 1-221.

Gill KS, Chapman AH, Weston MJ. The changing face of emphysematous cholecystitis. Br J Radiol 1997; 70: 986-991.

Gleckman RA, al-Wawi M. A review of selective infections in the adult diabetic. Compr Ther 1999; 25: 109-113.

Golden SH, Peart-Vigilance C, Kao WH, et al. Perioperative glycemic control and the risk of infectious complications in a cohort of adults with diabetes. Diabetes Care 1999; 22: 1408-1414.

Gonzalez MH, Bochar S, Novotny J, et al. Upper extremity infections in patients with diabetes mellitus. J Hand Surg [Am] 1999; 24: 682-686.

Joshi N, Caputo GM, Weitekamp MR, et al. Infections in patients with diabetes mellitus. N Engl J Med 1999; 341: 1906-1912.

Patterson JE, Andriole VT. Bacterial urinary tract infections in diabetes. Infect Dis Clin North Am 1997; 11: 735-750.

Wan YL, Lo SK, Bullard MJ, et al. Predictors of outcome in emphysematous pyelonephritis. J Urol 1998; 159: 369-373.

Yaghan RJ, Al-Jaberi TM, Bani-Hani I. Fournier's gangrene: changing face of the disease. Dis Colon Rectum 2000; 43: 1300-1308.

Patients Receiving Corticosteroids

Infection ranks high among the complications of systemic corticosteroid therapy at doses >10 mg/day or at cumulative doses >700 mg. Inhaled corticosteroids pose a low risk of infection other than oral candidiasis (thrush). The likelihood of significant systemic absorption of inhaled corticosteroids can be minimized by using a spacer and by thoroughly rinsing the mouth after each use. A tuberculin skin test before beginning corticosteroid therapy is prudent, since therapy lasting longer than 2 weeks can cause the test result to be nonreactive.

Problems in Host Defenses

Corticosteroids predispose to serious infection in at least four ways:

- Impairment of polymorphonuclear function. The patient has impaired production of the factors associated with the acute inflammatory response, impaired chemotaxis, and reduced ability of phagocytic cells to kill intracellular bacteria.
- Impaired lymphocyte function. Prolonged corticosteroid therapy causes lymphocytopenia. Corticosteroids cause broad impairment of cell-mediated immunity, with reduced production of cytokines and impaired function of macrophages.
- Impairment of wound healing. Corticosteroids interfere with fibroblast function, collagen synthesis, and other processes associated with wound healing, thereby interfering with processes that normally serve to contain infection.
- Impairment of the patient's recognition of infection. The broad antiinflammatory properties of steroids often mask the symptoms and signs of serious infection, causing serious delay in recognition by the patient or the physician.

In addition, many of the conditions that require systemic corticosteroid therapy predispose to infection in their own right.

Clinical Infections

Infections complicating corticosteroid therapy can be divided into two types: infections caused by usual pathogens but made worse by the effect of corticosteroids, and infections caused by opportunistic pathogens. An example of the former is the effect of corticosteroids on peritonitis caused by bowel perforation, including diverticulitis. Opportunistic infections caused by corticosteroids are usually due to DNA viruses, intracellular bacteria, fungi, or parasites:

- Viruses. The herpesviruses—herpes simplex virus, varicella-zoster virus, Epstein-Barr virus, and cytomegalovirus (CMV) (see Chapter 20)—commonly cause problems in patients receiving corticosteroids. Other viral infections include papillomavirus and measles virus (which unlike the others is an RNA virus).

- Intracellular bacteria. The impaired ability of macrophages to destroy bacteria within phagocytic vacuoles leads to serious infection caused by *M. tuberculosis, L. monocytogenes, Nocardia* species, *Salmonella* species, *Brucella* species, and *Legionella pneumophila.*
- Fungi. Corticosteroids predispose to infection caused by *Cryptococcus neoformans* (including meningitis), candidiasis, regional mycoses (such as histoplasmosis and coccidioidomycosis), and infection caused by *Pneumocystis carinii* (now classified as a fungus rather than a protozoan).
- Parasites. The major examples are toxoplasmosis and strongyloidiasis.

Patients receiving corticosteroids sometimes experience a succession of opportunistic infections, which should be suspected even when symptoms would seem to have another, more common explanation.

 KEY POINTS

PATIENTS RECEIVING CORTICOSTEROIDS

⊃ Doses of prednisone (or the equivalent) of >10 mg/day or cumulative doses >700 mg are associated with risk of infection.

⊃ The low risk of systemic infection from inhaled corticosteroids can be further minimized by use of a spacer and by mouth rinsing after each use.

⊃ A tuberculin skin test before corticosteroid therapy begins is prudent for indications other than short-term (<2 weeks) use.

⊃ Corticosteroids often mask the symptoms and signs of infection caused by "usual" microorganisms.

⊃ Corticosteroids predispose to opportunistic infections, especially those caused by DNA viruses, intracellular bacteria, certain fungi, and parasites.

SUGGESTED READING

Anstead GM. Steroids, retinoids and wound healing. Adv Wound Care 1998; 11: 277-285.

McEvoy CE, Niewoehner DE. Adverse effects of corticosteroid therapy for COPD: a critical review. Chest 1997; 111: 732-743.

Segal BH, Sneller MC. Infectious complications of immunosuppressive therapy in patients with rheumatic diseases. Rheum Dis Clin North Am 1997; 23: 219-237.

Stuck AK, Minder CE, Frey FJ. Risk of infectious complications in patients taking glucocorticosteroids. Rev Infect Dis 1989; 11: 954-963.

Toogood JH. Side effects of inhaled corticosteroids. J Allergy Clin Immunol 1998; 102: 705-713.

Zoorob RJ, Cender D. A different look at corticosteroids. Am Fam Physician 1998; 58: 443-450.

Patients with Prosthetic Devices

The number of patients throughout the world with major prosthetic devices continues to increase rapidly, perhaps doubling every 10 years (Table 3-2). Infectious complications are, in general, divided into two groups: early-onset infections related to the implantation procedure, and late-onset infections. Late-onset infections can be caused by microorganisms of low virulence that are acquired during surgery or by pathogens that are acquired long after the surgery and find their way to the device, usually through the bloodstream.

TABLE 3-2
Incidence of Infection Related to Various Implants and Devices

Implant or device	Number used or implanted per year	Incidence of infection (%)	Morbidity and mortality
Total artificial hip	222,000	<1	7%-63% mortality associated with infection
Total knee arthroplasty	110,000	1-2	2.5% mortality; 80% nonfunctioning prosthesis
Cardiac pacemaker leads	115,000-130,000	2-11	2% mortality
Prosthetic heart valve	>100,000	1-4	34% mortality; 25%-30% major complications
Vascular graft	>60,000	≤3	40% mortality, 20%-30% amputation rate
Hemodialysis grafts		10	28% mortality
CNS shunts	>80,000	10-15	
Peripheral IV catheter	150 million–200 million	<0.1	15%-20% mortality
Central venous catheter		3-7	15%-20% mortality
Dental implants	436,000	15	

Modified from Anderson JM, Marchant RE. Biomaterials: factors favoring colonization and infection. In: Waldvogel FA, Bisno AL, eds. Infections Associated with Indwelling Medical Devices. 3rd ed., Washington, DC: ASM Press; 2000.
CNS, Central nervous system.

Problems in Host Defenses

Among the numerous microorganisms that sometimes infect prosthetic devices, coagulase-negative staphylococci are the most feared. A half century ago these diverse microorganisms, then lumped together as *Staphylococcus albus,* were thought to be nonpathogenic. The unique pathogenicity of coagulase-negative staphylococci, and especially *S. epidermidis,* involves three phases. First, the organisms adhere to the prosthetic material. Second, the organisms form a complex multilayer of cells covered with a poorly understood substance variably known as glycocalyx, biofilm, or extracellular slime. This "slime" protects the embedded bacteria from antimicrobial agents. Finally, the organisms undergo various metabolic changes that render them less susceptible to antibiotics. The nature of the infection often mandates complete removal of the device for cure, resulting in substantial morbidity and even mortality.

Clinical Infections

This section considers the infections of most concern to primary care clinicians.

Cardiac Pacemakers and Defibrillators

About 1% to 2% of cardiac pacemakers, as well as about 2% to 11% of implantable cardioverter-defibrillators (ICD devices), become infected even with good surgical practices. Early-onset infections (within 2 weeks of implantation) usually arise as perioperative complications and are likely to involve *S. aureus.* Late-onset infections (>2 weeks) are often caused by coagulase-negative staphylococci. Factors that predispose to infection include postoperative hematoma, diabetes mellitus, corticosteroid therapy, multiple revisions, and erosion of the skin. Infections of pacemaker or ICD pockets are more common than infections of the electrodes. Pocket infection is usually suspected on clinical grounds. Infection of cardiac pacemakers occasionally causes endocarditis, which should be suspected when the patient has fever, pulmonary lesions, or other major complications. Diagnosis of endocarditis is based largely on blood cultures, with a role for transesophageal echocardiography. Removal of the entire pacemaker or ICD system is often necessary for cure.

Prosthetic Heart Valves

Infections of prosthetic heart valves represent, by definition, endocarditis. Early-onset prosthetic valve endocarditis (within 60 days of implantation) accounts for 18% to 36% of cases and is caused mainly by coagulase-negative staphylococci (43% of cases), *S. aureus* (15% of cases), aerobic gram-negative bacilli (10% of cases), and fungi (6% of cases). Late-onset prosthetic valve endocarditis (beyond 60 days) is often caused by coagulase-negative staphylococci (28% of cases) or by *S. aureus,* but an equal number of cases are caused by streptococci or by enterococci. The incidence of early-onset prosthetic valve endocarditis is about 1% at centers where large numbers of prosthetic valves are implanted. The risk of late-onset prosthetic valve endocarditis is highest within 5 to 6 months of surgery. The overall risk is about 0.5% per year for mechanical mitral valves and up to 1% per year for other types of valves.

The clinical presentation of prosthetic valve endocarditis is similar to that of native valve endocarditis, with fever being the most common sign. Fungal endocarditis on prosthetic heart valves, most frequently caused by *C. albicans,* typically results in bulky vegetations that tend to cause embolic occlusion of large arteries. In about one third of patients with fungal prosthetic valve endocarditis, stroke is the initial event. Periannular extension of prosthetic valve endocarditis leads to myocardial abscesses, pseudoaneurysms, and fistulas. It has been proposed that the Duke criteria for diagnosis of endocarditis (see Chapter 6) be modified for patients with prosthetic heart valves to include newly diagnosed clubbing, splenomegaly, splinter hemorrhages, petechiae, elevation of the sedimentation rate or C-reactive protein level, microscopic hematuria, and the presence of peripheral or central vascular access lines. Patients with suspected prosthetic valve endocarditis should be admitted to the hospital. A combined medical and surgical approach to therapy is usually superior to medical therapy alone.

Patients with prosthetic heart valves should receive thorough instruction about the need for prophylactic antibiotics before procedures likely to cause transient bacteremia (see Chapter 26). Use of vascular access lines should be avoided whenever possible in these patients.

Studies indicate that endocarditis occurs in about 16% of patients with prosthetic heart valves who develop nosocomial bacteremia, and in about 11% of patients who develop nosocomial candidemia. Central lines for monitoring or parenteral hyperalimentation should be used with great care, if at all.

Vascular Grafts

Infection is a feared complication of reconstructive vascular surgery, with high mortality and morbidity. Early graft infection (within 2 months of surgery) often becomes apparent within the immediate postoperative period. Femoropopliteal bypass surgery carries the highest risk, especially when incision through the groin is necessary. Other risk factors include diabetes mellitus, postoperative ileus, postoperative UTI, and transient bacteremia. *S. aureus* is a common pathogen; others include streptococci and aerobic gram-negative bacilli. Late graft infection (>2 months after surgery) is frequently caused by *S. epidermidis,* reflecting low-level contamination during surgery. The risk of late graft infection from transient bacteremia decreases with time as the endothelial lining of the graft (neointima) develops and matures.

Symptoms and signs of graft infections include fever, swelling, erythema, sinus tract formation, and peripheral septic emboli. Some patients, especially those with early-onset infection caused by *S. aureus,* may show signs of sepsis. In others, especially those with late-onset infections of aortic grafts caused by microorganisms of low virulence, the infection may manifest itself as a subacute or chronic failure to thrive, with anorexia, weight loss, and anemia. Gastrointestinal bleeding sometimes heralds the development of a graft-enteric fistula. CT and MRI scans are probably similar in sensitivity for diagnosis of graft infections. Inflammatory changes, fluid, gas, or expanding soft tissue may be present around the graft; other findings include pseudoaneurysms and thickening of adjacent bowel. Radionuclide scans are reserved for cases in which the diagnosis is equivocal. Management consists of excision of the graft and aggressive antimicrobial therapy. Infected vascular grafts to the lower extremities carry mortality rates of 5% to 10% and amputation rates of 30% to 60%, while infected aortic grafts carry mortality rates of 25% to 75%. Although the overall rate of graft infection appears to be relatively low (mean about 3%, range 1.3% to 6%), patients referred for vascular reconstruction should be aware of this risk.

Hip Prostheses and Artificial Joints

Numerous technical innovations have made artificial joints a near-miraculous boon to an aging population, "adding life to years." Infections are uncommon, but morbidity and mortality are substantial (Table 3-2). Early-onset infections (within 3 months of implantation) are often caused by *S. aureus,* and late-onset infections (>3 months after implantation) by *S. epidermidis.* Symptoms and signs of late-onset infection include pain, subtle signs of inflammation, and loosening of the prosthesis. Plain x-ray films may confirm loosening of the prosthesis. Radionuclide scanning, and especially labeled leukocyte scintigraphy, is often used for diagnosis. Management is difficult and usually entails a revision arthroplasty.

Late-onset infection can reflect hematogenous seeding of the prosthesis, but the incidence of this phenomenon is unknown. Whether patients with prosthetic joints are at risk of infection during dental procedures has been the subject of much debate. The risk remains unproved. However, the American Dental Association and the American Academy of Orthopaedic Surgeons suggest prophylaxis for "high-risk" patients, using a single dose of amoxicillin, cephradine, or clindamycin.

Vascular Access Devices

Primary care clinicians should have a general familiarity with the risk of infection in patients with vascular access devices, since such devices are now frequently used in the ambulatory setting (see Chapter 26).

Peritoneal Dialysis Catheters

Infections can result from contamination of a peritoneal dialysis catheter during implantation, contamination of the dialysis tubing during manipulation, contamination of the dialysate, or perforation of the bowel. About 50% to 80% of cases are caused by staphylococci, 20% by gram-negative rods, and 10% by staphylococci. Fungi and mycobacteria cause occasional cases. The clinical presentation consists of fever and abdominal pain, and infection is further suggested by cloudy drainage. Analysis of dialysis effluent reveals a rise in the WBC count (from the normal value of $<5 \times 10^7$ WBCs per liter with a predominance of mononuclear cells to $>10^8$ WBCs per liter with a predominance of polymorphonuclear neutrophils [PMNs]). The peritoneal fluid can be inoculated into a blood culture system. Treatment is based on the clinical severity of the infection and the results of Gram stains and cultures. Severe abdominal pain or a mixed bacterial flora suggests perforation of the bowel, which should prompt evaluation by a surgeon. Many of these infections resolve with appropriate antimicrobial therapy, often given by the intraperitoneal route, but removal of the dialysis catheter is sometimes necessary.

The incidence of infections related to peritoneal dialysis catheters has declined in recent years owing to aggressive infection control measures. Prophylactic administration of vancomycin has been used in many nephrology practices but is now discouraged because of the association of this practice with *S. aureus* strains having reduced susceptibility to vancomycin. Mupirocin (Bactroban) has been used to treat staphylococcal nasal carriage in patients receiving peritoneal dialysis, and some nephrologists apply mupirocin continuously to the catheter exit site. However, this practice promotes the emergence of mupirocin-resistant staphylococci.

Cerebrospinal Fluid Shunts

Cerebrospinal fluid (CSF) shunts, especially ventriculoperitoneal shunts, are commonly used for relief of hydrocephalus caused by obstruction of CSF flow. Coagulase-negative staphylococci cause more than 50% of these infections. *S. aureus* causes a\bout 20% of shunt infections; other pathogens include streptococci, aerobic gram-negative bacilli, and anaerobic diphtheroid pathogens. Risk factors to shunt infection include age <1 year or >60 years, revision surgery, and previous external drainage. The predominant symptoms are fever, irritability, behavioral changes, and anorexia. Headache, nausea, and vomiting suggest increased intracranial pressure caused by obstruction of the shunt. Chronic, low-grade infection can result in glomerulonephritis owing to circulating immune complexes. Ventriculoatrial shunts carry the risk of tricuspid valve endocarditis. Diagnosis of CSF shunt infection is best made by culture of the reservoir, which is positive in >95% of cases. Blood cultures are usually positive (>90% of cases) in patients with ventriculoatrial shunts but are less frequently positive (<25% of cases) in patients with ventriculoperitoneal shunts. Antimicrobial therapy without removal of the shunt succeeds in <40% of cases, and removal of the shunt is therefore usually necessary.

Other Prosthetic Devices

Infections of intraocular lenses implanted after cataract extraction are fortunately rare. These infections are managed by ophthalmologists, often in consultation with infectious disease specialists. Infections complicate about 1% to 3% of breast implants; skin flora, including *S. epidermidis,* are the usual pathogens, but unusual pathogens, including *Mycobacterium fortuitum,* may be seen. Infections of penile prostheses (about 1% to 4% of implants) and artificial urinary sphincters (about 2% to 15% of implants) are most commonly due to gram-positive bacteria and usually necessitate removal of the device.

 KEY POINTS

PATIENTS WITH PROSTHETIC DEVICES

⊃ Infections related to prosthetic devices are, in general, classified as "early-onset" (infections acquired during surgery) and "late-onset" (infections caused by microorganisms of low virulence or acquired subsequent to surgery).

⊃ Coagulase-negative staphylococci are the most important pathogens causing infection related to prosthetic devices. Once attached to a prosthetic device, these bacteria cause the formation of a "slime layer" that renders them resistant to antimicrobial agents.

⊃ Vascular access devices such as central IV catheters should be used judiciously and with great care in patients with major devices such as prosthetic heart valves because of the potential for bacteremia (or fungemia) with seeding of the prosthesis.

⊃ Patients with prosthetic heart valves should receive prophylactic antibiotics before procedures likely to cause transient bacteremia (see Chapter 26).

⊃ When patients with prosthetic heart valves develop fever, blood cultures should be obtained with special care to avoid contamination by skin flora.

⊃ Infected aortic grafts can cause low-grade fever and failure to thrive with weight loss and anemia.

⊃ Infected total joint replacements often cause pain and loosening of the prosthesis. Whether patients who have had total joint replacements are at risk for infection during dental and other procedures is controversial.

SUGGESTED READING

Bayston R, Andrews M, Rigg K, et al. Recurrent infection and catheter loss in patients on continuous ambulatory peritoneal dialysis. Perit Dial Int 1999; 19: 550-555.

Chua JD, Wilkoff BL, Lee I, et al. Diagnosis and management of infections involving implantable electrophysiologic cardiac devices. Ann Intern Med 2000; 133: 604-608.

Gillespie WJ. Prevention and management of infection after total joint replacement. Clin Infect Dis 1997; 25: 1310-1317.

Gordon SM, Serkey JM, Longworth DL, et al. Early onset prosthetic valve endocarditis: the Cleveland Clinic experience 1992-1997. Ann Thorac Surg 2000; 69: 1388-1392.

Klug D, Lacroix D, Savoye C, et al. Systemic infection related to endocarditis on pacemaker leads: clinical presentation and management. Circulation 1997; 95: 2098-2107.

Lamas CC, Eykyn SJ. Suggested modifications to the Duke criteria for the clinical diagnosis of native valve and prosthetic valve endocarditis: analysis of 118 pathologically proven cases. Clin Infect Dis 1997; 25: 713-719.

Palestro CJ, Torres MA. Radionuclide imaging in orthopedic infections. Semin Nuclear Med 1997; 27: 334-345.

Seeger JM. Management of patients with prosthetic vascular graft infection. Am Surg 2000; 66: 166-177.

Westenfelder GO, ed. Infections of prosthetic devices. Infect Dis Clin North Am 1989; 3: 187-373.

Patients with Alcoholism or Liver Disease

Alcoholism is a common but often unrecognized problem in primary care practices. Chronic liver disease with cirrhosis is currently the tenth leading cause of death in the United States.

Problems in Host Defenses

Acute intoxication with alcohol predisposes to pneumonia by promoting aspiration and by blunting the pulmonary clearance of bacteria that reach the lungs. Chronic persisting drinking (alcoholism) causes a maturation arrest of PMNs in the bone marrow and depresses cell-mediated immunity, including macrophage function. The effects of alcoholism on humoral immunity are unsettled, but patients with alcoholism often respond poorly to vaccines, including pneumococcal vaccine. Cirrhosis is associated with impaired cell-mediated immunity and also with impairment of the reticuloendothelial system in the liver, which normally serves to remove bacteria and other particulate matter from the portal circulation. Patients are therefore predisposed to spontaneous bacteremia and bacterial peritonitis (see later discussion). Poor living conditions, poor hygiene, and malnutrition further predispose patients suffering from alcoholism or cirrhosis to a variety of infections.

Clinical Infections

Pneumonia is the most common life-threatening infection in patients with alcoholism, whose age-specific mortality rates are two to seven times those of patients without alcoholism. *S. pneumoniae* is the usual cause. Patients with leukopenia (the ALPS syndrome; see Chapter 11) have a poor prognosis. *Klebsiella pneumoniae,* although uncommon, should be considered if a patient has alcoholism and pneumonia because the course is often fulminant, especially when bacteremia is present. Classically, *K. pneumoniae* causes upper lobe consolidation with a bulging fissure. Other important causes of acute bacterial pneumonia in patients with alcoholism include *H. influenzae, Staphylococcus aureus,* and in some geographic areas *L. pneumophila.* Recurrent pneumonia is relatively among patients with alcoholism.

Lung abscess and anaerobic pleuropulmonary infection caused by extensive aspiration of "mouth flora" bacteria is much more common in patients suffering from alcoholism than in the general population. Onset of symptoms is typically more gradual compared to pneumococcal pneumonia. Poor oral hygiene with extensive dental plaque formation and carious teeth is usually found on physical examination. A foul odor to the breath is highly suggestive of anaerobic pleuropulmonary disease. Gram stain of sputum shows multiple bacterial morphologies. The usual pathogens include peptostreptococci, *Prevotella melaninogenicus, Fusobacterium* species, and sometimes *B. fragilis.* Patients with lung abscess usually respond to treatment with appropriate antibiotics (e.g., clindamycin), but patients with pleural involvement (empyema) usually require tube thoracostomy.

Tuberculosis occurs in patients with alcoholism at rates up to 10 times those of persons without alcoholism, to the extent that in some populations more than one half of patients with newly diagnosed TB also have this disease. However, the frequency of pneumonia and lung abscess in persons with alcoholism sometimes causes the possibility of TB to be overlooked, which exposes other persons, including health care workers, to the disease. Hence, the clinician should adopt a liberal policy toward respiratory isolation and obtaining AFB smears and cultures. Patients with alcoholism and TB should be treated using directly observed therapy (see Chapter 22).

Spontaneous bacterial peritonitis (more accurately called "primary peritonitis," as distinguished from peritonitis secondary to intraabdominal disease including bowel perforation) occurs in up to one third of patients with cirrhosis and ascites at some point during their illnesses. Studies suggest that peritonitis is present in 8% to 27% (mean, about 15%) of persons with cirrhosis and ascites who are admitted to the hospital. Originally, spontaneous bacterial peritonitis was described as an acute illness with abrupt onset. More recent studies indicate that the presentation is often subtle, so that spontaneous bacterial peritonitis should be suspected whenever fever or abdominal pain develops in a patient with cirrhosis and ascites. Altered mental status (hepatic encephalopathy) is present in more than one half of patients. Diagnosis is by paracentesis, and the disease is generally defined by the presence in ascitic fluid of >250 PMNs/mm^3 combined with a positive culture. Most cases (92%) are due to a single microorganism. Gram-negative rods account for the majority of cases, with *E. coli* being the most common isolate; gram-positive cocci, especially streptococci, account for nearly 25% of cases. Anaerobic bacteria are uncommon. Patients whose ascitic fluid shows >500 PMNs/mm^3 but whose ascitic fluid cultures are sterile should be treated for spontaneous bacterial peritonitis; the term "culture-negative neutrocytic ascites" has been used for this situation. Cefotaxime (2 g IV q8h for 5 days, in persons with normal renal function) is commonly used in this situation. Ceftriaxone (which, however, undergoes hepatic metabolism with biliary excretion that can lead to biliary sludge) and β-lactam/β-lactamase inhibitor combinations may be useful but have not been specifically studied. Fluoroquinolones may be useful in patients with allergy to β-lactam antibiotics, and some patients may be candidates for outpatient treatment with an oral quinolone. Oral quinolones (such as norfloxacin) have been used for prophylaxis against this infection, but prolonged use promotes emergence of resistant bacteria and is therefore controversial.

Spontaneous bacteremia (a better term would be "primary bacteremia") without peritonitis is also common in patients with alcoholism. It is presumed that bacteria, usually aerobic gram-negative rods and most commonly *E. coli,* enter the portal circulation from the intestinal tract and fail to be cleared by the liver for the reasons discussed previously. Management is similar to that of spontaneous bacterial peritonitis.

Many other infections have been associated with alcoholism. Cellulitis of the lower extremities is a common problem in persons with alcoholism, ascites, and peripheral edema. *Vibrio vulnificus* septicemia (see Chapter 7) should be considered whenever cellulitis is found in a person with alcoholism and a history of ingesting raw oysters. Acute bacterial meningitis is associated with a higher mortality and tends to be overlooked in persons with alcoholism, pneumonia, and depressed sensorium. *S. pneumoniae* is the usual cause of bacterial meningitis in persons with alcoholism, but other causative agents, including *L. monocytogenes,* should be kept in mind. Limited data suggest that endocarditis may be more common in persons with alcoholism. Diphtheria, usually cutaneous (see Chapter 15), has been described in persons with alcoholism and poor living conditions. Pancreatic abscess should be considered when a patient with alcoholism has clinical deterioration, fever, nausea, vomiting, or abdominal pain 1 to 4 weeks after recovering from acute pancreatitis. Patients with alcoholism are also at increased risk for viral infections, notably HIV, hepatitis B, and hepatitis C. The combination of alcoholism and hepatitis C increases the likelihood of rapid progression to cirrhosis (see Chapter 13).

▶ KEY POINTS

PATIENTS WITH ALCOHOLISM OR LIVER DISEASE
⊃ Acute alcohol intoxication promotes aspiration and impairs pulmonary clearance; sustained use of alcohol (alcoholism) depresses bone marrow production of PMNs and impairs cell-mediated immunity; and cirrhosis impairs reticuloendothelial function.
⊃ Acute alcohol intoxication predisposes to bacterial pneumonia, lung abscess, anaerobic pleuropulmonary disease, and pancreatic abscess.
⊃ Patients with alcoholism have the additional risks of tuberculosis, gram-negative bacterial infection, legionnaire's disease, and meningitis caused by *L. monocytogenes.*

⊃ Patients with cirrhosis of the liver have the additional risks of spontaneous bacteremia and spontaneous bacterial peritonitis, with *E. coli* being the usual pathogen in both instances.

SUGGESTED READING
Conn HO, Rodés J, Navasa M. Spontaneous Bacterial Peritonitis: The Disease, Pathogenesis, and Treatment. New York: Marcel Dekker; 2000.
Jong GM, Hsiue TR, Chen CR, et al. Rapidly fatal outcome of bacteremic *Klebsiella pneumoniae* pneumonia in alcoholics. Chest 1995; 107: 214-217.
Menon KVN, Kamath PS. Managing the complications of cirrhosis. Mayo Clin Proc 2000; 75: 501-509.
Navasa M, Rimola A, Rodes J. Bacterial infections in liver disease. Semin Liver Dis 1997; 17: 323-333.
Such J, Runyon BA. Spontaneous bacterial peritonitis. Clin Infect Dis 1998; 27: 669-676.
Westphal J-F, Jehl F, Vetter D. Pharmacological, toxicologic, and microbiological considerations in the choice of initial antibiotic therapy for serious infections in patients with cirrhosis of the liver. Clin Infect Dis 1994; 18: 324-335.

Injecting Drug Users

Injecting drug use involves complex behavior patterns that not only predispose to infection but also make diagnosis and treatment more difficult. The culture of drug use includes persons who profit from the sale of drugs and syringes, "hit doctors" (people who help others inject), and commercial sex workers. Injecting drug use notoriously predisposes to HIV infection, hepatitis, and endocarditis, but skin and soft tissue infections are now the most common reason for hospitalization.

Problems in Host Defenses

S. aureus nasal colonization is possibly more common in injecting drug users. Drug users frequently treat themselves with antibiotics, predisposing to the emergence of resistant bacterial strains, including MRSA. Studies of the effect of injecting drug use on leukocyte function, humoral immunity, and cell-mediated immunity have borne inconclusive results.

Clinical Infections

Viral infections are common and problematic. Injecting drug use is now the most common means of HIV transmission in the United States. Some researchers have correlated HIV transmission in these patients with sexual promiscuity. Hepatitis A is more common among drug users and is occasionally transmitted by injection rather than poor hygiene, the usual cause. Hepatitis B is also more common and can be made worse by coinfection or superinfection with hepatitis D virus (delta agent). Most injecting drug users with hepatitis B, however, show a favorable clinical course with clearance of hepatitis B surface antigen and development of anti-HBs antibody (see Chapter 13). About 65% to 90% of injecting drug users are infected with hepatitis C virus that, unlike hepatitis A or hepatitis B, usually results in chronic infection. The combination of alcoholism with chronic hepatitis B or hepatitis C predisposes to severe liver disease. The prevalence of infection by either of the human T-cell lymphotropic viruses (HTLV-1 and HTLV-2) is increasing in drug users, but the long-term significance is unclear.

Skin and soft tissue infections are now the most common indication for hospitalization of injecting drug users in the United States. The usual syndromes are cellulitis, subcutaneous abscess, skin ulcers, necrotizing fasciitis, and pyomyositis. These infections often occur at unusual sites, as drug users search for previously unused veins for injection. *S. aureus* is the most common pathogen. *Streptococcus pyogenes* (group A streptococci) and *Clostridium* species can cause severe infection with systemic toxicity. Contamination of drugs, needles, and paraphernalia with saliva can lead to infections caused by "mouth flora" organisms including α-hemolytic streptococci, *Eikenella corrodens,* and anaerobic bacteria. Aerobic gram-negative rods are frequently isolated as well, and many of these infections are polymicrobial. Tetanus and wound botulism (see Chapter 6) occasionally occur. Necrotizing fasciitis (see Chapter 6) is becoming an increasingly important problem in these patients. The diagnosis can be difficult, especially since a major clue to the diagnosis of necrotizing fasciitis—severe pain with a paucity of physical findings—is understandably misinterpreted as drug-seeking behavior.

Infections of peripheral veins and arteries are common in injecting drug users and often lead to metastatic infection elsewhere. Sclerosis of the more accessible veins in the upper extremities prompts drug users to seek other injection sites, including the femoral artery and axillary arteries and the jugular veins. Hit doctors in "shooting galleries" maintained for this purpose often show skill and resourcefulness at finding out-of-the-way veins for injection. Syndromes related to injection include septic thrombophlebitis, mycotic aneurysm, infected hematoma, and traumatic arteriovenous fistula with infection. The latter lesion is often found in the left groin of right-handed drug users. *S. aureus* is the usual pathogen isolated from these infections, but *P. aeruginosa* and numerous other bacterial species are also encountered. Infection of arteries and veins commonly causes bacteremia, which leads to such metastatic infections as endocarditis, septic arthritis, osteomyelitis, splenic abscess, endophthalmitis, and central nervous system (CNS) infection.

Septic arthritis and osteomyelitis are also more common in injecting drug users. Hematogenous osteomyelitis often involves the spine, most commonly in the lumbar area. *S. aureus* is the usual pathogen, but others are streptococci, *P. aeruginosa,* and gram-negative rods. The left knee is the most common site of septic arthritis, but other sites are the wrist, shoulder, hip, sacroiliac joints, and unusual locations such as the sternoclavicular joints, costochondral joints, and symphysis pubis. *P. aeruginosa* has been prominently associated with septic arthritis at these unusual locations.

Endocarditis is a major problem in drug users. The classic presentation consists of a flulike illness with bilateral patchy pulmonary infiltrates caused by *S. aureus* endocarditis involving the tricuspid or pulmonic valve (right-sided endocarditis). Cardiac murmurs are unimpressive or absent. This form of endocarditis usually responds well to appropriate therapy provided the patient is not critically ill at the time of diagnosis. Some data suggest that endocarditis involving the mitral or aortic valve (left-sided endocarditis) is now occurring more frequently in drug users. In women, involvement of the mitral valve may even be more common than involvement of the tricuspid valve. Left-sided endocarditis carries a less favorable prognosis than right-sided endocarditis. Endocarditis in drug users is sometimes caused by unusual microorganisms and may also be polymicrobial. As in other patients with endocarditis, blood cultures are the key to accurate diagnosis. Patients with suspected endocarditis should be admitted to the hospital.

CNS infections in injecting drug users most often result from endocarditis. Examples are brain abscess and subdural empyema. Spinal epidural abscess (see Chapter 6) should be suspected when an injecting drug user seeks treatment for back pain and focal neurologic symptoms. Unusual infections include aspergillosis affecting the CNS and intramedullary spinal cord abscess.

Pneumonia is more common in injecting drug users and can be difficult to distinguish from pulmonary edema, septic pulmonary embolism, drug-induced bronchospasm, and talc granulomatosis. *S. pneumoniae* and oral anaerobic bacteria ("mouth flora aspiration pneumonia") are common causes of bronchogenic pneumonia. *S. aureus* and *P. aeruginosa* are more likely to cause pneumonia of hematogenous origin. Injecting drug users are at risk for tuberculosis because of their lifestyles. Recent studies indicate that monetary incentives promote compliance with tuberculin skin testing and treatment of latent tuberculosis infection in these patients.

 KEY POINTS

INFECTIONS IN INJECTING DRUG USERS

⊃ Injecting drug use is now the most common means of HIV transmission in the United States.

⊃ Hepatitis A, B, C, and D are all more common in injecting drug users. Up to 90% of injecting drug users are infected with hepatitis C.

⊃ *S. aureus* is the most commonly encountered bacterial pathogen in injecting drug users, but infections caused by group A and other streptococci, *P. aeruginosa* and other gram-negative rods, anaerobic bacteria, fungi, and *M. tuberculosis* are also common in this population. Unprescribed antibiotic use in drug users predisposes to drug-resistant bacteria, including MRSA.

⊃ Skin and soft tissue infections in injecting drug users include cellulitis, abscesses, cellulitis, and necrotizing fasciitis. Necrotizing fasciitis can be a difficult diagnosis in injecting drug users, since a principal clue—severe localized pain with a paucity of physical findings—is easily attributed to drug-seeking behavior.

⊃ Infections of peripheral arteries and veins, which are often in atypical locations, include septic thrombophlebitis, mycotic aneurysm, infected hematoma, and traumatic arteriovenous fistula.

⊃ Bloodborne (hematogenous) infections include septic arthritis, osteomyelitis, endocarditis, splenic abscess, brain abscess, and endophthalmitis.

⊃ Septic arthritis often occurs in unusual locations such as the sternoclavicular joints, costochondral joints, and symphysis pubis. Osteomyelitis often involves the spine. Persistent low back pain can also be the presenting symptom of spinal epidural abscess.

⊃ Endocarditis most commonly involves the right side of the heart and is evidenced by the triad of fever, septic pulmonary emboli, and *S. aureus* bacteremia. However, left-sided endocarditis is becoming more common, especially in women.

⊃ CNS infections include brain abscess, meningitis, ruptured mycotic aneurysm, and spinal epidural abscess.

⊃ Pneumonia is more common in injecting drug users. Bronchogenous pneumonia is often due to *S. pneumoniae* or anaerobic ("mouth flora") bacteria. Hematogenous pneumonia is often caused by *S. aureus* or *P. aeruginosa.*

SUGGESTED READING

Callahan TE, Schecter WP, Horn JK. Necrotizing soft tissue infection masquerading as cutaneous abscess following illicit drug injection. Arch Surg 1998; 133: 812-817.

Contoreggi C, Rexroad VE, Lange WR. Current management of infectious complications in the injecting drug user. J Subst Abuse Treat 1998; 15: 95-106.

Doherty MC, Garfein RS, Monterroso E, et al. Correlates of HIV infection among young adult short-term injection drug users. AIDS 2000; 14: 717-726.

Friedman SR, Furst RT, Jose B, et al. Drug scene roles and HIV risk. Addiction 1998; 93: 1403-1416.

Hagan H. Hepatitis C transmission dynamics in injection drug users. Subst Use Misuse 1998; 33: 1197-1212.

Lorvick J, Thompson S, Edlin BR, et al. Incentives and accessibility: a pilot study to promote adherence to TB prophylaxis in a high-risk community. J Urban Health 1999; 76: 461-467.

Passaro DJ, Werner SB, McGee J, et al. Wound botulism associated with black tar heroin among injecting drug users. JAMA 1998; 279: 859-863.

Patients with Lymphoma, Leukemia, and Other Malignancies

Patients in whom malignant disease has been diagnosed are usually under the care of an oncologist. Those with fever and granulocytopenia nearly always require hospitalization. This discussion therefore focuses mainly on infection as a presenting manifestation of lymphoma, leukemia, or other malignancies.

Problems in Host Defenses

Malignancies variably damage mucosal barriers, obstruct ducts and other passages, induce negative nitrogen balance, and inflict specific impairments on the immune system. Patients with multiple myeloma, and also patients with chronic lymphocytic leukemia, may lack the ability to produce antigen-specific antibodies (B-cell immunity). Patients with lymphoreticular malignancies often have impairment of the component of T-cell immunity for containment and elimination of intracellular pathogens by mononuclear phagocytes (monocyte-macrophages). The extent of T-cell dysfunction is proportional to the stage of the underlying cancer. The common malignancies in this setting are Hodgkin's disease, non-Hodgkin's lymphomas, and lymphocytic leukemias; rare diseases in this category include adult T-cell leukemia lymphoma (ATLL) and hairy cell leukemia.

Clinical Infections

Infections by encapsulated bacteria occur with increased frequency in patients with impaired humoral (B-cell) function. A classical association is that of pneumococcal pneumonia with multiple myeloma and chronic lymphocytic leukemia. Infections caused by *H. influenzae* also occur in these patients. Recurrent pneumonia in the same anatomic location should raise the suspicion of endobronchial lung cancer.

The association of *Streptococcus bovis* bacteremia with carcinoma of the colon is well known; this organism has also been associated with leukemia. Similarly, *Clostridium septicum* bacteremia has a strong association with malignancy. Patients with *C. septicum* bloodstream infection occasionally have gangrene distal to the site of infection ("distant myonecrosis").

Pyogenic bacterial infection with sepsis can be the presenting manifestation of acute leukemia. Patients with leukemia and granulocytopenia often become septic from ulcerations in the distal small bowel ("typhlitis"). *Corynebacterium jeikeium* is an important cause of vascular access line infections in granulocytopenic patients with malignancy.

Infections related to impaired T-cell immunity in patients with malignancy include the following:

■ Intracellular bacteria. *L. monocytogenes* (most commonly as meningitis), *Salmonella* species (bacteremia, sometimes complicated by metastatic infection), *Nocardia asteroides* (pneumonia and brain abscess), *M. tuberculosis* (pulmonary or disseminated), nontuberculous mycobacteria (such as *M. avium* complex and *M. kansasii),* *Legionella* species, and, less commonly, *Rhodococcus equi* and *Brucella* species.

■ Fungi. *Cryptococcus neoformans* (usually as meningitis), *Candida* species (mucocutaneous candidiasis), *P. carinii* (pneumonia), *Aspergillus* species, and, less commonly, endemic mycoses *(Histoplasma capsulatum, Coccidioides immitis,* and, possibly, *Blastomyces dermatitidis),* the agents of hyalohyphomycosis, and dematiaceous molds (see Chapter 21).

■ Viruses. Varicella-zoster virus (most commonly as shingles, but occasionally as disseminated infection or atypical presentations), cytomegalovirus (most commonly as a diffuse interstitial pneumonia), herpes simplex virus types 1 and 2, influenza virus, parainfluenza viruses, and respiratory syncytial virus. Less common viral infections include adenoviruses, Epstein-Barr virus, human herpesviruses 6 and 7, and JC virus (the agent of progressive multifocal leukoencephalopathy).

■ Parasites. *Toxoplasma gondii* (most commonly as brain abscess, encephalitis, or pneumonia) and, less commonly, *Strongyloides stercoralis* (pulmonary hyperinfection syndrome) and *Cryptosporidium, Cyclospora, Microsporidia,* and *Leishmania* species (see Chapter 23).

Herpes zoster (varicella-zoster virus reactivation) occurs with increased frequency in persons with Hodgkin's disease and other lymphomas, and its occurrence at an early age should suggest this possibility. In about 25% of patients with Hodgkin's disease, varicella-zoster virus is reactivated at some point during their illness, and the disease is occasionally manifested as pneumonitis or encephalitis or rarely as abdominal pain suggesting an acute abdomen. Mycobacterial infection, including tuberculosis, occurs with increased frequency in patients with Hodgkin's disease. The presentation may be atypical, sometimes involving multicentric infiltrates in the lower regions of the lung with sparing of the apices. Fever and nights sweats are absent in up to 20% of patients with Hodgkin's disease who have disseminated tuberculosis. Patients with lymphomas, ATLL, and hairy cell leukemia are also at risk of disseminated infection because of *Mycobacterium avium* complex.

 KEY POINTS

PATIENTS WITH LYMPHOMA, LEUKEMIA, AND OTHER MALIGNANCIES

⊃ Malignancies variably damage mucosal barriers, obstruct ducts and other passages, induce negative nitrogen balance, and inflict specific impairments on the immune system.

⊃ Infections that should raise the possibility of underlying malignancy include recurrent bacterial pneumonia in the same anatomic location (lung cancer), meningitis caused by *Cryptococcus neoformans* or *L. monocytogenes* (lymphoma), herpes zoster at a young age (lymphoma), frequent or severe pneumococcal infection (multiple myeloma, chronic lymphocytic leukemia), and otherwise unexplained bacteremia caused by *Salmonella* species, *S. bovis,* or *C. septicum.*

SUGGESTED READING

Safdar A, Armstrong D. Infections in patients with neoplastic diseases. In: Shoemaker WC, Grenvik M, Ayers SM, et al., eds. Textbook of Critical Care. 4th ed., Philadelphia: W.B. Saunders Company; 2000: 715-726.

Patients with Spinal Cord Injuries

About 10,000 persons in the United States survive spinal cord injuries each year. More than 200,000 persons in the United States are now living with this disability. Since their life expectancies steadily approach those of other persons, primary care clinicians are likely to encounter such patients in their practices.

Problems in Host Defenses

Recent data suggest that injury to the upper spinal cord (T10 or higher), by destroying the sympathetic outflow tracts, may adversely affect the immune system. In general, however, little convincing evidence has shown that spinal cord injury per se harms phagocyte, B-lymphocyte, or T-lymphocyte function. The major problems in host defenses are evident:

■ Neurogenic bladder, often accompanied by incontinence, the need for intermittent or indwelling urinary catheters, and ureterovesical reflux, predisposing to UTI

■ Weakness of the diaphragm and intercostalis muscles (in persons with cervical or high thoracic lesions of the spinal cord), predisposing to pneumonia

■ Immobility, predisposing to pressure sores (decubitus ulcers), which in turn predispose to osteomyelitis

■ Loss of sweating and muscular activity below the level of the lesion, causing impairment of heat dissipation and heat generation, respectively

More subtle problems include impaired gastrointestinal motility (which can promote aspiration), cholelithiasis (which has an increased incidence in these patients), malnutrition (which can in turn impair T-cell function), and renal failure (sometimes caused by amyloidosis related to chronic infection).

Clinical Infections

Lack of pain sensation below the level of the lesion makes early diagnosis of infection difficult. In some recently injured persons with quadriplegia, prolonged fever develops without obvious cause ("quadriplegic fever"). Impaired ability to dissipate heat is generally believed to cause self-limited episodes of fever that resolve within hours to a few days. However, patients with more prolonged fever should be assumed to have a treatable infection or noninfectious problem unless an extensive search suggests otherwise. Noninfectious problems cause about one fifth of febrile episodes in these patients, with deep vein thrombosis usually the most important consideration. Some patients have more than one possible source of fever.

UTI (see Chapter 14) causes substantial morbidity in persons with spinal cord injury even though improved methods of urinary drainage have dramatically reduced the rate of life-threatening complications. Use of intermittent catheterization not only reduces the incidence of bacteriuria, but also reduces the risk of complications from chronic indwelling catheterization such as squamous metaplasia of the bladder (which can progress to carcinoma), changes in the bladder wall (thickening, fibrosis, and formation of diverticula), prostatic abscess, fistulae in the penis and scrotum, and formation of urinary tract calculi. Preliminary data suggest that deliberate bladder colonization with a relatively avirulent *E. coli* strain (bacterial interference therapy) may reduce the frequency of symptomatic UTI. At present, asymptomatic bacteriuria remains common and is polymicrobial in about one half of patients. Bacteriuria caused by *Proteus mirabilis* and other urea-splitting bacteria promotes formation of struvite calculi. Treatment of asymptomatic bacteriuria predisposes to infection caused by antibiotic-resistant microorganisms and yeasts and is therefore discouraged. Since bacteriuria is so common in patients with UTI, fever should not be attributed to UTI without consideration of other possibilities. Clues to the diagnosis of pyelonephritis include high fever, systemic toxicity, and leukocyte casts in the urinary sediment. Recent data suggest that fluoroquinolones may be more effective than trimethoprim-sulfamethoxazole in relieving infection and eradicating bacterial biofilms on urinary bladder epithelial cells.

Pneumonia (see Chapter 11) is the leading infectious cause of death in patients with spinal cord injuries, even though it accounts for <10% of all infections. Pneumonia occurs most often in the left lower lobe and is frequently associated with atelectasis, which makes accurate radiographic diagnosis difficult. Pneumonia can be caused by "mouth flora" bacteria acquired by aspiration or by specific pathogens such as *S. pneumoniae.* Inability to cough effectively compromises the obtaining of a sputum specimen for Gram stain and culture. Pulmonary thromboembolism, estimated to occur in about 5% of persons with spinal cord injury, should be considered a possible cause of fever and pulmonary infiltrates, especially if hypoxemia is present. Ventilation-perfusion lung scans are often nondiagnostic because of atelectasis. Spiral CT scanning of the chest may be helpful when large emboli are present.

Decubitus ulcers (see Chapter 15) are a major cause of morbidity in patients with spinal cord injuries. They generally occur over dependent areas such as the sacrum, ischial tuberosities, and greater trochanter. Complications include cellulitis, abscesses, osteomyelitis, and bacteremia. Bone biopsy is often necessary to establish a definitive diagnosis of osteomyelitis. Decubitus ulcers usually have a polymicrobial flora that includes both aerobic and anaerobic bacteria. *B. fragilis* is a major cause of bacteremia in patients with decubitus ulcers; other etiologies include *S. aureus,* enterococci, and aerobic gram-negative bacilli. Decubitus ulcers are often colonized with antibiotic-resistant microorganisms such as MRSA and vancomycin-resistant enterococci. The proverbial "ounce of prevention" remains the best strategy, since treatment of infected decubitus ulcers is usually long and arduous and requires the services of a plastic surgeon.

Recognition of infections that occur in able-bodied persons, including such conditions as acute appendicitis or diverticulitis, can be difficult in patients with spinal cord injury, again because of the lack of pain sensation. Therefore the liberal use of blood cultures, other laboratory tests, and imaging procedures is usually prudent. Vertebral osteomyelitis (see Chapter 15) occurs more commonly in patients with spinal cord injury, with a relative risk seven-fold that of a general hospital population. The presence of pleural effusions or of a paraspinous mass on x-ray examination is an important clue to the correct diagnosis.

Determining the dosage of antimicrobial agents that have a relatively low therapeutic index (i.e., therapeutic dose to toxic dose) can be a problem with patients who have spinal cord injuries. Extracellular fluid volume (ECFV) is usually higher than would be predicted on the basis of weight. Creatinine clearance is usually lower than would be predicted on the basis of weight and the serum creatinine level. Because of the expanded ECFV, the prescriber should usually err toward a higher-than-usual dose of aminoglycoside antibiotics or vancomycin. Because of the possibility that the serum creatinine level may not accurately reflect renal function, however, the prescriber should err toward more frequent measurements of serum drug levels (see Chapter 19).

KEY POINTS

PATIENTS WITH SPINAL CORD INJURIES

⊃ Evaluation of fever and infection is often difficult because of lack of pain sensation.
⊃ Patients who are quadriplegic from a recent injury occasionally have prolonged fever for no apparent reason ("quadriplegic fever"), but in general, fever in these patients should be presumed to be due to a specific infection or noninfectious etiology, such as deep vein thrombosis.
⊃ Bacteriuria is extremely common, and therefore fever should not be attributed to UTI unless other possibilities have been considered.

⊃ Clean intermittent catheterization should be used for urinary drainage whenever possible.
⊃ Pneumonia is now the leading infectious cause of death in patients with spinal cord injuries and can be difficult to diagnose because of the presence of atelectasis.
⊃ Pulmonary thromboembolism should be considered a possible cause of fever, pulmonary infiltrates, or hypoxemia.
⊃ Decubitus ulcers can cause osteomyelitis of the underlying bone; frequently harbor drug-resistant organisms, including MRSA; and are a major source of bacteremia.
⊃ Determining the dosage of antibiotics with low therapeutic indices (e.g., aminoglycosides, vancomycin) can be difficult because (1) the extracellular fluid volume is usually greater than would be predicted on the basis of weight, and (2) the creatinine clearance is usually lower than would be predicted on the basis of weight and the serum creatinine level.

SUGGESTED READING

Esclarín De Ruz A, García Leoni E, Herruzo Cabrera R. Epidemiology and risk factors for urinary tract infection in patients with spinal cord injury. J Urol 2000; 164: 1285-1289.

Frisbie JH, Gore RL, Strymish JM, et al. Vertebral osteomyelitis in paraplegia: incidence, risk factors, clinical picture. J Spinal Cord Med 2000; 23: 15-22.

Gilman TM, Brunnemann SR, Segal JL. Comparison of population pharmacokinetic models for gentamicin in spinal cord–injured and able-bodied patients. Antimicrob Agents Chemother 1993; 37: 93-99.

Hull R, Rudy D, Donovan W, et al. Urinary tract infection prophylaxis using *Escherichia coli* 83972 in spinal cord injured patients. J Urol 2000; 163: 872-877.

Montgomerie JZ. Infections in patients with spinal cord injuries. Clin Infect Dis 1997; 25: 1285-1292.

Mylotte JM, Kahler L, Graham R, et al. Prospective surveillance for antibiotic-resistant organisms in patients with spinal cord injury admitted to an acute rehabilitation unit. Am J Infect Control 2000; 28: 291-297.

Segal JL, Brunnemann SR. Clinical pharmacokinetics in patients with spinal cord injuries. Clin Pharmacokinet 1989; 17: 109-129.

Weld KJ, Dmochowski RR. Effect of bladder management on urological complications in spinal cord injured patients. J Urol 2000; 163: 768-772.

West DA, Cummings JM, Longo WE, et al. Role of chronic catheterization in the development of bladder cancer in patients with spinal cord injury. Urology 1999; 53: 292-297.

Organ Transplant Recipients

Medical teams assuming care for organ transplantation must have detailed expertise in the diagnosis and management of infectious complications. The increasing frequency of transplantation makes a general familiarity with these infections desirable for primary care clinicians.

Problems in Host Defenses

Medications used to prevent transplant rejection also predispose to infection. Thus prednisone, cyclosporine, FK-506 (tacrolimus), and rapamycin all inhibit the ability of cytotoxic T lymphocytes to mount a microbe-specific response. This effect predisposes especially to infections caused by DNA viruses, fungi, and mycobacteria (see the earlier discussion of corticosteroids). Antilymphocyte antibodies and cytotoxic drugs such as azathioprine (Imuran) and cyclophosphamide (Cytoxan) not only inhibit T-lymphocyte function but also tend to reactivate latent viral infection.

Clinical Infections

During the first month after transplantation, recipients are vulnerable to wound infections, pneumonia, and intravenous line–related infections caused by the same pathogens that cause these infections in other postoperative patients. Hepatitis and herpes simplex virus infection may also develop.

Between 1 and 6 months after transplantation, viral infections become the major problem. The herpesviruses are the most important agents, and among these CMV is by far the most notorious. Three patterns of CMV disease are recognized in transplant recipients: (1) primary infection, in which a CMV-seronegative patient receives an organ from a CMV-positive donor; (2) reactivation of infection, in which a CMV-seropositive patient reactivates his or her own virus while receiving immunosuppressive therapy; and (3) superinfection, in which a CMV-seropositive patient receives latently infected cells from a CMV-positive donor. CMV damages the transplanted organ to a much greater extent than native organs. CMV myocarditis thus becomes a severe disease in heart transplant recipients, CMV hepatitis in liver transplant recipients, and CMV pneumonia in lung transplant recipients. Other important viruses during this period are varicella-zoster virus, Epstein-Barr virus, hepatitis viruses, and papovaviruses. Patients are also at risk of fungal infections, including aspergillosis and *P. carinii* pneumonia, *Nocardia* species infections, tuberculosis, and toxoplasmosis.

Beyond 6 months after transplantation the frequency and types of infection depend on how well the patient is doing. In general, about 80% of patients have good allograft function and require only maintenance immunosuppression. These patients are at risk mainly for the infections prevalent in the general community, such as influenza, pneumococcal pneumonia, and UTI. About 10% of patients have chronic viral infections. These patients are at risk for virus-related complications, such as cirrhosis from hepatitis B, lymphoproliferative disorder from Epstein-Bar virus, and squamous cell carcinoma from human papillomavirus. About 10% of patients do poorly, require high-dose immunosuppression, and are at risk for major opportunistic infections by such pathogens as *Cryptococcus neoformans, L. monocytogenes, P. carinii,* and *Aspergillus* species. Cryptococcal meningitis often occurs without an apparent inciting event. Herpes zoster can occur at any time following transplantation and may be disseminated (see Chapter 7). Hepatitis C can become a significant problem years after transplantation, as chronic hepatitis slowly but inexorably leads to clinical liver disease, including cirrhosis.

To some extent, transplantation-related infections are organ specific:

- Kidney transplants. The urinary tract is the most common site of infection (about 40% of infections), often because of technical complications from the procedure. CMV tends to be less of a problem than in heart, heart-lung, and liver transplants.

- Heart and heart-lung transplants. Deep fungal infections are relatively common and often severe.
- Liver transplants. Infection rates are high, and most deaths are due to infection. Serious bacterial infections often occur within the first 2 weeks. Deep fungal infections are more common than after other solid organ transplants.
- In one large compilation of data, mortality caused by infection during the first year after transplantation was nil after kidney transplantation, 13% after heart transplantation, 19% after heart-lung transplantation, and 23% after liver transplantation. Patients considering or undergoing transplantation should have a general appreciation of these risks.

 KEY POINTS

ORGAN TRANSPLANT RECIPIENTS

⊃ The medications necessary for preventing transplant rejection also predispose to infection.

⊃ During the first month after transplantation, patients are at risk mainly for the same types of infection that affect other postoperative patients.

⊃ Between 1 and 6 months after transplantation, patients are at risk mainly for viral infections, of which CMV is by far the most notorious.

⊃ Beyond 6 months after transplantation the risk of infection correlates with how well the patient is doing with the transplant. Patients who have well-functioning allografts while receiving low-dose maintenance immunosuppressive medication are at risk mainly for the types of infection that cause disease in the general population.

⊃ At present, mortality from infection is low after kidney transplantation, moderate (about 13%) after heart transplantation, and high (about 23%) after liver transplantation.

SUGGESTED READING

Dummer JS, Ho M. Infections in solid organ transplant recipients. In: Mandell GL, Bennett JE, Dolin R, eds. Mandell, Douglas, and Bennett's Principles and Practice of Infectious Diseases. 5th ed., Philadelphia: Churchill Livingstone; 2000: 3148-3159.
Patel R, Paya CV. Infections in solid-organ transplant recipients. Clin Microbiol Rev 1997; 10: 86-124.

Primary Immunodeficiency Syndromes Manifested in Adulthood

Primary immunodeficiency syndromes usually manifest themselves as frequent infections during childhood (see Chapter 4). An occasional adult with a serious infection gives a history of frequent infections during childhood, providing the clue to a primary immunodeficiency syndrome that was overlooked. Examples include chronic granulomatous disease of childhood and the hyperimmunoglobulinemia E–recurrent infection syndrome (Job's syndrome); in both cases a history of frequent "boils" during childhood may provide the diagnostic clue.

Three primary immunodeficiency syndromes that may be seen first in adulthood are, in order of importance, common variable immunodeficiency, deficiency of late-acting complement components, and selective IgA deficiency. Recommended tests for initial screening are summarized in Table 3-3.

Common Variable Immunodeficiency

The term "common variable immunodeficiency" refers to a heterogeneous group of disorders characterized by impaired antibody production. No specific genetic etiology has been established, although several patterns of inheritance have been described. The syndrome has no sex predilection. The prevalence is estimated to be between 1 in 50,000 and 1 in 200,000 persons. Common variable immunodeficiency usually manifests itself during the second or third decade of life with recurrent sinopulmonary infections such as otitis media, sinusitis, bronchitis, and pneumonia. The usual pathogens are encapsulated bacteria such as *S. pneumoniae* and *H. influenzae*. Some patients also have chronic enteric infections by *Giardia lamblia* or other pathogens. Diagnosis is established by measuring serum immunoglobulin levels. IgG levels are low, and the levels of IgM and IgA may be decreased as well. Intravenous immune globulin (IVIG) is useful for these

patients, who are also at risk for gastric carcinoma, autoimmune diseases, a syndrome resembling sarcoidosis, and lymphoproliferative diseases, including lymphoma.

Late-Acting Complement Deficiencies

Persons with deficiency of a late-acting complement component (notably C6 and C7) are at markedly increased risk for systemic infection with neisserial bacteremia caused by *N. meningitidis* or *N. gonorrhoeae*. Serum complement should be measured in all patients with two or more episodes of neisserial bacteremia.

Selective IgA Deficiency

Selective IgA deficiency is the most common primary immunodeficiency disorder, with an estimated prevalence of 1 in 300 to 1 in 700 persons. Most affected persons are asymptomatic, but a few seek medical attention because of recurrent upper respiratory tract, pulmonary, or gastrointestinal infections. About 20% of persons with IgA deficiency, including many who are symptomatic, also have IgG subclass deficiency (typically IgG_2 or IgG_4). Persons with selective IgA deficiency may have an increased incidence of allergies, autoimmune diseases, asthma, inflammatory bowel disease,

TABLE 3-3
Major Elements of the Immune System and Diagnostic Tests for Immune Deficiency

Element	Main function	Clinical characteristics of infection	Types of microorganism involved	Diagnostic tests
B-lymphocyte system (humoral immunity)	Antibody production	Recurrent sinopulmonary infections	Encapsulated bacteria	Quantitative immunoglobulin levels (IgG, IgA, IgM); IgG subclass titers; specific antibody titers after immunization*; bone marrow examination
T-lymphocyte system (cell-mediated immunity)	T-cell cytotoxicity; immune regulation	Infections caused by opportunistic pathogens	DNA viruses, intracellular bacteria, fungi (including *Pneumocystis carinii*), parasites	CBC with differential (absolute lymphocyte count); quantitation of $CD4^+$ and $CD8^+$ lymphocytes; skin testing with an "anergy panel"†
Complement system	Factors that promote the inflammatory response, phagocytosis, and antibody function	Pyogenic bacteria	*Neisseria meningitidis; Neisseria gonorrhoeae; Streptococcus pneumoniae*	Whole complement activity (CH_{50}); measurement of specific components‡
Phagocytic system	Innate or nonspecific immunity; phagocytosis	Recurrent skin and visceral abscesses; gingivitis	*Staphylococcus aureus; Pseudomonas aeruginosa; Aspergillus* species	White blood cell morphology; Nitroblue tetrazolium test§; immunoglobulin E level; chemotaxis assay

*For example, one can measure antibody titers against specific *Streptococcus pneumoniae* serotypes before and after giving the pneumococcal polysaccharide vaccine.
†Anergy panels consist of skin test antigens to which most persons are expected to show a response. Examples include mumps virus, *Candida*, *Trichophyton*, and endemic fungi (e.g., *H. capsulatum*, *C. immitis*). Further testing of T-lymphocyte function usually requires a specialized laboratory.
‡Whole complement level is used as a screen for deficiency of one or more components. Deficiency of late-acting components is specifically associated with recurrent neisserial infections (see text).
§The nitroblue tetrazolium test is used as a screen for disorders of PMN function, notably chronic granulomatous disease of childhood. Further testing requires a specialized laboratory.

and transfusion reactions (owing to the IgE response to trace levels of IgA in transfused blood products). There is no specific treatment unless IgG subclass deficiency is present, in which case IVIG may be useful. Persons with selective IgA deficiency should be warned against the risk of transfusion. When transfusion is necessary to correct anemia, washed packed red blood cells should be used.

 KEY POINTS

PRIMARY IMMUNODEFICIENCY SYNDROMES MANIFESTED IN ADULTHOOD

➲ Common variable immunodeficiency, which affects between 1 in 50,000 and 1 in 200,000 persons, usually is manifested as recurrent sinopulmonary infections during the second or third decade of life. The diagnosis is established by measurement of serum immunoglobulin levels.

➲ More than one episode of bacteremia caused by *N mening-itidis* or *N. gonorrhoeae* suggests deficiency of a late-acting complement component (C6 or C7).

➲ Selective IgA deficiency, present in 1 in 300 to 1 in 700 persons, is usually asymptomatic but can be evidenced by recurrent upper respiratory or gastrointestinal infections. There is no specific treatment unless IgG subclass deficiency is also present. Washed packed red blood cells should be used when anemia must be corrected by transfusion in persons with selective IgA deficiency.

SUGGESTED READING

Buckley RH. Primary immunodeficiency diseases due to defects in lymphocytes. N Engl J Med 2000; 343: 1313-1324.

Buckley RH, Schiff RI. The use of intravenous immune globulin in immunodeficiency diseases. N Engl J Med 1991; 325: 110-117.

Burrows PD, Cooper MD. IgA deficiency. Adv Immunol 1997; 65: 245-276.

Figueroa J, Andreoni J, Densen P. Complement deficiency states and meningococcal disease. Immunol Res 1993; 12: 295-311.

Hammarstrom L, Vorechovsky I, Webster D. Selective IgA deficiency (SigAD) and common variable immunodeficiency (CVID). Clin Exper Immunol 2000; 120: 225-231.

Orren A. Screening for complement deficiency. Methods Molecular Biol 2000; 150: 139-158.

Rosen FS, Cooper MD, Wedgwood RJ. The primary immuno-deficiencies. N Engl J Med 1995; 333: 431-440.

Sandler SG, Mallory D, Malamut D, et al. IgA anaphylactic trans-fusion reactions. Transfusion Med Rev 1995; 9: 1-8.

Spickett GP, Farrant J, North ME, et al. Common variable immuno-deficiency: how many diseases? Immunol Today 1997; 18: 325-328.

Special Populations

Some patients are at high risk of infection because of demographic or socioeconomic factors or because of lifestyle choices.

Homeless Persons

The more than 13 million homeless persons in the United States include not only men with alcoholism, but also women, adolescents, and even families with children. Psychiatric disorders and substance abuse are common in this population. Studies suggest that males, whites, and substances abusers are at special risk for death from infections or other causes and that nonfluency in English is also a risk factor. Outbreaks of pneumococcal pneumonia occur in homeless shelters, as do outbreaks of meningococcal disease and tuberculosis. Persons who frequent homeless shelters should be targeted for tuberculin skin testing (see Chapter 22). Homeless persons, especially runaway adolescents, are at high risk of HIV infection. Poor hygiene and living conditions also predispose the homeless to parasitic infestation, periodontal disease, and common skin infections such as cellulitis. Recent data indicate that homeless persons are especially susceptible to arboviral encephalitis and to trench fever (*Bartonella henselae* and *Bartonella quintana*).

Immigrants

About 1 million persons immigrate to the United States each year, usually from developing countries. Depending to some extent on the country of origin, immigrants are at high risk for tuberculosis; parasitic infections, including malaria; and sexually transmitted diseases, including HIV disease. Many immigrants have not been properly immunized and are therefore at risk for viral diseases such as chickenpox and rubella.

Incarcerated Persons

Persons who are incarcerated are at high risk for tuberculosis and HIV disease. These sometimes work in concert. Recently, a large outbreak of tuberculosis in a prison was traced to a person with HIV disease who had been admitted to a hospital with fever and normal chest x-ray findings. Sexually transmitted diseases of all types are relatively common in the prison setting.

Occupational and Recreational Exposures

Occupations of various types can pose unique risks of infection. Eponymous examples include fish handler's disease (*Erysipelothrix rhusiopathiae;* see Chapter 15) and wool sorter's disease (anthrax; see Chapter 6). Recreational activities that pose unique risks include exploring caves (histoplasmosis and also rabies transmitted by bats), camping in certain geographic areas (tickborne illnesses and giardiasis), and keeping pet birds (psittacosis). Bloodborne pathogens can be transmitted by contact sports. In recent years concern has been expressed that such fads as tattooing and body piercing can result in transmission of hepatitis C and other viruses, as well as abscesses caused by streptococci and anaerobic bacteria.

 KEY POINTS

SPECIAL POPULATIONS

➲ Homeless persons are at high risk for pneumococcal pneumonia, tuberculosis, meningococcal disease, HIV disease, and many other infections. Homeless persons should be targeted for tuberculin skin testing.

➲ Immigrants from developing countries are at increased risk for tuberculosis, sexually transmitted diseases, and parasitic diseases, including malaria. Immunization status should be reviewed carefully.

➲ Incarcerated persons are at high risk for tuberculosis and sexually transmitted diseases, including HIV disease.

➲ Various occupations and recreational pursuits pose unique infectious risks. Of current concern is transmission of hepatitis C by tattooing and body piercing.

SUGGESTED READING

Ackerman LK. Health problems of refugees. J Am Board Fam Pract 1997; 10: 337-348.

Booth RE, Zhang Y, Kwiatkowski CF. The challenge of changing drug and sex risk behaviors of runaway and homeless adolescents. Child Abuse Negl 1999; 23: 1295-1306.

Cunningham NM. Lymphatic filariasis in immigrants from developing countries. Am Fam Physician 1997; 55: 1199-1204.

Curtis AB, Ridzon R, Novick LF, et al. Analysis of *Mycobacterium tuberculosis* transmission patterns in a homeless shelter outbreak. Int J Tuberc Lung Dis 2000; 4: 308-313.

Hwang SW, Lebow JM, Bierer MF, et al. Risk factors for death in homeless adults in Boston. Arch Intern Med 1998; 158: 1454-1460.

Kitchen LW. Case studies in international medicine. Am Fam Physician 1999; 59: 3040-3044.

Marks SM, Taylor Z, Burrows NR, et al. Hospitalization of homeless persons with tuberculosis in the United States. Am J Pub Health 2000; 90: 435-438.

Mast EE, Goodman RA. Prevention of infectious disease transmission in sports. Sports Med 1997; 24: 1-7.

Rangel MC, Sales RM, Valeriano EN. Rubella outbreaks among Hispanics in North Carolina: lessons learned from a field investigation. Ethn Dis 1999; 9: 230-236.

4

Special Issues in Pediatrics

GEORGE S. KOTCHMAR, JR., JAMES R. STALLWORTH, C. WARREN DERRICK, JR.

Children are different from adults in many ways, including these:

■ Age-related changes in immune status (e.g., the "sluggish" immunology of neonates)
■ Age-related changes in anatomy (e.g., the physis [growth plate] is traversed by transepiphyseal blood vessels in children <18 months of age, predisposing to septic arthritis as a complication of osteomyelitis)
■ Age-related differences in the sensitivity of diagnostic tests (e.g., young children with Epstein-Barr virus infection are likely to be heterophil antibody negative, while neonates with osteomyelitis often have false-negative radionuclide bone scans)
■ Age-related differences in clinical presentation (e.g., occult bacteremia of childhood and pseudoparalysis of limb in neonatal osteomyelitis)

■ Impact of child care centers (e.g., risk of respiratory infections caused by pneumococcal strains that are nonsusceptible to penicillins and cephalosporins)
■ Impact of immigration and international adoption

The purpose of this chapter is to present an approach to children with suspected infections and to discuss infections in children that are common, unique, or likely to have serious consequences. Textbooks given entirely to pediatric infectious diseases are listed below. For primary care clinicians who see substantial numbers of children, we strongly recommend the "Red Book," which is updated every 3 years; it can be obtained from the Publications Section of the American Academy of Pediatrics (telephone: 1-888-227-1770).

SUGGESTED READING

American Academy of Pediatrics, Committee on Infectious Diseases. 2000 Red Book: Report of the Committee on Infectious Diseases. 25th ed., Elk Grove Village, Ill: American Academy of Pediatrics; 2000. (This publication is commonly known as the "Red Book.")
Feigin RD, Cherry JD, eds. Textbook of Pediatric Infectious Diseases. 4th ed., Philadelphia; W.B. Saunders Company; 1998.
Isaacs D, Moxon RE, eds. A Practical Approach to Pediatric Infections. New York: Churchill Livingstone; 1996.
Katz SL, Gershon AA, Hotez PJ, eds. Krugman's Infectious Diseases of Children. 10th ed., St. Louis: Mosby–Year Book; 1998.
Long SS, Pickering LK, Prober CG, eds. Principles and Practice of Pediatric Infectious Diseases. New York: Churchill Livingstone; 1997.
Nelson JD, Bradley JS. Nelson's 2000-2001 Pocket Book of Pediatric Antimicrobial Therapy. 14th ed., Philadelphia: Lippincott Williams and Wilkins; 2000.
Remington JS, Klein JO, eds. Infectious Diseases of the Fetus and Newborn Infant. 5th ed., Philadelphia: W.B. Saunders Company; 2001.
Siberry GK, Iannone R, eds. The Harriet Lane Handbook: A Manual for Pediatric House Officers. 15th ed., St. Louis: Mosby; 2000.
Steele RW, ed. The Clinical Handbook of Pediatric Infectious Disease. 2nd ed., New York: Parthenon Publishing; 2000.

Immunizations (see also Chapter 25)

Maintaining an up-to-date immunization status is pivotal to preventing specific infections in children. Ensuring immunization can be time consuming, especially since about 25% of parents believe that vaccines might weaken the child's immune system, and an equal percentage of parents believe their children are already receiving too many "shots." Primary care clinicians must be familiar with current recommendations and also with the rationale.

The first 2 years of life are the most critical in ensuring adequate immunization. In the past two decades, immunization against *Haemophilus influenzae* type b, hepatitis A and B, *Strep-*

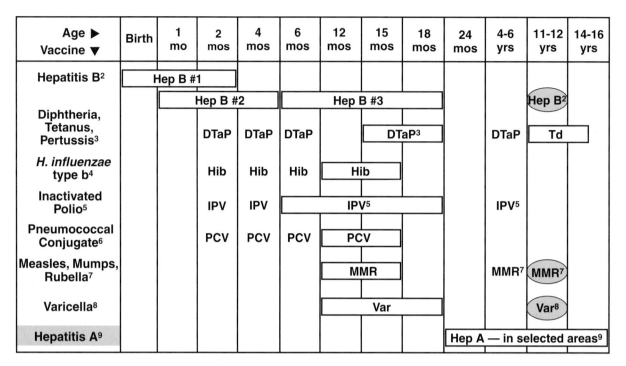

Age ▶ Vaccine ▼	Birth	1 mo	2 mos	4 mos	6 mos	12 mos	15 mos	18 mos	24 mos	4-6 yrs	11-12 yrs	14-16 yrs
Hepatitis B[2]		Hep B #1									Hep B[2]	
			Hep B #2			Hep B #3						
Diphtheria, Tetanus, Pertussis[3]			DTaP	DTaP	DTaP		DTaP[3]			DTaP	Td	
H. influenzae type b[4]			Hib	Hib	Hib	Hib						
Inactivated Polio[5]			IPV	IPV		IPV[5]				IPV[5]		
Pneumococcal Conjugate[6]			PCV	PCV	PCV	PCV						
Measles, Mumps, Rubella[7]						MMR				MMR[7]	MMR[7]	
Varicella[8]						Var					Var[8]	
Hepatitis A[9]									Hep A — in selected areas[9]			

FIG. 4-1 Current recommendations for routine immunization in children through 18 years of age.[1] (From American Academy of Pediatrics, Committee on Infectious Diseases. Recommended childhood immunization schedule—United States, January-December 2001. Pediatrics 2001; 107: 202-204.)

NOTES

[1] Licensed combination vaccines may be used whenever any components of the combination are indicated and its other components are not contraindicated. Manufacturers' package inserts should be consulted for details. Additional immunization can be obtained from the National Immunization Program Home Page (http://www.cdc.gov/nip) or from the National Immunization Hotline (in English at 1-800-232-2522; in Spanish at 1-800-232-0233).

[2] *Hepatitis B vaccine: Infants born to HBsAg-negative mothers* should receive the 1st dose of hepatitis B (Hep B) vaccine by age 2 months. The 2nd dose should be at least 1 month after the 1st dose. The 3rd dose should be given at least 4 months after the 1st dose and at least 2 months after the 2nd dose, but not before 6 months of age for infants. *Infants born to HBsAg-positive mothers* should receive hepatitis B vaccine and also hepatitis B immune globulin (HBIG), 0.5 mL, within 12 hours of birth at separate sites. The 2nd dose of Hep B is recommended at 1 to 2 months of age and the 3rd dose at 6 months of age. *Infants born to mothers whose HBsAg status is unknown* should receive Hep B within 12 hours of birth. Maternal blood should be drawn at the time of delivery to determine the mother's HBsAg status; if the HBsAg test is positive, the infant should receive HBIG as soon as possible (no later than 1 week of age). *All children and adolescents* who have not been immunized against hepatitis B should begin the series during any office visit. Special efforts should be made to immunize children who were born in or whose parents were born in countries with moderate or high endemicity of hepatitis B.

[3] *DtaP (diphtheria and tetanus toxoids and acellular pertussis vaccine):* The 4th dose of DtaP may be administered as early as 12 months of age, provided 6 months have elapsed since the 3rd dose and the child is unlikely to return at age 15 to 18 months. Td (tetanus and diphtheria toxoids) is recommended at 11 to 12 years of age if at least 5 years have elapsed since the last dose of DTP, DtaP, or DT. Subsequent routine Td boosters are recommended every 10 years.

[4] *Haemophilus influenzae type b (Hib) conjugate vaccines.* Three Hib conjugate vaccines are licensed for infant use. If PRP-OMP (Pedvax-HIB or ComVax [Merck]) is administered at 2 and 4 months of age, a dose at 6 months is not required. Because clinical studies in infants have shown that using some combination products may induce a lower immune response to the Hib vaccine component, DtaP/Hib combination products should not be used for primary immunization in infants at 2, 4, or 6 months of age, unless FDA-approved for these ages.

[5] *Inactivated polio vaccine (IPV):* An all-IPV schedule is recommended for routine childhood polio vaccination in the United States. All children should receive four doses of IPV at 2 months, 4 moths, 6 to 18 months, and 4 to 6 years of age. Oral polio vaccine (OPV) should be used only in selected circumstances (see MMWR 2000; 49[RR-5]: 1-22).

[6] *Pneumococcal conjugate vaccine (PCV):* Heptavalent PCV is recommended for all children 2 to 23 months of age. It also is recommended for certain children 24 to 59 months of age (see MMWR 2000; 49[RR-9]: 1-35).

[7] *Measles-mumps-rubella (MMR) vaccine:* The 2nd dose of MMR vaccine is recommended routinely at 4 to 6 years but may be administered during any visit, provided at least 4 weeks have elapsed since receipt of the 1st dose and that both doses are administered beginning at or after 12 months of age. Children who have not previously received the second dose should complete the schedule by the 11- to 12-year-old visit.

[8] *Varicella (Var) vaccine:* Varicella vaccine is recommended at any visit on or after the first birthday for susceptible children, i.e., those who lack a reliable history of chickenpox (as judged by a health care provider) and who have not been immunized. Susceptible persons 13 years of age or older should receive two doses, given at least 4 weeks apart.

[9] *Hepatitis A (HepA) vaccine:* Hep A vaccine is recommended for use in selected states and/or regions and for certain high-risk groups. Local public health authorities can be consulted (see MMWR 1999; 48 [RR-12]: 1-37).

tococcus pneumoniae, and varicella-zoster virus has been added to the vaccine armamentarium. Smallpox has been eradicated as a human pathogen, and eradication of poliomyelitis is expected in the near future. These tremendous strides were made possible by the attentiveness of primary care clinicians. The current immunization schedule for children is summarized in Figure 4-1. Wide use of the new conjugate pneumococcal vaccine has the potential to reduce dramatically the incidence of invasive pneumococcal disease in children and also, to a lesser extent, the incidence of acute otitis media (see Chapter 25). The American Academy of Pediatrics (AAP), Advisory Committee on Immunization Practices (ACIP) of the Centers for Disease Control and Prevention (CDC), and American College Health Association recommend the quadrivalent meningococcal A, C, Y, and W-135 polysaccharide vaccine for college students, particularly freshmen living in dormitories (who have a two- to five-fold increased risk of meningococcal disease). At least 60% of cases among dormitory students are potentially preventable. Detailed recommendations for new and current vaccines indicated for use during infancy, childhood, and adolescence are given in the *2000 Red Book,* AAP (http://www.aap.org), and ACIP (http://www.cdc.gov/nip) statements on specific vaccines, and the respective manufacturers' package inserts. Updated recommendations also appear each year in the January issue of *Pediatrics.*

SUGGESTED READING

Advisory Committee on Immunization Practices (ACIP). Preventing pneumococcal disease among infants and young children. MMWR 2000; 49 (RR-9): 1-35.

Advisory Committee on Immunization Practices (ACIP). Prevention and control of meningococcal disease, and meningococcccal disease and college students. MMWR 2000; 49 (RR-7): 1-20.

American Academy of Pediatrics, Committee on Infectious Diseases. Meningococcal disease prevention and control strategies for practice-based physicians (Addendum: recommendations for college students). Pediatrics 2000; 106: 1500-1504.

Eskola J, Kilpi T, Palmu A, et al. Efficacy of a pneumococcal conjugate vaccine against acute otitis media. N Engl J Med 2001; 344: 403-409.

Feikin DR, Lezotte DC, Hamman RF, et al. Individual and community risks of measles and pertussis associated with personal exemptions to immunization. JAMA 2000; 284: 3145-3150.

Gellin BG, Maibach EW, Marcuse EK. Do parents understand immunizations? A national telephone survey. Pediatrics 2000; 106: 1097-1102.

Gellin BG, Schaffner W. The risk of vaccination—the importance of "negative" studies (editorial). N Engl J Med 2001; 344: 372-373.

Giebink GS. The prevention of pneumococcal disease in children. N Engl J Med 2001; 345: 1177-1183.

Lutwick LI, Rubin LG, eds. Childhood immunizations 2000. Pediatr Clin North Am 2000; 47: 269-485.

General Approach to Children with Suspected Infection, by Age

Age is a key determinant of the approach to a child with suspected infection. Other important determinants are sex, race, immunization status, psychosocial situation, and living environment.

Infants

Infants (children <1 year of age) are especially vulnerable to infectious diseases for reasons that include the following:

- Immature immune systems
- Lack of pathogen-specific immunoglobulins
- Decreased ability to localize infections (particularly in infants <3 months of age)
- Anatomically small respiratory passages and orifices (e.g., eustachian tube and larynx)
- Rapid growth of young cells
- Child care centers

Because of this special vulnerability, fever (>100.4° F [38° C]) must always be taken seriously in an infant <3 months of age.

Fever

Fever >100.4° F (38° C) in an infant <1 month of age should usually prompt a sepsis workup with admission to the hospital. The sepsis workup includes a complete blood count (CBC), lumbar puncture, blood culture(s), urinalysis, and urine culture; when there is an abnormal breathing pattern or auscultatory findings on examination of the chest, a chest x-ray examination is also performed. After these studies are obtained, systemic antimicrobial therapy is initiated.

Fever in children between 1 and 3 months of age calls for a modified sepsis workup based on the physical examination, the Yale observation score (Table 4-1), and the results of screening laboratory tests such as the white blood cell (WBC) count (Figure 4-2).

Fever in children between 3 and 36 months of age without localization of symptoms is usually caused by a viral infection that has not yet declared itself. However, fever >102° F (39° C) raises the possibility of bacteremia or a potentially serious focus of infection. In these children, nonspecific screening tests such as the WBC count, absolute neutrophil count, absolute band count, erythrocyte sedimentation rate (ESR), and C-reactive protein (CRP) are often used to direct the clinician toward appropriate management (Figure 4-3). Blood cultures are usually indicated for febrile children between 3 and 36 months of age with a temperature >102° F without localization of symptoms. This is particularly true if the WBC count is >15,000/mm³ with a predominance of neutrophils, since the risk of bacteremia is five-fold higher than in children with a normal WBC count. Other than bacteremia, the most common source of fever in males <6 months of age and females <2 years of age is urinary tract infection. Therefore urine cultures, in addition to blood cultures, are indicated for these patients. For most of these patients with temperature >102° F and elevated WBC count, empiric therapy with ceftriaxone at 50 mg/kg/day given IM should be instituted after culture results are obtained. The patient should be reevaluated within 24 hours for consideration of a second injection of ceftriaxone and oral antibiotic therapy (amoxicillin-clavulanate or a third-generation cephalosporin) for 7 to 10 days.

Congenital Infections (see also Chapter 5)

The so-called TORCHES infections (toxoplasmosis, rubella, cytomegalovirus, herpes, and syphilis) in neonates continue to be of concern. Human immunodeficiency virus (HIV) infection must now be added to this list. Although each congenital infection has special presentations and organ system involvement, common presentations should alert the primary care physician to the possibility of a congenital infection:

- Small for gestational age
- Failure to thrive

TABLE 4-1
Yale Observation Scale

Observation item	SCORE		
	1 (Normal)	3 (Moderate impairment)	5 (Severe impairment)
Quality of cry	Strong with normal tone, or content and not crying	Whimpering or sobbing	Weak or moaning or high pitched
Reaction to stimulation by parent	Cries briefly, then stops, or content and not crying	Cries off and on	Continual cry or hardly responds
State variation	If awake, stays awake, or if asleep and stimulated, wakes up quickly	Eyes close briefly while awake or awakes with prolonged stimulation	Falls to sleep or will not rouse
Color	Pink	Pale extremities or acrocyanosis	Pale or cyanotic or mottled or ashen
Hydration	Skin and eyes normal and mucous membranes moist	Skin and eyes normal and mouth slightly dry	Skin doughy or tented, dry mucous membranes, sunken eyes
Response (talk, smile) to social overtures	Smiles or alerts (<2 months)	Brief smile or alerts briefly (<2 months)	No smile or face anxious, dull, expressionless, or no alerting (<2 months)

Interpretation: The total number of points is determined from the six observation items. A score >10 points indicates increased likelihood of serious infection.

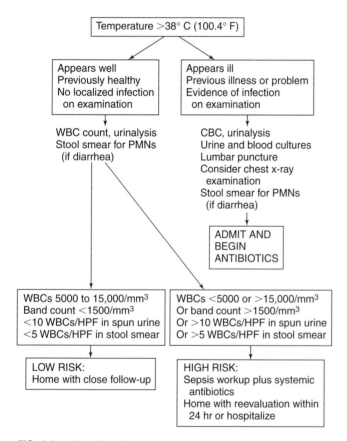

FIG. 4-2 Algorithm for management of an infant 1 to 3 months of age with a temperature >100.4° F (38° C).

- Thermoregulatory instability
- Hypotonia
- Hepatosplenomegaly

If a neonate has several of these presentations, the possibility of a congenital infection should be considered and specific diagnostic tests should be ordered. Suspected vertical transmission of HIV is discussed in the final section of this chapter.

Group B Streptococcal Infections (see also Chapter 5)

Early-onset (first 7 days of life) and late-onset (beyond 7 days) group B streptococcal infections are of special consideration during the neonatal period. These infections include sepsis (early) and meningitis (late) with subsequent high morbidity and mortality. The use of prophylactic antibiotics (ampicillin) in at-risk pregnant women has significantly reduced the frequency of early-onset infection in neonates (see Chapter 5 for further discussion). Infants of mothers who are known vaginal carriers of group B streptococci and who have not been treated before or during parturition should be considered for empiric ampicillin therapy. Careful monitoring of infants for late-onset disease is indicated for any infant born to an at-risk mother regardless of the therapeutic history.

Neonatal Sepsis and Meningitis

During the first few months of life, infants are at risk for meningitis and other serious infections caused by organisms inherently related to parturition. During infancy, bacteremia carries a high risk of meningitis and is more likely to result in meningitis, presumably because of immaturity of the blood-brain barrier. Organisms that commonly cause sepsis and meningitis within the first 6 weeks of life include group B

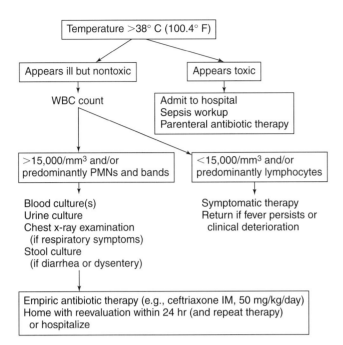

FIG. 4-3 Algorithm for management of a child 3 to 36 months of age >102° F (39° C).

streptococci, *Listeria monocytogenes,* and *Escherichia coli.* Empiric antimicrobial therapy should cover these organisms and also the bacteria that commonly cause sepsis and meningitis in older children: *S. pneumoniae, H. influenzae,* and *Neisseria meningitidis.*

Afebrile Pneumonia Syndrome

In addition to the usual organisms that cause pneumonia in children (*S. pneumoniae, Staphylococcus aureus, H. influenzae,* respiratory syncytial virus [RSV], and adenoviruses), a special group of agents is responsible for the so-called afebrile pneumonia syndrome in young infants. These include *Chlamydia trachomatis,* cytomegalovirus (CMV), and *Ureaplasma urealyticum. Pneumocystis carinii* was initially implicated in this syndrome but is now thought to cause disease almost exclusively in infants with HIV disease. Infants with the afebrile pneumonia syndrome are usually indolent and have cough, tachypnea, or conjunctivitis followed by a variable degree of respiratory compromise. Fever is usually absent, and radiographs show diffuse or patchy interstitial infiltrates. Chlamydial conjunctivitis should be treated with systemic antibiotics to prevent the development of pneumonia.

Maternal Human Immunodeficiency Virus Infection

Neonates born to mothers infected with the HIV agent are at risk for acquiring the virus during parturition. Advances in the management of the mother and infant during delivery have decreased the likelihood of transmission from 30% to less than 10%. Current management options include elective cesarean section and antiretroviral therapy (usually azidothymidine [AZT]) before the onset of labor and membrane rupture (antepartum and intrapartum), followed by AZT therapy in the neonate. Since the virus can be transmitted via breast milk, breast-feeding should not be an option for an HIV-infected mother. Follow-up of all infants born to

HIV-infected women should continue for 18 months to ensure HIV-negative antibody status, since passive maternal antibody can persist in an infant for this period of time.

KEY POINTS

INFANTS (CHILDREN <1 YEAR OF AGE)

⊃ Fever >100.4° F (38° C) in an infant <1 month of age should prompt consideration of a sepsis workup and admission to the hospital.

⊃ Fever in an infant between 1 and 3 months of age suggests the need for a modified sepsis workup based on physical examination, the Yale observation score, and the results of screening laboratory tests.

⊃ Fever in children between 3 and 36 months of age without localizing symptoms or signs is usually due to a viral infection that has not declared itself. However, fever >102° F (39° C) in children in this age group raises the possibility of bacteremia or a focus of serious infection and therefore calls for screening tests.

⊃ Congenital infection by one of the TORCHES agents or HIV is suggested by low birth weight, failure to thrive, thermoregulatory instability, hypotonia, or hepatosplenomegaly.

⊃ Common causes of neonatal sepsis and meningitis include group B streptococci, *E. coli,* and *L. monocytogenes.*

⊃ The afebrile pneumonia syndrome presents with cough, tachypnea, or conjunctivitis with a variable degree of respiratory compromise. The usual pathogens are *C. trachomatis,* cytomegalovirus, and *U. urealyticum.*

⊃ Chlamydial conjunctivitis should be treated with systemic antibiotics to prevent the development of pneumonia.

⊃ Infants born to HIV-infected mothers should be followed for 18 months to ensure antibody-negative status.

Toddlers and Preschoolers

The frequency of common viral and bacterial infections peaks between the ages of 1 and 3 years because of lack of specific antibody memory, anatomically small respiratory orifices and passages, and increased exposure to potential pathogens primarily through child care. The mean number of respiratory infections during these years ranges from six to 12 per toddler per year according to various studies. These high numbers are due in part to daily contact with infected cohorts in child care centers. The number of young children in child care has significantly increased because of the increase in working mothers (from 35% in 1970 to 69% in 1997).

Viral Versus Bacterial Infections

Despite the marked increase in the frequency of suppurative otitis media during the past two decades, viral infections still account for the vast majority of infections affecting young children. Rhinoviruses and adenoviruses account for most of the upper respiratory infections (URIs) in toddlers, with respiratory syncytial virus and parainfluenza virus causing croup, bronchiolitis, and pneumonia. Common bacterial agents affecting young children are *S. pneumoniae, H. influenzae, M. catarrhalis, S. aureus,* group A β-hemolytic streptococci (*Streptococcus pyogenes*; GAS), and *E. coli* (Table 4-2).

TABLE 4-2
Common Infections of Toddlers and Preschool Children

Syndrome	Usual viral agents	Usual bacterial agents
Otitis media	? Adenoviruses, respiratory syncytial virus	*Streptococcus pneumoniae, Haemophilus influenzae* (nontypeable), *Moraxella catarrhalis; Staphylococcus aureus;* group A streptococci
Pharyngitis	Adenoviruses, rhinoviruses	Group A streptococci, group C streptococci
Rhinitis	Adenoviruses, rhinoviruses	None
Croup	Respiratory syncytial viruses, parainfluenza viruses	None
Conjunctivitis	Adenoviruses, coxsackie A	*S. pneumoniae, H. influenzae, Haemophilus aegypti, S. aureus,* group A streptococci
Bronchiolitis (<3 years)	Respiratory syncytial virus, parainfluenza viruses	None
Impetigo and other skin infections	None	Group A streptococci, *S. aureus*
Gastroenteritis	Rotaviruses, adenoviruses, caliciviruses, astroviruses	*Campylobacter jejuni, Escherichia coli, Yersinia* species, *Salmonella* species, *Shigella* species
Urinary tract infections	Adenoviruses	*E. coli*

Fever

Unlike the neonate and young infant, the young child has a relatively intact immune system and can localize infections quite well. Febrile responses to seemingly trivial infections (common cold, otitis media) are common and expected in the young infant. However, fever >103.2° F (39.5° C) is associated with increased risk of occult pneumococcal bacteremia and should lead to appropriate evaluation (CBC, acute-phase reactants, blood cultures) when indicated. Since fever is so common in most childhood infections, fever alone (unless >103.2° F) is not an indication for extensive laboratory evaluation. As stated previously, most febrile illnesses in young children are due to viral agents. Localized infections (e.g., rhinorrhea, otitis media, or croup) in children can usually be diagnosed and managed without laboratory or radiologic evaluation. In febrile patients without localization, CBC and acute-phase reactants (ESR, CRP) may be useful in differentiating bacterial from viral etiologies. Urinary tract infections are notorious for producing fever without other symptoms in young children. Therefore urinalyses and urine cultures are commonly performed if a febrile young child has no localized symptoms. Diarrhea is also commonly seen in young children with nongastrointestinal infection (e.g., otitis media, urinary tract infections, and sepsis). This underscores the pediatric axiom, "Always perform a complete examination of children regardless of the chief complaint" *(in order not to overlook an unexpected source of infection).*

 KEY POINTS

TODDLERS AND PRESCHOOLERS

- ⊃ Common viral and bacterial infections have a peak incidence between 1 and 3 years of age because of lack of specific antibodies, anatomically small orifices and passages, and exposure in child care centers.
- ⊃ Viruses account for the majority of infections in this age group, but common bacterial agents include *S. pneumoniae, H. influenzae, M. catarrhalis,* group A streptococci, and *E. coli.*
- ⊃ Fever is common and to be expected in the young infant, even with trivial infections.
- ⊃ Fever >103.2° F (39.5° C) is associated with a increased risk for occult pneumococcal bacteremia and should prompt appropriate laboratory studies (CBC, acute-phase reactants, blood cultures).
- ⊃ Urinary tract infection often causes fever without other symptoms in young children.
- ⊃ Diarrhea often accompanies infections outside the gastrointestinal tract in this age group.
- ⊃ A complete examination should always be performed on children regardless of the chief complaint.

Grade-Schoolers and Preadolescents

Children between the ages of 6 and 11 years are generally healthy. Many of the common childhood diseases have been experienced, infections relating to small orifices such as otitis media and croup are much less common, and immunologic memory to specific infectious agents and serotypes has increased. Respiratory illnesses make up the bulk of infections in this age group, followed by gastroenteritis, skin and soft tissue infections, and viral exanthems. On the average, preadolescents have four to six acute, self-limiting infections per year.

Respiratory Infections

Although the common cold accounts for most of the respiratory infections in preadolescence, viral or streptococcal pharyngitis is seen with some regularity. In contrast to infants and preschool children, preadolescents seldom have fever as a symptom accompanying mild upper respiratory symptoms. However, fever often accompanies streptococcal or adenoviral pharyngitis. Acute laryngitis and bronchitis are common during the winter months and are usually of viral etiology (notably parainfluenza viruses and adenoviruses). Sinusitis is common but difficult to diagnose, even when x-ray examination or limited computed tomographic (CT) scans are used. Clinically important acute sinusitis is usually caused by common bacteria (*S. pneumoniae, H. influenzae,* and *M. catarrhalis*). By preadolescence, acute otitis media is almost a rarity. However, diffuse external otitis ("swimmer's ear") is common during the summer months (see Chapter 10).

Gastroenteritis

Gastroenteritis is common in preadolescents and is usually of viral origin. During the winter, rotaviruses are by far the usual cause. In the summer, enteric adenoviruses are common. Bacterial pathogens occasionally cause gastroenteritis, usually self-limited. Stool cultures are indicated mainly when diarrheal stools contain blood and mucus (dysentery). Bloody diarrhea should prompt consideration of Shiga toxin–producing *E. coli* because of the potential for hemolytic-uremic syndrome (see Chapter 12). The mainstay of treatment is fluid and electrolyte replacement. Use of antiperistaltic medications, especially the opiates, should be avoided in children.

Skin and Soft Tissue Infections

Since preadolescents are usually very active in the outdoors, skin infections are common, especially during the warmer months. Impetigo (streptococcal and staphylococcal) is common, and soft tissue infections following trauma are also seen (Chapter 15).

Of particular note is the almost epidemic occurrence of tinea capitis in preadolescents, especially African-American children. About 80% of these infections are caused by *Trichophyton tonsurans.* Topical antifungal medications are ineffective for tinea capitis, which requires systemic antifungal therapy. Microsize griseofulvin is given orally, 15 to 20 mg/kg/day (maximum, 1 g) once daily, optimally after a meal containing fat. Treatment is usually for 4 to 6 weeks and should be continued 2 weeks beyond clinical resolution.

 KEY POINTS

GRADE-SCHOOLERS AND PREADOLESCENTS

⊃ Children between 6 and 11 years of age are generally healthy but have about four to six self-limited infections per year.

⊃ Sinusitis is prevalent but difficult to diagnose. Clinically important sinusitis is usually of bacterial etiology.
⊃ Acute otitis media is almost a rarity, but diffuse external otitis ("swimmer's ear") is common.
⊃ Diarrhea is usually of viral origin and self-limited. Bloody diarrhea warrants investigation.
⊃ Use of antiperistaltic drugs, especially the opiates, should be avoided in children.

Adolescents

Infections in adolescents and young adults are generally similar to those in preadolescents, but less frequent. Acute respiratory infections (common cold, pharyngitis) account for the majority of them. Gastroenteritis is still a common problem in this age group and, as with younger children, is usually of viral origin. Acne is the major skin infection occurring in this population, although soft tissue infections are also seen. However, special concerns are particular to this age group.

Mononucleosis Syndromes

Infectious mononucleosis caused by the Epstein-Barr virus (EBV) is of special concern during adolescence. Cytomegalovirus (CMV) and occasionally other agents such as *Toxoplasma gondii* can cause a similar clinical picture. Mononucleosis should be suspected when an adolescent is being seen for exudative pharyngitis, lymphadenitis, or a flu-like illness and the rapid streptococcal test (RST) or throat culture for group A streptococci is negative (see Chapter 8).

Sexually Transmitted Disease

Since sexual activity is a prevalent part of some adolescents' behaviors, sexually transmitted diseases are a special concern for any sexually active teenager. With the advent of HIV and acquired immunodeficiency syndrome (AIDS) in the mid-1980s, the possible price for unprotected sexual activity has reached a higher level. About 50% of new HIV infections in the United States now occur in persons between 13 and 24 years of age. Along with the increase in HIV cases in the adolescent population, gonorrhea, chlamydial infection, and syphilis are showing significant increases. During routine health maintenance visits, care must be taken to educate adolescents and preadolescents regarding these risks.

KEY POINTS

ADOLESCENTS

⊃ Infectious mononucleosis should be suspected if an adolescent has exudative pharyngitis, lymphadenitis, or a flulike illness.
⊃ Sexually transmitted diseases, including HIV, are of major concern, and care must be taken to educate adolescents and preadolescents about risk-taking behaviors.

SUGGESTED READING

American Academy of Pediatrics. Committee on Pediatric AIDS and Committee on Adolescents. Adolescents and human immunodeficiency virus infection: the role of the pediatrician in prevention and intervention. Pediatrics 2001; 107: 188-190.

Baraff LJ. Management of fever without source in infants and children. Ann Emerg Med 2000; 36: 602-614.

Baraff LJ, Bass JW, Fleisher GR, et al. Practice guideline for the management of infants and children 0 to 36 months of age with fever without source. Agency for Health Care Policy and Research. Pediatrics 1993; 92: 1-12.

Jaskiewicz JA, McCarthy CA. Evaluation and management of the febrile infant 60 days of age or younger. Pediatr Ann 1993; 22: 477-480, 482-483.

Kuppermann N. Occult bacteremia in young febrile children. Pediatr Clin North Am 1999; 46: 1073-1109.

McCarthy PL, Klig JE, Kennedy WP, et al. Fever without apparent source on clinical examination, lower respiratory infections in children, and enterovirus infections. Curr Opin Pediatr 2000; 12: 77-95.

Peter J, Ray CJ. Infectious mononucleosis. Pediatr Rev 1998; 19: 276-279.

Slater M, Krug SE. Evaluation of the infant with fever without source: an evidence based approach. Emerg Med Clin North Am 1999; 17: 97-126.

Upper Respiratory Tract Infections: The Problem of Judicious Antibiotic Use

About three fourths of antibiotic prescriptions in the ambulatory care setting are written for one of five upper respiratory tract infections: otitis media, the common cold, acute bronchitis, sore throat, and sinusitis. Each year, 25 to 30 million courses of antimicrobials are prescribed for otitis media, 17 million courses for the common cold (or "nonspecific URI"), 16 million courses for acute bronchitis, 13 million courses for sore throat, and 13 million courses for sinusitis. Application of evidence-based principles suggests that about half of these courses of antimicrobial therapy are unnecessary. Children treated with antimicrobial agents are at increased risk of becoming carriers of drug-resistant bacteria, including *S. pneumoniae* (three to six times more likely) and *H. influenzae*. Of greater concern, invasive pneumococcal infection caused by penicillin-resistant strains is strongly associated with recent antibiotic therapy. Studies indicate that children with invasive disease caused by antibiotic-resistant pneumococci were 3.5 to 9.3 times more likely to have received a recent course of oral antibiotics than similar children with invasive infections caused by drug-susceptible pneumococcal strains.

In recent years, drug-nonsusceptible *S. pneumoniae* strains (DNSSP) have increased markedly in frequency (see Chapter 1). These strains exhibit reduced susceptibility not only to penicillin G but also to cefotaxime, ceftriaxone, and other antimicrobials. Nonsusceptible strains most often show intermediate resistance to penicillin G, with a minimum inhibitory concentration (MIC) of 0.1 to 1 μg/mL. However, highly resistant strains (MIC ≥ 2 μg/mL) are also becoming more common. In many geographic areas, 40% to 50% of isolates obtained from normally sterile body sites in children exhibit reduced susceptibility to penicillin G. About 50% of isolates with reduced susceptibility to penicillin G also exhibit reduced susceptibility to cefotaxime or ceftriaxone. The problem extends to other commonly used antibiotics as well. According to recent data compiled by the CDC, resistance to macrolides occurs in 31% of pneumococcal strains with intermediate resistance to penicillin G and in 60% of pneumococcal strains with high-level resistance to penicillin G. Similarly, resistance to trimethoprim-sulfamethoxazole (TMP/SMX) occurs in 49% of pneumococcal strains with intermediate resistance to penicillin G and in 91% of pneumococcal strains with high-level resistance to penicillin G. In contrast to pneumococcal resistance to β-lactam antibiotics, which can be overcome by raising the antibiotic concentration to a high level, pneumococcal resistance to macrolides and TMP/SMX tends to be absolute. Fluoroquinolone antibiotics are now commonly used to treat drug-resistant pneumococcal infections in adults but are contraindicated in children because of their potential effects on cartilage. For all of these reasons the progressive emergence of DNSSP threatens to limit the therapeutic options for common childhood infections.

The importance of *S. pneumoniae* as a cause of invasive infection cannot be overemphasized. According to the Active Bacterial Surveillance System maintained by the CDC, *S. pneumoniae* accounts each year for 23.8 cases of invasive disease per 100,000 population, far exceeding the rates for group B streptococci (6.2 per 100,000), group A streptococci (3.6 per 100,000) and *Neisseria meningitidis* (1.3 per 100,000). Children 12 months of age have a six-fold increased risk for invasive pneumococcal disease, and persons with AIDS have a 30-fold increased risk. Each year, *S. pneumoniae* causes 7 million cases of acute otitis media, 50,000 cases of bacteremia, 100,000 to 135,000 cases of pneumonia requiring hospitalization, and 3000 cases of meningitis. Risk factors for pneumococcal infection include young age, acquisition of new serotypes, exposure to secondhand cigarette smoke, exposure to sibling younger than school age, attendance at a child care center, history of frequent otitis media, and recent antibiotic exposure. Of these, the latter three are the most important and the latter two have also been identified as risk factors for carriage of multidrug-resistant *S. pneumoniae*. Risk factors for invasive pneumococcal disease include history of recurrent otitis media (up to nine-fold increase) and attendance in a child care center (up to 36-fold increase). Infants typically acquire their first pneumococcal serotype by age 6 months and sometimes carry up to four serotypes simultaneously. Pneumococcal acquisition occurs most often during the winter months, and 15% of acquisitions result in clinical disease. Nearly 30% of infants have a pneumococcal infection by 2 years of age.

During the first 2 years of life, children receive antibiotics on an average of 45 to 50 days each year. Antibiotic use, whether or not medically justified, contributes to the development of resistant bacteria, including the common respiratory pathogens of childhood (*S. pneumoniae*, *H. influenzae*, and *Moraxella catarrhalis*). Failures of antimicrobial therapy are more common in patients infected with drug-resistant bacteria. In response to this major societal issue, guidelines have been developed and adopted by the AAP, the American Academy of Family Physicians, and the CDC (Table 4-3). Specific issues are discussed in the following section.

Caretaker Expectations

Parents often make requests for unnecessary antibiotics, and telling them the child "has a virus" fails to reassure them. A recent study indicated that 84% of parents would accept a physician's decision not to prescribe antibiotics for a febrile illness if the physician took the time to explain why he or she was not prescribing them. The following approach can be used when parents insist on antibiotics for a viral illness:

TABLE 4-3
Key Principles of Judicious Antibiotic Use in Pediatric Upper Respiratory Infections

Syndrome	Principle
Serous otitis media with effusion	Serous otitis media with effusion should be distinguished from acute otitis media. Antibiotics are not indicated for initial treatment of serous otitis media. Persistent effusion after acute otitis media is to be expected and does not require treatment.
Group A streptococcal pharyngitis	Diagnosis of group A streptococcal pharyngitis should be based on a laboratory test in conjunction with clinical and epidemiologic findings. Antibiotic treatment should not be given without documentation of group A streptococci or other bacterial pathogens.
Common cold	Antibiotics should not be given for the common cold. Purulent rhinitis frequently accompanies the common cold and is not a separate indication for antibiotic treatment.
Suspected sinusitis	Antibiotic treatment in suspected sinusitis should be limited to children with prolonged nonspecific upper respiratory signs and symptoms (>10 days) or more severe upper respiratory tract findings (e.g., fever ≥102° F [39° C], facial swelling, or facial pain).
Acute cough or bronchitis	Children who have an illness characterized by acute cough or bronchitis and do not have chronic lung disease warrant antibiotic therapy only for certain specific indications (e.g., pertussis, *Mycoplasma pneumoniae* infection).

(1) deal with their anxieties and tell them what their child does not have; (2) tell the parents what their child does have; (3) tell the parents what to expect, that is, the natural history based on your diagnosis; (4) explain to the parents how to treat the illness, and if the child goes to child care, tell them when the child can go back; (5) reassure the parents that your door is always open and under what conditions they should bring their child back.

 KEY POINTS

UPPER RESPIRATORY TRACT INFECTIONS: THE PROBLEM OF JUDICIOUS ANTIBIOTIC USE

⊃ About 75% of courses of antimicrobials prescribed in ambulatory settings are for one of five URIs: otitis media, the common cold, acute bronchitis, sore throat, and sinusitis. About one half of antibiotic prescribing for URI is inappropriate according to evidence-based guidelines.
⊃ DNSSP strains have increased dramatically in recent years, becoming a major public health issue. DNSSP strains are commonly resistant to macrolides and TMP/SMX as well, which limits the therapeutic options in children (especially since fluoroquinolones and tetracyclines are contraindicated during childhood). Antimicrobial therapy in children predisposes them to colonization by DNSSP and other drug-resistant bacteria.
⊃ Conservative use of antimicrobial agents combined with immunization offers the best chance to limit the further spread of drug-resistant childhood pathogens. When antibiotics are not indicated, adequate reassurance of parents often requires a thorough explanation.

SUGGESTED READING
Bauchner H, Pelton SI, Klein JO. Patients, physicians and antibiotic use. Pediatrics 1999; 103: 395-401.
Dowell SF, ed. Centers for Disease Control and Prevention and the American Academy of Pediatrics. Principles of judicious use of antimicrobial agents for pediatric upper respiratory tract infections. Pediatrics 1998; 101 (Suppl): 161-184.
Henderson M, Rubin E. Misuse of antimicrobials in children with asthma and bronchiolitis: a review. Pediatr Infect Dis J 2001; 20: 214-215.
Marcy SM. When as patient insists on antibiotics for a virus. Am Fam Physician 1999; 59: 687-688.

Upper Respiratory Tract Infections: Diagnosis and Treatment

This section addresses specific issues pertaining to the five most common upper respiratory tract infections affecting children (for further discussion of these syndromes, see Chapter 10).

The Common Cold (Viral Rhinosinusitis)

Colds, including mucopurulent rhinitis, are almost always caused by viral infections. Antibiotic therapy is unnecessary and potentially harmful. Inappropriate antibiotic use increases the risk of colonization with resistant organisms, and any subsequent invasive infection may be unresponsive to standard antibiotic treatment. The evidence accumulated to date suggests that antibiotics are not particularly effective in preventing bacterial complications of viral infections. Mucopurulent rhinitis, among the most common symptoms of the cold, is not an indication for antimicrobial treatment, having no more effect than placebo.

Acute Otitis Media

Diagnosis of acute otitis media is based on the presence of middle ear effusion, loss of landmarks, or a bulging tympanic membrane with evidence of inflammation. Acute otitis media is often self-limited. Antibiotics, compared with placebo, improve the recovery rate by 14%, measured as clinical improvement and bacterial eradication. Bacteriologic studies indicate the presence of *S. pneumoniae* in 40% of cases, *H. influenzae* in 25%, and *M. catarrhalis* in 10%, with cultures being sterile in 25% of cases. The frequency of spontaneous resolution varies according to the microorganism, with 79% for *M. catarrhalis,* 48% for nontypeable *H. influenzae,* but only 19% for *S. pneumoniae* and *S. pyogenes.* A standard 10-day course of antibiotics is therefore recommended for children <2 years of age and for older children with underlying medical conditions, including craniofacial abnormalities, chronic or recurrent otitis media, or perforation of the tympanic membrane. A shortened course of antibiotics may be appropriate for the majority of older children with acute otitis media. Children up to 2 years of age are at increased risk for treatment failure, even with conventional dosages.

Treatment recommendations for initial therapy include high-dose amoxicillin (80 to 90 mg/kg/day) (Table 4-4). These recommendations are based on the observation that no currently available oral antibiotic provides better activity against DNSSP strains. High-dose amoxicillin provides drug concentrations in the middle ear that achieve reasonably high cure rates against pneumococcal strains with reduced susceptibility to penicillin G. Patients who are not improved 3 to 5 days after initial therapy and who are therefore defined as treatment failures require second-line drugs active against DNSSP and also against β-lactamase–producing strains of *H. influenzae* and *M. catarrhalis.* Such agents include high-dose oral amoxicillin-clavulanate (80 to 90 mg/kg/day of the amoxicillin component with the 7:1 formulation to reduce incidence of diarrhea), oral cefuroxime axetil, or intramuscular ceftriaxone (3 consecutive days). Other cephalosporins such as cefpodoxime or cefdinir might be reasonable alternatives, but prospective studies eval-

uating these drugs as second-line therapy for acute otitis media in children are lacking at present. The macrolides, TMP/SMX, and erythromycin-sulfisoxazole are not listed in Table 4-4 because of poor efficacy against DNSSP. Erythromycin-sulfisoxazole, clarithromycin, and azithromycin are appropriate alternatives for penicillin-allergic patients. Myringotomy should be considered for severe cases or recurrent treatment failure. For DNSSP strains resistant to many antibiotics, the use of clindamycin, rifampin, or other agents in consultation with an infectious disease consultant should be considered. Other potential second-line regimens could be considered on the basis of in vitro and pharmacodynamic data, even though definitive studies are unavailable; these include high-dose amoxicillin plus a highly β-lactamase–stable drug such as cefixime.

Antibiotic prophylaxis should be reserved for patients with well-defined, distinct episodes of recurrent acute otitis media. The benefit of prophylactic treatment tended to be greater when sulfisoxazole was used for this purpose, when treatment was continued for <6 months, or when the population being studied had a high rate of recurrence. Cephalosporins have not been shown to be effective for prophylaxis. Amoxicillin is more likely than sulfisoxazole to promote colonization with DNSSP and β-lactamase–producing bacterial strains. Other preventive measures found to be effective in reducing the burden of recurrent acute otitis media include encouraging breast-feeding, eliminating smoking in the home, encouraging sleep in the supine position, discouraging pacifier use, reducing child care attendance (and when possible parents should choose small-group programs), giving influenza vaccine (which has been shown to reduce the incidence of acute otitis media in children, especially those in child care centers), and giving the current 23-valent pneumococcal vaccine to children >2 years of age who are still having problems with acute otitis media. A pneumococcal conjugate vaccine is

TABLE 4-4

Management of Acute Otitis Media: Recommendations from the Drug-Resistant *Streptococcus pneumoniae* Therapeutic Working Group

Antibiotics in prior month?	Day 0	Clinical treatment failure by day 3	Clinical treatment failure by day 10 to 28
No	Amoxicillin, high-dose amoxicillin*	High-dose amoxicillin-clavulanate,† cefuroxime axetil, ceftriaxone‡	Same as day 3
Yes	High-dose amoxicillin, high-dose amoxicillin-clavulanate,† cefuroxime axetil	Ceftriaxone, clindamycin,§ tympanocentesis	High-dose amoxicillin-clavulanate, cefuroxime axetil, ceftriaxone, tympanocentesis

Modified from Dowel SF, Butler J, Giebing FS, et al. Acute otitis media: management and surveillance in an era of pneumococcal resistance—a report from the Drug-Resistant *Streptococcus pneumoniae* Therapeutic Working Group. Pediatr Infect Dis J 1999; 18: 1-9.
*High-dose amoxicillin: 80 to 90 mg/kg/day in divided doses q12h.
†High-dose amoxicillin-clavulanate: same high dose of amoxicillin with 6.4 mg/kg/day of clavulanate (i.e., amoxicillin 40 to 45 mg/kg/day *plus* amoxicillin-clavulanate, 40 to 45 mg/kg/day).
‡IM ceftriaxone should be given as three 50 mg/kg doses on consecutive days.
§Clindamycin is not effective against *Haemophilus influenzae* or *Moraxella catarrhalis*. A second drug such as a sulfonamide or a β-lactamase–stable cephalosporin should be added.

now available for children 6 weeks of age or older. A three-dose primary series of the pneumococcal conjugate vaccine reduces the incidence of invasive pneumococcal disease by 97%, but the impact on acute otitis media is less dramatic. Studies thus far indicate that the pneumococcal conjugate vaccine reduces the overall incidence of acute otitis media by about 7%, reduces the number of patients with frequent recurrences by 10% to 21%, and reduces the need for tympanostomy tube replacements by 20%. Capsular transformation of drug-resistant serotypes in vivo may have major implications for these new vaccines. In some patients, DNSSP persists even when the colonizing or infecting *S. pneumoniae* is of a new serotype.

Acute Sinusitis

Acute bacterial sinusitis complicates 0.5% to 5% of cases of viral URI. In 1992 an estimated 26 million cases of URI occurred in the United States, which would therefore be predicted to have caused 0.13 to 1.3 million cases of acute bacterial sinusitis. However, 13 million antibiotic prescriptions were written for acute sinusitis during 1992, suggesting that overdiagnosis and overtreatment of acute bacterial sinusitis are rampant. Moreover, about 60% of episodes of acute bacterial sinusitis resolve or improve spontaneously without antimicrobial therapy. The need for strict criteria for diagnosis and treatment is obvious.

Clinical criteria for the diagnosis of acute bacterial sinusitis in children include (1) 10 to 14 days of daytime cough and nasal discharge *without improvement*, or (2) fever ≥102° F (39° C) *and* purulent rhinorrhea ≥3 to 4 days. About 80% of children with either of these criteria have abnormal maxillary sinuses on x-ray examination. About 70% of children with clinical criteria for sinusitis and abnormalities on x-ray examination have positive cultures for bacteria on aspirates obtained by puncture of the maxillary sinus. These data suggest, then, that about 56% of children who meet the clinical criteria for acute bacterial sinusitis actually have the disease as defined by positive cultures. When the disease is defined on the basis of prolonged symptoms (symptoms lasting 10 to 30 days), *S. pneumoniae* is isolated in about 30% of cases, *H. influenzae* in 20%, and *M. catarrhalis* in 20%, and the remaining 30% of cultures are sterile.

Up to 20% of children with uncomplicated viral URI have rhinorrhea or cough on day 10, but at that point the signs and symptoms are improving. Treatment for acute bacterial sinusitis is not recommended for such patients. Empiric treatment for acute bacterial sinusitis is reserved for patients who meet either of the two clinical criteria stated previously. The oral antibiotic regimens recommended for the treatment of acute otitis media (Table 4-4) are also recommended for acute bacterial sinusitis, since the bacteriology is essentially the same. The optimum duration of antimicrobial therapy for children with acute bacterial sinusitis has received little systematic study. Few children have been studied in shortened-course trials. Most children treated for acute bacterial sinusitis show some improvement within 3 to 4 days, but about one third of children improve slowly and become symptom free only after 8 to 10 days of therapy. Relapse is relatively common. Therefore most authorities advise treatment for 7 days beyond resolution of signs and symptoms of acute sinusitis, which typically results in 10 to 18 days of total therapy.

Acute Pharyngitis

Clinical findings cannot reliably differentiate viral pharyngitis from pharyngitis caused by group A β-hemolytic streptococci (*S. pyogenes;* GABHS). Only about 12% of children with fever and exudative pharyngitis have GABHS by culture. Documentation of GABHS before treatment is therefore strongly recommended (see Chapter 10). A 10-day course of penicillin is recommended for GABHS pharyngitis owing to its low cost, narrow spectrum of activity, and proven efficacy. Preliminary data suggest that oral amoxicillin given as a single daily dose for 10 days is as effective as oral penicillin V given three times daily for 10 days. Intramuscular benzathine penicillin G is also appropriate therapy. Patients allergic to penicillin should be given oral erythromycin for 10 days. Other macrolides, namely clarithromycin for 10 days or azithromycin for 5 days, are also effective. A 10-day course of a first-generation (narrow-spectrum) oral cephalosporin is another acceptable alternative, especially in persons allergic to penicillin (but not immediate, anaphylactic-type hypersensitivity, since cross-reactivity is as high as 15%). To date, resistance of *S. pyogenes* to β-lactam antibiotics has not been identified. Resistance of *S. pyogenes* to macrolides has been observed but is uncommon in most areas of the United States. Children with recurrence of *S. pyogenes* pharyngitis shortly after completing a recommended 10-day course of treatment can be retreated with that antibiotic, given an alternative oral drug, or given an intramuscular dose of benzathine penicillin G. Alternative drugs include a cephalosporin, amoxicillin-calvulanate, clindamycin, erythromycin, or another macrolide.

Cough Illness and Bronchitis

Nonspecific cough illness or bronchitis seldom warrants antimicrobial therapy in children, regardless of the duration of symptoms or the presence of fever. In nine clinical trials, antibiotics did not prevent or decrease the severity of bacterial complications after viral respiratory tract infections. Cough illness or bronchitis does not include the specific clinical diagnosis of pneumonia, bronchiolitis, and asthma. In certain situations antibiotics may be appropriate for cough lasting more than 10 to 14 days. These situations include the presence of sinusitis or the presence of infection by *Mycoplasma pneumoniae* or *Bordetella pertussis* as determined by appropriate diagnostic studies. *M. pneumoniae* can cause bronchitis or pneumonia and prolonged cough, usually in children >5 years of age. Treatment consists of a macrolide or, in children 8 years of age or older, a tetracycline. Children with 4 to 8 weeks of cough merit investigation for a specific diagnosis including reactive airway disease, tuberculosis, foreign body aspiration, pertussis, cystic fibrosis or sinusitis. Children with underlying chronic pulmonary disease other than asthma may benefit from antibiotic treatment of acute exacerbations (Chapter 10).

 KEY POINTS

UPPER RESPIRATORY TRACT INFECTIONS: DIAGNOSIS AND TREATMENT

⊃ The common cold, including mucopurulent rhinitis, should not be treated with antibiotics.

○ Acute otitis media, diagnosed on the basis of a middle ear effusion with loss of anatomic landmarks and/or bulging of the tympanic membrane with evidence of inflammation, should be treated with antibiotics.

○ Pneumococcal conjugate vaccine has, thus far, shown a modest reduction in the frequency and severity of acute otitis media.

○ Acute bacterial sinusitis should be treated with antibiotics only if the clinical criteria are met: (1) 10 to 14 days of daytime cough and nasal discharge *without improvement* or fever ≥102° F (39° C) *and* purulent rhinorrhea lasting more than 3 to 4 days.

○ Streptococcal pharyngitis should be treated with antibiotics when the diagnosis has been confirmed by laboratory studies (rapid streptococcal antigen test or culture).

○ Nonspecific cough illness or bronchitis in children rarely warrants antibiotic therapy.

SUGGESTED READING

Bluestone CD, Klein JO, eds. Otitis Media in Infants and Children. 3rd ed. Philadelphia: W.B. Saunders Company; 2000.

Brooks I, Gooch WM, Jenkins SG, et al. Medical management of acute bacterial sinusitis: recommendations of a clinical advisory committee on pediatric and adult sinusitis. Ann Otol Rhinol Laryngol 2000; 182 (Suppl 2000—May): 2-20.

Dowell SF, Butler JC, Giebink GS, et al. Acute otitis media: management and surveillance in an era of pneumococcal resistance—a report from the Drug-resistant *Streptococcus pneumoniae* Therapeutic Working Group. Pediatr Infect Dis J 1999; 18: 1-9.

Parsons DS, ed. Pediatric sinusitis. Otolaryngol Clin North Am 1996; 29: 1-224.

Acute Infectious Diarrhea (see also Chapter 12)

About 5% of pediatric office visits are for gastrointestinal disorders, which includes 5 million cases of diarrhea each year in the United States. About 20% of these episodes prompt telephone consultations. In the United States each year about 220,000 children <5 years of age are hospitalized with diarrhea (about 10% of all hospitalizations in this age group) and an estimated 300 to 400 deaths are caused by diarrhea in children <1 year of age. Diarrhea of <2 weeks' duration is called *acute,* diarrhea of >2 weeks' duration is called *persistent,* and persistent diarrhea of >3 weeks' duration is called *chronic.* These adjectives are not helpful at the onset of diarrhea but may point to one or another etiology as the illness evolves. Acute diarrhea is usually infectious, is usually caused by a virus or a bacterial pathogen, and usually resolves within 7 days. In infants increased stool frequency does not necessarily indicate diarrhea. Formula-fed infants have up to seven stools per day, and breast-fed infants may have up to 12 stools per day. Dietary indiscretions, especially overfeeding and large fruit juice intake that includes sorbitol, fructose, and sucrose, may cause diarrhea. In infants diarrhea is defined by stools >10 g/kg/day. In children 4 years of age or older, diarrhea is defined by stools >200 g/day. In practice, an increase in both frequency and volume (or weight) of stools is observed.

Various pathogens cause diarrhea that is predominantly inflammatory or noninflammatory (see Chapter 12). Inflammatory diarrhea is by far the more serious, although noninflammatory diarrhea can be life threatening in infants because of its propensity to cause severe dehydration.

The classic clinical patterns of inflammatory versus secretory diarrhea are far from specific in distinguishing the etiology because of the overlap in disease manifestations. The epidemiology of a case may be more important in predicting its cause. Most episodes of diarrhea are of brief duration and respond to appropriate fluid and feeding therapy. Therefore a precise diagnosis is usually unimportant. However, bloody diarrhea indicating colitis should always prompt an attempt to establish the etiology (Figure 4-4). Clinical manifestations of diarrhea vary according to the etiology.

Shiga toxin–producing *E. coli* (STEC, also known as enterohemorrhagic *E. coli*) has become extremely important in pediatric practice, not because of its frequency but rather because of the severity of the complications. Of most concern is the hemolytic-uremic syndrome, now the most common cause of acute renal failure in children in the United States. Milder cases of hemolytic-uremic syndrome (*forme fruste*) occur, and other serious complications include rectal prolapse, rare cases of intestinal perforation, colonic necrosis, sepsis, and intussusception. STEC infection often begins as nonbloody diarrhea that later usually becomes bloody and is accompanied by severe abdominal pain. Fever, usually low grade, is present in less than one third of cases. STEC typically occurs in children <5 years of age. In cases of bloody diarrhea the laboratory should be directed to culture the stool specifically for *E. coli* O157:H7. Stool should be saved for possible testing for the presence of Shiga toxin as well, since the organism may not be of the O157:H7 serotype (see Chapter 12). *Because of the strong association of antibiotic therapy with hemolytic-uremic syndrome in children with STEC, antibiotics should not be given to most children with bloody diarrhea until STEC has been excluded.* Also, antimotility agents increase the risk for progression from hemorrhagic colitis to hemolytic-uremic

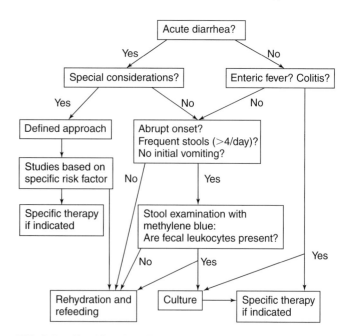

FIG. 4-4 Algorithm for diagnostic evaluation of acute diarrhea. (Modified from Radetsky M. Laboratory evaluation of acute diarrhea. Pediatr Infect Dis J 1986; 5: 230-238.)

syndrome, and their use should be avoided. Children infected with STEC should be kept out of child care until stool samples are culture negative. Up to 70% of family members of children with STEC and hemolytic-uremic syndrome have been found to have positive cultures, providing further evidence of the highly infectious nature of this agent.

Campylobacter species, notably *C. jejuni,* are the most common agents of bacterial diarrhea in the United States (about 2.1 million to 2.4 million cases each year) and worldwide. The diarrhea is watery in about two thirds of cases and bloody in about one third of cases. Complications include Guillain-Barré syndrome (about 1 in 1000 to 2000 cases), reactive arthritis, and erythema nodosum. Peaks of infection occur during the first year of life and in young adults. *Campylobacter* can cause crampy right lower quadrant abdominal pain resembling that of acute appendicitis. Erythromycin or azithromycin, if given early during the infection, shortens the duration of illness and prevents relapse. Treatment usually eradicates the organism from the stool within 2 to 3 days. If antimicrobial therapy is given for gastroenteritis, the recommended duration is 5 to 7 days.

Salmonella species are the most common cause of bacterial diarrhea in children <5 years of age, with a peak incidence within the first 6 months of life. Because therapy does not shorten the duration of disease, *antimicrobial therapy usually is not indicated* for patients with noninvasive (uncomplicated) gastroenteritis caused by nontyphoidal *Salmonella* species. Antimicrobial therapy (ampicillin, amoxicillin, TMP/SMX, cefotaxime, or ceftriaxone for susceptible strains) is recommended for *Salmonella* gastroenteritis with increased risk of invasive disease; such patients include infants <3 months of age and patients with malignant neoplasms, hemoglobinopathies, HIV infection, or other immunosuppressive illnesses or therapy; chronic gastrointestinal disease; or severe colitis. The duration of therapy in persons with normal host defenses is 5 to 7 days. Intravenous antibiotics and more prolonged therapy are recommended for invasive disease, including bacteremia. Resistance of *Salmonella* species to fluoroquinolones and third-generation cephalosporins is now being reported.

Shigella species are the classic cause of bacillary dysentery, manifested as high fever, headache, leukopenia, toxicity, and profuse watery diarrhea often followed by crampy abdominal pain, tenesmus, and bloody stools with mucus and polymorphonuclear leukocytes. Shigellosis occurs mainly between the ages of 6 months and 10 years, is highly infectious, and is the most common cause of outbreaks of bacterial diarrhea in child care centers. Complications include seizures (12% to 45% of patients), hallucinations, Ekiri syndrome (fulminant acute toxic encephalopathy), hemolytic-uremic syndrome (*Shigella dysenteriae* type 1), and rectal prolapse. Antimicrobial therapy (ampicillin, TMP/SMX, cefixime, ceftriaxone, cefotaxime, and azithromycin) is effective, and administration for 5 days is recommended. The oral route of therapy is acceptable except for seriously ill patients. If susceptibility is unknown, either parenteral ceftriaxone (children and adults) or a fluoroquinolone (adults) should be given. Infected children should be kept out of child care until stool samples are culture negative.

Yersinia species, more common in developed colder countries than in the United States, cause diarrhea most often in children <5 years of age. The diarrhea is bloody in about

10% of cases and is accompanied by fever and headache and occasionally by sore throat or frank pharyngitis. In addition to enterocolitis, *Yersinia* species can cause mesenteric lymphadenitis (pseudoappendicitis syndrome; see Chapter 12), reactive arthritis, septicemia (especially in patients with iron overload), and an unusual presentation that mimics Kawasaki disease. The clinical benefit of antibiotic therapy for enterocolitis or mesenteric lymphadenitis caused by *Yersinia* species has not been firmly established.

Aeromonas species, ubiquitous in the surface waters of the United States, including saltwater and chlorinated drinking water, have been associated with diarrhea in children <3 years of age. TMP/SMX has been used to prevent complications in patients with chronic diarrhea or in persons who are immunocompromised.

Viruses are the major cause of acute diarrhea in children. Diarrhea is typically watery and often accompanied by nausea and vomiting. Rotaviruses, the most important cause of dehydrating diarrhea worldwide, are common causes of diarrhea in children with a peak incidence between 3 and 15 months. In children <2 years of age, rotaviruses cause up to 70% of cases of diarrhea requiring admission to the hospital for correction of dehydration. Rotaviruses often cause outbreaks of diarrhea, especially in child care centers. The incidence is increased during the winter months. Diarrhea is usually self-limited, lasting 2 to 8 days. Rotavirus detection in stool by antigen assay is helpful, with the enzyme immunoassay (EIA) being more sensitive late in the course of the illness. False-positive and nonspecific test results can occur in neonates and in persons with underlying intestinal illness. Norwalk virus (a calicivirus) is the major cause of large epidemics of diarrhea, which is usually but not always accompanied by vomiting. Norwalk virus generally affects older children and exhibits no seasonal variation. Enteric adenoviruses, occurring mainly during the summer months, usually affect children <2 years of age and cause symptoms that last up to 14 days. Caliciviruses other than Norwalk virus usually affect children 3 months to 6 years of age, causing symptoms that last for 2 to 8 days.

Management Approach to Acute Infectious Diarrhea

Antimicrobials are appropriate for selected cases of acute diarrhea. Antibiotics are useful for treatment of colitis (after Shiga toxin–producing *E. coli* has been excluded) and enteric fever (e.g., typhoid fever). Antibiotics are also useful to reduce shedding of bacteria in persons who might be the source of outbreaks, such as diapered children in child care centers, institutionalized patients, and foodhandlers. With these principles in mind, it is possible to formulate a reasoned approach to the office evaluation of acute diarrhea, including the need for stool culture. A specific constellation of symptoms, combined with evaluation of stool for polymorphonuclear neutrophils (PMNs) using methylene blue, is highly useful for predicting which patients are likely to have bacterial diarrhea (Figure 4-4).

 KEY POINTS

STEPWISE EVALUATION OF THE PATIENT WITH DIARRHEA
⊃ Clinical questions: Abrupt onset? Frequent stools (more than four per day)? Absence of vomiting before onset of diarrhea?

➲ Interpretation: "Yes" to all three of the above questions suggests bacterial diarrhea (sensitivity, 86%; specificity, 60%; positive predictive value, 27%; negative predictive value, 96%). The probability of a positive stool culture for a bacterial pathogen is 27% if the answer is "yes" to all three questions, versus 4% if the answer is "no" to any of the three questions.

➲ Laboratory question: Does the stool specimen contain fecal leukocytes (>5 PMNs per high-power field [HPF] when a drop of stool with methylene blue added is examined microscopically)?

➲ Interpretation: When the answer is "yes" to all three clinical questions *and* fecal leukocytes are present, the likelihood of bacterial diarrhea is high (sensitivity, 74%; specificity, 94%; positive predictive value, 69%; negative predictive value, 95%; accuracy, 91%).

➲ When facilities are not available for microscopic examination of stool for PMNs using methylene blue, the stool should be tested for occult blood. A positive test for occult blood correlates with fecal PMNs in up to 90% of cases.

When historical information places the patient into one or another "special consideration" category (Figure 4-4), the appropriate diagnostic approach for such a patient should be pursued. For example, a patient who is immunocompromised should be evaluated for *Cryptosporidium;* a patient who has recently received antibiotics should be evaluated for *Clostridium difficile;* a person with a history of recent travel should be evaluated for *Entamoeba histolytica, Escherichia coli, Vibrio cholerae,* and *Giardia lamblia;* a person in child care or an institutional center should be evaluated for *G. lamblia* and *Cryptosporidium;* and a person who seems to be part of an outbreak should be evaluated for one of the agents of food poisoning (see Chapter 12). If none of the "special consideration" categories is applicable, the child should be screened for the two high-risk clinical syndromes: (1) a stool culture should be obtained when the child is febrile with watery, bloody stools, since the likelihood of finding a bacterial pathogen is high; and (2) if all three of the screening symptoms are present, even if the symptoms of dysentery are absent, a methylene blue examination of stool should be performed, and if it is positive for PMNs, a stool culture should follow. If the child belongs to neither high-risk group, further workup is of low yield. Rehydration with continued observation becomes the appropriate course.

Outpatient therapy for acute diarrhea includes supportive treatment, antibiotics for certain infections, and nonspecific antidiarrheal treatments. Oral rehydration therapy (ORT) is the preferred treatment for fluid and electrolyte losses caused by diarrhea in children who have *mild to moderate dehydration* (ORT carbohydrate to sodium ratio should not exceed 2:1). Intestinal transport of glucose and sodium is coupled physiologically, with this mechanism remaining intact during episodes of acute diarrhea, enabling ORT. The World Health Organization oral rehydration solution is available in packets (Jianas Brothers Packaging Company, 2533 SW Blvd., Kansas City, MO 64108) or can be prepared at home as follows: 3/4 teaspoon salt, 1 teaspoon baking soda, 4 tablespoons sugar, 1 cup orange juice, and 1 liter water. ORT with standard glucose electrolyte solutions containing 45 to 90 mEq/L of

sodium should be given for dehydration *over 4 hours* initiated with 5-ml aliquots every 1 to 2 minutes: 50 mL/kg for mild dehydration and 100 mL/kg for moderate dehydration over 4 hours. Also, replacement of stool losses, at 10 mL/kg for each stool, and emesis requires the addition of appropriate amounts of solution to the total. Children who have diarrhea without dehydration should continue to be fed age-appropriate diets (breast milk or formula; for an older infant, foods high in simple sugars, sweetened tea, juices, soft drinks, and fatty foods should be avoided, and complex carbohydrates—rice, wheat, potatoes, bread, cereals—and lean meats, including chicken, yogurt, fruits, and vegetables should be encouraged). If dehydration is present, feeding should be restarted as soon as rehydration has been accomplished. For diarrhea present >3 days, reducing substance testing may be considered; if greater than 1%, lactose-free formula or oral rehydration solution for 24 hours may be considered. *Generally, pharmacologic agents should not be used to treat acute diarrhea and antimotility agents should never be used in acute infectious colitis.* Most children with acute enteritis should not receive antibiotics until *E. coli* O157:H7 infection has been ruled out.

Close monitoring and reassessment of hydration are required. Indications for admission to the hospital include bacteremia, metastatic focus of infection with bacterial diarrhea, a toxic clinical appearance, electrolyte abnormalities, inability of the family to follow ORT guidelines, intractable vomiting, inability to drink, ileus, alteration in consciousness, and severe dehydration, including circulatory insufficiency (10% to 15% dehydration). Patients in whom STEC is suspected should be hospitalized with enteric precautions and observed for onset of hemolytic-uremic syndrome. Any abnormal laboratory tests suggesting hemolytic-uremic syndrome should prompt consultation with a nephrologist.

 KEY POINTS

ACUTE INFECTIOUS DIARRHEA

➲ Acute infectious diarrhea is a common problem in office practice and accounts for about 10% of hospitalizations in children <5 years of age.

➲ When children have diarrhea, the following questions should be asked: Was the onset abrupt? Are the stools frequent (more than four per day)? Was vomiting absent before onset of diarrhea? "Yes" answers to all three questions suggest bacterial diarrhea rather than diarrhea of viral origin.

➲ Combining the above clinical questions with microscopic examination of stool for PMNs using methylene blue increases the ability to predict which children have bacterial diarrhea.

➲ Children with bloody diarrhea should be evaluated for Shiga toxin–producing strains of *E. coli* (STEC, also known as enterohemorrhagic *E. coli*).

➲ Antibiotics should not be prescribed for most children with diarrhea until STEC has been excluded, since antibiotic therapy now seems to be a major risk factor for hemolytic-uremic syndrome.

➲ Antimotility agents should not be given to children who might have acute infectious colitis.

➲ ORT is the mainstay of treatment of acute infectious diarrhea in children.

SUGGESTED READING

DeWitt TG, Humphrey KF, McCarthy P. Clinical predictors of acute bacterial diarrhea in young children. Pediatrics 1985; 76: 551-556.

Northrup RS, Flanigan TP. Gastroenteritis. Pediatr Rev 1994; 15: 461-472.

Pickering LK, ed. Diarrheal disease. Semin Pediatr Infect Dis 1994; 5: 1-250.

Provisional Committee on Quality Improvement, Subcommittee on Acute Gastroenteritis. Practice parameter: the management of acute gastroenteritis in young children. Pediatrics 1996; 97: 424-435.

Radetsky M. Laboratory evaluation of acute diarrhea. Pediatr Infect Dis 1986; 5: 230-238.

Wong CS, Jelacic S, Habeeb RL, et al. The risk of hemolytic uremic syndrome after antibiotic treatment of *Escherichia coli* O157:H7 infections. N Engl J Med 2000; 342: 1930-1936.

Bone and Joint Infections (see also Chapter 15)

Bone and joint infections are uncommon in children, but serious consequences make rapid recognition and treatment critical to optimal outcome.

Osteomyelitis

Osteomyelitis in children is usually of hematogenous origin, affects the metaphysis of tubular bones, and is typically caused by *S. aureus* (90% of cases). Septic arthritis of the adjacent joint is sometimes present. Clinical manifestations usually include abrupt onset of bone or joint pain with fever, local "point tenderness," and increased heat, although not all of these signs are necessarily present. The child may refuse to bear weight on or move the involved extremity ("pseudoparalysis in an infant"). Focal tenderness is greater than local findings would suggest, although as the infection progresses, swelling, warmth, and erythema of the overlying skin may be noted. An infant with osteomyelitis may have a septic appearance. Tuberculosis and fungal infection are more insidious.

Differential diagnosis includes cellulitis or pyomyositis; septic arthritis; malignancy; trauma, including periostitis or subperiosteal hematoma in child abuse; sickle cell vasoocclusive crisis with bone infarction; bone cyst; and congenital syphilis. Cellulitis usually differs from osteomyelitis in that the soft tissue findings are greater than the disability, tenderness is greater than pain and may be significantly greater than the soft tissue findings would suggest, tenderness is diffuse rather than localized over the metaphysis, and a skin break may be present. Septic arthritis usually differs from osteomyelitis in that the joint is immobile (rather than having some mobility), the maximal findings are at the joint rather than over the metaphysis, and findings are present on both sides of the joint rather than only over one joint-to-metaphysis interface. Malignancy usually differs from osteomyelitis in that the onset is insidious or subacute and the tenderness and swelling tend to be diffuse rather than focal. Also, malignancy tends to affect bones at random sites, without special predilection for the metaphysis.

Diagnostic studies reveal an elevated ESR in 90% of cases (mean 40 to 60 mm/hr with normalization in about 3 weeks after peaking 3 to 5 days after initiation of therapy). The CRP level is elevated in 98% of cases (mean 8.3 mg/L with normalization in about 1 week after peaking on day 2 after initiation of therapy). Peripheral WBC and platelet counts may be elevated or normal. A specific bacterial etiology is confirmed in 50% to 80% of cases when multiple specimens, such as blood cultures (positive in more than one half of patients), bone aspirates, and bone biopsy specimens obtained at the time of decompression, are obtained. Imaging studies should include conventional radiographs, which still play an important role, including the exclusion of fracture or malignancy in some instances. Plain radiographs reveal inflammation, destruction, and new bone formation, as follows: (1) within 3 days of symptom development, deep soft tissue swelling and loss of visible tissue planes; (2) within 7 to 21 days, subperiosteal abscesses with periosteal elevation and new bone formation; (3) within 10 to 21 days, bone destruction with lytic lesion; and (4) after 30 days, sclerosis. Ultrasound has been used successfully in some centers. Radionuclide scanning has a sensitivity of 80% to 100% (technetium-99m bone scan) and permits an early diagnosis (within 3 to 5 days) in older children. The sensitivity of radionuclide scanning is less in younger infants, and radionuclide scanning is not recommended for neonates (32% sensitivity). Magnetic resonance imaging (MRI) may be the best imaging technique for bone, with a reported sensitivity for detection of osteomyelitis of 92% to 100% (distinction by T1/T2-weighted image). MRI may be particularly useful in differentiating cellulitis from osteomyelitis, outlining anatomy for surgery, and evaluating chronic osteomyelitis.

Subsets of children with osteomyelitis include the following:

- Neonatal osteomyelitis, which is often manifested as nonspecific symptoms. Pseudoparalysis is sometimes present. Results of radionuclide bone scans, WBC count, and ESR are often normal. The development of an osteolytic bone lesion by 10 to 12 days, seen on plain x-ray examination, is often the key to diagnosis.
- Vertebral osteomyelitis and diskitis, which are less common in children than in adults and may present in an indolent fashion. Symptoms are nonspecific and include pain in the back, chest, abdomen, or lower extremities, refusal to walk, and limp. MRI is the imaging procedure of choice.
- Pelvic osteomyelitis, which involves mainly the ileum and ischium bones. Most patients have fever, gait abnormality, and pain in the hip, groin, or buttocks.
- Osteochondritis of the foot complicating nail puncture wounds (see Chapter 15).
- Osteomyelitis in children with sickle cell disease, which is often due to *Salmonella* species (up to 70% of cases), as well as *S. aureus* and other bacteria. Osteomyelitis is often difficult to distinguish from vasoocclusive crisis. Factors that suggest infection include fever >102° F (39° C), toxic appearance, absolute band count >500 cells/mm³, and significant elevation of the ESR. If fever and bone pain are not improved after supportive care for vasoocclusive crisis, a diagnostic needle aspiration should be performed.

Delays in diagnosis compromise the eventual outcome. Suspected osteomyelitis in children usually calls for hospitalization and consultation with an orthopedic surgeon.

Septic Arthritis

Pyogenic arthritis, which has a peak incidence in children <3 years of age, usually results from hematogenous spread of microorganisms to the highly vascular synovium of the joint space. Clinical manifestations often resemble those of osteomyelitis, but localization of the infection is usually more obvious than in osteomyelitis. Typical clinical findings are erythema, swelling, local pain, warmth, and immobility of the affected joint. Swelling is often associated with extreme loss of motion. The child assumes a posture that decreases motion and provides maximal opportunity for distention of the affected joint. Pseudoparalysis may be present in infants or in the upper extremities of older children. Pyogenic arthritis of the hip can be difficult to diagnose because often there is no obvious joint swelling and the child may exhibit only nonspecific symptoms and signs. The child with arthritis of the hip typically demonstrates flexion, abduction, and external rotation to distend the joint. Septic arthritis in children is monoarticular in about 90% of patients. The knee is the most frequently affected joint, followed by the hip, ankle, and shoulder.

Differential diagnosis includes trauma (hemarthrosis, torn meniscus), collagen-vascular disease (juvenile rheumatoid arthritis, systemic lupus erythematosus), inflammatory bowel disease, hemophilia, leukemia, villonodular synovitis, tumors (hemangioma, neuroblastoma), and Legg-Calvé-Perthes disease or slipped femoral epiphysis. When caused by a virus (rubella, hepatitis B, mumps, varicella, parvovirus B19, HIV, EBV, enterovirus), septic arthritis is usually first evidenced as symmetric small joint involvement with modest fluid and modest loss of motion. Lyme disease usually involves the knee, shoulder, or elbow joints with significant large effusions, although the child does not appear ill; loss of joint motion is minor, and the enlarged joint is not significantly hot or erythematous. Reactive arthritis is usually polyarticular with involvement of large joints, especially those of the lower extremities, and with other diagnostic clues such as a recent episode of diarrhea. Microorganisms associated with reactive arthritis include *Shigella flexneri*, *Salmonella* species, *Yersinia enterocolitica*, *Campylobacter* species, *C. trachomatis*, group A *Streptococcus*, *Neisseria gonorrhoeae*, and *N. meningitidis*.

The presence of transient synovitis should be considered in patients whose clinical features are consistent with septic arthritis but seem relatively mild. Transient synovitis typically occurs in preschool-age children (mean 5 years, range 3 to 8 years). Symptoms include posturing of the involved limb in flexion and external rotation, or a unilateral limp. Fever, if present, is usually low grade. An upper respiratory tract infection may be associated with the synovitis. The ESR is ≤30 mm/hr, and aspiration of the joint produces <5 mL of synovial fluid, containing fewer than 1000 WBCs/mm³. Although considerable overlap exists between the presentations of septic arthritis and transient synovitis, 97% of children with septic arthritis have a temperature >99.6° F (37.5° C) and an ESR >20 mm/hr. The course of transient synovitis is, by definition, self-limited.

Diagnostic studies in cases of suspected septic arthritis should include aspiration of joint fluid to obtain a specimen and to relieve pressure. In an adolescent patient or when there is reason to suspect sexual abuse, specimens are also obtained from the urethra or cervix, throat, skin lesions, and rectum for *N. gonorrhoeae* isolation. The ESR and CRP are usually significantly elevated (mean values 44 to 65 mm/hr and 9 mg/L, respectively). Blood cultures are positive in 40% of cases, and joint fluid cultures are positive in 50% to 60% of cases; overall, a bacterial etiology is established in about 60% to 70% of cases. Radiography is rarely helpful in establishing the diagnosis or in differentiating between infectious and noninfectious arthritis.

S. aureus is a common cause of septic arthritis in all age groups. In children <3 months of age, group B streptococci and gram-negative bacilli, including *E. coli*, should be considered.

In children >3 months of age, possibilities include group A streptococci, *S. pneumoniae*, *H. influenzae* type b, and *Kingella kingae* (in children <5 years of age; isolation of *K. kingae* is enhanced if synovial fluid is inoculated directly into liquid blood culture media and cultures are incubated for 7 days). In sexually active children and adolescents, including all children >12 years of age, *N. gonorrhoeae* should be considered. *Salmonella* species occasionally cause septic arthritis in infants, and *N. meningitidis* occasionally causes septic arthritis in children.

Children with suspected septic arthritis should usually be admitted to the hospital for aggressive intravenous antimicrobial therapy and consultation with an orthopedic surgeon.

KEY POINTS

BONE AND JOINT INFECTIONS IN CHILDREN
⊃ Osteomyelitis and septic arthritis in children are usually of hematogenous origin. *S. aureus* is the most common pathogen.
⊃ Osteomyelitis typically affects the metaphysis of tubular bones. Variants include vertebral osteomyelitis, pelvic osteomyelitis, and osteochondritis after puncture wounds of the foot.
⊃ Septic arthritis most commonly involves the knee, followed by the hip, ankle, and shoulder.
⊃ Suspicion of osteomyelitis or septic arthritis is usually an indication for hospitalization and consultation with an orthopedic surgeon. Delays in initiating appropriate treatment can seriously compromise normal skeletal development and function.

SUGGESTED READING
Abbasi S, Orlicek SL, Almohsen I, et al. Septic arthritis and osteomyelitis caused by penicillin and cephalosporin-resistant *Streptococcus pneumoniae* in a children's hospital. Pediatr Infect Dis J 1996; 15: 78-83.

Fernandez M, Carrol CL, Baker CJ. Discitis and vertebral osteomyelitis in children: an 18-year review. Pediatrics 2000; 105: 1299-1304.

Jacobs R. *Pseudomonas* osteochondritis complicating puncture wounds of the foot in children. Semin Pediatr Infect Dis 1997; 8: 250-253.

Jaramillo D, Treves ST, Kasser JR, et al. Osteomyelitis and septic arthritis in children: appropriate use of imaging to guide treatment. AJR 1995; 165: 399-403

Nelson JD. Acute osteomyelitis in children. Infect Dis Clin North Am 1990; 4: 513-522.

Nelson JD. Toward simple but safe management of osteomyelitis. Pediatrics 1997; 99: 883-884.

Roy DR. Osteomyelitis. Pediatr Rev 1995; 16: 380-384.

Shetty AK, Gedalia A. Septic arthritis in children. Rheum Dis Clin North Am 1998; 24: 287-304.

Yagupsky P, Bar-Ziv Y, Howard CB, et al. Epidemiology, etiology, and clinical features of septic arthritis in children younger than 24 months. Arch Pediatr Adolesc Med 1995; 149: 537-540.

Common or Unique Problems in Children: Some Salient Features

Viral Exanthems (see also Chapter 7)

The term "exanthem" is used to describe a rash associated with a systemic illness. Although certain bacteria and rickettsiae can cause exanthems (e.g., meningococcemia, Rocky

Mountain spotted fever, scarlet fever, and ehrlichiosis; see Chapter 7), viruses are the most common causes of exanthems in children. Historically the common exanthems of childhood have been numbered 1 through 6, as follows: first disease (measles), second disease (scarlet fever), third disease (rubella), fourth disease (staphylococcal scarlet fever and staphylococcal scalded skin syndrome, also called Filatov-Dukes disease), fifth disease (erythema infectiosum), and sixth disease (roseola infantilis).

Rubeola ("Red Measles") (see also Chapter 7)

Universal immunization has made measles a sporadic disease in developed countries. When it occurs, it is often associated with recent vaccination and an atypical presentation of milder symptoms with a petechial rash. In 1997 only 138 cases of confirmed measles cases were reported in the United States. Complications of measles include pneumonia, encephalitis, mesenteric lymphadenitis, and subacute sclerosing panencephalitis. The latter complication, which is rare, occurs 2 to 10 years after the measles infection.

Rubella ("German Measles") (see also Chapter 7)

Rubella is a mild illness with minimal respiratory symptoms and low-grade fever. In contrast to rubeola, the maculopapular rash is nonconfluent and lasts for only 3 to 4 days. The hallmark of rubella is the associated lymphadenopathy, which, although generalized, is particularly prominent in the posterior cervical and occipital areas. Although a mild and almost insignificant disease of childhood, rubella is notorious for its propensity to cause serious defects in the developing fetus (see Chapter 5). Since many viral exanthems can mimic rubella, any pregnant woman exposed to a child or adult with a viral exanthem should have her rubella immune status checked. The importance of universal immunization against rubella cannot be overemphasized.

Roseola (Exanthem Subitum)

Roseola, or exanthem subitum, is one of the classic childhood exanthems identified at the turn of the 20th century. It was not until the 1980s that the etiologic agents, human herpesviruses 6 and 7 (HHV-6 and HHV-7), were identified.

Classically, roseola occurs in infancy, after an incubation period of 10 days, with high fever (up to 140° F [40° C]) for 2 to 4 days followed by diminution or cessation of the fever and the onset of a maculopapular rash, which begins on the face or trunk and quickly spreads to other parts of the body. The rash typically lasts for 2 to 5 days. During the febrile phase the infants are listless or irritable and may have associated cough, lymphadenopathy, diarrhea, edematous eyelids, or bulging fontanel. Significant complications include seizures (8% to 10%) and (rarely) encephalitis. HHV-7 infections are said to involve older children (18 to 36 months of age) and are more frequently associated with seizures than HHV-6 infections.

Erythema Infectiosum (Fifth Disease) (see also Chapters 5 and 7)

Erythema infectiosum, or fifth disease (so named because it was the fifth of the childhood exanthems to be identified), is a mild childhood illness caused by parvovirus B19. It is characterized by malar erythema ("slapped cheek" appearance) that spreads to the extremities and trunk, becoming reticulated and occasionally pruritic. Few constitutional symptoms are associated with erythema infectiosum. It is most commonly seen in children under 10 years of age. Typically, the rash disappears in 4 to 5 days, only to reappear multiple times within a 4- to 6-week period when nonspecific stimuli (sunlight, temperature, emotional stress) occur. Parvovirus B19 has a propensity to infect and lyse erythroid precursor cells and thus interfere with normal red blood cell (RBC) production. This effect is greatly exaggerated in the infected young fetus because of shortened RBC survival and rapidly expanding RBC volume. The result may be severe anemia and fetal hydrops, which can be fatal. Management of parvovirus B19 infection during pregnancy is discussed in Chapter 5. Parvovirus B19 infection in healthy adults can cause arthritis and rash (see Chapter 7). Parvovirus B19 is an important cause of aplastic crisis in patients with hemoglobinopathy, advanced HIV disease, or other conditions that require increased production of RBCs.

Varicella (Chickenpox) (see also "Disseminated Herpes Zoster" in Chapter 7)

Historically, varicella has been one of the most ubiquitous of the common childhood infections. Caused by the varicella-zoster virus, varicella (or chickenpox) infected an estimated 4 million patients (mostly children) each year before the advent of the vaccine in 1995. The lesions start as erythematous macules, which quickly become vesicles and then pustules and later crust over. The hallmark of varicella is the presence of lesions in all of the various stages of development (in contrast to smallpox, in which the lesions are at the same stage of development at any given time). In addition to the exanthem, mucous membranes are often involved and lesions sometimes extend down the esophagus into the stomach and even the lower intestine. Although systemic manifestations are usually mild, the rash is intensely pruritic. The so-called hemorrhagic varicella (with hemorrhagic lesions adjacent to the pox lesions) is occasionally seen and, despite its frightening appearance, is no more severe than the usual chickenpox. Treatment of uncomplicated infection in the normal, nonpregnant host is entirely symptomatic. Acyclovir can be used to treat complicated infections or immunocompromised patients. Acyclovir has been shown to be efficacious in preventing the clinical expression of chickenpox in children exposed to varicella even if given up to 10 days after exposure.

Maternal infection in the perinatal period (between 4 days before birth and 3 days after birth) carries a risk of severe infection in the neonate, with varying reports of mortality incidence. Neonates with perinatal exposure should be given passive immunity with varicella-zoster immune globulin (VZIG).

Other complications of varicella-zoster infections include the fetal varicella syndrome—atrophy of an extremity, cicatricial lesions, central nervous system (CNS) damage, and eye anomalies. This rare fetal wastage syndrome occurs with severe maternal varicella during the first half of pregnancy (see Chapter 5). Varicella encephalitis is uncommon but potentially lethal, with a mortality rate of 5% to 20%. Cerebellar ataxia is more common but carries an excellent prognosis. Varicella pneumonia is the third most common complication and occurs mainly in adults or immunocompromised children.

Of considerable concern is bacterial superinfection of the pox lesions. Usually caused by group A β-hemolytic streptococci (GABHS) or *S. aureus*, cellulitis is a frequent complication. More recently, necrotizing fasciitis, a rapidly progressive cellulitis caused by GABHS, has become prominent in the lay and scientific literature—underscoring the need for universal vaccination. Treatment of necrotizing fasciitis is a medical emergency and includes two antibiotics (e.g., a β-lactamase-resistant antistaphylococcal antibiotic plus clindamycin) with aggressive débridement to prevent fatal tissue necrosis (see Chapter 6). Recent data suggest that NSAIDs do not predispose children with varicella to necrotizing fasciitis.

With the universal use of a live attenuated varicella vaccine (Varivax) in the United States since 1996, varicella has already shown a significant decrease in incidence and expectations are that this ubiquitous childhood disease will soon be a rare occurrence.

Enteroviral Exanthems

The enteroviruses, particularly echovirus, coxsackie A, and enterovirus 71, are responsible for a variety of childhood exanthems:

- Herpangina, caused by coxsackie A and occasionally by coxsackie B, is characterized by 1- to 4-mm vesicles on the uvula and soft palate. Fever usually lasts for 1 to 4 days and is accompanied by sore throat. Recovery occurs in about 1 week.
- Hand-foot-and-mouth disease, caused by coxsackie A16, is characterized by small vesicles in the anterior part of the mouth and also on the palms and the plantar surfaces of the feet. Like herpangina, it is accompanied by low-grade fever and sore throat, with recovery usually taking place within a week.
- Nonspecific exanthems are caused by echoviruses (notably types 70 and 71) and coxsackie A viruses. These exanthems are typically rubella-like, maculopapular eruptions that are often generalized. Low-grade fever and mild constitutional symptoms are usually present.

These exanthems tend to occur in outbreaks, and diagnosis is usually made on clinical presentation. Occasionally, potentially serious complications have been reported with these enteroviral infections (aseptic meningitis, myocarditis).

 KEY POINTS

VIRAL EXANTHEMS

- ↻ Rubeola ("red measles") is now rare in the United States. When it occurs, it is most often associated with recent vaccination and is manifested as mild symptoms and a petechial rash.
- ↻ Rubella ("German measles") remains an important cause of birth defects and is preventable by vaccine.
- ↻ Roseola (exanthem subitum), caused by human herpesviruses 6 and 7 (HHV-6 and HHV-7), can cause seizures and rarely encephalitis.
- ↻ Erythema infectiosum ("fifth disease"), caused by parvovirus B19, produces a mild illness in children but can cause fetal loss and, in persons with hematologic disorders, aplastic crisis.
- ↻ Varicella (chickenpox) is prone to bacterial superinfection, which, when caused by group A β-hemolytic streptococci, can result in necrotizing fasciitis.
- ↻ Enteroviral exanthems cause nonspecific, discrete or lacy, maculopapular rashes involving the trunk, extremities, and sometimes the face. Complications include aseptic meningitis and myocarditis.

SUGGESTED READING

Cherry JD. Contemporary infectious exanthems. Clin Infect Dis 1993; 16: 199-205.

Gable EK, Liu G, Morrell DS. Pediatric exanthems. Primary Care 2000; 27: 353-369.

Lesko SM, O'Brien KL, Schwartz B, et al. Invasive group A streptococcal infection and nonsteroidal anti-inflammatory drug use among children with primary varicella. Pediatrics 2001; 107: 1108-1115.

Sawyer, MH. Enterovirus infections: diagnosis and treatment. Pediatr Infect Dis J 1999; 18: 1033-1040.

Weisse ME. The fourth disease, 1900-2000. Lancet 2001; 357: 299-301.

Fever of Undetermined Origin (see also Chapter 1)

Fever of undetermined origin (FUO) is defined as persistent fever of at least 101° F (38.3° C) for 3 weeks after at least 1 week of intensive investigation without an identifiable source. True FUO is uncommon in children. Diseases that often went undiagnosed in the past commonly yield their identities now that better diagnostic tools are available. Infectious diseases continue to be the most common causes of FUO in childhood, followed by connective tissue diseases and neoplasms. In a prospective study of about 150 children with prolonged fever and FUO, conducted between 1990 and 1996, the diagnosis was established in 58% of cases. The most common infectious disease diagnoses were EBV infection (15%), osteomyelitis (10%), bartonellosis (5%) and UTIs (4%). Three of seven patients with confirmed *Bartonella henselae* infection had FUO and no ultrasonographic findings compatible with hepatosplenic involvement; two patients had FUO and hepatosplenic involvement. Evaluation of a child with true FUO should include consultation with an infectious disease specialist and diagnostic testing guided by abnormalities suggested by history, physical examination, and routine laboratory testing.

SUGGESTED READING

Arisoy SE, Correa AG, Wagner ML, et al. Hepatosplenic cat-scratch disease in children: selected clinical features and treatment. Clin Infect Dis 1999; 28: 778-784.

Chantada G, Casak S, Plata JD, et al. Children with fever of unknown origin in Argentina: an analysis of 113 Cases. Pediatr Infect Dis J 1994; 13: 260-263.

Gartner JC. Fever of unknown origin. Adv Pediatr Infect Dis 1992; 7: 1-24.

Isaacman DJ, Shults J, Gross TK, et al. Predictors of bacteremia in febrile children 3 to 36 months of age. Pediatrics 2000; 106: 977-982.

Jacobs RF, Schutze GE. *Bartonella henselae* as a cause of prolonged fever and fever of unknown origin in children. Clin Infect Dis 1998; 26: 80-84.

Park JW. Fever without source in children: recommendations for outpatient care in those up to 3. Postgrad Med 2000; 107: 259-266.

Thomas KT, Feder HM, Lawton AR, et al. Periodic fever syndrome in children. J Pediatr 1999; 135: 15-21.

Fever and Lymphadenopathy (see also Chapter 8)

In pediatrics, lymphadenopathy may be part of many disease processes, including local or generalized infection. Lymphadenitis, on the other hand, reflects inflammation or infection of the node(s). The particular nodes involved and the age of the child yield clues to diagnostic possibilities. A history of animal exposure often provides the crucial information. Supraclavicular lymphadenopathy warrants a more aggressive diagnostic approach to rule out malignancy.

Outpatient management of lymphadenopathy and lymphadenitis depends on the likely underlying process. Enlargement of the cervical lymph nodes most commonly represents a response to a viral process.

S. aureus and *S. pyogenes* cause about 65% to 89% of cases of acute unilateral cervical adenitis in young children. Treatment options include amoxicillin–clavulanic acid, cephalexin, clindamycin, and erythromycin. Follow-up is important to rule out abscess formation, which would require surgical intervention. A Mantoux skin test is important and may help in the diagnosis not only of tuberculosis (typically >15 mm of induration in children), but also of nontuberculous mycobacterial infection (typically <10 mm of induration), both of which have subacute presentations (see Chapter 22). Anaerobic organisms can infect lymph nodes. The recovery of these organisms, especially from cervical nodes, strongly suggests periodontal disease. Other diagnostic tests such as throat culture, complete blood count, and ultrasound or CT study of the neck may be helpful.

In the appropriate clinical setting, other disease processes should be considered for a child with fever and regional lymphadenopathy, such as cat scratch disease caused by *B. henselae* (see Chapter 8). This disease can also manifest itself as meningoencephalitis, oculoglandular disease (Parinaud's syndrome), microabscesses of liver or spleen, or osteolytic bone lesions. Treatment options available for lymphadenitis are azithromycin, ciprofloxacin, erythromycin, gentamicin, clarithromycin, rifampin, and TMP/SMX, although only one well-controlled randomized trial, using azithromycin, has shown a clear benefit. Rifampin should be included in a regimen for the hepatosplenic form of cat scratch disease. Toxoplasmosis, EBV, CMV, brucellosis, histoplasmosis, tularemia, and *Yersinia* infection can present with lymphadenopathy and fever. Appropriate serologic tests and cultures should be performed to confirm these diagnoses.

SUGGESTED READING

Chesney PJ. Cervical adenopathy. Pediatr Rev 1994; 15: 276-285.

Hickey SM, Strasburger VC. What every pediatrician should know about infectious mononucleosis in adolescents. Pediatr Clin North Am 1997; 44: 1541-1556.

Schutze GE. Diagnosis and treatment of *Bartonella henselae* infections. Pediatr Infect Dis J. 2000; 19: 1185-1187.

Skin and Soft Tissue Infections (see also Chapter 15)

Impetigo (see also Chapter 15)

Impetigo is a ubiquitous feature of summertime childhood infections, particularly in the hot, humid climate of the southern United States. Streptococcal impetigo (caused by group A β-hemolytic streptococci [GABHS]) follows minor skin trauma (chiefly mosquito bites) and is characterized by pustules that evolve into "honey-crusted" scablike lesions associated with regional adenitis. Staphylococcal impetigo (bullous impetigo), on the other hand, causes large bullae on the intact skin of young children from the toxin-secreting phage II staphylococci. However, in the past several decades staphylococci have been commonly associated with the classic "streptococcal" im-

petigo, and therapy for both forms therefore necessitates antistaphylococcal antibiotics (e.g., cephalexin, erythromycin) for 10 days. Complications of streptococcal impetigo include lymphangitis, cellulitis, and, rarely, necrotizing fasciitis (often associated with varicella infection). Acute poststreptococcal glomerulonephritis can be a significant problem if nephritogenic strains of GABHS are present in the community.

Cellulitis (see also Chapter 15)

Cellulitis is defined as localized inflammation of the skin and subcutaneous tissue. Increased heat, erythema, and tenderness are the early signs. Cellulitis is commonly seen in children after penetrating wounds or other skin trauma in which the affected areas are not properly cleansed. Organisms are usually *S. aureus* or GABHS; appropriate therapy consists of an antistaphylococcal antibiotic. Cellulitis in the genitoanal area may be caused by gram-negative bacilli. Buccal and facial cellulitis was formerly due to *H. influenzae* type b, but with the universal use of Hib vaccine this has become a rarity.

Necrotizing Fasciitis (see also Chapter 6)

Necrotizing cellulitis and fasciitis result when the organism causing local cellulitis is unusually virulent and begins dissecting through adjacent tissue planes in a rapid and unrelenting fashion. The result is massive tissue necrosis, progressing to gangrene, limb loss, and possibly death. As noted previously, necrotizing fasciitis is closely associated with varicella and is most often caused by GABHS. Any patient with clinical varicella who shows signs of early cellulitis should be admitted to the hospital for intensive intravenous antibiotic therapy. Recent data suggest that treatment with high-dose clindamycin (given in part to reduce toxin production) combined with a β-lactam antibiotic and surgery when indicated is the optimum regimen for GABHS infections.

Pustules, Furuncles, and Abscesses (see also Chapter 15)

Most often caused by *S. aureus,* pustules, furuncles, and abscesses are common in children of all ages. Pustules are conical, pus-containing elevations on the skin. They are usually 1 to 5 mm in diameter. A furuncle is a large pustule, usually about 1 cm in diameter (carbuncles are deeper lesions that can be viewed as coalescences of furuncles with multiple openings). Abscesses are large (>1 cm), deeper collections of pus that are usually walled off by a capsule. Antistaphylococcal antibiotic therapy and warm compresses are indicated for all of these, and incision and drainage are the mainstay of treatment for furuncles and deep abscesses. Recurrent furunculosis is usually the result of chronic nasal carriage of the offending staphylococcus with "ping-ponging" back and forth among family members. Elimination of the carriage state is somewhat difficult and controversial, but a topical antistaphylococcal antibiotic in the nares of identified carriers or prophylactic oral antistaphylococcal antibiotics have been used with success. Persistent recurrence should alert the physician to the possibility of defects in neutrophil function, including the recurrent infection–hyperimmunoglobulinemia E syndrome (Job's syndrome, named after the boil-plagued Biblical character).

Fungal Infections (see also Chapter 15)

Fungal infections of the skin are more common in younger children than in older children and adults. Diaper rash and stomatitis (thrush) caused by *Candida albicans* are ubiquitous problems in neonates and young infants but should be viewed with concern in older children unless they have been receiving continual antibiotic therapy or using inhaled steroids.

Tinea capitis is particularly common in African-American children, and >80% of these infections are due to *T. tonsurans,* which unlike most other causes of ringworm does not fluoresce under Wood's light. Relative resistance to griseofulvin has occurred in recent years, necessitating an increase in the recommended dosage from 15 mg/kg/day to 20 to 25 mg/kg/day. Newer oral agents such as itraconazole and terbinafine are being evaluated for therapy but have not yet been approved for use in children.

Tinea corporis is most often due to *Trichophyton* species and is sensitive to most topical antifungal therapies, including clotrimazole, ketoconazole, and terbinafine.

SUGGESTED READING

Blumer JL, Lemon E, O'Horo J, et al. Changing therapy for skin and soft tissue infections in children: have we come full circle? Pediatr Infect Dis J 1987; 6:117-122.

Leyden, JJ, ed. Update on tinea capitis and new antifungal therapies. Pediatr Infect Dis J 1999; 18 (Suppl): 180-216.

Zimbelman J, Palmer A, Todd J. Improved outcome of clindamycin compared with beta-lactam antibiotic treatment for invasive *Streptococcus pyogenes* infection. Pediatr Infect Dis J 1999; 18(12): 1096-1100.

Croup, Epiglottitis, and Bacterial Tracheitis (see also Chapters 6, 10, and 11)

Croup (laryngotracheobronchitis) is a common childhood viral illness caused primarily by parainfluenza and RSV and typically seen in the fall or winter. Children with croup are usually between 6 months and 4 years of age. Fever, stridor, and a barking cough herald the onset. Coryza is sometimes present. Respiratory distress is worse at night, and the disease can last up to 10 days. *Not all respiratory stridor, however, is caused by viral croup.* Acute epiglottitis, bacterial tracheitis, subglottic hemangiomas, and gastroesophageal disease with aspiration are a few of the entities that can mimic viral croup. Epiglottitis has become a rare disease because of immunization against *H. influenzae* type b. Bacterial tracheitis, caused by *S. aureus* and other bacteria, can be a complication of viral croup. Epiglottitis and bacterial tracheitis often manifest themselves by high fever, drooling, and signs and symptoms of systemic illness and respiratory distress.

"Typical viral croup" is a clinical diagnosis. Anteroposterior and lateral inspiratory neck films aid in the diagnosis but are often obtained to rule out acute epiglottitis or retropharyngeal abscess. When these latter conditions are suspected in an acutely ill child, however, airway management takes priority over imaging procedures. Strategies for outpatient management of croup include hydration, corticosteroids, and inhaled racemic epinephrine. Current evidence regarding the value of mist therapy is inconclusive. In the emergency room setting dexamethasone 0.6 mg/kg IM (maximal dose, 10 mg) or 0.15 to 0.6 mg/kg PO is currently recommended. No good comparative studies of oral versus parenteral corticosteroids for croup have been published. Nebulized budesonide (2 mg) may have a role in the management of croup, but more data are needed before definitive recommendations can be made. In addition, 0.05 mL/kg of 2.25% racemic epinephrine aerosol can be used, keeping in mind that rebound may occur after the medication is withdrawn. Viral croup should be distinguished from spasmodic croup. Although similar in presentation, spasmodic croup lacks fever and symptoms of URI. Also, spasmodic croup occurs predominantly at night. No treatment is indicated for spasmodic croup, although induced vomiting has been associated with symptom abatement.

SUGGESTED READING

Cressman WR, Myer CM. Diagnosis and management of croup and epiglottitis. Pediatr Clin North Am 1994; 41: 265-276.

Malhotra A, Krilov LR. Viral croup. Pediatr Rev 2001; 22: 5-11.

Pertussis (Whooping Cough)

In pediatrics, pertussis caused by *Bordetella pertussis* is seen in very young children who have not received pertussis vaccine. The disease also occurs in older adolescents and adults whose immunity to pertussis may have waned. The incubation period is 7 to 10 days. Three clinical phases of pertussis have been defined. The first phase consists of rhinorrhea, conjunctivitis, and mild cough. The second phase, about 2 weeks after onset of symptoms, features the typical paroxysmal coughing with inspiratory "whoop." Apnea and cyanosis may occur during the second phase. The final phase, which can last up to 2 months after onset of symptoms, involves persistent cough that gradually wanes. The CBC in pertussis usually shows marked lymphocytosis. Isolation of *B. pertussis* from nasopharyngeal secretions remains the "gold standard" for diagnosis. A positive direct immunofluorescent antibody test supports the diagnosis, with a specificity of about 95%. Polymerase chain reaction (PCR) assays are now available.

The treatment of choice is erythromycin 40 to 50 mg/day PO in four divided doses for 14 days. However, therapy has not been shown to shorten the course of pertussis. Its chief value is preventing the spread of the organism. The newer macrolides offer an alternative treatment for 5 to 7 days; however, efficacy is unproved. Supportive treatment such as nebulized β-agonists or steroids can be used to reduce coughing paroxysms, but their benefit is questionable. It is generally recommended that young children with documented pertussis nonetheless complete a schedule of diphtheria-tetanus-pertussis vaccinations.

Complications of pertussis include seizures, pneumonia, encephalopathy, and death. Other organisms that can produce a pertussis-like syndrome are *Bordetella parapertussis, M. pneumoniae, Chlamydia pneumoniae,* and adenoviruses.

SUGGESTED READING

Edwards KM. Pertussis in older children and adults. Adv Pediatr Infect Dis 1997; 13: 49-77.

Gordon M, Davies HD, Geld R. Clinical and microbiologic features of children, presenting with pertussis to a Canadian pediatric hospital during an eleven-year period. Pediatr Infect Dis J 1994; 13: 617-622.

Hewlett EL. Pertussis: current concepts of pathogenesis and prevention. Pediatr Infect Dis J 1997; 16 (Suppl 4): S78-S84.

Muller FM, Hoppe JE, Wirsing von Konig CH. Laboratory diagnosis of pertussis: state of the art in 1997. J Clin Microbiol 1997; 35: 2435-2443.

Bronchiolitis (see also Chapter 11)

Bronchiolitis typically occurs in young children (<3 years of age) and is usually viral in etiology. Respiratory syncytial virus (RSV) heads the list of potential pathogens, and parainfluenza types l, 2, and 3 and adenovirus are also significant causative viruses. Cough, tachypnea, wheezing, and fever are common presenting complaints. The diagnosis is based on clinical examination, with rales a frequent auscultatory finding. Chest x-ray examination reveals overdistention with increased interstitial markings. An RSV ELISA nasal washing can aid in confirming RSV as the causative agent. Treatment is generally supportive, with antipyretics and hydration as mainstays. Bulb suctioning of the nasal passages helps to improve airway patency. Solid evidence supports the use of aerosolized epinephrine, and studies have given fair support to the use of β_2 agonists. Evaluation of the use of inhaled corticosteroids is ongoing. Hypoxemia and dehydration are indications for hospitalization. Inhaled ribavirin for RSV infection has generally fallen from favor, and any decision to use it in severe RSV infections should be made in consultation with an infectious disease specialist (see Chapter 20).

Palivizumab (Synagis) is a monoclonal antibody given intramuscularly each month during the RSV season to prevent this disease. The AAP has developed guidelines for selecting infants and children to receive this treatment. For certain patients an alternative prophylactic option, RSV-IVIG, should be considered. Only limited data on cost-benefit analyses of these two treatment strategies are available. Neither of these preparations is recommended for children with cyanotic congenital heart disease.

In children 2 weeks to 3 months of age the afebrile pneumonias mimic typical bronchiolitis (see earlier discussion). Erythromycin 50 mg/kg/day in divided doses for 2 weeks shortens the duration of *C. trachomatis* pneumonia and also the duration of nasopharyngeal shedding. *Chlamydia, Ureaplasma,* and CMV are agents to be considered in the diagnosis of pneumonia. Reactive airway disease, myocarditis, and congestive heart failure resulting from undiagnosed congenital heart disease should also be considered in the differential diagnosis.

SUGGESTED READING

American Academy of Pediatrics, Committee of Infectious Diseases and Committee of Fetus and Newborn. Prevention of respiratory syncytial virus infections: indications for the use of Palivizumab and update on the use of RSV-IGIV. Pediatrics 1998; 102: 1211-1216.

Tang N, Want E. Bronchiolitis. Clinical Evidence 2000; 173-181.

The Medical Letter on Drugs and Therapeutics. *Synagis* revisited. Med Lett 2001; 43: 13-14.

Welliver R. Bronchiolitis: etiology and management. Semin Pediatr Infect Dis 1998; 9: 154-162.

Pneumonia (see also Chapter 11)

The causes of pneumonia in children are age related. In young infants pneumonia is often of viral etiology and unaccompanied by fever ("afebrile pneumonia syndrome"; see preceding discussion). In toddler, preschool, and school-aged children pneumonia is uncommon and, when it occurs, usually of viral or pneumococcal etiology. *M. pneumoniae* is a common cause of pneumonia in older children and adolescents.

The diagnosis of pneumonia in children is usually made on clinical grounds with or without x-ray examination. Cultures, although often indicated, are seldom helpful—particularly in younger children. Sputum is not obtainable from young children, and blood cultures seldom establish the diagnosis (<20% of patients with pneumococcal pneumonia have positive blood cultures). Diagnostic transthoracic lung puncture or bronchial aspiration is occasionally performed, but these procedures are invasive and require technical expertise. Throat cultures are without value, having little correlation with the pulmonary pathogen.

The classic presentations of viral and bacterial pneumonias differ (see Chapter 11). Viral pneumonia (interstitial pneumonia) begins insidiously, often after a URI, and is associated with tachypnea, generalized wheezing, and fine, diffuse rales on auscultation of the chest. Bacterial pneumonia (parenchymal pneumonia), when caused by *S. pneumoniae,* often begins abruptly with high fever, systemic toxicity, localized intercostal retractions, and evidence of lobar consolidation on auscultation of the chest. Considerable overlap, however, may exist in the presentations of viral or "atypical" pneumonia and bacterial pneumonia.

Pneumonia in Infants

Although pneumococcal and staphylococcal pneumonias occur in young infants, the more common agents are RSV and adenoviruses. The so-called afebrile pneumonia syndrome in young infants is usually due to RSV, *C. trachomatis, U. urealyticum,* or rarely *Pneumocystis carinii.* These patients are often afebrile and have progressively worsening tachypnea, with or without expiratory wheezing, cough, and x-ray changes consistent with diffuse interstitial infiltrates. DNA probe is probably the best diagnostic test at present for *C. trachomatis* respiratory infection, and PCR is useful for diagnosis of *U. urealyticum* infection. Diagnosis of *P. carinii* is difficult at best, with PCR the best diagnostic test (although not widely available). TMP/SMX is the usual drug of choice for *P. carinii* infection in infants, and macrolides are used for *U. urealyticum* and *C. trachomatis* infections.

Pneumonia in Young Children

In preschool and school-aged children viral agents account for most of the episodes of pneumonia. RSV is common in children <3 years old, and adenoviruses in preschool- and grade school–age children. Pneumococcal pneumonia is seen in this age group, and the diagnosis is most often based on clinical and x-ray presentations. Penicillin G is still the drug of choice for pneumococcal pneumonia except in areas of significant penicillin resistance, where a third-generation cephalosporin or vancomycin or both must be considered.

Pneumonia in Older Children and Adolescents

Adenoviral, *C. pneumoniae,* and pneumococcal pneumonia are seen in older children and adolescents, but *M. pneumoniae* is probably the most common cause of pneumonia in this age group. Mycoplasmal pneumonia has a subacute onset, prominent extrapulmonary features, and minimal chest signs with diffuse, bilateral patchy infiltrates seen on x-ray examination. Treatment is with a macrolide or, in children >8 years of age, a tetracycline.

Special Considerations

Tuberculosis can appear at any age and should be considered, along with fungi, when history or x-ray findings (such as hilar lymphadenopathy or cavitary lesions) are suggestive. Staphylococcal pneumonia occurs occasionally, especially in infants, and should be suspected in a toxic-appearing child with empyema or air-containing infiltrates (pneumatoceles). Pneumonias caused by gram-negative bacilli are rare in children and, when present, suggest an immunodeficiency disorder such as HIV infection.

SUGGESTED READING

Cohen GJ. Management of infections of the lower respiratory tract in children. Pediatr Infect Dis J 1987; 6: 317-323.

Correa A. Diagnostic approach to pneumonia in children. Semin Respir Infect 1996; 11: 131-138.

Heiskanen-Kosma T, Korppi M, Jokinin C, et al. Etiology of childhood pneumonia: serologic results of a prospective, population-based study. Pediatr Infect Dis J 1998; 17: 986-991.

McCracken GH Jr. Diagnosis and management of pneumonia in children. Pediatr Infect Dis J 2000; 19: 924-928.

Schidlow D, Callahan C. Pneumonia. Pediatr Rev 1996; 17: 300-309.

Conjunctivitis (see also Chapter 9)

Viruses, especially adenoviruses and enteroviruses, cause the majority of cases of conjunctivitis in children, particularly in day care settings. Nontypeable *H. influenzae, Haemophilus aegyptius, S. aureus, M. catarrhalis,* and *S. pneumoniae* head the list of bacterial causes of conjunctivitis. *C. trachomatis* and *N. gonorrhoeae* are important causes of neonatal conjunctivitis, and herpes simplex virus occasionally infects the newborn eye. Bacterial conjunctivitis, manifested by mucopurulent discharge, is rare in children >5 years of age.

Conjunctivitis is usually self-limited. Topical ciprofloxacin, tobramycin, Sodium Sulamyd, and combinations containing polymyxin B can be used for 5 to 7 days in children with suspected bacterial disease. Issues of cost-effectiveness and delays in identification of the microorganism discourage the use of routine eye cultures. Definitive diagnosis of conjunctivitis caused by *C. trachomatis* is based on isolation of the organism in tissue culture. An eye scraping is used for this purpose, since the organism is an obligate intracellular pathogen. PCR for *C. trachomatis* is more sensitive than DNA probe or culture, direct fluorescent antibody tests, or enzyme immunoassays. A presumptive diagnosis of chlamydial conjunctivitis can be based on finding the characteristic intracellular inclusions on a Giemsa-stained smear of conjunctival exudates. Gonococcal conjunctivitis is treated with eye irrigations and systemic therapy with ceftriaxone 25 to 50 mg/kg/day, not to exceed 125 mg/day, IM or IV, usually in the hospital setting. Patients with suspected conjunctivitis caused by herpes simplex virus should be referred promptly to an ophthalmologist because of the risk of corneal perforation.

Conjunctivitis is highly contagious. Children should be allowed to remain in school or day care once an indicated therapy is implemented. However, careful handwashing and minimizing close contact with others is required.

Pharyngitis caused by adenoviruses is often associated with conjunctivitis (hence, "pharyngoconjunctival fever"), as is acute otitis media caused by *H. influenzae*. Other infectious diseases that can have conjunctivitis as part of the symptom complex are leptospirosis, Kawasaki disease, *Yersinia* infection, tularemia, Lyme disease, and cat scratch disease (conjunctivitis with preauricular lymphadenitis is known as the oculoglandular syndrome or Parinaud's syndrome). Many noninfectious diseases should be included in the differential diagnosis of conjunctivitis and red eye. In pediatric practice, these include especially juvenile rheumatoid arthritis, allergy, and contact lens use.

SUGGESTED READING

Chung C, Cohen E. Conjunctivitis. Clinical Evidence, June 2000, pp 305-310.

Gigliotti F. Acute conjunctivitis. Pediatr Rev 1995; 16: 203-207

Urinary Tract Infection (see also Chapter 14)

Urinary tract infection (UTI) encompasses a range of diagnostic possibilities from urethritis-epididymitis to pyelonephritis. Approach to diagnosis and treatment depends on anatomic location and the patient's age and gender.

Significant bacteriuria in children is defined as the presence of >1000 CFUs/mL of bacteria in a specimen obtained by suprapubic bladder puncture, >10,000 CFUs/mL in a specimen obtained by catheterization, and >100,000 CFUs/mL of a single microorganism in a clean-catch specimen. Smaller numbers of bacteria may be significant in patients with pyelonephritis. *E. coli* is by far the most common organism associated with childhood UTI. Gram stain of spun urine sediment is highly sensitive for UTI. The diagnosis is supported by the presence of pyuria (>5 to 10 WBCs/HPF in spun sediment) and by a positive dipstick test for leukocyte esterase and nitrite.

Symptoms and signs of UTI differ according to age. They include fever without apparent source, failure to thrive, and a symptom complex of vomiting, diarrhea, dysuria, and flank pain. Uncircumcised males have a higher incidence of UTI during the first year of life.

Children with UTI should be evaluated for possible voiding dysfunction. The extent of the workup depends largely on the history, age, and sex. Imaging studies are recommended for all males with UTI, all females <4 years of age, and prepubertal females with pyelonephritis or frequent recurrences of UTI. Options for the initial imaging study include ultrasound, CT scan, intravenous pyelography, and renal scan, each with its advantages and disadvantages. Renal ultrasound is the least invasive. The dimercapto–succinic acid (DMSA) renal scan is an excellent way to document renal scarring. Voiding cystourethrogram (VCUG) is used to evaluate the urethra, the bladder, and the presence or absence of vesicoureteral reflux. Radionuclide cystography, compared with VCUG, gives less radiation exposure but also less anatomic detail. The radionuclide cystogram can be used as a screening tool or as a way to document resolution of the problem after intervention. The identification of vesicoureteral reflux warrants antibiotic prophylaxis and possible referral to a urologist, depending on the severity and frequency of UTI. Vesicoureteral reflux has a genetic component, and therefore screening is recommended for siblings <4 years of age of patients found to have this disorder.

Treatment options for an acute UTI include TMP (8 to 12 mg/kg/day)/SMX (40 to 60 mg/kg/day) or cefixime (8 mg/kg/day) for 10 to 14 days. Recent studies validate treatment of pyelonephritis on an outpatient basis with ceftriaxone intramuscularly initially, followed by oral medication.

However, neonates with UTI and older children with marked toxicity should be admitted to the hospital for parenteral therapy and fluid support. Patients with recurrent UTI should be given prophylactic antimicrobial therapy with TMP/SMX at 2 mg/kg/day (based on the TMP component) for a minimum of 6 to 12 months. Nitrofurantoin 1 to 2 mg/kg/day is an acceptable alternative.

SUGGESTED READING

American Academy of Pediatrics. Committee on Quality Improvement. Subcommittee on Urinary Tract Infection. Practice parameter: the diagnosis, treatment and evaluation of the initial urinary tract infection in febrile infants and children. Pediatrics 1999; 103: 843-852.

Dick P, Feldman W. Routine diagnostic imaging for childhood UTI: a systemic overview. J Pediatr 1996; 128: 15-22.

Hellerstein S. Long-term consequences of urinary tract infections. Curr Opin Pediatr 2000; 12: 125-128.

Hoberman A, Wald ER, Hickey RW, et al. Oral versus initial intravenous therapy for UTI in young febrile children. Pediatrics 1999; 104: 79-86.

Lohr J, ed. Pediatric urinary tract infections. Pediatr Ann 1999; 28: 639-699.

Kawasaki Disease (see also Chapter 7)

Kawasaki disease is a dramatic disorder of unknown etiology typically seen in children between 1 and 5 years of age and defined as fever of 5 or more days' duration with at least four of the following signs: (1) bulbar conjunctivitis sparing the limbus; (2) changes in the lips and oral cavity; (3) abnormalities of the extremities with swelling of the palms and soles; (4) polymorphous rash; and (5) cervical lymphadenopathy. Arteritis of the coronary arteries with formation of aneurysms is the major complication and the focus of preventive intervention. Young African-American males have the highest rate of complications. Atypical cases that do not meet the above criteria have been reported. Patients with suspected Kawasaki disease should usually be hospitalized and evaluated by a consultant.

Infections Related to Out-of-Home Child Care

Approximately 13 million children <5 years of age, representing almost two thirds of preschool children in the United States, participate in a child care program. Promoting the growth of child care programs are changes in family dynamics (about 75% of mothers now participate in the workforce) and the demonstrated value of preschool education. Grouping of children in child care centers often consists of infants (<12 months of age), toddlers (13 to 35 months of age), preschoolers (36 to 59 months of age), and school-age children (5 to 12 years of age). Major types of out-of-home child care facilities are small-family child care (private residence with fewer than 6 unrelated children), large-family child care (private residence with 7 to 12 children), center child care (nonresidential facility with ≥13 children), and sick child care (specialized program for mildly ill children excluded from regular child care). Most infants and toddlers receive out-of-home care in small- and large-family child care settings, which are sometimes licensed but not usually regulated; preschoolers are primarily enrolled in center child care programs, which are licensed and regulated by the states.

Infants, toddlers, and young children who are cared for in groups have increased rates of certain infectious diseases and increased risks for acquiring antibiotic-resistant organisms. The differences in the number of infections between children in child care and those in home care tend to disappear after children have been in child care for more than 3 years. Control and prevention of infection in out-of-home child care programs are influenced by several factors: caregivers' personal hygiene and immunization status, environmental sanitation, food-handling procedures, ages and immunization status of children, ratio of children to caregivers, physical space and quality of facilities, and frequency of antibiotic use in children in child care. Child care programs should require that all children and staff receive age-appropriate immunizations and routine health care. The most important factor for reducing transmission of disease in child care programs is appropriate and thorough handwashing. Children infected in child care may transmit infection not only within the group, but also within their households and community.

Infectious Diseases and Agents in Out-of-Home Child Care

Some infectious agents potentially associated with child care settings and their modes of transmissions are summarized in Table 4-5. Risk factors for infection in out-of-home child care centers include early childhood (because children in diapers have relative immunologic naïveté, require more hands-on contact by care providers, and have not developed good hygiene and sanitation habits), inadequate numbers of staff, frequent staff turnover, education lapses by the staff, poor handwashing practices by the staff (often because of frequent crisis intervention), entry of new children into the center, and failure to isolate children with diarrhea. Contamination of the environment, food, or water facilitates spread of agents such as rotaviruses, hepatitis A virus, *G. lamblia* cysts, and *Cryptosporidium parvum* oocysts. Also promoting infection is the propensity of children to explore the environment and to "share" secretions. In one child care center the rate of fecal contamination of toys and other objects was found to be 17% on an average day and 38% during an outbreak of diarrhea. Children's "hand-to-mouth behaviors," according to age and frequency per hour, were determined to be as follows: from 1 to 12 months of age, 64 times per hour; from 13 to 24 months of age, 34 times per hour; and from 31 to 48 months of age, 8 times per hour.

The incidences of many infectious diseases are increased in the child care setting. Notable examples are hepatitis A and diarrhea of diverse origins; acute otitis media; invasive bacterial disease caused by *S. pneumoniae, N. meningitidis,* and *H. influenzae* type b, and herpesvirus infections (CMV, herpes simplex, and varicella-zoster virus). Less conclusive evidence suggests increased incidences of sinusitis, pharyngitis, pneumonia, aseptic meningitis caused by enteroviruses, and skin diseases such as impetigo, scabies, pediculosis, and ringworm. Only a few cases of hepatitis B transmission in the child care setting have been documented, and no cases of HIV transmission have been documented. A few instances of necrotizing fasciitis caused by group A β-hemolytic streptococci have been reported. Because of the rarity of subsequent cases and the low risk, in general, of invasive group A streptococcal disease in children, prophylaxis after a single case is not recommended in child care facilities. *Local or state health authorities should be notified of any communicable diseases involving children or staff in a child care setting.*

TABLE 4-5
Modes of Transmission of Infectious Agents in Child Care Settings

	Respiratory transmission	Fecal-oral transmission	Person-to-person contact via skin	Contact with blood or urine
Bacteria	*Haemophilus influenzae* type b, *Streptococcus pneumoniae*, *Neisseria meningitidis*, *Streptococcus pyogenes*, *Bordetella pertussis*, *Mycobacterium tuberculosis*	*Campylobacter* species, *Salmonella* species, *Shigella* species, *Clostridium difficile*	*S. pyogenes*, *Staphylococcus aureus*	
Viruses	Influenza A and B, parainfluenza viruses, respiratory syncytial virus, parvovirus B19, rhinoviruses, adenoviruses, measles, rubella, varicella-zoster virus	Enteroviruses, hepatitis A virus, rotaviruses, caliciviruses, astroviruses, enteric adenoviruses	Herpes simplex viruses, varicella-zoster virus	Cytomegalovirus, hepatitis B virus, hepatitis C virus, herpes simplex viruses, human immunodeficiency virus*
Parasites		*Cryptosporidium parvum*, *Giardia lamblia*, *Enterobius vermicularis*	*Pediculus capitis*, *Sarcoptes scabiei*, *Trichophyton* species, *Microsporon* species	

Modified from Wald ER. Infections in child care environments. In: Burg FD, Wald ER, Ingelfinger JR, et al., eds. Gellis & Kagan's Current Pediatrics Therapy. 16th ed., Philadelphia: W.B. Saunders Company; 1999; 202-208.
*Transmission in the child care setting by casual contact has not been documented.

Enteric diseases such as diarrhea in the child care setting are generally associated with close personal contact and poor hygiene. Hepatitis A is often asymptomatic in young children. Only about 10% of children <6 years of age with hepatitis A have symptoms, compared with about 50% of children 6 to 14 years of age and about 80% to 90% of persons >14 years of age, most of whom are adult contacts of asymptomatic younger children. Child care programs account for about 14% of identified sources of hepatitis A infection in the community. Hepatitis A in a parent or other family member of a child in day care may be the initial manifestation of an outbreak. Appropriate control measures include enhanced emphasis on handwashing, intramuscular administration of immune globulin, and active immunization with the hepatitis A vaccine. Major causes of outbreaks of diarrhea in child care centers include rotaviruses, enteric adenoviruses, astroviruses, caliciviruses, *Shigella*, *E. coli* O157:H7, *G. lamblia*, and *Cryptosporidium parvum*. Asymptomatic excretion (high for *Giardia*, rotavirus, and enteric adenovirus) is common, with newly enrolled children having an increased susceptibility. The most common causes of outbreaks of diarrhea are rotaviruses, other enteric viruses, and *G. lamblia*. The most worrisome causes of outbreaks are Shiga toxin–producing *E. coli* (STEC, notably *E. coli* O157:H7) and *Shigella* species because of the potential for complications, including the hemolytic-uremic syndrome. Cultures remain positive for *E. coli* O157:H7 for an average of 17 to 29 days (range 2 to 62 days), with up to 90% of children having positive cultures at 21 days.

Respiratory tract infections in child care settings include both invasive bacterial pathogens and viruses commonly prevalent in the community. The relative risk for acute otitis media among infants and toddlers in child care is 2 to 3.6 compared with those who remain at home. The relative risk for invasive pneumococcal disease is 10 to 36 compared with children who remain at home. During the winter months the carriage rate of drug-nonsusceptible *S. pneumoniae* is often 50% to 75% in child care settings. Contributing to this high rate of DNSSP carriage is the high use of antibiotics among children attending child care centers. Studies indicate that at any given time about 36% of children <3 years of age in child care centers are receiving antibiotics, compared with <10% of children <3 years of age who are in small- or large-family child care settings.

Bloodborne transmission of viruses can occur but is uncommon. Limited data indicate that the child who is a hepatitis B carrier poses minimal risk to other children, provided the infected child behaves normally and there are no risk factors for transmission of bloodborne agents. Such risk factors include biting behavior, frequent scratching, generalized dermatitis, and bleeding problems. The risk of transmission of HIV infection to children in the child care setting seems to be negligible even when biting behavior is present. However, and especially because the potential risk of transmission cannot be denied, admission of a child who is known to be either a hepatitis B carrier or HIV infected should be assessed by the child's physician and the program director, sometimes in consultation with public health authorities, if one or more potential risk factors for transmission of bloodborne agents is present.

Inclusion and Exclusion in Child Care Settings

Consensus recommendations for inclusion or exclusion in child care settings have been established by the AAP and the American Public Health Association (APHA) (Box 4-1). These

BOX 4-1
Consensus Recommendations for Exclusion from Child Care Settings

SYMPTOMS
- Illness that prevents the child from participating comfortably in program activities
- Illness that results in a greater need than the child care staff can provide without compromising the health and safety of the other children
- Any of the following conditions: fever, unusual lethargy, irritability, persistent crying, difficulty breathing, or other signs of possible severe illness
- Diarrhea (defined as an increased number of stools compared with the child's normal pattern, with increased stool water or decreased form), or stools that contain blood, mucus, *Escherichia coli* O157:H7, or *Shigella* species, until the diarrhea has resolved, *Shigella* infection has been adequately treated, or there have been two negative stool cultures
- Vomiting two or more times during the previous 24 hours, unless the vomiting is determined to be due to a noncommunicable condition and the child is not in danger of dehydration
- Mouth sores associated with an inability of the child to control his or her saliva, unless the child's physician or local health department authority states that the child is not infected
- Rash with fever or behavior change until a physician has determined that the illness is not due to a communicable disease

SPECIFIC DISEASES
- Purulent conjunctivitis (defined as pink or red conjunctiva with white or yellow eye discharge, often with matted eyelids after sleep and eye pain or redness of the eyelids or of the skin surrounding the eye), until examined by a physician or approved for readmission, with or without treatment
- Streptococcal pharyngitis, until 24 hours after treatment has been initiated
- Tuberculosis, until the child's physician or local health department authority states that the child is noninfectious
- Impetigo, until 24 hours after treatment has been initiated
- Ringworm, until the morning after therapy has been given
- Head lice (pediculosis), until the morning after the first treatment
- Pinworms, until the morning after therapy has been given
- Scabies, until after the treatment has been completed
- Varicella, until all the lesions have dried and crusted (usually 6 days)
- Pertussis, until 5 days of appropriate therapy has been completed (the total course of treatment is 14 days)
- Measles, until 4 days after the onset of rash
- Mumps, until 9 days after the onset of parotid gland swelling
- Hepatitis A infection, until 1 week after the onset of the illness or jaundice, provided symptoms are mild or until passive immunoprophylaxis (immune serum globulin) has been administered to appropriate children and staff in the program, as directed by the responsible health department

Modified from Wald ER. Infections in child care environments. In: Burg FD, Wald ER, Ingelfinger JR, et al., eds. Gellis & Kagan's Current Pediatrics Therapy. 16th ed., Philadelphia: W.B. Saunders Company; 1999; 202-208.

recommendations reflect both the potential for secondary cases and the understanding that children with moderate to severe illness are unable to participate in the usual activities and may require more individual attention than the staff can provide. When an outbreak of communicable disease has been identified in a child care setting, any child who is determined to be contributing to the transmission of the illness may have to be excluded until the risk is no longer present.

Medical conditions that permit inclusion of children in child care programs include (1) infections that have been adequately treated; (2) minor illnesses, including diarrhea, that are attributed to dietary changes or medication; (3) rash without fever or behavioral changes; (4) upper respiratory symptoms such as rhinorrhea or mild cough when fever is not present; (5) recurrent herpes simplex infection of mucous membranes or skin; (6) nonpurulent conjunctivitis (pink conjunctiva with a clear, watery discharge without fever, eye pain, or eyelid redness); (7) asymptomatic shedding of certain potential pathogens, including group A β-hemolytic streptococci, *Salmonella* species, CMV, *G. lamblia* (without diarrhea), chronic hepatitis B, HIV (provided the child exhibits safe behavior), and parvovirus B19 (erythema infectiosum, provided the child is immunocompetent); and (8) a positive tuberculin skin test without disease or provided effective treatment has been instituted and the child has been cleared by a physician.

 KEY POINTS

INFECTIONS RELATED TO OUT-OF-HOME CHILD CARE
- Children in child care centers are at increased risk of acute otitis media, diarrheal disease, and other common infections of early childhood.
- At a given time about 36% of children in child care centers may be taking antibiotics, which contributes to the high risk of carriage of drug-nonsusceptible *S. pneumoniae*.
- The differences in infection rates between children in child care centers and those who remain at home largely disappear after the child has been in a child care center for >3 years.
- Outbreaks of infectious disease in child care centers should be reported to public health authorities.
- Consensus recommendations for exclusion of children from child care centers have been issued by the AAP and the APHA.

SUGGESTED READING
American Academy of Pediatrics. Children in out-of-home child care. In: Pickering LK, ed. 2000 Red Book: Report of the Committee on Infectious Diseases. 25th ed. Elk Grove Village, IL: American Academy of Pediatrics; 2000: 105-119.

Churchill RB, Pickering LK. Infection control challenges in child care centers. Infect Dis Clin North Am 1997; 11: 347-365.

Donowitz LG, ed. Infection Control in the Child Care Center and Preschool. 4th ed., Philadelphia: Lippincott Williams and Wilkins, 1999.

Holmes SJ, Morrow AL, Pickering LK. Child care practices: effects of social changes on epidemiology of infectious diseases and antibiotic resistance. Epidemiol Rev 1996; 18: 10-28.

Pickering LK, ed. Infections in day care centers. Semin Pediatr Infect Dis 1990; 1: 181-292.

Robinson J. Infectious diseases in schools and childcare facilities. Pediatr Rev 2001; 22: 39-46.

Infectious Diseases in Immigrants and Foreign Adoptees

Each year about 15,000 internationally adopted children (16,339 in 1999) immigrate to the United States. About 90% of international adoptees now come from Asia (especially China, Korea, India, Cambodia, the Philippines, and Vietnam), Central and South America (especially Guatemala and Colombia), and Eastern Europe (especially Russia, Romania, and Ukraine). Approximately 50% of internationally adopted children now come from the former Soviet Union and Eastern Europe. About 250,000 immigrant children enter the United States each year, usually as relatives of persons already living in the United States; they come from the countries mentioned above and also from North America, especially Mexico. Any person entering the United States as a permanent resident must undergo a medical examination in the country of origin by a physician approved by the U.S. consul before an immigration visa is issued. However, this examination is usually limited to screening for serious physical and mental defects and for certain contagious diseases (syphilis, lymphogranuloma venereum, gonorrhea, chancroid, granuloma inguinale, HIV infection, active tuberculosis, and infectious leprosy) and is therefore not a comprehensive assessment of the child's health. HIV and syphilis serologic tests and chest x-ray examination are performed on applicants 15 years of age or older. For international adoptees there is no standardized examination; therefore documentation of the child's health varies considerably. Children applying for orphan visas must undergo the standard medical examination required for a visa. The only requirement for parents is an agreement that children <10 years of age become fully immunized after arrival in the United States.

As just described, the extent of medical evaluation and intervention before arrival in the United States differs between refugee children and internationally adopted children. Most refugees have undergone organized screening in camps. Serious diseases have usually been identified, and preventive health care has been initiated. However, most international adoptees have not undergone organized health screening. Adoptees' illnesses are often unidentified, and moreover, medical testing may be inaccurate or falsified and preventive health care may have been delayed. Thus medical evaluation of international adoptees is extremely variable and frequently unreliable.

Infectious diseases, often asymptomatic, are found in up to 60% of foreign adoptees, depending on the country of origin. These include the following:

- Bacterial diseases: tuberculosis, typhoid fever, melioidosis, leprosy, syphilis, and enteric infection by *Campylobacter, Salmonella, Shigella,* or *Yersinia* species
- Viral diseases: hepatitis A, B, C, and D; HIV; and CMV
- Protozoal diseases: amebiasis, giardiasis, toxoplasmosis, and malaria
- Helminth diseases: ascariasis, hookworm, schistosomiasis, strongyloidiasis, tapeworm (including cysticercosis), trichuriasis, filariasis, liver flukes, and lung flukes
- Arthropod diseases: lice and scabies

Other medical conditions include abnormalities of vision and hearing, nutritional deficiencies, growth and developmental retardation, and congenital anomalies.

Medical Assessment After Arrival in the United States

International adoptees should undergo thorough evaluation within 2 weeks of entering the United States. Although the likelihood of various infections depends largely on the country of origin, the following are recommended for all adopted and immigrant children:

- Hepatitis B serologic tests, including HBsAg, anti-HBs, and anti-HBc, irrespective of the results of screening tests in the country of origin

- HIV serologic tests, consisting of ELISA in children >18 months of age and both ELISA and HIV DNA PCR in children <18 months of age, irrespective of whether testing was done in the country of origin
- Tuberculin skin testing, consisting of 5 tuberculin units of purified protein derivative using the Mantoux intradermal test method (prior receipt of bacille Calmette-Guérin vaccine is not a contraindication, nor does it modify interpretation of the test result)
- Stool examination for ova and parasites (three specimens with at least 1 week between specimens, collected into containers with preservative if possible)
- Syphilis serologic tests (rapid plasma reagin or Venereal Disease Research Laboratory, irrespective of a laboratory report or history of treatment given in another country)
- Complete blood count with RBC indices
- Dipstick urinalysis
- Screening examinations for vision, hearing, and dental problems
- Developmental examination

Hepatitis C serologic testing is recommended for children from China, Russia, Eastern Europe, and Southeast Asia, as well as for children with a history of blood product transfusion, maternal injecting drug use, or elevated aminotransferase level. Some specific concerns are summarized in Table 4-6. Diseases such as typhoid fever, leprosy, melioidosis, filariasis, liver fluke infection, and malaria are encountered infrequently in foreign adoptees compared with refugee children. Routine screening for these diseases is not recommended. However, such findings as fever, splenomegaly, respiratory tract symptoms, anemia, or eosinophilia should prompt appropriate evaluation.

Immunization

According to new ACIP guidelines, reimmunization is usually the simplest approach for international adoptees from developing countries. When a question exists concerning whether vaccines were given or were immunogenic, the best course is usually to give them again. When adoptive parents are concerned about "extra injections," judicious use of serologic testing may clarify certain issues. Recent data indicate that many children coming to the United States from other countries lack protective antibody levels even when records indicate that they have received the vaccines. Vaccination records from such areas as Eastern Europe, Russia, and China, especially those pertaining to children who were in orphanages, may not accurately reflect protection because of unreliability of the records, lack of vaccine potency, or malnutrition. Guidelines specific for adoptees (as opposed to other immigrants) are published within the 2001 general recommendations for childhood immunizations in the CDC's *Morbidity and Mortality Weekly Report;* the recommendations include a table listing individual vaccines. International adoptees should receive vaccines according to schedules recommended for children born in the United States. Catch-up immunization schedules are published in the AAP *Red Book* and are also available at state and local health departments. In general, written records may be considered valid if the vaccines, date of administration, number of doses, intervals between doses, and age of the patient at the time of immunization are comparable to the current U.S. schedule. However, recent studies reveal that vaccination certificates may not necessarily equate to protection against diphtheria and tetanus.

TABLE 4-6
Some Infectious Diseases of Importance in Refugees and International Adoptees

Disease or infectious agent	Comments
Hepatitis B	The incubation period may be prolonged. Consideration should be given to a repeated evaluation 6 months after adoption. Children who are HbsAg positive should usually be evaluated by a specialist and should have an annual follow-up examination. Household contacts of children who are HbsAg positive should be immunized against hepatitis B virus.
Hepatitis C	Children infected with hepatitis C virus should usually be evaluated by a specialist. They should also be considered for hepatitis A vaccine and counseled about the need to avoid alcohol use during early adolescence, since alcohol use puts them at high risk for progression to cirrhosis.
Hepatitis D (delta agent)	Hepatitis D virus is found only in combination with hepatitis B. Any child who is HbsAg positive for 6 months should have a one-time screen for hepatitis D virus. Most children with hepatitis C virus originate from Eastern Europe, Africa, Mediterranean countries, South America, or the Middle East.
Cytomegalovirus	Cytomegalovirus is excreted by about one half of foreign adoptees. Adoptive parents should be counseled about cytomegalovirus with instructions on the importance of appropriate handwashing after contact with urine, diapers, and respiratory tract secretions. Adoptive mothers contemplating pregnancy after adoption should have their own cytomegalovirus immunity status determined (which is preferable to considering the foreign adoptee a possible source for infection).
HIV	As of 1998, most identified HIV-infected foreign adoptees had come from Russia, Romania, Cambodia, Vietnam, and Panama. Results of HIV antibody tests in the countries of origin should not be considered reliable.
Measles	Measles outbreaks in the United States are now nearly always traced to imported cases. Newly arrived foreign adoptees with fever and rash should be carefully evaluated. All immigrating children with measles should receive an injection of vitamin A because of the high rate of accompanying malnutrition.
Tuberculosis	The rates of tuberculosis in foreign adoptees are 8 to 13 times those in children born in the United States. The initial evaluation does not exclude tuberculosis, since the risk remains high for 5 years after arrival in the United States. If the child is asymptomatic and the Mantoux skin test is nonreactive, routine chest x-ray examination is not warranted. When there is a strong reason to suspect tuberculosis exposure but the Mantoux skin test shows <10 mm of induration, the Mantoux skin test should be repeated because a significant number of foreign adoptees exhibit anergy.
Syphilis	Children from tropical countries may have a false-positive rapid plasma reagin (or Venereal Disease Research Laboratory) test for syphilis because of another spirochetal disease such as yaws or pinta. Positive screening test results should be further evaluated with one of the treponemal tests (see Chapter 16).
Intestinal pathogens	Intestinal pathogens are identified in 15% to 35% of foreign adoptees. Since complete eradication does not always occur with therapy, children with enteric symptoms that develop months to years after adoption should be evaluated carefully for intestinal parasites.
Cysticercosis	Cysticercosis of the central nervous system may have a long incubation period. Unexplained neurologic symptoms or signs (e.g., focal nonfebrile seizures) should prompt evaluation (e.g., computed tomography or magnetic resonance imaging).
Malaria	Malaria should be suspected whenever unexplained high fever occurs in a child from a country known to be a site for malaria (see Chapter 24).

HIV, Human immunodeficiency virus.

 KEY POINTS

INFECTIOUS DISEASES IN IMMIGRANTS AND FOREIGN ADOPTEES

⊃ Most refugees have undergone organized screening in camps, with the result that serious infections have usually been identified and preventive health care has been initiated.

⊃ Most adoptees have not undergone organized screening. Medical illnesses are frequently unidentified, medical testing may be inaccurate or falsified, and preventive health care may be lacking.

⊃ Up to 60% of international adoptees are found to have infectious diseases, often asymptomatic.

⊃ All refugees and international adoptees should undergo systematic screening examinations.

⊃ Diseases such as hepatitis B, tuberculosis, and CNS cysticercosis may be come apparent only months to years after arrival in the United States.

⊃ Vaccination records pertaining to international adoptees are frequently unreliable.

⊃ When the immunization status of an international adoptee is in question, reimmunization using current U.S. schedules is nearly always the best course. Determination of antibody titers may be a reasonable alternative for selected children.

SUGGESTED READING

Albers LH, Johnson DE, Hostetter MK, et al. Health of children adopted from the former Soviet Union and Eastern Europe: comparison with preadoptive medical records. JAMA 1997; 278: 922-924.

American Academy of Pediatrics. Medical Evaluation of Internationally Adopted Children for Infectious Diseases. In: Pickering LD, ed. 2000 Red Book: Report of the Committee on Infectious Diseases. 25th ed. Elk Grove Village, Ill: American Academy of Pediatrics; 2000: 148-152.

Hostetter MK. Infectious diseases in internationally adopted children: findings in children from China, Russia, and Eastern Europe. Adv Pediatr Infect Dis 1999; 14: 147-161.

Talbot EA, Moore M, McCray E, et al. Tuberculosis among foreign-born persons in the United States, 1993-1998. JAMA 2000; 284: 2894-2900.

Children with Recurrent Infections

During the first 5 years of life, normal, healthy children experience an average of eight episodes of respiratory illnesses and one to two episodes of gastroenteritis annually. Between birth to 2 years of age, the number of otitis media episodes annually ranges from none to six. During the school years, the number of respiratory illnesses per year drops from six to eight in grade schoolers to four to five in adolescents. The numbers are increased for children in child care and those exposed to indoor air pollutants such as tobacco smoke. These data are helpful to the physician in dealing with parents' concerns about an "excessive" number of respiratory infections in their children.

The timing and approach to evaluating a child with recurrent infections should be determined only after the frequency, type, and duration of infections have been established and it has been decided that they probably are excessive and cannot be explained by reasons other than possible immunodeficiency. Once a breech in the host defense system is suspected as the cause of the recurrent infections, a systematic evaluation should be undertaken based on the most likely etiologies.

Nonimmunologic Causes

Involvement of a single organism suggests an anatomic defect or foreign body. Examples include recurrent urinary tract infection or repeated episodes of pneumonia involving the same lobe. Appropriate studies in these examples include imaging studies (ultrasonography and voiding cystourethrogram) and direct visualization (bronchoscopy).

Secondary Immunodeficiencies (see also Chapter 3)

Patients with underlying health problems are often susceptible to recurrent or chronic infections. These problems include malnutrition, malignancies, and HIV infection.

Primary Immunodeficiencies

Recognition of patients with primary immunodeficiency can be difficult, primarily because this condition is uncommon. Clues to possible diagnoses include characteristic clinical and laboratory presentations (e.g., recurrent *Candida* infection in Wiskott-Aldrich syndrome), infections with unusual organisms (e.g., *Serratia marcescens, Mycobacterium avium* complex), infections with encapsulated bacteria (e.g., *S. pneumoniae, N. meningitidis),* and recurrent or persistent pyogenic infections (e.g., *S. aureus, Aspergillus* species).

Evaluating Patients with Recurrent Infections (see also Chapter 3)

Before launching into an exhaustive workup for recurrent infections, the practitioner must be careful to ascertain reasons other than host defense aberrations for frequent infections (e.g., patients with recurrent lower respiratory tract infections should be evaluated for cystic fibrosis or chronic aspiration). Immunodeficiencies should be suspected in the following situations:

■ Unusual organisms cause infections (*S. marcescens* in suppurative lymphadenitis).

■ Infections are caused by organisms usually of low pathogenicity.

■ Infections are unusually severe or protracted or frequent.

■ Infections recur multiple times after appropriate therapy (staphylococcal abscesses in chronic granulomatous disease of childhood).

■ Infections are unusual for age (thrush in an older child or adolescent).

■ Infections usual for age are associated with unusual complications.

■ Infections occur at multiple body sites.

Physical findings that raise the possibility of immunodeficiency include the following:

■ Failure to thrive or small size for age

■ Absence or paucity of lymphoid tissue

■ Chronic, unexplained dermatitis (i.e., eczema)

■ Chronic periodontal disease

Typical clinical presentations of the primary immunodeficiency disorders, which nearly always become apparent during childhood, are as follows:

■ B-lymphocyte disorders (impaired humoral immunity): recurrent sinopulmonary infections, recurrent sepsis, CNS infection, and malabsorption (pathogens include *S. pneumoniae, H. influenzae, S. aureus,* enteroviruses, and the oral polio vaccine)

■ T-lymphocyte disorders (impaired cell-mediated immunity): persistent thrush, chronic diarrhea, chronic or recurrent skin and mucous membrane infections, recurrent respiratory disease, recurrent sepsis, and failure to thrive (pathogens include certain intracellular bacteria, DNA viruses, mycobacteria, fungi, or parasites)

■ Complement disorders: infections caused by encapsulated bacteria (especially *S. pneumoniae, H. influenzae,* and *N. meningitidis*) and also autoimmune disorders

■ Phagocytic disorders (impaired PMN function): abscesses involving the skin and various internal organs, mouth ulcers, and delayed response to antimicrobial therapy (pathogens include *S. aureus;* gram-negative bacilli such as *S. marcescens, Pseudomonas aeruginosa,* and *Klebsiella* species; and *Aspergillus* species; some infections are polymicrobial)

Although patients with suspected immunologic disorders are often referred to an immunologist, the primary care physician can initiate certain screening laboratory tests (see Table 3-3).

SUGGESTED READING

Fischer A. Primary immunodeficiency diseases: an experimental model for molecular medicine. Lancet 2001; 357: 1863-1869.

Fleisher TA, Ballow M, eds. Primary immune deficiencies: presentation, diagnosis, and management. Pediatr Clin North Am 2000; 6: 1197-1446.

Lekstrom-Himes JA, Gallin JI. Immunodeficiency diseases caused by defects in phagocytes. N Engl J Med 2000; 343: 1703-1714.

Owayed AF, Campbell DM, Wang EE. Underlying causes of recurrent pneumonia in children. Arch Pediatr Adolesc Med 2000; 154:190-194.

Puck JM. Primary immunodeficiency diseases. JAMA 1997; 278: 1835-1841.

Human Immunodeficiency Virus Infection in Children

HIV is now one of the most common causes of immunodeficiency in children. First reported in 1982, AIDS had by 1997 become the 11th leading cause of death in U.S. children 1 to 4 years of age.

In recent years the knowledge of the pathogenesis of pediatric HIV infections, its natural history, and its treatment (role of viral load as a marker of disease progression and the clinical use of antiretroviral agents for management of HIV-infected children and pregnant women) has advanced considerably. In the United States HIV infection has evolved from a rapidly progressive, fatal disease to a chronic lifelong infection in which a moderately effective therapy prolongs survival. Many affected children now survive into adolescence, and the long-term prognosis for at least some of these children may be good with highly active antiretroviral therapy (HAART). However, HIV disease is in general more aggressive in children than in adults. Children are likely to have impaired growth, lethal *P. carinii* pneumonia (PCP), and CNS disease. In about one fourth of children born with HIV infection, AIDS-defining disease develops within the first year of life. Other children have a slower progression to AIDS (mean time to AIDS >5 years). The management of HIV infection has been dramatically altered with the development of HAART, measurement of viral load, and availability of prophylactic medications to prevent select opportunistic infections. A total of 16 antiretroviral agents have been approved by the U.S. Food and Drug Administration, 11 of which have been approved for use in pediatrics.

The pathogenesis of HIV infection and the general virologic and immunologic principles underlying the use of antiretroviral therapy are similar for all HIV-infected patients (see Chapter 17). Unique considerations in pediatrics include the following:

- Infection acquired through perinatal exposure
- In utero exposure to AZT and other antiretroviral medications in many perinatally infected children
- Differences in the diagnostic evaluation of perinatal infection, based in large measure on the presence of maternally derived antibodies
- Differences in the interpretation of immunologic markers (Table 4-7)

- Changes in pharmacokinetic parameters with age, brought about by the continuing development and maturation of organ systems involved in drug metabolism and clearance
- Differences in the clinical and virologic manifestations of perinatal HIV infection related to the occurrence of primary infection in growing, immunologically immature persons
- Special considerations associated with adherence to complicated drug regimens in children and adolescents

Management of pediatric HIV infection is rapidly evolving and increasingly complex. Whenever possible, management should be directed by a physician whose primary interest lies in this area. If this is not possible, such experts should be consulted regularly. Updated guidelines issued by the Working Group on Antiretroviral Therapy and Medical Management of HIV-Infected Children, convened by the National Pediatric and Family HIV Resource Center, the Health Resources and Service Administration, and the National Institutes of Health, can be obtained at the HIV/AIDS Treatment Information Service Website (http://www.hivatis.org).

Reduction of Perinatal HIV Transmission (see also Chapter 17)

About 25% to 30% of perinatal transmissions occur during gestation (in utero), about 70% to 75% occur during delivery, and some cases result from breast-feeding. In the absence of preventive therapy, the risk of transmission from an HIV-infected mother to a non–breast-fed infant in the United States is about 25%. Maternal risk factors for vertical transmission include failure to receive AZT preventive therapy, prolonged rupture of membranes, vaginal delivery, low birth weight or prematurity, chorioamnionitis or placental inflammation, firstborn twins, maternal injecting drug use, bloody amniotic fluid, breast-feeding, and maternal AIDS or advanced HIV infection as defined by a low CD4 lymphocyte count and a high plasma viral load. The risk of vertical transmission can be reduced by these measures:

- AZT therapy given before delivery (shown to reduce transmission from 25% to 8% in a large-scale trial; later observational studies suggest reduction of transmission to as low as 4% to 5%)
- Delivery by elective cesarean section before rupture of membranes and onset of labor (shown to reduce transmission to 1% to 2% if the mother also received antiretroviral therapy; however, cesarean section is recommended only when obstetrically indicated)
- Aggressive HAART therapy for pregnant women (recent data indicate that perinatal transmission among women with undetectable plasma viral loads is <1%)

Pregnancy should not preclude the use of optimal combination antiretroviral therapy. Indeed, combination therapy (HAART) should be given during pregnancy, labor, and delivery. Current categories for use in pregnancy are as follows (see Chapter 5 for definition of categories):

- Category B: didanosine, saquinavir, ritonavir, and nelfinavir
- Category C: most of the remaining antiretrovirals, including efavirenz (which is best avoided because it has caused birth defects in primates)
- Category D: hydroxyurea (cytotoxic and therefore contraindicated)

The three-part AZT regimen reported in 1994 by the Pediatric AIDS Clinical Trials Group (Protocol 076) is as follows:

TABLE 4-7

Immunologic Categories of Human Immunodeficiency Virus Infection in Children Less Than 13 Years of Age Based on Age-Related CD4 Lymphocyte Counts and Percentage of Total Lymphocytes*

	AGE OF CHILD					
	<12 MONTHS		1-5 YEARS		6-12 YEARS	
Immunologic category	CD4/mm³	Percent†	CD4/mm³	Percent†	CD4/mm³	Percent†
1. No evidence of immunosuppression	≥1500	≥25	≥1000	≥25	≥500	≥25
2. Evidence of moderate immunosuppression	750-1499	15-24	500-999	15-24	200-499	15-24
3. Severe immunosuppression	<750	<15	<500	<15	<200	<15

From Centers for Disease Control and Prevention. 1994 revised classification system for human immunodeficiency virus infection in children less than 13 years of age. MMWR 1994; 43 (RR-12): 1-10.

*Immunologic categories (1, 2, and 3) are based on the CD4 count and percentage, as shown here. Clinical categories are as follows:
- Category N: asymptomatic (no signs or symptoms attributed to HIV infection, or only one of the conditions listed below in category A).
- Category A: mildly symptomatic (two or more of the following conditions, but none of the conditions listed in category B and no AIDS-defining condition): lymphadenopathy [nodes ≥0.5 cm at more than two sites, bilateral lymphadenopathy being considered as a single site], hepatomegaly, splenomegaly, dermatitis, parotitis, or recurrent or persistent upper respiratory tract infection, sinusitis, or otitis media).
- Category B: moderately symptomatic (for example, any of the following conditions: anemia [hemoglobin <8 g/dL], neutropenia [WBC <1000/mm³]; or thrombocytopenia [<100,000/mm³] persisting ≥30 days); bacterial meningitis, pneumonia, or sepsis (single episode); oropharyngeal candidiasis (thrush) persisting >2 months in children >6 months of age; cardiomyopathy; cytomegalovirus infection with onset before 1 month of age; recurrent or chronic diarrhea; hepatitis; recurrent herpes simplex virus (HSV) stomatitis (more than two episodes within 1 year); HSV bronchitis, pneumonitis, or esophagitis with onset before 1 month of age; herpes zoster (shingles) involving at least two distinct episodes or more than one dermatome; leiomyosarcoma; lymphoid interstitial pneumonia or pulmonary lymphoid hyperplasia complex; nephropathy; nocardiosis; persistent fever lasting >1 month; toxoplasmosis with onset before 1 month of age; and disseminated varicella (complicated chickenpox).
- Category C: severely symptomatic (patients with an acquired immunodeficiency syndrome (AIDS)-defining condition, as given in the 1987 CDC surveillance case definition for AIDS in children, with the exception of lymphoid interstitial pneumonia (which is a category B condition).

The immunologic and clinical categories are then combined. For example, a patient is 1-N if the CD4 count is normal and there are no symptoms, while a patient is 3-C if the CD4 count is extremely low and severe symptoms and signs of AIDS are present.

†CD4⁺ lymphocytes as a percentage of the total lymphocyte count.

(1) antepartum AZT beginning after 14 weeks' gestation (100 mg 5 times daily; alternative regimens are 200 mg t.i.d. or 300 mg b.i.d.) and continuing until onset of labor; (2) intrapartum AZT given IV (2 mg/kg loading dose over 1 hour followed by 1 mg/kg/hour by IV infusion until delivery); and (3) postpartum AZT given to the newborn infant, 2 mg/kg every 6 hours and given as a syrup, beginning within 8 to 12 hours of birth. AZT is given to the infant for 6 weeks if the HIV DNA PCR test on the infant is negative. The dose of AZT is adjusted for weight gain, as needed, and the infant's hematocrit is determined at baseline, at 4 weeks, at completion of AZT therapy, and at 3 months of age. If the infant cannot tolerate AZT by the oral route, IV therapy (1.5 mg/kg every 6 hours) can be used. Doses recommended for premature infants vary, and a specialist should be consulted. *AZT should be offered for all newborns if exposure is recognized before 7 days of age even if their mothers did not receive AZT.*

For women receiving antiretroviral therapy ante partum or before pregnancy, adding or substituting AZT should be considered if this drug is not part of the regimen. AZT and d4T should not be given concomitantly. AZT prophylaxis alone is recommended for the occasional woman who, although HIV infected, has a normal CD4 lymphocyte count and a low or undetectable viral load and who therefore does not require

therapy. Various regimens alternative to the standard AZT regimen described have been evaluated for HIV-infected women who are in labor and have not received antiretroviral therapy. To date, none of these regimens has been shown to be superior to the standard AZT regimen. Regimens that have been studied include nevirapine and lamivudine (3TC). Clinicians treating HIV-infected pregnant women are encouraged to report their data to a confidential national registry kept for this purpose: Antiretroviral Pregnancy Registry, 1410 Commonwealth Drive, Wilmington, NC (telephone 1-800-258-4263; fax 1-800-800-1052).

Diagnosis of HIV Infection in Children and Management of a Child Born to an HIV-Infected Mother

A child <18 months of age is considered to be infected if positive results are obtained on two separate occasions (excluding cord blood) from one or more of the following HIV detection tests: HIV culture; HIV PCR (DNA detection is recommended as the virologic method of choice; RNA detection seems to have equal or superior sensitivity and specificity, but data are limited regarding its use for diagnostic purposes); or HIV p24 antigen test (in a child ≥1 month of age). A child <18 months of age is also considered to infected if he or she meets the criteria for AIDS based on the 1987 surveillance case definition.

A child ≥18 months of age is considered to be infected if shown to be HIV antibody positive by repeated reactive enzyme immunoassay (EIA) and a confirmatory test (e.g., Western blot or immunofluorescence assay), or if he or she meets any of the test criteria for a child <18 months of age.

A perinatally exposed child is defined as one who was born to an HIV-infected mother but who does not meet the preceding criteria, even if seropositive by EIA and a confirmatory test during the first 18 months of life (since these test results could reflect maternally derived antibodies), or one whose HIV antibody test results are unknown.

A seroreverter is a child, born to a mother known to be HIV infected, who has been documented as HIV antibody negative (by two or more negative EIA tests performed at 6 to 18 months of age or by one negative EIA test after 18 months of age), *or* who has no other laboratory evidence of infection *and* who has not had an AIDS-defining condition.

Management of an infant born to an HIV-infected mother should ideally include consultation with a specialist in pediatric HIV disease. Components include the following:

- At birth, obtain a CBC and HIV DNA PCR while initiating AZT therapy. If the mother's treatment regimen included a protease inhibitor, additional laboratory studies should include a differential blood count and measurement of bilirubin, alanine aminotransferase, and plasma glucose. The perinatally exposed child is at risk for other potential infections, including hepatitis B, hepatitis C, CMV, syphilis, tuberculosis, gonorrhea, and *C. trachomatis* infection.
- During the early neonatal period evaluate for complications of prematurity, feeding intolerance, poor weight gain, drug withdrawal syndrome, developmental delay, and inconsistent care provision resulting from demands on the mother's health needs.
- At 2 to 3 weeks of age, obtain CBC and HIV DNA PCR (especially if not done at birth)
- At 6 weeks of age, obtain a CBC and HIV DNA PCR. If the HIV DNA PCR test is negative, discontinue AZT. If the child is HIV infected or if the HIV status is indeterminate, start PCP prophylaxis with TMP/SMX, 75 mg/m² of body surface area per dose b.i.d. (based on the TMP component) 3 times per week (Monday, Wednesday, and Friday), continuing through at least 12 months of age. Treatment can be discontinued if the child is shown convincingly to be uninfected.
- At 4 months of age, obtain CBC, HIV DNA PCR, and quantitative immunoglobulin levels (IgG, IgA, IgM); consider quantitation of CD4 lymphocyte subsets (e.g., CD4$^+$ and CD8$^+$ lymphocytes).
- At 12 months of age, and again at 18 months of age, obtain HIV antibody tests if the patient is uninfected or is of antibody-indeterminate status in order to document the disappearance of maternally derived antibody.

HIV infection is reasonably excluded by two or more negative virologic tests, provided two of the tests are performed at age ≥1 month, with at least one performed at ≥4 months of age. Two or more negative HIV immunoglobulin G (IgG) antibody tests performed at age ≥6 months with an interval of at least 1 month between the tests reasonably excludes HIV infection among children with no clinical evidence of HIV infection. HIV infection can be definitively excluded if HIV IgG antibody is negative in the absence of hypogammaglobulinemia at age 18 months and if the child has no clinical symptoms of HIV infection and negative HIV virologic assays.

Clinical Manifestations, Treatment, and Management of HIV Infection in Children

The CDC classification system for children <13 years of age outlines various categories based on immunologic status (Table 4-7), infections, and clinical status. Clinical manifestations most typically seen early in HIV-infected infants include oral candidiasis, hematologic abnormalities, hepatomegaly, splenomegaly, generalized lymphadenopathy, and a subtle growth delay. Sinusitis and otitis media tend to recur or persist, whereas viral respiratory infections are more often symptomatic, severe, and prolonged. As immune function wanes, advanced HIV disease develops and AIDS-defining opportunistic infections and malignancies begin to occur. Manifestations include failure to thrive; recurrent and severe bacterial infection; *P. carinii* pneumonia (the most common AIDS-defining opportunistic infection in North America and Europe); other opportunistic infections, including those caused by DNA viruses, fungi, mycobacteria, and parasites; recurrent or persistent diarrhea; hepatitis; CNS disease, including developmental delay that can be progressive; persistent unexplained fever; lymphoid interstitial pneumonitis; parotitis; and lymphomas. The more rapid progression of HIV in children compared with adults is explained, at least in part, by the immaturity of the neonatal immune system. About 20% to 25% of children with HIV infection are classified as "rapid progressors" on the basis of onset of HIV-related symptoms within the first year of life. The remaining children are "slow progressors," in whom, however, symptoms usually appear by 4 to 6 years of age. The HIV viral load (see Chapter 17) after the first month of life correlates with the rapidity of disease progression.

Criteria for initiation of antiretroviral therapy, which are continuing to evolve, include the following:

- All HIV-infected infants <12 months of age should be treated, irrespective of immunologic, virologic, or clinical status.
- All HIV-infected infants and children with evidence of immune suppression, as indicated by the CD4$^+$ lymphocyte count or percentage (Table 4-7), should be treated.
- All children with clinical symptoms related to HIV infection should be treated.

Treatment should also be considered in HIV-infected children >1 year of age who are asymptomatic and who have normal immune status. Recommendations for specific antiretroviral regimens continue to updated on the basis of new drugs and results of ongoing clinical trials (for the most recent recommendations, refer to http://www.hivatis.org).

Combination therapy with three or more drugs is the current standard of care. Adherence to prescribed schedules is critical. The duration of response is short when the patient misses even 20% to 25% of doses. Effective therapy should reduce the viral load to an undetectable level, accompanied by good growth and development with absence of HIV-related complications. Monitoring of treatment involves evaluation at least every 3 months, to include clinical assessment, immune status (CD4 count), viral load, and evidence of drug toxicity.

Immunization recommendations for children with known or suspected HIV disease include the following:

- Inactivated vaccines as scheduled for routine immunization (Figure 4-1)

- Inactivated polio vaccine (IPV) rather than OPV for both patients and also for household contacts
- Yearly influenza immunization before the influenza season, beginning as early as 6 months of age
- Pneumococcal conjugate vaccine, as recommended in Figure 4-1, and also Pneumovax at 2 and 5 years of age
- Measles-mumps-rubella (MMR) vaccine, as determined by the degree of immunosuppression, as shown in Table 4-7. The child is a candidate for MMR vaccination if asymptomatic (class M) or mildly symptomatic (class A) with no evidence of immunosuppression (category 1) or evidence of moderate immunosuppression (category 2). Immunization is initiated at 12 months of age with a second dose as soon as 1 month later to ensure early conversion

Varicella vaccine should be considered for class N1 or A1 (Table 4-7) and with CD4 lymphocyte counts $\geq$25% of total lymphocytes; two doses are given 3 months apart.

KEY POINTS

HUMAN IMMUNODEFICIENCY VIRUS INFECTION IN CHILDREN

- ➲ HIV is now one of the most common causes of severe immunodeficiency in children. In 1997, HIV was the 11th leading cause of death in the United States in children between 1 and 4 years of age.
- ➲ HIV is a more aggressive disease in children than in adults, at least in part because of the immaturity of the neonatal immune system.
- ➲ The risk of perinatal transmission from an HIV-infected mother to her infant is about 25% unless preventive therapy is given. Preventive therapy with a standard AZT protocol reduces transmission to 8% or lower. Highly active antiretroviral therapy (HAART) that reduces the mother's viral load to an undetectable level reduces the risk of transmission to <1%.

- ➲ Infants born to HIV-infected mothers should be monitored for evidence of infection through 18 months of age, since maternally derived antibodies make serologic diagnosis difficult. The HIV DNA PCR test helps determine the infant's need for antiretroviral therapy.
- ➲ Consultation with a specialist in pediatric HIV disease is advised for all infants born of HIV-infected mothers and for all infants and children shown to have HIV infection.
- ➲ Updated recommendations for perinatal prophylaxis against HIV transmission and also for HIV treatment regimens can be obtained from the Working Group on Antiretroviral Therapy and Medical Management of HIV-infected Children at http://www./hivatis.org.

SUGGESTED READING

American Academy of Pediatrics. Pediatric HIV Infection: A Compendium of AAP Guidelines on Pediatric HIV infection. Elk Grove, Ill: American Academy of Pediatrics; 1999.

Centers for Disease Control and Prevention. Report of the NIH Panel to Define Principles of Therapy of HIV Infection. Guidelines for the use of antiretroviral agents in pediatric HIV infection. MMWR 1998; 47 (RR-4): 1-43 (updated at http://www.hivatis.org).

Centers for Disease Control and Prevention. Revised recommendations for HIV screening of pregnant women. MMWR 2001; 50 (RR-19): 59-86.

Gortmaker Sl, Hughes M, Cervia J, et al. Effect of combination therapy including protease inhibitors on mortality among children and adolescents inflected with HIV-1. New Eng J Med 2001; 345: 1522-1528.

Mayer KH, ed. HIV/AIDS 2000. Infect Dis Clin North Am 2000; 14: 791-1032.

Rogers MF, ed. HIV/AIDS in infants, children, and adolescents. Pediatr Clin North Am 2000; 47: 1-267.

Working Group on Antiretroviral Therapy and Medical Management of Infants, Children and Adolescents with HIV Infection. Antiretroviral therapy and medical management of pediatric HIV infection and 1997 USPHS/IDSA report on the prevention of opportunistic infections in persons infected with the human immunodeficiency virus. Pediatrics 1998; 102: 999-1085.

5 Special Issues in Obstetrics

JULIE Y. LO, JEANNE S. SHEFFIELD, SUSAN M. COX

The extent to which primary care clinicians assume responsibility for pregnant patients varies considerably, but all primary care clinicians should be familiar with certain principles. Women of childbearing age, especially those who are not in monogamous relationships, should be counseled regularly about sexual and reproductive hygiene. They should be encouraged to report any symptoms suggestive of sexually transmitted disease (STD; see Chapter 16). Low-grade or subclinical gonococcal and chlamydial infection can damage the fallopian tubes, causing infertility or tubal pregnancy. Chlamydial infection is of great concern as a "silent epidemic" of infertility. Current recommendations of the Centers for Disease Control and Prevention (CDC) include screening for *Chlamydia trachomatis* at least annually for all sexually active females under 20 years of age and annual screening of women 20 years or older with one or more risk factors for *Chlamydia,* such as new or multiple sex partners and lack of barrier contraception. Syphilis, human immunodeficiency virus (HIV) infection, and genital herpes simplex virus infection can be devastating to the fetus and newborn. All women of childbearing age should also be immunized against rubella and varicella (see Chapter 25) if they have not been naturally infected with these viruses. In this chapter we present an overview of prevention and management of infections during pregnancy and also an in-depth discussion of three infections: urinary tract infection (UTI), chorioamnionitis, and endometritis.

SUGGESTED READING

Faro S, Soper D, eds. Infectious Diseases in Women. Philadelphia: W.B. Saunders Company; 2000.
Gilstrap LC, Faro S, eds. Infections in Pregnancy. New York: Wiley-Liss; 1990.
Tuomala RE, Cox SM, eds. Infections in obstetrics. Infect Dis Clin North Am 1997; 11:1-244.

Screening

Preconception Screening

The optimal time to assess, manage, and treat potential pregnancy complications is before conception. Knowledge of a woman's prior infectious diseases can assist in the prevention of various congenital infections by providing information about her immune status and the need for vaccination or appropriate medical therapy. Vaccines are available for rubella, hepatitis B, and varicella. Preconception treatment of HIV, tuberculosis, and infections caused by *Neisseria gonorrhoeae, C. trachomatis,* and *Treponema pallidum* is optimal for preventing or decreasing complications during pregnancy. In addition, cytomegalovirus and toxoplasmosis screening may be indicated so the patient can be advised to avoid particular risk factors for the respective disease processes.

Prenatal Screening

All patients receiving routine prenatal care should have certain basic laboratory tests:
- Urine culture
- Serologic tests: rubella titer, serologic test for syphilis (rapid plasmin reagin [RPR]), hepatitis B surface antigen (HBsAg), and HIV antibody test (enzyme-linked immunosorbent assay [ELISA], with Western blot confirmation if reactive)
- Screening tests for *N. gonorrhoeae* and *C. trachomatis* (cervix), using culture or nonculture methods

Documented HIV infection, injecting drug use, or unusual travel history warrants additional screening laboratory tests, discussed later in the chapter.

SUGGESTED READING

American Academy of Pediatrics and American College of Obstetricians and Gynecologists. Guidelines for Perinatal Care, 4th ed., Washington, DC: American College of Obstetricians and Gynecologists; 1997: 207-249.

American College of Obstetricians and Gynecologists. Gonorrhea and chlamydial screening. Tech Bull No. 190; March 1994.

Use of Antimicrobials During Pregnancy and Nursing

Recommendations for drug use in pregnancy generally are based on five categories defined in 1979 by the U.S. Food and Drug Administration (FDA; Table 5-1). All antimicrobial agents cross the fetoplacental barrier to some extent. None of the currently available antimicrobial agents are considered to be entirely safe in pregnancy (i.e., in category A) on the basis of large-scale, well-controlled clinical trials. The β-lactam antibiotics (penicillins, cephalosporins, and others with the apparent exception of ticarcillin) and erythromycin (other than the estolate form, which should not be used during pregnancy) are usually considered the safest drugs during all stages of pregnancy. Metronidazole (Flagyl) can be used with reasonable safety during the later stages of pregnancy but is potentially teratogenic during the first trimester. The sulfonamides can be used with reasonable safety during the early stages of pregnancy, but their use should be avoided at term because of risk of jaundice and hemolytic anemia in the newborn. Trimethoprim-sulfamethoxazole (Bactrim, Septra, and others), although widely used for treatment of UTI, should be avoided if possible during pregnancy. Tetracyclines should seldom if ever be used during pregnancy because of their effect on developing bones and teeth. Despite the numerous uncertainties and potential toxicities associated with the use of antimicrobial agents during pregnancy, most patients can be treated with reasonable safety using currently available drugs. Examples in which pregnancy limits the choices are syphilis in a penicillin-allergic patient and Rocky Mountain spotted fever. In the former situation, desensitization to penicillin G in the hospital setting is often required. For Rocky Mountain spotted fever during pregnancy, chloramphenicol is generally preferred to spare the fetus the toxicity of tetracycline on bones and teeth; however, doxycycline would be preferred near term to avoid the "gray baby" syndrome caused by chloramphenicol.

Nearly all antimicrobials are secreted into breast milk in measurable quantities. In theory this exposure could cause the neonate to be sensitized; however, this possibility remains largely unproved. Sulfonamides should not be given to mothers who are nursing premature infants, since even small amounts of the drug can displace enough bilirubin from albumin-binding sites to cause kernicterus. The sulfonamides and nalidixic acid, if given to infants with G6PD deficiency, can cause hemolysis. Tetracyclines appear to be safe for nursing mothers, since calcium in breast milk binds to the tetracyclines to form a chelate that will not be absorbed by the infant's gastrointestinal tract.

SUGGESTED READING

Briggs GG, Freeman RK, Yaffe SJ. Drugs in Pregnancy and Lactation. 5th ed., Baltimore: Williams & Wilkins; 1998.

Gilstrap LC III, Little BB, eds. Drugs and Pregnancy. 2nd ed., New York: Chapman & Hall; 1998.

Vaginitis in Pregnancy

The most common complaint that prompts women to seek medical attention is vulvovaginitis (for in-depth discussion, see Chapter 16). Fortunately, the etiologic agents responsible for vulvovaginitis can commonly be identified in the office or clinic setting by microscopic examination.

Candida Vulvovaginitis During Pregnancy

Pregnancy predisposes to vulvovaginal candidiasis (VVC) by several mechanisms, including increased vaginal glycogen content. Imidazole preparations are currently the mainstay of therapy. These include miconazole (Monistat), clotrimazole (Gyne-Lotrimin or Mycelex G), butoconazole (Femstat), tioconazole (Vagistat), and ketoconazole (Nizoral). Miconazole has been shown to be superior to nystatin for treatment of VVC during pregnancy. VVC seldom affects the fetus adversely, although there have been rare cases of acute chorioretinitis and intraamniotic infection caused by *Candida albicans*. Occasionally, oropharyngeal candidiasis is identified in the newborn and is thought to be due to colonization of the newborn's alimentary tract during passage through the birth canal. The attack rate for such candidiasis has been estimated to be as high as 50%, but this infection is rarely identified in the nursery.

Trichomoniasis in Pregnancy

Trichomonas vaginalis is usually a sexually transmitted pathogen. Trichomoniasis has no unique association with pregnancy, but trichomoniasis is sufficiently common (20% of all women during their lifetimes) that the condition is frequently seen during pregnancy. The standard treatment is metronidazole, either 2 g PO as a single dose or 500 mg PO b.i.d. for 5 to 7 days. Metronidazole is an FDA category B drug and has no reported teratogenic effects. However, many clinicians avoid prescribing metronidazole during the first trimester because of theoretical concerns about teratogenicity. To prevent reinfection, treatment of all sexual partners is highly recommended. Trichomoniasis is prevented through abstinence or practice of safe sex methods, using a latex condom each time intercourse occurs and with every partner. Importantly, a woman should limit her number of sexual partners to avoid reinfection with trichomoniasis, as well as other STDs. Cases of trichomoniasis clinically resistant to metronidazole have been reported (see Chapter 16). Treatment of such cases remains problematic, and unfortunately, no alternative therapies are available.

Occasionally trichomoniasis is passed on to an infant at the time of birth. The infant will have fever, and vaginal infection may develop in young girls who were infected at birth. In isolated reports *Trichomonas* has been associated with abortion, preterm labor, and premature rupture of the membranes, although a causative relationship has not been proved. In a recent multicenter, placebo-controlled trial of 617 asymptomatic women with *T. vaginalis* (identified on cultures at 16 to 32 weeks), treatment with metronidazole actually increased the risk of preterm birth. Thus screening for asymptomatic infection is *not* recommended.

Text continued on p.93

TABLE 5-1
Safety of Antimicrobial Agents During Pregnancy

Category	Drug	Comments
A (considered safe on the basis of controlled studies in humans)	None	
B (considered reasonably safe on the basis of little or no demonstrated fetal risk in humans and animals)	**ANTIBACTERIAL DRUGS**	
	Ampicillin-sulbactam (Unasyn)	
	Azithromycin (Zithromax)	Harmless in animals; inadequate data in humans.
	Aztreonam (Azactam)	Harmless in animals except at very high doses; caution in use advised during pregnancy.
	Cephalosporins	Harmless in animals; inadequate data in humans with some of the newer drugs.
	Clindamycin	No apparent risk in humans on basis of extensive experience. Use with caution.
	Erythromycins (other than the estolate preparation)	Erythromycin estolate can cause hepatotoxicity during pregnancy. Use only when clearly indicated.
	Meropenem (Merrem)	Harmless in animals. Use only when clearly indicated.
However,	Metronidazole (Flagyl)	In animal studies, fetal toxicity has been associated with parenteral use. There is no clear evidence of teratogenicity in humans. because of the theoretic risk of teratogenicity, many clinicians prefer to avoid prescribing metronidazole during the first trimester.
	Nitrofurantoin (Macrodantin)	*Contraindicated near term;* can cause hemolytic anemia in neonates; also causes hemolytic anemia in patients with G6PD deficiency.
	Penicillins (including preparations with clavulanic acid)	Harmless in animals.
	Piperacillin-tazobactam (Zosyn)	
	Rifabutin (Mycobutin)	
	Ticarcillin-clavulanate (Timentin)	Although Timentin is considered category B, there is possible evidence that ticarcillin may be teratogenic.
	ANTIFUNGAL DRUGS	
	Amphotericin B	Harmless in animals.
	Clotrimazole	
	Nystatin	
	ANTIVIRAL DRUGS OTHER THAN ANTIRETROVIRALS	
	Famciclovir (Famvir)	Some teratogenicity in animals at high doses; use only when clearly indicated.
	Valacyclovir (Valtrex)	No teratogenicity in animals.

Continued

TABLE 5-1—cont'd
Safety of Antimicrobial Agents During Pregnancy

Category	Drug	Comments
	ANTIRETROVIRAL DRUGS	
	Didanosine (DDI; Videx)	No teratogenicity in animals; use only when clearly indicated.
	Nelfinavir (Viracept)	No teratogenicity in animals; use only when clearly indicated.
	Ritonavir (Norvir)	No teratogenicity in animals; use only when clearly indicated.
	Saquinavir (Invirase; Fortovase)	No teratogenicity in animals; use only when clearly indicated.
	ANTIPARASITIC DRUGS	
	Niclosamide	Harmless in animals.
	Praziquantel (Biltricide)	Generally harmless in animals but increased abortion rates.
Category C (use with caution during pregnancy and only when the need justifies the risk; evidence of toxicity in animals, and inadequate data regarding humans)	**ANTIBACTERIAL DRUGS**	
	Clarithromycin (Biaxin)	Teratogenicity in animals.
	Dapsone	No adverse effects are reported, but use with caution.
	Gentamicin	*Use only for life-threatening infections.*
	Imipenem-cilastatin (Primaxin)	*Use only for life-threatening infections.*
	Quinolones (Cipro, Levaquin, many others)	*Generally contraindicated during pregnancy.* Arthropathy has developed in immature animals, with erosion of the joint cartilage.
	Rifampin (Rifadin)	
	Sulfonamides	*Avoid during the last trimester (risk of hemolytic anemia and jaundice) and use with caution during other stages.* Little toxicity has been shown during second and third trimesters with extensive use. High doses in animals have caused cleft palate and bone abnormalities.
	Ticarcillin (Ticar)	Ticarcillin has been shown to be teratogenic in rodents.
	Trimethoprim (Proloprim)	*Use with caution if at all during pregnancy because of effect on folic acid metabolism.* Teratogenic in animals at doses 40 times the usual human dose.
	Trimethoprim-sulfamethoxazole (TMP/SMX; Bactrim; Septra)	*Use with caution if at all during pregnancy and avoid during the last trimester* (see sulfonamides and trimethoprim, above).
	Vancomycin	Few data are available. Use only when clearly indicated.
	ANTIFUNGAL DRUGS	
	Fluconazole (Diflucan)	Embryotoxic and teratogenic in animals; use with caution if at all in humans.
	Flucytosine (Ancobon)	Use only when clearly indicated. May suppress bone marrow when used with amphotericin B.
	Itraconazole (Sporanox)	Same as fluconazole.
	Ketoconazole	Same as fluconazole.

TABLE 5-1—cont'd
Safety of Antimicrobial Agents During Pregnancy

Category	Drug	Comments
	Miconazole	*Do not use the vaginal preparation during the first trimester unless absolutely essential for the patient's welfare.*
ANTIVIRAL DRUGS OTHER THAN ANTIRETROVIRAL DRUGS		
	Acyclovir (Zovirax)	Has caused chromosomal damage in animals at high doses. Recommended for use of life-threatening disease only by CDC. Use for treatment or prevention of genital herpes simplex infection during pregnancy is discouraged.
	Amantadine (Symmetrel)	Embryotoxic and teratogenic in animals. Should be used with great caution if at all during pregnancy.
	Cidovir (Vistide)	Use only when clearly indicated.
	Foscarnet (Foscavir)	Has caused skeletal abnormalities in animals. Should be used only when clearly indicated.
	Ganciclovir (Cytovene)	Embryotoxic and teratogenic in animals. Should be used only when necessary.
	Interferon alfa (Alferon-N; Roferon-A)	Has increased abortions. Should be used only when necessary.
	Rimantadine (Flumadine)	Embryotoxic. Should be used only when necessary.
	Vidarabine	Teratogenic; fetal abnormalities; maternal toxicity. Should be used only when necessary.
ANTIRETROVIRAL DRUGS*		
	Delavirdine (Rescriptor)	Teratogenic in animals when given in high doses.*
	Efavirenz (Sustiva)	Teratogenic in primates. Use should be avoided in pregnancy if all possible.*
	Indinavir (Crixivan)	No clear evidence of teratogenicity in animals.*
	Lamivudine (3TC; Epivir)	Embryotoxic in rabbits; no clear evidence of teratogenicity.*
	Nevirapine (Viramune)	No clear evidence of teratogenicity. Reporting use to registry is encouraged.*
	Stavudine (d4T; Zerit)	Embryotoxic in rodents; no clear evidence of teratogenicity.*
	Zalcitabine (ddC; Hivid)	Teratogenic in animals when used in high doses.*
	Zidovudine (AZT; Retrovir)	Teratogenic in animals, and transplacental carcinogenesis has occurred in animals given high doses.*
ANTIPARASITIC DRUGS		
	Albendazole (Albenza; Zentel)	Teratogenic in animals; use only when clearly indicated.
	Atovaquone (Mepron)	Little or no evidence of teratogenicity in animals; use only when clearly indicated.
	Chloroquine (Aralen)	Accumulates in melanin of fetal eyes in animals. Recommended by CDC and WHO for malaria prophylaxis when risk of exposure outweighs risk of toxicity.

Continued

TABLE 5-1—cont'd
Safety of Antimicrobial Agents During Pregnancy

Category	Drug	Comments
	Furazolidone (Furoxone)	Should not be given to nursing mothers because of risk of hemolytic anemia.
	Mebendazole (Vermox)	Embryotoxic and teratogenic in animals. Should be used with caution, especially during the first trimester.
	Mefloquine (Lariam)	Embryotoxic and teratogenic in animals. Accepted by CDC as being generally safe during the second and third trimesters. When used for prophylaxis against malaria, CDC recommends contraception during administration of the drug and for 2 months after its discontinuation.
	Oxamniquine (Vansil)	Generally contraindicated during pregnancy.
	Paromomycin (Humatin)	Few data; considered to be probably safe during pregnancy.
	Pentamidine	Spontaneous abortion has been reported in humans, but a causal relationship has not been established. Aerosolized pentamidine should be avoided during pregnancy and also when pregnancy is being planned or anticipated.
	Primaquine	Theoretically, could cause hemolytic anemia in a G6PD-deficient fetus. CDC therefore recommends chloroquine for malaria until after delivery, at which time primaquine can be given to consolidate therapy.
	Pyrantel pamoate (Antiminth; Pin-Rid)	Avoid in pregnancy if at all possible.
	Pyrimethamine (Daraprim)	Teratogenic in animals. Indicated for treatment of toxoplasmosis during pregnancy.
	Pyrimethamine plus sulfadoxine (Fansidar)	May be used with caution for prophylaxis in situations where there is an unavoidable risk of chloroquine-resistant falciparum malaria.
	Quinidine gluconate (Quinaglute)	May be indicated for treatment of life-threatening falciparum malaria and is preferable to quinine for this purpose (see below).
	Thiabendazole (Mintezol)	Little or no evidence of teratogenicity in animals; use only when clearly indicated.
Category D (use with extreme caution during pregnancy, since there is evidence of risk to the human fetus)	**ANTIBACTERIAL DRUGS**	
	Aminoglycosides other than gentamicin	Congenital deafness has been reported after use of streptomycin during pregnancy. Use only when clearly necessary.
	Chloramphenicol (Chloromycetin)	*Contraindicated in late pregnancy and labor* owing to risk of gray baby syndrome.
	Tetracyclines (including doxycycline)	*Contraindicated during pregnancy.* Both impairment of skeletal development and discoloration of teeth and enamel hyperplasia are well documented.
	ANTIFUNGAL DRUGS	
	Griseofulvin	Contraindicated during pregnancy.
	ANTIVIRAL DRUGS OTHER THAN ANTIRETROVIRAL DRUGS	
	None in this category	

TABLE 5-1—cont'd
Safety of Antimicrobial Agents During Pregnancy

Category	Drug	Comments
	ANTIRETROVIRAL DRUGS	
	None in this category	
	ANTIPARASITIC DRUGS	
	Trimetrexate (Neutrexin)	
Category X (do not use during pregnancy, as the risk far outweighs the potential benefit on the basis of studies in animals or experience in humans)	**ANTIBACTERIAL DRUGS**	
	None in this category	
	ANTIFUNGAL DRUGS	
	None in this category	
	ANTIVIRAL DRUGS	
	None in this category	
	ANTIPARASITIC DRUGS	
	Iodoquinol (Diquinol; Yodoxin)	
	Quinacrine	
	Quinine	Teratogenic effects and stillbirths have been reported. Quinidine gluconate rather than quinine is now recommended for life-threatening falciparum malaria during pregnancy.

Data from Physicians' Desk Reference, 2000. Montvale, NJ: Medical Economics Company; 1999; Bartlett JG. 2000 Pocket Book of Infectious Disease Therapy. Philadelphia: Lippincott Williams & Wilkins; 2000; Schlager SI. Clinical Management of Infectious Diseases: A Guide to Diagnosis and Therapy. Baltimore: Williams & Wilkins; 1998.
CDC, Centers for Disease Control and Prevention; *G6PD,* glucose-6 phosphate dehydrogenase; *WHO,* World Health Organization.
*Physicians are encouraged to report the use of these drugs during pregnancy, as well as any adverse reactions, to Antiretroviral Pregnancy Registry, P.O. Box 13398, Research Triangle Park, NC 27709-3398 (telephone 1-800-258-4263 or 1-919-483-947; fax 1-800-800-1052). This registry is a collaborative effort among pharmaceutical firms to determine the safety of these drugs in pregnancy. Reports are anonymous in that patients' names are not requested.

Bacterial Vaginosis in Pregnancy

Bacterial vaginosis (BV), formerly called nonspecific vaginitis or *Gardnerella* vaginitis, has no unique predisposition during pregnancy, but as with trichomoniasis, the disease is sufficiently prevalent (10% to 25% of women in obstetric/gynecologic clinic populations) that it is often encountered during pregnancy. Metronidazole is the drug of choice for symptomatic infections. Current CDC recommendations for metronidazole are 250 mg PO t.i.d. for 7 days or one applicator full (5 g) of 0.75% gel (MetroGel) intravaginally twice a day for 5 days. Alternative regimens are metronidazole 2 g PO as a single dose or clindamycin 300 mg PO b.i.d. for 7 days (reservations about metronidazole during pregnancy are discussed in the preceding section).

BV is associated with several adverse pregnancy outcomes, including spontaneous abortion, preterm birth, preterm labor, premature rupture of the membranes, postpartum endometritis, postcesarean wound infections, and amniotic fluid infections. Clearly, women who are symptomatic during pregnancy should be treated to decrease the likelihood of these pregnancy complications. However, no recommendations have been issued for screening of asymptomatic women during pregnancy or treatment to prevent these complications. In fact, recent literature suggests that treatment of asymptomatic BV does not reduce the likelihood of preterm birth or adverse perinatal outcomes. Currently, women at high risk for preterm birth (low maternal prepregnancy weight [<50 kg] or prior history of preterm birth) should be screened and treated if BV is detected.

KEY POINTS

VAGINITIS DURING PREGNANCY

○ VVC seldom affects the fetus adversely, although rare cases of acute chorioamnionitis and intraamniotic infection caused by *C. albicans* have been reported. Miconazole is superior to nystatin for treatment of VVC during pregnancy.

○ In rare cases trichomoniasis is transmitted from mother to infant at birth, causing fever in the infant. Metronidazole is the drug of choice.

○ BV during pregnancy is associated with adverse pregnancy outcomes. Symptomatic women with BV should be treated. Metronidazole is the drug of choice.

○ Metronidazole is now considered reasonably safe for use during pregnancy. Many clinicians prefer to avoid use of metronidazole during the first trimester because of the theoretical risk of teratogenicity.

SUGGESTED READING

Centers for Disease Control and Prevention. 1998 guidelines for treatment of sexually transmitted diseases. MMWR 1998; 47 (RR-1) :1-111.

Cotch MF, Pastorek JG II, Nugent RP, et al. The Vaginal Infections and Prematurity Study Group. *Trichomonas vaginalis* associated with low birth weight and preterm delivery. Sex Transm Dis 1997; 24: 353-360.

Eschenbach DA. Bacterial vaginosis. In: Hitchcock PJ, MacKay HT, Wasserheit JN, Binder R, eds. Sexually Transmitted Diseases and Adverse Outcomes of Pregnancy. Washington, DC: ASM Press; 1999: 103-123.

Hillier SL, Nugent RP, Eschenbach DA, et al. The Vaginal Infections and Prematurity Study Group. Association between bacterial vaginosis and preterm delivery of a low-birth-weight infant. N Engl J Med 1995; 333: 1737-1742.

Meis PJ, Goldenberg RL, Mercer B, et al. The NICHD Maternal-Fetal Medicine Units Network. The preterm prediction study: significance of vaginal infections. Am J Obstet Gynecol 1995; 173: 1231-1235.

Wolner-Hanssen P. Trichomoniasis. In: Hitchcock PJ, MacKay HT, Wasserheit JN, Binder R, eds. Sexually Transmitted Diseases and Adverse Outcomes of Pregnancy. Washington, DC; ASM Press; 1999: 103-123.

Mucopurulent Cervicitis in Pregnancy

N. gonorrhoeae and *C. trachomatis,* the major causes of mucopurulent cervicitis, are both associated with preterm labor, premature rupture of the membranes, and disease in newborn infants such as ophthalmia neonatorum.

Gonorrhea in Pregnancy

Gonorrhea (see Chapters 7 and 16) continues to be highly prevalent in the United States, with about 600,000 cases occurring each year. Gonococcal infection during any trimester may have deleterious effects on pregnancy outcome. For this reason routine prenatal screening is strongly recommended. Women in whom *N. gonorrhoeae* is detected at the time of delivery are more likely to have preterm delivery, premature rupture of the membranes, chorioamnionitis, and postpartum infection. Gonococcal ophthalmia neonatorum may develop in newborns of infected mothers, and therefore prophylactic ther-

apy is recommended. Recommended one-dose treatments for uncomplicated gonococcal infections during pregnancy include ceftriaxone 125 mg IM and cefixime 400 mg PO. *Quinolones (e.g., ciprofloxacin or ofloxacin) should not be used.* Spectinomycin (2 g IM as a single dose) is the recommended treatment for patients with history of severe allergy to cephalosporins. Patients with gonorrhea should be treated for possible coinfection with *C. trachomatis* (for regimens, see the following text).

Chlamydial Infection in Pregnancy

Infection by *C. trachomatis,* the most prevalent STD in the United States, is often asymptomatic but is a major risk factor for infertility and also for HIV infection (see Chapter 16). Chlamydial infection during pregnancy has been associated with premature rupture of membranes and preterm labor. There have also been occasional reports of stillbirth and presumed intraamniotic infections. However, the major complications of chlamydial infection during pregnancy result from perinatal exposure of the neonate to the mother's infecting cervix, causing ophthalmia neonatorum or pneumonia resulting from *C. trachomatis.* Recommended treatment for chlamydial infection during pregnancy is erythromycin 500 mg PO q.i.d. for 7 days or amoxicillin 500 mg PO t.i.d. for 7 days. Azithromycin 1 g PO as a single dose is a potential alternative, but the safety and efficacy of azithromycin in pregnant and lactating women have not been rigorously established. Repeat testing, via culture, is recommended 3 weeks after therapy because of unknown efficacy of these treatments. *The tetracyclines, including doxycycline, and erythromycin estolate should not be used during pregnancy.*

 KEY POINTS

MUCOPURULENT CERVICITIS IN PREGNANCY

○ Gonococcal and chlamydial infections are associated with premature rupture of membranes, preterm labor, and disease such as ophthalmia neonatorum in the newborn.

○ Screening for these pathogens at the first prenatal visit should be routine. Gonococcal and chlamydial infection should also be considered when a pregnant women has symptoms of cervicitis or vaginitis.

○ All pregnant patients with gonorrhea should also be treated with erythromycin or amoxicillin for possible coinfection by *C. trachomatis.* Azithromycin is a potential alternative; tetracyclines, including doxycycline, should be avoided.

○ Because the efficacy of erythromycin and amoxicillin is unclear and probably less than that of doxycycline, follow-up cultures for *C. trachomatis* should be obtained 3 weeks after treatment.

SUGGESTED READING

Centers for Disease Control and Prevention. 1998 guidelines for treatment of sexually transmitted diseases. MMWR 1998; 47 (RR-1) :1-111.

Goldenberg RI, Andrews WW, Yuan AC, et al. Sexually transmitted disease and adverse outcomes of pregnancy. Clin Perinatol 1997; 24:23-41.

Jones RB. Chlamydial infection. In: Hitchcock PJ, MacKay HT, Wasserheit JN, Binder R, eds. Sexually Transmitted Diseases and Adverse Outcomes of Pregnancy. Washington, DC: ASM Press; 1999: 195-208.

Genital Ulcer Disease in Pregnancy

The major genital ulcer diseases in the United States, syphilis and herpes simplex virus infection, assume great importance during pregnancy.

Syphilis

Syphilis (see Chapters 7 and 16), caused by the motile spirochete *T. pallidum,* reached a recent low of 2.6 cases per 100,000 persons in 1998. Likewise, congenital syphilis has decreased to 20.6 cases per 100,000 live births. Risk factors associated with maternal syphilis include young age, African-American or Hispanic ethnicity, single status, low socioeconomic status, inadequate prenatal care, prostitution, and substance abuse. The cervical changes associated with pregnancy, including eversion, hyperemia, and friability, increase the risk of spirochete entry. Fetal acquisition most commonly occurs transplacentally, although syphilis may also be acquired across the fetal membranes or through direct contact at delivery. The risk of fetal infection increases as pregnancy advances, but infection may occur throughout gestation.

Pregnancy has little effect on the clinical course of syphilis, which is staged as primary, secondary, latent, or tertiary (see Chapter 16). Syphilis, however, has a major impact on pregnancy. Preterm delivery, stillbirth, spontaneous abortion, neonatal demise, and congenital infection are all increased. Secondary syphilis poses the highest risk to the fetus because of the level of spirochetemia. Maternal syphilis is commonly diagnosed on the basis of a nontreponemal serologic screening test, with a treponemal serologic test used for confirmation. Pregnant women are screened at the initial visit, at 28 to 32 weeks, and again at delivery with either the RPR or the Venereal Disease Research Laboratory (VDRL) nontreponemal test. About 1% of positive results are false positive for one reason or another. Therefore a positive RPR or VDRL must be confirmed with one of the treponemal tests (e.g., fluorescent treponemal antibody–absorbed [FTA-ABS] or microhemagglutination–*Treponema pallidum* [MHA-TP]).

Congenital syphilis was the most common cause of stillbirth before routine prenatal screening was instituted. Early congenital syphilis manifests itself in the first 2 years of life. Common findings are hepatosplenomegaly, rash, anemia and thrombocytopenia, osteochondritis, periostitis, rhinitis, and central nervous system (CNS) involvement. Evaluation of a neonate born to a mother with untreated or recently treated syphilis should include physical examination and placental histologic tests. Late congenital syphilis often manifests itself near adolescence as Hutchinson's teeth, interstitial keratitis, mental retardation, seizures, eighth nerve deafness, saddle nose deformity, frontal bossing, and saber shins. Congenital syphilis is one of the only STDs infecting neonates that can be prevented or treated in utero.

Penicillin G remains the drug of choice for the treatment of syphilis in pregnancy. The 1998 CDC guidelines recommend 2.4 million units IM of benzathine penicillin G for primary, secondary, and early latent syphilis (some experts recommend repeating this dose a week later). Late latent syphilis or syphilis of unknown duration is treated with benzathine penicillin G 2.4 million units IM weekly for three doses. No other antimicrobial agent is recommended in pregnancy. If a woman reports a penicillin allergy, a skin test for major or minor determinant antigens of penicillin should be performed. If the patient is reactive, penicillin desensitization is undertaken (see suggested readings). Up to 50% of women treated for early-stage syphilis will have a systemic reaction called the Jarisch-Herxheimer reaction. Although this reaction is transient with only mild constitutional symptoms, preterm labor and fetal distress may complicate treatment of the pregnant woman. Follow-up of the pregnant woman after treatment is very important. Serologic testing is performed monthly to ensure that reinfection has not occurred. Treatment failure is rare.

Herpes Simplex Virus Infection

Herpes simplex viruses type 1 and, less commonly, type 2 cause genital herpes. Routine prenatal screening for herpes simplex virus (HSV) by culture or serology is not recommended at this time. However, both HSV-1 and HSV-2 can cause congenital herpes, and therefore the clinician should remain vigilant for this possibility.

Rarely, congenital herpes infection is acquired by transplacental passage. More commonly, neonatal herpes is acquired by cervical or lower genital contact at delivery. The infected neonate may be asymptomatic; have localized findings such as skin, eye, or CNS lesions; or, most dramatically, have disseminated infection. The risk of neonatal infection correlates with the stage of maternal infection; the risk is up to 50% with maternal primary infection but only 4% or less if the mother has recurrent disease at delivery. Asymptomatic viral shedding to date has little association with neonatal infection. Currently, cesarean delivery is recommended if the patient has prodromal or active maternal disease. This approach to antenatal management prevents most but not all cases of neonatal herpesvirus infection.

Chancroid

Infection by *Haemophilus ducreyi,* although common in many developing nations, is now rare in the United States (see Chapter 16). The disease is manifested as a painful genital ulcer, often accompanied by tender inguinal lymphadenopathy. The diagnosis is usually based on clinical findings after syphilis and herpes simplex virus infection have been rigorously excluded. Treatment during pregnancy consists of erythromycin base, 500 mg PO q.i.d. for 7 days.

Human Papillomavirus Infection

Between 20% and 40% of reproductive-age women are infected with human papillomavirus (HPV; see Chapter 16). Condylomata acuminata or genital warts frequently increase in size and number during pregnancy for unknown reasons. These lesions often improve or disappear post partum. Treatment is reserved for women with extensive condylomata that may obstruct the vaginal canal, leading to excessive bleeding after vaginal delivery. Treatment regimens safe to use in pregnancy include 10% to 90% trichloroacetic acid (TCA) applied to the affected area once a week, cryotherapy laser ablation, and, rarely, surgical debulking. Podophyllin resin, imiquimod cream, interferon, and 5-fluorouracil cream are not recommended in pregnancy. Neonatal infection from HPV is rare. Laryngeal papillomatosis has been reported in children exposed to HPV-6 or HPV-11 at delivery. Whether cesarean delivery is protective is not known at this time; it is currently not recommended.

 KEY POINTS

GENITAL ULCER DISEASE IN PREGNANCY

⊃ Syphilis: Cervical changes during pregnancy increase the risk of spirochete entry. Pregnancy has little impact on the clinical course of syphilis, but syphilis has a major impact on pregnancy. Pregnant women should be screened for syphilis (by RPR) at the first prenatal visit, at 28 to 32 weeks, and again at delivery.

⊃ HSV infection: Routine screening for HSV is not recommended, but the clinician should be vigilant for this possibility. The risk of neonatal infection is up to 50% during maternal primary infection. Cesarean section is recommended when prodromal or active maternal disease is present.

⊃ HPV infection: Neonatal transmission is rare. Treatment is reserved for women with extensive condylomata.

SUGGESTED READING

Brown ZA. Genital herpes and pregnancy. In: Hitchcock PJ, MacKay HT, Wasserheit JN, Binder R, eds. Sexually Transmitted Diseases and Adverse Outcomes of Pregnancy. Washington, DC: ASM Press; 1999: 245-258.

Centers for Disease Control and Prevention. 1998 guidelines for treatment of sexually transmitted diseases. MMWR 1998; 47 (RR-1) :1-111.

Centers for Disease Control and Prevention. Congenital syphilis—United States 1998. MMWR 1999; 48: 757-761.

Donders GG. Treatment of sexually transmitted bacterial diseases in pregnant women. Drugs 2000; 59: 477-485.

Genc M, Ledger WJ. Syphilis in pregnancy. Sex Transm Infect 2000; 76: 73-79.

Scott LL. Prevention of perinatal herpes: prophylactic antiviral therapy. Clin Obstet Gynecol 1999; 42:134-148.

Sheffield JS, Wendel GD Jr. Syphilis in pregnancy. Clin Obstet Gynecol 1999; 42: 97-106.

Wendel GD, Stark BJ, Jamison RB, et al. Penicillin allergy and desensitization in serious infections during pregnancy. N Engl J Med 1985; 312:1229-1232.

Congenital Infections in Pregnancy
Cytomegalovirus Infection

Cytomegalovirus (CMV) remains the most common cause of perinatal infection in the United States, infecting 0.5% to 2% of all neonates (0.1% are symptomatic). About 55% of reproductive-age women in high socioeconomic classes are seropositive, compared with 85% of women in the lower socioeconomic classes. Between 1% and 4% of susceptible women acquire a primary CMV infection during pregnancy. Most of these women are asymptomatic; a mononucleosis-like illness develops in only 15% (see Chapter 8). Diagnosis is made by a four-fold increase in IgG serologic titers using acute and convalescent sera. An IgM serologic test is available but at this time is not always reliable. No treatment is necessary for maternal disease in an immunocompetent woman.

Congenital CMV infection risks and manifestations vary depending on the maternal serologic status. A primary maternal infection is associated with a 40% transmission rate to the fetus overall; the transmission risk is highest in the third trimester, but the clinical severity is worse in the first half of pregnancy. Between 10% and 15% of infected fetuses have clinically apparent disease at birth, and 90% of these have long-term sequelae. The 85% to 90% of infected infants who do not have clinically apparent disease at birth have different outcomes; only 5% to 15% of these infants have long-term sequelae. Recurrent maternal disease carries a 0.5% to 1% risk of congenital infection, and only 1% or less of these infants have clinically apparent disease. Congenital CMV may manifest itself as low birth weight, microcephaly, intracranial calcifications, chorioretinitis, hearing deficits, motor and mental retardation, hepatosplenomegaly, anemia, and thrombocytopenia. Some of these findings may be detected by prenatal sonography. Prenatal diagnosis is, however, best performed by use of amniotic fluid for viral culture or, more recently, polymerase chain reaction (PCR). Fetal blood sampling is not necessary for the diagnosis but will provide information on hematologic and hepatic enzyme abnormalities. Negative testing does not always exclude fetal infection, nor does positive testing equal fetal infection. No effective in utero treatment for congenital CMV infection has been approved. For this reason, and also because positive serologic test results do not always indicate active CMV disease, routine prenatal screening for CMV antibodies is not recommended.

Rubella

Rubella or German measles (see Chapter 7) is one of the most teratogenic infections known. Fortunately, since the introduction of the rubella vaccine, the incidence of rubella and congenital rubella syndrome has decreased substantially. In the majority of women infected with rubella a rash and constitutional symptoms develop approximately 1 week after viremia develops. These resolve with rare long-term sequelae. Antibody formation occurs 1 to 2 weeks later. IgM antibodies may persist for up to a year. Reinfection, in the presence of low levels of IgM, has also been reported. Because of this, accurate diagnosis of maternal disease is difficult.

Transmission rates to the fetus vary with the onset of maternal infection. About 80% of infants born to mothers with primary rubella infection acquired during the first 12 weeks of gestation are infected. This decreases to 54% by 13 to 14 weeks and to 25% by the end of the second trimester. The clinical manifestations of congenital rubella syndrome also vary depending on the stage of organogenesis. Possible manifestations include chromosomal abnormalities, bony changes, hepatosplenomegaly, hepatitis, sensorineural deafness, cataracts, glaucoma, heart defects, CNS abnormalities, intrauterine growth restriction, thrombocytopenia, and anemia. These infants are also at risk for type I diabetes and progressive panencephalitis in later years.

No treatment is available. Vaccination is the mainstay for rubella prevention. All women should be screened for rubella and vaccinated if necessary before pregnancy. Pregnancy should be avoided for 3 months after vaccination because of the *theoretical* risk of congenital rubella syndrome, since the vaccine consists of a live virus. Pregnant women should have prenatal screening for rubella immunity, and those who are not immune should have vaccination performed post partum.

Parvovirus B19 Infection

Parvovirus B19, the only parvovirus associated with human disease, causes erythema infectiosum (fifth disease) in children but can also cause rash and arthritis in adults (see Chapter 7). The virus shows tropism for erythroid precursors and essentially shuts down red blood cell production for a limited time. About 40% of adults are susceptible to parvovirus B19 infection, and the risk of infection after a close exposure is 25% to 50%. Whereas infected children typically have a rash and erythroderma of the face ("slapped cheek" rash), adults are frequently asymptomatic. Clinical features in adults include rashes of different types (see Chapter 7), arthralgias or arthritis, anemia, thrombocytopenia, and constitutional symptoms. The viremia peaks 5 to 7 days before the onset of symptoms, and therefore transmission to the fetus typically occurs before clinically apparent maternal disease. Diagnosis of maternal disease is based on the demonstration of IgM antibodies, which may be detected for 1 to 4 months.

Congenital parvovirus B19 infection is associated with an increased risk of spontaneous abortion and a fetal loss rate of 2% to 10% (up to 15% if infection occurs during the second trimester). Parvovirus B19 now causes about 15% of cases of nonimmune hydrops fetalis, which results from temporary arrest of red blood cell production. If the fetus becomes infected and hydrops develops, spontaneous resolution is possible if the fetus survives the initial insult. Surviving infants are thought not to be at risk for congenital anomalies. Intrauterine transfusion has been shown to improve outcome, depending on the severity of fetal anemia at diagnosis.

Women who have been exposed to parvovirus B19 and develop clinical features of infection or who have a fetus with nonimmune hydrops should be carefully evaluated. Our approach to the assessment of these women is summarized in Figure 5-1.

Toxoplasmosis

Toxoplasma gondii (see Chapters 8, 17, and 23), a protozoan transmitted in infected cat feces, in raw or undercooked meat (beef, pork, or wild mammals), and transplacentally, causes about 400 to 4000 cases of congenital disease in the United States each year. About 70% of women in the United States lack antibodies to *T. gondii* and are therefore susceptible. Maternal infection is often asymptomatic. Fever, arthralgias, myalgias, fatigue, and occasionally lymphadenopathy may occur (see Chapter 8). Diagnosis can be difficult. Serologic

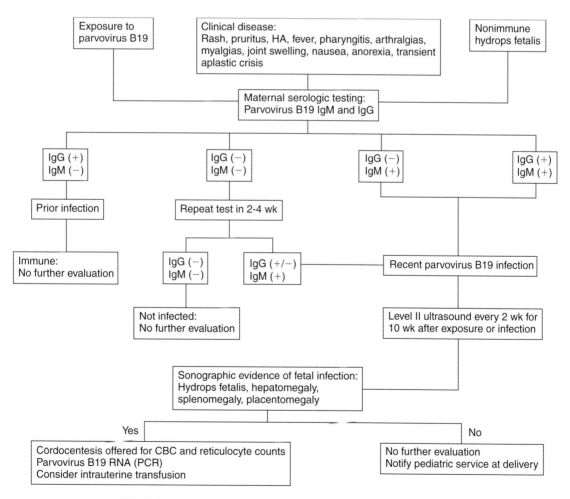

FIG. 5-1   Management of parvovirus B19 infection during pregnancy.

testing can be performed but may be difficult to interpret. Positive IgM serologic results should be confirmed by a reference laboratory, since false-positive results are relatively common. Acute and convalescent IgG titers are useful. At this time prenatal screening for toxoplasmosis is not recommended. The American College of Obstetricians and Gynecologists (ACOG) does recommend preconceptional counseling. In theory the risk of toxoplasmosis might be reduced by advising women who lack antibodies to *T. gondii* to wear gloves when changing cat litter or while gardening and to avoid eating meat that is not gray in the center (including game, such as venison).

The overall risk of transmission of maternal toxoplasmosis to the fetus is about 50%, but this varies by trimester: 10% during the first trimester, 25% to 30% during the second trimester, and 60% during the third trimester. However, fetal infection is more virulent the earlier it is acquired. About 25% of neonates with congenital infection actually have signs or symptoms of toxoplasmosis at birth. These include hepatosplenomegaly, low birth weight, anemia, thrombocytopenia, intracranial calcifications, hydrocephaly, and microcephaly. Long-term sequelae include chorioretinitis, hearing loss, and mental retardation. Diagnosis of a congenitally infected fetus involves sonography and PCR testing of the amniotic fluid.

Toxoplasmosis is one of the only congenital infections that can be at least partially treated in utero (syphilis being the other major example). Pyrimethamine and sulfadiazine cross the placenta and alter both maternal and fetal infection. Spiramycin, available from the FDA, is effective for maternal disease but does not cross the placenta. Both regimens *may* attenuate maternal disease, *may* decrease transmission rate, and *may* reduce fetal sequelae. No regimen to date can prevent all cases of congenital toxoplasmosis.

Listeria Monocytogenes Infection (Listeriosis)

Listeria monocytogenes is an unusual cause of congenital infection. It is transmitted by contaminated foods such as undercooked meats, delicatessen meats, soft cheeses, and unpasteurized milk. It is transmitted to a fetus across the placenta. Although immunocompetent persons may be infected, they rarely become seriously ill. However, pregnant women and immunocompromised persons, including newborns, are much more likely to have serious illness. Pregnant women may have a mild, flulike illness with gastrointestinal symptoms, fever, and muscle aches. Nervous system involvement is manifested as headache, stiff neck, seizures, or confusion. Diagnosis is based on a careful history, symptoms, and a positive blood culture. Serologic testing is also available.

Congenital infection is possible with a reported increase in preterm labor and meconium passage. Early-onset neonatal sepsis has an associated mortality rate of 50%. Prompt maternal antimicrobial therapy with ampicillin and gentamicin is often effective in preventing fetal infection.

Varicella-Zoster Virus Infection

Varicella-zoster virus is one of the most contagious of all viral infections, with a 60% to 90% rate of transmission to susceptible individuals (see Chapter 7). Fortunately, more than 95% of adults have serologic evidence of immunity and a vaccine is now available. The infection is detected in only 0.1 to 0.4 per 1000 pregnant women each year in the United States. Adult varicella (chickenpox), especially in the pregnant woman, tends to be more serious than childhood infection, with a higher rate of pneumonia and death (>2%). Maternal zoster infection, or "shingles," is no different from the infection in nonpregnant women, and no cases of congenital infection have been reported. The diagnosis of maternal varicella is usually clinical. Serologic evaluation is also useful; antibodies usually develop within 1 to 2 weeks of infection.

Fetal infection manifests itself two ways: congenital infection and neonatal infection. Congenital infection occurs in up to 2% of maternal varicella infections *before* 20 weeks (highest risk is at 13 to 20 weeks). Congenital malformations include cerebral cortical atrophy, cardiac malformations, hydronephrosis, chorioretinitis, cutaneous lesions (cicatricial skin scarring), and limb hypoplasia. Fetal infection after 20 weeks may manifest as cutaneous lesions. Neonatal infection occurs secondary to exposure of the fetus or newborn 5 days before delivery to 2 days post partum before protective maternal antibodies develop. Neonatal infection produces the highest mortality rates, which are associated with disseminated visceral and CNS disease.

Treatment of active maternal disease with acyclovir in the first 24 hours may decrease the duration of lesions and *possibly* fetal transmission. A pregnant woman who is exposed to varicella and does not have a history of chickenpox should be tested for immune status. If she is not immune, varicella-zoster immune globulin (VZIG) should be given within 96 hours of exposure. This may attenuate maternal infection but does not necessarily prevent fetal infection. The maternal dose of VZIG is 125 units/10 kg up to 625 units. VZIG should also be given to a neonate if varicella infection developed in the mother between 5 days before delivery and 2 days post partum. The varicella vaccine now available uses a live attenuated virus and is contraindicated in pregnancy.

KEY POINTS

CONGENITAL INFECTIONS

- ⊃ Cytomegalovirus infection: Routine prenatal screening for CMV antibodies is not recommended. However, primary CMV infection occurs in 1% to 4% of all pregnancies, and about 0.1% of neonates have symptomatic infection. Prenatal diagnosis of CMV disease is best made on the basis of viral culture or PCR of amniotic fluid.
- ⊃ Rubella: All women should be screened for rubella and vaccinated if necessary before pregnancy, which should be avoided for 3 months after vaccination. The risk of congenital rubella is 80% if primary rubella is acquired during the first 12 weeks of gestation.
- ⊃ Parvovirus B19: This virus causes about 15% of cases of nonimmune hydrops fetalis and is associated with an overall risk of spontaneous abortion of 2% to 10%. Women who have been exposed to parvovirus B19 (fifth disease in children) should be evaluated according to an algorithm (Figure 5-1).
- ⊃ Toxoplasmosis: About 70% of women in the United States lack antibodies to *T. gondii* and are therefore vulnerable to infection during pregnancy. The risk of infection to the fetus increases from 10% during the first trimester to 60% during the third trimester, but fetal infection is more virulent the earlier it is acquired.

⊃ *Listeria monocytogenes* infection: Serious illness is more likely to develop in pregnant women and immunocompromised persons, including newborns. Early-onset neonatal sepsis caused by *L. monocytogenes* has an associated mortality rate of 50%.

⊃ Varicella-zoster virus infection: Women who develop varicella (chickenpox) during pregnancy are at risk of pneumonia and death (>2%). Pregnant women who are not immune and who have been exposed to a person with varicella should be given VZIG within 96 hours of exposure. The current varicella vaccine, consisting of a live attenuated virus, is contraindicated during pregnancy.

SUGGESTED READING

American College of Obstetricians and Gynecologists. Management of herpes in pregnancy. Pract Bull No. 8, October 1999.

American College of Obstetricians and Gynecologists. Perinatal viral and parasitic infections. Pract Bull No. 20, September 2000.

Crino JP. Ultrasound and fetal diagnosis of perinatal infection. Clin Obstet Gynecol 1999; 42: 71-80.

Daffos F, Forestier F, Capella-Pavlovsky M, et al. Prenatal management of 746 pregnancies at risk for congenital toxoplasmosis. N Engl J Med 1988; 381:271-275.

Demmler GJ. Infectious Disease Society of America and Centers for Disease Control. Summary of a workshop on surveillance for congenital cytomegalovirus disease. Rev Infect Dis 1991; 13: 315-329.

Ely JW, Yankowitz J, Bowdler NC. Evaluation of pregnant women exposed to respiratory viruses. Am Fam Physician 2000; 61: 3065-3074.

Enders G, Miller E, Cradock-Watson J, et al. Consequences of varicella and herpes zoster in pregnancy: prospective study of 1739 cases. Lancet 1994; 343: 1548-1551.

Helfgott A. TORCH testing in HIV-infected women. Clin Obstet Gynecol 1999; 42: 149-162.

Newton ER. Diagnosis of perinatal TORCH infections. Clin Obstet Gynecol 1999; 42: 59-70.

Piper JM, Wen TS. Perinatal cytomegalovirus and toxoplasmosis: challenges of antepartum therapy. Clin Obstet Gynecol 1999; 42: 81-96.

Rodis JF. Parvovirus infection. Clin Obstet Gynecol 1999; 42: 107-120.

Viral Hepatitis in Pregnancy

Pregnancy does not appear to increase the risk of maternal mortality from viral hepatitis with the exception of hepatitis E (see Chapter 13). However, hepatitis viruses are sometimes transmitted to the fetus.

Hepatitis A occurs in about 1 in 1000 pregnancies in the United States. Although hepatitis A can be fatal, it does not result in chronic residua for the mother or her infant.

Hepatitis B is the form of hepatitis most frequently transmitted to the fetus in the United States. Acute hepatitis B occurs in about 1 to 2 in every 1000 pregnancies. Chronic hepatitis B infection (defined by a positive blood test for HBsAg) is present in 5 to 15 of every 1000 pregnancies and is more prevalent among certain ethnic groups and among injecting drug users. Most perinatal transmissions (85% to 95%) result from intrapartum exposure to contaminated blood and genital tract secretions. The remaining transmissions result from hematogenous transplacental dissemination, breast-feeding, and close contact. The frequency of transplacental transmission varies depending on the presence of HBeAg and the gestational age at the time of infectivity. The blood of patients with hepatitis B who test positive for HBeAg but negative for the corresponding antibody (anti-HBe) is highly infectious. The overall transplacental transmission rate for HBsAg-positive women is about 10% if HBeAg is absent but about 90% if HBeAg is present. Similarly, hepatitis B is acquired by about 10% of infants born to mothers infected during the first trimester but by about 80% to 90% of infants born to mothers with acute hepatitis B contracted during the third trimester. Prevention of hepatitis B can be achieved by the administration of hepatitis B immune globulin (HBIG) and hepatitis B vaccine at the time of delivery, followed by two injections within the first 6 months of life.

Hepatitis C is transmitted from about 2% to 8% of infected women to their infants. The hepatitis C viral load (hepatitis C viral RNA measured by PCR; see Chapter 13) within the maternal blood influences the probability of vertical transmission to the infant. Transmission increases substantially with concomitant HIV infection (from an average of about 5% to 15%). Breast-feeding has to date not been associated with vertical transmission of hepatitis C. Recent data suggest that mother-to-infant transmission of hepatitis C occurs mainly around the time of delivery. It has been suggested, but not confirmed as a standard of care, that cesarean section may be indicated for women who have hepatitis C virus infection with high viral loads.

Hepatitis D virus requires hepatitis B virus for replication and expression. Ultimately up to 25% of chronic carriers of hepatitis B virus become coinfected with the hepatitis D virus, which can be transmitted to the fetus.

Hepatitis E infection resembles hepatitis A but is uncommon in the United States. Hepatitis E during pregnancy is a severe disease with substantial maternal mortality (see Chapter 13).

SUGGESTED READING

Centers for Disease Control and Prevention. Recommendations for prevention and control of hepatitis C virus (HCV) infection and HCV-related chronic disease. MMWR 1998; 47(RR-19):1-39.

Eriksen NL. Perinatal consequences of hepatitis C. Clin Obstet Gynecol 1999; 42:121-133.

Gibb DM, Goodall RL, Dunn DT, et al. Mother-to-child transmission of hepatitis C virus: evidence for preventable peripartum transmission. Lancet 2000; 356: 904-907.

Other Infections in Pregnancy

Among the numerous infections that occasionally occur during pregnancy, four deserve special comment: malaria, tuberculosis, group A streptococcal infection, and group B streptococcal infection.

Malaria

Malaria should always be suspected in a returning traveler with fever. The common antimalarial drugs are not contraindicated in pregnancy (Table 5-1). Chloroquine is the treatment of choice for all forms of malaria except chloroquine-resistant falciparum infection. The CDC recommends intravenous quinidine for the treatment of falciparum malaria during pregnancy. For prophylaxis, physicians advocate chloroquine (300 mg of base PO once a week, beginning 1 to 2 weeks before departure and continuing until 4 weeks after leaving the endemic area). Travel to chloroquine-resistant areas should be postponed until the second trimester, and then mefloquine prophylaxis should be started. Several possible vaccines are being investigated.

Pregnancy enhances the severity of falciparum malaria. The presence of the disease process may adversely affect pregnancy outcomes. The incidence of spontaneous abortions and preterm labor is increased. Fetal loss and stillbirths may be related to placental and fetal infection, in which the parasites have an affinity for decidual vessels. The incidence of congenital malaria is estimated to be 0.39% in infants of immune mothers but may be as high as 10% in infants of nonimmune mothers.

Tuberculosis

Tuberculosis (see Chapter 22) occurs in up to 0.1% of pregnancies in certain endemic areas. Clinical manifestations of active tuberculosis in pregnancy resemble those observed in nonpregnant patients and include cough with minimal sputum production, low-grade fever, hemoptysis, and weight loss. Chest x-ray examination reveals a variety of infiltrative patterns with possible pulmonary cavitation or mediastinal lymphadenopathy. Miliary or miliary-meningeal tuberculosis occurs rarely and can be a fulminant illness. With initiation of prenatal care, pregnant women at high risk for tuberculosis should be screened with a purified protein derivative (PPD) skin test. Women with a positive PPD skin test must be evaluated for active tuberculosis with a thorough physical examination for extrapulmonary disease and a chest x-ray examination once they are beyond the first trimester.

Treatment regimens for tuberculosis are based on the presence or absence of active disease and, in the absence of active disease, the duration of PPD positivity. In women with a known recent conversion (2 years) to a positive PPD and no evidence of active disease, recommended therapy is isoniazid (INH) 300 mg/day, starting after the first trimester and continuing for 6 to 9 months. Women less than 35 years of age with an unknown or prolonged duration of PPD positivity should receive isoniazid 300 mg/day for 6 to 9 months after delivery. Some physicians advise that therapy be delayed until after delivery.

Treatment of active tuberculosis in pregnancy should begin immediately, optimally in consultation with the local health department and with knowledge about the likelihood of drug-resistant *M. tuberculosis* strains. Today's fortified regimen, recommended for most patients who are *not* pregnant and in whom drug-resistant strains are a reasonable possibility, consists of a four-drug regimen with INH, rifampin, ethambutol (EMB), and pyrazinamide (PZA). INH, EMB, and rifampin have been used extensively during pregnancy with relatively few adverse effects. In animal studies, which often use high doses, INH can be embryocidal, EMB can be teratogenic, and rifampin has caused congenital abnormalities (cleft palate, spina bifida) and embryotoxicity. In humans rifampin has been associated with isolated cases of fetal abnormalities and with postnatal hemorrhage when given during the last few weeks of pregnancy. PZA is used in much of the world for

tuberculosis in pregnancy. In the United States, however, data concerning its teratogenicity are believed to be inadequate and PZA is therefore considered a category C drug in pregnancy. When the presence of INH-resistant strains is considered unlikely, two regimens can be endorsed: INH (300 mg/day) plus EMB (15 mg/kg/day) for 18 to 24 months, or INH plus rifampin (600 mg/day) for 6 to 9 months. Pyrazinamide (vitamin B_6) supplementation, 50 mg/day, is essential for patients receiving INH. Antituberculous agents not recommended for use in pregnancy include ethionamide, streptomycin, capreomycin, kanamycin, cycloserine, and, as noted previously, PZA. Because of the increasing problem of drug-resistant tuberculosis throughout the world, including the United States (see Chapter 22), in vitro susceptibility testing of *M. tuberculosis* isolates is strongly recommended.

Failure to diagnose and treat congenital or neonatal tuberculosis results in significant morbidity and mortality. Infection can be acquired hematogenously in the liver or lungs or by aspiration of infected secretions at delivery. Infants with congenital tuberculosis usually do not show evidence of disease for several days to weeks after delivery. Signs and symptoms are nonspecific and include respiratory distress, fever, poor feeding, lethargy, failure to thrive, lymphadenopathy, abdominal distention, and hepatosplenomegaly. Culture results of biopsy specimens from liver, skin or peripheral lymph nodes, spinal fluid, urine, bone marrow, middle-ear fluid, or tracheal aspirates provide definitive diagnosis of congenital or neonatal tuberculosis.

Active tuberculosis in a neonate should be treated with INH and rifampin immediately upon diagnosis. Multidrug therapy with INH, rifampin, streptomycin, and PZA is recommended for drug-resistant organisms. If appropriate therapy is given, most long-term morbidity can be avoided. Infants born to women with active tuberculosis at the time of delivery should receive INH preventive therapy (10 mg/kg/day) until the maternal disease has been inactive for 3 months. Newborns are quite susceptible to tuberculosis; therefore many physicians propose isolation from the mother suspected of having active disease. If an infant born to a woman with active disease is not treated, the risk of disease is 50% during the first year of life.

Group B Streptococcal Disease

Streptococcus agalactiae, more commonly known as the group B streptococcus (GBS), is part of the normal vaginal flora. During the 1960s and 1970s it became apparent that GBS was a major cause of maternal morbidity and both morbidity and mortality among infected infants. The disease was extensively studied, and as a result of preventive strategies the rate of neonatal infection continues to decline—from 1.7 per 1000 live-born infants in 1993 to <0.6 per 1000 live-born infants in 1998. However, about 20,000 neonatal cases still occur in the United States each year. Risk factors for neonatal GBS include maternal colonization with the organism, prolonged rupture of membranes, preterm delivery, and maternal GBS bacteriuria. Colonization rates are higher among African-Americans, adolescents, and persons of lower socioeconomic status.

The maternal spectrum of disease includes UTIs such as asymptomatic bacteriuria, cystitis, and pyelonephritis, as well as genital tract infections such as chorioamnionitis, septicemia, and postpartum endometritis. About 20% to 30% of women are asymptomatic carriers of GBS.

Neonatal GBS disease assumes two forms: early-onset disease (75% to 80% of cases) and late-onset disease (20% to 25% of cases). Early-onset disease, attributed to maternal colonization, occurs during the first week of life and generally during the first 24 to 48 hours. Septicemia, pneumonia, and meningitis are among the complications. Clinical findings include respiratory distress, apnea, grunting, tachypnea, cyanosis, hypotension, lethargy, poor feeding, temperature instability, pallor, tachycardia, jaundice, and abdominal distention. Late-onset neonatal disease occurs between 7 days and 12 weeks of age and is generally found in term infants. These infants have fever, irritability, lethargy, and meningitis. Only 50% of late-onset disease occurs in infants of women colonized with GBS.

Diagnosis of asymptomatic genital tract colonization is made by traditional culture methods. The rapid tests that use growth enhancement and immunologic methods are unreliable and nonspecific. Appropriate culture techniques require obtaining a swab from the lower vagina and perianal areas. The perianal culture is important, since colonization is usually greater in this area than in the vagina. Selective media containing Todd-Hewitt broth, sheep blood, nalidixic acid, and gentamicin are used so that the growth of the streptococci is not masked by overgrowth of other bacteria.

Symptomatic infections in pregnancy caused by GBS should be treated with penicillin or ampicillin. The prevention of neonatal GBS infection includes intrapartum antibiotic prophylaxis. Currently both ACOG and the CDC support the use of intrapartum antibiotic prophylaxis based on clinical risk factors for preterm labor. These risk factors include gestational age of <37 weeks, premature rupture of membranes at <37 weeks, ruptured membranes >18 hours previously, prior birth of a child with GBS disease, or maternal fever during labor >100.4° F (38° C). The CDC recommends the use of either of two strategies to prevent early-onset GBS disease. The first strategy is based on late prenatal cultures, obtained between 35 to 37 weeks as a primary risk determinant. The second strategy is based solely on clinical risk factors. Women in labor with a positive culture or risk factors are treated with intrapartum antibiotics. Intrapartum prophylaxis includes use of penicillin G, 5 million units initially and then 2.5 million units every 4 hours until delivery, or ampicillin 2 g initially and then 1 g every 4 hours until delivery. Regardless of the strategy adopted by the obstetric provider, not all cases of early-onset GBS disease will be prevented.

The CDC provides an algorithm for the management of newborns whose mothers received intrapartum antimicrobial prophylaxis for GBS. Simply put, newborns are observed for signs and symptoms of infection, then treated accordingly.

Group A Streptococcal Disease

Streptococcus pyogenes, more commonly known as the group A streptococcus (GAS), is the classic cause of childbed sepsis. Recently there has been a serious resurgence of life-threatening invasive GAS infections. An estimated 10,000 cases of invasive GAS infection now occur in the United States each year, or 3.7 cases per 100,000 population. Major manifestations include necrotizing fasciitis and the streptococcal toxic shock syndrome (see Chapter 6). Invasive dis-

eases during the puerperium that have been reported recently include bacteremia and shock. Frequently, invasive GAS infection during pregnancy necessitates hysterectomy. Penicillin G (or ampicillin) remains the mainstay of pregnancy.

 KEY POINTS

OTHER INFECTIONS IN PREGNANCY

⊃ Malaria: Pregnancy enhances the severity of falciparum malaria, and this disease may adversely affect pregnancy outcome. Malaria should be considered whenever a returning traveler has a fever.

⊃ Tuberculosis: Pregnant women at high risk should undergo tuberculin skin testing (PPD). Tuberculosis can be a severe disease during pregnancy, and failure to diagnose and treat congenital or neonatal tuberculosis results in significant morbidity and mortality.

⊃ Group B streptococcal (GBS) disease: About 20,000 cases of neonatal GBS disease, which can be life threatening, occur in the United States each year. Maternal disease caused by GBS can also be serious. Two preventive strategies are currently endorsed: (1) obtaining vaginal and perianal cultures between 35 and 37 weeks of gestation, and (2) evaluating clinical risk factors. By either strategy, women who are identified as definite or likely GBS carriers are given intrapartum prophylaxis with penicillin G or ampicillin.

⊃ Group A streptococcal (GAS) disease: Invasive GAS infection during pregnancy can cause bacteremia and shock and may necessitate hysterectomy.

SUGGESTED READING

American College of Obstetricians and Gynecologists. Prevention of early-onset group B streptococcus disease in newborns. Committee on Obstetric Practice, Committee Opinion No. 173, June 1996.

American Thoracic Society. Treatment of tuberculosis and tuberculosis infection in adults and children. Am J Respir Crit Care Med 1994; 149: 1359-1374.

Hulbert TV. Congenital malaria in the United States: report of a case and review. Clin Infect Dis 1992; 14: 922-926.

Udagawa H, Oshio Y, Shimizu Y. Serious group A streptococcal infection around delivery. Obstet Gynecol 1999; 94: 153-157.

Urinary Tract Infection in Pregnancy

UTI is common during pregnancy and symptomatic in the majority of patients. However, physiologic changes during pregnancy predispose to pyelonephritis. Pyelonephritis occurs in 20% to 40% of pregnant patients with untreated asymptomatic bacteriuria. Also, about 70% to 80% of cases of pyelonephritis during pregnancy occur in women with a history of asymptomatic bacteriuria. The overall incidence of pyelonephritis during pregnancy can be reduced from 4% to 0.8% by a policy of routine prenatal screening with urine cultures and treatment of asymptomatic bacteriuria. An understanding of the mechanisms, diagnosis, and treatment of UTIs in pregnancy is important to any physician involved in maternal health care.

Presentation and Progression
Cause

Risk factors for UTI during pregnancy include sexual activity, increasing age, parity, sickle cell disease or trait (with associated renal parenchymal damage), lower socioeconomic status, prior UTIs, diabetes mellitus, and functional or anatomic urinary tract abnormalities. Asymptomatic bacteriuria ($>10^5$ CFUs/mL of a single pathogen in a patient without UTI symptoms; see Chapter 14) occurs in 2% to 10% of pregnancies and is the most important risk factor.

Less than 1% of pregnant women with sterile urine cultures on first prenatal screen eventually have asymptomatic bacteriuria during the remainder of the pregnancy. About two thirds of cases of pyelonephritis during pregnancy occur in women with prior asymptomatic bacteriuria. In a classic study, Kass determined that 20% to 40% of pregnant women who received placebo treatment for asymptomatic bacteriuria subsequently had pyelonephritis, whereas no pregnant woman who received effective antimicrobial treatment later had pyelonephritis.

During pregnancy, mechanical factors and progesterone transform the ureters from thin, muscular, peristaltic, one-way conduits to standing, relatively static columns of fluid. Mechanical compression by the gravid uterus during the second half of pregnancy causes proximal ureteral dilatation. The right ureter is especially affected because of dextrorotation of the uterus. Bladder changes, including decreased tone, increased filling capacity, incomplete emptying, and change in position, may occur and predispose to vesicoureteral reflux. Moreover, nonmechanical changes in intrinsic urinary tract defenses are altered in pregnancy. The chemical composition of the urine itself is enriched in pregnancy with such products as glucose, amino acids, and degraded hormones, providing a medium that facilitates bacterial growth.

The bacteria frequently isolated are gram-negative bacilli, notably the Enterobacteriaceae and especially *Escherichia coli* (63% to 80% of cases). Other pathogens include *Klebsiella pneumoniae, Proteus mirabilis, Enterobacter* species, and group B streptococci. *Pseudomonas aeruginosa, Serratia, Citrobacter,* and *Candida* species are rarely isolated from healthy pregnant women.

Presentation

Although pyelonephritis may occur during any trimester of pregnancy, 90% of cases develop during the second and third trimesters.

Early treatment of cystitis does not always prevent its progression to pyelonephritis. The onset of lower urinary tract symptoms often coincides with the appearance of signs and symptoms of upper tract involvement. The presentation of pyelonephritis in pregnant women includes fever, chills, nausea, vomiting, and manifestations of upper urinary tract disease, such as costovertebral angle pain and tenderness. Anorexia and nausea and vomiting resulting in signs of dehydration are common symptoms of pyelonephritis. On physical examination, renal involvement is usually unilateral, with a right-sided predominance 50% of the time. Signs and symptoms are bilateral in about 25% of cases.

Diagnosis

Initial evaluation of women with suspected pyelonephritis includes a complete history and physical examination (including vital signs), urinalysis, complete blood cell count, serum creatinine level, and electrolytes. In the presence of sepsis or high fever ($>102.2°$ F [$39°$ C]), blood samples should be drawn for culture. If fetal tachycardia and uterine contractions are present, chorioamnionitis must be considered and excluded.

The diagnosis, based on symptoms and clinical findings, is confirmed by urinalysis and urine culture. Either a midstream clean-catch or catheterized urine specimen should be obtained. Although catheterization is highly accurate, it should be used with caution because bacteria can be introduced into the bladder. Specimens obtained in the office must be delivered promptly to the microbiology laboratory or refrigerated immediately. A delay of more than 2 hours will cause a falsely elevated bacterial count.

Pyuria on urinalysis is suggestive but not diagnostic of pyelonephritis. The diagnosis can be made before a positive urine culture if bacteria are identified on microscopic examination of a Gram stain of an unspun specimen or if >50 white blood cells (WBCs) per high-power field (HPF) are found in a spun specimen. In addition, casts and red blood cells can be identified in the sediment. A well-mixed, unspun urine specimen that contains >5 bacteria/HPF correlates with a urine culture of $>10^5$ CFUs/mL and can be used to confirm the clinical diagnosis. Urine cultures are characteristically positive for a uropathogen ($>10^5$ CFUs/mL), but a negative culture may not exclude the diagnosis if the woman has received antimicrobial therapy. Even a single dose of an antimicrobial drug may render the urine sterile. Blood cultures are positive in about 10% of women with pyelonephritis.

Treatment
Methods

Hospitalization is recommended for most patients to treat sepsis, ensure hydration, and monitor for signs of preterm labor. Vigorous intravenous hydration with crystalloid solution is used to establish a diuresis of 30 to 60 mL of urine per hour. An indwelling Foley catheter is rarely needed but may be required for adequate monitoring of urine output. Seriously ill patients or those with sepsis may require invasive hemodynamic monitoring. Options for parenteral antimicrobial therapy include a cephalosporin (e.g., cefazolin, cefuroxime, or ceftriaxone), a penicillin derivative (e.g., mezlocillin or piperacillin), ampicillin-sulbactam, or the combination of ampicillin and gentamicin. Ampicillin is no longer recommended as monotherapy for pyelonephritis because gram-negative bacilli, including many *E. coli* strains, have acquired resistance. If aminoglycosides are used, levels should be monitored because the safety of these drugs in pregnancy has never been determined (see Chapter 19).

Expected Response

Clinical response to intravenous antimicrobial therapy usually occurs within 72 to 96 hours. Bacteremia, identified in 10% to 20% of cases, does not mandate prolonged intravenous therapy. Initial parenteral antimicrobial therapy is continued until the patient is afebrile for 48 hours and symptoms have improved. Oral administration of a susceptibility-guided antimicrobial agent is then continued for 5 to 10 days. After therapy, follow-up cultures should be obtained in 2 weeks to determine whether bacteriuria is resolved.

Recurrent acute pyelonephritis is common without antimicrobial suppression (23% versus 2.7%). In general, the organism identified in the initial episode will be responsible for all subsequent episodes. With recurrent pyelonephritis, review of the previous urine culture and sensitivity results will aid in the selection of the most appropriate antibiotics.

The goal of antimicrobial therapy is complete elimination of bacteria from the urinary tract. Once antimicrobial therapy and intravenous hydration have been initiated, clinical resolution usually occurs within 72 hours. After the patient remains afebrile for 24 to 48 hours, appropriate oral antimicrobial therapy should be instituted for a total of 7 to 10 days.

Suppressive therapy is recommended during the remainder of the pregnancy. Suppression is accomplished with the administration of nitrofurantoin macrocrystals, 100 mg taken orally at bedtime. Women not receiving suppressive therapy require frequent clinical evaluation and urine cultures.

Complications

Acute pyelonephritis during pregnancy can result in serious maternal and fetal complications. As many as 25% of women with severe infection have a component of multiorgan involvement, suggesting that pregnant women may be more susceptible to endotoxin-mediated organ damage. Urine concentrating ability and creatinine clearance are often decreased during the infection. Renal insufficiency, occurring in up to 18% of patients, is usually transient, but chronic pyelonephritis and chronic renal failure can occur despite adequate treatment. Anemia (Hematocrit <30%) is found in up to 25% of patients with acute pyelonephritis. Septic shock is a rare complication, usually associated with gram-negative bacteremia (observed in 10% to 15% of patients). Respiratory insufficiency, one of the most significant complications of acute pyelonephritis, occurs in 2% to 8% of affected pregnant women. The extent of respiratory insufficiency ranges from mild respiratory distress to pulmonary failure caused by endotoxin-induced alveolar capillary membrane injury. Furthermore, aggressive hydration and use of tocolytics, such as terbutaline and magnesium sulfate, may contribute to the development of pulmonary edema. Development of dyspnea, tachypnea, hypoxemia, or cyanosis typically occurs once the patient has been admitted to the hospital and therapy is initiated. Deterioration in respiratory symptoms should prompt a thorough investigation, including chest-x ray examination and arterial blood gas measurements. In one study women in whom acute respiratory distress syndrome developed had higher temperatures, elevated serum creatinine levels, severe anemia, thrombocytopenia, leukocytosis, and radiographic evidence of pulmonary infiltrates. Because of the level of critical care required, consultation and comanagement with intensive care service personnel are appropriate. Prompt recognition and appropriate therapy can offer an excellent prognosis to the mother and fetus.

Acute pyelonephritis has been associated with an increase in low birth weight and preterm delivery. Before routine prenatal screening and treatment the incidence of preterm delivery of affected pregnant women was 20% to 50%. Endotoxin affecting the prostaglandin pathway may provoke myometrial contractility or exert destructive effects on the vasculature of the uterus and placenta, leading to preterm labor and delivery.

When to Refer

The need to hospitalize all pregnant women with pyelonephritis has been challenged in recent years. Nonpregnant women with pyelonephritis are effectively treated as outpatients. In one recent study of women at less than 24 weeks' gestation, outpatient therapy with intramuscular administration of ceftriaxone was found to be as effective as inpatient therapy with intravenously administered cefazolin. However, candidates for outpatient management of pyelonephritis in pregnancy should be selected judiciously. They should be relatively healthy, have no sign of sepsis, have no confounding complications of pregnancy, and be able to tolerate oral fluids. Other contraindications to ambulatory therapy include recurrent upper urinary tract disease, concurrent preterm labor, uncertain diagnosis, and a poor record of compliance. Liberalizing the criteria for outpatient therapy may lead to serious consequences, such as respiratory distress and preterm delivery. Institution of antimicrobial therapy in women with pyelonephritis may result in increased uterine activity, which is most likely the result of the release of endotoxin.

Indications for complete urologic evaluation are failure of a patient to show clinical response after 72 hours of antimicrobial therapy despite the organism's sensitivity to the antimicrobial therapy and bacterial persistence after initial urine culture. Radiologic evaluation of the urinary tract is warranted to exclude renal abscesses, calculi, or an obstruction. Sonography is the preferred method of diagnosis, although the sensitivity of ultrasound for detecting calculi is limited. If the diagnosis is in doubt after the initial examination, a limited exposure intravenous pyelogram should be obtained. Sonography and magnetic resonance imaging are the methods of choice for evaluating suspected renal nephronia and perinephric abscess. Either problem may require surgical intervention.

 KEY POINTS

URINARY TRACT INFECTION IN PREGNANCY

⊃ Acute pyelonephritis occurs in 1% to 2% of pregnant women, with 70% to 80% of cases occurring in women with a history of asymptomatic bacteriuria.

⊃ Ureteral obstruction and stasis affect the progression of bacteriuria in pregnancy.

⊃ *E. coli* is the uropathogen most commonly isolated in women with pyelonephritis.

⊃ Clinical signs and symptoms are fever, chills, nausea, vomiting, lower urinary tract symptoms (dysuria, frequency, and urgency), and costovertebral angle tenderness.

⊃ Renal involvement is usually unilateral, with a right-sided predominance (>50%).

⊃ Treatment includes intravenous hydration and parenteral antimicrobial therapy (ampicillin-gentamicin) or a cephalosporin.

⊃ Approximately 90% of affected patients respond to antimicrobial therapy within 72 hours.

⊃ Long-term antimicrobial suppression or close monitoring and treatment of bacteriuria may prevent recurrence.

⊃ UTI in pregnancy is associated with multiple organ dysfunction, including endotoxemia and shock, anemia and thrombocytopenia, renal insufficiency, and respiratory distress syndrome.

⊃ UTI in pregnancy is associated with fetal growth restriction, prematurity, and fetal death.

SUGGESTED READING

Connolly A, Thorp JM Jr. Urinary tract infections in pregnancy. Urol Clin North Am 1999; 26: 779-787.

Cox SM, Shelburne P, Mason R, et al. Mechanisms of hemolysis and anemia associated with acute antepartum pyelonephritis. Am J Obstet Gynecol 1991; 164: 587-590.

Faro S, Fenner DE. Urinary tract infections. Clin Obstet Gynecol 1998; 41: 744-754.

McDermott S, Callaghan W, Szwejbka L, et al. Urinary tract infections during pregnancy and mental retardation and developmental delay. Obstet Gynecol 2000; 96: 113-119.

Millar LK, Cox SM. Urinary tract infections complicating pregnancy. Infect Dis Clin North Am 1997;11:13-26.

Millar LK, Wing DA, Paul RH. Outpatient treatment of pyelonephritis in pregnancy: a randomized controlled trial. Obstet Gynecol 1995; 86: 560-564.

Patterson TF, Andriole VT. Detection, significance and therapy of bacteriuria in pregnancy. Infect Dis Clin North Am 1997; 11: 593-608.

Towers CU, Kaminskas CM, Garite TG. Pulmonary injury associated with antepartum pyelonephritis: can patients at risk be identified? Am J Obstet Gynecol 1991; 164: 974-980.

Wing DA. Pyelonephritis. Clin Obstet Gynecol 1998; 41: 515-526.

Chorioamnionitis

Acute chorioamnionitis and intraamniotic infection are regularly encountered intrapartum complications of pregnancy. These terms are frequently used interchangeably, but they are not synonymous entities. Intraamniotic infection describes the clinical syndrome of an infection involving the amniotic cavity, amniotic fluid, membranes, placenta, or uterus and diagnosed on the basis of maternal and fetal clinical manifestations. Chorioamnionitis is an infection that involves the amniotic cavity and its membranes and is diagnosed histologically by detecting bacteria and leukocytes between the chorion and amnion. Chorioamnionitis is used in this discussion to describe the clinical entity, although histologic diagnosis may or may not have been documented. Both chorioamnionitis and intraamniotic infection are associated not only with significant maternal morbidity and mortality, but also with significant neonatal morbidity and mortality.

Chorioamnionitis is more commonly associated with preterm labor and delivery; however, it complicates 0.5% to 2% of term pregnancies. The incidence of chorioamnionitis is reported to range from 0.5% to 10.5%, reflecting different obstetric populations, mode of diagnosis (histologic versus clinical), and obstetric management. Chorioamnionitis accounts for 10% to 40% of febrile morbidity cases in the peripartum period and is associated with 20% to 40% of early neonatal sepsis and pneumonia. The incidences of respiratory distress syndrome, neonatal sepsis, seizures during the first 24 hours of life, intraventricular hemorrhage, and periventricular leukomalacia are significantly increased in very low birth weight infants (<1500 g) delivered of mothers with clinical chorioamnionitis. This observation suggests that chorioamnionitis somehow predisposes very low birth weight infants to neurologic damage. In term infants, however, short-term neurologic morbidity manifesting as seizures appears to be related to labor complications rather than to chorioamnionitis.

Chorioamnionitis is also associated with an increase in maternal pelvic infections, sepsis, and death. Similarly, neonatal septicemia, pneumonia, and adverse neurologic outcomes are more common in pregnancies complicated by chorioamnionitis. Early diagnosis and appropriate treatment are paramount to minimize fetal risks and other adverse sequelae for the mother and neonate.

Presentation and Progression

Cause

Risk factors for chorioamnionitis include young age, nulliparity, bacterial vaginosis (BV), bacterial colonization of the cervix, meconium-stained amniotic fluid, number of digital cervical examinations during labor, internal fetal monitoring, preterm labor, duration of labor, and ruptured membranes. The two most common associations are BV and preterm premature ruptured membranes. BV, prenatally and antenatally, in term pregnancies increases the risk of intraamniotic infection by as much as seven-fold. Women with evidence of BV during the second and third trimesters have a two-fold increased risk of chorioamnionitis. Meconium-stained amniotic fluid, a potential marker of microbial invasion of the amniotic fluid cavity, is associated with a four-fold increased incidence of chorioamnionitis.

Rupture of membranes before labor, term or preterm, is the single most common risk factor. Preterm premature rupture of membranes results in a 10-fold increased risk of chorioamnionitis. Chorioamnionitis is usually polymicrobial. The number of microorganisms in the amniotic fluid depends on the concentration of microorganisms within the cervix and vagina, the rate of ascent into the amniotic cavity, and the replication rate of the microorganisms. Group B streptococci and *E. coli* are the aerobic organisms most commonly associated with chorioamnionitis. Anaerobic microorganisms are commonly present when chorioamnionitis complicates preterm births. *Ureaplasma urealyticum, Mycoplasma hominis, Candida tropicalis, P. aeruginosa,* and *Salmonella typhi* have also been implicated in the pathogenesis of chorioamnionitis.

Chorioamnionitis sometimes results from hematogenous spread of microorganisms to the amniotic cavity. Microorganisms can also be introduced iatrogenically at the time of invasive procedures. Infection occurs in approximately in 0.6% of patients undergoing percutaneous umbilical blood sampling and 0.01% of patients undergoing amniocentesis. Infection has been found in 1% to 2% of patients undergoing elective cervical cerclage placement and up to 39% of patients undergoing emergency cerclage after advanced cervical dilation and prolapse of membranes.

Presentation

Chorioamnionitis may complicate up to 2% of term pregnancies, but it is more commonly associated with preterm labor and delivery. Early diagnosis of clinical chorioamnionitis is challenging because the clinical signs and symptoms occur relatively late and may be quite subtle. Although the criteria used in the diagnosis are neither sensitive nor specific, a high level of suspicion must be maintained to avoid delay in diagnosis.

The presentation of clinical chorioamnionitis includes fever (≥99° F [37.8° C]), maternal tachycardia, uterine tenderness, ruptured membranes, foul-smelling amniotic fluid, and maternal leukocytosis. The most significant and constant finding is maternal fever, which is considered the hallmark for diagnosis. Nearly all pregnant patients with documented chorioamnionitis are febrile (95% to 100%). Fetal manifestations may include a nonreassuring fetal heart rate pattern, such as fetal tachycardia and decreased variability. When the presentation is intrapartum fever and ruptured membranes, chorioamnionitis must be immediately considered, especially in the absence of other sources of infection.

Diagnosis

Chorioamnionitis is a clinical diagnosis, but it is ultimately confirmed histologically. Chorioamnionitis is diagnosed when the intrapartum temperature is $\geq 99°$ F (37.8° C) and two or more of the following conditions exist: maternal tachycardia (pulse >100 beats/min), fetal tachycardia (fetal heart tone >160 beats/min), uterine tenderness, foul odor of the amniotic fluid, or maternal leukocytosis (WBC count >15,000/mm³). A variety of combinations of these criteria may be present in patients with chorioamnionitis.

Leukocytosis, elevated C-reactive protein level, and positive blood cultures may help in the diagnosis of chorioamnionitis. In one study leukocytosis (WBC count >15,000/mm³) was found in 63% of pregnant women with infection; however, labor alone may result in an elevated WBC count. An elevated level of C-reactive protein, an acute-phase reactant, may also be found in pregnancies complicated by chorioamnionitis. Bacteremia occurs in about 10% of patients with chorioamnionitis.

Amniotic fluid, collected via aspiration with an intrauterine pressure catheter or by transabdominal amniocentesis, can be evaluated for leukocyte concentration, leukocyte esterases, glucose concentration, cytokines, prorenin and renin, organic acid by-products of bacterial metabolism, and bacteria through Gram stain and culture. Elevated leukocyte counts and leukocyte esterase levels in amniotic fluid are found in the majority of women with clinical chorioamnionitis. Detection of amniotic fluid leukocytes is considered to be of little diagnostic value. Amniotic fluid leukocyte esterase, however, provides more dependable information about the presence of chorioamnionitis. The relationship between amniotic fluid glucose level and chorioamnionitis is equivocal. In the presence of moderate amniotic fluid leukocytosis, low glucose concentrations (normal defined as <20 mg/dL) are common. The combination of Gram stain of the amniotic fluid and aerobic and anaerobic culture is the best method for confirming the diagnosis of chorioamnionitis. Gram staining of amniotic fluid is used as an adjunctive rapid diagnostic test for chorioamnionitis. The identification of microorganisms on HPF of unspun amniotic fluid is considered a positive finding, but the correlation between a positive Gram stain and clinical chorioamnionitis remains unclear. In one study the sensitivity and specificity of a positive Gram stain in predicting clinical infection were 78% and 81%, respectively. Bacterial culture of amniotic fluid may provide useful information; however, the 48- to 72-hour delay for the results limits the clinical application. Once again, positive bacterial growth may not be associated with clinical chorioamnionitis. In one study 17 of 90 women in labor at term had positive bacterial cultures of amniotic fluid, but only one of these 17 women showed clinical signs of clinical chorioamnionitis. Although not recommended as a basis for clinical management, positive cultures can guide the management of postpartum endometritis (discussed later in the chapter).

Histologic evaluation of the placenta, membranes, and umbilical cord provides retrospective diagnosis of chorioamnionitis. On gross examination the infected membranes may appear opaque and friable. As the leukocyte exudate accumulates, the membrane surfaces may turn yellow. In addition, the placenta is sometimes malodorous. Microscopic examination reveals an acute inflammatory reaction with polymorphonuclear leukocytes, eosinophils, and macrophages. Maternal leukocytes migrate from the intervillous space, and fetal leukocytes from the fetal vessels on the surface of the placenta. Both maternal and fetal leukocytes appear to migrate toward the amniotic cavity. Unfortunately, histologic confirmation of chorioamnionitis does not necessarily correlate with the diagnosis of intraamniotic infection or clinical chorioamnionitis. Histologic chorioamnionitis is detected in 11% to 16% of full-term pregnancies, whereas clinical signs of chorioamnionitis are reported in 1% to 29% of full-term pregnancies. In one study histologic chorioamnionitis was found in more than one half of low birth weight deliveries despite the absence of clinical signs of infection.

Treatment

When the diagnosis of chorioamnionitis has been made, appropriate management consists of parenteral antimicrobial therapy and delivery of the fetus. Broad-spectrum antibiotic therapy is used, since the infection is nearly always polymicrobial. The following are appropriate regimens:

- For combination therapy: ampicillin or penicillin plus gentamicin, sometimes with the addition of clindamycin; vancomycin plus gentamicin; or cefazolin plus gentamicin
- For monotherapy: a cephalosporin (cefoxitin or a third-generation cephalosporin), an extended spectrum penicillin (mezlocillin, piperacillin, ticarcillin-clavulanate, piperacillin-tazobactam, or ampicillin-sulbactam); or erythromycin

The physician must take into consideration that about 20% of women with chorioamnionitis are colonized with anaerobic organisms; thus the addition of an antimicrobial with good anaerobic coverage may be necessary. Other authorities recommend empiric anaerobic coverage only for women undergoing operative delivery. When dual therapy (ampicillin-gentamicin) was compared with triple therapy (ampicillin-gentamicin-clindamycin), no difference was found in the frequency of pelvic infections after vaginal delivery; however, with triple therapy the incidence of postpartum endometritis after cesarean delivery was lower. No differences in neonatal morbidity and mortality were noted.

Antimicrobial therapy should be given as soon as chorioamnionitis is diagnosed. Previously a delay in antimicrobial therapy was supported to allow time to obtain antimicrobial-free blood specimens from the neonate for cultures; however, several studies show a significant advantage of immediate intrapartum therapy over postpartum therapy. In one study neonatal sepsis (especially from group B streptococci) occurred in 4.7% of cases in which postpartum therapy was given versus no cases in which immediate intrapartum therapy was initiated. In a prospective randomized trial, pneumonia and sepsis developed in 32% of the neonates who received postpartum therapy but in none of the neonates whose mothers were treated intrapartum. Length of hospitalization was also decreased in mothers who were treated intrapartum.

With appropriate antimicrobial therapy for clinical chorioamnionitis, there is no critical time period in which delivery must be accomplished to decrease maternal and neonatal complications. Intervals greater than 12 hours, however, may have an impact on neonatal morbidity.

Chorioamnionitis is associated with dysfunctional labor patterns, resulting in an increased incidence in cesarean deliveries. The cesarean delivery rate in pregnancies complicated by chorioamnionitis is 35% to 40%. However, chorioamnionitis is not an indication for operative delivery. If a cesarean delivery is indicated, the standard transperitoneal low transverse uterine incision is appropriate. In the past, some researchers recommended extraperitoneal cesarean delivery to decrease maternal infection–related complications by avoiding contamination of the peritoneal cavity. This technique is no longer used because of technical difficulty and the higher surgical morbidity and similar infectious morbidity as compared with the transperitoneal approach.

If the patient is receiving dual therapy (ampicillin-gentamicin) and requires a cesarean delivery, clindamycin is added empirically at the time of operative delivery to decrease postcesarean endometritis, pelvic abscess, and septic pelvic thrombophlebitis. Generally, the antimicrobial agents are continued post partum until the patient remains afebrile for 24 to 48 hours.

Complications

Maternal complications of chorioamnionitis include dysfunctional labor, cesarean delivery, bacteremia, sepsis, endometritis, and wound infection. Neonatal complications include stillbirth, pneumonia, sepsis, intraventricular and periventricular hemorrhage, and cerebral palsy. Various studies on chorioamnionitis have shown an increased requirement for oxytocin augmentation and higher doses of oxytocin to achieve an adequate contraction pattern. Labor progression may be slow. Analysis of the impact of chorioamnionitis on labor progression, depending on the time of diagnosis of chorioamnionitis and oxytocin augmentation, led to the conclusion that clinical chorioamnionitis after oxytocin augmentation of labor might be a harbinger of labor dystocia.

The incidence of a postpartum infection is directly related to the route of delivery. Women who undergo a cesarean delivery are at increased risk for postpartum infection. The frequency of postpartum infection is further heightened with a concurrent diagnosis of chorioamnionitis. In one study postpartum infection was diagnosed in 48% of patients who underwent a cesarean delivery compared with 11% of patients who underwent a vaginal delivery.

Regardless of gestational age, in the presence of chorioamnionitis there is an increased incidence in neonatal morbidity and mortality associated with infection. Prematurity potentially makes the infant more susceptible to infection, which magnifies the risk of infectious complications in infants born to mothers with chorioamnionitis. The most common infection-related complications are pneumonia (≤23%) and sepsis (≤21%), the risk for which may be altered by maternal antimicrobial therapy. Infants weighing <2500 g have an increased rate of sepsis when compared with term infants (16% versus 4%). In addition to having a higher risk for infectious morbidity, the preterm infant of a mother with chorioamnionitis is at greater risk for respiratory distress syndrome, intraventricular hemorrhage, seizures, periventricular

leukomalacia, cerebral palsy, necrotizing enterocolitis, and neonatal death than a preterm infant born to a mother without chorioamnionitis. Term infants who have been exposed to maternal infection also seem to be more prone to periventricular leukomalacia, resulting in cerebral palsy.

Although a rare event, the most devastating adverse fetal outcome with chorioamnionitis is death. In the investigation of the death of a preterm infant, it may be difficult to determine whether infection or complications of prematurity were the cause.

 KEY POINTS

CHORIOAMNIONITIS

- ⊃ Chorioamnionitis is more commonly associated with preterm labor and delivery; however, it complicates 0.5% to 2% of term pregnancies.
- ⊃ Chorioamnionitis accounts for 10% to 40% of febrile morbidity cases in the peripartum period.
- ⊃ Premature rupture of membranes before labor, term or preterm, is the single most common risk factor for chorioamnionitis.
- ⊃ Chorioamnionitis is generally polymicrobial
- ⊃ Clinical signs and symptoms of chorioamnionitis are fever, maternal tachycardia, uterine tenderness, ruptured membranes, foul-smelling amniotic fluid, and fetal tachycardia.
- ⊃ Chorioamnionitis is a clinical diagnosis, ultimately confirmed histologically.
- ⊃ Treatment of chorioamnionitis includes broad-spectrum antimicrobials (ampicillin-aminoglycoside) and delivery of the fetus. Antimicrobial therapy is continued until the patient remains afebrile for 24 to 48 hours.
- ⊃ Chorioamnionitis is associated with dysfunctional labor patterns, maternal pelvic infections, sepsis, and death.
- ⊃ Chorioamnionitis is associated with neonatal septicemia, pneumonia, and adverse neurologic outcomes.

SUGGESTED READING

Alexander JM, Gilstrap LC, Cox SM, et al. Clinical chorioamnionitis and the prognosis for very low birth weight infants. Obstet Gynecol 1998; 91: 725-729.

Alexander JM, McIntire DM, Leveno KJ. Chorioamnionitis and the prognosis for term infants. Obstet Gynecol 1999; 94: 274-278.

Casey BM, Cox SM. Chorioamnionitis and endometritis. Infect Dis Clin North Am 1997; 11: 203-222.

Chapman SJ, Owen J. Randomized trial of single-dose versus multiple-dose cefotetan for the postpartum treatment of intrapartum chorioamnionitis. Am J Obstet Gynecol 1997; 177: 831-834.

Grether JK, Nelson KB. Maternal infection and cerebral palsy in infants of normal birth weight. JAMA 1997; 278: 207-211.

Mark SP, Croughan-Minihane MS, Kilpatrick SJ. Chorioamnionitis and uterine function. Obstet Gynecol 2000; 95: 909-912.

Parilla BV, McDermott TM. Prophylactic amnioinfusion in pregnancies complicated by chorioamnionitis: a prospective randomized trial. Am J Perinatol 1998; 15: 649-652.

Seaward PG, Hannah ME, Myhr TL, et al. International multicentre term prelabor rupture of membranes study: evaluation of predictors of clinical chorioamnionitis and postpartum fever in patients

with prelabor rupture of membranes at term. Am J Obstet Gynecol 1997; 177: 1024-1029.
Turnquest MA, How HY, Cook CR, et al. Chorioamnionitis: is continuation of antibiotic therapy necessary after cesarean section? Am J Obstet Gynecol 1998; 179: 1261-1266.

Endometritis

Pelvic infection is the most commonly encountered postpartum complication of infection. It is defined as infection of the endometrium or decidua with extension into the myometrium, parametrial tissues, or ovarian and pelvic vessels. Depending on the extent of bacterial invasion, the resultant infection is termed metritis, endometritis, endomyometritis, or endomyoparametritis. Regardless of the degree of invasion, many practitioners use the term "endometritis" or "metritis" to describe this postpartum complication.

Route of delivery and patient's socioeconomic status greatly influence the occurrence of puerperal endometritis. The likelihood of endometritis after vaginal delivery is less than 3%, whereas after cesarean delivery the risk ranges from 15% to 95%, reflecting obstetric populations (private versus indigent) and use of prophylactic antibiotics.

Pelvic infection should be considered when a woman has postpartum fever in the absence of another identifiable source of infection. Endometritis that develops despite the use of prophylactic antibiotics may be associated with significant postpartum morbidity. Sequelae include phlegmons, septic pelvic vein thrombophlebitis, pelvic abscess, and wound infection with dehiscence.

Presentation and Progression
Cause

Postpartum endometritis is usually polymicrobial and results from an ascending infection. Generally two or three organisms indigenous to the cervicovaginal flora are involved. Both aerobic and anaerobic organisms have been isolated from the uterus or decidua in women with puerperal endometritis.

In women with early postpartum endometritis (i.e., within the first 48 hours after delivery), gram-positive facultative microorganisms account for 40% of endometrial and 25% of blood culture isolates. Group B streptococci (15% of cases), the most frequently identified gram-positive aerobic organisms, are associated with high fever immediately after delivery. Other classic signs or symptoms of endometritis may be absent. *Enterococcus faecalis* (10%), viridans streptococci, *Staphylococcus aureus,* and *Staphylococcus epidermidis* are also sometimes present. *E. faecalis* is rarely the sole pathogen but rather is usually isolated with other aerobic and anaerobic bacteria.

Gram-negative facultative organisms account for 22% of endometrial and 21% of blood culture isolates from women with early postpartum endometritis. *Gardnerella vaginalis* (54%) and *E. coli* (30%) are the most commonly identified gram negative organisms. In the clinical setting of postpartum sepsis, *E. coli* should be strongly suspected. Other gram-negative microorganisms, such as *Enterobacter aerogenes, Klebsiella pneumoniae,* and *Proteus mirabilis,* have also been detected.

Anaerobic bacteria account for 38% of endometrial and 54% of blood isolates from women with postpartum endo-

metritis. Peptostreptococci and peptococci are the most common anaerobic gram-positive isolates, whereas *Bacteroides bivius* is the most common anaerobic gram-negative isolate. *Clostridium perfringens* and *Fusobacterium* species are other anaerobic microorganisms implicated in endometritis. *C. trachomatis* is associated with late-onset postpartum endometritis (i.e., 3 days to 6 weeks after delivery); however, this organism is occasionally isolated in early postpartum endometritis (4%). Antimicrobial regimens selected to treat puerperal endometritis are not effective against *Chlamydia;* thus an endometrial specimen for culture should be obtained from women with late-onset endometritis. Genital mycoplasmas (76%), *M. hominis,* and *U. urealyticum* are commonly detected in women with puerperal infections, but their precise role in endometritis remains unclear.

Administration of prophylactic antimicrobial agents (e.g., a cephalosporin) before cesarean delivery alters the cervicovaginal flora, which influences the organisms isolated in women with postpartum endometritis. Although susceptible microorganisms are less likely to be identified, cephalosporin prophylaxis increases the detection of enterococci and *Enterobacter* by three-fold and 15-fold, respectively, and decreases the detection of *Proteus* species. Ampicillin prophylaxis leads to an increase in the detection of *Mycoplasma, Klebsiella,* and *E. coli.* Postpartum endometritis is usually a polymicrobial infection, but after intraoperative prophylaxis, endometritis caused by a single pathogen is more common. In addition, if postoperative endometritis develops despite appropriate prophylaxis, the woman should not be treated with the same antimicrobial because of the increased likelihood of resistant organisms and wound infections.

The pathogenesis of puerperal endometritis involves an intricate relationship between host defense mechanisms, size of bacterial inoculum, and bacterial virulence. Socioeconomic and general health status of the women influences the host defense mechanisms, which may predispose women to postpartum infection. The number of vaginal examinations, duration of labor, and time since rupture of membranes affect the size of the bacterial inoculum. Bacterial virulence depends on the microorganism isolated from the cervicovaginal flora. In addition, wound ischemia after an operative delivery and serosanguineous fluid provide an ideal environment for infection. Some women, however, do not become infected regardless of the presence of the above-mentioned factors.

Risk Factors

The route of delivery (i.e., cesarean versus vaginal) is the most important determinant in the development of puerperal endometritis. Protracted labor, prolonged rupture of membranes, and multiple vaginal examinations are the major risk factors associated with endometritis. The presence of bacterial vaginosis, prenatally and antenatally, can predispose women to postpartum infection. Internal monitoring, manual extraction of the placenta at the time of cesarean delivery, anesthesia, adolescence, maternal anemia, obesity, and indigent socioeconomic status can, furthermore, influence the occurrence of endometritis.

Endometritis occurs in less than 3% of vaginal deliveries; however, the incidence ranges between 15% and 95% of cesarean deliveries depending on the patient's clinical status. A distinction exists between the low- and high-risk groups.

Low-risk groups include women undergoing a scheduled repeat cesarean delivery who have not entered labor and have intact fetal membranes. High-risk factors include labor greater than 6 hours, prolonged time since rupture of membranes (>6 hours), numerous cervical examinations, and diagnosis of chorioamnionitis. Although postcesarean endometritis occurs in 5% to 6% of low-risk women, it complicates the postoperative course of 22% to 85% of high-risk women.

The duration of labor is a significant factor in postpartum endometritis. Typically, protracted labor results in multiple vaginal examinations and increases the bacterial colonization of the lower uterine segment. In one study frequent examinations were associated with a 2.2-fold increased risk of postcesarean endometritis. That vaginal examinations introduce indigenous cervicovaginal flora into the intraamniotic cavity is well established; in addition, uterine contractions may produce a vacuum that draws pathogens into this space. The length of time after rupture of the membrane has also been correlated with the development of puerperal endometritis. In one study all women whose membranes had been ruptured for more than 6 hours had positive amniotic fluid cultures, and puerperal endometritis developed in 95% of these women.

Internal fetal heart rate monitors may be a minor risk factor for postpartum endometritis. The presumption is that microorganisms gain access to the uterine cavity via the fetal monitors. Available data on this association are conflicting. In general, fetal monitoring is required in high-risk states, that is, slow labor or failure to progress, both of which are clear risk factors for endometritis.

Presentation

Endometritis usually (but not always) is accompanied by fever and should always be considered in the differential diagnosis of puerperal fever. Besides fever ($\geq$100.4° F [38° C]), postpartum endometritis may manifest itself with maternal tachycardia, lower abdominal pain, uterine tenderness, decreased bowel sounds, foul-smelling lochia, or leukocytosis. Uterine tenderness may be the major clue to endometritis in an afebrile patient.

Puerperal fever should never be ignored in the postoperative and postpartum period. On the first postpartum day, low-grade temperatures (100.4° to 101° F [38° to 38.3° C]) that resolve spontaneously may be the result of dehydration, atelectasis, reaction to infusion of fetal proteins, or transient bacteremia. Persistent low-grade temperatures, however, should be appropriately evaluated; untreated infection may result in significant maternal morbidity.

Diagnosis

The diagnosis of endometritis is based on clinical signs and symptoms, including fever, uterine tenderness, lower abdominal pain, foul-smelling lochia, and maternal leukocytosis. Group A and group B streptococcal infection, however, may be manifested as high fever without other classic signs and symptoms of endometritis. A complete history and physical examination (including an evaluation of possible risk factors and a complete pelvic examination) are essential to differentiate postpartum endometritis from other sources of postpartum morbidity, such as urinary tract infections, viral syndrome, pneumonia, mastitis, and phlebitis.

Laboratory studies that may be beneficial include a CBC, aerobic and anaerobic blood cultures, and endometrial cultures. Although leukocytosis may be indicative of infection, it is frequently observed in noninfected women during labor and post partum. Bacteremia occurs in 10% to 30% of patients with early postpartum endometritis. Organisms isolated from blood cultures represent a portion of the aerobic and anaerobic organisms cultured from the uterine cavity or decidua in patients with endometritis.

Transcervical aerobic and anaerobic endometrial cultures may identify the causative microorganisms of the infectious process. Gram stain of endometrial fluid can be used as a rapid adjunctive test, especially if hemolytic streptococci or clostridia are suspected. A specimen acquired from the endometrial cavity with an unprotected transcervical swab or catheter, however, is frequently contaminated with endogenous lower genital tract flora. Double-lumen protected swabs, double-lumen protected brushes with a protective polyethylene glycol plug, and a triple-lumen protected aspirator have been created to minimize cervicovaginal contamination. Because of the difficulty in obtaining endometrial cultures and the 72-hour delay until results are available, most physicians initiate antimicrobial therapy without obtaining a culture. In most cases patients will respond to empiric therapy. For patients who do not respond to conventional therapy, endometrial cultures may guide the selection of an appropriate antimicrobial regimen.

Treatment
Methods

After other sources of infection are eliminated, parenteral antimicrobial therapy should be initiated immediately for postpartum endometritis. Since endometritis is polymicrobial from endogenous cervicovaginal flora, broad-spectrum antimicrobial agents are appropriate as an initial line of therapy. However, no consensus has been reached on the most efficacious therapeutic regimen.

The combination of ampicillin with an aminoglycoside is 95% effective in postpartum endometritis after vaginal delivery, but identical therapy is only 64% to 78% effective after cesarean delivery. With postcesarean endometritis the combination of clindamycin and an aminoglycoside provides excellent coverage in 90% to 95% of patients and markedly reduces the incidence of major infectious complications, such as pelvic abscesses or septic pelvic thrombophlebitis.

The replacement of clindamycin for ampicillin for postcesarean endometritis increases coverage of *Bacteroides* species, which are usually penicillin resistant; however, the clindamycin-gentamicin combination is not effective against enterococci, which may occur in patients who receive cephalosporin prophylaxis. For better synergistic coverage for enterococci, penicillin or ampicillin is added to the regimen.

During the last two decades a trend toward the use of single-agent therapy has emerged because of the advantages of less toxicity and theoretically less pharmacy and nursing time required for administration. Because of the polymicrobial nature of endometritis, broad-spectrum second- and third-generation cephalosporins, semisynthetic extended-spectrum penicillins, and combinations of β-lactam and β-lactamase inhibitors have been used. Drugs that have been studied as single-agent therapy include cefamandole, cefoxitin, cefotetan, cefoperazone, piperacillin, mezlocillin, ticarcillin-clavulanate, ampicillin-sulbactam, and ciprofloxacin. In general these agents are efficacious in 80% to 90% of patients. Although no single agent provides activity against the entire bacterial spectrum plus *C. trachomatis,* most of these drugs have sufficient aerobic and anaerobic activity to warrant consideration of their use. However, the limitations of clinical trials are such that the efficacy of drugs such as the β-lactams for monotherapy is often unknown or poorly defined in situations in which they are likely to be used, such as the treatment of endometritis in patients in whom antibiotic prophylaxis has failed. Recently investigators attempted to decrease the incidence of postpartum endometritis by using chlorhexidine vaginal washes during labor. Unfortunately, the likelihood of endometritis was the same in the control and treatment groups.

The intent of antimicrobial therapy is the eradication of causative microorganisms from the endometrial cavity. With the initiation of intravenous therapy a rapid clinical response can be anticipated. Although the patient may be improved clinically, she must remain afebrile for 24 to 48 hours before discontinuation of treatment. Oral antimicrobial agents after parenteral treatment have proved unnecessary.

Complications

Most patients respond during the initial 72 hours of antimicrobial therapy, but women who do not improve clinically may have organisms that are resistant or not covered by the empiric therapy. Despite adequate antimicrobial therapy, patients may continue to have persistent fever because of cellulitis, abdominal wound infection, phlegmon, pelvic abscess, septic pelvic thrombophlebitis, a nongenital source of infection (e.g., mastitis), connective tissue disease, or drug fever.

Wound infections require drainage and aggressive débridement two or three times a day. With persistent fever, abdominal and pelvic computed tomographic scans can detect phlegmon, pelvic abscesses, and septic thrombophlebitis, which will eventually respond to the continuation of broad-spectrum antimicrobial therapy with an emphasis on anaerobic coverage. Hysterectomy should be considered only for women with evidence of uterine myonecrosis.

 KEY POINTS

ENDOMETRITIS

⊃ The likelihood of postpartum endometritis after a vaginal delivery is less than 3%, whereas after cesarean delivery the risk ranges from 15% to 95%.

⊃ Postpartum endometritis is generally polymicrobial.

⊃ Clinical signs and symptoms include fever, maternal tachycardia, lower abdominal pain, uterine tenderness, decreased bowel sounds, foul-smelling lochia, and maternal leukocytosis.

⊃ Diagnosis is based on clinical signs and symptoms.

⊃ Treatment includes broad-spectrum antimicrobials (ampicillin-aminoglycoside for vaginal delivery or clindamycin-aminoglycoside for cesarean delivery). Antimicrobial agents should be continued until the patient remains afebrile for 24 to 48 hours.

⊃ Endometritis is associated with phlegmons, septic vein thrombophlebitis, pelvic abscess, and wound infection with dehiscence.

SUGGESTED READING

Casey BM, Cox SM. Chorioamnionitis and endometritis. Infect Dis Clin North Am 1997;11: 203-222.

Gall S, Koukol DH. Ampicillin/sulbactam vs. clindamycin/gentamicin in the treatment of postpartum endometritis. J Reprod Med 1996; 41:575-580.

Lasley DS, Eblen A, Yancey MK, et al. The effect of placental removal method on the incidence of postcesarean infections. Am J Obstet Gynecol 1997; 176: 1250-1254.

Monga M, Oshiro BT. Puerperal infections. Semin Perinatol 1993; 17: 426-431.

Newton ER, Wallace PA. Effects of prophylactic antibiotics on endometrial flora in women with postcesarean endometritis. Obstet Gynecol 1998; 92: 262-268.

Rouse DJ, Hauth JC, Andrews WW, et al. Chlorhexidine vaginal irrigation for the prevention of peripartal infection: a placebo-controlled randomized clinical trial. Am J Obstet Gynecol 1997; 176: 617-622.

6

Infectious Disease Emergencies

CHARLES S. BRYAN

From time to time the primary care clinician will face as an emergency a disease or syndrome with which he or she has little or no previous experience. The outcome will vary from triumph to tragedy. In the preparation of this book, a survey was conducted among fellows of the Infectious Diseases Society of America to determine what infectious diseases were especially problematic for primary care clinicians. Bad outcomes, measured as death, disability, or litigation, were particularly likely to occur in cases of necrotizing fasciitis and spinal epidural abscess—diseases that are distinctly uncommon in primary

care (Table 6-1). The goal of this chapter is to review some of the common and uncommon emergencies posed by acute infectious diseases. The differential diagnoses of fever and rash (see Chapter 7), rhinocerebral mucormycosis and malignant otitis externa (see Chapter 3), and infectious aspects of traumatic wounds (see Chapter 26) are discussed elsewhere. Infections involving the central nervous system (CNS) are discussed here, since these nearly always warrant hospitalization or referral. Some classic presentations are summarized in Table 6-2.

SUGGESTED READING

Brillman JC, Quenzer RW. Infectious Diseases in Emergency Medicine. 2nd ed., Philadelphia: Lippincott-Raven; 1998.

Davis LE, Kennedy PGE, eds. Infectious Diseases of the Nervous System. Oxford: Butterworth-Heinemann; 2000.

Lutwig LI, ed. Infectious disease emergencies. Infect Dis Clin North Am 1996; 10: 693-937.

Roberts R. Management of patients with infectious diseases in an emergency department observation unit. Emerg Med Clin North Am 2001; 19: 187-207.

Scheld WM, Whitley RJ, Durack DT, eds. Infections of the Central Nervous System. 2nd ed., Philadelphia: Lippincott-Raven, 1997.

Talan DA. Infectious disease issues in the emergency department. Clin Infect Dis 1996; 23: 1-14.

Sepsis Syndrome: Differential Diagnosis of the Flulike Illness

The syndrome of fever, malaise, myalgias, and other constitutional complaints is common in primary care practice. When localizing symptoms and physical findings are few and no rash is seen, patients are often presumed to have a "flulike illness" or "viral syndrome." Some, however, have treatable life-threatening disease. Examples are septicemia caused by *Staphylococcus aureus* or aerobic gram-negative rods, septic abortion, endocarditis, and Rocky Mountain spotted fever. The clinician's task is to determine which patients require close observation, special laboratory studies, and empiric antimicrobial therapy.

Presentation and Progression
Cause

Microorganisms have diverse effects on human cells and tissues, but the concept of a "final common pathway" leading to refractory shock continues to evolve (Figures 6-1 and 6-2). At the molecular level, researchers focus especially on a large number of cytokines (peptide hormones that act on cells) released in response to various insults. The best-studied interaction involves the endotoxin molecule (specifically, the lipid A moiety of a complex lipopolysaccharide) of gram-negative bacteria

TABLE 6-1
Frequency of Diseases in Which Mistakes Made by Primary Care Physicians Resulted in Serious Consequences*

Condition	No. (%) of positive responses	Condition	No. (%) of positive responses
Necrotizing soft tissue infection	112 (64)	Brain abscess	58 (33)
Spinal epidural abscess	96 (55)	Toxic shock syndrome	58 (33)
Sepsis syndrome	95 (54)	Asplenia (failure to vaccinate)	57 (33)
Endocarditis	94 (54)	Rocky Mountain spotted fever	54 (31)
Meningococcal disease	89 (51)	Travel-related problem§	54 (31)
Tuberculosis	84 (48)	Acute epiglottitis	35 (20)
Herpes simplex encephalitis	82 (47)	Pelvic inflammatory disease	32 (18)
Antibiotic toxicity†	82 (47)	Clostridial syndrome ‖	31 (18)
Pneumonia	80 (46)	*Haemophilus influenzae* meningitis	29 (17)
Pneumococcal meningitis	80 (46)	Sphenoid sinusitis	22 (13)
Intraabdominal sepsis	59 (34)	Cavernous sinus thrombosis	21 (12)
AIDS-related problem‡	58 (33)	Miscellaneous¶	32 (18)

AIDS, Acquired immunodeficiency syndrome.
*From a survey of fellows of the Infectious Diseases Society of America (IDSA).
METHOD: A survey instrument was mailed to 600 IDSA fellows. The survey listed 23 diagnoses (shown here) and asked the recipients to checkmark the diagnoses in which, in their experience, a mistake made by a physician acting in a primary care capacity had led to death, disability, or litigation. The rate of response to the survey was 30%. These data do not indicate the actual incidence of mistakes made in primary care (which some data indicate is relatively low). Rather, they indicate pitfalls in diagnosis and disease management as seen from the perspective of infectious disease specialists, who are usually consulted on especially difficult cases.
†Antibiotics most frequently named were the aminoglycosides (ototoxicity and nephrotoxicity) and the sulfonamides (Stevens-Johnson syndrome).
‡AIDS-related problems included failure to suspect and diagnose human immunodeficiency virus disease and to recognize its complications.
§Travel-related problems were dominated by malaria, which was often misdiagnosed as a "viral syndrome."
‖Clostridial syndromes included gas gangrene, *Clostridium difficile* colitis, and *Clostridium septicum* disease in the setting of malignancy.
¶Miscellaneous problems included babesiosis, blastomycosis, chronic fatigue syndrome, cryptococcosis, dengue shock syndrome, diabetic foot ulcer, ehrlichiosis, enterococcal infection, frontal sinusitis with osteomyelitis, histoplasmosis (disseminated), Kawasaki disease, listeriosis, Lyme disease, malignant otitis externa, mucormycosis, Pott's disease, and pulmonary infarction.

and human mononuclear cells, but it is now clear that gram-positive bacteria and other types of microorganisms cause shock by similar mechanisms.

Presentation

Certain definitions can facilitate the understanding of what happens during acute infections:

- Sepsis denotes clinical evidence of infection plus a host response: fever (temperature >100.4° F [38° C]) or hypothermia (temperature <96.8° F [36° C]), tachycardia (heart rate >90 beats/min), tachypnea (respiratory rate >20 breaths/min or $PaCO_2$ <32 mm Hg, and both quantitative and qualitative changes in circulating white blood cells (WBCs) (>12,000 cells/mm³ or <4000 cells/mm³ or >10% immature [band] forms).
- Sepsis syndrome denotes sepsis plus evidence of impaired organ perfusion. Evidence of impaired organ perfusion in the primary care setting includes altered mental status,

decreased urine output, and low oxygen saturation by pulse oximetry. Lactic acidosis may also be present.
- Severe sepsis denotes sepsis associated with organ dysfunction, hypoperfusion, or hypotension. Hypoperfusion abnormalities include oliguria and altered mental status. Hypotension is defined as systolic blood pressure <90 mm Hg or a falloff >40 mm Hg from baseline in the absence of other causes of hypotension.
- Septic shock is defined as sepsis with hypotension despite adequate fluid resuscitation, along with perfusion abnormalities such as lactic acidosis, oliguria, or acute alteration in mental status.

Many clinicians still use the older term "septicemia," which denotes the presence of microorganisms in the blood (as confirmed by culture) plus clinical evidence of sepsis. The concept of a systemic inflammatory response syndrome expresses the notion that the body responds in certain ways to a wide variety of insults. Thus, for example, shock with acute

TABLE 6-2
Some Classic Presentations of Infectious Disease Emergencies

Presentation	Cause
Severe localized pain over a seemingly trivial skin or soft tissue lesion, with marked systemic toxicity, in a patient who may have been taking nonsteroidal antiinflammatory drugs	Necrotizing fasciitis
Same patient as above, with bullae, watery discharge, or crepitance over an extremity that feels "heavy" to the patient	Clostridial myonecrosis (gas gangrene)
Listlessness and poor feeding in an infant or young child	Meningitis caused by *Listeria monocytogenes, Haemophilus influenzae* type b, or *Streptococcus pneumoniae*
Fever, headache, stiff neck, nausea, and vomiting in a previously healthy college student	Meningitis caused by *Neisseria meningitidis*
Fever, headache, and altered mental status in an older adult with a red tympanic membrane, paranasal sinus tenderness, or an abnormal chest examination	Meningitis caused by *Streptococcus pneumoniae*
Low-grade fever and altered mental status in a frail elderly nursing home resident	Meningitis caused by *S. pneumoniae, L. monocytogenes,* or an aerobic gram-negative rod
Lethargy, fever, and symptoms and signs pointing to the temporal lobe such as impaired speech	Encephalitis caused by herpes simplex virus, type 1
Overwhelming sepsis in a patient with a scar over the left upper quadrant of the abdomen	Overwhelming postsplenectomy infection syndrome, most commonly caused by *S. pneumoniae* or *H. influenzae*
Shock, multiorgan failure, and diffuse erythroderma in a young woman	Staphylococcal toxic shock syndrome
Shock, multiorgan failure, and localized skin infection with severe pain in a middle-aged person of either sex	Streptococcal toxic shock syndrome
Fever with abdominal and back pain in an older person with risk factors for atherosclerosis and a recent history of self-limited diarrhea	Mycotic aneurysm of the abdominal aorta caused by *Salmonella* species
Fever and localized back pain progressing to weakness of the lower extremities, with impaired bowel or bladder function	Spinal epidural abscess, most often caused by *Staphylococcus aureus*
Ascending flaccid paralysis in a young girl who has just returned from vacation in a wooded area	Tick paralysis
Fever, toxicity, and exquisite pain in the groin in a young man who has just returned from a camping trip in New Mexico	Bubonic plague
Fever with "flulike illness" in a patient complaining of the "worst headache ever," who has been in a tick habitat	Rocky Mountain spotted fever
Fever with "flulike illness" in an injecting drug user, with patchy bilateral infiltrates on chest x-ray examination	Acute staphylococcal endocarditis on tricuspid or pulmonic valves
Fever with "flulike illness" in an older person, with history or physical findings of valvular heart disease and evidence of heart failure	Acute staphylococcal endocarditis on aortic or mitral valves
Fever with "flulike illness" in a person with known cirrhosis, who has recently eaten raw oysters; skin lesions suggesting cellulitis with or without bullae are noted	Sepsis caused by *Vibrio vulnificus*

Continued

TABLE 6-2—cont'd
Some Classic Presentations of Infectious Diseases Emergencies

Presentation	Cause
Sore throat with difficulty breathing; patient may be leaning forward and drooling; pharynx relatively normal on examination	Acute epiglottitis
Returning traveler with high fever, headache, and systemic toxicity	Malaria caused by *Plasmodium falciparum*
Severe headache with facial pain or pain localized over the vertex in a patient with history of "sinus trouble"	Sphenoid sinusitis
Fever with rebound tenderness anywhere over the abdomen and bandemia on peripheral blood smear	Acute abdomen (causes include cholecystitis, pancreatitis, appendicitis, diverticulitis, and perforated viscus)
Personality change, impaired speech, lethargy, and confusion in a patient with no obvious underlying illness or exposure	Herpes simplex virus encephalitis
Fever with relative bradycardia, bilateral patchy pulmonary infiltrates, and mild elevation of aminotransferase levels and with a history of exposure to wild rabbits or other animals	Tularemia
Fever, chills, headaches, and pneumonia or tender lymphadenopathy with history of out-of-doors exposure in the southwestern United States	Plague
"Flulike illness" progressing to hypotension and pulmonary edema in a patient with out-of-doors exposure in the southwestern United States	Hantavirus pulmonary syndrome
Ascending flaccid paralysis in a young girl who has been in a tick habitat	Tick paralysis
Symmetric cranial nerve palsies and descending paralysis in a patient with dilated pupils and a dry mouth with furrowed tongue	Botulism

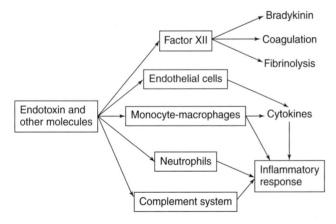

FIG. 6-1 Endotoxin (present in gram-negative bacterial cell walls) and other molecules (present in gram-positive bacteria and other types of microorganisms) interact with the numerous molecules in the blood and on the surfaces of various cells. If unchecked, these interactions lead to severe sepsis and then to refractory septic shock.

respiratory distress syndrome and renal failure can result from conditions as diverse as Rocky Mountain spotted fever and acute hemorrhagic pancreatitis.

Staphylococcal septicemia sometimes is manifested as an undifferentiated flulike illness, and this presentation can be especially treacherous when influenza A is prevalent in a community. The illness often begins abruptly with chills and generalized "aching all over," which is sometimes localized to the joints. Physical examination is often unrevealing. Endocarditis (discussed later in the chapter) is relatively common in this setting (≥10% of cases). Some patients have occult abscesses or osteomyelitis. Patients with *S. aureus* bacteremia can progress rapidly through the stages of sepsis, sepsis syndrome, severe sepsis, septic shock, and refractory septic shock.

Diagnosis

The clinician has three tasks: (1) to find clues by history and physical examination suggesting one or another specific, treatable infectious disease; (2) to determine whether the patient's general appearance, underlying condition, or findings on complete blood count (such as marked bandemia

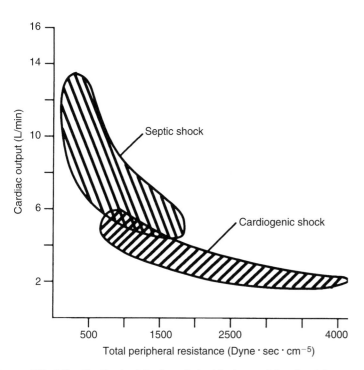

FIG. 6-2 Septic shock is characterized by low peripheral resistance and variable cardiac output, in contrast to cardiogenic shock (low cardiac output and variable peripheral resistance). The hemodynamic profiles of established shock caused by gram-negative and gram-positive bacteria are similar. (Modified from Wiles JB, Cerra FB, Siegel JH, et al. The systemic septic response: does the organism matter? Crit Care Med 1980; 8: 55-60.)

or thrombocytopenia) warrant admission to the hospital; and (3) to ensure close follow-up.

First, the clinician should search for an alternative diagnosis by careful if targeted history (Table 6-3) and physical examination (Table 6-4) before assigning a diagnosis of nonspecific "viral syndrome." Did the illness begin suddenly or gradually? Is the headache the patient's worst ever, and is it localized in any way? Does the "aching all over" specifically involve the joints? Has the patient been in a tick habitat? Vital signs must be carefully obtained. The clinician should personally obtain the heart rate and the respiratory rate. Tachypnea, which can be subtle, often indicates respiratory compensation to lactic acidosis, a marker that the patient has progressed from sepsis to the sepsis syndrome. What symptoms and signs are atypical for influenza or whatever "virus" seems to be circulating in the community? Answers to these questions can be lifesaving.

Second, the clinician must estimate the margin for error should the diagnosis of nonspecific "viral syndrome" prove incorrect. Younger patients with no underlying disease often tolerate septicemia remarkably well. However, the margin for error is small in older patients and those with "ultimately fatal underlying disease," defined as any condition likely to result in death within 5 years if untreated. Does the patient "look sick"—that is, appear toxic? Is there a history of "cold chills" (cold chills increase the likelihood of serious illness)? What does the peripheral blood show? If possible, the clinician should personally examine the peripheral blood, looking especially for toxic changes in the neutrophils and for thrombocytopenia.

Finally, if there are no clues to an alternative diagnosis and hospitalization does not seem to be indicated, the clinician should arrange for close follow-up. The patient should be advised to contact the office in the event of any worsening of his or her condition. It is often advisable to give the patient an appointment within the next several days, with the request that the appointment be canceled ahead of time if the condition improves. The clinician should be sure to follow up personally on any laboratory results that are pending when the patient leaves the office. The patient should be instructed to avoid sedatives of any kind, including such preparations as Fiorinal. Antipyretics should be used judiciously, if at all. Arranging for an early morning "buddy check" by the patient's parent, spouse, or roommate is often worthwhile (see Appendix 3). The clinician should remember that rare patients progress with great and unexpected rapidity from sepsis to sepsis syndrome to severe sepsis to refractory septic shock, with fatal outcome.

Some causes of abrupt onset of nonhemorrhagic shock in a previously healthy person are summarized in Table 6-5, and most of these are discussed later in the chapter.

Natural History
Expected Outcome

In the preantibiotic era, untreated staphylococcal and streptococcal septicemia carried mortality rates of 80% or higher.

Treatment
Methods

Treatment depends on the presumptive diagnosis. Some regimens for suspected septicemia are summarized in Appendix 2. Case-fatality rates of 30% to 35% for *Staphylococcus aureus* septicemia continue to be reported.

Expected Response

Response to treatment is highly variable and depends on the eventual diagnosis and the patient's age and underlying condition.

When to Refer

Patients with sepsis syndrome should be hospitalized. Hospitalization, if only for brief observation, should be considered for patients with sepsis who have severe underlying diseases.

 KEY POINTS

SEPSIS SYNDROME: DIFFERENTIAL DIAGNOSIS OF THE FLULIKE ILLNESS

⊃ Sepsis is now defined as evidence of infection *plus* a systemic response manifested by at least two of the following: fever or hypothermia; tachycardia (heart rate >90 beats/min); tachypnea (respiratory rate >20 breaths/min); and changes in the peripheral white blood cells (WBC count >12,000 or <4000, or >10% band forms on differential count).

⊃ Sepsis syndrome is now defined as sepsis *plus* evidence of altered organ perfusion with at least one of the following: altered mentation, oliguria, hypoxemia, or elevated lactate level.

TABLE 6-3
History: Questions to Ask of the Patient with Acute Undifferentiated "Flulike" Illness

Question	Implications and examples
Onset: Was it sudden or gradual?	A sudden onset is more likely to indicate an acute, treatable disease.
Headache: Is it the worst you've ever had?	Infectious causes of "worst headache ever" include Rocky Mountain spotted fever, meningitis, brain abscess, and sphenoid sinusitis.
Nausea: Is it severe, and have you vomited?	Nausea and vomiting sometimes indicate raised intracranial pressure, especially if the vomiting is forceful or "projectile."
Bowel habits: Any constipation or diarrhea?	Diarrhea does not necessarily indicate "gastroenteritis." It can be a nonspecific manifestation of septicemia. Patients with typhoid fever often have constipation rather than diarrhea.
Dyspnea: Do you feel short of breath?	Dyspnea may be a subtle clue to heart failure or to lactic acidosis from sepsis syndrome.
Pain: Do you have *any* localized pain or discomfort?	Localized pain—for example, over the spine—may indicate a localized pathologic condition such as a staphylococcal abscess or vertebral osteomyelitis.
Dysuria: Do you have burning on urination?	Patients with "upper UTI" symptoms (pyelonephritis) often have "lower UTI" symptoms as well.
Drugs: What drugs, including nonprescription drugs, have you taken within the past month?	Drugs are an important cause of undifferentiated fever. It is frequently worthwhile to look up all of the unusual side effects of the patient's drugs in the *Physician's Desk Reference.*
Prior illnesses: Have you ever had anything like this before?	Some patients will recall a similar infectious illness. Others may have diseases such as sickle cell anemia or familial Mediterranean fever that may not have been diagnosed.
Heart: Have you ever been told you have a murmur?	Undifferentiated fever with heart failure suggests that endocarditis should be considered.
Tick habitats and rural areas: Have you been out in the woods or exposed to ticks or wild animals?	Patients with Rocky Mountain spotted fever and other vectorborne diseases often do not recall a specific bite. Tularemia can manifest itself as a nonspecific "typhoidal" illness.
Family and friends: Has anyone been sick recently?	Disease transmission may be from person to person or from a common source.
Pregnancy: Is it possible that you may be pregnant, or have been pregnant recently?	Patients may be reluctant to volunteer a history of recent illegal abortion despite life-threatening sepsis, including gas gangrene of the uterus.
Sexual exposures: Have you had a new sex partner? Are you at risk for HIV?	Syphilis and gonorrhea can manifested themselves as undifferentiated flulike illness. The acute retroviral syndrome is an important cause of fever during the early (antibody-negative) stage of HIV infection.
Travel: Where have you been lately?	Exotic travel histories sometimes prove to be red herrings, but even travel within the United States may be significant (e.g., coccidioidomycosis in the Southwest and in southern California).
Pets: What animals do you keep?	Psittacosis can present as an undifferentiated flulike illness. Dogs often have ticks capable of transmitting Rocky Mountain spotted fever.

HIV, Human immunodeficiency virus; *UTI,* urinary tract infection.

TABLE 6-4
Physical Examination: Signs and Symptoms to Look for in the Patient with Undifferentiated "Flulike" Illness

Sign or symptom	Implications and examples
General appearance: Does the patient look "toxic"?	The primary care clinician who knows the patient well is uniquely prepared to make this subjective observation.
Vital signs: Do these meet the definitions of "sepsis"?	Pay close attention to the blood pressure, heart rate, and respiratory rate. Obtain pulse oximetry ("the fifth vital sign") if available.
Hands: Does the patient have splinter hemorrhages in the nail beds, Osler's nodes, or a palmar rash?	The nail beds and fingers may be the first clues to endocarditis. Palmar rashes occur in Rocky Mountain spotted fever and secondary syphilis.
Skin: Does the patient have a rash? Are there needle tracks suggesting injecting drug use? Are there embedded ticks?	For example, the petechiae of meningococcemia and the rose spots of typhoid fever may be few and far between (see Chapter 7 for a thorough discussion of fever and rash).
Head: Does the patient have tenderness over the paranasal sinuses? Are the temporal arteries palpable and tender?	Infection of the frontal, ethmoid, or sphenoid sinuses sometimes has life-threatening consequences. Temporal arteritis is an important cause of fever, although seldom of acute "flulike" illness.
Ears: Does the patient show any evidence of otitis media?	Otitis media can be the clue to sepsis from *S. pneumoniae* or *H. influenzae.*
Eyes: Does the patient have conjunctival hemorrhages or suffusion? Are there focal lesions in the retina?	Hemorrhages in the palpebral conjunctivae suggest endocarditis or meningococcemia. Conjunctival suffusion occurs in leptospirosis. Careful funduscopic examination may reveal Roth spots (endocarditis) or choroidal tubercles (miliary tuberculosis).
Oral cavity: What is the state of the patient's dental hygiene? Are any teeth tender? Are there exudates, ulcerations, or other lesions?	Dental abscess is an occasional cause of unexplained fever. Sharp, "punched-out" ulcers occur in disseminated histoplasmosis. Hairy leukoplakia or thrush may be the clues to previously undiagnosed HIV infection.
Neck: Does the patient have any palpable lymph nodes, especially in the supraclavicular or scalene areas? Is the thyroid tender? Is the trachea tender?	Palpable lymph nodes often assume diagnostic significance (see Chapter 8). Subacute thyroiditis can present as a febrile illness, and rare patients have thyroid abscess. The pathogens causing "atypical pneumonia" (see Chapter 11) often cause tracheal tenderness.
Spine and back: Does the patient have any localized tenderness over the vertebrae, costovertebral angles, or sacroiliac joints?	Vertebral osteomyelitis is an important cause of unexplained fever, which can present acutely with septicemia. Costovertebral angle tenderness suggests pyelonephritis. Septic arthritis sometimes affects the sacroiliac joints, especially in injecting drug users.
Chest: What is the nature of the respiratory excursions? Are there localized findings in the lung fields?	Deep breathing or rapid, shallow breathing may indicate that the patient has heart failure, diffuse pulmonary disease, or lactic acidosis. Localized rales and egophony (e→a change) can be early clues to pneumonia.
Precordium: Is there murmur, friction rub, or gallop?	Listen especially for the diastolic murmur of aortic regurgitation and for systolic murmurs at the base (aortic stenosis) and apex (mitral regurgitation). A friction rub may indicate acute pericarditis. A ventricular gallop (S_3) suggests heart failure and hence a narrow margin for error (see text).
Abdomen: Are bowel sounds present? Is ascites present? Is there any localized tenderness? Is there rebound accentuation? Is the liver or spleen enlarged?	Especially in elderly patients, perforation of the stomach or bowel can cause acute peritonitis, which can occur initially as the sepsis syndrome. Patients with ascites are at high risk of spontaneous bacterial peritonitis and bacteremia (see Chapter 3).

Continued

TABLE 6-4—cont'd
Physical Examination: Signs and Symptoms to Look for in the Patient with Undifferentiated "Flulike" Illness

Sign or symptom	Implications and examples
Extremities: Does the patient have localized pain over any muscles, bones, or joints?	Localized muscle pain occasionally provides the clue to polyarteritis nodosa, which can have an acute onset as unexplained fever. Anterior thigh pain can be a nonspecific response to septicemia. Localized pain over bones and joints suggests septic arthritis or osteomyelitis.
Genitalia: Does the patient have any sores or ulcers? Is testicular tenderness present?	The painless chancres of syphilis may be in subtle locations, especially in women. Testicular tenderness is sometimes the clue to polyarteritis nodosa.
Pelvic examination: Does the patient have a discharge from the cervix? Is the cervix normal?	Lacerations of the cervix suggest septic abortion, and this physical finding may be lifesaving. Any discharge should be evaluated for gonococci and *Chlamydia* by culture or enzyme-linked assay.

⤳ When examining a patient with a nonspecific flulike illness, the clinician has three tasks: (1) to find clues by history and physical examination suggesting one or another specific, treatable infectious disease; (2) to determine whether the patient's general appearance, underlying condition, or findings on complete blood count (such as marked bandemia or thrombocytopenia) warrant admission to the hospital; and (3) to ensure close follow-up.

⤳ Septicemia caused by *S. aureus* often manifests itself as a severe flulike illness. The source is frequently found to be a localized abscess, osteomyelitis, or endocarditis.

SUGGESTED READING

Abraham E, Matthay MA, Dinarello CA, et al. Consensus conference definitions for sepsis, septic shock, acute lung injury, and acute respiratory distress syndrome: time for a reevaluation. Crit Care Med 2000; 28: 232-235.

Balk RA. Pathogenesis and management of multiple organ dysfunction or failure in severe sepsis or septic shock. Crit Care Clin 2000; 16: 337-352.

Dhainaut JF, Thijs LG, Park G, eds. Septic Shock. London: W.B. Saunders; 2000.

Hardaway RM. A review of septic shock. Am Surg 2000; 66: 22-29.

Jindal N, Hollenberg SM, Dellinger RP. Pharmacologic issues in the management of septic shock. Crit Care Clin 2000; 16: 233-249.

Rangel-Frausto MS, Pittet D, Costigan M, et al. The natural history of the systemic inflammatory response syndrome (SIRS): a prospective study. JAMA 1995; 273: 117-123.

Simon D, Trenholme G. Antibiotic selection for patients with septic shock. Crit Care Clin 2000; 16: 215-231.

Staphylococcal and Streptococcal Toxic Shock Syndromes

The staphylococcal and streptococcal toxic shock syndromes now rank prominently among the causes of sudden onset of nonhemorrhagic shock in previously healthy patients (Table 6-6).

Presentation and Progression
Cause

The toxic shock syndromes are caused by strains of group A streptococci (*S. pyogenes*) and *S. aureus* that produce unique toxins. These toxins function as superantigens; that is, they cause T lymphocytes to produce and release massive quantities of cytokines, resulting in widespread tissue damage, shock, and multiple organ system failure.

Staphylococcal toxic shock syndrome came to the attention of the general public as a disease affecting young women during menstruation. Some nonmenstrual cases have been associated with rhinoplasty and other surgical procedures in which nasal packing or Teflon stents are used to close off spaces. Other nonmenstrual cases are associated with sites of staphylococcal colonization and disease, such as skin infections, decubitus ulcers, or pneumonia. Influenza predisposes to staphylococcal pneumonia and toxic shock syndrome. Streptococcal toxic shock syndrome is usually associated with an obvious site of infection, with skin infections—ranging in severity from cellulitis to necrotizing fasciitis—being the most common.

In both streptococcal and staphylococcal toxic shock syndrome, patients have an acute illness characterized by fever, hypotension, tachycardia, and tachypnea. Prodromal symptoms vary according to the pathogen and the clinical setting (Table 6-6). Staphylococcal toxic shock syndrome is usually preceded by a short flulike illness with chills, malaise, and generalized aching before the onset of fever and lethargy. Diarrhea is common. Confusion may also be present, causing patients to fail to grasp the seriousness of their illness. A flulike prodrome is less common in streptococcal toxic shock syndrome. These patients are more likely to have symptoms of localized infection, typically on an extremity, accompanied by severe pain.

Diagnosis

Staphylococcal and streptococcal toxic shock syndromes are clinical diagnoses. In streptococcal toxic shock the causative organism is more likely to be isolated from blood cultures or from cultures of clinically apparent sites of infection. A diagnostic

TABLE 6-5
Causes of Abrupt Onset of Nonhemorrhagic Shock in a Previously Healthy, Nonhospitalized Patient

Cause	Distinctive features
Rocky Mountain spotted fever	Severe headache ("the worst ever") and petechial rash that begins distally; history of tick exposure; thrombocytopenia. The rash is often absent, especially early in the course of the disease ("Rocky Mountain spotless fever").
Meningococcemia	Petechial rash beginning on extremities or axillary folds. The illness often progresses rapidly, with shock occurring within several hours of the onset of symptoms.
Overwhelming postsplenectomy infection	History of splenectomy or disease predisposing to functional asplenia. A history of minor respiratory illness may be obtained. Microorganisms are often seen on peripheral blood smear or buffy coat preparation.
Staphylococcal toxic shock syndrome	Tampon use or packing of a closed space (e.g., nasal packing); clinical evidence of staphylococcal infection; diffuse or localized erythroderma.
Streptococcal toxic shock syndrome	Evidence of streptococcal skin infection, most often in an extremity, with severe localized pain.
Gram-negative sepsis with shock	Evidence of a localized infection is usually present. Community-acquired, life-threatening sepsis caused by gram-negative rods in a patient without severe underlying disease is uncommon.
Staphylococcal septicemia with shock	Staphylococcal septicemia may originate from endocarditis or from an occult abscess. The disease can be manifested as a "flulike" illness with generalized aching and progress rapidly to refractory septic shock.
Acute endocarditis	Acute endocarditis of the aortic or mitral valve, especially when caused by *Staphylococcus aureus,* can damage valve leaflets, chordae tendineae, or papillary muscles, causing acute heart failure with pulmonary edema.
Hantavirus pulmonary syndrome	After what seems to be a nonspecific "viral syndrome," shock and pulmonary edema abruptly develop. A history of out-of-doors exposure (notably in the Four Corners area of the Southwest but also elsewhere) can be obtained.
Heatstroke	A history of heavy exertion in a hot, humid environment suggests heatstroke as the cause of fever, confusion, shock, and renal failure.
Addisonian crisis	Adrenal insufficiency should always be considered as a possible cause of unexplained shock. Simultaneous diagnosis and treatment can be accomplished by measuring the plasma cortisol level, giving adrenocorticotropic hormone (to stimulate the adrenal glands) and dexamethasone (as replacement therapy), and repeating the plasma cortisol measurement 1 hour later.

hallmark of staphylococcal toxic shock syndrome is desquamation of the skin occurring during the second week of the illness.

Natural History
Expected Outcome

Mortality associated with staphylococcal toxic shock syndrome is low (<3%). Some patients, however, are prone to recurrent symptoms. Streptococcal toxic shock syndrome has a much higher mortality rate.

Treatment
Methods

Treatment of toxic shock syndrome should not be attempted in the outpatient setting, apart from obtaining appropriate initial studies and ordering the first dose of antibiotic. Empiric treatment of staphylococcal toxic shock syndrome

consists of high-dose nafcillin or oxacillin (2 g IV q4h). Empiric treatment of streptococcal toxic shock syndrome consists of high-dose penicillin G (24 million units IV daily assuming normal renal function). Mounting evidence supports the addition of clindamycin 900 mg IV q8h, especially for streptococcal toxic shock syndrome, with the rationale that clindamycin suppresses toxin synthesis. Supportive therapy includes aggressive management of the symptoms and signs of shock. Neutralization of toxin by immune globulin therapy has also been recommended for these syndromes.

Expected Response

Response is variable. Mortality remains high, especially with streptococcal toxic shock syndrome (Table 6-6), even with appropriate treatment.

TABLE 6-6
Features of Staphylococcal and Streptococcal Toxic Shock Syndromes

Feature	Staphylococcal toxic shock syndrome	Streptococcal toxic shock syndrome
Pathogen	*Staphylococcus aureus*	*Streptococcus pyogenes* (group A streptococcus)
Recognized toxins	Toxic shock syndrome toxin I; staphylococcal enterotoxin B; others	Streptococcal pyrogenic exotoxins A and B; others
Peak age and sex	15 to 30 years, most often in women	Most often between 20 and 50 years, either sex
Predisposing factors	Tampons; ? NSAIDs	Streptococcal skin infection related to cuts, burns, bruises, or varicella; ? NSAIDs
Prodrome	Flulike illness of 2 to 3 days' duration is usually present before the onset of shock	Flulike illness is present in about 20% of patients; the first symptom is more likely to be abrupt, severe pain
Tissue necrosis	Rare	Common
Severe localized pain	Rare	Common
Diffuse erythroderma	Common	Uncommon
Hypotension	100%, by definition	100%, by definition
Renal failure	Common	Common
Positive blood cultures	Uncommon	60% of cases
Mortality	<3%	30% to 70%

Modified from Stevens DL. The toxic shock syndromes. Infect Dis Clin North Am 1996; 10: 727-746.
NSAIDs, Nonsteroidal antiinflammatory drugs.

When to Refer

Patients with either staphylococcal or streptococcal toxic shock syndrome should be admitted to the hospital.

SUGGESTED READING

Andrews M-M, Parent EM, Barry M, et al. Recurrent nonmenstrual toxic shock syndrome: clinical manifestations, diagnosis, and treatment. Clin Infect Dis 2001; 32: 1470-1479.

Crossley KB, Archer GL, eds. The Staphylococci in Human Disease. New York: Churchill Livingstone; 1997.

Kain KC, Schulzer M, Chow AW. Clinical spectrum of nonmenstrual toxic shock syndrome (TSS): comparison with menstrual TSS by multivariate discriminant analyses. Clin Infect Dis 1993; 16: 100-106.

Stevens DL. Streptococcal toxic-shock syndrome: spectrum of disease, pathogenesis, and new concepts in treatment. Emerg Infect Dis 1995; 1: 69-78.

Stevens DL, Kaplan EL, eds. Streptococcal Infections: Clinical Aspects, Microbiology, and Molecular Pathogenesis. New York: Oxford University Press; 2000.

Sepsis in the Asplenic Patient

Healthy persons without spleens are at lifetime risk—estimated at 5%—for overwhelming sepsis. Primary care practitioners must (1) carefully consider the indications for elective splenectomy, (2) make sure that splenectomized persons have received appropriate vaccines (see Chapter 25), (3) counsel splenectomized persons about the early warning symptoms of sepsis, and (4) take prompt action whenever an asplenic person is seen with fever.

Presentation and Progression
Cause

The spleen is of strategic importance to the immune system when the body lacks previous experience with a microorganism. Overwhelming infection can occur in persons who lack functioning spleens for any reason: congenital asplenia, "functional" asplenia (seen in such diverse conditions as sickle cell anemia, acute alcoholism, chronic graft-versus-host disease, amyloidosis, and various chronic inflammatory diseases), and previous splenectomy. The highest incidence of overwhelming infection occurs in patients who have undergone splenectomy for lymphoma or for other hematologic conditions such as hereditary spherocytosis, congenital anemias, and thalassemia. Patients are most vulnerable to overwhelming infection within the first 2 years of splenectomy, but the risk is lifelong.

The usual pathogens in sepsis of an asplenic patient are the encapsulated pyogenic cocci that require type-specific antibody for successful phagocytosis by leukocytes. *Streptococcus pneumoniae* accounts for 50% to 90% of infections and about 60% of deaths in asplenic patients. *Haemophilus influenzae* may account for nearly one third of the mortality. *Neisseria meningitidis* is also important. The syndrome has furthermore been associated with a wide variety of gram-positive and gram-negative bacteria. I have seen a fatal case, caused by *Salmonella enteritidis,* as the initial manifestation of HIV infection in an asplenic patient. Unusual but well-publicized causes include *Capnocytophaga canimorsus* (see Chapter 26) after dog bites and *Babesia microti* (babesiosis; see Chapter 7) after tick bites in endemic areas.

Presentation

Most patients have a short prodrome of nonspecific symptoms. These may include chills, headache, malaise, and symptoms pointing to the abdomen such as nausea, vomiting, diarrhea, and abdominal pain. Symptoms of pneumonia (cough, chest pain) and meningitis may also be present. The short prodrome is followed by symptoms and signs of severe sepsis. Assessment of vital signs often reveals fever, tachycardia, hypotension, and tachypnea. The patient may appear anxious, delirious, or stuporous. Rapid deterioration is the rule rather than the exception.

Diagnosis

Sepsis should be suspected whenever an asplenic person shows symptoms and signs of an infectious illness. Symptoms suggesting "viral syndrome" or "gastroenteritis" should not cause postponement of aggressive treatment. Empiric therapy takes priority over diagnostic deliberation. Microorganisms are often seen on examination of a random peripheral blood smear, which implies truly massive bacteremia ($>10^6$ organisms/mL). The yield is increased by examining the buffy coat. Studies to be performed in most cases include blood cultures, complete blood count and electrolyte panel, urine culture, sputum culture, chest x-ray examination, and lumbar puncture for analysis and culture of the cerebrospinal fluid (CSF).

Natural History
Expected Outcome

The full-blown syndrome is probably fatal in all cases without treatment.

Treatment
Methods

When sepsis in association with asplenia is suspected, the following approach is recommended: (1) note the exact time; (2) order *immediate* antibiotic therapy, requesting documentation of the exact time therapy is given; and (3) obtain blood for culture and other studies just before starting antibiotic administration. If facilities for blood cultures are not available, giving the first dose of antibiotics takes priority. For most patients initial therapy should consist of 2 g of ceftriaxone (for children 50 mg/kg). If the possibility of highly resistant *S. pneumoniae* is a concern (see Chapter 11), 1 g of vancomycin (for children 30 mg/kg) should be given in addition to ceftriaxone. Clindamycin and quinine are recommended for overwhelming babesiosis, a situation in which exchange transfusions may also be useful.

Expected Response

The reported mortality is up to 75% even with appropriate treatment.

When to Refer

When sepsis in association with asplenia is suspected, patients should be given immediate therapy and then hospitalized.

KEY POINTS

SEPSIS IN THE ASPLENIC PATIENT

- ⊃ In persons who are anatomically or functionally asplenic for any reason, sepsis is frequently devastating, with mortality up to 75% even with appropriate treatment.
- ⊃ The lifetime risk of overwhelming postsplenectomy infection is about 5%. The risk is greatest during the first 2 years after splenectomy.
- ⊃ *S. pneumoniae* causes about 60% of deaths in asplenic patients with sepsis. *H. influenzae* is the second-leading pathogen. Also important are *N. meningitidis,* various gram-positive and gram-negative bacteria, *Capnocytophaga canimorsus* (after dog bites), and babesiosis (in endemic areas). When the diagnosis is suspected, appropriate antibiotic therapy—usually ceftriaxone with or without vancomycin—should be started at once.
- ⊃ Asplenic persons should be immunized against *S. pneumoniae, H. influenzae* type b, and *N. meningitidis* groups A, C, Y, and W135 (see Chapter 25).
- ⊃ Asplenic persons should be counseled about the need to seek medical attention promptly for any sign of sepsis. Empiric self-treatment with antibiotics should be considered especially when such persons travel to remote areas.

SUGGESTED READING
Holdsworth RJ, Irving AD, Cuschieri A. Postsplenectomy sepsis and its mortality rate: actual versus perceived risks. Br J Surg 1991; 78: 1031-1038.

Lynch AM, Kapila R. Overwhelming postsplenectomy infection. Infect Dis Clin North Am 1996; 10: 693-707.

Meningococcemia

Meningococcemia with or without meningitis is one of the few infectious diseases capable of killing a previously healthy person within hours. It affects mainly children, adolescents, and young adults but can occur at any age. The initial symptoms are nonspecific, and the diagnosis is frequently delayed.

Presentation and Progression
Cause

N. meningitidis is a normal colonizer of the human upper respiratory tract, its only known reservoir (see Chapter 1). To cause invasive disease, the organisms must first penetrate the respiratory mucosa, a process facilitated by viral or mycoplasmal respiratory tract infection or by cigarette smoking (including exposure of young children to passive smoke). Once in the bloodstream, the organisms must evade the serum bactericidal system to multiply and cause disease. Most if not all of the disease manifestations are now understood as the host response to endotoxin, which is mainly the release of cytokines and other inflammatory mediators by monocytes, macrophages, and endothelial cells. The end-stage results are shock, disseminated intravascular coagulation, and multiple organ system failure.

Host defense against invasive meningococcal disease depends mainly on serum bactericidal activity, which requires complement and serogroup-specific antibody. The highest attack rates occur in patients with impaired serum bactericidal activity. Sporadic meningococcal disease occurs most frequently in young children who have yet to develop antibodies against *N. meningitidis*. In one study 90% of cases occurred in children <2 years of age. Patients with deficiencies of the late-acting complement components (C5 to C9) form another high-risk group. Although this condition is uncommon, up to 60% of patients with such complement deficiencies have at least one episode of invasive meningococcal disease during their lifetimes, and up to one half of individuals with such episodes have a second episode. Also predisposing to meningococcal disease are asplenia (see preceding discussion), immunoglobulin deficiency, and acquired complement deficiencies (e.g., in systemic lupus erythematosus, end-stage liver disease, the nephrotic syndrome, and protein-losing enteropathy).

Presentation

The mean age of meningococcal disease in the general population is about 3 years; however, the mean age for the first episode of meningococcal disease in persons with deficiency of late-acting complement components is about 17 years. There is often a prodromal upper respiratory tract infection. This is followed by a flulike illness with fever, chills, malaise, generalized aching (myalgias, arthralgias), headache, nausea, and vomiting. In some patients meningococcemia develops with rapid progression to shock; others have meningitis with or without meningococcemia.

Diagnosis

Meningococcemia should be considered in any patient with fever and petechiae, the differential diagnosis of which is discussed in Chapter 7. However, the presenting symptoms are often subtle. For this reason the "buddy check" (see Appendix 3) is advisable for persons who *might* have early meningococcal disease but for whom the index of suspicion is too low to recommend hospitalization. Petechial rash, which eventually occurs in up to 60% of patients and which becomes purpuric in severe cases, is the telltale finding (Figure 6-3). The petechiae usually begin on the distal parts of the extremities (ankles and wrists), in the axillary folds, or in places exposed to pressure, as by the elastic straps of underwear. Later, petechiae spread to the trunk and can involve the conjunctivae. The palms, soles, and face are usually spared. The rash is sometimes macular or maculopapular rather than petechial.

As is so often the case, the key to diagnosis is a high index of suspicion. Blood cultures are the definitive test. Commercially available rapid serologic tests are reasonably sensitive for detecting the polysaccharide antigens of serogroups A, C, Y, and W135. Unfortunately, these tests, which can be performed on body fluids, including CSF and urine, are relatively insensitive for detecting serogroup B, which is a common cause of sporadic meningococcal disease in the United States.

Natural History

Untreated meningococcemia with shock is fatal in nearly 100% of cases. Expressions of the disease with a better prognosis include chronic meningococcemia with rash and arthritis (resembling the gonococcal arthritis-dermatitis syndrome) and occult, self-limited bacteremia in children.

Treatment
Methods

Ceftriaxone (or cefotaxime) is the first-line drug for initial therapy before the availability of blood culture results, since penicillin G—the more specific agent—lacks coverage against other common bacteria (e.g., *H. influenzae* and the common Enterobacteriaceae) that could also be involved. The dose of ceftriaxone is 50 mg/kg/day for infants and children and 2 g/day for adults. If Rocky Mountain spotted fever is considered a possibility, the patient should be given doxycycline (see later discussion). Giving the cephalosporin first is prudent because of the potential antagonism between the two drugs (see the discussion of antagonism between antibiotics in Chapter 19).

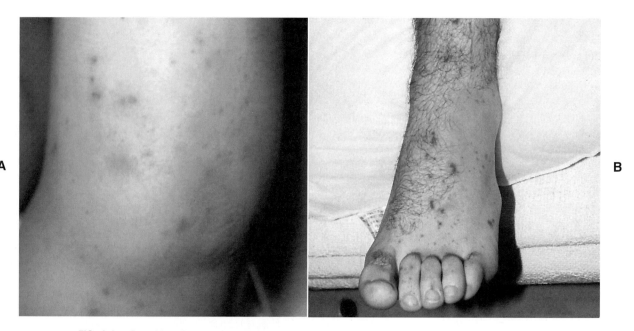

A

B

FIG. 6-3 Petechiae, **A,** over the elbow and, **B,** diffusely over the lower extremities in two patients with meningococcemia. Rapid deterioration with shock can occur in patients with this finding. The rash of meningococcemia, unlike that of Rocky Mountain spotted fever (see Figure 7-17), usually spares the palms and soles.

Treatment also involves dealing with contacts. Few diseases evoke the concern bordering on hysteria that ensues after a case of meningococcemia has been recognized. Prophylaxis is indicated for four groups: household contacts (defined as those who frequently eat and sleep in the same dwelling), intimate contacts (those who have had direct contact with respiratory secretions, as through kissing or mouth-to-mouth resuscitation), small children in nurseries or day care centers, and the patient himself or herself if treated with penicillin G. Penetration of penicillin G into the nasopharyngeal secretions, even during high-dose therapy, is insufficient to ensure eradication of the carrier state. However, ceftriaxone 250 mg IM for adults or 125 mg IM for children has been shown to eradicate the carrier state in 96% of cases. Ciprofloxacin 500 mg as a single dose has replaced rifampin 10 mg/kg or up to 600 mg every 12 hours as the drug of choice for prevention of secondary cases except during pregnancy (when ceftriaxone is the drug of choice) and for children under 18 years of age (for additional discussion, see Chapter 26).

Expected Response

The mortality rate for meningococcemia is up to 10% despite antibiotic therapy, and up to 30% with the fulminant form of the disease. In children the mortality was found to be about 90% if three or more of the following factors were present: onset of petechiae <12 hours before admission to the hospital, hypotension (systolic blood pressure <70 mm Hg), absence of meningitis (<20 leukocytes/mm³ of CSF), absence of leukocytosis (WBC count <10,000/mm³), and normal sedimentation rate (<10 mm/hr). Mortality was 9% if two or fewer of these factors were present. Symptoms and signs of shock, disseminated intravascular coagulation, and organ system failure—for example, stupor or coma, thrombocytopenia, and metabolic acidosis—also portend a poor prognosis. Current research on prognostic factors centers on measurement of cytokine levels.

When to Refer

Patients in whom meningococcemia is strongly suspected should be admitted to the hospital, preferably after administration of the first dose of antibiotic.

 KEY POINTS

MENINGOCOCCEMIA

- ⊃ Meningococcemia can cause death within hours. Therefore a high index of suspicion should be maintained when a patient has a nonspecific flulike illness with fever, myalgias, arthralgias, headache, malaise, nausea, and vomiting.
- ⊃ Up to 90% of cases occur in children under 2 years of age, and the median age for all patients with meningococcemia is about 3 years.
- ⊃ Deficiency of a late-acting complement component should be suspected in older patients with meningococcal disease.
- ⊃ A petechial rash, found in up to 60% of patients, appears first on the ankles, wrists, axillary folds, and points of pressure (as from elastic).
- ⊃ The "buddy check" (see Appendix 3) is recommended for patients who *might* have meningococcal disease, but the likelihood is not great enough to justify hospitalization.
- ⊃ Ceftriaxone (or cefotaxime) is currently the drug of choice for initial therapy.

- ⊃ Patients whose disease might be Rocky Mountain spotted fever should be given doxycycline, ideally started after the first dose of a cephalosporin has been administered.
- ⊃ Intimate contacts, household contacts, and young children who have been exposed to meningococcal disease should receive prophylaxis.

SUGGESTED READING

Centers for Disease Control and Prevention. Prevention and control of meningococcal disease and meningococcal disease in college students. Recommendations of the Advisory Committee on Immunization Practices (ACIP). MMWR 2000 (RR-7): 1-20.

Diaz PS. The epidemiology and control of invasive meningococcal disease. Pediatr Infect Dis J 1999; 18: 633-634.

Rosenstein NE, Perkins BA, Stephens DS, et al. Meningococcal disease. N Engl J Med 2001; 344: 1378-1388.

van Deuren M, Brandtzaeg P, van der Meer JW. Update on meningococcal disease with emphasis on pathogenesis and clinical management. Clin Microbiol Rev 2000; 13: 144-166.

Rocky Mountain Spotted Fever

Rocky Mountain spotted fever is a generalized infection of the vascular endothelium caused by *Rickettsia rickettsii* and transmitted by ticks. The name is misleading, since the disease no longer occurs mainly in the Rocky Mountains and the telltale rash is often absent, especially when the patient is first seen ("Rocky Mountain spotless fever"). Failure to suspect and treat this tickborne illness can have disastrous consequences.

Presentation and Progression
Cause

R. rickettsii is an intracellular bacterium belonging to the rickettsiae. *Dermacentor andersoni,* the Rocky Mountain wood tick, transmits the disease in the western United States. *Dermacentor variabilis,* the American dog tick, transmits the disease in the South Atlantic and west south central regions, where the disease is now more prevalent. The painless tick bite often goes unnoticed, and history of tick exposure may therefore be lacking. The organisms pass from the skin to the bloodstream and then to vascular endothelial cells, leading to widespread tissue injury.

Presentation

Rocky Mountain spotted fever begins as a nonspecific flulike illness with fever, headache, and myalgia after an incubation period of 2 to 14 days (median 7 days) after a tick bite. The headache is typically severe and often described as the worst the patient has ever experienced. Fever eventually exceeds 102° F (38.9° C) in more than 90% of patients but may be low grade when the patient is first seen. Most patients have myalgia. Nausea, vomiting, abdominal pain and tenderness, and diarrhea often direct attention to the abdomen.

Rash occurs by the end of the third day of the illness in about one half of patients and eventually occurs in 84% to 91% of patients. Rash is less often present in older patients and in African-American patients. The rash is typically maculopapular, petechial, or both; often central petechiae are seen within maculopapules. It begins most frequently on the wrists and ankles. Involvement of the palms and soles, although considered classic, often appears late in the illness or not at all.

The WBC count is usually within normal limits, but a shift to the left is typically present. Thrombocytopenia is a common finding and may suggest the diagnosis. Disseminated intravascular coagulation can be seen in unusually severe cases. Hyponatremia is found in about one half of patients, and elevated levels of various enzymes (including serum glutamic oxaloacetic transaminase, lactate dehydrogenase, and creatine phosphokinase) are common. Lumbar puncture, if performed because of headache and meningismus, shows pleocytosis in about one third of patients that may be predominantly polymorphonuclear or lymphocytic. The CSF protein level may be increased, but the glucose level is usually normal.

Diagnosis

Rocky Mountain spotted fever should be suspected in any patient with a generalized flulike illness and prominent headache in an endemic area during the late spring and summer months, when the disease is most prevalent. A history of tick exposure should be sought but is frequently absent. Although the disease occurs most often in children, young adults, or woodsmen, it can develop in anyone, including the elderly, and occasional cases occur throughout the year in endemic areas. Furthermore, the disease can crop up in unusual places, as evidenced by its recent appearance in New York City.

The diagnosis is usually suggested by the characteristic rash (see Figure 7-17). Confirmation is carried out most often by retrospective serologic tests using one or more of several available methods. The organisms can often be demonstrated in skin biopsy specimens in laboratories equipped for this purpose. Culture is usually not attempted, and the polymerase chain reaction (PCR) has not proved to be sufficiently sensitive.

Natural History
Expected Outcome

Untreated, Rocky Mountain spotted fever has a 20% mortality rate. Mortality is higher in older patients and among those with shorter incubation periods. In some patients, especially African-American males with glucose-6-phosphate dehydrogenase (G6PD) deficiency, the disease has a fulminant course in which death occurs within 5 days of the onset of symptoms. More commonly death occurs during the second week of the illness as a result of organ failure, which may reflect involvement of the CNS (encephalopathy, seizures), kidneys (acute renal failure), and lungs (interstitial and alveolar infiltrates, pleural effusion, noncardiogenic pulmonary edema—in summary, features of the acute respiratory distress syndrome). Fulminant purpura with peripheral gangrene may also occur. The prognosis may be worse in older patients and in men.

Treatment
Methods

Doxycycline 100 mg b.i.d. PO or IV (for patients with severe illness or with nausea and vomiting) is currently the treatment of choice except for young children and pregnant women. In the latter patients chloramphenicol has been considered the drug of choice. However, since toxicity of the tetracyclines to the fetus and young child is dose related, the case can be made that a short course of doxycycline carries less risk than a course of chloramphenicol (which is associated with a risk of fatal bone marrow aplasia in about 1 in 25,000 to 1 in 40,000 recipients). The newer quinolones such as ciprofloxacin are effective in vitro and in animal models and may become approved for Rocky Mountain spotted fever. *R. rickettsii* is resistant to the macrolides (such as erythromycin), trimethoprim-sulfamethoxazole (TMP/SMX), the β-lactam antibiotics, and the aminoglycosides.

Expected Response

The introduction of effective drug therapy lowered the mortality of Rocky Mountain spotted fever to about 3% to 4%, but deaths still occur, especially when presumptive diagnosis and treatment are delayed.

When to Refer

Patients with severe Rocky Mountain spotted fever should be hospitalized.

 KEY POINTS

ROCKY MOUNTAIN SPOTTED FEVER

⊃ Rocky Mountain spotted fever often occurs as an undifferentiated flulike illness. The characteristic rash appears during the first 3 days of illness in only about one half of patients and never appears in some patients.

⊃ The diagnosis should be suspected during an acute febrile illness with *any* of the following features: unusually severe headache, endemic area, occurrence during the spring or summer months, or history of a tick exposure.

⊃ Doxycycline 100 mg b.i.d. is currently the drug of choice for most patients.

SUGGESTED READING

Archibald LK, Sexton DJ. Long-term sequelae of Rocky Mountain spotted fever. Clin Infect Dis 1995; 20: 1122-1125.

Cale DF, McCarthy MW. Treatment of Rocky Mountain spotted fever in children. Ann Pharmacother 1997; 31: 492-494.

Drage LA. Life-threatening rashes: dermatologic signs of four infectious diseases. Mayo Clin Proc 1999; 74: 68-72.

Helmick CG, Bernard KW, D'Angelo LJ. Rocky Mountain spotted fever: clinical, laboratory, and epidemiological features of 262 cases. J Infect Dis 1984; 150: 480-488.

Thorner AR, Walker DH, Petri WA Jr. Rocky Mountain spotted fever. Clin Infect Dis 1998; 27: 1353-1359.

Acute Bacterial Meningitis

Acute bacterial meningitis is a medical emergency variably characterized by fever, headache, meningismus (stiff neck), nausea, vomiting, and altered mental status. In about 15% of patients and especially in young children and elderly patients, the presentation is subtle. Gastrointestinal symptoms may predominate, leading to a misdiagnosis of gastroenteritis. Delayed diagnosis invites tragic consequences.

Presentation and Progression
Cause

The three main causes of community-acquired bacterial meningitis beyond the neonatal period are *S. pneumoniae, H. influenzae* type b, and *N. meningitidis*. These organisms have in common the ability to colonize the nasopharynx and elude host defenses by virtue of their polysaccharide capsules. Widespread vaccination of young children against *H. influenzae* type b now makes this form of meningitis uncommon. *N. meningitidis* is a relatively common cause in children, adolescents, and young adults. *S. pneumoniae* causes meningitis in all age groups, is the most common cause in older adults, and is a frequent cause in persons with a history of basilar skull fracture. *Listeria monocytogenes* is an important cause in neonates and in patients who are elderly, debilitated, or immunosuppressed (e.g., patients with lymphomas or receiving corticosteroids). Aerobic gram-negative rods are important causes of meningitis in neonates, elderly patients, and patients who have undergone neurosurgical procedures.

Presentation

The presentation is to some extent age dependent. In infants the main symptoms are listlessness, poor feeding, and altered breathing patterns. The frail elderly with meningitis may show a decline in awareness. Meningitis caused by *L. monocytogenes* or aerobic gram-negative rods usually has a less dramatic, more subacute onset than meningitis caused by *S. pneumoniae, H. influenzae* type b, or *N. meningitidis.* When any of the "big three" bacteria cause meningitis in a previously healthy younger person, the symptoms usually prompt immediate medical attention. However, the history sometimes suggests a nonspecific flulike illness that gradually worsened over several days to a week. In this setting close attention must be paid to the potential significance of any combination of headache, nausea, and vomiting.

S. pneumoniae is the most common cause of community-acquired bacterial meningitis when all age groups are taken into account (Figure 6-4). Older patients with pneumococcal meningitis—unlike younger patients with *H. influenzae* or meningococcal meningitis—frequently have underlying conditions such as alcoholism or neurologic disease to which altered consciousness can be easily attributed. However, patients with pneumococcal meningitis—again, unlike younger patients with *H. influenzae* or meningococcal meningitis—frequently have a clinically apparent site of infection elsewhere, such as otitis media, sinusitis, pneumonia, or—rarely—endocarditis.

Diagnosis

The clinician should think immediately of meningitis when patients seek treatment for some combination of fever, headache, stiff neck, nausea or vomiting, and altered consciousness. None of these symptoms is sufficiently sensitive, however, to exclude meningitis by its absence. In adults the overall sensitivity is about 50% for headache and about 30% for nausea and vomiting. The absence of fever, stiff neck, and altered mental status allows the practitioner to exclude meningitis with 99% to 100% confidence.

Physical examination should target the following areas: (1) the skin, looking for the petechial rash of meningococcemia; (2) the tympanic membranes, looking for evidence of otitis media as a portal of entry for pneumococcal meningitis; (3) the optic discs, looking for evidence of papilledema as a relative contraindication to lumbar puncture (pulsations in the central retinal veins effectively exclude increased intracranial pressure); and (4) signs of meningeal irritation. Meningeal irritation can be assessed by at least four tests, all of which can be performed briefly and are therefore recommended:

- Anterior neck flexion. With the patient supine, the examiner asks the patient to flex the head forward ("Put your head on your chest"). Alternatively, the patient is asked to put his or her head between the knees. Neck stiffness is present when the patient experiences pain on anterior flexion.
- Kernig's sign. With the patient supine and the hip flexed at 90 degrees, the knee is extended. Kernig's sign is present when the patient experiences pain or resistance in the lower back or posterior thigh. This test can also be performed with the patient in the sitting position.
- Brudzinski's sign. With the patient supine, the examiner holds the patient's head and flexes it so that the chin touches the chest. Brudzinsksi's sign is present when the patient flexes the knees and hips in response to this maneuver.
- Jolt test. The patient is asked to turn his or her head from side to side at a frequency of two to three rotations per second (Figure 6-5). The jolt sign is present when this maneuver worsens the patient's headache.

Kernig's and Brudzinski's signs have high specificity but low sensitivity for the diagnosis of meningitis. Jolt accentuation of headache has been determined to have a 97% sensitivity and 60% specificity; a recent review also concluded that the test has a positive likelihood ratio of 2.2 and a negative likelihood ratio of zero. It has been suggested that absence of the jolt sign essentially excludes meningitis. More experience is needed to establish this point with a reasonable degree of certainty.

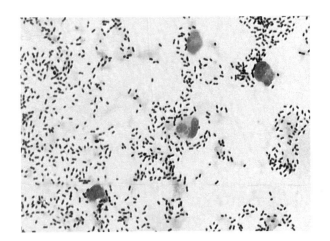

FIG. 6-4 Pneumococcal meningitis, with myriad gram-positive diplococci on Gram stain of cerebrospinal fluid.

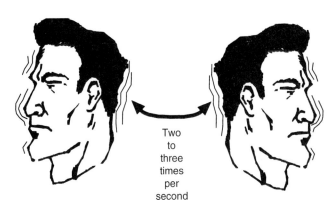

Two to three times per second

FIG. 6-5 Jolt test. Jolt accentuation of headache by rapid turning of the head was reported to have a 97% sensitivity and 60% specificity for cerebrospinal fluid pleocytosis. (Based on information from Uchihara T, Tsukagoshi H. Jolt accentuation of headache: the most sensitive sign of CSF pleocytosis. Headache 1991; 31: 167-171.)

When meningitis is suspected, lumbar puncture should be performed. The current tendency to postpone lumbar puncture until a localized intracranial lesion has been excluded by computed tomography (CT) or magnetic resonance imaging (MRI) is unfortunate because a delay of several hours in the institution of therapy can be crucial to the outcome. *When the illness is acute and no localizing neurologic signs or evidence of papilledema is present, the risk-benefit ratio for lumbar puncture weighs heavily in favor of going ahead with the procedure.* CSF should be obtained for leukocyte count, differential count, glucose level, and protein content (collectively, these four parameters are known as the CSF formula) and also for culture. The CSF formula is not diagnostic but can be extremely helpful, as follows:

- Acute bacterial meningitis. A leukocyte count >1000/µL with a predominance of polymorphonuclear neutrophils, a low glucose level (<40 mg/dL or <40% of the blood glucose), and a high protein content (>150 mg/dL) are highly characteristic.
- Viral ("aseptic") meningitis. The leukocyte count is usually <1000/µL with <50% polymorphonuclear neutrophils in the differential count, a normal glucose level, and a normal or slightly elevated protein content (exceptions to these rules are discussed later under "Aseptic Meningitis").
- Fungal or tuberculous meningitis (chronic meningitis). The leukocyte count is usually <500/µL with <50% polymorphonuclear neutrophils, a low glucose level, and an elevated protein content.
- Parameningeal infection (such as brain abscess). The leukocyte count is usually <1000/µL with <50% polymorphonuclear neutrophils, a normal glucose level, and a normal or elevated protein content.

An extra tube of CSF should be saved, since additional studies may be indicated if the initial tests are nondiagnostic.

Natural History
Expected Outcome

Untreated, meningococcal and pneumococcal meningitides are probably uniformly fatal. Survivors of *H. influenzae* meningitis in the preantibiotic era often spent the remainder of their lives in institutions for the severely retarded.

Treatment
Methods

When patients have an acute onset of fever, headache, and some combination of stiff neck, nausea, or vomiting, *the practitioner should note the exact time and attempt to have the first dose of an appropriate antibiotic given within 30 minutes.* At present, appropriate initial therapy for most patients is a single dose of a third-generation cephalosporin (ceftriaxone or cefotaxime, 2 g). Vancomycin is recommended for adults to cover the possibility of penicillin-nonsusceptible *S. pneumoniae,* and ampicillin is added for older patients to cover the possibility of *L. monocytogenes* (see Appendix 2). The optimum strategy is to request simultaneously a lumbar puncture tray and a 2-g dose of ceftriaxone or cefotaxime. Optimally the antibiotic is given just after completion of the lumbar puncture. If lumbar puncture cannot be performed immediately, the antibiotic should be administered and lumbar puncture done as soon as possible.

Expected Response

Early diagnosis and treatment of *H. influenzae* and meningococcal meningitis usually result in survival without residua. However, *H. influenzae* meningitis causes numerous complications such as subdural effusions and deafness, and meningococcal meningitis with or without meningococcemia can be a fulminant illness. Pneumococcal meningitis still carries a mortality rate of about 30%, and survivors often have neurologic sequelae.

When to Refer

Patients with suspected acute bacterial meningitis should receive the first dose of antibiotic as soon as possible and then be admitted to the hospital. Some recommendations for initial empiric therapy are summarized in Appendix 2.

 KEY POINTS

ACUTE BACTERIAL MENINGITIS

- ⊃ Acute bacterial meningitis usually manifests itself with some combination of fever, headache, meningeal signs (such as stiff neck), and evidence of brain dysfunction (nausea, vomiting, altered consciousness), but the illness can be subtle, especially in preschool children and the elderly.
- ⊃ Acute gastroenteritis and "viral syndrome" are common misdiagnoses.
- ⊃ The jolt test (accentuation of headache by rapid turning of the head from side to side) may have 99% to 100% sensitivity for acute bacterial meningitis and can therefore be used, in conjunction with other symptoms and signs, for excluding the diagnosis with reasonable certainty.
- ⊃ The diagnosis of pneumococcal meningitis—the most common type of acute bacterial meningitis in adults—is often delayed because of comorbid conditions such as alcoholism, neurologic disease, or pneumonia.
- ⊃ When meningitis is suspected and the patient has no localizing neurologic signs and no papilledema, lumbar puncture should be performed. The practitioner should not delay lumbar puncture while awaiting the results of an imaging study (such as a CT or MRI scan of the brain).
- ⊃ Antimicrobial therapy (e.g., ceftriaxone 2 g IV) is ideally given within 30 minutes of the patient's arrival at the health care facility.

SUGGESTED READING

Andes DR, Craig WA. Pharmacokinetics and pharmacodynamics of antibiotics in meningitis. Infect Dis Clin North Am 1999; 13: 595-618.

Attia J, Hatala R, Cook DJ, et al. Does this adult patient have acute meningitis? JAMA 1999; 282: 175-181.

Booy R, Kroll JS. Bacterial meningitis and meningococcal infection. Curr Opin Pediatr 1998; 10: 13-18.

Coyle PK. Overview of acute and chronic meningitis. Neurol Clin 1999; 17: 691-710.

Rajnik M, Ottolini MG. Serious infections of the central nervous system: encephalitis, meningitis, and brain abscess. Adolesc Med 2000; 11: 401-425.

Schaad UB, ed. Bacterial meningitis. Infect Dis Clin North Am 1999; 13: 515-755.

Spach DH, Jackson LA. Bacterial meningitis. Neurol Clin 1999; 17: 711-735.

Aseptic Meningitis, Chronic Meningitis, and Other Causes of Cerebrospinal Fluid Pleocytosis

Numerous causes exist for fever, headache, focal neurologic signs and symptoms, and CSF pleocytosis. The more common ones are discussed here because of the need to distinguish these diverse syndromes and specific diseases from acute bacterial meningitis.

Aseptic Meningitis (Viral Meningitis)

The term "aseptic meningitis" was introduced during the 1930s to describe a self-limited condition characterized by headache, mild nuchal rigidity, and predominantly lymphocytic CSF pleocytosis. The term has been used synonymously with "viral meningitis," but it is now recognized that the aseptic meningitis syndrome has many possible causes, including drugs.

Presentation and Progression

Cause. Surveillance reports suggest that aseptic meningitis affects about 1 in 10,000 persons each year; mild cases go unrecognized, and the true incidence is unknown. Rigorous attempts to isolate or identify viruses are successful in the majority of cases (55% to 70%). Enteroviruses are by far the most common causes in the United States (85% to 95% of cases in which a virus is identified). Aseptic meningitis caused by enteroviruses occurs mainly during the summer and fall. Infants and young children are most commonly affected. Some of the enteroviruses can cause a rash. Aseptic meningitis occurs in up to 30% of patients with mumps, often without evidence of salivary gland disease. The lymphocytic choriomeningitis virus causes aseptic meningitis with a relatively intense CSF pleocytosis. This virus is transmitted by rodents such as hamsters, mice, and rats; hence the disease occurs especially in pet owners, laboratory workers, and persons living in substandard housing. Arboviruses such as the St. Louis encephalitis virus can cause a syndrome resembling aseptic meningitis more than encephalitis (these terms are relative, since patients with meningitis usually have some brain involvement and patients with encephalitis usually have some meningeal involvement). Herpes simplex virus (HSV) type 2 often causes aseptic meningitis (in contrast to HSV type 1, which more often causes encephalitis; see later discussion). Finally, aseptic meningitis is a common manifestation of the acute retroviral syndrome caused by HIV.

Aseptic meningitis can punctuate the course of many systemic bacterial, rickettsial, mycoplasmal, spirochetal, and parasitic infections. Aseptic meningitis occurs in syphilis, especially secondary syphilis. Aseptic meningitis is a prominent feature of Lyme disease (neuroborreliosis). Leptospirosis can cause an aseptic meningitis syndrome during either or both of the two phases of the disease: the acute infectious phase or the secondary phase during which manifestations are presumed to be the result of circulating immune complexes. CSF pleocytosis can occur during the course of bacterial endocarditis as the result of emboli, immune complex encephalitis, or possibly mycotic aneurysm. Drugs are being reported increasingly as a cause of aseptic meningitis. These include not only drugs used in chemotherapy (such as azathioprine) but also commonly used drugs such as nonsteroidal antiinflammatory drugs (NSAIDs), antimicrobial agents (especially TMP/SMX and its separate components and occasionally ciprofloxacin, penicillin, and isoniazid [INH]),

ranitidine, and carbamazepine (in patients with underlying connective tissue diseases).

Presentation. Onset is usually abrupt with headache and mild nuchal rigidity, but the more severe manifestations of acute bacterial meningitis such as stupor and coma do not occur.

Diagnosis

A presumptive diagnosis of aseptic meningitis can be made when a patient with no history of recent antibiotic therapy seeks medical treatment for a headache and mild nuchal rigidity and is found to have low-grade CSF pleocytosis, predominantly lymphocytic, with normal CSF glucose and protein levels. The diagnosis is confirmed by the clinical course, since a self-limited course distinguishes the illness from chronic meningitis (e.g., tuberculous meningitis and cryptococcal meningitis). Problems arise when either the clinical course or the CSF formula is atypical for aseptic meningitis. Some of the agents of aseptic meningitis (notably mumps and lymphocytic choriomeningitis) may cause a low CSF glucose content.

In occasional patients the disease begins with headache, mild nuchal rigidity, and low-grade CSF pleocytosis with a predominance of polymorphonuclear neutrophils. When the history and physical examination reveal no other signs or symptoms pointing to acute bacterial meningitis and the patient does not look especially "sick," the clinician faces a dilemma. Should the patient be hospitalized and committed to a 7- to 10-day course of treatment for presumed acute bacterial meningitis? Or should the patient be sent home? A third option is to observe the patient closely without treatment and repeat the lumbar puncture in 4 to 6 hours. The second lumbar puncture reveals CSF with a predominance of lymphocytes, thus pointing to nonbacterial infection. Recently PCR has been shown to be effective for early, specific diagnosis of enterovirus infection of the CNS.

All patients with aseptic meningitis should be screened for syphilis with a Venereal Disease Research Laboratory (VDRL) test of both serum and CSF. An extra tube of CSF should be saved because the patient could have one of the causes of chronic meningitis and further studies may be necessary. Viral cultures of CSF can be attempted but are unnecessary in daily practice.

Natural History

Expected Outcome. By definition, aseptic meningitis is self-limited. Typically improvement begins within 3 days, and most patients can return to their usual activities within 7 to 10 days.

Treatment

Treatment of aseptic meningitis is symptomatic. Use of parenteral antibiotics appropriate for acute bacterial meningitis is the prudent course when the latter disease cannot be excluded with confidence. If, for example, lumbar puncture is performed in the office setting but the CSF must be sent elsewhere for analysis, administration of one dose of ceftriaxone may be appropriate while awaiting the results.

When to Refer

Hospitalization is indicated for patients with unusually severe headache and other symptoms, especially when acute bacterial meningitis cannot be excluded with confidence at the time of initial presentation.

KEY POINTS

ASEPTIC MENINGITIS

⊃ Aseptic meningitis is a self-limited syndrome characterized by headache, mild nuchal rigidity, and CSF pleocytosis.

⊃ Viruses, notably enteroviruses, are the usual cause.

⊃ The disease occurs most often in infants and young children during the summer and fall.

⊃ Occasional patients show predominantly neutrophilic pleocytosis in the CSF. Acute bacterial meningitis can be excluded in such patients if a second lumbar puncture, performed 4 to 6 hours after the first and without intervening antimicrobial therapy, shows conversion of the CSF to predominantly lymphocytic pleocytosis.

⊃ PCR facilitates early, specific diagnosis of enteroviral infection of the CNS.

⊃ Syphilis should always be excluded by performing a VDRL test on serum and CSF.

⊃ Although the aseptic meningitis syndrome is usually of viral etiology, numerous other causes are possible. These include bacterial, rickettsial, mycoplasmal, spirochetal, and parasitic infections; systemic illnesses such as systemic lupus erythematosus; and drugs.

⊃ An extra tube of CSF should be saved, since rare patients prove to have chronic meningitis rather than self-limited disease.

SUGGESTED READING

Jolles S, Sewell WA, Leighton C. Drug-induced aseptic meningitis: diagnosis and management. Drug Safety 2000; 22: 215-226.

Moris G, Garcia-Monco JC. The challenge of drug-induced aseptic meningitis. Arch Intern Med 1999; 159: 1185-1194.

Norris CM, Danis PG, Gardner TD. Aseptic meningitis in the newborn and young infant. Am Fam Physician 1999; 59: 2761-2770.

Ramers C, Billman G, Hartin M, et al. Impact of a diagnostic cerebrospinal fluid enterovirus polymerase chain reaction test on patient management. JAMA 2000; 283: 2680-2685.

Spanos A, Harrell FE Jr, Durack DT. Differential diagnosis of acute meningitis: an analysis of the predictive value of initial observations. JAMA 1989; 262: 2700-2707.

Chronic Meningitis

The term "chronic meningitis" was introduced during the 1970s to embrace a large number of illnesses causing meningoencephalitis (fever, headache, lethargy, confusion, nausea, vomiting, stiff neck) and CSF abnormalities (predominantly lymphocytic pleocytosis, elevated protein level, and often low glucose level) lasting at least 4 weeks. Tuberculosis and cryptococcosis are the most common causes in the United States.

Presentation and Progression

Cause. Etiologies are both infectious and noninfectious. The former include tuberculosis, fungal diseases (cryptococcosis, coccidioidomycosis, histoplasmosis, blastomycosis, candidiasis, and sporotrichosis), spirochetal diseases (syphilis and Lyme disease), brucellosis, and parasitic infections (*Acanthamoeba* and *Angiostrongylus cantonensis*). The latter include tumors, sarcoidosis, granulomatous angiitis, Behçet's disease, and uveomeningoencephalitis. Some patients are given the diagnosis "chronic benign lymphocytic meningitis," and in other cases a satisfactory diagnosis is never reached. Chronic meningitis is often a component of diseases manifested mainly as encephalitis

(e.g., subacute sclerosing panencephalitis caused by the measles virus) or as focal lesions of the CNS (e.g., toxoplasmosis).

Presentation. The onset is typically insidious but can be acute, mimicking bacterial meningitis or aseptic meningitis. Patients often give a history of symptoms that began a week to several weeks before and include headache, fever (which can be low grade), lethargy, and nausea. If a diagnosis is not made and treatment instituted, the illness steadily progresses, although the course is sometimes characterized by remissions and exacerbations.

Diagnosis

The key to diagnosis of chronic meningitis is early suspicion and lumbar puncture. An ample volume of CSF should be saved, since a large number of studies may be necessary. Initial studies of CSF should include cryptococcal antigen, VDRL, PCR for *Mycobacterium tuberculosis,* acid-fast bacillus and fungal cultures (each preferably on 3 to 5 mL of CSF), and cytospin cytology. Patients should also have a tuberculin skin test, chest x-ray examination, and imaging of the brain (CT or MRI with gadolinium enhancement). Additional studies should be targeted on the basis of a thorough history and physical examination (both of which may need to be repeated carefully) and the results of initial laboratory tests. For example, travel or residence in the southwestern United States suggests coccidioidomycosis, tick exposures in New England or elsewhere suggest Lyme disease, and eosinophilia in the CSF suggests *Coccidioides,* parasites, lymphoma, or chemicals.

Natural History

Expected Outcome. If untreated, tuberculous and cryptococcal meningitis is nearly always fatal. In previously healthy persons cryptococcal meningitis can cause a subtle, extremely indolent illness that culminates in dementia. Prognosis for other forms of chronic meningitis is variable.

Treatment

Treatment depends on the etiology. In some patients with tuberculous meningitis, treatment on a presumptive basis is prudent.

When to Refer

Most patients with chronic meningitis require hospitalization or referral.

 KEY POINTS

CHRONIC MENINGITIS

⊃ Chronic meningitis is a syndrome that has diverse etiologies and is characterized by signs and symptoms of meningoencephalitis with CSF abnormalities lasting at least 4 weeks.

⊃ Causes in the United States include tuberculosis, cryptococcosis, regional mycoses (such as coccidioidomycosis and histoplasmosis), syphilis, and Lyme disease.

⊃ Most patients require hospitalization or referral.

SUGGESTED READING

Bonington A, Strang JI, Klapper PE, et al. Use of Roche AMPLICOR *Mycobacterium tuberculosis* PCR in early diagnosis of tuberculous meningitis. J Clin Microbiol 1998; 36: 1251-1254.

Smith JE, Aksamit AJ Jr. Outcome of chronic idiopathic meningitis. Mayo Clin Proc 1994; 69: 548-556.

Swartz MN. "Chronic meningitis"—many causes to consider. N Engl J Med 1987; 317: 957-959.

Wilhelm C, Ellner JJ. Chronic meningitis. Neurol Clin 1986; 4: 115-141.

Yechoor VK, Shandera WX, Rodriguez P, et al. Tuberculous meningitis among adults with and without HIV infection. Arch Intern Med 1996; 156: 1710-1716.

Other Causes of Cerebrospinal Fluid Pleocytosis

CSF pleocytosis has numerous causes, of which partially treated bacterial meningitis is perhaps the most important to the primary care clinician. Patients who receive oral antibiotics early in the course of acute bacterial meningitis may show temporary improvement, and the CSF pleocytosis may shift from predominantly neutrophilic to predominantly lymphocytic. The CSF protein level usually remains high, helping to distinguish this entity from more benign conditions. PCR may prove highly useful for establishing the diagnosis of partially treated bacterial meningitis. Diagnosis of parameningeal infections, discussed further later in the chapter, usually hinges on the history, physical examination, and appropriate imaging studies. Tumors may cause lymphocytic pleocytosis, sometimes with a low CSF glucose level. Seizures may cause mild CSF pleocytosis, which tends to be predominantly neutrophilic after alcohol-related seizures and predominantly lymphocytic after seizures caused by stroke. Rare patients have recurrent meningitis, the causes of which include leaking cyst contents from craniopharyngioma or epidermoid cyst, systemic lupus erythematosus, and an unusual condition known as Mollaret's meningitis. Drugs are being recognized increasingly as a cause of CSF pleocytosis; examples are NSAIDs and various antibiotics such as TMP/SMX, trimethoprim, sulfonamides, penicillin, and INH.

SUGGESTED READING

Ni H, Knight AI, Cartwright K, et al. Polymerase chain reaction for diagnosis of meningococcal meningitis. Lancet 1992; 340: 1432-1434.

Prokesch RC, Rimland D, Petrini JL Jr, et al. Cerebrospinal fluid pleocytosis after seizures. South Med J 1983; 76: 322-327.

Tedder DG, Ashley R, Tyler KL, et al. Herpes simplex virus infection as a cause of benign recurrent lymphocytic meningitis. Ann Intern Med 1994; 121: 334-338.

Townsend GC, Scheld WM. Infections of the central nervous system. Adv Intern Med 1998; 43: 403-447.

Encephalitis Caused by Herpes Simplex and Other Viruses

Viral encephalitis is a life-threatening process characterized clinically by altered consciousness and frequently by focal neurologic signs, seizures, and other abnormalities. HSV-1 is the most important cause of sporadic viral encephalitis in the United States, although it accounts for only about 10% to 20% of the estimated 20,000 cases of encephalitis that occur each year. Prompt diagnosis is crucial because, in contrast to most of the other forms of viral encephalitis, specific treatment is available.

Presentation and Progression

Cause

The major causes of viral encephalitis are the herpes simplex viruses, the arboviruses, mumps, measles, and varicella-zoster virus. About 95% of cases of encephalitis caused by herpes simplex are caused by HSV-1, and the remainder by HSV-2. About 70% of these cases result from reactivation of latent infection, and about 30% result from primary infection. Why encephalitis develops in occasional patients infected by this common virus remains a mystery. Most severely affected patients are immunologically normal; indeed an intact immune system may be required for full expression of the disease, since immunocompromised patients tend to have a milder course. Little or no evidence has been found for person-to-person transmission or influence by environmental factors. By contrast, arboviral infections causing encephalitis are carried by mosquitoes and ticks.

Presentation

Viral encephalitis, including HSV encephalitis, affects persons of all ages. Symptoms and signs of HSV encephalitis usually begin suddenly, in contrast to the usual subacute onset of the other forms of viral encephalitis. The first symptoms sometimes consist of behavioral abnormalities such as hypomania, elevated mood, and the Kluver-Bucy syndrome (loss of normal emotional responses such as anger and fear with hypersexuality). Lethargy progresses rapidly to confusion, stupor, and coma. Fever is usually present and may be high. Herpes labialis is present in less than 10% of cases, and its presence or absence has no diagnostic significance.

The most characteristic symptoms and signs of encephalitis caused by HSV-1 are attributed to the affinity of the virus for the medial temporal and inferior frontal lobes. This is manifested as some combination of speech impairment, bizarre behavior, and olfactory and gustatory hallucinations. Other localizing neurologic symptoms and signs, such as hemiparesis, ataxia, or cranial nerve palsies, are also seen. Focal seizures may occur.

Diagnosis

Temporal lobe involvement can be demonstrated by imaging procedures (CT or MRI scan) or by electroencephalography (EEG). MRI scans are more sensitive and specific than CT scans, especially during the early phases of the disease (Figure 6-6). The EEG shows focal abnormalities in more than 80% of cases. Lumbar puncture usually discloses red blood cells in the CSF, which reflects the necrotizing nature of the disease. The white blood cell count, glucose level, and protein content in CSF are variable, and occasionally all of these parameters are within normal limits. The most important specific test on CSF is the PCR for HSV-1 DNA. Reported to be up to 98% sensitive and 100% specific, PCR has replaced brain biopsy as the diagnostic procedure of choice.

Many diseases can mimic herpes simplex encephalitis. These include vascular disease, brain abscess or subdural empyema, toxic encephalopathy, tuberculosis, fungal infections (especially cryptococcosis and mucormycosis), tumor, subdural hematoma, and connective tissue diseases. Whether to perform brain biopsy before starting empiric therapy for herpes simplex encephalitis in less-than-classic cases has been debated for many years. Many authorities recommend brain biopsy. In practice, and especially in nonacademic settings, many neurosurgeons are reluctant to perform the procedure and therefore empiric therapy with acyclovir (see later discussion) is often given even when the probability that HSV is the causative agent is relatively low.

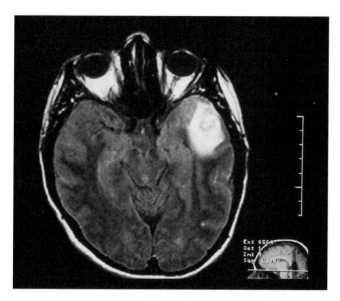

FIG. 6-6 Encephalitis caused by herpes simplex virus involving the left temporal lobe on magnetic resonance image in a 38-year-old woman who had had a seizure. (Courtesy of Dr. Charles Shissias.)

Natural History
Expected Outcome

The natural history of encephalitis caused by HSV-1 was well characterized before the introduction of effective antiviral therapy. Coma developed in about 85% of patients, seizures in up to 60%, and aphasia in about 20%. Mortality was about 70%, and survivors had a high prevalence of neurologic residua.

Treatment
Methods

Acylovir 10 mg/kg IV q8h for 10 to 14 days is the treatment of choice for HSV encephalitis and should be started as soon as possible when this diagnosis is suspected.

Expected Response

The introduction of acyclovir lowered the mortality of HSV encephalitis from 70% to 19%. However, only about 38% of patients return to normal function.

When to Refer

HSV encephalitis is a medical emergency, and hospitalization is indicated. Patients with encephalitis caused by arboviruses or as part of systemic infectious disease should usually be admitted to the hospital.

 KEY POINTS

ENCEPHALITIS CAUSED BY HERPES SIMPLEX AND OTHER VIRUSES

⊃ Of the many causes of sporadic viral encephalitis, HSV-1 is the most important and the most life threatening.
⊃ HSV encephalitis usually begins with fever and lethargy and progresses rapidly to stupor and coma.
⊃ Involvement of the temporal and frontal lobes is manifested clinically by impaired speech, bizarre behavior, and hallucinations and can be shown by CT or MRI scan and by EEG.

⊃ The CSF commonly shows red blood cells, reflecting the nature of the process.
⊃ Detection of HSV-1 DNA in CSF by PCR is up to 98% sensitive and 100% specific for HSV encephalitis and has replaced brain biopsy as the diagnostic procedure of choice.
⊃ Acyclovir 10 mg/kg IV q8h should be started in any patient in whom HSV-1 encephalitis is suspected on clinical grounds.

SUGGESTED READING

Atkins JT. HSV PCR for CNS infections: pearls and pitfalls. Pediatr Infect Dis J 1999; 18: 823-824.

Domingues RB, Tsanaclis AM, Pannuti CS, et al. Evaluation of the range of clinical presentations of herpes simplex encephalitis by using polymerase chain reaction assay of cerebrospinal fluid samples. Clin Infect Dis 1997; 25: 86-91.

Dupuis O, Audibert F, Fernandez H, et al. Herpes simplex virus encephalitis in pregnancy. Obstet Gynecol 1999; 94:810-812.

Falcone S, Post MJ. Encephalitis, cerebritis, and brain abscess: pathophysiology and imaging findings. Neuroimaging Clin North Am 2000; 10: 333-353.

Leonard JR, Moran CJ, Cross DT III, et al. MR imaging of herpes simplex type 1 encephalitis in infants and young children: a separate pattern of findings. AJR 2000; 174: 1651-1655.

Rappole JH, Derrickson SR, Hubalek Z. Migratory birds and spread of West Nile virus in the Western Hemisphere. Emerg Infect Dis 2000; 6: 319-328.

Sauerbrei A, Eichhorn U, Hottenrott G, et al. Virological diagnosis of herpes simplex encephalitis. J Clin Virol 2000; 17: 31-36.

Whitley RJ, Lakeman F. Herpes simplex virus infections of the central nervous system: therapeutic and diagnostic considerations. Clin Infect Dis 1995; 20: 414-420.

Brain Abscess, Subdural Empyema, and Intracranial Epidural Abscess

The term "parameningeal infection" (literally, "beside the meninges") encompasses several syndromes that require prompt diagnosis and usually surgical drainage. Examples are brain abscess, subdural empyema, septic thrombosis of the dural sinuses, and epidural abscess (both intracranial and spinal). Newer imaging studies (CT and MRI) simplify the diagnosis.

Presentation and Progression
Cause

Brain abscess is usually caused by spread from a contiguous focus of infection or hematogenous spread from a distant site of infection. Examples of the former are sinusitis (mainly frontal and ethmoid), otitis media or mastoiditis, dental sepsis, and penetrating injury or neurosurgery; examples of the latter are congenital heart disease with a right-to-left shunt, hereditary hemorrhagic telangiectasia with pulmonary arteriovenous fistulas, suppurative pulmonary infection, endocarditis, and opportunistic infections arising in immunocompromised patients. Brain abscess can also complicate head trauma. Streptococci, both aerobic and anaerobic, are the usual isolates, but other aerobic and anaerobic bacteria are often present. Unusual microorganisms such as fungi and *Toxoplasma gondii* cause brain abscess mainly in the severely immunocompromised (see Chapter 17).

Subdural empyema, which is less common than brain abscess, arises most often (60% to 70%) as an extension from sinusitis, especially frontal sinusitis. Otitis media with or without mastoiditis is the other major cause. Cases also result from trauma or surgery. Streptococci and especially anaerobic streptococci are again the most common isolates, but staphylococci (notably *S. aureus*) and aerobic gram-negative rods are also encountered. Intracranial epidural abscess, which is rare, has similar predisposing causes and similar microbiologic characteristics.

Presentation

Brain abscess is usually manifested as some combination of headache, fever, focal neurologic deficit, nausea or vomiting, seizures, nuchal rigidity, and papilledema. However, the presenting symptoms often evolve slowly and are nonspecific. Headache is the most common symptom (70% of patients) and can be localized or generalized. Fever is present in slightly less than one half of adults. Altered mental status and hemiparesis are the most common focal neurologic signs. Neurologic signs frequently predict the site of disease: for example, bizarre behavior with frontal lobe abscess; speech abnormalities with temporal lobe abscess; ataxia, nausea, and nystagmus with cerebellar abscess; and visual field cuts with temporal, parietal, or occipital lobe abscess. Symptoms and signs of the predisposing disease, such as sinusitis, otitis media, dental sepsis, or pulmonary disease, are often but not always present.

Subdural empyema usually evolves more rapidly than brain abscess. Typically symptoms suggestive of sinusitis or of otitis media are followed within days to several weeks by fever, severe headache, and neck pain (meningismus) and then by altered mental status and focal neurologic signs, sometimes with seizures. Intracranial epidural abscess, on the other hand, usually develops slowly over weeks or even months. Nonspecific symptoms give way to symptoms of increased intracranial pressure (nausea, vomiting, headache, altered mental status) and focal neurologic signs.

Diagnosis

MRI with gadolinium enhancement is now the diagnostic procedure of choice for all three conditions. Contrast-enhanced CT scans are usually effective, especially in the diagnosis of brain abscess.

Natural History
Expected Outcome

Untreated, all three conditions are probably uniformly fatal. Before the introduction of antibiotics, neurosurgical intervention had lowered the mortality for brain abscess to between 40% and 80%.

Treatment
Methods

Treatment of all three conditions consists of aggressive parenteral antibiotic therapy and neurosurgical drainage. Empiric antimicrobial therapy recommendations for brain abscess vary according to the predisposing position. Empiric therapy for most patients includes high-dose penicillin G, a cephalosporin (ceftriaxone or cefotaxime), and metronidazole. Vancomycin should be included in the initial regimen for subdural empyema and for brain abscess in which sinusitis appears to be the predisposing condition.

Expected Response

The reported mortality for brain abscess now ranges from zero to 30% and the mortality for subdural empyema from 6% to 20%. Many patients, especially those with subdural empyema, are left with a neurologic deficit.

When to Refer

Patients with any of the three conditions should be hospitalized.

 ## KEY POINTS

BRAIN ABSCESS, SUBDURAL EMPYEMA, AND INTRACRANIAL EPIDURAL ABSCESS

⊃ Brain abscess often evolves slowly and with nonspecific symptoms. The classic triad—headache, fever, and focal neurologic signs—is present in less than one half of cases.

⊃ Subdural empyema usually results from sinusitis or otitis media and evolves rapidly. Most patients have fever, headache, and nuchal rigidity (meningismus).

⊃ Intracranial epidural abscess, which is now rare, is often secondary to sinusitis and should be suspected especially when headache with nausea or vomiting gradually develops in patients with frontal sinusitis.

⊃ MRI is now the imaging procedure of choice for all three of these conditions.

SUGGESTED READING

Dill SR, Cobbs CG, McDonald CK. Subdural empyema: analysis of 32 cases and review. Clin Infect Dis 1995; 20: 372-386.

Dolan RW, Chowdhury K. Diagnosis and treatment of intracranial complications of paranasal sinus infections. J Oral Maxillofac Surg 1995; 53: 1080-1087.

Heilpern KL, Lorber B. Focal intracranial infections. Infect Dis Clin North Am 1996; 10: 879-898.

Mathisen GE, Johnson JP. Brain abscess. Clin Infect Dis 1997; 25: 763-781.

Septic Cavernous Sinus Thrombosis

Septic thrombosis of the large dural sinuses that provide venous drainage to the brain is a rare but life-threatening cause of severe headache. Diagnosis is usually delayed. The three major syndromes are cavernous sinus thrombosis, lateral sinus thrombosis, and superior sagittal sinus thrombosis. This section focuses on the most common of these syndromes, septic cavernous sinus thrombosis.

Presentation and Progression
Cause

Facial infections, most often nasal furuncles, precede about one half of cases of cavernous sinus thrombosis. Sphenoid sinusitis accounts for about 30% of cases and dental infections about 10%; the remainder of cases originate from otitis media, mastoiditis, or other localized infections. *S. aureus* is the most common etiologic agent and the usual cause of cavernous sinus thrombosis resulting from facial infections or sphenoid sinusitis. *S. pneumoniae* and other streptococci are the source of some cases, and anaerobic bacteria sometimes cause the condition, especially when it is due to dental infection or other forms of sinusitis. Diabetes mellitus is possibly a risk factor.

Presentation

Most patients with cavernous sinus thrombosis have severe, progressive, unilateral, retroorbital and frontal headache. The illness usually evolves over several days, but in some cases the headache is subacute or chronic. Migraine is a common misdiagnosis. Subsequent symptoms include unilateral swelling of the orbit, diplopia, and drowsiness. Rapid progression of the disease leads to proptosis, chemosis, papilledema, and ophthalmoplegia. Close examination often reveals decreased sensation over the forehead, nose, upper cheek and lip, and cornea and, on ophthalmoscopic examination, papilledema or dilated and tortuous retinal veins.

Diagnosis

Severe unilateral headache with orbital swelling suggests the possibility of septic cavernous thrombosis, which then must be distinguished from other conditions. Orbital cellulitis is the most common problem in differential diagnosis. Other possibilities include blepharitis, intraorbital abscess, trauma, tumors (meningioma and nasopharyngeal carcinoma), and several rare vascular diseases. The CSF is usually but not always abnormal. CSF pleocytosis is present in about two thirds of cases, and in about one third the CSF formula suggests bacterial meningitis (see earlier discussion). Neurodiagnostic imaging—currently high-resolution CT with enhancement or MRI with enhancement—is the diagnostic procedure of choice.

Expected Outcome

If untreated, septic cavernous sinus thrombosis is nearly uniformly fatal.

Treatment
Methods

Appropriate initial intravenous antibiotic therapy consists of high-dose nafcillin or oxacillin (2 g q4h) plus a third-generation cephalosporin such as ceftriaxone 1 g q12h or cefotaxime 2 g q4-6h plus—if sinusitis or dental infection is suspected as the source—metronidazole 500 to 750 mg q8h. Some authorities recommend high-dose corticosteroids (e.g., dexamethasone 10 mg q6h) *after* antibiotic therapy is under way. Sphenoid sinusitis, if present, should be drained surgically (see later discussion). Some authorities recommend aggressive anticoagulant therapy with heparin.

Expected Response

The overall mortality even with aggressive treatment is about 30%, and another 30% have serious residua such as hemiparesis, blindness, and hypopituitarism.

When to Refer

All patients with suspected septic cavernous sinus thrombosis should be hospitalized.

 KEY POINTS

SEPTIC CAVERNOUS SINUS THROMBOSIS

⊃ Septic cavernous sinus thrombosis usually begins with severe, progressive, unilateral, retroorbital and frontal headache.
⊃ Unilateral orbital swelling, an early sign of the disease, must be distinguished from uncomplicated orbital cellulitis.

⊃ Late findings include proptosis, chemosis, papilledema, and ophthalmoplegia.
⊃ Mortality without treatment is nearly 100%, and delays in diagnosis are common.
⊃ Neuroimaging studies (enhanced CT or MRI) distinguish cavernous sinus thrombosis from other conditions.
⊃ Patients with suspected cavernous sinus thrombosis should be hospitalized.
⊃ Pimples and furuncles in the "dangerous area" of the nose and face should be squeezed or massaged with great care if at all.

SUGGESTED READING

DiNubile MJ. Septic thrombosis of the cavernous sinuses. Arch Neurol 1988; 45: 567-572.

Gerszten PC, Welch WC, Spearman MP, et al. Isolated deep cerebral venous thrombosis treated by direct endovascular thrombolysis. Surg Neurol 1997; 48: 261-266.

Southwick FS, Richardson EP Jr, Swartz MN. Septic thrombosis of the dural venous sinuses. Medicine (Baltimore) 1986; 65: 82-106.

Sphenoid Sinusitis

Acute sphenoid sinusitis is a life-threatening cause of "the worst headache ever." Diagnosis requires a high index of suspicion and CT scan of the paranasal sinuses.

Presentation and Progression
Cause

The sphenoid sinuses and their venous drainage are intimately related to the same structures that surround the cavernous sinus (see earlier discussion): the brain, pituitary gland, carotid artery, and several cranial nerves. Infection of the sphenoid sinuses can occur in the setting of chronic sinusitis or acute pansinusitis or can be an isolated event with no apparent cause. Cocaine snorting may be a risk factor.

Presentation

Although the classic headache of sphenoid sinusitis is localized to the vertex of the skull, other pain patterns are more common. Unilateral facial pain is sometimes caused by irritation of one or more branches of the fifth cranial nerve. The pain can also radiate to the temporal or occipital areas or can be a severe, generalized, "pancephalic" headache. Other clinical signs of sinusitis, such as nasal drainage or postnasal drip, are variably present.

Diagnosis

Diagnosis of sphenoid sinusitis is based on imaging studies. The sphenoid sinuses can be seen on lateral radiographs of the skull but are better visualized by CT scan.

Natural History
Expected Outcome

Opacification of the sphenoid sinus can be an unanticipated finding on CT scan of the brain and of little or no clinical consequence. However, sphenoid sinusitis with extension of the disease process into surrounding structures carries a high morbidity and mortality. Complications include stroke with hemiparesis, meningitis, brain abscess, subdural empyema, and pituitary apoplexy.

Treatment
Methods
Empiric antibiotic therapy should be the same as that described previously for septic cavernous vein thrombosis (e.g., nafcillin or oxacillin plus ceftriaxone or cefotaxime plus metronidazole). The sphenoid sinuses should be drained surgically.

Expected Response
Morbidity and mortality are reduced by appropriate therapy for this uncommon condition but remain high.

When to Refer
Patients with suspected acute sphenoid sinusitis should usually be hospitalized.

 KEY POINTS

SPHENOID SINUSITIS
⊃ Sphenoid sinusitis is a potentially lethal cause of "the worst headache ever."
⊃ As classically described, pain is over the vertex of the skull. However, facial pain in the fifth nerve distribution, temporal-occipital pain, and severe generalized headache are also common.
⊃ Accurate diagnosis of sphenoid sinusitis can be made only with appropriate imaging studies.
⊃ Hospitalization for aggressive antibiotic therapy and surgical drainage is mandatory.

SUGGESTED READING
Lew D, Southwick FS, Montgomery WW, et al. Sphenoid sinusitis: a review of 30 cases. N Engl J Med 1983; 309: 1149-1154.
Oruckaptan HH, Akdemir P, Ozgen T. Isolated sphenoid sinus abscess: clinical and radiological failure in preoperative diagnosis; case report and review of the literature. Surg Neurol 2000; 53: 174-177.
Sethi DS. Isolated sphenoid lesions: diagnosis and management. Otolaryngol Head Neck Surg 1999; 120: 730-736.
Turgut S, Ozcan KM, Celikkanat S, et al. Isolated sphenoid sinusitis. Rhinology 1997; 35: 132-135.

Spinal Epidural Abscess
The classic presentation of spinal epidural abscess is fever and back pain that progress to weakness of the lower extremities with impaired bowel or bladder function and then to paralysis. The correct diagnosis is seldom made at the first patient encounter.

Presentation and Progression
Cause
As seen in primary care practice, spinal epidural abscess is usually a complication of vertebral osteomyelitis or diskitis (see Chapter 15). Bacteria gain access to the spine through hematogenous dissemination. Most abscesses are posterior to the spinal cord, although below the level of the L1 vertebra some of them are anterior to the cord. *S. aureus* is the most common microorganism and is found in more than 60% of cases (>90% of cases in some series), but aerobic gram-negative rods, streptococci, *M. tuberculosis,* and other organisms are major causes of the disease. Spinal epidural abscess also occurs as a complication of spinal surgery, trauma, drug use, or spinal anesthesia.

Presentation
Many patients first have a flulike illness with fever, malaise, and—especially if *S. aureus* is the causative organism—myalgias. As the abscess expands, severe, localized back pain develops, often accompanied by nerve root pain. Weakness in the extremities then develops along with sensory changes and functional impairment of the bladder or bowel or both.

Diagnosis
Fever and localized back pain suggest vertebral osteomyelitis or diskitis; the appearance of weakness in this setting strongly suggests spinal epidural abscess. Other diseases to consider are herpes zoster, meningitis, and metastatic tumor. Gadolinium-enhanced MRI is now the procedure of choice. CT scanning with gadolinium contrast is also useful but in general provides less information than MRI scanning. Blood cultures are positive in about 60% of cases.

Natural History
Expected Outcome
Untreated, spinal epidural abscess progresses to complete progression of the spinal cord with permanent paralysis.

Treatment
Methods
Treatment in most cases consists of surgical drainage, preferably within 24 hours of admission to the hospital, followed by appropriate antibiotic therapy for at least 4 weeks.

Expected Response
Prognosis generally hinges on promptness of diagnosis and adequacy of surgical drainage. Morbidity and mortality remain high.

When to Refer
Patients with suspected spinal epidural abscess should be hospitalized.

 KEY POINTS

SPINAL EPIDURAL ABSCESS
⊃ Spinal epidural abscess is suggested by fever, localized back pain, and signs of cord compression.
⊃ *S. aureus* is the usual organism, but many cases are caused by aerobic gram-negative rods, other bacteria, and *M. tuberculosis.*
⊃ Suspicion of this diagnosis should prompt imaging of the spine with MRI or CT.
⊃ Early diagnosis and effective surgical drainage are usually crucial to a successful outcome.

SUGGESTED READING
Akalan N, Ozgen T. Infection as a cause of spinal cord compression: a review of 36 spinal epidural abscess cases. Acta Neurochir 2000; 142: 17-23.
Baker AS, Ojemann RG, Swartz MN, et al. Spinal epidural abscess. N Engl J Med 1975; 293: 463-468.
Mackenzie AR, Laing RB, Smith CC, et al. Spinal epidural abscess: the importance of early diagnosis and treatment. J Neurol Neurosurg Psychiatry 1998; 65: 209-212.

Rigamonti D, Liem L, Sampath P, et al. Spinal epidural abscess: contemporary trends in etiology, evaluation, and management. Surg Neurol 1999; 52: 189-196.

Torda AJ, Gottlieb T, Bradbury R. Pyogenic vertebral osteomyelitis: analysis of 20 cases and review. Clin Infect Dis 1995; 20: 320-328.

Tung GA, Yim JW, Mermel LA, et al. Spinal epidural abscess: correlation between MRI findings and outcome. Neuroradiology 1999; 41: 904-909.

Infective Endocarditis

Infective endocarditis—the term now preferred to "bacterial endocarditis," since microorganisms other than bacteria sometimes cause the disease—is uniformly fatal without adequate treatment. Unfortunately, the diagnosis can be masked by prior antibiotic therapy. The primary care clinician's task is to know when to suspect endocarditis, when to request blood cultures, when to order special studies such as echocardiography, and when to refer patients for hospitalization because of the suspicion of endocarditis caused by highly destructive organisms such as *S. aureus*.

Presentation and Progression
Cause

The term "infective endocarditis" usually refers to infection of the heart valves, but other surfaces can be affected, such as the endocardium adjacent to a ventricular septal defect. "Endarteritis" refers to an identical process affecting a large blood vessel, such as a patent ductus arteriosus. In any case pathogenesis requires two events: damage to the endothelial surface and the presence of microorganisms in the bloodstream. Formation of platelet-fibrin thrombi on heart valves and other endothelial surfaces may be a relatively common event in persons with preexisting cardiac abnormalities and can also be induced by hemodynamic stress or by the "chunks of junk" that traverse the veins of injecting drug users. Microorganisms whose presence in the bloodstream would usually be a transient phenomenon (e.g., after a dental procedure) find in the bland thrombi a privileged sanctuary to which host defenses have little or no access.

The diverse clinical manifestations of endocarditis reflect four phenomena: (1) The continuous multiplication of microorganisms causes their constant presence in the bloodstream in most instances. Fever and other constitutional symptoms result, and highly virulent bacteria such as *S. aureus* can cause severe sepsis progressing to septic shock. (2) Pieces of the vegetations can break off and cause the transport of septic emboli to the lungs (in patients with right-sided endocarditis) or to the brain, coronary arteries, kidneys, spleen, skin, and other organs (in patients with left-sided endocarditis). (3) Antibodies made in response to microorganisms in the bloodstream promote formation of circulating antigen-antibody complexes (immune complexes), which can cause disease manifestations such as arthritis, cerebritis, and glomerulonephritis. (4) Destruction of heart valves, myocardium, and other tissue can cause heart failure, which is now the most important cause of death in certain types of endocarditis, or arrhythmias.

Viridans streptococci are historically the most common causes of endocarditis, although staphylococci have been more common in some of the recently published series. Viridans streptococci usually enter the bloodstream from the oral cavity. The viridans streptococci are a diverse group of bacteria (see Chapter 1); *S. sanguis* and *S. mutans* are the most common in

cases of endocarditis. Enterococci cause up to 18% of cases, typically affecting young women with gynecologic or obstetric problems and older men with genitourinary problems. *S. bovis,* a group D streptococcus that resides in the intestine, is an important cause of endocarditis and is often associated with carcinoma or villous adenoma of the colon. *S. aureus* causes up to about one third of cases of endocarditis in some localities. Coagulase-negative staphylococci and fungi are usually found in patients with prosthetic heart valves. Fastidious gram-negative bacteria collectively known as the "HACEK group" occasionally cause a form of endocarditis that is not only difficult to diagnose but also associated with large, bulky vegetations that can cause embolic occlusion of large arteries. The acronym stands for *Haemophilus* species, *Actinobacillus actinomycetemcomitans, Cardiobacterium hominis, Eikenella corrodens,* and *Kingella* species. Numerous other microorganisms occasionally cause endocarditis, such as anaerobic bacteria, *Coxiella burnetii* (Q fever), and *Chlamydia psittaci.*

Presentation

Although classification of endocarditis as "acute," "subacute," and "chronic" has been largely abandoned in favor of the more general term "infective endocarditis," knowledge of the typical time frames associated with the various pathogens remains useful. *S. aureus* typically causes "acute" endocarditis. In younger patients the characteristic triad consists of *S. aureus* bacteremia, patchy bilateral pulmonary infiltrates, and evidence of injecting drug use by history or by the presence of needle tracks. A murmur of tricuspid or pulmonic regurgitation is sometimes present. In older patients the characteristic triad consists of *S. aureus* bacteremia, peripheral embolic phenomena, and clinically evident heart disease manifested as murmurs, arrhythmias, or heart failure. When caused by destruction of a valve or rupture of a papillary muscle, heart failure can progress rapidly. Viridans streptococci are more commonly associated with a subacute course. When first seen, patients have vague complaints that may suggest a "viral syndrome." If the disease is unrecognized, patients continue to have low-grade fever and malaise punctuated by such events as transient cerebral ischemic attack (embolism to the CNS), transient left upper quadrant pain (embolism to the spleen), and hematuria (embolism to the kidneys). Endocarditis caused by the HACEK organisms or by fungi can follow a more indolent course; embolic occlusion of a large artery sometimes brings the patient to medical attention. Overall, about 90% of patients with endocarditis have fever, 85% have a heart murmur, more than 50% manifest embolic phenomena if carefully sought, and about 20% to 50% have mucocutaneous manifestations of one kind or another. The latter include splinter hemorrhages (Figure 6-7), pustular purpura (Figure 6-8), petechiae (typically found in the conjunctivae, buccal mucosa, palate, or extremities; Figures 6-9 and 6-10), Janeway lesions (hemorrhagic, painless plaques usually found on the palms or soles; Figure 6-11), and Osler's nodes (small, painful, nodular lesions usually found on the pads of the fingers or toes; Figure 6-12). Other manifestations include progressive anemia, delirium, intracranial hemorrhage from mycotic aneurysms, and renal failure.

Diagnosis

Blood cultures are the key to early diagnosis of endocarditis. For this reason, when endocarditis is suspected or patients have a cardiac lesion that notably predisposes to endocarditis,

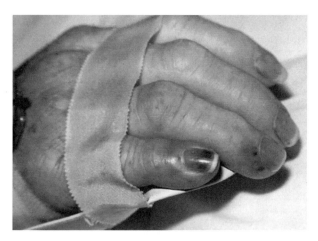

FIG. 6-7   Large splinter hemorrhage in the nail bed of the fifth finger in a patient with acute staphylococcal endocarditis.

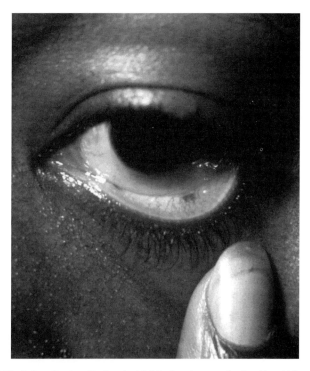

FIG. 6-9   Conjunctival petechial lesion in a patient with viridans streptococcal endocarditis.

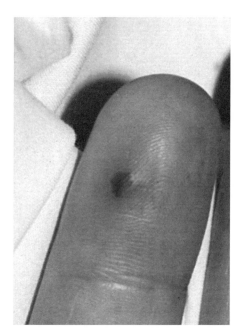

FIG. 6-8   Pustular lesion ("purulent purpura") on the fingertip of a patient with staphylococcal endocarditis.

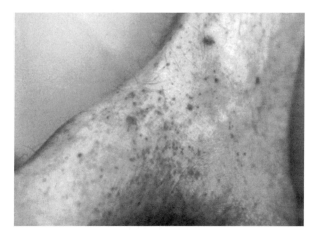

FIG. 6-10   Numerous petechiae on the lower extremity of a patient with endocarditis caused by *Pseudomonas aeruginosa*.

blood cultures should be obtained before antibiotics are administered. The recently introduced "Duke criteria" take into account the emerging role of echocardiography, especially transesophageal echocardiography (TEE), in the diagnosis of the disease (Table 6-7).

When endocarditis caused by *S. aureus* is suspected in a patient with an acute illness, hospitalization is usually the best course. When endocarditis is considered a possibility in the differential diagnosis of a subacute or chronic illness, it is often more judicious to obtain blood cultures on an outpatient basis while arranging for close follow-up. Occasional patients who are eventually proved to have endocarditis present thorny diagnostic problems. Streptococci with unusual growth requirements ("nutritionally deficient streptococci," now known as *Abiotrophia* species),

HACEK organisms, *Brucella* species, fungi, *C. burnetii*, and other diverse microorganisms are associated with so-called culture-negative endocarditis. Diagnosis of these cases usually requires referral or close consultation with a good microbiology laboratory.

Natural History
Expected Outcome

If untreated, endocarditis is uniformly fatal.

Treatment
Methods

Treatment of endocarditis typically requires 4 to 6 weeks of parenteral antimicrobial therapy. Shorter courses of therapy (2 weeks) may be appropriate for some cases of viridans

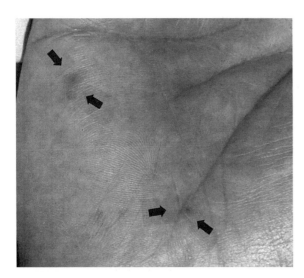

FIG. 6-11 Janeway lesions (painless erythematous lesions) on the palm of a patient with endocarditis.

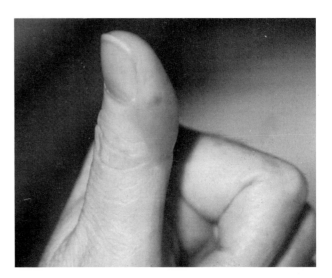

FIG. 6-12 Osler's node on the thumb of a patient with staphylococcal endocarditis.

streptococcal endocarditis and for right-sided *S. aureus* endocarditis in injecting drug users. Some regimens are summarized briefly elsewhere in the book (see Appendix 2). When streptococci are determined to be the cause of endocarditis, the susceptibility (minimum inhibitory concentration [MIC]) of the organism to penicillin G must be determined. Many patients with endocarditis ($\geq 25\%$) require surgery for valve replacement or valvuloplasty.

Expected Response

Most patients with uncomplicated endocarditis caused by penicillin-sensitive (MIC <0.2 μg/mL) viridans streptococci are cured with appropriate drug therapy. Current mortality is about 20% for endocarditis caused by penicillin-resistant streptococci and enterococci, about 40% for endocarditis caused by *S. aureus,* and greater than 50% for endocarditis complicated by acute aortic regurgitation.

When to Refer

Patients with endocarditis should nearly always be hospitalized for appropriate diagnosis and treatment. Optimum management of complicated cases requires close collaboration among cardiologists, cardiac surgeons, and infectious disease specialists.

 KEY POINTS

INFECTIVE ENDOCARDITIS

⊃ Endocarditis should be suspected when a patient has fever accompanied by a heart murmur, but the manifestations can be quite diverse.

⊃ The manifestations of endocarditis are caused by (1) continuous presence of microorganisms in the bloodstream, (2) embolism from the vegetations, (3) circulating immune complexes, and (4) destruction of cardiac tissue, causing heart failure or arrhythmias.

⊃ Blood cultures are the cornerstone to diagnosis. The newer "Duke criteria" for endocarditis take into account the value of echocardiography.

⊃ Patients with a recent onset of symptoms and signs consistent with endocarditis caused by *S. aureus* should be hospitalized.

⊃ If a patient has a subacute or chronic illness consistent with endocarditis, a reasonable approach is to obtain serial blood cultures and monitor the patient closely on an outpatient basis.

⊃ Patients with endocarditis should probably be hospitalized initially for evaluation and antimicrobial therapy.

SUGGESTED READING

Bayer AS, Bolger AF, Taubert KA, et al. Diagnosis and management of infective endocarditis and its complications. Circulation 1998; 98: 2936-2948.

Mylonakis E, Calderwood SB. Infective endocarditis in adults. N Engl J Med 2001; 345: 1318-1330.

Vlessis AA, Bowling SF, eds. Endocarditis: A Multidisciplinary Approach to Modern Treatment. Armonk, NY: Futura Publishing Company; 1999.

Wilson WR, Karchmer AW, Dajani AS, et al. Antibiotic treatment of adults with infective endocarditis due to streptococci, enterococci, staphylococci and HACEK microorganisms. JAMA 1995; 274: 1706-1713.

Pericarditis and Myocarditis

Pericarditis and myocarditis are uncommon problems in primary care and have overlapping clinical features. When these conditions are suspected, referral to a cardiologist is usually necessary.

Presentation and Progression
Cause

Both pericarditis and myocarditis have been associated with a large number of viruses and bacteria, as well as with fungi and parasites. In the United States most cases are eventually called "idiopathic" and presumed to be caused by viruses. Enteroviruses, especially the coxsackieviruses, are frequently associated with both diseases. Other viruses reported to cause both pericarditis and myocarditis are influenza viruses, echo-

TABLE 6-7
"Duke Criteria" for the Diagnosis of Endocarditis*

Aspect	Criteria
Major criteria	1. *Positive blood cultures:* typical microorganism for endocarditis from two separate blood cultures (viridans streptococci, *Streptococcus bovis,* or HACEK group†) or community-acquired *Staphylococcus aureus* or enterococci in the absence of a primary focus, *or* persistently positive blood cultures for any microorganism (i.e., from blood cultures drawn more than 12 hours apart), *or* all of three or the majority of four or more separate blood cultures, with first and last specimens drawn at least 1 hour apart 2. *Evidence of endocardial involvement:* Findings on echocardiogram positive for infective endocarditis (oscillating intracardiac mass on valve or supporting structures or in the path of regurgitant jets, or on iatrogenic devices, in the absence of an alternative anatomic explanation), *or* abscess, *or* new partial dehiscence of prosthetic valve, *or* new valvular regurgitation
Minor criteria	*Predisposition:* predisposing heart condition or intravenous (injecting) drug use *Fever:* ≥100.4° F (38° C) *Vascular phenomena:* arterial embolism, septic pulmonary infarcts, mycotic aneurysm, intracranial hemorrhage, Janeway lesions *Immunologic phenomena:* glomerulonephritis, Osler's nodes, Roth spots, rheumatoid factor *Echocardiogram:* findings consistent with infective endocarditis but not meeting the major criteria above *Microbiologic evidence:* positive blood culture but not meeting major criteria above, *or* serologic evidence of active infection with organism consistent with infective endocarditis
Definite endocarditis on clinical grounds	Both major criteria, or one major and three minor criteria, or five minor criteria
Definite endocarditis based on pathologic specimen	*Microorganisms* demonstrated by culture or histologic tests in a vegetation, or in a vegetation that has embolized, or in an intracardiac abscess; *or pathologic lesions:* vegetation of intracardiac abscess present, confirmed by histologic tests showing active endocarditis
Possible endocarditis	Findings consistent with infective endocarditis that fall short of criteria for *definite* endocarditis, but that preclude *rejection* of diagnosis
Rejection of diagnosis	Firm alternative diagnosis explaining evidence of infective endocarditis, *or* resolution of endocarditis syndrome with antibiotic therapy for 4 days or less, *or* no pathologic evidence of infective endocarditis at surgery or autopsy, after antibiotic therapy for 4 days or less

Modified from Durack DT, Lukes AS, Bright DK, et al. New criteria for diagnosis of infective endocarditis. Am J Med 1994; 96: 200-209.
*Using the two major and six minor criteria, the clinician determines whether endocarditis is "definite," "possible," or "rejected."
†For definition of HACEK organisms, see text.

viruses, adenoviruses, mumps, Epstein-Barr virus, varicella-zoster virus, cytomegalovirus, and hepatitis B. Other systemic bacterial infections—for example, meningococcemia, staphylococcal or streptococcal bacteremia, or *Legionella pneumophila* infection—can similarly involve the myocardium, pericardium, or both. Myocarditis occurs in about 30% of persons infected with *Trypanosoma cruzi* (the cause of Chagas' disease), which is endemic in parts of Latin America. *Mycobacterium tuberculosis* is an extremely important cause of pericarditis, which can also be caused by the agents of "regional mycosis" (i.e., histoplasmosis, blastomycosis, and coccidioidomycosis) encountered in the United States.

Presentation

Acute idiopathic or viral pericarditis usually causes substernal chest pain, which is made worse by breathing and swallowing and is relieved by leaning forward. Fever is present in about 60% of patients, and many patients give a history of flulike illness with cough, malaise, myalgias, and arthralgias. Acute bac-

terial pericarditis (purulent pericarditis) usually occurs in the setting of severe bacterial infection in a patient with marked toxicity. Tuberculous pericarditis is sometimes an acute illness but more commonly begins gradually with vague chest pain and some combination of night sweats, weight loss, cough, and dyspnea. Myocarditis can also manifest itself as chest pain, but more commonly the diagnosis is considered as a cause of heart failure or arrhythmias in a previously healthy person or during the course of an obvious systemic viral or bacterial infection.

Diagnosis

Acute pericarditis is strongly suggested by the finding of a three-component pericardial friction rub, present in about 50% of cases. Constrictive pericarditis, as found in tuberculosis, is suggested by the finding of a paradoxic pulse (marked fall in systolic blood pressure with inspiration) and by Kussmaul's sign (distention of the neck veins during inspiration). In patients with large pericardial effusions the heart sounds are distant and blood pressure is often low.

Physical examination of patients with myocarditis may show tachycardia, arrhythmia, and ventricular gallop (S_3).

Suspicion of either pericarditis or myocarditis or presence of any of the signs mentioned should prompt an electrocardiogram. About 50% of patients with acute pericarditis show characteristic ST segment elevations without changes in the QRS morphology (i.e., the patient has no pathologic Q waves). As the ST segments return to baseline, T-wave flattening and then inversion occur. Patients with large pericardial effusions often show reduced QRS voltage and electrical alternans (i.e., the QRS axis changes from beat to beat). Patients with myocarditis typically have nonspecific ST segment and T-wave changes. As in pericarditis, ST segment elevations can be followed by T-wave inversions, without the development of pathologic Q waves. The development of Q waves, abnormal QRS complexes, or left bundle branch block in myocarditis portends a fulminant course and risk of sudden death.

Echocardiography is extremely useful in both conditions. In pericarditis the clinician looks for pericardial effusions and thickening; in myocarditis, changes in the myocardium, impaired systolic function, and wall motion abnormalities are sought. CT scans sometimes provide additional data in pericarditis, and some evidence suggests that MRI may be useful in the diagnosis of idiopathic or viral myocarditis. The diagnosis of pericarditis can be secured in most cases by open pericardial biopsy, although this procedure may lead to the precise etiology and does not suffice to exclude tuberculosis as a possible cause. The diagnosis of myocarditis can often be established by endomyocardial biopsy, but the necessity for this procedure in most cases is unclear.

Natural History
Expected Outcome

Acute idiopathic ("viral") pericarditis and acute idiopathic ("viral") myocarditis often have self-limited courses. Both conditions can lead to intractable heart failure.

Treatment
Methods

Treatment of idiopathic ("viral") pericarditis and myocarditis is symptomatic. Prednisone should not be given to patients with acute myocarditis because of clinical and experimental evidence that it can lead to rapid deterioration. Some authorities believe that prednisone should also be withheld from patients with acute pericarditis because many of these patients have a component of myocarditis as well. In severe cases both conditions can be treated surgically. For pericarditis this may entail creation of a pericardial window for drainage or pericardiectomy. For end-stage myocarditis the only cure is heart transplantation.

Expected Response

The response is variable and is generally poorer for myocarditis than for pericarditis.

When to Refer

Patients with suspected pericarditis or myocarditis should usually be referred to a cardiologist. Acutely ill patients should be hospitalized.

 KEY POINTS

PERICARDITIS AND MYOCARDITIS

- ⊃ Pericarditis and myocarditis are uncommon problems in primary care and have overlapping clinical and pathologic features.
- ⊃ A majority of cases of pericarditis and myocarditis are considered idiopathic and presumed to be of viral etiology.
- ⊃ Acute idiopathic (viral) pericarditis is suggested by chest pain, a pericardial friction rub, and ST segment elevations on the electrocardiogram, but not all of these features are necessarily present.
- ⊃ Tuberculosis should be considered in every case of acute pericarditis.
- ⊃ Myocarditis is suggested by unexplained heart failure or arrhythmias, either in a previously healthy person or during the course of a systemic infection.
- ⊃ Most patients with acute idiopathic ("viral") pericarditis or pericarditis recover completely.
- ⊃ Steroids should not be given to patients with acute myocarditis and are not recommended at present for patients with acute pericarditis because of the possibility of a myocardial component to their disease.

SUGGESTED READING

Arsan S, Mercan S, Sarigül A, et al. Long-term experience with pericardiectomy: analysis of 105 consecutive cases. Thorac Cardiovasc Surg 1994; 42: 340-344.

Brodison A, Swann JW. Myocarditis: a review. J Infect 1998; 37: 99-103.

Mason JW. Myocarditis. Adv Intern Med 1999; 44: 293-310.

Mercé J, Sagristá-Sauleda J, Permanyer-Miralda G, et al. Should pericardial drainage be performed routinely in patients who have a large pericardial effusion without tamponade? Am J Med 1998; 105: 106-109.

Pawsat DE, Lee JY. Inflammatory disorders of the heart: pericarditis, myocarditis, and endocarditis. Emerg Med Clin North Am 1998; 16: 665-681.

Peters NS, Poole-Wilson PA. Myocarditis—continuing clinical and pathologic confusion. Am Heart J 1991; 121: 942-947.

Aortitis and Mycotic Aneurysm

Mycotic aneurysm of the aorta is most commonly caused by nontyphoidal *Salmonella* species. Mortality is high if the disease is unrecognized.

Presentation and Progression
Cause

Gastroenteritis resulting from ingestion of *Salmonella* (see Chapter 12) probably causes a transient bacteremia in many patients that usually resolves without treatment. However, these organisms have an affinity for atherosclerotic plaques. Multiplication in atherosclerotic plaques leads to weakening of the aortic wall and formation of an aneurysm.

Presentation

The usual patient is an older adult, most commonly a man, with risk factors for significant atherosclerosis such as diabetes mellitus or hypertension. Some affected patients have underlying peptic ulcer disease, treatment of which usually raises the gastric pH, thereby lowering the patient's resistance to ingested *Salmonella* organisms. Others have a condition that impairs the ability of macrophages to clear the bloodstream of *Salmonella,* such as cirrhosis or a condition requiring immunosuppressive drugs. Onset of symptoms is commonly insidious. In a recent study the average duration of symptoms was about 1 month (range of 1 day to 6 months). At the time of initial examination nearly all patients have fever and pain in the abdomen, back, or both. Results from three clinical series suggest that mycotic aneurysm develops in about 10% of persons >50 years of age with *Salmonella* bacteremia of the non-*typhi* type.

Diagnosis

The diagnosis of aortitis with or without mycotic aneurysm is made most easily by CT scan with contrast enhancement. The diagnosis can also be based on arteriography (Figure 6-13). Most aneurysms are found in the abdominal aorta, typically below the renal arteries. The thoracic aorta is involved in about 17% of patients. Blood cultures are usually positive (85% of patients), and stool cultures are frequently positive (64% of patients). Definitive diagnosis is made at surgery.

Natural History
Expected Outcome

Aortitis with aortic aneurysm is probably uniformly fatal without treatment. Rupture of the aneurysm is the usual cause of death.

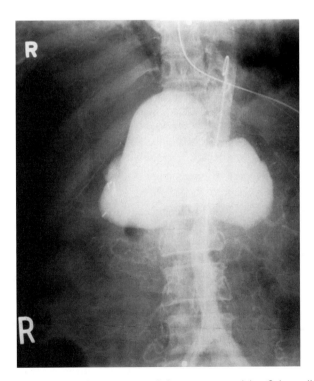

FIG. 6-13 Mycotic aneurysm of the aorta caused by *Salmonella* species in a patient with underlying atherosclerosis. This aneurysm was unresectable, and the patient died. Treatment of *Salmonella* gastroenteritis in older patients is recommended because of the possibility of this occurrence.

Treatment
Methods

Optimum treatment requires early surgical intervention and long-term suppressive antibiotic therapy.

Expected Response

The mortality from aortitis caused by *Salmonella* is about 60%. In a recent review, mortality was 36% for patients treated with a combined medical and surgical approach but 96% for patients treated only medically.

When to Refer

Recognition of mycotic aneurysm necessitates prompt referral for resection.

 KEY POINTS

AORTITIS AND MYCOTIC ANEURYSM
- ⊃ Mycotic aneurysm should be suspected when an older patient with risk factors for atherosclerosis seeks treatment for fever and pain in the back or abdomen.
- ⊃ *Salmonella* species are the usual cause.
- ⊃ Mycotic aneurysm occurs in about 10% of persons >50 years of age with *Salmonella* bacteremia; antimicrobial therapy is therefore recommended.
- ⊃ Cure requires urgent resection of the aneurysm and long-term suppressive drug therapy.

SUGGESTED READING
Benenson S, Raveh D, Schlesinger Y, et al. The risk of vascular infection in adult patients with nontyphi *Salmonella* bacteremia. Am J Med 2001; 110: 60-63.

Bronze MS, Shirwany A, Corbett C, et al. Infectious aortitis: an uncommon manifestation of infection with *Streptococcus pneumoniae.* Am J Med 1999; 107: 627-630.

Sessa C, Farah I, Voirin L, et al. Infected aneurysms of the infrarenal abdominal aorta: diagnostic criteria and therapeutic strategy. Ann Vasc Surg 1997; 11: 453-463.

Soravia-Dunand VA, Loo VG, Salit IE. Aortitis due to *Salmonella*: report of 10 cases and comprehensive review of the literature. Clin Infect Dis 1999; 29: 862-868.

von Segesser LK, Vogt P, Genoni M, et al. The infected aorta. J Card Surg 1997; 12 (Suppl 2): 256-260.

Acute Epiglottitis (Supraglottitis)

Acute epiglottitis (or supraglottitis) is a life-threatening cellulitis of the epiglottis and adjacent structures. It occurs mainly in children, is usually caused by *Haemophilus influenzae,* and has the potential for sudden, complete obstruction of the airway. It is a medical emergency and must be distinguished from croup.

Presentation and Progression
Cause

H. influenzae type b is the usual pathogen in both children and adults, but occasional cases result from *S. pneumoniae, S. aureus* (including methicillin-resistant strains), streptococci, *Haemophilus paraphrophilus,* and numerous bacterial species and viruses. The incidence of the disease in children has decreased markedly since the introduction of the

H. influenzae type b conjugated vaccine. Epiglottitis can also be a noninfectious illness caused by allergic reactions, physical agents, or the smoking of recreational drugs or may occur as a complication of tonsillectomy. The process consists of a diffuse cellulitis of the supraglottic tissues (hence "supraglottitis" may be the more accurate term).

Presentation

The onset in children is usually sudden with fever, dysphonia, dysphagia, and difficulty breathing. The child characteristically leans forward and drools, with tentative respirations. Adults are more likely to have a severe sore throat, odynophagia, and a sensation of airway obstruction.

Diagnosis

The major differential diagnosis in children is croup. Croup usually has a more gradual onset, often preceded by an upper respiratory infection. Also, children with croup prefer to lie supine and typically do not have drooling or dysphagia. Patients with epiglottitis (unlike those with croup) seldom have a barking cough or aphonia.

The diagnosis can be made by observing a "thumb sign" (i.e., swelling causes the epiglottis to resemble a thumb, whereas the normal epiglottis resembles a finger). In children, however, vigorous attempt to visualize the epiglottis can precipitate airway obstruction or vagally mediated cardiopulmonary arrest and sending the patient for x-ray studies can be a fatal error because complete airway obstruction can develop within minutes.

Natural History
Expected Outcome

In children the mortality from acute epiglottitis with airway obstruction is 80%. Mortality is much lower in adults (<5% in some series).

Treatment
Methods

Children with suspected epiglottis should undergo emergency endotracheal intubation. Most authorities agree that attempts to confirm the diagnosis ahead of time by laryngoscopy or x-ray examination are ill advised, as is observation alone when evidence of airway obstruction is seen. When epiglottitis is suspected in adults, however, obtaining a lateral radiograph of the neck or performing direct or indirect laryngoscopy is appropriate. All patients should be treated with ceftriaxone or cefotaxime as initial therapy.

Expected Response

Most patients improve within 12 to 48 hours.

When to Refer

All patients with acute epiglottitis should be hospitalized.

▶ KEY POINTS

ACUTE EPIGLOTTITIS (SUPRAGLOTTITIS)
- Acute epiglottitis is a life-threatening cellulitis of the epiglottis and adjacent tissues, usually caused by *H. influenzae* type b.
- At onset children commonly have fever, dysphonia, dysphagia, and difficulty breathing. Characteristically the child leans forward and drools.
- When there is strong evidence that a child has acute epiglottitis, the airway should be secured with an endotracheal tube as soon as possible.
- Adults with acute epiglottitis have a sore throat and odynophagia. In adults, in contrast to children, an attempt should usually be made to confirm the diagnosis by visualization of the epiglottis or obtaining a lateral radiograph of the neck.

SUGGESTED READING

Andreassen UK, Baer S, Nielsen TG, et al. Acute epiglottitis—25 years experience with nasotracheal intubation, current management policy, and future trends. J Laryngol Otol 1992; 106: 1072-1075.

Damm M, Eckel HE, Jungehulsing M, et al. Management of acute inflammatory childhood stridor. Otolaryngol Head Neck Surg 1999; 121: 633-638.

Franz TD, Rasgon BM, Quesenberry CP. Jr. Acute epiglottitis in adults: analysis of 129 cases. JAMA 1994; 272: 1358-1360.

Freeman L, Wolford R. Acute epiglottitis caused by methicillin-resistant *Staphylococcus aureus* in adults. Clin Infect Dis 1998; 26: 1240-1241.

Musharrafieh UM, Araj GF, Fuleihan NS. Viral supraglottitis in an adult: a case presentation and literature update. J Infect 1999; 39: 157-160.

Rothrock SG, Pignatiello GA, Howard RM. Radiologic diagnosis of epiglottitis: objective criteria for all ages. Ann Emerg Med 1990; 19: 978-982.

Schamp S, Pokieser P, Danzer M, et al. Radiological findings in acute adult epiglottitis. Eur Radiol 1999; 9: 1629-1631.

Wagle A, Jones RM. Acute epiglottitis despite vaccination with *Haemophilus influenzae* type b vaccine. Paediatr Anaesth 1999; 9: 549-550.

Soft Tissue Infections of the Head and Neck

Several distinctive syndromes of life-threatening deep cervical infection are best understood in terms of the complex anatomy of the fascial layers, spaces, and potential spaces of that region (Table 6-8 and Figure 6-14). These syndromes were more common before the antimicrobial era but are still occasionally encountered in primary care.

Presentation and Progression
Cause

Deep infections of the head and neck usually begin when bacteria indigenous to the mouth or oropharynx gain access to deeper tissues and fascial planes by way of dental infection, severe tonsillitis or pharyngitis, or perforation caused by foreign bodies such as fish bones or chicken bones.

Presentation

Ludwig's angina arises from the floor of the mouth, often as a result of infection involving the second or third mandibular molars. Presenting symptoms are fever, difficulty eating and swallowing, and a brawny or "woody" swelling in the submandibular space. Patients complain of difficulty eating and swallowing. The mouth is often held open and the tongue pushed upward to the palate. The basic problem is a rapidly spreading cellulitis that can progress to airway obstruction and asphyxia.

Lateral pharyngeal space infection arises from dental infection, otitis media, mastoiditis, parotitis, tonsillitis, or pharyngitis. Patients with involvement of the anterior compartment have

TABLE 6-8
Deep Infections of the Head and Neck

Syndrome	Anatomy	Usual microorganisms	Physical examination
Submandibular space infection (Ludwig's angina)	From the mucosa of the floor of the mouth superiorly to the muscular and fascial attachments of the hyoid bone inferiorly	Aerobic and anaerobic streptococci; staphylococci; anaerobic gram-negative rods such as *Prevotella melaninogenicus*	Swelling of the tongue; "woody," usually symmetric submandibular swelling
Lateral pharyngeal space infection	An inverted cone bounded superiorly by the sphenoid bone and inferiorly by the hyoid bone and divided into anterior and posterior compartments by the hyoid process; the posterior compartment contains the carotid sheath	Same as above	Swelling and tenderness of the lateral aspect of the neck often present when the anterior compartment is involved
Retropharyngeal space infection	Bounded anteriorly by the pharynx and posteriorly by the prevertebral fascia, this space communicates potentially with the lateral pharyngeal space	Same as above, with anaerobic bacteria being invariably present	Retropharyngeal swelling is sometimes apparent on examination of the oral cavity; extension into the lateral pharyngeal space causing lateral neck swelling
Cervical prevertebral space infection	Bounded anteriorly by the prevertebral fascia and posteriorly by the cervical spine	*Staphylococcus aureus;* other aerobic bacteria	Localized tenderness over the cervical spine; a bulge in the posterior pharyngeal mucosa sometimes apparent
Acute epiglottitis (supraglottitis)	Epiglottis and surrounding supraglottic tissues	*Haemophilus influenzae;* less commonly other microorganisms or physical agents	Edematous, cherry-red epiglottis
Septic thrombophlebitis of the internal jugular vein (Lemierre syndrome)	Internal jugular vein, which lies within the carotid sheath	*Fusobacterium* species, usually *F. necrophorum*	Tenderness at the angle of the jaw and along the sternocleidomastoid muscle

fever, chills, and dysphagia accompanied by severe pain, trismus, and swelling with tenderness just below the angle of the mandible. Patients with involvement of the posterior compartment have sepsis. Involvement of the posterior compartment causes less pain but is more treacherous; extension to the larynx can cause respiratory obstruction, and extension into the carotid sheath can cause erosion of the internal carotid artery and thrombosis of the internal jugular vein.

Retropharyngeal space infection arises as an extension from infection in the lateral pharyngeal space, from infection involving the retropharyngeal lymph nodes, or from perforation of the pharynx by a foreign body. Fever, chills, dysphagia, dyspnea, and neck pain are common presenting complaints. Examination may reveal bulging of the posterior pharyngeal wall, and spread to the lateral pharyngeal space causes swelling, usually localized to one side of the neck. Again, extension into the carotid sheath is possible. Cervical prevertebral space infection, which is less common, usually occurs as a complication of osteomyelitis involving the cervical spine. The associated prevertebral abscess is usually contained by the prevertebral fascia,

and therefore the external neck swelling characteristic of lateral pharyngeal and retropharyngeal space infections does not occur.

Septic thrombophlebitis of the internal jugular vein, known as Lemierre syndrome, arises by extension of any oropharyngeal or odontogenic infection into the carotid sheath. Presenting symptoms are fever, chills, prostration, and tenderness along the sternocleidomastoid muscle. This syndrome is most commonly caused by *Fusobacterium necrophorum,* an anaerobic gram-negative rod capable of producing severe sepsis. The full syndrome is characterized by septic pulmonary emboli and sometimes by metastatic infection in distant organs.

Diagnosis

Soft tissue infections of the head and neck are usually suggested by the history and by localized swelling on physical examination, but at times the presentation can be subtle. Easily overlooked physical findings include localized tenderness over the cervical spine (prevertebral space infection caused by osteomyelitis) and tenderness along the sternocleidomastoid (Lemierre syndrome). Lateral x-ray examination of the cervical

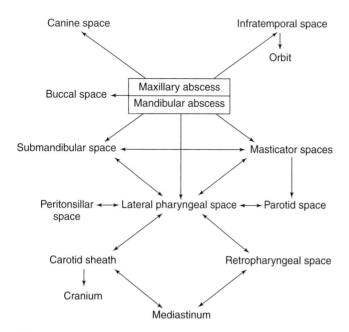

FIG. 6-14 Relationships of the spaces and potential spaces formed by the fascial layers of the head and neck, with typical locations of various abscesses. (From Ingrid K, Blomquist IK, Bayer AS. Life-threatening deep fascial space infections of the head and neck. Infect Dis Clin North Am 1998; 2: 237-264.)

spine shows widening of the retropharyngeal space in patients with retropharyngeal and prevertebral space infections (the two spaces cannot be distinguished on plain radiographs). Newer imaging procedures (CT and MRI) greatly facilitate precise anatomic diagnosis. Blood cultures should be obtained and are usually positive in Lemierre syndrome.

Natural History
Expected Outcome

Complications of soft tissue infections of the head and neck include respiratory obstruction and asphyxiation (especially with Ludwig's angina and infection of the lateral pharyngeal or retropharyngeal spaces), thrombosis of the internal vein, erosion of the internal carotid artery, extension into the mediastinum, and severe sepsis. Untreated, all of these syndromes carry high mortality rates.

Treatment
Methods

Treatment is high-dose parenteral antibiotic therapy appropriate for anaerobic and aerobic bacteria. In most cases surgical drainage is performed.

When to Refer

All patients with deep soft tissue infections of the head and neck should be hospitalized.

 KEY POINTS

SOFT TISSUE INFECTIONS OF THE HEAD AND NECK
- Ludwig's angina is manifested as symmetric, "woody" submandibular swelling that can rapidly progress to respiratory obstruction and asphyxiation.

- Lateral pharyngeal space infection can cause swelling of the lateral aspect of the neck or respiratory obstruction and complications related to carotid sheath extension.
- Retropharyngeal space infection is characterized by fever, chills, dysphagia, and dyspnea accompanied by retropharyngeal swelling and often by extension into the lateral pharyngeal space.
- Osteomyelitis of the cervical spine, which is rare, is manifested as sepsis, pain in the neck, and prevertebral swelling caused by abscess.
- Septic thrombophlebitis of the internal jugular vein (Lemierre syndrome) is characterized by systemic toxicity with septic emboli to the lungs and elsewhere.

SUGGESTED READING
Brook I. The swollen neck: cervical lymphadenitis, parotitis, thyroiditis and infected cysts. Infect Dis Clin North Am 1988; 2: 221-236.

Chow AW. Life-threatening infections of the head and neck. Clin Infect Dis 1992: 14: 991-1002.

Shindo ML, Nalbone VP, Dougherty WR. Necrotizing fasciitis of the face. Laryngoscope 1997; 107: 1071-1079.

Whitesides L, Cotto-Cumba C, Myers RA. Cervical necrotizing fasciitis of odontogenic origin: a case report and review of 12 cases. J Oral Maxillofac Surg 2000; 58: 144-151.

Zeitoun IM, Dhanarajani PJ. Cervical cellulitis and mediastinitis caused by odontogenic infections: report of two cases and review of literature. J Oral Maxillofac Surg 1995; 53: 203-208.

Necrotizing Infections of Skin, Fascia, and Muscle

Necrotizing infections of skin, fascia, and muscle form a diverse group of syndromes that have in common the urgent need to begin antibiotic therapy and to seek surgical consultation. These syndromes should be considered whenever tissue injury to the skin or subcutaneous tissue is accompanied by any combination of blebs, bullae, crepitance, dusky coloration, marked swelling, disproportionate pain, or systemic toxicity. Necrotizing fasciitis caused by group A streptococci has received the greatest attention in recent years as "the flesh-eating bacteria syndrome," but many processes fit into this broad category.

Presentation and Progression
Cause

Diverse etiology and confusing nomenclature characterize the necrotizing infections (Table 6-9). These infections are often but not always preceded by some form of trauma or surgery. The causative bacteria can be placed in three broad categories: mixed aerobic and anaerobic, group A streptococcal, and clostridial.

Mixed aerobic and anaerobic infection accounts for up to 47% of cases. The syndromes include nonclostridial anaerobic cellulitis, synergistic necrotizing cellulitis, cervical necrotizing fasciitis, and type I necrotizing fasciitis. All of these syndromes—and also Fournier's gangrene, which can be viewed as a subset of type I necrotizing fasciitis that involves the perineum, the lower abdominal wall, the gluteal area, and (in males) the scrotum and penis—are more common in patients with diabetes mellitus.

Group A streptococci (*S. pyogenes*) cause type II necrotizing fasciitis, previously known as "streptococcal gangrene." This form of necrotizing fasciitis has become much more common in recent years, probably because of an increased frequency of streptococcal strains (notably M types 1 and 3)

TABLE 6-9
Necrotizing Infections of Skin, Fascia, and Muscle

Category	Examples	Usual organisms	Clinical features
Necrotizing cellulitis	Clostridial cellulitis, nonclostridial anaerobic cellulitis	*Clostridium perfringens*	Cutaneous and subcutaneous gas is prominent. There is usually a history of recent trauma or surgery.
	Meleney's synergistic gangrene	*Staphylococcus aureus* and microaerophilic streptococci	An indolent ulcer slowly expands within the superficial fascia. There is usually a history of recent surgery.
	Synergistic necrotizing cellulitis	Mixed aerobic and anaerobic bacteria	The cellulitis is usually found on the perineum or lower extremities, especially in patients with diabetes mellitus
Necrotizing fasciitis	Necrotizing fasciitis, type I	Mixed aerobic and anaerobic bacteria	A deep-seated subcutaneous infection. The skin may or may not be involved. Occurs most often as a postoperative infection. Patients with diabetes mellitus or peripheral vascular disease are especially predisposed.
	Cervical necrotizing fasciitis	Mixed aerobic and anaerobic bacteria	See "Soft Tissue Infections of the Head and Neck."
	Fournier's gangrene	Mixed aerobic and anaerobic bacteria	A rapidly spreading infection with severe pain, involving the perineum and often the anterior abdominal wall and gluteal area. Involvement of the scrotum and penis is prominent in males. Most patients have diabetes mellitus.
	Necrotizing fasciitis, type II	*Streptococcus pyogenes* (group A streptococcus)	Severe pain and systemic toxicity characterize "streptococcal gangrene" (see text).
Necrotizing infection of muscle	Anaerobic myonecrosis (gas gangrene)	*Clostridium* species, most often *C. perfringens*	Severe pain, sometimes with "heaviness" of a limb, is followed by edema, discoloration of the skin, bullae, and systemic toxicity.
	Pyomyositis	*S. aureus*; rarely *S. pyogenes* or gram-negative rods	Systemic toxicity with muscle pain and swelling is present, often (20% to 50%) preceded by blunt trauma.

that produce pyrogenic exotoxins (see Chapter 1). Many of the cases occur in young, previously healthy persons, who often give a history of blunt or penetrating trauma, childbirth, varicella (chickenpox), or injecting drug use. It has been suggested but not proved that NSAIDs predispose to this infection and mask its severity (Figure 6-15).

Clostridial infection of skin and soft tissues is responsible for two clinical syndromes: clostridial cellulitis (anaerobic cellulitis) and clostridial myonecrosis (true gas gangrene). The presence of clostridial species in wounds often represents simple contamination and is of no clinical consequence. Clostridia multiply and cause disease in tissue environments made anaerobic by ischemia, necrosis, or foreign bodies. *Clostridium perfringens,* which produces at least 12 identified toxins, is the most common cause of necrotizing infection, but other species (e.g., *C. novyi, C. histolyticum,* and *C. septicum*) are also important.

The preceding categories are by no means exhaustive. *V. vulnificus* can cause necrotizing soft tissue infection in wounds exposed to saltwater, and *Aeromonas hydrophila* can do the same in wounds exposed to freshwater (see Chapter 15). Meleney's synergistic gangrene, for example, is a rare but distinctive infection in which *S. aureus* and microaerophilic streptococci combine to cause a relentlessly progressive wound infection. In some studies *Pseudomonas aeruginosa* has been found to play an important role in Fournier's gangrene, a necrotizing infection of the perineum and, in men, of the external genitalia.

Presentation

Clostridial cellulitis, nonclostridial anaerobic cellulitis, and synergistic necrotizing cellulitis are by definition more superficial than infections of muscle and fascia and therefore easier to diagnose. Clostridial cellulitis usually occurs as a

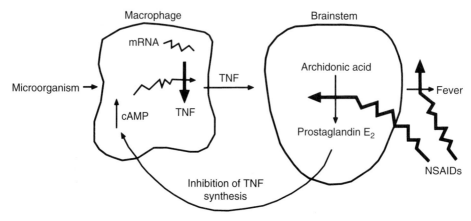

FIG. 6-15 Hypothesis advanced by Dr. Dennis L. Stevens to explain the frequent association between use of nonsteroidal antiinflammatory drugs (NSAIDs) and necrotizing fasciitis. Under normal circumstances, infection incites macrophages to produce tumor necrosis factor (TNF). In the brainstem, increased synthesis of prostaglandin E$_2$ causes "feedback inhibition" of further TNF synthesis by macrophages. NSAIDs have two treacherous effects: (1) they blunt the febrile response and also the skin manifestations of fasciitis, thereby masking the severity of the illness; yet (2) they promote further uncontrolled production of TNF. Although this hypothesis has not been verified by randomized control trials, withholding NSAIDs from patients with musculoskeletal pain seems reasonable when a benign diagnosis is not clear cut. (Modified from Stevens DL. Could noninflammatory drugs [NSAIDs] enhance the progression of bacterial infections to toxic shock syndrome? Clin Infect Dis 1995; 21: 977-980.)

superficial, spreading infection 3 or more days after trauma or surgery. Gas is present in the skin, causing crepitus that is usually striking. Pain and systemic toxicity tend to be relatively mild. Nonclostridial anaerobic cellulitis, usually encountered in patients with diabetes mellitus, is caused by a combination of aerobic and anaerobic components. A foul odor is often present. Synergistic necrotizing cellulitis differs from necrotizing fasciitis type I in that the process is confined to the skin rather than extending into fascia, muscle, and fat. Diabetes mellitus is frequently present, and the infection usually occurs on the perineum or lower extremities.

Necrotizing fasciitis is defined by fascial necrosis with widespread undermining of the skin. It typically begins with nonspecific symptoms such as localized pain and high fever. Localized pain may be the only evidence of inflammation when the patient is first seen. Pain and toxicity disproportionate to the local skin findings on physical examination should suggest the diagnosis. Pain may be minimal or absent in patients with diabetes mellitus who have peripheral neuropathy. Pain may also be relatively minor in patients who are convalescing from trauma, surgery, or childbirth. Erythema usually develops within 24 to 48 hours and often darkens with a reddish purple hue. Other suggestive features are crepitation, local anesthesia, vesicles, and bullae. Patients with necrotizing fasciitis are usually in a toxic state with tachycardia, tachypnea (indicating respiratory compensation for metabolic acidosis), and hypotension.

Clostridial myonecrosis, commonly known as gas gangrene, is a fulminant, necrotizing infection of muscle with marked toxicity caused by toxin-producing clostridial strains, notably *C. perfringens*. Up to 3000 cases occur in the United States each year, some of which are related to trauma or surgery and some of which are spontaneous. The spontaneous form often occurs in patients with cancer and is frequently caused by *C. septicum*. Pain is often the initial complaint. When the infection affects an extremity, patients often note

that the limb feels heavy. The skin becomes dark and often mottled, with edema and multiple bullae. Crepitus, although often present, is usually less marked than in clostridial cellulitis. The patient has marked systemic toxicity with fever, tachycardia, tachypnea, and a sense of impending doom. Hemolytic anemia, caused by the effect of circulating toxin on red blood cells, can be severe.

All of the preceding infections are usually accompanied by leukocytosis with a shift to the left. The creatinine phosphokinase and serum creatinine levels are often elevated in more severe cases.

Diagnosis

The task in primary care is to suspect the presence of necrotizing skin, fascial, or muscle infection rather than to make an accurate diagnosis in one or another of the above categories. Clinical features such as dusky coloration, marked swelling, crepitance, bullae, and disproportionate pain or systemic toxicity should prompt institution of therapy and consultation with a surgeon. In one study leukocytosis (WBC count >15,400/mm^3) and hyponatremia (serum sodium level <135 mmol/L) were useful parameters for distinguishing between necrotizing fasciitis and other soft tissue infections. Surgical exploration is usually necessary to define the level of tissue involvement. Punch biopsy with examination of frozen sections can confirm the diagnosis of deep necrotizing infection, but because of the possibility of sampling error it does not suffice to exclude the diagnosis. An incision down to the fascia is followed by an attempt to pass a probe along the fascial plane. Biopsies reveal necrosis and leukocyte infiltration in the deeper dermis and fascial plane. Imaging studies (plain radiography, CT, MRI) can be helpful, especially if they show soft tissue gas. In fulminant cases, however, definitive surgical débridement should not be postponed.

Natural History
Expected Outcome

Before the antibiotic era, necrotizing fasciitis and clostridial myonecrosis were frequent causes of battlefield infections and were nearly always fatal. With the possible exception of the most superficial of these infections, patients are unlikely to survive without some combination of antibiotic therapy and aggressive surgical débridement or amputation.

Treatment
Methods

Parenteral antibiotic therapy should be instituted and a surgeon consulted. Initial high-dose antibiotic therapy appropriate for most anticipated pathogens would include ampicillin-sulbactam or ticarcillin-clavulanate plus clindamycin. Clindamycin is recommended not only because of its activity against most anaerobic bacteria but also because, as a potent inhibitor of protein synthesis, it limits further toxin production.

Expected Response

Reported mortality rates for necrotizing fasciitis range from 9% to 74% (average about 30%). Current mortality for clostridial myonecrosis is about 20%, but amputation is frequently required. Mortality for patients with necrotizing fasciitis of the male genitalia (Fournier's gangrene) is also about 20%.

When to Refer

Patients with suspected necrotizing infection of the skin, fascia, or muscle should be admitted to the hospital for antibiotic therapy and urgent surgical consultation.

 KEY POINTS

NECROTIZING INFECTIONS OF SKIN, FASCIA, AND MUSCLE

⊃ Necrotizing infections of the skin, fascia, and muscle are a diverse group of conditions that have in common the need for prompt antimicrobial therapy and surgical consultation.

⊃ Suggestive clinical features include blebs, bullae, crepitance, dusky coloration, marked swelling (with edema out of proportion to erythema), disproportionate pain, or systemic toxicity.

⊃ Imaging studies (e.g., MRI) help in the diagnosis, but surgical exploration is usually necessary to define the type of infection.

⊃ Removal of all involved tissue by wide débridement or amputation is often necessary to prevent death or major disability.

⊃ Appropriate initial antibiotic therapy should give broad coverage of aerobic and anaerobic bacteria.

⊃ Patients with diabetes mellitus are especially predisposed to aggressive soft tissue infections caused by a mixture of aerobic and anaerobic bacteria.

⊃ NSAIDs possibly predispose patients to necrotizing fasciitis and toxic shock syndrome caused by group A streptococci.

SUGGESTED READING

Dahm P, Roland FH, Vaslef SN, et al. Outcome analysis in patients with primary necrotizing fasciitis of the male genitalia. Urology 2000; 56: 31-35.

Elliott D, Kufera JA, Myers RA. The microbiology of necrotizing soft tissue infections. Am J Surg 2000; 179: 361-366.

File TM Jr, Tan JS, DiPersio JR. Group A streptococcal necrotizing fasciitis: diagnosing and treating the "flesh-eating bacteria syndrome." Cleve Clin J Med 199; 65: 241-249.

Fontes RA Jr, Ogilvie CM, Miclau T. Necrotizing soft-tissue infections. J Am Acad Orthop Surg 2000; 8: 151-158.

Leitch HA, Palepu A, Fernandes CM. Necrotizing fasciitis secondary to group A streptococcus: morbidity and mortality still high. Can Fam Physician 2000; 46: 1460-1466.

Lewis RT. Soft tissue infections. World J Surg 1998; 22: 146-151.

Ma LD, Frassica FJ, Bluemke DA, et al. CT and MRI evaluation of musculoskeletal infection. Crit Rev Diagn Imaging 1997; 38: 535-568.

Stevens DL. Streptococcal toxic shock syndrome associated with necrotizing fasciitis. Annu Rev Med 2000; 51: 271-288.

Wall DB, Klein SR, Black S, et al. A simple model to help distinguish necrotizing fasciitis from nonnecrotizing soft tissue infection. J Am Coll Surg 2000; 191: 227-231.

Zerr DM, Alexander ER, Duchin JS, et al. A case-control study of necrotizing fasciitis during primary varicella. Pediatrics 1999; 103: 783-790.

Falciparum Malaria

Malaria (see also Chapters 23 and 24) is an important infectious disease worldwide but an uncommon disease in the United States, where nearly all cases are imported. Almost all deaths from the disease are caused by *Plasmodium falciparum*. At its onset falciparum malaria is an undifferentiated flulike illness. Patients have usually traveled abroad (most often to Africa) within the previous 2 months. Severe malaria is defined as falciparum malaria with complications such as CNS involvement (altered consciousness, seizures), renal involvement (acute renal failure), respiratory distress, hypotension, hypoglycemia, generalized bleeding, or jaundice. Severe malaria is uniformly fatal without treatment. The mortality with appropriate treatment remains about 20%. When falciparum malaria has been diagnosed, the Centers for Disease Control and Prevention (CDC) can be contacted for assistance with management; the telephone number is 770-488-7788 or 404-639-2888. Intravenously administered quinidine, which requires cardiac monitoring, is the drug of choice for most patients in the United States.

Tick Paralysis

Tick paralysis is an ascending flaccid paralysis usually affecting young girls and curable by removal of the tick, which is often found hiding in the hair.

Presentation and Progression
Cause

Tick paralysis is caused by neurotoxins secreted in the saliva of female ticks during attachment and feeding. About 40 species of ticks have been associated with the disease. In the northwestern United States most cases have been caused by *Dermacentor andersoni* (the Rocky Mountain wood tick); in the southeastern United States most cases have been caused by *D. variabilis* (the American dog tick). Most reported cases have occurred in young children, typically girls. Adults are thought to be affected less often because their larger body mass dilutes the impact of the neurotoxin. A history of living, hiking, or camping in a wooded rural area is nearly always obtained.

Presentation

The initial symptoms are nonspecific and include irritability, fatigue, and localized pain or paresthesias. Within 24 hours flaccid paralysis ascends to the upper extremities. This is followed by bulbar paralysis with such symptoms as dysphagia, dysarthria, and cranial nerve paralyses. Sensory function is spared. If unrecognized, the disease progresses to paralysis of the respiratory muscles, leading to death. Patients are afebrile, and studies of the peripheral blood, blood chemistry, or CSF show no abnormalities.

Diagnosis

Diagnosis is made by recognition of the tick and its removal, which usually results in prompt recovery. The tick is most commonly found hiding in the hair; the hairline on the back of the neck of a young girl is the classic location. When the diagnosis is suspected, the entire body should be examined for ticks.

Differential diagnosis includes Guillain-Barré syndrome, acute polyneuropathy caused by porphyria, poliomyelitis, acute necrotic myelopathy, botulism, myasthenia gravis, periodic paralysis, diphtheria, insecticide poisoning, porphyria, spinal cord lesions, solvent paralysis, cerebellar ataxia, and hysteria.

Natural History
Expected Outcome

The reported mortality rate is 10% to 12%.

Treatment
Methods

The tick is grasped near its point of attachment with a forceps or tweezers. Care should be taken to apply even pressure and to remove the tick with a steady pull in order to avoid separating its body from its mouth parts. Hands should be washed promptly with soap and water. If the tick is to be removed by hand, gloves should be worn.

Expected Response

Most patients make a full recovery. Recognition of tick paralysis by practicing physicians now makes death a rarity.

When to Refer

Referral is unnecessary provided the disease is recognized before respiratory paralysis ensues.

 KEY POINTS

TICK PARALYSIS
- Tick paralysis should be suspected in any patient with ascending flaccid paralysis of unknown cause.
- Most cases occur in young girls, with the tick found most often in the scalp or hairline.
- Removal of the tick usually enables a full recovery from an otherwise fatal illness.

SUGGESTED READING

Dworkin MS, Shoemaker PC, Anderson DE Jr. Tick paralysis: 33 human cases in Washington State, 1946-1996. Clin Infect Dis 1999; 29: 1435-1439.

Felz MW, Smith CD, Swift TR. A six-year-old girl with tick paralysis. N Engl J Med 2000; 342: 90-94.

Tetanus

Tetanus annually affects more than 100 persons in the United States and is a significant problem in developing nations. The disease has four forms, as follows: generalized tetanus, which causes trismus or "lockjaw"; localized tetanus, which causes rigidity of muscles at or near the site of the causative organism (*Clostridium tetani*); cephalic tetanus, which affects the muscles innervated by the cranial nerves; and neonatal tetanus, which originates in the umbilical stump of infants whose mothers are inadequately immunized. Most cases in the United States now occur in older persons, especially women.

Presentation and Progression
Cause

All of the manifestations of tetanus are attributed to a toxin, tetanospasmin, produced by *C. tetani* after its introduction into a wound. *C. tetani* is a gram-positive, tennis racket–shaped anaerobic bacillus capable of surviving indefinitely in the environment in its spore form. Injuries leading to tetanus are often trivial and indeed are inapparent or not remembered by the patient in about one fourth of cases. The precise mechanism by which tetanospasmin disrupts the nervous system remains unknown, but clearly it blocks neurotransmitter release, mainly from inhibitory neurons. Removal of the inhibitory influence on excitatory neurons causes the rigidity and spasms that define the disease. Tetanospasm also has a major effect on the autonomic nervous system, causing a hypersympathetic state explained in part by loss of the normal inhibition to catecholamine release by the adrenal glands.

Presentation

Generalized tetanus most often begins with rigidity of the masseter muscles, which causes "lockjaw" with trismus and risus sardonicus (a sinister-looking, unintentional smile). This is followed by generalized spasms with opisthotonos (arching of the back, flexing of the arms, and extension of the legs). Spasms can cause death by airway obstruction or spasm of the diaphragm. Localized tetanus affecting muscles other than those supplied by the cranial nerves (cephalic tetanus) is usually a milder form of the disease but can progress to generalized tetanus. Neonatal tetanus usually begins with weakness and failure to thrive, followed by rigidity and spasms.

Diagnosis

Tetanus is a clinical diagnosis. Most but not all patients lack protective titers of antitetanus antibodies, but laboratory tests neither confirm nor exclude the diagnosis of tetanus. The most frequent diagnosis to exclude is dystonic reaction to neuroleptic drugs (such as phenothiazines) or other central dopamine antagonists. Facial spasms and expressions in patients with dystonic reactions often resemble tetanus. Patients with dystonic reactions tend to turn the head laterally during spasms (which is rare in patients with tetanus) and often respond rapidly to therapy with diphenhydramine (Benadryl) or benztropine. Strychnine poisoning can be confused with tetanus, and therefore blood and urine samples should be obtained for assays for strychnine. Dental infections can cause trismus but not the other manifestations of tetanus.

Natural History
Expected Outcome

The mortality from tetanus currently ranges from 6% in cases of mild tetanus to greater than 90% in neonatal tetanus. In severe generalized tetanus, mortality remains about 30% to 60% even with specialized care.

Treatment
Methods

The mainstays of therapy are passive immunization with human tetanus immune globulin, administration of benzodiazepines for symptomatic relief of spasms, and attempted control of the hyperadrenergic state with drugs that block both α- and β-adrenergic function. The role of antimicrobial therapy in tetanus is unclear. Waiting for the results of tests for strychnine should not delay therapy, since the initial treatments for tetanus and strychnine poisoning are similar.

Expected Response

Effective treatment shortens the duration of the disease and lowers the mortality rate.

When to Refer

Patients with suspected tetanus should be hospitalized.

 KEY POINTS

TETANUS

➲ In the United States, tetanus, a preventable disease, now affects mainly older persons and especially older women.
➲ The portal of entry is often trivial and overlooked.
➲ Dystonic reactions to neuroleptic drugs and other central dopamine antagonists can resemble tetanus; however, patients with dystonic reactions tend to show lateral neck turning and to respond to diphenhydramine or benztropine.
➲ Strychnine poisoning resembles tetanus, and therefore patients with suspected tetanus should have blood and urine samples tested for strychnine.
➲ Patients with suspected tetanus should be hospitalized. Mortality remains high.

SUGGESTED READING

Boyles CS, Mills MH, Trupiano P. Tetanus: critical implications for nursing. Crit Care Nurse 1998; 18: 44-49.

Ernst ME, Klepser ME, Fouts M, et al. Tetanus: pathophysiology and management. Ann Pharmacother 1997; 31: 1507-1513.

Farrar JJ, Yen LM, Cook T, et al. Tetanus. J Neurol Neurosurg Psychiatry 2000; 69: 292-301.

Tobias JD. Anesthetic implications of tetanus. South Med J 1998; 91: 384-387.

Botulism

Botulism, caused by an extremely potent neurotoxin produced by *Clostridium botulinum,* affects about 110 persons in the United States each year *but could occur more widely as a result of bioterrorism.* Four forms of the disease are currently recognized: infant botulism, which accounts for about 72% of recent cases; foodborne botulism (25% of cases); wound botulism (3% of cases); and adult infectious botulism (rare). The hallmark of botulism consists of cranial nerve palsies and symmetric descending weakness. Early suspicion of the disease is mandatory to prevent death from respiratory paralysis.

Presentation and Progression
Cause

C. botulinum, widely distributed in nature, is a gram-positive, spore-forming, strictly anaerobic bacillus. The spores, although heat resistant, are destroyed by a temperature of 248° F (120° C) sustained for 5 minutes. The organism is capable of causing localized infections, including abscesses, but disease manifestations are nearly always caused by its neurotoxin. Eight types of botulinum toxin based on antigenic differences are currently recognized. Types A and B commonly cause foodborne botulism and wound botulism, types A, B, and F commonly cause infant botulism, and type E is often associated with botulism attributed to fish products. Once in the body, botulinum toxin spreads from the bloodstream to presynaptic nerve terminals, where it irreversibly blocks the release of acetylcholine.

Presentation

All forms of botulism feature bilateral cranial nerve palsies and descending paralysis, but the clinical features vary according to the mode of acquisition (i.e., the form of botulism) and to a lesser extent according to the type of toxin.

Infant botulism, caused by multiplication of *C. botulinum* in the neonatal gastrointestinal tract, often begins with failure to thrive, irritability, weak cry, drooling, and hypotonia. Dry mucous membranes, fecal and urinary retention, and a labile blood pressure are often present early in the course of the disease and reflect involvement of the autonomic nervous system. Foodborne botulism, caused by ingestion of preformed toxin, similarly begins with nonspecific symptoms such as dry mouth, sore throat, nausea, vomiting, diarrhea, and abdominal pain. The symptoms typically develop 12 to 36 hours (range several hours to 1 week) after ingestion of inadequately cooked food. Wound botulism, caused by wound contamination with *C. botulinum,* usually lacks prodromal symptoms. Adult infectious botulism is similar to infant botulism in its cause and presentation but is rare, since the normal flora of the adult gastrointestinal tract resists colonization by *C. botulinum.*

Diagnosis

Botulism should be suspected in any patient with symmetric peripheral nerve palsies and descending paralysis. Suggestive exposure histories include the ingestion of raw honey (in cases of infant botulism) or home-canned vegetables and the use of injected drugs, especially "black tar" heroin (wound botulism). Clinical features that are variably present and support the diagnosis are blurred vision, diplopia, dilated pupils, dry mouth with furrowed tongue, dysphagia, and weakness of the upper and lower extremities. Although the toxin enters the CNS, most patients are mentally alert and responsive, at least when first seen. Fever is a feature of the disease only in wound botulism. In contrast to tetanus, sympathetic hyperreactivity does not occur and therefore the heart rate is normal or even slow and the blood pressure remains normal.

The differential diagnosis of botulism includes tick paralysis (see earlier discussion), myasthenia gravis and the Lambert-Eaton syndrome (both of which usually evolve more slowly and lack autonomic symptoms and signs), the Miller Fisher variant of acute inflammatory polyneuropathy (which, unlike classic Guillain-Barré syndrome, often begins with cranial nerve palsies; however, there is prominent ataxia that does not occur in botulism), magnesium intoxication, organophosphate poisoning, brainstem infarction, and diphtheria. Sepsis, meningitis, and encephalitis should be considered, especially in the differential diagnosis of infant botulism. When botulism is suspected, the patient should be admitted to the hospital and health authorities should be contacted. Serum should be obtained for assays for botulinum toxin. Stool samples and any implicated food should be obtained for toxin assays and anaerobic culture.

Natural History
Expected Outcome

The mortality from botulism was greater than 60% before the advent of modern methods of critical care.

Treatment
Methods

Aggressive critical care with mechanical ventilation now enables patients with botulism to survive. Recovery, brought about by the sprouting of new presynaptic nerve terminals, may require several months. Equine serum trivalent botulism antitoxin is available from the CDC.

Expected Response

Because botulism is rare, diagnosis of a sporadic case is often delayed. Data suggest that the mortality rate is 25% for the first case caused by an outbreak but only about 4% for subsequent cases. Mortality is higher in older persons. Survivors often have psychological residua.

When to Refer

All patients in whom botulism is strongly suspected should be hospitalized.

 KEY POINTS

BOTULISM

- Symmetric cranial nerve palsies and descending motor paralysis are common to all forms of botulism.
- Other suggestive features of botulism are blurred vision, diplopia, dilated pupils, dry mouth, mental alertness, normal or slow heart rate with normal blood pressure, and lack of sensory defects other than blurred vision.
- Conditions that can mimic botulism include stroke, Guillain-Barré syndrome, myasthenia gravis, diphtheria, and organophosphate poisoning.
- Infant botulism, now the most common form of the disease in the United States, often begins with weakness, including weak cry, feeding problems, irritability, and hypotonia.
- Foodborne botulism usually causes symptoms within 36 hours of the ingestion of preformed toxin.

- Fever can be present in wound botulism but is absent in the other forms of the disease.
- When botulism is suspected, patients should be hospitalized because of the danger of respiratory obstruction or respiratory arrest.
- For advice about botulism, the CDC can be contacted at 404-639-2206 (Monday through Friday, 8 AM to 4:30 PM) or 404-639-2888 (all other times).

SUGGESTED READING

Cherington M. Clinical spectrum of botulism. Muscle Nerve 1998; 21: 701-710.

Shapiro RL, Hatheway C, Swerdlow DL. Botulism in the United States: a clinical and epidemiologic review. Ann Intern Med 1998; 129: 221-228.

Plague

Plague remains endemic in areas of the American Southwest, as well as in other countries. It should be suspected whenever a patient with unexplained fever and toxicity gives a history of outdoors activities in any of the Four Corners states (Arizona, Colorado, New Mexico, and Utah) or southern California. Plague could also result from bioterrorism. Prompt initiation of antibiotic therapy dramatically lowers the mortality.

Presentation and Progression
Cause

Yersinia pestis, the causative bacillus, resides among rodents and is transmitted from rodent to rodent or from rodent to a human by various fleas. Although rats continue to be the most important reservoirs in most countries where plague remains endemic, the major reservoirs in the United States are ground squirrels, rock squirrels, and prairie dogs. Humans usually acquire the disease when bitten by fleas that have previously fed on infected rodents. The disease can also be acquired by exposure (direct contact or inhalation) to infected animal tissues or fluids or by contact with a person with the pneumonic form of the disease. In addition, cases in the United States have now been traced to exposure to domestic cats with pneumonia or submandibular abscesses.

Presentation

In the United States a majority of cases (about 60%) occur in persons under 20 years of age. Bubonic plague, the most common form of the disease, usually begins with sudden onset of fever, chills, and headache followed within 24 hours by intense localized pain that corresponds to an infected lymph node (bubo). The femoral and inguinal nodes are most often affected, but involvement of the axillary and cervical nodes is also common. Symptoms rapidly progress toward prostration, seizures, hypotension, and shock. High-grade bacteremia (i.e., large numbers of bacilli in the blood) is present in advanced cases, but the term "septicemic plague" is usually reserved for cases of plague without an obvious bubo. Pneumonic plague is usually caused by hematogenous seeding of the lungs from a bubo but occasionally occurs as a result of inhalation. Symptoms include cough, chest pain, and hemoptysis; the radiographic pattern varies from patchy bronchopneumonia to dense consolidation. Plague can manifest itself as meningitis, pharyngitis, and gastroenteritis.

Diagnosis

Accurate diagnosis is made by obtaining a smear and culture from an aspirate of a bubo. The technique for aspiration involves injecting a small amount (about 1 mL) of sterile saline without preservative into the involved node by use of a 10-mL syringe and a 19- or 20-gauge needle and then aspirating back until the saline in the syringe becomes blood tinged (see Chapter 15). *Y. pestis* can be isolated from blood cultures in many cases of bubonic plague and in virtually all cases of septicemic plague and can be isolated from sputum in cases of pneumonic plague. A retrospective diagnosis of plague can be made serologically by use of paired serum samples obtained during the acute and convalescent phases.

Natural History
Expected Outcome

The mortality for plague without treatment is estimated to be greater than 50%.

Treatment
Methods

Streptomycin is the drug of choice; the dose is 30 mg/kg of body weight per day in two divided doses. In recent years streptomycin has sometimes been difficult to obtain; gentamicin and tobramycin are also probably effective (based on in vitro susceptibility tests and their similarities to streptomycin) but have not been rigorously studied.

Expected Response

Streptomycin has lowered the mortality for plague to less than 5%. Mortality tends to be much higher in patients with septicemic plague because of delays in diagnosis. Unless treatment is begun within 24 hours of the onset of symptoms, plague pneumonia remains fatal in nearly 100% of cases.

When to Refer

Patients with plague should probably be hospitalized.

 KEY POINTS

PLAGUE
- ⊃ Plague should be suspected as a cause of unexplained fever with systemic toxicity in anyone with outdoors exposure in the southwestern United States during the spring, summer, and fall.
- ⊃ A majority of patients are young (below the age of 20), but persons of any age can be affected.
- ⊃ Bubonic plague, the most common form of the disease, begins with fever and headache, soon followed by intense pain over infected lymph nodes.
- ⊃ The septicemic and pneumonic forms of the disease carry high mortality unless empiric therapy is promptly initiated.
- ⊃ Streptomycin is the drug of choice.

SUGGESTED READING

Gage KL, Dennis DT, Orloski KA, et al. Cases of cat-associated human plague in the Western US, 1977-1998. Clin Infect Dis 2000; 30: 893-900.

Inglesby TV, Dennis DT, Henderson DA, et al. Working Group on Civilian Biodefense. Plague as a biological weapon: medical and public health management. JAMA 2000; 283: 2281-2290.

Madon MB, Hitchcock JC, Davis RM, et al. An overview of plague in the United States and a report of investigations of two human cases in Kern County, California, 1995. J Vector Ecol 1997; 22: 77-82.

Parmenter RR, Yadav EP, Parmenter CA, et al. Incidence of plague associated with increased winter-spring precipitation in New Mexico. Am J Trop Med Hyg 1999; 61: 814-821.

Anthrax

Previously rare in the United States, anthrax assumed enormous importance for primary care clinicians in the wake of the terrorist attacks of September 2001. The inhalational form of the disease is rapidly fatal.

Presentation and Progression
Cause

Bacillus anthracis is a gram-positive, spore-forming bacillus that primarily infects herbivorous animals. The organism produces a toxin consisting of three proteins, the most harmful of which is known as lethal factor. Humans become infected by exposure to infected animals or their products or as a result of deliberate dissemination of the spores. Human-to-human transmission does not seem to occur.

Presentation

The three major forms of anthrax are cutaneous, gastrointestinal, and inhalational. Cutaneous anthrax ("malignant pustule"), which accounts for about 95% of naturally occurring cases, begins as a pruritic papule that ulcerates, becomes surrounded by vesicles, and evolves into a painless, depressed black eschar. Lymphangitis and lymphadenopathy are sometimes present.

Gastrointestinal anthrax usually follows the ingestion of undercooked meat and is manifested as gastroenteritis. This form has not been recognized in the United States.

Inhalational anthrax develops after the deposition of aerosolized spores into the lungs, where they are taken up by macrophages and transported to hilar and mediastinal lymph nodes. Underlying lung disease, alcoholism, and previous irradiation therapy appear to be risk factors. The disease is usually biphasic. The initial phase, lasting 1 to 4 days, begins insidiously with variable symptoms such as fever, chills, malaise, weakness, dyspnea, nonproductive cough, nausea and vomiting, abdominal pain, and chest pain or precordial discomfort. Some patients recover briefly before progressing to the second phase, which is characterized by rapid onset of deterioration with acute dyspnea, fever, diaphoresis, and in many cases meningismus and septic shock.

Diagnosis

Cutaneous anthrax should be considered in the differential diagnosis of a cutaneous ulcer, especially on an exposed area such as the arm, hand, face, or neck. The black eschar is highly characteristic. Ecthyma gangrenosum (see Chapter 7) has a similar appearance but usually occurs in patients with serious underlying disease. In rare cases tularemia (see Chapter 8), plague, and staphylococcal disease can be confused with cutaneous anthrax. *B. anthracis* can be identified by Gram stain and culture of material obtained from vesicular fluid with use of a sterile swab.

Inhalational anthrax in its early stages cannot be distinguished from viral upper respiratory infection. However, rhinorrhea (the hallmark of the common cold) is not a feature of anthrax. Nasopharyngeal swab cultures for *B. anthracis* may be useful for surveillance purposes, but their value for excluding clinical disease is unclear. Anthrax should be considered in the differential diagnosis of acute onset of severe respiratory distress in a previously healthy person. Chest x-ray examination characteristically shows lobulated mediastinal widening caused by massive lymphadenopathy. Hemorrhagic mediastinitis occurs in up to one half of patients and is characterized by delirium progressing to coma. Blood cultures are usually positive for *B. anthracis*.

Natural History

Cutaneous anthrax carries a 10% case-fatality rate without treatment. Inhalational anthrax is almost uniformly fatal.

Treatment
Methods

High-dose IV penicillin G (see Chapter 19) is the traditional treatment of choice for anthrax. For anthrax associated with bioterrorism, current CDC guidelines (available at www.cdc.gov) and health departments should be consulted because of the possibility of bioengineered strains that are resistant to multiple antibiotics. At the time of this writing, initial treatment of bioterrorism-associated inhalational anthrax consists of IV ciprofloxacin (400 mg q12h for adults, including pregnant women; 10 to 15 mg/kg q12h for children) or doxycycline (100 mg IV q12h for adults, including pregnant women, and for children >8 years of age and weighing >45 kg; 2.2 mg/kg q12h for younger or smaller children). For cutaneous anthrax, initial oral therapy similarly consists of ciprofloxacin (500 mg q12h for adults; 10 to 15 mg/kg q12h for children) or doxycycline (100 mg IV q12h for adults, including pregnant women, and for children >8 years of age and weighing >45 kg; 2.2 mg/kg q12h for younger or smaller children). Levofloxacin (500 mg q24h) and ofloxacin (400 mg q12h) are probably acceptable alternatives, although fewer data are available. Clindamycin, erythromycin, and amoxicillin may also be useful. *B. anthracis* is characteristically resistant to third-generation cephalosporins and to TMP/SMX.

Expected Response

Cutaneous anthrax nearly always responds to appropriate therapy. The prognosis of advanced inhalational anthrax is poor even with appropriate therapy.

When to Refer

Suspicion of anthrax should prompt notification of health authorities. Hospitalization is indicated for any evidence of systemic toxicity.

 KEY POINTS

ANTHRAX
- The three major forms are cutaneous, gastrointestinal (not reported in the United States), and inhalational.

- Cutaneous anthrax is characterized by a pruritic papule that becomes vesiculopustular and then evolves into a painless, depressed black eschar with edema.
- Inhalational anthrax is usually a biphasic illness. The first phase resembles a viral upper respiratory infection. The second phase is the rapid onset of dyspnea, fever, diaphoresis, cyanosis, and in many cases meningismus with septic shock.
- Lobulated mediastinal widening caused by massive lymphadenopathy is highly characteristic of inhalational anthrax.
- Hospitalization should be considered for all but the mildest cases, and health authorities should be notified.
- Updated information about bioterrorism-associated anthrax can be obtained at www.cdc.gov.

SUGGESTED READING

Inglesby TV, Henderson DA, Bartlett JG, et al. Working Group on Civilian Biodefense. Anthrax as a biological weapon: medical and public health management. JAMA 1999; 281: 1735-1745.

Jernigan JA, Stephens DS, Ashford DA, et al. Bioterrorism-related inhalational anthrax: the first 10 cases reported in the United States. Emerg Infect Dis 2001, 7: 933-944.

Mayer TA, Bersoff-Matcha S, Murphy C, et al. Clinical presentation of inhalational anthrax following bioterrorism exposure: report of 2 surviving patients. JAMA 2001; 286: 2549-2553.

Shafazand S, Doyle R, Ruoss S, et al. Inhalational anthrax: epidemiology, diagnosis, and management. Chest 1999; 116: 1369-1376.

Hantavirus Pulmonary Syndrome

First described in 1993 as a cluster of cases of severe pneumonia acquired in the Four Corners region of the southwestern United States, disease caused by Hantaviruses has now been described in many other parts of the United States. This illness carries a 50% case-fatality rate.

Presentation and Progression
Cause

The major cause of the Hantavirus pulmonary syndrome in the United States is a recently described Hantavirus called the Sin Nombre virus. Related Hantaviruses include the Bayou virus in Texas and Louisiana, the New York virus in New York and Rhode Island, and the Black Creek Canal virus in Florida. Other Hantaviruses cause disease in South America.

Transmission of the disease to humans seems to occur mainly by inhalation of aerosolized excreta of rodents, which provide the key reservoir for Hantaviruses. Rodents implicated to date include the deer mouse (*Peromyscus maniculatus*) in the southwestern United States, the white-footed mouse (*Peromyscus leucopus*) in the northeastern United States, the rice rat (*Oryzomys palustris*) in Louisiana, and the cotton rat (*Sigmodon hispidus*) in Florida. Person-to-person transmission has not been observed in the United States but has not been entirely excluded, since such transmission was strongly suspected in several instances of Hantavirus disease in Argentina.

The disease has an incubation period of about 3 weeks. The virus appears to attack endothelial cells and platelets in a way that causes widespread capillary leak.

Presentation

The first symptoms are usually fever, malaise, and myalgia, sometimes accompanied by headache and gastrointestinal symptoms. This prodrome resembles numerous viral syndromes. Cough is not necessarily present. About 3 to 6 days after the onset of prodromal symptoms, a rapid onset of hypotension with pulmonary edema occurs. Within 48 hours nearly all patients have evidence of pulmonary edema on chest x-ray examination, with rapid progression that includes significant pleural effusions. Laboratory studies show marked leukocytosis with a left shift and hemoconcentration. Thrombocytopenia may be present, and the partial thromboplastin time may be prolonged.

Diagnosis

The key to diagnosis is a high index of suspicion when a patient who has had outdoor exposure seeks treatment for illness characterized by hypotension and pulmonary edema. Vector histories might include exploring poorly ventilated spaces such as caves or seldom-used buildings. Confirmation is usually made by demonstrating Hantavirus-specific IgM antibodies; this test is considered diagnostic. Acute and convalescent serologic tests show a four-fold rise in IgG titers to Hantaviruses.

Natural History
Expected Outcome

The case-fatality rate is about 50%.

Treatment
Methods

No treatment has been proved effective. A trial of ribavirin therapy is under way.

Expected Response

Treatment has not yet been shown to be effective. The literature should be watched.

When to Refer

Suspected Hantavirus pulmonary infection demands immediate hospitalization, aggressive supportive care, and notification of health authorities.

 KEY POINTS

HANTAVIRUS PULMONARY SYNDROME

↪ The Hantavirus pulmonary syndrome was initially described in the Four Corners area of the American Southwest but has now been reported from a majority of states and also from Canada and Latin America.

↪ The prodrome lasts 3 to 6 days and resembles a nonspecific viral illness with fever, malaise, and myalgias.

↪ The illness usually is manifested as hypotension and pulmonary edema.

↪ Hantavirus pulmonary syndrome resembles many of the atypical pneumonias in its presentation.

↪ Although the diagnosis can be confirmed by demonstrating IgM antibodies to Hantaviruses, the key to diagnosis is a high index of suspicion for anyone likely to have been exposed to aerosolized rodent excreta.

↪ The case-fatality rate is 50%, making immediate hospitalization mandatory.

↪ Updated information can be obtained from the CDC website (www.cdc.gov).

SUGGESTED READING

Crowley MR, Katz RW, Kessler R, et al. Successful treatment of adults with severe Hantavirus pulmonary syndrome with extracorporeal membrane oxygenation. Crit Care Med 1998; 26: 409-414.

Duchin JS, Koster F, Peters CJ, et al. Hantavirus pulmonary syndrome: a clinical description of 17 patients with a newly recognized disease. N Engl J Med 1994; 330: 949-955.

Khan AS, Khabbaz RF, Armstrong LR, et al. Hantavirus pulmonary syndrome: the first 100 US cases. J Infect Dis 1996; 173: 1297-1303.

Vitek CR, Breiman RF, Ksiazek TG, et al. Evidence against person-to-person transmission of Hantavirus to health care workers. Clin Infect Dis 1996; 22: 824-826.

Bioterrorism

Growing concern about bioterrorism (the use of biologic agents against civilian populations) prompted the U.S. government to develop a comprehensive, coordinated defense strategy, which proved well founded when anthrax spores were disseminated by mail after the terrorist attacks of September 11, 2001. Primary care clinicians are crucial to the recognition of bioterrorism, since—in contrast to terrorism with chemical or physical agents—affected persons are usually widely dispersed before disease manifestations appear.

Presentation and Progression
Cause

Potential agents of bioterrorism have been grouped into three categories:

■ Category A: organisms that are easily disseminated from a central source or transmitted from person to person, cause high mortality, require special action for public health response, and often disrupt society. These include the agents of smallpox, anthrax, plague, tularemia, botulism, and certain viral hemorrhagic fevers (such as Ebola, Marburg, and Argentine hemorrhagic fevers and Lassa fever).

■ Category B: organisms that are moderately easy to disseminate, cause low mortality but considerable morbidity, and pose difficulties in recognition. These include the agents of salmonellosis, shigellosis, cholera, cryptosporidiosis, hemorrhagic colitis (*Escherichia coli* O157:H7), Q fever, brucellosis, glanders, and viral encephalitis.

■ Category C: organisms that could be bioengineered in the future with the potential for high morbidity and mortality and a major impact on public health. These include multidrug-resistant tuberculosis, yellow fever, Hantaviruses, tickborne hemorrhagic fever viruses, tickborne encephalitis virus, and nipah virus.

Diagnosis

Bioterrorism should be suspected whenever clinicians encounter either a large number of cases of severe illness in previously healthy persons or a single case of a rare infectious disease. Other clues are higher morbidity and mortality than would be expected with a common disease or treatment, failure of a common disease to respond to the usual therapy, disease with an unusual geographic or seasonal distribution, outbreaks of unexplained disease among animals that precede or accompany severe illness in humans, and outbreaks associated with common exposures or ventilation systems.

Smallpox is diagnosed on the basis of the characteristic painful, pustular rash. The individual pustules of smallpox resemble those of chickenpox, but the rash of smallpox differs from that of chickenpox in two crucial ways. First, the pustules appear simultaneously (whereas in chickenpox the pustules appear in waves or crops). Second, the pustules are concentrated most heavily on the face and in the pharynx (whereas in chickenpox they usually start on the chest and back). The virus can be identified by electron microscopy, but no diagnostic procedures are readily available.

Inhalational anthrax (discussed previously) is a biphasic illness, with the first phase resembling a viral upper respiratory infection and the second phase consisting of hemorrhagic mediastinitis with shock. Widening of the mediastinum, seen in advanced cases, is highly characteristic of anthrax. Pneumonic plague (discussed previously) manifests itself as fulminant bronchopneumonia. Blood and sputum cultures reveal gram-negative bacilli. Tularemia (see Chapter 8) is characterized by patchy bilateral pneumonia with high fever, relative bradycardia, and elevations of aspartate aminotransferase and alanine aminotransferase levels. Botulism (discussed previously) should be considered in all cases of bilateral, symmetric cranial nerve palsies with descending paralysis. Viral hemorrhagic fevers vary in their presentation, which includes fever, pharyngitis, retrosternal pain, cough, other systemic and localizing symptoms, and proteinuria. Marburg and Ebola viruses often cause encephalitis, diffuse bleeding, and, later, shock. Lassa virus and the agents of South American hemorrhagic fevers (Argentine, Bolivian, and Venezuelan) cause, in fatal cases, a capillary leak syndrome with hypotension, peripheral vasoconstriction, edema, and mucosal hemorrhages.

When to Refer

Suspicion of bioterrorism mandates urgent notification of public health authorities. The diseases associated with bioterrorism nearly always require referral and may require hospitalization.

 KEY POINTS

BIOTERRORISM

- ⊃ Victims of bioterrorism are usually widely dispersed because infectious agents—unlike chemical and physical agents— require an incubation period before causing disease. Primary care clinicians therefore form a crucial line of defense.
- ⊃ Category A agents of potential bioterrorism include the organisms that cause smallpox, anthrax, plague, tularemia, botulism, and certain viral hemorrhagic fevers.
- ⊃ Bioterrorism should be suspected when clinicians encounter a large number of previously healthy persons with severe illnesses or a single person with a rare infectious disease.
- ⊃ Smallpox should be suspected when what appears to be "adult chickenpox" features pustules that evolve simultaneously and are concentrated especially on the face.
- ⊃ Inhalational anthrax should be suspected when a fulminant flulike illness develops in previously healthy persons in a community. Widening of the mediastinum, seen in advanced cases, is highly characteristic, and blood cultures may reveal gram-positive bacilli.
- ⊃ Pneumonic plague should be suspected when fulminant bronchopneumonia develops in previously healthy persons in a community.
- ⊃ Suspicion of bioterrorism mandates urgent notification of public health authorities.

SUGGESTED READING

Franz DR, Jahrling PB, Friedlander AM, et al. Clinical recognition and management of patients exposed to biological warfare agents. JAMA 1997; 278: 399-411.

Henderson DA. The looming threat of bioterrorism. Science 1999; 283: 1279-1282.

Henderson DA, Inglesby TV, Bartlett JG, et al. Working Group on Civilian Biodefense. Smallpox as a biological weapon: medical and public health management. JAMA 1999; 281: 2127-2137.

Inglesby TV, O'Toole T, Henderson DA. Preventing the use of biological weapons: improving response should prevention fail. Clin Infect Dis 2000; 30: 926-929.

Khan AS, Morse S, Lillibridge S. Public-health preparedness for biological terrorism in the USA. Lancet 2000; 356: 1179-1182.

7

Fever with Rash and Other Skin Lesions

SHARON J. LONGSHORE, CHARLES CAMISA

The patient's history often provides important clues. Recent travel, place of permanent residence, recreational activities, sexual practices, type of employment, ill contacts, season of the year, past medical history, immune status, recreational drug use, ingestion of certain foods, and drug exposure are all pertinent aspects of the history. Associated systemic symptoms and time course of the disease help to complete the clinical picture. The physical examination is of paramount importance (Table 7-1). Accurate description of the cutaneous morphology allows categorization and quick reference. This requires a familiarity with basic dermatologic terms and descriptions (Tables 7-2 and 7-3).

Perhaps the most important skill in diagnosing potentially life-threatening diseases associated with fever and rash is recognizing that a patient is critically ill. Supportive care is essential in all of these diseases. When specific physical findings are lacking, the history will direct empiric therapy until confirmatory testing is complete. The diseases discussed in this chapter are arranged from the most frequently life-threatening to the seldom life-threatening infectious diseases associated with fever and rash. This arrangement mimics the thought process of the astute clinician, who rules out the most dangerous diagnosis when presented with an unknown clinical situation. When this is done, treatment of potentially dangerous infectious diseases is not delayed.

SUGGESTED READING

Aly R, Maibach HI. Atlas of Infections of the Skin. New York: Churchill Livingstone; 1998.

Braverman IM. Skin Signs of Systemic Disease. 3rd ed., Philadelphia: W.B. Saunders Company; 1998.

Sanders CV, Lopez FA. Cutaneous manifestations of infectious diseases: approach to the patient with fever and rash. Trans Am Clin Climat Assoc 2001; 112: 235-252.

Sanders CV, Nesbitt LT, eds. The Skin and Infection: A Color Atlas and Text. Baltimore: Williams & Wilkins, 1995.

Ecthyma Gangrenosum and Pseudomonas Septicemia

Skin lesions in septicemia arise by at least five mechanisms:
- Disseminated intravascular coagulation and coagulopathy—for example, in sepsis caused by gram-negative and gram-positive bacteria
- Invasion of blood vessel walls—for example, in ecthyma gangrenosum, Rocky Mountain spotted fever, meningococcemia, disseminated candidiasis, *Aspergillus* infection, and mucormycosis

Most previously healthy patients with an acute fever and rash have benign viral exanthems, but how does the clinician adequately rule out potentially dangerous diseases? An awareness of the clinical presentation of life-threatening infections associated with fever and rash expedites treatment and reduces morbidity and mortality.

TABLE 7-1
Clues to Diagnosis: Unique Cutaneous Manifestations on Physical Examination

Unique cutaneous manifestation	Associated diagnoses
Painless, indurated ulcer with a central necrotic black eschar	Ecthyma gangrenosum, *Pseudomonas* septicemia
Palpable purpura and petechiae	Meningococcemia, purpura fulminans
Large, hemorrhagic bullae	*Vibrio vulnificus* infection
Nikolsky's sign*	Staphylococcal scalded skin syndrome, toxic epidermal necrolysis
Osler's nodes, Janeway lesions, splinter hemorrhages	Infective endocarditis
Blanching, erythematous macules on the wrists and ankles	Rocky Mountain spotted fever
Erythema chronicum migrans	Lyme disease
Erythema marginatum	Acute rheumatic fever
Condylomata lata	Secondary syphilis
Grouped vesicles on an erythematous base	Herpes zoster

*Nikolsky's sign: rupture and separation of the upper part of the dermis induced by light stroking of the skin.

TABLE 7-2
Definitions of Dermatologic Terms Used to Describe Primary Lesions

Term	Definition
Macule	A circumscribed, flat area of perceptible color change ≤1 cm in size
Papule	A circumscribed, solid, elevation above the skin surface, ≤1 cm in size
Plaque	A plateaulike elevation above the skin surface, >1 cm in size
Nodule	A palpable, rounded lesion with depth
Pustule	A rounded, superficial cavity of the skin with a purulent exudate
Crust	A lesion caused by drying fluid (e.g., from ruptured vesicles)
Vesicle	A circumscribed, elevated, superficial fluid-filled cavity, ≤1 cm in size
Bulla*	An elevated, superficial, fluid-filled cavity, >1 cm in size
Petechia*	A nonblanching lesion caused by a small hemorrhage into the skin
Ecchymosis	An extensive, deep hemorrhage into the skin

*In everyday speech the plural forms bullae and petechiae are used more commonly. "Bullous lesion" and "petechial lesion" are used to describe individual lesions. The distinction between a vesicle and a small bulla is arbitrary; some authorities use 0.5 cm rather than 1 cm as the cut-off.

- Immune complex formation with vasculitis—for example, endocarditis, disseminated gonococcal disease, typhoid fever, and meningococcemia (later phases)
- Embolism—for example, endocarditis and, rarely, mycotic aneurysm

- Toxin formation—for example, toxic shock syndrome, scarlet fever

Ecthyma gangrenosum is especially important to recognize, since it provides an early clue to severe infection caused by *Pseudomonas aeruginosa* and less commonly to infection

TABLE 7-3
Cutaneous Morphology of Diseases Associated with Fever and Rash

Type of lesion	Treatable infectious causes	Infectious causes without specific treatment	Noninfectious causes (with or without fever)
Macules and papules (nonpurpuric)	Primary HIV infection, leptospirosis, disseminated gonococcal infection, Lyme disease, typhoid fever, typhus, *Mycoplasma pneumoniae* infection, acute rheumatic fever, secondary syphilis, ehrlichiosis, early Rocky Mountain spotted fever, early meningococcemia, chronic meningococcemia (rare), trichinosis (rare), toxoplasmosis (rare), leprosy (rare)	Rubeola, rubella, parvovirus B19 infection (fifth disease), enteroviral infection, human herpesvirus 6 infection, adenovirus infection, Epstein-Barr virus infection (mononucleosis)	Erythema multiforme, erythema marginatum, allergy, dermatomyositis, systemic lupus erythematosus, serum sickness
Petechiae, purpuric macules, and papules	Meningococcemia, purpura fulminans, disseminated candidiasis, infective endocarditis, Rocky Mountain spotted fever, babesiosis, epidemic typhus, rat-bite fevers, acute rheumatic fever, tularemia (rare), plague (rare), congenital syphilis (rare), disseminated histoplasmosis (rare), miliary tuberculosis (rare), brucellosis (rare), *Vibrio vulnificus* infection (rare), leptospirosis (rare)	Enteroviral infection, dengue, rubella, hepatitis, Epstein-Barr virus infection	Hypercoagulable states, thrombocytopenia, Henoch-Schönlein purpura, allergy, hypersensitivity vasculitis (palpable purpura), systemic lupus erythematosus, acute rheumatic fever, amyloidosis, hyperglobulinemia, scurvy
Vesicles, bullae, and pustules	Ecthyma gangrenosum (see text), *Vibrio vulnificus* infection, varicella-zoster virus infection (chickenpox, shingles, and disseminated herpes zoster), disseminated gonococcal infection, herpes simplex virus infection, staphylococcal septicemia, rickettsialpox	Parvovirus B19 infection (fifth disease), enteroviral infection	Erythema multiforme bullosum, pemphigus, pemphigoid, porphyria cutanea tarda, allergy, plant dermatitis
Papules and plaques	Blastomycosis, coccidioidomycosis, cryptococcosis, histoplasmosis, Lyme disease		Allergy, psoriasis, eczema, lymphoma, Sézary syndrome, pityriasis rubra
Diffuse erythema with subsequent desquamation	Toxic shock syndrome, staphylococcal scalded skin syndrome, Kawasaki disease (mucocutaneous lymph node syndrome), scarlet fever	Stevens-Johnson syndrome, toxic epidermal necrolysis	Exfoliative dermatitis
Urticaria	*Mycoplasma pneumoniae* infection, Lyme disease	Hepatitis (especially prodrome of hepatitis B), adenoviral infection, enteroviral infection, Epstein-Barr virus infection, HIV infection	Idiopathic, cholinergic urticaria, cold urticaria, allergy, vasculitis, malignancy

Modified in part from Schlossberg D, Shulman JA. Differential Diagnosis of Infectious Diseases. Baltimore: Williams & Wilkins; 1996: 133-161.
HIV, Human immunodeficiency virus.

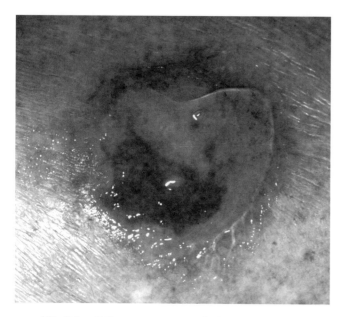

FIG. 7-1   Ecthyma gangrenosum in the ulcerated stage.

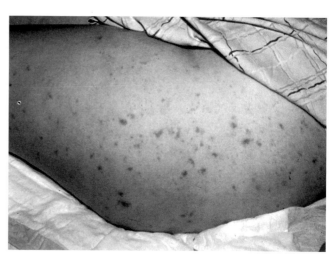

FIG. 7-2   Meningococcemia: petechial papules on the thigh of a child.

by other bacteria and fungi. The characteristic skin lesion of ecthyma gangrenosum, seen in 1% to 6% of patients with *Pseudomonas* septicemia, is usually encountered in severely immunocompromised persons, especially patients undergoing chemotherapy for cancer. However, ecthyma gangrenosum and pseudomonal sepsis occasionally occur in previously healthy infants and children.

The initial skin lesions of ecthyma gangrenosum are erythematous to purpuric macules, hemorrhagic vesicles, bullae, or nodules. They rapidly progress to a painless, indurated ulcer (Figure 7-1) with a central necrotic black eschar and surrounding erythema. The most common sites of distribution are the axillae and anogenital regions. Diagnosis is confirmed by blood and tissue cultures. Histologic examination and culture of punch biopsy specimens obtained from patients with sepsis and skin lesions are often invaluable. Suspicion of ecthyma gangrenosum and pseudomonal septicemia mandates hospitalization. Mortality remains high (30% to 70%) even with aggressive treatment.

 KEY POINTS

ECTHYMA GANGRENOSUM AND PSEUDOMONAS SEPTICEMIA

⊃ Ecthyma gangrenosum is classically associated with *Pseudomonas* septicemia but also occurs in sepsis caused by other microorganisms. Most patients are severely immunocompromised, but ecthyma gangrenosum and pseudomonal sepsis occasionally occur in previously healthy persons, including infants and young children.

⊃ The characteristic skin lesion is an erythematous macule, bulla, or nodule, which rapidly forms an indurated ulcer with a central necrotic black eschar.

⊃ Mortality from ecthyma gangrenosum and *Pseudomonas* septicemia remains high despite treatment.

SUGGESTED READING

Agger WA, Mardan A. *Pseudomonas aeruginosa* infections of intact skin. Clin Infect Dis 1995; 20: 302-308.

Mull CC, Scarfone RJ, Conway D. Ecthyma gangrenosum as a manifestation of *Pseudomonas* sepsis in a previously healthy child. Ann Emerg Med 2000; 36: 383-387.

Sevinsy LD, Viecens C, Ballesteros DO, et al. Ecthyma gangrenosum: a cutaneous manifestation of *Pseudomonas aeruginosa* sepsis. J Acad Derm 1993; 29: 104-106.

Meningococcemia and Purpura Fulminans

As discussed in Chapter 6, meningococcemia is a life-threatening illness caused by the gram-negative diplococcus *Neisseria meningitidis*. The infection is characterized by fever, rash, myalgias, arthralgias, headache, and hypotension. Petechiae are the most common lesions, but macular, maculopapular, urticarial, and hemorrhagic vesicular lesions also occur. The petechiae are initially distributed on the wrists, ankles, and axillae. Later in the course of disease nearly the entire body surface area may be involved, with a predilection for the lower extremities (Figure 7-2). The petechiae may progress to palpable purpura, a finding that strongly suggests meningococcal infection. Purpuric and confluent ecchymotic lesions may occur with acute, fulminant disease.

Purpura fulminans is defined as an acute illness with rapidly progressive disseminated purpura and hypotensive shock, which occurs most commonly in children. It may be seen with meningococcemia or other bacterial infections. Diffuse cutaneous and visceral hemorrhage commonly develops and frequently leads to surgical débridement, amputation, and even death. Symmetric petechiae and purpura of the skin and mucous membranes appear suddenly. Bullae with progression to necrosis may also be present.

SUGGESTED READING

Darmstadt GL. Acute infectious purpura fulminans: pathogenesis and medical management. Pediatr Dermatol 1998; 15: 169-183.

Vibrio Vulnificus Infection

Vibrio vulnificus infection ranges in severity from localized wound infections to septicemia and septic shock. These infections are reported throughout the United States, especially on the Gulf Coast. Expedient diagnosis and treatment are essential to prevent morbidity and mortality, which occur frequently.

Presentation and Progression
Cause

Vibrio vulnificus is an invasive, marine, gram-negative bacillus found in warm seawater. It has been isolated from the Gulf of Mexico, the Pacific and Atlantic oceans, and the waters of Hawaii, Utah, and Massachusetts. The organism is found in oysters, crabs, clams, and mussels. Most cases (>90%) have been associated with ingestion of oysters 1 to 3 days before clinical presentation. Cirrhosis is the major risk factor for *V. vulnificus* septicemia. Other predisposing factors are iron overload states (e.g., hemochromatosis or hemolytic anemia), immunosuppressive drug therapy, human immunodeficiency virus (HIV) disease, chronic renal failure, and malignancy.

Presentation

Symptoms begin abruptly with chills and fever, often followed by hypotension. The typical skin lesions usually appear within 36 hours of the initial symptoms. Most patients give a history of ingesting raw shellfish within the previous week. The characteristic skin findings are large bullae filled with hemorrhagic fluid (Figure 7-3). Other associated skin manifestations are necrotic ulcers, necrotizing fasciitis, vasculitis, pustules, petechiae, purpura, generalized papules or macules, gangrene, urticaria, and an erythema multiforme–like rash. The skin lesions are usually on the extremities, especially the lower extremities. Sepsis develops rapidly, so early recognition is essential.

Localized wound infections may also occur after direct exposure of soft tissue to *V. vulnificus* through new or preexisting wounds after submersion in seawater. Local cellulitis and pain are followed quickly by fever, bullous lesions with vasculitis, and later frank tissue necrosis. Necrotizing fasciitis caused by *V. vulnificus* differs from that caused by *Streptococcus pyogenes* (see Chapter 6) in that it is more likely to occur during the summer months and to be associated with edema and subcutaneous hemorrhage, but is less likely to be associated with superficial necrosis of the skin.

Diagnosis

Vibrio infection must be diagnosed clinically to expedite initiation of therapy. Blood and wound cultures confirm the diagnosis. In septicemia, blood cultures are positive in 97% of patients.

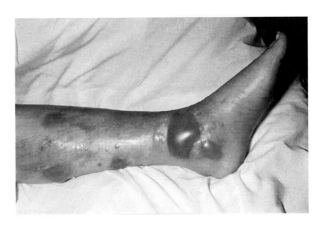

FIG. 7-3 *Vibrio vulnificus* infection: cutaneous hemorrhage in a patient with liver disease who had eaten oysters. (Courtesy of Dr. Charles V. Sanders.)

Natural History
Expected Outcome

The mortality of patients with *V. vulnificus* septicemia is greater than 50% and increases to greater than 90% if septic shock occurs. *V. vulnificus* now accounts for about 90% of deaths caused by seafood in the United States.

Treatment
Methods

Doxycycline 100 mg IV or PO b.i.d. should be initiated immediately. Some clinicians use a third-generation cephalosporin in combination with doxycycline. Ciprofloxacin is an alternative agent. Aminoglycosides, commonly used to treat patients with sepsis, are unreliable against *V. vulnificus*. Supportive care includes fluid replacement, close monitoring, and wound débridement.

Expected Response

Despite early administration of antibiotics, mortality from *V. vulnificus* infections remains high (about 33%). Patient education about the risks of infection from eating raw shellfish is essential, especially for those who are immunocompromised.

When to Refer

Patients with suspected *V. vulnificus* infections should be hospitalized for intravenous and supportive care.

 KEY POINTS

VIBRIO VULNIFICUS INFECTION

- ⊃ *V. vulnificus* septicemia should be expected whenever skin lesions (erythema followed by necrosis) occur within 1 to 3 days of the ingestion of oysters.
- ⊃ Risk factors for severe infection include cirrhosis and other chronic diseases, iron overload states, and immunosuppression.
- ⊃ The characteristic skin findings of *V. vulnificus* septicemia are large bullae filled with hemorrhagic fluid, usually on the lower extremities.

⊃ *V. vulnificus* also causes severe infection, including necrotizing fasciitis, in wounds that have been exposed to saltwater.

⊃ Suspicion of *V. vulnificus* should prompt hospitalization and intravenous administration of antibiotics.

SUGGESTED READING

Fujisawa N, Yamada H, Kohda H, et al. Necrotizing fasciitis caused by *Vibrio vulnificus* differs from that caused by streptococcal infection. J Infect 1998; 36: 313-316.

Kumamoto KS, Vukich DJ. Clinical infections of *Vibrio vulnificus*: a case report and review of the literature. J Emerg Med 1998; 16: 61-66.

Shapiro RL, Altekruse S, Hutwagner L, et al. Vibrio Working Group. The role of Gulf Coast oysters harvested in warmer months in *Vibrio vulnificus* infections in the United States, 1988-1996. J Infect Dis 1998; 178: 752-759.

Strom MS, Paranjpye RN. Epidemiology and pathogenesis of *Vibrio vulnificus*. Microbes Infect 2000; 2: 177-188.

Toxic Shock Syndrome

Toxic shock syndrome is an acute febrile illness associated with a scarlatiniform and later desquamating rash, hypotension, and multiorgan abnormalities. The two most common etiologic agents are *Staphylococcus aureus* and *S. pyogenes*. The disease is characterized by the sudden onset of high fever, vomiting, diarrhea, headache, hypotension, oliguria, and shock. Generalized, scarlatiniform, blanching macules and patches appear early in the illness and fade within a few days. Other skin findings are a papulopustular eruption, petechiae, and bullae. Desquamation starts on the hands and feet about 1 to 2 weeks after the onset of illness. Mucosal involvement is manifested as a strawberry tongue (diffuse erythema of the tongue with prominent papillae) and conjunctival injection. Other features of toxic shock syndrome are covered extensively in Chapter 6.

Staphylococcal Scalded Skin Syndrome

Staphylococcal scalded skin syndrome is a toxin-mediated epidermolytic skin disease primarily affecting newborns and infants. The most common causative agent is *S. aureus*. The initial skin finding is a diffuse, ill-defined erythema with a fine sandpaper appearance. Within a period of hours, the skin becomes tender and the outermost layers of the epidermis begin to peel. Nikolsky's sign, extension of blisters with pressure on the skin, is present. The skin changes are most impressive in perineal and periumbilical locations. Affected patients require aggressive care in an intensive care unit.

Stevens-Johnson Syndrome and Toxic Epidermal Necrolysis

Erythema multiforme minor (EM minor), Stevens-Johnson syndrome (SJS), and toxic epidermal necrolysis (TEN) represent a spectrum of bullous disease. EM minor is the mildest and most common of the three disorders. It does not typically cause systemic disease, and the skin findings usually resolve in 1 to 6 weeks. SJS and TEN may be classified by the extent of involvement of the total body surface area. SJS may be defined as mucosal exfoliation and widespread purpuric macules and epidermal detachment limited to less than 10% of the body surface area. Transitional SJS-TEN and TEN are defined in the same manner except that 10% to 30% and greater than 30% of the body surface area are involved, respectively. This section concentrates on SJS and TEN, since they lead to considerable morbidity and mortality.

Presentation and Progression
Cause

SJS often follows drug exposure or *Mycoplasma* infection. TEN nearly always occurs after drug exposure. Antibiotics implicated as causative agents of SJS and TEN are penicillins, cephalosporins, sulfonamides, fluoroquinolones, vancomycin, rifampin, and ethambutol. Recently erythromycin was implicated as well. The mechanism for the severe reactions is unknown.

Presentation

The skin findings of SJS are preceded by a prodromal illness of fever, myalgias, malaise, pharyngitis, and headache. A

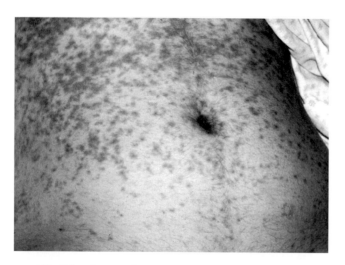

FIG. 7-4 Stevens-Johnson syndrome: morbilliform rash.

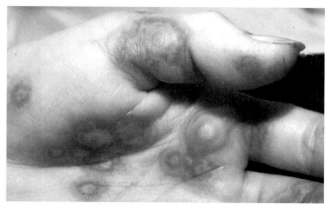

FIG. 7-5 Stevens-Johnson syndrome: target or iris lesions on the palm.

morbilliform rash (Figure 7-4) occurs initially, followed by vesicles and bullae on or near large erythematous macules and plaques. Target lesions may be present (Figure 7-5). Bullae may become hemorrhagic, and erosions are common. Epidermal detachment is limited to less then 10% of the body surface area. Erosions and blisters of mucous membrane surfaces, which occur early in the reaction, involve two or more of the following: oropharynx, including the lips (Figure 7-6); eyes; urethra; and genitalia.

High, spiking fevers accompany the prodromal illness of TEN. Generalized erythema is followed by the appearance of macules with dark centers and large bullae. Widespread epidermal detachment (Figure 7-7) peaks at 2 to 3 days from the onset of illness. Nikolsky's sign, the spread of blisters with lateral pressure, can be elicited on physical examination. Mucosal lesions may be severe. Affected individuals may complain of photophobia, gastrointestinal disturbances, respiratory distress, and painful micturition as a result of generalized erosions.

Diagnosis

Diagnostic criteria for SJS include the following:
- An acute, self-limited illness of less than 6 weeks' duration
- Prodromal symptoms
- Symmetrically distributed target and atypical target lesions
- Progression of some lesions to bullae
- Epidermal detachment
- Severe, extensive mucosal involvement of more than two mucosal surfaces
- Characteristic histopathologic findings

The diagnosis of TEN is based on a similar clinical and histopathologic picture that typically involves a larger body surface area. Helpful laboratory tests are complete blood count with differential, erythrocyte sedimentation rate, urinalysis, chest x-ray examination, serologic assays for *Mycoplasma,* blood cultures, and urine cultures.

Natural History
Expected Outcome

The mortality rates of SJS and TEN are 5% and 30%, respectively. The most common cause of death is sepsis. Possible serious long-term sequelae include a Sjögren-like sicca syndrome, cutaneous scarring, photophobia, visual impairment, eruptive nevi, nail loss, phimosis, and vaginal stenosis.

Treatment
Methods

Early diagnosis is important. Studies have shown that the mortality from SJS and TEN may be lowered by discontinuing offending drugs when blisters or erosions occur in the course of a drug eruption.

Supportive measures are essential in the treatment of SJS and TEN. Any new or unnecessary medications should be discontinued, and antibiotic therapy for *Mycoplasma pneumoniae* infection should be started, if indicated. Systemic corticosteroid therapy remains controversial but may be beneficial in the early stages of disease. Prophylactic antibiotics to prevent infection may also be useful.

Expected Response

Response to treatment generally requires 3 to 6 weeks or more.

When to Refer

In general, individuals with SJS and TEN should be hospitalized for adequate monitoring and supportive care.

KEY POINTS

STEVENS-JOHNSON SYNDROME AND TOXIC EPIDERMAL NECROLYSIS
- ⊃ Erythema multiforme, SJS, and TEN represent a continuum of disease characterized by epidermal detachment.
- ⊃ SJS is associated with drug exposure and *Mycoplasma* infection. TEN is almost always associated with drug exposure.
- ⊃ Antibiotics known to cause SJS and TEN are penicillins, cephalosporins, sulfonamides, fluoroquinolones, vancomycin, rifampin, ethambutol, and erythromycin.
- ⊃ The characteristic skin findings of SJS and TEN are vesicles and bullae on or near large erythematous macules and plaques. Target lesions are common.

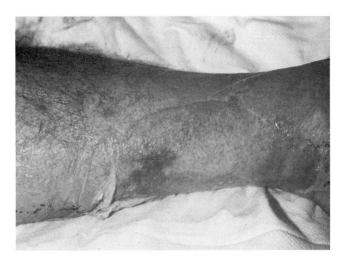

FIG. 7-6   Stevens-Johnson syndrome: typical hemorrhagic crust on the vermilion border of the lips.

FIG. 7-7   Toxic epidermal necrolysis: epidermal detachment demonstrated by Nikolsky's sign.

⊃ Mortality rates of SJS and TEN are 5% and 30%, respectively. To reduce the mortality of SJS and TEN, practitioners should discontinue drugs whenever blisters or erosions occur as part of a drug eruption.

⊃ Patients with SJS and TEN should be hospitalized for adequate supportive treatment.

SUGGESTED READING

Garcia-Doval I, LeCleach L, Bocquet H, et al. Toxic epidermal necrolysis and Stevens-Johnson syndrome: does early withdrawal of causative drugs decrease the risk of death? Arch Dermatol 2000; 136: 323-327.

Ledesma GN, McCormack PC. Erythema multiforme. Clin Dermatol 1986; 4: 70-80.

Lerner LH, Qureshi AA, Reddy BV, et al. Nitric oxide synthase in toxic epidermal necrolysis and Stevens-Johnson syndrome. J Invest Dermatol 2000; 114: 196-199.

Roujeau JC. Treatment of severe drug eruptions. J Dermatol 1999; 26: 718-722.

Tripathi A, Ditto AM, Grammer LC, et al. Corticosteroid therapy in an additional 13 cases of Stevens-Johnson syndrome: a total series of 67 cases. Allergy Asthma Proc 2000; 21: 101-105.

Wolkenstein PE, Roujeau JC, Revuz J. Drug-induced toxic epidermal necrolysis. Clin Dermatol 1998; 16: 399-409.

Infective Endocarditis

Infective endocarditis (see Chapter 6) results from infection of the heart valves, most commonly by streptococci and staphylococci. The clinical presentation often includes fever, rash,

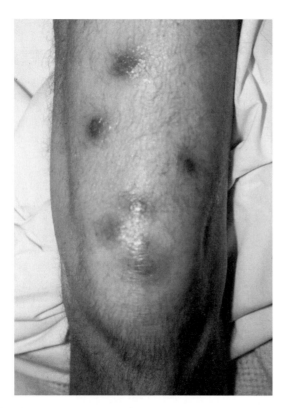

FIG. 7-8 Disseminated candidiasis on the leg of an immunosuppressed patient.

fatigue, weight loss, and a changing heart murmur. Cutaneous lesions of infective endocarditis are petechiae, purpura, Osler's nodes, Janeway lesions, and splinter hemorrhages. Petechiae are the most common mucocutaneous manifestation of infective endocarditis. These small, red, nonblanching macules are frequently distributed on the heels, legs, shoulders, oral mucosa, and conjunctiva. Nonpalpable or palpable purpura may also be present. Osler's nodes are erythematous, painful macules, papules, or nodules on the tips of the fingers, palms, and soles. Janeway lesions are similar to Osler's nodes; however, they are distributed more proximally on the palms and soles and are painless. Splinter hemorrhages are red, brown, or black linear lesions under the nail plate. These lesions should be sought in every patient with unexplained fever (see Chapters 1 and 6).

Systemic Infection by Fungi and Higher Bacteria

Skin lesions sometimes provide the vital clue to diagnosis of systemic fungal infections (see Chapter 21) and infections by certain higher bacteria (nocardiosis and actinomycosis).

Disseminated Candidiasis

Disseminated candidiasis (see Chapter 21), a potentially fatal illness, is most frequently encountered in patients with a hematologic malignancy or immunocompromised state. This disease should be suspected in a febrile patient who is deteriorating rapidly despite treatment with broad-spectrum antibiotics. Blood cultures are sometimes sterile even when disseminated lesions are present in such organs as the brain, heart, lungs, kidneys, spleen, and liver. The diagnosis thus requires a high index of clinical suspicion. Ophthalmoscopic examination may disclose characteristic retinal lesions (*Candida* endophthalmitis). The clinician should also search for telltale skin lesions, biopsy of which may yield the correct diagnosis. Skin lesions consist of erythematous papules and 0.5- to 1-cm nodules, distributed on the trunk and extremities (Figure 7-8). Mortality remains high even with aggressive treatment.

North American Blastomycosis

North American blastomycosis (see Chapter 21), a fungal infection endemic to the Mississippi and Ohio river basins, is

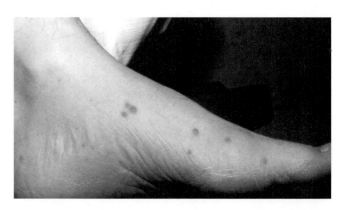

FIG. 7-9 Blastomycosis: inflammatory papules on the foot.

asymptomatic in nearly one half of patients. Pulmonary symptoms usually predominate. Extrapulmonary lesions can occur in the larynx (sometimes misdiagnosed as squamous cell carcinoma), bone, and genitourinary tract, including the prostate gland. Skin disease, however, is the most common extrapulmonary manifestation and may provide the clue to more extensive disease. Inflammatory papules (Figure 7-9), pustules, and nodules with crusts enlarge to form hyperkeratotic plaques with central ulceration or scarring (Figure 7-10). The skin lesions are located most frequently on the face and extremities. Visualization of broad-based budding yeasts of *Blastomyces dermatitidis* on potassium hydroxide (KOH) mounts of pus, skin scrapings, or sputum provides a rapid method for presumptive diagnosis before definitive results of fungal culture.

Histoplasmosis

Histoplasmosis (see Chapter 21), which is also endemic to the Ohio and Mississippi river valleys, is usually asymptomatic but sometimes causes symptomatic pulmonary disease and disseminated infection. Dissemination is more common in the elderly, infants, and immunocompromised patients, including persons with advanced HIV disease. Patients with disseminated histoplasmosis often have fever and weight loss. Skin lesions include ulcers, papules, plaques, purpura, abscesses, and nodules. Mucosal ulcerations in the oral cavity (Figure 7-11) are highly characteristic and are found in about one half of patients with the chronic progressive form of disseminated histoplasmosis. The clinical appearance of these ulcers, which may occur on the tongue, buccal mucosa, palate, larynx, gums, or lips, often suggests cancer. Hence a high index of clinical suspicion is required. Identification of the intracellular yeasts of *Histoplasma capsulatum* within macrophages provides a presumptive diagnosis.

Coccidioidomycosis

Coccidioidomycosis (see Chapter 21) is a systemic fungal infection endemic to the southwestern United States and parts of Central and South America. In many patients coccidioidomycosis is an asymptomatic pulmonary infection.

Other patients may have mild symptoms, but erythema multiforme or erythema nodosum develops during the acute infection. Dissemination, which may occur during the first few months of the infection, is more common in immunocompromised persons. The skin, bone, joints, and central nervous system may be involved. Skin findings include granulomatous papules, nodules, plaques, or ulcers, frequently located on the head (Figure 7-12). Papulopustular lesions have also been described. Diagnosis is based on direct examination of sputum, bronchial aspirates, blood, pus, and cerebrospinal fluid (CSF) for spore-containing spherules of *Coccidioides immitis* on KOH mount. Fungal culture is the method for definitive diagnosis. Treatment of disseminated coccidioidomycosis must be initiated early to prevent significant morbidity and mortality.

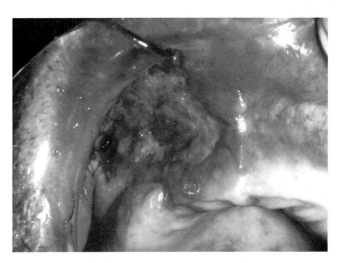

FIG. 7-11 Histoplasmosis of the oral cavity. (From Allen CM, Blozis CG. Oral mucosal lesions. In: Cummings CW, Frederickson JM, Harker LA, et al., eds. Otolaryngology–Head and Neck Surgery. 3rd ed., St. Louis: Mosby; 1998.)

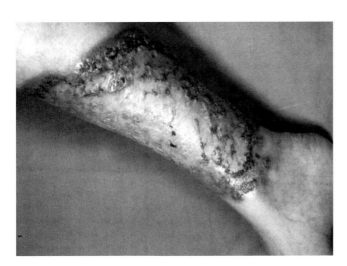

FIG. 7-10 Blastomycosis: annular verrucoid plaque with central scarring on the leg.

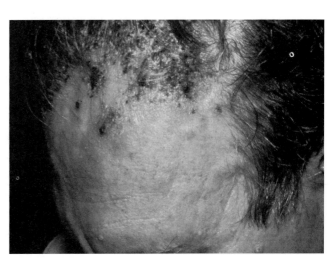

FIG. 7-12 Coccidioidomycosis disseminated to the scalp and face.

Cryptococcosis

Cryptococcosis (see Chapter 21) is another systemic fungal infection that affects primarily the lungs but sometimes occurs as disseminated disease, especially meningitis in immunocompromised persons. Skin lesions include papules, plaques, nodules (Figure 7-13), ulcers, palpable purpura, cellulitis (see Chapter 15), and pyoderma gangrenosum–like ulcers. Papules may resemble molluscum contagiosum. The typical location is the head and neck. Rarely, primary cutaneous cryptococcosis has been reported. Diagnosis of disseminated cryptococcosis is commonly based on an antigen detection assay using latex agglutination on blood or CSF. In addition, direct microscopy with India ink or nigrosin mounts allows observation of the budding encapsulated yeast of *Cryptococcus neoformans*. Definitive diagnosis is made by culture.

Nocardiosis

Nocardia species belong to a diverse group of aerobic higher bacteria, known as actinomycetes, that typically appear on Gram stains as branching, beaded, filamentous gram-positive structures (Figure 7-14). These bacteria are widely present in the environment and sometimes cause skin lesions afte minor wounds. Another cutaneous manifestation consists of a lymphocutaneous syndrome (see Chapter 8), usually caused by *Nocardia brasiliensis* and clinically resembling sporotrichosis. The *Nocardia asteroides* complex of bacteria is commonly associated with systemic disease. Pulmonary infection is the usual manifestation and includes a spectrum ranging from subacute pneumonia to chronic cavitary disease with extension to contiguous tissues. Disseminated nocardiosis, which occurs most commonly in severely immunocompromised persons, causes abscesses in numerous organs, including the brain, eyes, kidneys, bone, and heart. Skin lesions sometimes provide the key to diagnosis (Figure 7-15). When nocardiosis is suspected, the laboratory should be informed because the organism is sometimes overlooked on routine culture.

Actinomycosis

Actinomycosis is caused by a variety of anaerobic or microaerophilic bacteria, of which *Actinomyces israelii* is generally considered the most important. Current thinking favors the notion that actinomycosis is usually a polymicrobial infection arising from the patient's normal flora. Orocervicofacial disease accounts for about one half of cases of actinomycosis and usually occurs as a soft tissue swelling of the head and neck, classically at the angle of the jaw ("lumpy jaw"). Abscesses and draining sinus tracts are the hallmarks of actinomycosis but are not always present. A purplish red or bluish hue to the overlying skin is characteristic. Diagnosis can sometimes be made by demonstration of the characteristic grains or "sulfur granules" in pus. One method is to place the pus in a glass tube containing saline solution; the sulfur granules will adhere to the walls of the tube. On microscopic examination, sulfur granules are seen as conglomerations of microorganisms (Figure 7-16). The diagnosis of actinomycosis is frequently overlooked. Often, it is made when sulfur granules are discovered in histologic sections of tissue removed because of suspicion of cancer. The other major forms of actinomycosis are (1) thoracic disease, accounting for about

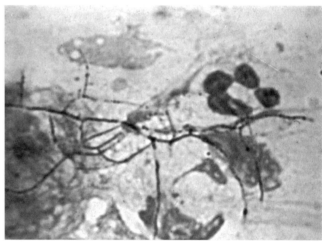

FIG. 7-14 The branching, beaded, gram-positive filaments of *Nocardia* species can be identified by Gram stain and are usually acid fast. (Courtesy of Dr. Charles S. Bryan.)

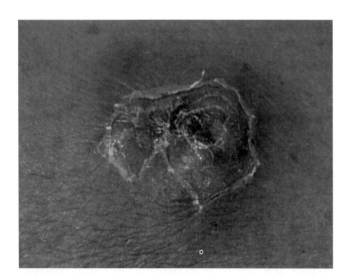

FIG. 7-13 Cryptococcosis disseminated to the skin as volcanic nodules.

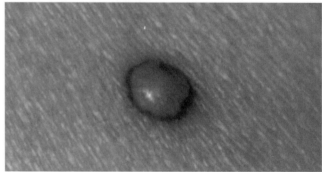

FIG. 7-15 Vesicular lesion in a patient with disseminated nocardiosis. (Courtesy of Dr. Charles S. Bryan.)

15% of cases and manifested as an indolent pneumonia with frequent pleural involvement; (2) abdominal disease, accounting for about 20% of cases and usually manifested as an abscess or mass lesion suggestive of carcinoma; and (3) pelvic disease, often associated with intrauterine contraceptive devices. Disseminated actinomycosis also occurs and can involve the heart, brain, kidneys, and skin.

KEY POINTS

SKIN INFECTION BY FUNGI AND HIGHER BACTERIA

⊃ Skin lesions can provide an important clue to the diagnosis of systemic fungal disease and also to disease caused by higher bacteria (nocardiosis and actinomycosis).

⊃ In disseminated candidiasis the characteristic skin lesions are erythematous papules and nodules on the trunk and extremities.

⊃ In North American blastomycosis the characteristic lesions are papules and nodules that enlarge to form ulcerated or scarred plaques on the face and extremities.

⊃ In disseminated histoplasmosis the skin lesions include ulcers, papules, plaques, nodules, and purpura. Ulcers in the oral cavity occur in about one half of patients with the progressive disseminated form of the disease.

⊃ In coccidioidomycosis the skin lesions include papules, nodules, plaques, and ulcers.

⊃ In nocardiosis the skin lesions may be part of disseminated disease in severely immunocompromised patients.

⊃ In actinomycosis, draining sinus tracts containing grains or "sulfur granules" enable diagnosis of this often-overlooked infection.

Durden FM, Elewski B. Cutaneous involvement with *Cryptococcus neoformans* in AIDS. J Am Acad Dermatol 1994; 30: 844-888.

Grossman ME, Silvers DN, Walther RR. Cutaneous manifestations of disseminated candidiasis. J Am Acad Dermatol 1980; 2: 111-116.

Lerner PI. Nocardiosis. Clin Infect Dis 1996; 22: 891-905.

Quimby SR, Connolly SM, Winkelmann RK, et al. Clinicopathologic spectrum of specific cutaneous lesions of disseminated coccidioidomycosis. J Am Acad Dermatol 1992; 26: 79-85.

Weil M, Mercurio MG, Brodell RT, et al. Cutaneous lesions provide a clue to mysterious pulmonary process: pulmonary and cutaneous North American blastomycosis infection. Arch Dermatol 1996; 132: 822-825.

Rocky Mountain Spotted Fever

Rocky Mountain spotted fever is a potentially dangerous disease caused by the tickborne bacterium *Rickettsia rickettsii* (see Chapter 6). The classic triad of symptoms is fever, headache, and rash. The skin findings are initially small, blanching, erythematous macules on the wrists and ankles (Figure 7-17). Within a week the rash becomes maculopapular and deep red to violaceous. It spreads to involve the face, arms, legs, and trunk. The lesions become hemorrhagic and are no longer blanchable.

Acute Retroviral Syndrome (Primary Human Immunodeficiency Virus Infection)

Acute infection with HIV type 1 causes a transient illness lasting about 2 weeks and often unrecognized (see Chapters 8 and 17). Nonspecific skin lesions appear in 40% to 80% of patients and include painless, nonpruritic, erythematous macules and papules up to 1 cm in diameter on the face and trunk.

SUGGESTED READING

Bonifaz A, Cansela R, Novales J, et al. Cutaneous histoplasmosis associated with acquired immunodeficiency syndrome (AIDS). Int J Dermatol 2000; 39: 35-38.

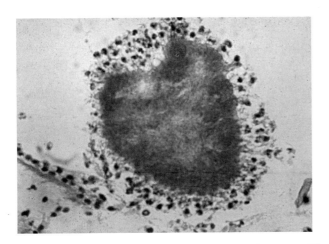

FIG. 7-16 Sulfur granule surrounded by polymorphonuclear neutrophils in a case of actinomycosis. (Courtesy of Dr. Charles S. Bryan.)

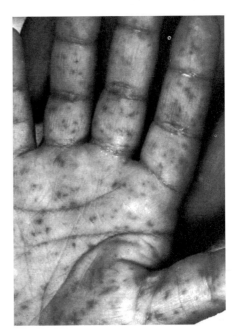

FIG. 7-17 A petechial rash on the palms and soles is highly suggestive of Rocky Mountain spotted fever. However, this finding is present in fewer than one half of patients and often appears only after the fifth day of the illness.

A morbilliform exanthem of the trunk is particularly characteristic (Figure 7-18). Mucocutaneous ulcerations and palatal erythematous papules may also occur. The presence of risk factors should prompt laboratory evaluation. Antibodies are not present during this stage of HIV infection. Diagnosis depends on demonstrating viral RNA by the polymerase chain reaction (PCR; see Chapter 17).

Kawasaki Disease

Kawasaki disease, first described in 1967, is a systemic vasculitis of unknown cause but generally presumed to be of infectious etiology. Up to 5000 cases occur each year in the United States, mainly in young children, in whom it has become an important cause of acquired heart disease. The disease was formerly known as the mucocutaneous lymph node syndrome.

Presentation and Progression
Cause

The etiology is unknown. Recent data suggest a role for bacterial superantigens (see "Toxic Shock Syndrome," Chapter 6). Perhaps the most compelling evidence for the superantigen theory is the response of the disease to intravenous therapy with high-dose immune globulin. Small epidemics occur, but person-to-person spread remains undocumented.

Presentation

Kawasaki disease is most common during the second year of life. About 80% of affected patients are under 4 years of age. Onset is usually dramatic with high, spiking fever followed by conjunctivitis and then by dramatic changes involving the lips, oral mucosa, skin, extremities, and lymph nodes (Box 7-1). The rash, which usually begins shortly after the onset of fever, typically consists of raised, deep red plaques distributed over the trunk and extremities and concentrated especially in the perineal area. The rash can also be maculopapular (morbilliform) with target lesions, diffusely erythematous (scarlatiniform), or even pustular. Cervical lymphadenopathy is present in about 70% of patients. Features that strongly suggest Kawasaki disease during the acute illness include erythema of the lips with fissuring and cracking (Figure 7-19), a strawberry tongue, and edema of the palms of the hands and soles of the feet (Figure 7-20). Affected patients are typically irritable and may have a variety of other manifestations, including arthralgias, heart failure (see later discussion), aseptic meningitis, pneumonia, and urethritis with sterile pyuria. The white blood cell count is usually elevated with bandemia. Thrombocytosis often appears during the second week of the illness and may be extreme (platelet count >1 million/mm^3). Abnormalities of liver function tests (especially the alkaline phosphatase test) are common, and the gallbladder is often distended.

Diagnosis

In the absence of a single definitive test, diagnosis is based on criteria published by the Centers for Disease Control and Prevention (CDC; Box 7-1). Desquamation that begins around the nail beds and may extend to involve the entire palms and soles occurs during recovery and helps to confirm the diagnosis. The full diagnostic criteria are not met in up to 10% of patients; these patients, who are most often young infants, are said to have atypical Kawasaki disease.

Natural History

Without treatment, Kawasaki disease is usually a triphasic illness: (1) fever lasting 7 to 14 days and accompanied by dramatic mucocutaneous findings and lymphadenopathy; (2) a subacute phase lasting 2 to 4 weeks, characterized especially by irritability, arthritis, and thrombocytosis; and (3) convalescence. Up to 3% of patients have recurrences, usually within a few weeks of the first episode.

The major complications involve the heart. About 50% of patients have evidence of myocarditis during the acute illness, manifested as tachycardia, gallop rhythm, and occasionally heart failure. Other cardiac complications during the acute phase are aortic regurgitation, mitral regurgitation, and cardiac conduction abnormalities. Aneurysmal dilatation of the coronary arteries occurs in about 20% of untreated patients.

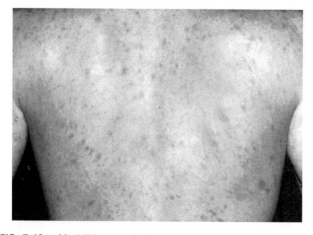

FIG. 7-18   Morbilliform rash in a patient with the acute retroviral syndrome. (Courtesy of Dr. Charles S. Bryan.)

BOX 7-1
CDC Diagnostic Criteria for Kawasaki Disease

A. Fever of at least 5 days' duration (100% of patients)
B. Presence of at least four of the following five conditions
  1. Bilateral conjunctivitis (85%)
  2. Any of the following changes involving the lips and oral mucosa (90%)
    a. Dry, red, fissured lips
    b. Strawberry tongue
    c. Oropharyngeal erythema
  3. Any of the following changes involving the extremities (75%)
    a. Erythema of the palms and soles
    b. Edema of the hands and feet
    c. Periungual desquamation
  4. Polymorphous rash (80%)
  5. Cervical lymphadenopathy with at least one node >1.5 cm in diameter (80%)
C. No other known disease process that explains the illness

CDC, Centers for Disease Control and Prevention.

Coronary thrombosis with sudden death occurs in >2% of patients, often during the subacute phase of the illness when thrombocytosis is common.

Treatment
Methods

High-dose intravenous immune globulin (IVIG), usually given as a single dose of 2 g/kg over 10 to 12 hours, has become the standard therapy based on randomized studies in Japan and the United States. Therapy also includes aspirin 80 to 100 mg/kg/day until the 14th day of illness and then 3 to 5 mg/kg/day. In patients with coronary artery aneurysms, aspirin is continued indefinitely or for 1 year after the aneurysms have been shown to be resolved. The American Heart Association has issued guidelines for long-term management of patients with Kawasaki disease.

Expected Response

Clinical symptoms and signs usually respond dramatically to IVIG. More important, IVIG given within the first 10 days of illness reduces the incidence of coronary artery aneurysms from about 20% to about 3% to 4%.

When to Refer

Patients with Kawasaki syndrome should usually be referred to a pediatrician or cardiologist knowledgeable about the disease. Echocardiography should be performed initially and should be repeated 3 to 6 weeks after IVIG therapy to determine the duration of aspirin therapy.

 KEY POINTS

KAWASAKI DISEASE

⊃ Kawasaki disease is a systemic vasculitis of unknown (but presumed infectious) etiology mainly affecting young children.
⊃ About one half of patients have myocarditis during the acute illness.
⊃ In about 20% of untreated patients, aneurysmal dilatation of the coronary arteries develops.

⊃ About 1% to 2% of untreated patients die suddenly from coronary thrombosis and myocardial infarction, usually during the 2nd to 4th weeks of the illness when marked thrombocytosis is common.
⊃ Diagnostic criteria include fever, bilateral conjunctivitis, dramatic changes in the lips and oral mucosa, polymorphous rash, edema of the hands and feet, cervical lymphadenopathy, and—during recovery—periungual desquamation that may involve the entire palms and soles.
⊃ Patients with Kawasaki disease should usually be referred to a consultant for evaluation and therapy.

SUGGESTED READING

Dajani AS, Taubert KA, Takahashi M, et al. Guidelines for long-term management of patients with Kawasaki disease. Report from the Committee on Rheumatic Fever, Endocarditis, and Kawasaki Disease. Council on Cardiovascular Disease in the Young, American Heart Association. Circulation 1994; 89: 916-922.

Laupland KB, Dele Davies H. Epidemiology, etiology, and management of Kawasaki disease: state of the art. Pediatr Cardiol 1999; 20: 177-183.

Meissner HC, Leung DY. Superantigens, conventional antigens and the etiology of Kawasaki syndrome. Pediatr Infect Dis J 2000; 19: 91-94.

Rowley AH, Shulman ST. Kawasaki syndrome. Clin Microbiol Rev 1998; 11: 405-414.

Rowley AH, Shulman ST. Kawasaki syndrome. Pediatr Clin North Am 1999; 46: 313-329.

Taubert KA, Shulman ST. Kawasaki disease. Am Fam Physician 1999; 59: 3093-3102, 3107-3108.

Leptospirosis

Leptospirosis occasionally occurs in the United States and should be considered in the differential diagnosis of unexplained fever. Outbreaks have been associated with farming,

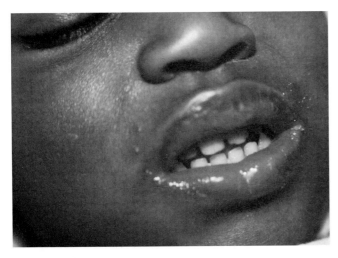

FIG. 7-19 Erythema and fissuring of the lips in a child with Kawasaki disease. (Courtesy of Dr. Charles S. Bryan.)

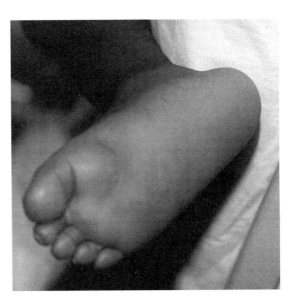

FIG. 7-20 Edema of soles of feet in a child with Kawasaki disease. (Courtesy of Dr. Charles S. Bryan.)

ranching, freshwater swimming, white-water rafting, and hunting. Clinical syndromes range from subclinical infection to life-threatening illness.

Presentation and Progression
Cause

The etiologic agent of leptospirosis is the spirochete *Leptospira interrogans,* of which at least 218 serovars have been identified. Humans are infected by direct exposure to animals, the reservoirs of the spirochete, or exposure to water or soil contaminated with animal urine. The organism enters the body through abraded skin, mucous membranes, or conjunctiva. After penetrating skin or mucous membranes, the spirochete invades the bloodstream.

Presentation

After an incubation period of 7 to 12 days, fever, chills, headache, nausea, vomiting, abdominal pain, and myalgias develop. The most common sign of infection is conjunctival injection. Skin lesions may include macules, papules, wheals, or purpura, usually distributed on the trunk. The duration of the initial illness, the septicemic phase, is 3 to 7 days. After an asymptomatic period of several days a low-grade fever, aseptic meningitis, rash, uveitis, and hepatosplenomegaly develop. This immune phase lasts from a few days to several weeks.

Two distinguishable syndromes of leptospirosis have been described. Anicteric leptospirosis has distinct septicemic and immune stages. Icteric leptospirosis, or Weil's syndrome, is the more severe form of leptospirosis. The septicemic and immune stages of illness are often less distinct in this form. Icteric leptospirosis is characterized by hepatic, renal, and vascular abnormalities. Fever, jaundice, hypotension, hemorrhage, congestive heart failure, azotemia, and circulatory collapse may occur.

Diagnosis

The diagnosis of leptospirosis is generally based on the observation of a four-fold increase in antibody titers between the acute and convalescent phases of illness. The most reliable test is the microscopic agglutination test, which is available in the United States through the CDC. In addition, blood and CSF should be sent for culture during the first 10 days of illness, and urine culture should be performed after the second week of illness. Culture of the organism is slow and difficult.

Natural History
Expected Outcome

Icteric leptospirosis is associated with a poorer outcome than anicteric. Mortality may be as high as 40% to 50%.

Treatment
Methods

Supportive therapy is required for dehydration, hypotension, hemorrhage, and renal failure. Whether antimicrobial agents significantly modify the course of leptospirosis is unclear. However, a current consensus holds that mild leptospirosis should be treated with doxycycline 100 mg PO twice daily, ampicillin 500 to 750 mg IV every 6 hours, or amoxicillin 500 mg PO every 6 hours. Moderate to severe leptospirosis should be treated with penicillin G 20 to 24 million units IV

daily by continuous or intermittent infusion. Doxycycline 200 mg PO once weekly is used for prevention of leptospirosis in individuals who have been exposed to settings with increased risk for infection, such as farmers of domestic livestock.

Expected Response

Antibiotic treatment has been found to reduce the duration of illness and prevent renal involvement of leptospirosis. Complete resolution is expected with anicteric leptospirosis. The overall mortality of leptospirosis with supportive therapy is 5% to 10%.

When to Refer

Patients with icteric leptospirosis should be hospitalized for intravenous administration of antibiotics and supportive therapy.

 KEY POINTS

LEPTOSPIROSIS

⊃ Symptoms and signs of leptospirosis are headache, fever, myalgias, nausea, vomiting, aseptic meningitis, hepatosplenomegaly, jaundice, azotemia, hypotension, conjunctival injection, and rash.

⊃ The skin findings in leptospirosis are macules, papules, wheals, and purpura on the trunk.

⊃ Leptospirosis infection includes septicemic and immune stages.

⊃ Mortality may be as high as 50%. Anicteric leptospirosis typically resolves. Icteric leptospirosis has higher morbidity and mortality.

⊃ Mild leptospirosis is treated with oral doxycycline. Moderate to severe leptospirosis requires intravenously administered penicillin.

SUGGESTED READING

Campagnolo ER, Warwick MC, Marx HL Jr, et al. Analysis of the 1998 outbreak of leptospirosis in Missouri in humans exposed to infected swine. J Am Vet Med Assoc 2000; 216: 676-682.

Farr RW. Leptospirosis. Clin Infect Dis 1995; 21: 1-8.

Lomar AV, Diament D, Torres JR. Leptospirosis in Latin America. Infect Dis Clin North Am 2000; 14: 23-39.

Disseminated Gonococcal Infection

Although the overall incidence of gonorrhea in the United States is declining, the disease remains a highly prevalent sexually transmitted disease (see Chapter 16). Disseminated gonococcal infection, also called the arthritis-dermatitis syndrome, develops in about 1% to 2% of patients. Characteristic skin findings are small erythematous macules, which progress to vesicles or pustules on an erythematous base. Petechiae and hemorrhagic bullae may also develop (Figure 7-21). Typically the skin lesions are concentrated on the distal extremities near the involved joint. Ceftriaxone is currently the drug of choice. Most patients should be hospitalized for diagnosis and initial therapy.

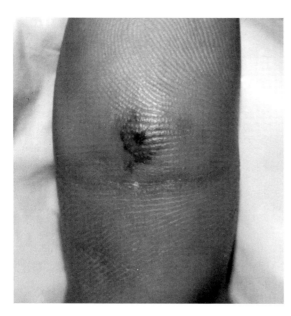

FIG. 7-21 Gonococcemia: hemorrhagic blister with surrounding erythema on the thumb.

Lyme Disease

Lyme disease takes its name from Lyme, Connecticut, where an epidemic of what was thought to be juvenile rheumatoid arthritis took place during the 1970s. Lyme disease has become the most common vectorborne disease in the United States. Two U.S. epidemics are occurring:

- An epidemic of multistage, multisystem disease, mainly in the southern parts of New England, the eastern parts of the mid-Atlantic states, and the upper Midwest, with a smaller focus along the northern Pacific coast. About 90% of confirmed cases in the United States have come from eight states: Connecticut, Rhode Island, New York, New Jersey, Delaware, Pennsylvania, Maryland, and Wisconsin.
- An epidemic of hysteria and overdiagnosis with a considerably wider geographic distribution, fueled by the news media, the Internet, and patients' understandable desire to secure a diagnosis for nonspecific symptoms. One observer has facetiously called this epidemic "lime disease."

A confident diagnosis of Lyme disease can be made when typical symptoms occur in a patient documented to have the characteristic skin lesion, erythema migrans. The diagnosis should rarely if ever be based on currently available serologic tests in the absence of highly suggestive symptoms and objective signs of the disease.

Presentation and Progression
Cause

Lyme disease is caused by the spirochete *Borrelia burgdorferi*, which is transmitted to humans in the United States by ticks of the *Ixodes* family. *Ixodes scapularis* (the black-legged tick or "deer tick," formerly known as *Ixodes dammini*) transmits the disease in the eastern United States, while *Ixodes pacificus* (the western black-legged tick) assumes importance in the Midwest. Both ticks are found in wooded areas. Their life cycles are dependent on rodents

(notably the white-footed mouse) and larger mammals (notably deer). During feeding the tick acquires the spirochete from an infected host. The spirochete stays in the tick's midgut until the tick feeds a second time. Then it penetrates the gut and invades the tick's salivary glands. Transmission of the spirochete to the host is achieved through the tick's saliva, usually after 48 hours of attachment. The tick bite is painless and often goes unrecognized.

At this writing there is much interest in the possibility that spirochetes other than *B. burgdorferi* cause an illness similar to Lyme disease, including an erythema migrans–like rash. One candidate is *Borrelia lonestari,* considered a possible cause of the emerging southern tick-associated rash illness (STARI).

Presentation

Lyme disease is characterized by three stages, the features of which may overlap (Table 7-4). The first stage is an acute onset of fever, rash, fatigue, headache, and lymphadenopathy. Erythema migrans (also called erythema chronicum migrans) is the classic skin lesion. It usually appears about a week (range 3 to 32 days) after the tick bite, most often as a solitary lesion on the trunk, groin, thigh, or axilla. It begins as an erythematous macule, which transforms into a papular lesion and then into an annular plaque, or target lesion (Figure 7-22). The lesion is characteristically large, with a median diameter of about 15 cm (range 3 to 68 cm). The outer borders are usually red to bright red. The central portion may become indurated, vesicular, and crusted. Multiple lesions may occur with multiple bite sites.

The second stage of Lyme disease, which begins several days to weeks after the initial, localized infection, is caused by hematogenous dissemination of the spirochete. This may result in multiple (up to 100) erythema migrans lesions, which are usually annular, smaller than the original lesion, and without indurated centers. They can occur anywhere except the palms of the hands and soles of the feet. Other manifestations of the second stage are facial nerve palsy (often bilateral), lymphocytic meningitis, asymmetric oligoarticular arthralgia or arthritis, motor or sensory polyradiculopathy, and fluctuating heart block. A firm, painless, bluish red nodular skin lesion known as borrelial lymphocytoma is seen mainly in Europe when the disease is caused by spirochetes other than *B. burgdorferi* (such as *Borrelia afzelii* and *Borrelia garinii*).

The third stage of the disease, which occurs more than a year after the initial infection, is dominated by chronic oligoarticular arthritis. In some patients a mild subacute encephalopathy or a polyneuropathy develops. A skin lesion accompanying the third stage in Europe and Africa and occurring mainly with *B. afzelii* infection is acrodermatitis chronica atrophicans, which begins months to years after the initial infection as a bluish red discoloration of the skin. The lesion may progress to nontender nodules and bands and then to atrophy. Other manifestations of Lyme disease are optic neuritis, retinal detachment, a multiple sclerosis–like demyelinating illness, and spastic paraparesis.

Diagnosis

The definitive diagnosis of Lyme disease is based on isolation of the spirochete from the affected patient. Unfortunately, this technique has very low yield. The most important component of diagnosis is a high index of clinical suspicion. The importance of documenting erythema migrans cannot be

TABLE 7-4
The Three Overlapping Stages of Lyme Disease

Stage	Manifestations	Comment
Stage 1 (early localized)	Erythema migrans	A characteristic rash that occurs in the majority (currently thought to be 75% to 90%) of patients and is the most specific diagnostic criterion for the disease
Stage 2 (early disseminated)	Multiple or secondary erythema migrans lesions	Lesions are smaller than the primary erythema migrans lesions, are generally annular, and lack indurated centers
	Lymphocytic meningitis	Presents as headache with neck stiffness, pain, or "pressure"
	Cranial neuropathy, especially eighth nerve paralysis (Bell's palsy)	Bell's palsy, which can be bilateral, may be the presenting manifestation of the disease
	Other neurologic abnormalities	These include motor and sensory radiculoneuritis, mononeuritis multiplex, myelitis, and mild encephalitis
	Fluctuating atrioventricular heart block	Cardiac involvement occurs in about 5% of patients, most often as first-degree, Wenckebach, or complete heart block; this is usually short lived (<6 weeks), and permanent pacemakers are seldom necessary
	Asymmetric oligoarticular arthralgia and arthritis	Migratory arthralgia and arthritis usually affect only a few joints at a time and especially affect the knees, lasting a few hours to several days
	Borrelial lymphocytoma	A painless, firm, bluish red nodule usually found on the nipple or earlobe; seen in Europe but rare in the United States
	Conjunctivitis	Interstitial keratitis, iritis, choroiditis, and retinal detachment have also been described
	Hepatitis	Occurs in about 20% of patients and is usually mild
	Other	Miscellaneous symptoms and signs include malaise and fatigue, sore throat, nonproductive cough, regional or generalized lymphadenopathy, and splenomegaly
Stage 3 (late)	Chronic oligoarticular arthritis	Intermittent arthritis involving mainly the large weight-bearing joints, especially the knees, develops in 60% of patients
	Mild, subacute encephalopathy	Manifestations include disturbances of memory, language, mood, and sleep
	Polyneuropathy	Usually manifested as a distal sensory polyneuropathy; however, nerve conduction studies often show diffuse axonal neuropathy involving both proximal and distal nerve segments
	Acrodermatitis chronica atrophicans	A skin lesion seen mainly in Europe; it begins with red violaceous lesions

overemphasized. Especially in nonendemic areas, where clinical experience with this lesion may be lacking, a photograph of skin lesions suggestive of erythema migrans should be obtained for future documentation.

A diagnosis of Lyme disease can be made with confidence when a patient with a history of tick exposure in an endemic area has well-documented erythema migrans and other features of the disease (Table 7-4). Serologic testing is insensitive

in patients with erythema migrans (early localized Lyme disease, stage I) because the immune response develops slowly.

Serologic tests are commonly used to confirm the diagnosis in patients who lack a clear history of erythema migrans. Usually an enzyme-linked immunosorbent assay (ELISA) is used to detect IgM and IgG antibodies to *B. burgdorferi* and positive results are confirmed by the Western blot (immunoblot) method. IgM antibodies usually appear 3 to 4 weeks after the initial

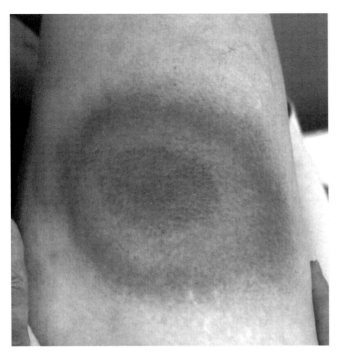

FIG. 7-22 Lyme disease: classic lesion of erythema chronica migrans.

infection and peak at about 6 to 8 weeks. However, they may persist even after antibiotic treatment, and therefore the presence of IgM antibodies does not necessarily indicate recently acquired Lyme disease. IgG antibodies appear about 6 to 8 weeks after the initial infection and peak in 4 to 6 months. Causes of false-positive ELISA tests for *B. burgdorferi* are autoimmune diseases such as systemic lupus erythematosus, viral infections such as varicella, and other spirochetal infections such as syphilis and leptospirosis, but many patients have false-positive results for reasons that are unclear.

Who should undergo serologic testing for Lyme disease? According to a position paper published by the American College of Physicians, testing is indicated mainly (perhaps only) when the pretest probability of Lyme disease is between 20% and 80%. When the pretest probability is >80%, treatment is usually indicated because the drugs of choice (notably doxycycline and amoxicillin) are relatively safe and inexpensive. When the pretest probability is <20%, the likelihood that a positive test result is a false positive rather than a true positive is high (see Chapter 1). Many patients with symptoms consistent with chronic fatigue syndrome, fibromyalgia, depression, or somatization disorder become obsessed with the results of their serologic tests and insist on (and often receive) prolonged courses of treatment, including intravenous ceftriaxone. Simultaneous measurement of antibodies to *B. burgdorferi* in serum and CSF, as an index to intrathecal antibody production, has been used to diagnosis Lyme disease of the central nervous system (neuroborreliosis), but the sensitivity of this approach seems to be low, at least in the United States, and the results can be difficult to interpret.

PCR can be used to demonstrate *B. burgdorferi* DNA in skin biopsy specimens, blood, CSF, and synovial fluid. To date, PCR has been of greatest usefulness in the diagnosis of

Lyme arthritis (85% sensitivity). Sensitivity has been <40% in patients with early neuroborreliosis. Other tests, including a urine antigen test, have been developed, but for the most part these have not been standardized.

Natural History
Expected Outcome
Studies of the natural history of Lyme disease in the United States, based on patients who had clear-cut early Lyme disease, including erythema migrans, and who did not receive treatment, indicate the development of cardiac involvement in about 5%, chronic arthritis in 11%, and overt neurologic disease in about 15%. Thus Lyme disease is a self-limited disorder more often than not. Long-term follow-up of the original patients with Lyme disease indicates that sequelae occurred mainly in patients who had facial palsy during the acute stage and who did not receive antibiotics. The general health of the other patients did not differ significantly from that of control subjects. However, the potential for significant cardiac, neurologic, musculoskeletal, and other abnormalities cannot be dismissed.

Treatment
Methods
Recommended drug regimens vary according to the manifestations of the disease (Table 7-5). Temporary pacing may be necessary for transient heart block.

Expected Response
Most patients respond well to treatment, without complications. The diagnosis should probably be questioned when symptoms persist or recur in patients who lack a clear, documented history of erythema migrans. However, in some patients with well-documented Lyme disease a symptom complex known as chronic Lyme disease or the post–Lyme disease syndrome develops after treatment. Manifestations include impaired memory, loss of concentration, sleep disorders, myalgias, arthralgias, and fatigue. The basis for this symptom complex is unknown, and whether patients benefit from a second course of treatment is not clear.

When to Refer
Patients with moderate to severe cardiac and neurologic involvement should be hospitalized for intravenous antibiotics and monitoring. Patients with more severe manifestations of the disease (stages II and III) may benefit from referral to a rheumatologist, cardiologist, neurologist, or infectious disease specialist. Primary care clinicians and their patients should be wary of persons (whether physicians and nonphysicians) who offer novel diagnostic and therapeutic approaches to Lyme disease that have not been published in the standard, peer-reviewed medical literature.

 KEY POINTS

LYME DISEASE
⊃ Lyme disease is now the most common vectorborne disease in the United States. It usually occurs during the summer months in persons who have been exposed to a tick habitat.

TABLE 7-5
Treatment of Lyme Disease

Stage or disease manifestation	Drug	Dose for children <8 Years	Dose for adults and children >8 years
Early localized or early disseminated (stages I and II), including multiple erythema migrans lesions, isolated facial nerve palsy with normal CSF, and mild carditis	Doxycycline	Not recommended	100 mg b.i.d. for 21 days
	Amoxicillin (± probenecid)	20 to 40 mg/kg/day in 3 divided doses for 21 days	500 mg q.i.d. for 21 days
	Cefuroxime axetil	250 mg b.i.d. for 21 days	500 mg b.i.d. for 21 days
Meningitis, facial nerve palsy with abnormal CSF, severe neurologic disease, severe carditis, and persistent or recurrent arthritis (stages II and III)	Ceftriaxone	50 to 80 mg/kg/day IV for 14 to 21 days	2 g/day IV for 14 to 21 days
	Penicillin G	250,000 to 400,000 units/kg/day for 10 to 21 days*	20 to 24 million units/day for 14 to 21 days*
Arthritis, early or late	Doxycycline	Not recommended	100 mg b.i.d. for 28 days
	Amoxicillin (± probenecid)	40 mg/kg/day in divided doses 3 times daily for 28 days	500 mg q.i.d. for 28 days
	Ceftriaxone	50 to 80 mg/kg/day for 10 to 21 days	2 g/day for 14 to 28 days
	Penicillin G	250,000 to 400,000 units/kg/day for 10 to 21 days*	20 to 24 million units/day for 14 to 28 days*

CSF, Cerebrospinal fluid; *IV*, intravenous.
*Most authorities recommend penicillin G therapy in divided doses (e.g., q4h); in our opinion, continuous infusion may be more cost effective.

⊃ Eight states—Connecticut, Rhode Island, New York, New Jersey, Delaware, Pennsylvania, Maryland, and Wisconsin—account for 91% of confirmed cases in the United States. Cases have been reported from most areas of the United States, and the endemic range of the disease may be slowly expanding. However, caution should be exercised when patients who have not been exposed to ticks in endemic areas have symptoms and signs consistent with but not highly suggestive of Lyme disease.

⊃ The three stages of Lyme disease feature a wide range of overlapping clinical manifestations involving the skin, joints, heart, central and peripheral nervous systems, lymph nodes, and numerous organs.

⊃ Erythema migrans, the classic skin lesion of Lyme disease, is a targetoid plaque usually found on the trunk or lower extremities and >5 cm in diameter. Erythema migrans occurs in about 75% to 90% of patients with Lyme disease.

⊃ Early lesions of erythema migrans can be confused with other skin lesions such as an insect bite, cellulitis, nummular eczema, tinea, or granuloma inguinale. When the diagnosis is in doubt in an otherwise asymptomatic patient, observation of the rash for several days without treatment may be useful. Rapid expansion of the lesion suggests erythema migrans.

⊃ Serologic confirmation is unnecessary in patients with erythema migrans and other typical features of the disease. These patients should be treated for Lyme disease. With successful treatment, antibodies often do not appear. Serologic testing for Lyme disease should be discouraged for patients with nonspecific symptom complexes such as chronic fatigue or fibromyalgia. Serologic testing is most useful for patients who have a pretest probability between 20% and 80%. Testing patients with a lower pretest probability often yields false-positive results, prompting unnecessary treatment.

⊃ Uncomplicated Lyme disease is treated with oral doxycycline or amoxicillin.

⊃ Lyme disease usually responds satisfactorily to appropriate therapy. There is little or no basis for repeated or prolonged courses of therapy.

SUGGESTED READING

Barbour AG, Maupin GO, Teltow GJ, et al. Identification of an uncultivable *Borrelia* species in the hard tick *Amblyomma americanum*: possible agent of a Lyme disease–like illness. J Infect Dis 1996; 173: 403-409.

Edlow JA. Lyme disease and related tick-borne illnesses. Ann Emerg Med 1999; 33: 680-693.

Kalish RA, Kaplan RF, Taylor E, et al. Evaluation of study patients with Lyme disease, 10-20-year follow-up. J Infect Dis 2001; 183: 453-460.

Nichol G, Dennis DT, Steere AC, et al. Test-treatment strategies for patients suspected of having Lyme disease: a cost-effectiveness analysis. Ann Intern Med 1998; 128: 37-48.

Shapiro ED, Gerber MA. Lyme disease. Clin Infect Dis 2000; 31: 533-542.

Steere AC. Lyme disease. N Engl J Med 2001; 345: 115-125.

Typhus

Typhus is categorized into epidemic typhus, murine typhus, and scrub typhus. This discussion is limited to epidemic typhus and murine typhus, which occur in the United States. Both forms of typhus typically cause an uncomplicated flulike illness. In rare cases the infection is life threatening.

Presentation and Progression
Cause

Epidemic typhus was associated with the human body louse until 1975, when *Rickettsia prowazekii* was isolated from the southern flying squirrel. The vector for transmission to humans is presumed to be squirrel lice or fleas. The flying squirrel is found in the eastern United States. Epidemic typhus has been reported in North Carolina, Virginia, West Virginia, Georgia, Tennessee, Massachusetts, and Pennsylvania. The infection is most common in rural environments during the winter months.

Murine typhus, or endemic typhus, is caused by *Rickettsia typhi* and the ELB agent, a newly recognized rickettsia. The vectors for transmission to humans are the rat flea, rat louse, and cat flea. Murine typhus is endemic in Central America, Mexico, and the Rio Grande Valley of southern Texas. This infection occurs in seaboard regions during the summer months.

Presentation

Epidemic typhus begins with malaise, which is followed by the abrupt onset of severe headache, fever, and myalgias. On the fifth day of illness erythematous, blanchable macules form in the axillary folds and on the upper trunk. Later, maculopapular and petechial lesions develop on the trunk and extremities. The face, palms, and soles are typically spared.

Murine typhus also develops as a flulike illness with the abrupt onset of fever, malaise, and headache. The rash, which appears on about the fifth day of illness, may be macular, maculopapular, papular, petechial, or morbilliform. It is distributed over the trunk and extremities.

Diagnosis

The diagnosis of epidemic and murine typhus is confirmed by a four-fold increase between acute and convalescent specific antibody titers, as measured by microimmunofluorescent and plate microagglutination tests.

Natural History
Expected Outcome

The course of both epidemic and murine typhus is generally uncomplicated. Possible complications of epidemic typhus are gangrene and cerebral thrombosis with neurologic deficits. Rarely the infection is life threatening. Rare complications of murine typhus are neuropsychiatric abnormalities, seizures, renal insufficiency, respiratory failure, and jaundice. The case-fatality rate is less than 5%.

Treatment
Methods

Treatment of epidemic and murine typhus is the same. For uncomplicated infection, doxycycline 100 mg PO is given twice daily for 7 days or until 4 days after the patient becomes afebrile. Chloramphenicol 500 mg PO four times daily is an alternative treatment. For complicated infections doxycycline and chloramphenicol may be given intravenously.

Expected Response

Patients recover fully from the infection without sequelae except in very rare cases.

When to Refer

Only complicated cases of epidemic and murine typhus require hospitalization for intravenous antibiotics.

 KEY POINTS

TYPHUS
- Epidemic and murine typhus are the two types of typhus infection seen in the United States.
- The onset of typhus is characterized by headache, malaise, myalgias, fever, and rash.
- Cutaneous findings of epidemic typhus are erythematous, blanchable macules in the axillae and on the upper trunk. As the disease progresses, maculopapular and petechial lesions develop on the trunk and extremities.
- Murine typhus is associated with a macular, papular, maculopapular, morbilliform, or petechial skin eruption over the trunk and extremities.
- The diagnosis of typhus is confirmed by serologic tests.

SUGGESTED READING
Azad AF, Beard CB. Rickettsial pathogens and their arthropod vectors. Emerg Infect Dis 1998; 4: 179-186.

Raoult D, Roux V, Ndihokubwayo JB, et al. Jail fever (epidemic typhus) outbreak in Burundi. Emerg Infect Dis 1997; 3: 357-360.

Roux V, Raoult D. Body lice as tools for diagnosis and surveillance of reemerging diseases. J Clin Microbiol 1999; 37: 596-599.

Acute Rheumatic Fever

The incidence and prevalence of acute rheumatic fever had been declining in the United States until the mid-1980s, when several outbreaks were reported. Recognition of acute rheumatic fever, which is mainly a disease of childhood, is important for prevention of long-term sequelae.

Presentation and Progression
Cause

Acute rheumatic fever is thought to result from an abnormal immune response to an upper respiratory tract infection caused by *Streptococcus pyogenes*. Other group A streptococcal infections, such as soft tissue infections, do not cause acute rheumatic fever.

Presentation

Streptococcal pharyngitis precedes the onset of acute rheumatic fever by about 1 to 3 weeks. The onset of illness is usually subtle with fever, malaise, and weight loss. Gradually the disease progresses to involve the heart, central nervous system, joints, and skin. Migratory polyarthritis of the large joints is the most common manifestation of acute rheumatic fever. Cardiac involvement occurs in about 50% of patients. Pancarditis, associated with a systolic or diastolic heart murmur, is often present. Sydenham's chorea is a rare and late sign of disease.

The classic cutaneous manifestations of acute rheumatic fever are erythema marginatum and subcutaneous nodules. Erythema marginatum (Figure 7-23) appears early in the illness and typically precedes joint involvement. Erythematous, annular or polycyclic macules appear on the trunk and extremities and spread rapidly. The macules may have pale or slightly pigmented centers. Subcutaneous nodules are firm, painless nodules, which occur over the extensor surfaces of the elbows, knees, wrists, vertebrae, and occiput.

Diagnosis

The diagnosis of acute rheumatic fever is based on the modified Jones criteria, as follows:

- Major criteria include polyarthritis, carditis, chorea, erythema marginatum, and subcutaneous nodules.
- Minor criteria include arthralgias, fever, elevated erythrocyte sedimentation rate, elevated C-reactive protein level, and prolonged PR interval on electrocardiogram.
- Evidence of preceding streptococcal infection includes a positive throat culture, a positive rapid streptococcal antigen test, or an increased titer of antistreptococcal antibodies.
- A diagnosis of rheumatic fever is based on the fulfillment of two major criteria, or of one major criterion and two minor criteria, plus evidence of preceding streptococcal infection.

Some patients whose illnesses do not fulfill the Jones criteria are said to have poststreptococcal reactive arthritis (see Chapter 15). Whether these latter patients are at risk for chronic heart disease has not been settled.

Natural History
Expected Outcome

Morbidity and mortality from acute rheumatic fever are secondary to the cardiac effects. Prognosis is related to the number of recurrent attacks and valvular damage. Mortality is quite rare.

Treatment
Methods

The recommended treatment for acute rheumatic fever is a single dose of benzathine penicillin G 1.2 million units IM. An alternative is penicillin V 250 mg PO every 8 hours for 10 days. For patients allergic to penicillin, erythromycin 20 to 40 mg/kg/day divided in four doses daily should be given for 10 days.

Symptomatic treatment is based on the organ system involved. Salicylates are useful for the arthritis. Aspirin 100 mg/kg/day for children and 6000 to 8000 mg/day for adults may be given. Severe carditis is treated with prednisone.

Antibiotic prophylaxis should be used to prevent recurrences. Therapeutic options are benzathine penicillin G 1.2 million units intramuscularly every 4 weeks, penicillin V 250 mg PO every 12 hours, sulfadiazine 1 g PO once daily, or erythromycin 250 mg PO twice daily. Secondary prophylaxis should be continued for 5 years or until 18 years of age in patents without carditis and for 10 years or until 25 years of age in patients with carditis.

Prophylaxis for bacterial endocarditis is essential before dental or surgical procedures in patients with known rheumatic heart disease (see Chapter 26). This preprocedure prophylaxis should be given in addition to the routine secondary prophylaxis.

Expected Response

Most patients respond well to treatment for the acute illness. Prevention is extremely important in their future management.

When to Refer

The decision to admit patients with acute rheumatic fever to the hospital is based on the overall clinical picture.

 KEY POINTS

ACUTE RHEUMATIC FEVER

- ⊃ Streptococcal pharyngitis precedes the onset of acute rheumatic fever by 1 to 3 weeks.
- ⊃ Migratory polyarthritis is the most common symptom of illness.
- ⊃ The classic skin findings of acute rheumatic fever are erythema marginatum and subcutaneous nodules.
- ⊃ The modified Jones criteria are used for the clinical diagnosis of acute rheumatic fever.
- ⊃ Secondary prevention is an important aspect of treatment.
- ⊃ Morbidity and mortality from acute rheumatic fever are due largely to its effects on the heart.

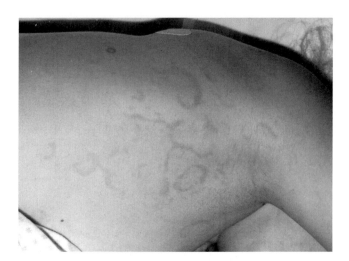

FIG. 7-23 Erythema marginatum (acute rheumatic fever): evanescent red annular and polycyclic macules.

SUGGESTED READING

Alsaeid K, Majeed HA. Acute rheumatic fever: diagnosis and treatment. Pediatr Ann 1998; 27: 295-300.

Bitar FF, Hayek P, Obeid M, et al. Rheumatic fever in children: a 15 year experience in a developing country. Pediatr Cardiol 2000; 21: 119-122.

Cunningham MW. Pathogenesis of group A streptococcal infections. Clin Microbiol Rev 2000; 13: 470-511.

Thatai D, Turi ZG. Current guidelines for the treatment of patients with rheumatic fever. Drugs 1999; 57: 545-555.

Secondary Syphilis

Manifestations of syphilis, caused by the spirochete *Treponema pallidum,* are divided into three stages (see Chapter 16). Secondary syphilis is an important consideration in the differential diagnosis of fever and rash, since treatment during this stage prevents long-term complications.

Secondary syphilis is often manifested as a flulike illness with headache, pharyngitis, fever, malaise, and generalized lymphadenopathy. Painless mucocutaneous lesions then occur in a symmetric, generalized distribution. The morphology of the rash varies according to the duration of the infection. The rash begins as red, blanching, nonpruritic macules. The most common locations are the trunk, shoulders, extremities, and flexor surfaces of the arms and forearms. Notably, this stage of the rash spares the face, palms, and soles. The macules are replaced in about 2 weeks with a coppery-red maculopapular eruption in a similar distribution but also on the face, palms, and soles (Figures 7-24 and 7-25). Mucous patches (Figure 7-26) may arise on mucous membranes. They are slightly elevated, flat-topped, round to oval macules or

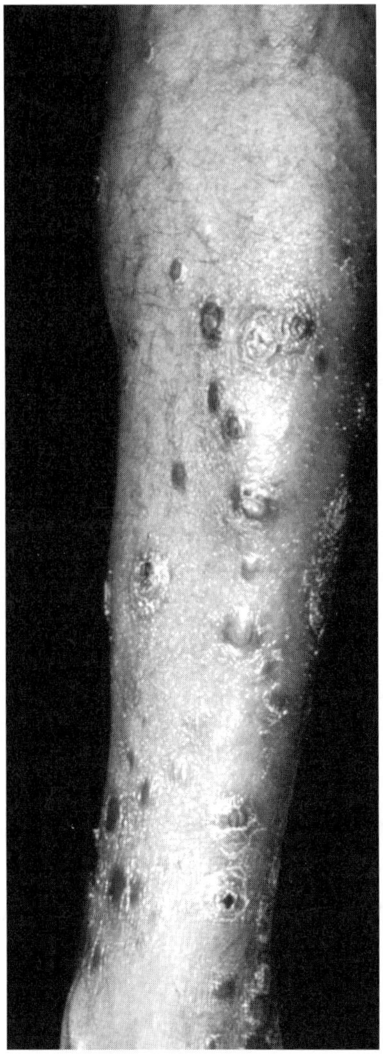

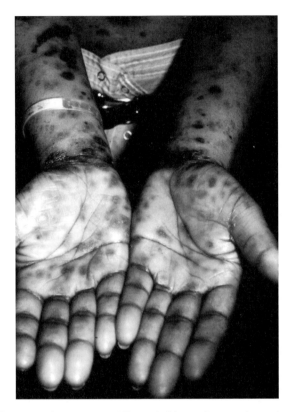

FIG. 7-25 Secondary syphilis: typical hyperpigmented macules on the palms.

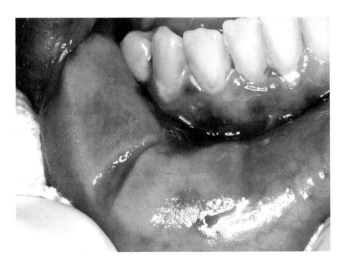

FIG. 7-24 Secondary syphilis: generalized rupioid lesions on the legs.

FIG. 7-26 Secondary syphilis: mucous patches on the labial mucosa.

papules with a central shallow ulcer covered by a gray-white membrane. Later cutaneous lesions tend to be darker red papules involving the palms and soles. Follicular involvement causes a moth-eaten alopecia. On moist areas, such as the mouth, groin, and intertriginous areas, the papules coalesce to form condylomata lata. These are red to pale, flat-topped, moist papules and nodules. Finally, pustules may form from softened papules. Cutaneous lesions of secondary syphilis resolve spontaneously in 2 to 10 weeks, but recurrence is common.

Nontreponemal serologic tests (rapid plasma reagin and Venereal Disease Research Laboratory tests) are nearly always positive in secondary syphilis, in contrast to the other stages of the disease. Spirochetes can also be demonstrated by dark-field microscopy of material taken from papules and mucous patches. Tertiary syphilis develops in about one third of untreated persons. Therefore a high index of suspicion of secondary syphilis in all patients with a rash is important, especially since the rash is easily confused with other skin diseases, including pityriasis rosea and psoriasis.

Disseminated Herpes Zoster

Disseminated herpes zoster is a more diffuse form of the acute dermatomal infection "shingles." It is common in patients with malignancy, HIV infection, or an underlying immunodeficiency.

Presentation and Progression
Cause

Herpes zoster is caused by the varicella-zoster virus, a double-stranded DNA virus. Primary infection with varicella-zoster virus produces varicella, or chickenpox (see Chapter 4). Reactivation of the virus results in herpes zoster, or shingles.

Presentation

In an immunocompetent host, herpes zoster is almost always localized to a dermatomal cutaneous distribution. Patients have pain followed by grouped vesicles on an erythematous base (Figure 7-27).

In immunocompromised patients herpes zoster may become disseminated. Dissemination occurs days after the onset of localized lesions. It may be limited to the skin or spread to the viscera. Cutaneous lesions may include grouped vesicles on an erythematous base, pustules, hemorrhagic bullae, large ulcers, and verrucous, hyperkeratotic plaques on an ulcerated base (Figure 7-28). Symptoms include headache, malaise, and fever.

Diagnosis

The diagnosis of disseminated herpes zoster is made immediately on the basis of a positive Tzanck smear or within 24 hours via direct fluorescent antibody testing. Viral cultures and skin biopsy are less efficient but more sensitive.

Natural History
Expected Outcome

Significant morbidity and mortality are associated with disseminated infection. Gastrointestinal, pulmonary, and neurologic complications may occur. Varicella-zoster pneumonitis, retinal necrosis, progressive leukoencephalitis, and cerebral vasculitis are possible complications.

Treatment
Methods

The recommended treatment for disseminated herpes zoster is IV acyclovir 10 to 12 mg/kg/day q8h for at least 7 days.

Expected Response

Patients may have greater morbidity with disseminated herpes zoster, but the mortality rate remains low.

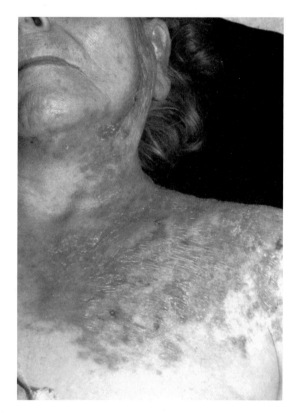

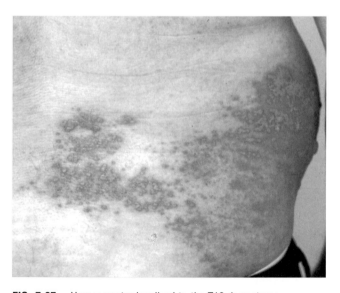

FIG. 7-27   Herpes zoster localized to the T12 dermatome.

FIG. 7-28   Herpes zoster disseminated to the scalp, face, neck, chest, and arm.

When to Refer

All patients with disseminated herpes zoster should be hospitalized for intravenous administration of acyclovir.

 KEY POINTS

DISSEMINATED HERPES ZOSTER

⊃ Disseminated herpes zoster is more common in patients with malignancy, HIV infection, and other immunocompromised states.

⊃ Skin findings in disseminated herpes zoster are grouped vesicles on an erythematous base, pustules, hemorrhagic bullae, large ulcers, and verrucous, hyperkeratotic plaques on an ulcerated base.

⊃ Complications of infection involve the gastrointestinal, pulmonary, and neurologic systems.

⊃ Diagnosis is based on Tzanck smear or direct fluorescent antibody testing.

⊃ Treatment is with intravenously administered acyclovir.

SUGGESTED READING

Cohen JI, Brunell PA, Straus SE, et al. Recent advances in varicella-zoster virus infection. Ann Intern Med 1999; 130: 922-932.

McCrary ML, Severson J, Tyring SK. Varicella-zoster virus. J Am Acad Dermatol 1999; 41: 1-14.

Babesiosis

Babesiosis is a tickborne disease caused by a protozoan parasite. Endemic areas in the United States include the coastal areas of Massachusetts, islands near New York City, Rhode Island, and Connecticut. Cases have also been reported in Maryland, Virginia, Georgia, Indiana, Wisconsin, Minnesota, California, and Washington. The infection rate is highest from May to September.

The majority of infections are asymptomatic, but in rare cases severe illness occurs. Clinical infection is typically more severe in patients with asplenia, age over 40 years, and immunosuppression.

Presentation and Progression
Cause

Babesial parasites are among the most common blood parasites worldwide. In the United States the most common etiologic agent is *Babesia microti,* a protozoan. The tick vector is *Ixodes scapularis.* After transmission occurs by the bite of the tick, the protozoa enter erythrocytes of the human and multiply. Transmission also occurs in utero, during delivery, and from blood transfusion.

Presentation

Most cases of babesiosis in the United States are asymptomatic. Patients seldom recall the tick bite. Between 1 and 4 weeks after the bite, fever, myalgias, nausea, headache, abdominal pain, sweating, and emotional lability slowly develop. The skin findings may include petechiae, purpura, or ecchymoses. If lesions similar to erythema migrans are seen, a simultaneous infection of Lyme disease is likely because the two diseases have the same tick vector. Other frequent signs of illness are hepatomegaly, splenomegaly, dark urine, and jaundice.

Possible complications of illness are severe hemolysis, respiratory distress, hypotension, shock, disseminated intravascular coagulation, congestive heart failure, and renal failure. Death may rarely occur.

Diagnosis

The diagnosis of babesiosis is based on examination of the peripheral blood smear. A Giemsa-stained blood smear reveals intraerythrocytic ring forms resembling the ring forms of *Plasmodium falciparum.* In addition, indirect immunofluorescence is diagnostic of an acute infection if the titer is ≥1:256.

Natural History
Expected Outcome

Symptoms usually last for several weeks. Fatigue and malaise may persist. Rarely, the infection is fatal. Dense parasitemia involving up to 80% of red blood cells can cause massive hemolysis. Overwhelming infection is especially likely to occur in asplenic persons.

Treatment
Methods

Patients who are asymptomatic and immunocompetent do not require treatment. Patients with immunosuppression, asplenia, or severe clinical infection should receive clindamycin and quinine. Clindamycin 1.2 g IV b.i.d. or 600 mg PO t.i.d. plus quinine 650 mg PO t.i.d. is prescribed for 7 days of therapy. Recently, atovaquone 750 mg q12h plus azithromycin 500 mg on the first day, then 250 mg daily for 6 days was described as a well-tolerated alternative regimen for patients with less severe illness. Exchange transfusions may be needed for patients who are severely ill with a high level of parasitemia and hemolysis.

Expected Response

Most patients recover even without treatment. Rarely, death occurs in an immunosuppressed or asplenic patient.

When to Refer

Only patients with severe infection should be hospitalized.

 KEY POINTS

BABESIOSIS

⊃ Babesiosis in the United States is seen mainly in northeastern coastal areas between May and September.

⊃ In the United States babesiosis is caused by a protozoan, *B. microti.*

⊃ Most infections are subclinical.

⊃ In asplenic persons, babesiosis can cause a fulminant, rapidly fatal illness. Other patients at risk for severe disease include the elderly, the immunocompromised, and patients with HIV infection.

⊃ Skin findings may include petechiae, purpura, and ecchymoses.

⊃ Babesiosis is transmitted by the same tick (*I. scapularis*) that transmits Lyme disease and ehrlichiosis, and therefore coinfections occur.

⊃ Diagnosis is based on presence of the organisms on peripheral blood smear or on serologic tests.

⊃ Treatment is necessary only in the more severe clinical infections.

SUGGESTED READING

Hatcher JC, Greenberg PD, Antique J, et al. Severe babesiosis in Long Island: review of 34 cases and their complications. Clin Infect Dis 2001; 32: 1117-1125.

Homer MJ, Aguilar-Delfin I, Telford SR III, et al. Babesiosis. Clin Microbiol Rev 2000; 13: 451-469.

Krause PJ, Lepore T, Sikand VK, et al. Atovaquone and azithromycin for the treatment of babesiosis. N Engl J Med 2000; 343: 1454-1458.

Ehrlichiosis

Ehrlichiosis is an emerging tickborne illness first described in the United States in 1986, with two clinical types based on etiology. More than 1500 cases of human monocytic ehrlichiosis have been reported, mainly from southeastern, south central, mid-Atlantic, and western regions of the United States. The disease is often misdiagnosed as Rocky Mountain spotted fever. More than 600 cases of human granulocytic ehrlichiosis have been reported, with most of the patients having been infected in Minnesota, Wisconsin, Connecticut, New York, or New Jersey. The disease usually occurs during the late spring or summer. Ehrlichiosis is often subclinical but can manifest itself as an acute, life-threatening illness with encephalopathy, coagulopathy, and respiratory and renal failure.

Presentation and Progression
Cause

Ehrlichiae are obligate intracellular bacteria closely related to the rickettsiae. They reproduce within human leukocytes, forming characteristic mulberry-like structures known as morulae. At least 10 *Ehrlichia* species cause disease in various mammals. The etiologic agent of human monocytic ehrlichiosis is *Ehrlichia chaffeensis,* which is transmitted mainly by the Lone Star tick (*Amblyomma americanum*) in the southeastern and south central United States and by other tick vectors, including the American dog tick (*Dermacentor variabilis*), in the western and northwestern United States. The etiologic agent of human granulocytic ehrlichiosis is currently called the HGE agent for want of a definitive name but has been assigned to the *Ehrlichia phagocytophila* group of microorganisms. It is transmitted mainly by *I. scapularis* (the black-legged tick), *I. pacificus* (the western black-legged tick), and *I. ricinus* (the sheep tick, in western Europe). Transmission of human granulocytic ehrlichiosis and Lyme disease by the same ticks raises the possibility of dual infections, which indeed occur.

Presentation

Fever, headache, myalgias, chills, and malaise develop about a week after the tick bite. Other symptoms are nausea, vomiting, anorexia, diarrhea, abdominal pain, cough, and dyspnea. Confusion occurs in about one fifth of cases. Other neurologic signs are lethargy, broad-based gait, hyperreflexia, clonus, photophobia, cranial nerve palsies, seizures, and coma. The white blood cell count is normal or, in 50% to 60% of patients, low. Thrombocytopenia is common (60% or more of cases in most series). Levels of the hepatic aminotransferases (alanine aminotransferase and aspartate aminotransferase) are elevated in about 60% to 90% of cases, and abnormal renal function is especially common in human granulocytic ehrlichiosis. Life-threatening complications include respiratory failure, renal failure, hemorrhage, and opportunistic infection.

A transient rash occurs in about one third of patients with human monocytic ehrlichiosis and is more likely to occur in children. Several days after onset of symptoms, macules, papules, or petechiae develop on the trunk. Rash is less common in human granulocytic ehrlichiosis (2% to 11% in reported series). Some observers believe that rash is not a feature of human granulocytic ehrlichiosis and that the presence of a rash suggests coinfection with *B. burgdorferi* or another disease such as meningococcemia or Rocky Mountain spotted fever.

Ehrlichiosis has many features in common with Rocky Mountain spotted fever. These include peak incidence in late spring and summer; incubation about 1 week after a tick exposure; abrupt onset of a flulike illness with fever, chills, headache, and myalgia; complications such as encephalopathy, coagulopathy, and respiratory and renal failure in severe cases; thrombocytopenia; and elevation of the hepatic aminotransferase levels. On serologic examination, many disconfirmed cases of Rocky Mountain spotted fever (that is, cases with clinical features of the disease but in which serologic studies are negative) prove to be ehrlichiosis. Leukopenia is more common in patients with ehrlichiosis, and vasculitis—the major pathologic finding in Rocky Mountain spotted fever—does not occur.

Diagnosis

Examination of peripheral blood or buffy coat preparations reveals the characteristic morulae (mulberry-like clusters of microorganisms in the cytoplasm of leukocytes) in about 7% of patients with human monocytic ehrlichiosis and in 20% to 80% of patients with human granulocytic ehrlichiosis. However, the diagnosis is usually made serologically. Serologic tests for ehrlichiosis are not widely available, but they can be obtained through the CDC. The most sensitive confirmatory test is indirect immunofluorescent antibody detection using reagents specific for HME and HGE. Titers are detectable by the third week of illness. Diagnosis is based on a four-fold rise or fall in titer. Isolation of the organisms by culture of peripheral blood has been accomplished but is too cumbersome for practical use. PCR-based assays have been developed.

Natural History
Expected Outcome

Reported case-fatality rates are 2% to 5% for HME and 7% to 10% for HGE.

Treatment
Method

The treatment of choice is doxycycline 100 mg b.i.d. either PO or IV for 7 to 14 days. Chloramphenicol, the alternative drug for Rocky Mountain spotted fever, may not be effective treatment for ehrlichiosis.

Expected Response

Most patients recover fully without complication. Rarely, death occurs.

When to Refer

Patients with severe symptoms should be hospitalized for rapid initiation of intravenous antibiotics.

 ## KEY POINTS

EHRLICHIOSIS

⊃ Ehrlichiosis is a nonspecific febrile illness with fever, headache, chills, myalgias, and often a variety of gastro-intestinal, pulmonary, and neurologic symptoms and signs.

⊃ Rash occurs in about one third of patients with human monocytic ehrlichiosis, especially in children, and includes macules, papules, and petechiae.

⊃ Human monocytic ehrlichiosis is transmitted mainly by the Lone Star tick in the southeastern and south central United States and by other ticks, including the American dog tick, in the western and northwestern United States.

⊃ Human granulocytic ehrlichiosis is transmitted by *Ixodes* ticks—the same ticks that transmit Lyme disease and babesiosis, thus raising the possibility of dual infections. Rash is less common in human granulocytic ehrlichiosis. Some authorities believe that the presence of a rash suggests coinfection with *B. burgdorferi* or another diagnosis (e.g., meningococcemia or Rocky Mountain spotted fever).

⊃ Diagnosis is usually made serologically.

⊃ Doxycycline is the treatment of choice.

SUGGESTED READING

Bakken JS, Dumler JS. Human granulocytic ehrlichiosis. Clin Infect Dis 2000; 31: 554-560.

Fritz CL, Glaser CA. Ehrlichiosis. Infect Dis Clin North Am 1998; 12: 123-136.

Gershel JC. Human granulocytic ehrlichiosis presenting as abdominal pain. Pediatrics 2000; 106: 602-604.

McQuiston JH, Paddock CD, Holman RC, et al. The human ehrlichioses in the United States. Emerg Infect Dis 1999; 5: 635-642.

Ogden NH, Woldehiwet Z, Hart CA. Granulocytic ehrlichiosis: an emerging or rediscovered tick-borne disease? J Med Microbiol 1998; 47: 475-482.

Measles (Rubeola)

Measles is a highly contagious and sometimes life-threatening disease that has become uncommon in the United States since the introduction of live attenuated measles vaccine in 1963.

Presentation and Progression

Cause

The measles virus is a paramyxovirus containing a single strand of DNA. It is transmitted by droplets, by person-to-person contact, or less commonly by airborne spread. The attack rate in a susceptible population can exceed 95%. The virus invades respiratory epithelium and enters the blood, where it resides mainly in monocytes. A secondary viremia, attributed to necrosis of infected reticuloendothelial cells, leads to diffuse involvement of the lungs. Antibodies appear at about the same time as the generalized rash.

Presentation

Typical measles begins with fever, irritability, malaise, conjunctivitis, and evidence of respiratory infection such as a croupy cough. Within several days Koplik's spots—small, raised white or bluish gray lesions that resemble grains of salt or breadcrumbs on an erythematous base—appear on the buccal mucosa opposite the upper premolar and molar teeth. The characteristic nonpruritic maculopapular rash begins on the third or fourth day of illness, starting in the hairline and behind the ears and descending to the trunk and lower extremities. The temperature begins to fall when the rash reaches the distal lower extremities.

Atypical measles occurs in persons who received killed measles vaccine and were later exposed to wild measles virus. In contrast to typical measles, the rash begins peripherally. Also, a variety of rashes are encountered in atypical measles: urticarial, vesicular, or hemorrhagic in addition to more usual maculopapular rash.

Diagnosis

Typical measles is easily diagnosed on clinical grounds by clinicians who have experience with the disease. The sequence of fever, respiratory symptoms, Koplik's spots, and a generalized, nonpruritic maculopapular rash starting in the hairline and moving downward is highly characteristic. However, because the disease is now uncommon (<1000 cases in the United States each year), laboratory confirmation is usually desirable. An IgM ELISA test can be used to confirm the diagnosis; other serologic methods are the demonstration of a rising antibody titer on the basis of acute and convalescent serum and the demonstration of measles virus RNA using a reverse transcriptase PCR assay. Demonstration of multinucleated giant cells in cytologic studies of Koplik's spots or respiratory mucosal cells is highly suggestive of measles. Viral isolation provides the most definitive diagnosis but is technically difficult.

Natural History

Measles is usually a self-limited disease, with most of the symptoms resolving within 7 to 10 days of the onset of fever. Dangerous signs and symptoms include symptomatic pneumonia early in the clinical course, a petechial or hemorrhagic rash, and encephalitis.

Children may become extremely irritable and have febrile convulsions during the initial stage of the illness. In immunocompromised persons life-threatening disease can develop, including measles pneumonia without rash. Otherwise healthy adults with measles are more prone to complications than are children. In one large series 3% of adult military recruits had pneumonia requiring hospitalization, 30% had bacterial superinfection of the respiratory tract, 29% had otitis media, and 31% had abnormal liver function tests. Pregnant women are more susceptible to pneumonia, which can be severe, and are at risk for spontaneous abortion or premature delivery. Unlike rubella, measles does not cause congenital anomalies.

Pneumonia is a relatively common complication, when aggressively sought, but is frequently mild. Primary viral pneumonia (giant cell pneumonia) can lead to respiratory failure and death. Secondary bacterial infections of the respiratory tract are common. Measles suppresses tuberculin reactivity, and it is widely taught that measles worsens the course of tuberculosis. Postmeasles encephalitis occurs in about 1 in 1000 patients with measles, usually during the second week of illness; the mortality is 15%, and many of the survivors have residua. Subacute sclerosing panencephalitis, which occurs as a neurologic disease 7 to 10 years after an episode of measles in a young child (usually <2 years of age), is extremely rare (about 1 in 1 million cases) but uniformly fatal. Keratitis, evidenced as blurred vision, occurs rarely.

Treatment and Prevention
Methods

There is no specific treatment for measles, although large doses of vitamin A (200,000 IU PO daily for 2 days) have been reported to reduce the severity of measles in children. Since death often results from pneumonia, the question arises whether prophylactic antibiotic therapy is useful. The weight of available evidence suggests that antibiotics should be given only if clinical signs of pneumonia or other evidence of sepsis occurs. Immunization is discussed in Chapter 25.

When to Refer

Measles should be reported to health authorities. Patients with severe hemorrhagic disease, measles pneumonia, or measles encephalitis should usually be hospitalized.

 KEY POINTS

MEASLES (RUBEOLA)
⊃ Measles is one of the most highly communicable infectious diseases (attack rate of 95% or greater in susceptible persons).
⊃ After an 8- to 13-day incubation period, typical measles begins with fever and respiratory symptoms followed by the appearance of Koplik's spots and then by a maculopapular rash that starts in the hairline and moves downward toward to the lower extremities.
⊃ Koplik's spots, which are considered pathognomonic of measles, appear on the buccal mucosa opposite the upper molar and premolar teeth as raised white to bluish gray lesions resembling grains of salt on a red base.
⊃ The diagnosis of measles can be confirmed by an IgM ELISA, acute and convalescent serologic tests, or a reverse transcription PCR (RT-PCR) assay for measles virus RNA.
⊃ Atypical measles, which occurs in persons who received killed measles virus vaccine, begins peripherally and can be manifested as a variety of rashes (e.g., vesicular, pustular, or hemorrhagic) in addition to the characteristic maculopapular rash of typical measles.
⊃ Symptoms usually resolve within 7 to 10 days of onset of fever.

⊃ Complications of measles include severe hemorrhagic disease, viral pneumonia (giant cell pneumonia), secondary bacterial infections of the upper and lower respiratory tract, postinfectious encephalitis, subacute sclerosing panencephalitis, and keratitis.

SUGGESTED READING

Duclos P, Redd SC, Varughese P, et al. Measles in adults in Canada and the United States: implications for measles elimination and eradication. Int J Epidemiol 1999; 28: 141-146.

Gremillion DH, Crawford GE. Measles pneumonia in young adults: an analysis of 106 cases. Am J Med 1981; 71: 539-542.

Hersh BS, Tambini G, Nogueira AC, et al. Review of regional measles surveillance data in the Americas, 1996-1999. Lancet 2000; 355: 1943-1948.

Rubella (German Measles)

In 1941 the discovery of the relationship of maternal rubella to congenital anomalies made German measles, a mild exanthem of childhood, a major public concern. Rubella is now vaccine preventable, and therefore all women of childbearing age should know their immune status (see Chapter 5).

Presentation and Progression
Cause

The rubella virus is currently classified as a rubivirus in the Togaviridae family of RNA viruses. It is usually transmitted from infected persons by respiratory droplets. The pathogenesis is believed to resemble that of measles, including both primary and secondary viremias (see earlier discussion). As in measles, the characteristic rash occurs as serum antibodies make their appearance.

Presentation

Rubella in children is usually a mild or even subclinical infection. The disease begins with mild sore throat and conjunctivitis followed by a low-grade fever. The rash appears during the second or third day of the illness, typically starting on the face and moving downward. The rash usually consists of fine macules. Papules are unusual, and petechiae are rare. Petechial lesions (Forschheimer spots) are sometimes found on the soft palate. Cervical lymphadenopathy (posterior auricular, posterior cervical, and suboccipital) can be prominent, and splenomegaly is sometimes detected. Rubella in adults may have a more prominent prodrome with fever, malaise, and anorexia. Arthritis, typically involving the fingers, wrists, and knees, develops in one third of adult women with rubella.

Diagnosis

The clinical features of rubella seldom permit a specific diagnosis in individual patients. Therefore laboratory confirmation is often desirable. The current methods of choice are demonstration of IgM antibodies by ELISA or other methods or demonstration of a four-fold rise in antibody titer. Viral culture permits a specific diagnosis but is expensive and time consuming. In difficult situations, such as diagnosis of congenital rubella (see below), viral RNA can be demonstrated by RT-PCR or other molecular techniques. The presence of IgG antibodies to rubella indicates previous infection or successful immunization.

Natural History

Fever, if present, usually resolves within 24 hours of onset of the rash, and the rash usually begins to clear after 3 to 5 days.

Congenital rubella causes a wide spectrum of transient, permanent, and developmental problems. The severity of the disease correlates inversely with the time during gestation at which infection occurs. Thus infection acquired during the first 2 months of pregnancy carries a 65% to 85% risk of spontaneous abortion or multiple congenital defects. Manifestations of congenital rubella include low birth weight, hepatosplenomegaly, thrombocytopenic purpura, meningoencephalitis, mental retardation, and congenital anomalies such as microcephaly, cataract, retinopathy, patent ductus arteriosus, and pulmonic stenosis. Infants with congenital rubella shed large numbers of viral particles for many months.

Hemorrhagic complications occur in about 1 in 3000 cases of rubella and can be caused by thrombocytopenia, damage to blood vessels, or both. Rubella is thought to be one of the most common infectious causes of thrombocytopenic purpura, which in rare cases is the sole manifestation of the disease.

Encephalitis occurs in about 1 in 5000 cases, more commonly in adults than in children. The case-fatality rate is 20% to 50%, but survivors generally have no permanent residua. Rubella rarely causes mild hepatitis.

Reinfection can occur in persons who have been vaccinated or who have previously had rubella. However, such reinfections are generally mild and have not been conclusively shown to cause viremia sufficient to infect the fetus.

Treatment and Prevention

There is currently no specific treatment. Use of immune globulin for prevention or treatment of rubella during pregnancy has been largely abandoned because it does not seem to prevent viremia. The focus should be on prevention with the highly effective rubella vaccine (see Chapter 25).

When to Refer

When rubella is suspected during pregnancy, referral is often indicated, since diagnosis of congenital rubella in utero may be possible through placental biopsy or other techniques.

 KEY POINTS

RUBELLA (GERMAN MEASLES)
- ⊃ Rubella is a mild exanthem of childhood caused by an RNA virus. The clinical features of rubella are usually much less specific than those of measles. Laboratory confirmation is therefore desirable.
- ⊃ The typical rash consists of fine macules, beginning first on the face and then moving downward. Cervical lymphadenopathy is often prominent, but fever is usually low grade or absent.
- ⊃ Rubella is most conveniently diagnosed by the demonstration of IgM antibodies using ELISA or other methods.

- ⊃ Arthritis, especially of the fingers, wrists, and knees, occurs in up to one third of adult women with rubella.
- ⊃ Congenital rubella is most likely to complicate infection acquired during the first trimester of pregnancy.
- ⊃ Reinfection can occur in persons who have been vaccinated or who have previously had rubella, but such reinfections are generally mild.

SUGGESTED READING

Bar-Oz B, Ford-Jones L, Koren G. Congenital rubella syndrome: how can we do better? Can Fam Physician 1999; 45: 1865-1869.

Danovaro-Holliday MC, LeBaron CW, Allensworth C, et al. A large rubella outbreak with spread from the workplace to the community. JAMA 2000; 284: 2733-2739.

Rosa C. Rubella and rubeola. Semin Perinatol 1998; 22: 318-322.

Webster WS. Teratogen update: congenital rubella. Teratology 1998; 58: 13-23.

Parvovirus B19 (Fifth Disease, Erythema Infectiosum)

Parvovirus B19 causes a characteristic "slapped cheek" rash in children known as erythema infectiosum or fifth disease. Fifth disease is so called because historically the other common childhood exanthems were numbered 1 through 4 as follows: measles, scarlet fever, rubella, and chickenpox (a "sixth disease," roseola infantum or exanthem subitum, was subsequently added). The virus selectively infects red blood cell precursors, which can be disastrous in pregnant women, persons with high red blood cell turnover, and immunosuppressed persons.

Presentation and Progression
Cause

Parvovirus B19 is a tiny (Latin *parvum,* "small") DNA virus that infects mainly if not exclusively human red blood cell precursors. The virus seems to be spread mainly by respiratory transmission and is moderately to highly infectious, with secondary attack rates up to 50% in household contacts. Symptoms and signs of the disease are typically biphasic, reflecting an initial infectious (viremic) phase followed by a convalescent (immune complex–mediated) phase. In experimental studies parvovirus B19 infection has been shown to cause cessation of red blood cell production lasting 4 to 8 days.

Presentation

Parvovirus B19 infection is usually asymptomatic or subclinical. About 50% of persons by age 15, as well as more than 90% of elderly persons, have serologic evidence of past infection, usually without a history of the disease.

In children the disease develops most often between 5 and 14 years of age. In children the illness is characterized by the sequential appearance of (1) a nonspecific prodrome; (2) a nonspecific febrile illness that may include headache, coryza, nausea, and diarrhea; and (3) a striking, bright-red "slapped cheek" facial rash with relative sparing of the area around the mouth (circumoral pallor). Still later, a maculopapular rash develops over the trunk and extremities. Unusual features include a vesicopustular or purpuric rash and intense itching of the soles of the feet and arthralgia.

Adults, who may become infected at a rate of about 1.5% per year, seldom manifest the "slapped check" rash seen in children and are more likely to have arthralgia or frank arthritis—typically a symmetric polyarthralgia or polyarthritis affecting mainly the small joints of the hands and feet. As in rubella, joint symptoms are more common in women. Rashes encountered in adults can be maculopapular, purpuric, or lacy and reticular. Arthralgia or arthritis usually resolves within 3 weeks, but symptoms can persist for several months to even years, causing diagnostic confusion with rheumatoid arthritis.

Infection during pregnancy carries a risk of miscarriage and hydrops fetalis (see Chapter 5).

Severe, life-threatening anemia occurs in immunosuppressed patients and in patients with hemolytic disorders or other causes of "stressed bone marrow." Immunosuppressed patients, including patients with advanced HIV disease, are unable to clear the virus and thus have a sustained shutdown of red blood cell production. Aplastic crisis can develop in persons with increased need for red blood cell production as a result of hemoglobinopathy (e.g., sickle cell disease and thalassemia), hemolytic anemia (e.g., spherocytosis, autoimmune hemolytic anemia, and red blood cell enzymopathies), recent hemorrhage, or severe iron deficiency anemia.

The papular-purpuric gloves and socks syndrome is an unusual manifestation reported mainly in Europe and the Middle East and only rarely in the United States. The clinical features are fever, oral erosions, acral pruritus, edema, and petechiae.

Diagnosis

The diagnosis is usually confirmed by measuring IgM antibodies by ELISA or other methods. Parvovirus DNA can be demonstrated in blood by means of PCR, but positive PCR results in otherwise healthy persons limit the usefulness of this methodology. No convenient method has been developed for direct virus isolation, but the small viral particles can be demonstrated in serum by electron microscopy. IgG antibodies are of little or no diagnostic usefulness because of the high prevalence of such antibodies in normal persons.

Natural History

Parvovirus B19 infection is usually self-limited except in immunocompromised patients. Anecdotal reports suggest a possible association with a wide range of conditions, such as idiopathic (autoimmune) thrombocytopenic purpura, Henoch-Schönlein purpura, aseptic meningitis, encephalitis, brachial plexus neuropathy, myocarditis, hepatitis, and vasculitis. A possible role for parvovirus B19 in connective tissue diseases such as rheumatoid arthritis and systemic lupus erythematosus has been suggested.

Treatment and Prevention
Methods

Aplastic crisis caused by parvovirus B19 infection is treated with IVIG, usually at a dose of 0.4 g/kg for 5 days.

The question sometimes arises whether women in the early months of pregnancy should be excluded from working with children during epidemics of fifth disease. The current consensus is that they should not, based on the low overall risk (estimated to be early fetal loss in about 2 to 6 of every 1000

pregnancies and fetal death from hydrops fetalis in about 2 to 5 of every 10,000 pregnancies).

Expected Response

The response to IVIG is often dramatic.

When to Refer

Patients with severe hematologic manifestations of parvovirus B19 infection sometimes require hospitalization.

KEY POINTS

PARVOVIRUS B19 INFECTION (FIFTH DISEASE; ERYTHEMA INFECTIOSUM)

⊃ Parvovirus B19 infection is caused by a small DNA virus.

⊃ The disease is usually asymptomatic or subclinical; the prevalence of IgG antibodies is about 50% by age 15 and more than 90% among the elderly.

⊃ In children fifth disease is characterized by a bright-red, "slapped cheek" facial rash that develops shortly after a nonspecific febrile illness.

⊃ In adults, especially women, parvovirus B19 infection is often manifested as symmetric polyarthralgia or polyarthritis involving mainly the small joints of the hands and feet and sometimes accompanied by rash that can be maculopapular, purpuric, or lacy and reticular.

⊃ Parvovirus B19 infection in normal persons causes a shutdown of red blood cell production for 4 to 8 days.

⊃ Parvovirus B19 infection during pregnancy, especially during the second trimester, may cause hydrops fetalis or miscarriage. However, the overall risk to pregnant women is low.

⊃ As a cause of severe anemia caused by aplastic crisis, parvovirus B19 should be suspected in patients with advanced HIV disease, immunosuppression from any cause, or increased need for red blood cell production for such reasons as hemolytic anemia or hemoglobinopathy.

⊃ IVIG is the treatment of choice for aplastic crisis caused by parvovirus B19.

SUGGESTED READING

Cherry JD. Parvovirus infections in children and adults. Adv Pediatr 1999; 46: 245-269.

Gilbert GL. Parvovirus B19 infection and its significance in pregnancy. Commun Dis Intell 2000; 24 (Suppl): 69-71.

Miller E, Fairley CK, Cohen BJ, et al. Immediate and long term outcome of human parvovirus B19 infection in pregnancy. Br J Obstet Gynaecol 1998; 105: 174-178.

Smith PT, Landry ML, Carey H, et al. Papular-purpuric gloves and socks syndrome associated with acute parvovirus B19 infection: case report and review. Clin Infect Dis 1998; 27:164-168.

Summary

Some considerations in the differential diagnosis of fever and rash are summarized in Table 7-6.

TABLE 7-6
Some Major Diseases Associated with Fever and Rash

Disease	Morphology of rash	Distribution of rash	Diagnostic method	Treatment
Ecthyma gangrenosum and *Pseudomonas* septicemia	Erythematous to purpuric macules, hemorrhagic vesicles, bullae, nodules, painless ulcers with central necrotic, black eschar	Especially in axillae and anogenital regions	Blood culture; biopsy with tissue culture	Admit to hospital; aminoglycoside plus an antipseudomonal penicillin or antipseudomonal cephalosporin (e.g., ceftazidime or cefepime)
Meningococcemia and purpura fulminans	Petechiae, macules, papules, purpura (may become ecchymotic)	Generalized; especially on lower extremities; neck and face usually spared	Blood culture	Admit to hospital; penicillin G or third-generation cephalosporin (e.g., ceftriaxone)
Vibrio vulnificus infection	Large, hemorrhagic bullae are characteristic; also, cellulitis, lymphangitis	Especially on lower extremities	Blood and wound cultures	Admit to hospital; doxycycline plus ceftazidime; débridement often necessary
Staphylococcal toxic shock syndrome	Scarlatiniform rash (diffuse erythema), strawberry tongue; desquamation late in course	Generalized	Clinical assessment of diagnostic criteria	Admit to hospital; appropriate antibiotic (e.g., nafcillin); supportive care
Staphylococcal scalded skin syndrome	Diffuse, ill-defined erythema with fine sandpaper appearance; peeling of skin; Nikolsky's sign present	Generalized; especially in perineal and periumbilical regions (in neonates) and extremities (in older children)	Blood cultures	Admit to hospital; antistaphylococcal antibiotics (e.g., nafcillin)
Streptococcal toxic shock syndrome	Localized area of cellulitis or necrotizing fasciitis; sometimes generalized erythema as well	Localized or generalized	Clinical assessment; blood cultures; culture of local primary lesion if present; CT scan to evaluate for necrotizing fasciitis	Admit to hospital; penicillin G plus clindamycin
Disseminated candidiasis	Erythematous papules and nodules	Trunk and extremities	Blood and tissue cultures	Admit to hospital; amphotericin B or fluconazole
Stevens-Johnson syndrome	Macules, plaques, target lesions (both typical and atypical), vesicles, bullae, erosions and blisters of mucous membranes	Generalized	Fulfillment of clinical and histopathologic criteria	Admit to hospital; supportive care; discontinuation of unnecessary drugs; antibiotic therapy for *Mycoplasma pneumoniae* if indicated
Toxic epidermal necrolysis	Macules, target lesions, large bullae, severe mucosal erosions	Generalized; especially on trunk and proximal extremities	Fulfillment of clinical and histopathologic criteria	Same as for Stevens-Johnson syndrome
Infective endocarditis	Petechiae, purpura, Osler's nodes, Janeway lesions, splinter hemorrhages	Petechiae and purpura on heels, shoulders, legs, oral mucosa, conjunctivae; Osler's nodes on digits (especially pulps of fingers and toes); Janeway lesions on palms and soles; splinter hemorrhages on nail plates	Blood cultures; echocardiography; clinical presentation	Admit to hospital; appropriate antibiotic therapy

Continued

TABLE 7-6—cont'd
Some Major Diseases Associated with Fever and Rash

Disease	Morphology of rash	Distribution of rash	Diagnostic method	Treatment
Scarlet fever (usually *Streptococcus pyogenes* [group A streptococcus])	Diffuse erythema with punctate elevations ("sandpaper skin"); linear striations (Pastia's lines) of confluent petechiae (which can be demonstrated on arms by applying a tourniquet)	Generalized, with sparing of area around mouth ("circumoral pallor")	Clinical assessment; throat culture; blood cultures	Penicillin
North American blastomycosis	Inflammatory papules and nodules with crusts; hyperkeratotic plaques with central ulceration	Face and extremities	Blood culture; biopsy with tissue culture	Itraconazole or amphotericin B
Histoplasmosis	Ulcers, papules, plaques, purpura, abscesses, nodules, mucosal ulcerations	Generalized	Blood cultures; biopsy and tissue cultures	Itraconazole or amphotericin B
Coccidioidomycosis	Papules, nodules, plaques, ulcers, papulopustules	Head	Blood cultures; biopsy and tissue cultures	Fluconazole or amphotericin B
Cryptococcosis	Papules, plaques, nodules, palpable purpura, cellulitis, pyoderma gangrenosum–like ulcers	Head and neck	Blood and tissue cultures	Amphotericin B
Rocky Mountain spotted fever	Macules, papules; later becomes petechial	Wrists and ankles initially, then palms and soles; finally, centripetal spread to face, trunk, and more proximal aspects of extremities	Four-fold increase in antibody titers between acute and convalescent phases	Doxycycline
Primary HIV infection	Macules, papules, mucocutaneous ulcers, palatal papules	Face, trunk	HIV-1 RNA testing and HIV antibody testing (ELISA)	See Chapter 17
Leptospirosis	Macules, papules, urticaria (wheals), purpura	Trunk	Four-fold increase in antibody titers between acute and convalescent phases	Doxycycline or penicillin G
Disseminated gonococcal infection	Macules, papules, vesicles, and petechiae initially, which may evolve into hemorrhagic vesicopustules	Distal extremities, typically near an involved joint	Blood cultures; biopsy with tissue cultures; cultures of urethra, cervix, rectum, and pharynx	Ceftriaxone
Lyme disease	Macules, papules, erythema chronica migrans	Trunk, lower extremities; classically a single lesion but multiple lesions can be present	Serologic tests 4 to 6 weeks after onset	Doxycycline
Typhoid fever (*Salmonella typhi*)	Slightly raised pink macules that blanch on pressure (rose spots)	Trunk, anteriorly and posteriorly (typically in crops of about 10 to 20 lesions)	Blood cultures; urine and stool cultures; smear and culture of rose spots	Ciprofloxacin, trimethoprim-sulfamethoxazole, or third-generation cephalosporin (ceftriaxone or cefotaxime)

TABLE 7-6—cont'd
Some Major Diseases Associated with Fever and Rash

Disease	Morphology of rash	Distribution of rash	Diagnostic method	Treatment
Mycoplasma pneumoniae infection	Maculopapular or morbilliform rash most common; a variety of rashes can be seen, including urticaria, erythema multiforme (including Stevens-Johnson syndrome), erythema nodosum, and papulovesicular lesions	Variable	Four-fold increase in antibody titers between acute and convalescent phases, or demonstration of high IgM antibody titer	Doxycycline or a macrolide antibiotic (erythromycin, azithromycin, or clarithromycin)
Rat-bite fever caused by *Spirillum minus*	Maculopapular, later becoming petechial	Begins on abdomen; progresses to extremities; may involve palms and soles	Inoculation of blood or wound aspirate into mice or guinea pigs; dark-field examination of bite, rash, or aspirate from lymph node; RPR (VDRL) often false positive (50%)	Penicillin G
Rat-bite fever caused by *Streptobacillus moniliformis*	Maculopapular or petechial	Most extensive on extremities; typically around joints; may become generalized	Blood, wound, or joint fluid cultures; serologic tests may be helpful (four-fold increase in antibody titers between acute and convalescent phases)	Penicillin G
Epidemic typhus	Macules, papules, petechiae	Axillary folds, trunk, extremities (characteristically the face, palms, and soles are spared)	Four-fold increase in antibody titers between acute and convalescent phases	Doxycycline
Murine typhus	Macules, papules, morbilliform rash	Begins on inner surfaces of arms and axillae; quickly becomes generalized, involving especially the trunk (limited involvement of face, palms, and soles)	Four-fold increase in antibody titers between acute and convalescent phases	Doxycycline
Acute rheumatic fever	Macules, erythema marginatum, subcutaneous nodules	Erythema marginatum on trunk, extremities; subcutaneous nodules on extensor surfaces near joints	Fulfillment of Jones criteria	Benzathine penicillin G
Secondary syphilis	Macules, papules, mucous patches, condylomata lata; rash is sometimes pustular	Usually generalized, with involvement of palms and soles; sometimes confined to palms and soles or to face	RPR (VDRL) is nearly always positive in secondary syphilis (in contrast to other stages of syphilis); confirmed by FTA-ABS (or MHA-TP) assays; dark-field microscopy	Benzathine penicillin G

Continued

TABLE 7-6—cont'd
Some Major Diseases Associated with Fever and Rash

Disease	Morphology of rash	Distribution of rash	Diagnostic method	Treatment
Herpes zoster (shingles and disseminated herpes zoster)	Grouped vesicles on an erythematous base; hemorrhagic bullae; in disseminated form, large ulcers and plaques	Shingles has dermatomal distribution; disseminated herpes zoster is generalized	Tzanck smear or direct fluorescent antibody test	Acyclovir
Babesiosis	Petechiae, purpura, ecchymoses	Generalized	Giemsa-stained blood smear or indirect immunofluorescence	Clindamycin and quinine
Ehrlichiosis	Usually, macules and papules; may be petechial; diffuse erythema sometimes seen	Trunk	Four-fold increase in antibody titers between acute and convalescent phases; indirect immunofluorescence	Doxycycline
Kawasaki disease	Erythema (most often, raised, deep red, plaquelike eruption; sometimes morbilliform); swelling of hands and feet; involvement of mucous membranes (dry, fissured lips, strawberry tongue; oropharyngeal erythema; conjunctival suffusion; later, desquamation)	Generalized, especially on trunk and extremities; accentuation in perineal area	Clinical criteria with exclusion of other etiologies	Aspirin; IV immune globulin

CT, Computed tomography; *ELISA,* enzyme-linked immunosorbent assay; *FTA-ABS,* fluorescent treponemal antibody, absorbed; *HIV,* human immunodeficiency virus; *IV,* intravenous; *MHA-TP,* microhemagglutination–*Treponema pallidum; RPR,* rapid plasma reagin; *VDRL,* Venereal Disease Research Laboratory.

8

Fever and Lymphadenopathy

TONYA JAGNEAUX, GEORGE H. KARAM

Fever with lymphadenopathy is a frequent problem in primary care, with many potential causes, including malignancy. Fever and lymphadenopathy with the most common etiologies tend to run a benign course, and a noninvasive, low-cost evaluation that provides an accurate diagnosis is desired. In this chapter we address the more common causes of fever and lymphadenopathy, including appropriate testing, interventions, and treatment to be used depending on the clinical scenario and suspected diagnosis. Both infectious and noninfectious etiologies must be considered (Table 8-1). Tender lymph nodes or nodes >1.5 cm in diameter usually signify a pathologic process—that is, aspiration or biopsy of the node will show clear evidence of disease rather than a nonspecific reactive hyperplasia. Abnormalities in consistency include hard nodes, fluctuant nodes, and firm, rubbery nodes. When a diagnosis is not readily apparent on

the basis of the history, physical examination, and initial laboratory tests (including serologic tests) in a patient with significant lymphadenopathy, lymph node biopsy is frequently appropriate.

Overview of Infectious Causes of Lymphadenopathy

The nature and extent of further evaluation depend on the answers to a handful of questions. Does the patient have an exposure history, for example, to kittens (cat scratch disease), rabbits and other wild animals (tularemia), rosebushes or sphagnum moss (sporotrichosis), ingestion of undercooked venison (toxoplasmosis), or rodents in the southwestern United States (bubonic plague)? What are the associated symptoms and signs? Are skin abnormalities present? Is the lymphadenopathy localized or generalized? Generalized lymphadenopathy suggests one or another of the mononucleosis syndromes or a systemic disease such as tuberculosis, human immunodeficiency virus (HIV) infection, secondary syphilis, toxoplasmosis, or histoplasmosis. Localized lymphadenopathy raises many diagnostic possibilities, depending in part on what node or group of nodes is involved (Table 8-2).

Regional lymphadenopathy often correlates with inoculation of a microorganism through the skin. Lymphangitis—inflammation of lymphatic channels leading to a lymph node group—is sometimes apparent as visible red streaks in the skin. In the United States acute lymphangitis is usually caused by group A streptococci (see Chapter 15). *Staphylococcus aureus* and *Pasteurella multocida* occasionally cause acute lymphangitis with lymphadenopathy. Herpes simplex infection of the fingers (herpetic whitlow) often causes lymphangitis if attempts are made to probe or incise and drain the lesion. Filariasis is an important cause of acute lymphangitis in some developing countries (see Chapter 23). Chronic lymphangitis is more commonly a "lymphocutaneous syndrome" with subcutaneous nodules along the path of the lymphatic channels. The usual causes in the United States are *Sporothrix schenckii* (sporotrichosis) and *Mycobacterium marinum* infection.

Lymphadenopathy involving the head and neck is encountered on a daily basis in primary care. The clinician should identify the lymph node group involved (Figure 8-1). Anterior cervical lymphadenitis commonly results from group A streptococcal pharyngitis and other upper respiratory tract infections. Prominent anterior and posterior cervical lymphadenopathy is often found in infectious mononucleosis caused by the Epstein-Barr virus (EBV). Occipital lymphadenopathy can result from rubella but now is more likely to

TABLE 8-1
Principal Infectious and Noninfectious Causes of Lymphadenopathy in Primary Care*

Category	Causes
INFECTIOUS CAUSES	
Heterophil-positive mononucleosis	Epstein-Barr virus
Heterophil-negative mononucleosis	Cytomegalovirus, toxoplasmosis, human immunodeficiency virus, streptococcal pharyngitis, human herpesviruses 6, 7, and 8, acute hepatitis B, rubella, measles
Lymphocutaneous syndromes	Zoonoses: Lyme disease, tularemia, plague Bacterial lymphadenitis: *Staphylococcus aureus,* streptococci Mycobacterial lymphadenitis: *Mycobacterium tuberculosis,* nontuberculous mycobacteria Cat scratch disease Nodular lymphangitis: sporotrichosis, *Mycobacterium marinum, Nocardia brasiliensis* Sexually transmitted diseases: syphilis, lymphogranuloma venereum, herpes simplex, chancroid
NONINFECTIOUS CAUSES	
Autoimmune and granulomatous disorders	Systemic lupus erythematosus, rheumatoid arthritis, adult Still's disease, sarcoidosis
Hypersensitivity reactions	Drugs (prescription and nonprescription), injecting drug use, serum sickness
Neoplastic disorders	Lymphoma, leukemia, metastatic cancer

*For a comprehensive list of causes of lymphadenopathy, see Habermann TM, Steensma DP. Lymphadenopathy. Mayo Clin Proc 2000; 75: 723-732.

be the result of localized infection of the scalp. Prominent unilateral cervical lymphadenopathy in otherwise healthy young children is sometimes caused by nontuberculous mycobacteria (see Chapter 22). Cervical lymphadenopathy is an important component of Kawasaki disease (see Chapters 4 and 7). Rarely in the United States it can be caused by diphtheria. Preauricular lymphadenopathy is part of Parinaud's oculoglandular syndrome (see later discussion of cat scratch disease). Cervical masses caused by actinomycosis (see Chapter 7), usually ill defined and located over or just below the mandible, can be mistaken for lymphadenopathy. Supraclavicular lymph nodes often have great diagnostic significance even when <1.5 cm in diameter and are the most worrisome in terms of malignancy.

Axillary or epitrochlear lymphadenopathy is usually caused by pyogenic infection of the upper extremities, most often by group A streptococci and less commonly by *S. aureus.* Rarely, infection of the thumb or of the web space between the thumb and index finger can cause subpectoral lymphadenitis, which can in turn causes cellulitis over the lower chest and upper abdomen. The ulceroglandular form of tularemia can cause prominent epitrochlear lymphadenopathy that can be mistaken for cellulitis. Inguinal lymphadenopathy accompanied by a genital ulcer usually indicates a sexually transmitted disease. However, inguinal lymphadenopathy commonly results from pyogenic infection of the lower extremities. Occasionally, infection of the lower extremities, lower abdominal wall, or perineum causes suppurative iliac lymphadenitis, which can lead to a deep abscess adjacent to the psoas and iliac fascia on the posterior peritoneal wall. Early signs of such an abscess, which is usually caused by *S. aureus,* include limp, back pain, hip pain, and fever. Later

findings include fever with systemic toxicity, spasm of the rectus abdominis muscle, and a tightly flexed hip. Diagnosis is usually based on computed tomography, and surgical drainage combined with parenteral antibiotics is the treatment of choice.

In this chapter the major infectious causes of generalized lymphadenopathy precede a review of the infectious causes of regional lymphadenopathy.

SUGGESTED READING

Ellison E, LaPuerta P, Martin SE. Supraclavicular masses: results of a series of 309 cases biopsied by fine needle aspiration. Head Neck 1999; 21: 239-246.

Ferrer R. Lymphadenopathy: differential diagnosis and evaluation. Am Fam Physician 1998; 58: 1313-1320.

Habermann TM, Steensma DP. Lymphadenopathy. Mayo Clin Proc 2000; 75: 723-732.

Karadeniz C, Oguz A, Ezer U, et al. The etiology of peripheral lymphadenopathy in children. Pediatr Hematol Oncol 1999; 16: 525-531.

Kelly CS, Kelly RE Jr. Lymphadenopathy in children. Pediatr Clin North Am 1998; 45: 875-888.

Schlossberg D, Shulman JA. Localized and generalized lymphadenopathy. In: Schlossberg D, Schulman JA. Differential Diagnosis of Infectious Diseases. Baltimore: Williams & Wilkins; 1996: 227-259.

Heterophil-Positive Mononucleosis (Epstein-Barr Virus Mononucleosis)

Infectious mononucleosis is an extremely important disease in primary care. About 80% of cases are caused by EBV. These cases are commonly called heterophil-positive mononucleosis.

TABLE 8-2
Localized and Generalized Lymphadenopathy of Infectious Etiology

Nodal site	Area of drainage	Some principal considerations
Cervical	Oropharynx, upper respiratory tract, scalp, face, ear	Pharyngitis (diverse causes); mycobacterial lymphadenitis (both tuberculosis and nontuberculous mycobacteria); Kawasaki disease; localized infections of the scalp; rubella (occipital lymphadenopathy)
Supraclavicular	Chest, breast, abdomen	Granulomatous diseases including tuberculosis (supraclavicular and scalene lymph nodes often indicate malignancy)
Axillary	Upper extremities, breast	Localized infection of upper extremities; cat scratch disease
Subpectoral	Thumb, web space between thumb and index finger; axillary drainage area	When cellulitis or subpectoral abscess develops, presentation can suggest an intraabdominal infection
Epitrochlear	Fingers (middle, ring, little), medial aspect of hand, ulnar portion of forearm	Localized infection of upper extremities; cat scratch disease; sporotrichosis; herpetic whitlow
Inguinal and femoral	Lower extremities, genital area	Sexually transmitted disease; localized infection of lower extremities
Iliac	Lower abdominal wall; superficial and deep inguinal lymph nodes	Suppurative lymphadenitis with abscess formation, usually caused by *Staphylococcus aureus*; can be difficult to diagnose (see text)
All lymph nodes (generalized lymphadenopathy)	Blood and lymphatic circulatory systems	Heterophil-positive and -negative mononucleosis syndromes; human immunodeficiency virus infection; secondary syphilis; tuberculosis; histoplasmosis; brucellosis; tularemia; measles; dengue

Primary care clinicians should be thoroughly familiar with this disease, including its nuances.

Presentation and Progression
Cause
EBV is a DNA herpesvirus that attaches to receptors on various cells, including B lymphocytes and nasopharyngeal epithelial cells. The virus is transmitted through infected saliva during intimate contact. Incubation time between exposure and development of symptoms is usually about 1 month. Transmission has been reported after blood transfusion and after cardiopulmonary bypass, although cytomegalovirus rather than EBV is the usual cause of mononucleosis in these settings. About 50% of children in the United States become infected by 5 years of age and thereby acquire immunity. Seroconversion occurs more often among individuals of lower socioeconomic status and is more common in the southern United States than in other parts of the country. Patients of higher socioeconomic status and background tend to be exposed later in adolescence and young adulthood and therefore are more likely to have the full spectrum of symptoms.

Presentation
EBV infection is often subclinical. Clinical manifestations tend to be age dependent. Children are often asymptomatic and

rarely present the entire syndrome of infectious mononucleosis. They more commonly have mild pharyngitis or upper respiratory tract infection. Adolescents and young adults are the usual patients with the full-blown syndrome of infectious mononucleosis. In patients over 40 years of age, EBV is uncommonly diagnosed. This is partly explained by immunity, since about 90% to 95% of older adults have EBV antibodies. However, older patients with documented EBV infection are less likely than younger patients to present the classic symptoms of mononucleosis. Older patients are more likely to have fever, without lymphadenopathy or pharyngitis. They also have a higher frequency of hematologic and hepatic enzyme abnormalities, making the diagnosis more challenging and often prompting an extensive workup without consideration of EBV. Thus EBV mononucleosis should be considered in an adult with unexplained fever.

The syndrome of mononucleosis is characterized by fever, lymphadenopathy (about 94% of cases), pharyngitis (84%), splenomegaly (52%), a transient appearance of heterophil antibodies, and an atypical lymphocytosis. The classic distribution of lymphadenopathy is bilateral in the posterior cervical chains but may also include the anterior and submandibular chains. Patients typically manifest symptoms of headache, fatigue, malaise, and abdominal discomfort or full-

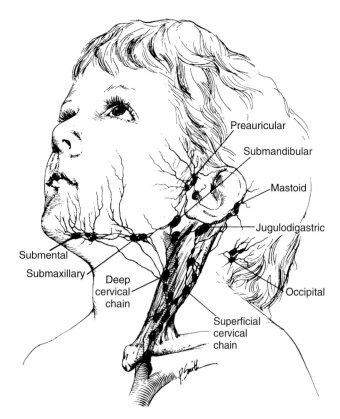

FIG. 8-1 Lymphatic drainage and lymph nodes of the head and neck. (From Butler KM, Baker CJ. Cervical lymphadenitis. In: Feigin RD, Cherry JD, eds. Textbook of Pediatric Infectious Diseases. 3rd ed., Philadelphia: W.B. Saunders Company; 1992; vol 3: 221.)

ness. Signs include enlarged tonsils with exudate, splenomegaly (52%), and hepatomegaly (12%). Palatal petechiae, unrelated to thrombocytopenia, are found in 25% to 60% of patients. A rash is present in about 5% of patients. The rash can be macular, petechial, or urticarial and can also resemble scarlet fever or erythema multiforme. A distinctive maculopapular exanthem frequently develops in patients who are treated with ampicillin or amoxicillin. The etiology of the rash is not clear, but it is not associated with an allergy to the β-lactam antibiotics administered. The predictability of this "ampicillin rash" in mononucleosis is such that it has been proposed (tongue-in-cheek) as a diagnostic test for the disease. Two- to three-fold elevations in levels of the hepatic aminotransferases (alanine aminotransferase [ALT] and aspartate aminotransferase [AST]) occur in 20% to 90% of cases, and they peak in weeks 2 to 3 of the illness.

Diagnosis

Patients with suspected infectious mononucleosis should have a complete blood count with peripheral smear and differential to assess for a lymphocytosis with atypical lymphocytes. The Monospot test identifies heterophil antibodies characteristic of an EBV infection. It carries a sensitivity of 70% to 92% and a specificity of 96% to 100%. Rarely the Monospot test is false positive in patients with lymphoma, hepatitis, or autoimmune disease. Positive Monospot tests were recently described in patients with the acute retroviral syndrome caused by HIV (discussed later in the chapter and also in Chapter 17). When the Monospot test is negative in a patient with suspected EBV virus mononucleosis, as occurs in about 10% of patients, more spe-

cific antibody testing may be indicated. Appropriate tests include assays for antibodies to viral capsid antigen IgG (VCA IgG), viral capsid antigen IgM (VCA IgM), and anti-EBV nuclear antigen (EBNA IgG) (Table 8-3). A positive VCA IgG and VCA IgM with a negative EBNA IgG are most indicative of an acute infection. Methods to detect and even quantify viral DNA in blood and tissues have also been developed but are seldom necessary in daily clinical practice.

Natural History
Expected Outcome

For the majority of affected persons infectious mononucleosis is a self-limited illness with no complications that resolves without therapy over a 2- to 3-week period.

Upper airway obstruction from massively enlarged tonsils occurs rarely and is probably the most common indication for admission to the hospital. Corticosteroids can prevent the need for emergency intubation. Spontaneous and trauma-induced splenic rupture occurs in 0.2% of cases, typically within the first 21 days of illness and most often during the second or third week. Rupture of the spleen should be suspected when abdominal pain, which may be insidious or sudden in onset, develops in a patient with mononucleosis. The course may rarely be complicated by antibody-mediated thrombocytopenia, neutropenia, and hemolytic anemia. Although rare in adults, fulminant hepatitis and encephalitis caused by a host immune response have been reported. Late and rare complications that are associated with EBV include lymphoproliferative disorders and malignancies such as Burkitt's lymphoma, Hodgkin's disease, and nasopharyngeal carcinoma.

A problem in primary care concerns patients with persistent fatigue and other constitutional symptoms after infectious mononucleosis. As is well known, some patients experience debilitating fatigue that can interfere with normal daily activities, including schoolwork. Nearly all patients make a full recovery over weeks to several months. In a recent study, baseline predictors for failure to recover at 6 months included female sex, a greater number of life events >6 months before the onset of EBV infection, and greater family support. The case definition of "chronic fatigue syndrome" (see Chapter 18) takes into account the common observation that some patients with infectious mononucleosis have a prolonged "postinfectious asthenia," which, however, nearly always resolves within 6 months. The idea that serologic markers for EBV, such as antibodies to EBV early antigens, are useful in the diagnosis of chronic fatigue syndrome has generally fallen into disrepute.

Treatment

Supportive care is the mainstay of therapy. Nonsteroidal antiinflammatory drugs or aspirin may be suggested for symptomatic relief of fever and myalgias. Rest and adequate hydration are also recommended, but strict bed rest is unnecessary. Athletically active patients should be counseled to avoid contact sports for 1 month after disease onset and longer if splenomegaly persists.

Corticosteroids are recommended for certain complications, including impending airway obstruction caused by tonsillar enlargement, severe thrombocytopenia, and severe hemolytic anemia. They may play a role in central nervous system involvement, myocarditis, and pericarditis. Antiviral therapy has no role in treatment of immunocompetent patients.

TABLE 8-3
Serologic tests for Infectious Mononucleosis Caused by Epstein-Barr Virus

Antibody test	Prevalence during course of EBV mononucleosis (%)	Time and duration of presence of antibodies in serum	Comments
Heterophil (Monospot)	90 to 95	Usually at clinical presentation; persist several weeks	May be false negative and rarely false positive; delayed appearance of heterophil antibodies correlates with more prolonged convalescence
IgM VCA	~100	At clinical presentation; persist 4 to 8 weeks	This test is extremely useful when diagnosis is in doubt or heterophil test is suspected to be false negative or false positive
IgG VCA	~100	Usually at clinical presentation; persist lifelong	Typically, peak titers occur near time of clinical presentation, so a four-fold rise can be demonstrated in only 10% to 20% of cases; more useful as a marker of past EBV infection
Anti-D early antigen	70	Peak 3 to 4 weeks after onset and persist 3 to 6 months	Patients with positive results tend to have more severe disease; found in patients with nasopharyngeal carcinoma attributed to EBV
Anti-R early antigen	Low	Appear about 2 weeks after onset; persist 2 months to >3 years	Patients with positive results tend to have unusually severe disease; found in patients with African Burkitt's lymphoma
EBV nuclear antigen	~100	Appear 3 to 4 weeks after onset; persist lifelong	Useful for diagnosis of heterophil-negative patients, especially when seen late in the illness
Anti-S (soluble complement-fixing antigens)	~100	Appear 3 to 4 weeks after onset; persist lifelong	

Modified from Schooley RT. Epstein-Barr virus (infectious mononucleosis). In: Mandell GL, Bennett JE, Dolin R, eds. Mandell, Douglas, and Bennett's Principles and Practice of Infectious Diseases. 5th ed., Philadelphia: Churchill Livingstone; 2000: 1599-1613.
EBV, Epstein-Barr virus.

When to Refer

Hospitalization is indicated for airway obstruction and splenic rupture. Specialist referral should be considered for complications of severe hematologic, myocardial, or nervous system involvement.

 KEY POINTS

HETEROPHIL-POSITIVE MONONUCLEOSIS (EPSTEIN-BARR VIRUS MONONUCLEOSIS)

⊃ The mononucleosis syndrome includes fever, pharyngitis, atypical lymphocytosis, and transient appearance of heterophil antibodies. Asymptomatic elevation of aminotransferases (AST, ALT) occurs in up to 90% of cases.

⊃ The Monospot test has a sensitivity of 70% to 92% and a specificity of 96% to 100%. When the Monospot test is negative, detection of antibodies to the viral capsid antigen (IgM VCA) can be extremely useful.

⊃ False-positive Monospot tests occur occasionally in such conditions as lymphoma, hepatitis, autoimmune disease, and the acute retroviral syndrome caused by HIV.

⊃ Complications that may require steroid therapy include airway obstruction, thrombocytopenia, and hemolytic anemia.

⊃ Rupture of the spleen, spontaneous or caused by trauma, should be suspected when abdominal pain develops in a patient with mononucleosis. Patients with mononucleosis should avoid contact sports until lymphadenopathy has subsided.

SUGGESTED READING

Auwaerter, PG. Infectious mononucleosis in middle age. JAMA 1999; 281: 454-459.

Bailey RE. Diagnosis and treatment of infectious mononucleosis. Am Fam Physician 1994; 281: 454-459.

Borer A, Gilad J, Haikin H, et al. Clinical features and costs of care for hospitalized adults with primary Epstein-Barr virus infection. Am J Med 1999; 107: 144-148.

Buchwald DS, Rea TD, Katon WJ, et al. Acute infectious mononucleosis: characteristics of patients who report failure to recover. Am J Med 2000; 109: 531-537.

Vidrih JA, Walensky RP, Sax PE, et al. Positive Epstein-Barr virus heterophile antibody tests in patients with primary human immunodeficiency virus infection. AM J Med 2001; 111: 192-194.

Heterophil-Negative Mononucleosis Syndromes: An Overview

Although it is thought that about 80% of mononucleosis cases are due to EBV, heterophil-negative mononucleosis has a number of causes (Table 8-1). Cytomegalovirus (CMV) accounts for a significant percentage of these cases, and toxoplasmosis also causes mononucleosis, although far less commonly. Several other disease syndromes can mimic the presentation of infectious mononucleosis. These include primary HIV infection, streptococcal pharyngitis, acute hepatitis B, and human herpesvirus 6 and 7 infections. Because of its relevance and impact on patient management, primary human immunodeficiency virus (HIV) infection will be discussed separately.

Cytomegalovirus Mononucleosis

CMV, the largest virus known to affect humans, was found to cause heterophil-negative mononucleosis in 1965 and is now considered the major cause of this syndrome. Patients with CMV mononucleosis tend to be older than those with EBV mononucleosis, with a median age in the thirties. CMV mononucleosis is an important cause of fever of unclear origin, especially in young adults.

Presentation and Progression
Cause

The human cytomegalovirus is a DNA virus of the human herpesvirus group. The virus is transmitted mainly by kissing, other forms of intimate contact, blood transfusion, and organ transplantation. In the United States 60% to 70% of adults eventually become infected. In some developing countries nearly 100% of persons become infected. Like other herpesviruses, CMV establishes latent virus infection after clinical recovery.

Presentation

Most cases of CMV infection are asymptomatic. The mononucleosis syndrome caused by CMV has several distinct features. Compared with heterophil-positive mononucleosis caused by EBV, CMV causes a more protracted febrile illness but less prominent pharyngitis and lymphadenopathy. CMV mononucleosis can occur as an undifferentiated "typhoidal" illness with few if any localizing manifestations. Pharyngeal exudates are uncommon. Mild maculopapular and rubella-like rashes sometimes occur. Rash is especially likely to develop in patients given ampicillin or amoxicillin.

Laboratory studies usually reveal relative lymphocytosis (>50% lymphocytes on differential blood count, of which 10% or more are atypical lymphocytes). Mild elevation of aminotransferase (AST, ALT) levels is common.

Diagnosis

Definitive diagnosis of CMV as the etiology of mononucleosis is difficult. CMV blood and urine cultures can be obtained but can identify only infection, not disease. A demonstration of a four-fold rise in complement fixation titers from acute to convalescent phases of the illness is accepted as diagnostic; however, this also occurs in asymptomatic individuals. The presence of CMV IgM is a more sensitive test for diagnosis than complement fixation but is less specific because these antibodies cross-react with acute EBV infection and the test remains positive for up to 6 months after the illness. A PCR assay for CMV DNA is proving extremely useful for diagnosis

and management of CMV disease in immunocompromised patients, including those with advanced HIV disease, but this method is seldom used in the diagnosis of CMV mononucleosis. With the appropriate clinical presentation and positive serologic tests, the assumption of CMV-induced mononucleosis can be made. Follow-up observation is necessary to ensure resolution of signs and symptoms.

Natural History

Patients with CMV mononucleosis generally recover uneventfully. Protracted fevers may occur. Occasionally, severe complications develop. These include interstitial pneumonia, clinical hepatitis with nausea and vomiting and granulomas on liver biopsy, meningoencephalitis, and myocarditis. Rarely, Guillain-Barré syndrome complicates CMV infection. In one series nearly 10% cases of Guillain-Barré syndrome were associated with CMV. Severe epidermolysis has been reported. CMV causes severe disease in patients with advanced HIV disease (see Chapter 17), is a major problem after organ transplantation (see Chapter 3), and is of concern in pregnancy because of its potential to cause fetal abnormalities (see Chapter 5).

Treatment
Methods

Antiviral drug therapy for CMV mononucleosis is seldom if ever indicated. Ganciclovir, foscarnet, and cidofovir are available for treatment of severe manifestations of CMV disease (see Chapter 20).

When to Refer

Referral in cases of CMV mononucleosis is indicated only for the rare patient with severe complications.

 KEY POINTS

CYTOMEGALOVIRUS MONONUCLEOSIS
- Heterophil-negative mononucleosis may be caused by CMV, a large DNA herpesvirus.
- Compared with heterophil-positive (EBV) mononucleosis, CMV mononucleosis is associated more with prominent and prolonged fever but less prominent exudates, pharyngitis, and lymphadenopathy.
- CMV mononucleosis is sometimes the reason for unexplained fever in otherwise healthy-appearing persons.
- Demonstration of IgM antibodies to CMV is the most cost-effective confirmatory diagnostic test. However, some cross-reactivity occurs with EBV mononucleosis, and IgM antibodies can remain persent for 6 months or longer.

SUGGESTED READING

Deyi YM, Goubau P, Bodeus M. False-positive IgM antibody tests for cytomegalovirus in patients with acute Epstein-Barr virus infection. Eur J Clin Microbiol Infect Dis 2000; 19: 557-560.

Ho M. Cytomegalovirus: Biology and Infection. 2nd ed., New York: Plenum; 1991.

Horwitz CA, Henle W, Henle G, et al. Clinical and laboratory evaluation of cytomegalovirus-induced mononucleosis in previously healthy individuals. Medicine (Baltimore) 1986; 65: 124-134.

Kano Y, Shiohara T. Current understanding of cytomegalovirus infection in immunocompetent individuals. J Dermatol Sci 2000; 22: 196-204.

Acute Retroviral Syndrome (Primary Human Immunodeficiency Virus Infection)

HIV, the cause of acquired immunodeficiency syndrome (AIDS), produces a syndrome resembling infectious mononucleosis in about 50% to 60% of patients between 1 and 6 weeks after exposure and initial infection.

Presentation and Progression
Cause

HIV transmission occurs via sexual intercourse, injecting drug use, or exposure to contaminated blood products. Common signs noted on examination include orthostatic hypotension, exanthems (see Chapter 7), pharyngitis, aphthous ulcers, exudative pharyngitis, thrush, lymphadenopathy, hepatosplenomegaly, genital and rectal ulcers, and neuropathy. The distribution of the lymphadenopathy is typically occipital, cervical, and axillary in location. Laboratory evaluation may reveal lymphopenia, lymphocytosis, atypical lymphocytes, elevated sedimentation rate, a negative Monospot test, elevated aminotransferase levels, and an elevated alkaline phosphatase level.

A high index of suspicion with attention to possible exposures is crucial to making the correct diagnosis. During acute infection a quantitative plasma HIV-RNA assay, with use of either polymerase chain reaction (PCR) or branched DNA (bDNA), has become the test of choice for diagnosis, with a sensitivity of 100% and specificity of 97% (occasional false-positive results occur). Antibody testing should be performed also with the understanding that seroconversion, detected by enzyme-linked immunosorbent assay (ELISA) and Western blot test, typically does not occur until 6 to 12 weeks after virus acquisition. However, having a negative baseline antibody test and later repeating the test confirms the time of seroconversion, and a positive antibody assay confirms the diagnosis. It is during this period before seroconversion that circulating virus is present in especially high titer.

Persistent generalized lymphadenopathy (PGL) may occur in 50% to 70% of HIV-infected individuals who have acute retroviral syndrome. PGL refers to lymphadenopathy present in two or more noncontiguous sites for greater than 3 to 6 months. Lymph node enlargement is thought to be caused by viral replication within the follicular cells of the node. Biopsy typically demonstrates follicular hyperplasia without evidence of organisms. The remainder of the patients enter the stage of clinical latent infection and remain asymptomatic for years. This period is followed by the stages of early symptomatic HIV, AIDS, and advanced HIV infection. Rapidly enlarging nodes and localized lymphadenopathy are not characteristic of HIV infection alone and should prompt an evaluation for another process of infection or malignancy. This evaluation should include a search for opportunistic pathogens. Fine-needle aspiration may be useful for diagnosing infection and should include Gram staining, cytopathologic tests, and acid-fast bacillus stains with culture. Occasionally with otherwise unexplained lymphadenopathy, lymph node biopsy is indicated to rule out lymphoma.

 KEY POINTS

ACUTE RETROVIRAL SYNDROME (PRIMARY HUMAN IMMUNODEFICIENCY VIRUS INFECTION)

⊃ Signs and symptoms of acute retroviral syndrome, which overlap with those of infectious mononucleosis, occur in more than half of patients newly infected with HIV.

⊃ The test of choice for diagnosis is the quantitative plasma HIV-RNA assay. Patients are highly infectious during the first few weeks after becoming infected because of high levels of viremia.

⊃ Primary antiretroviral therapy may be indicated (see Chapter 17), and referral to an infectious disease specialist should be considered.

SUGGESTED READING
Daar ES, Little S, Pitt J. Diagnosis of primary HIV-1 infection. Ann Intern Med 2001; 134: 25-29.

Schacker T, Collier AC, Hughes J, et al. Clinical and epidemiologic features of primary HIV infection. Ann Intern Med 1996: 125: 257-264.

Causes of Heterophil-Negative Mononucleosis Other Than Cytomegalovirus and Human Immunodeficiency Virus, Including Toxoplasmosis

The list of diseases that occasionally cause heterophil-negative mononucleosis continues to expand.

Presentation and Progression

Toxoplasma gondii is a common infectious agent that does not cause symptoms in most immunocompetent individuals. It is a rare cause of heterophil-negative mononucleosis characterized by a self-limited illness of fatigue, lymphadenopathy, and fever. Streptococcal pharyngitis, acute hepatitis B, rubella, and measles have signs and symptoms that overlap with the presentation of EBV and are discussed on that basis. Evidence suggests that several of the more recently identified human herpesviruses, known as HHV-6, HHV-7, and HHV-8, may cause a heterophil-negative mononucleosis syndrome. With HHV-6, patients have either four-fold rises in antibody titer or the presence of HHV-6 IgM. With HHV-7, patients have fever, pancytopenia, and hepatosplenomegaly, and the virus may be isolated. HHV-8 may also manifest itself as a mononucleosis syndrome, particularly in immunocompromised patients. It has been described as the cause of Castleman's disease, a lymphoproliferative illness with associated fever, hepatosplenomegaly, and impressive lymphadenopathy.

Presentation

With toxoplasmosis (see Chapter 23), lymphadenopathy is the predominant finding and can be regional or generalized without suppuration or ulceration. Pharyngitis and significant fevers are less common. Atypical lymphocytosis, if present, is typically mild. The lymphadenopathy that is present can persist or occur intermittently for up to a year. It is for this reason that a diagnosis of this self-limited illness is pursued.

About 10% to 20% of patients with acute hepatitis B virus infection have a serum sickness syndrome that lasts up to 2 weeks. Symptoms may include fever, rash, generalized lymphadenopathy, and arthralgias. Although elevations of aminotransferase levels are usually mild in mononucleosis, hepatitis B–related mononucleosis is associated with elevations up to 1000 to 2000 IU/L and hyperbilirubinemia.

Vaccination has reduced the incidence of rubella and measles. However, both can cause fever, rash, malaise, and an associated cervical lymphadenopathy. Their characteristic rashes begin on the face and progress down the body. Rubella can also be associated with splenomegaly, arthritis, thrombocytopenia, and hepatitis. Measles is typically associated with conjunctivitis, respiratory symptoms, and pathognomonic Koplik's spots (which have a bluish gray speck centered on an erythematous base).

Diagnosis

Patients with heterophil-negative mononucleosis syndromes should have a serum specimen drawn during the active course of their illness. The benefit of obtaining acute and convalescent serum is to potentially avoid lymph node biopsy when nodal enlargement persists for weeks or months. Patients' sera can be kept on reserve after it has been obtained during their acute illness, and when lymphadenopathy fails to resolve quickly, additional serologic studies can be sent along with a convalescent sample to confirm the etiology of a heterophil-negative mononucleosis syndrome.

The Sabin-Feldman dye test has been the traditional serologic method for diagnosis of toxoplasmosis. In recent years it has been largely replaced by the ELISA tests for IgG and IgM antibodies. In patients with lymphadenopathy caused by toxoplasmosis, IgM antibodies are usually present if the serum was obtained within 3 months of onset of symptoms. When the test for IgM antibodies yields equivocal, low-positive, or negative results, the diagnosis can be made by demonstrating IgG or IgA antibodies or by showing an acute pattern of response in a differential agglutination test. Use of this approach was found to be 100% sensitive for diagnosis of toxoplasmic lymphadenitis in one study.

If confirmation of diagnosis is not obtained, lymph node biopsy may reasonably be performed and usually reveals characteristic histologic features.

Natural History
Expected Outcome

Toxoplasmosis can be associated with persistent lymphadenopathy. Some patients with acute hepatitis B become chronic carriers of the virus and may be at risk for cirrhosis and hepatocellular carcinoma (see Chapter 13). The other diseases discussed here are usually self-limited.

Only supportive therapy is required for CMV, toxoplasmosis, hepatitis B, measles, and rubella, since they are self-limited diseases. The decision to initiate antibiotic therapy is based on isolating group A streptococci as the cause of the clinical presentation (see "Streptococcal Pharyngitis" in Chapter 10).

Complications

Toxoplasma has been implicated in chorioretinitis, pneumonitis, hepatitis, myocarditis, and myositis. Untreated streptococcal pharyngitis can result in acute rheumatic fever or, uncommonly, acute glomerulonephritis.

When to Refer

Referral in cases of heterophil-negative mononucleosis syndrome is necessary only for complications.

 KEY POINTS

CAUSES OF HETEROPHIL-NEGATIVE MONONUCLEOSIS OTHER THAN CYTOMEGALOVIRUS AND HUMAN IMMUNODEFICIENCY VIRUS INFECTION

➲ When a patient has what appears to be a mononucleosis syndrome or unexplained lymphadenopathy, obtaining a serum sample in the acute phase is good practice. This can later be compared with a convalescent serum sample to secure a diagnosis and avoid the necessity of lymph node biopsy.

➲ Toxoplasmosis occasionally causes a heterophil-negative mononucleosis. The predominant finding is lymphadenopathy. The diagnosis can nearly always be made on the basis of serologic demonstration of IgM antibodies in a specimen drawn within 3 months of onset of symptoms.

➲ Other causes of heterophil-negative mononucleosis include acute hepatitis B, rubella, measles, and infection by herpesvirus (HHV-6, HHV-7, or HHV-8).

SUGGESTED READING

Montoya JG, Remington JS. Studies on the serodiagnosis of toxoplasmic lymphadenitis. Clin Infect Dis 1995; 20: 781-789.
Zaharopoulos P. Demonstration of parasites in toxoplasma lymphadenitis by fine-needle aspiration cytology: report of two cases. Diagn Cytopathol 2000; 22: 11-15.

Lymphocutaneous Syndromes: Overview

The lymphocutaneous syndromes comprise multiple causes of lymphadenopathy that is typically localized with concurrent skin lesions or sites of inoculation. Key points in the history include inquiring about exposure, travel, and risk-related behavior. The physical examination should focus especially on the groups of nodes involved and the presence of skin lesions. Additional diagnostic testing and biopsy procedures may be indicated, and the need for them is based on the working diagnosis as determined by the presentation.

Cat Scratch Disease

Cat scratch disease is a slowly progressive, usually self-limited regional lymphadenitis that occurs mainly in children. History of contact with a cat, usually a kitten or a feral cat, is obtained in about 90% of cases. Some 25,000 cases occur in the United States each year, making cat scratch disease an important condition in primary care. The disease is usually benign, but serious complications can occur.

Presentation and Progression
Cause

Most cases are now attributed to *Bartonella henselae*, a slow-growing, fastidious gram-negative rod. Rare cases have been associated with other *Bartonella* species. *B. henselae* occurs in domestic and feral cats worldwide, especially in warmer climates. Asymptomatic bacteremia with *B. henselae* occurs in otherwise healthy cats. Cat-to-cat transmission takes place by way of the cat flea, *Ctenocephalides felis.* There is little or no evidence that the flea transmits the disease to humans. However, flea feces containing *B. henselae* can contaminate the claws of cats, which explains transmission by cat scratches. *B. henselae* has been linked not only to cat scratch disease but also to bacillary angiomatosis and visceral peliosis (conditions seen mainly in HIV-infected patients) and to cases of septicemia and endocarditis.

Presentation

Patients with cat scratch disease usually have tender, occasionally suppurative lymphadenopathy, typically in the cervical or axillary region. A single lymph node is involved in about one half of patients with "typical" cat scratch disease. The others have involvement of multiple nodes in a single node-bearing region or, in about one fifth of patients, lymphadenopathy at multiple sites. Additional history includes fever, malaise, and exposure to a cat, particularly a kitten, within the previous 3 to 10 days. The exposure may be subclinical without the patient's recollection of being bitten or scratched. Skin lesions from the actual encounter may be present, as well as symptoms of fever and malaise. Lesions appear as erythematous nodules or papules. Vesiculation, ulceration, and pustule formation can occur.

About 12% of cases are "atypical." Of these, about one half are Parinaud's oculoglandular syndrome. This is defined as granulomatous conjunctivitis with preauricular lymphadenitis. Other patients may have atypical pneumonia, granulomatous hepatitis, prolonged fever of unknown origin (described in children), encephalopathy, neuroretinitis, or osteomyelitis. Encephalopathy caused by *B. henselae* occurs rarely before the onset of lymphadenopathy and even in its absence. Clinical features include headache, restlessness, combativeness, seizures, stupor, coma, and focal neurologic signs. Most patients with encephalopathy have made a full recovery. Neuroretinitis caused by *B. henselae* usually manifests itself as acute or subacute unilateral loss of vision. Funduscopic examination reveals papilledema with stellate (star-shaped) macular exudates.

Diagnosis

The diagnosis is strongly suggested by the typical presentation of regional lymphadenopathy with a history of exposure to a young cat. Aspiration and drainage of the involved nodes may be both therapeutic and diagnostic; however, the organism is not easily isolated in culture or reliably identified through serologic testing. A positive antibody response to *B. henselae,* positive results of a Warthin-Starry stain of tissues, and a positive PCR assay all support the diagnosis in the appropriate clinical setting. Newer assays for detecting IgM and IgG antibodies to *B. henselae* are reported to have up to 95% sensitivity and 98% specificity, and thus serology has become the confirmatory method of choice. If cultures are performed, communication with laboratory personnel before submission of blood or tissue culture specimens is recommended to achieve the optimum diagnostic yield. A PCR assay for *B. henselae* DNA has been developed.

Natural History
Expected Outcome

The majority of patients recover uneventfully, with lymphadenopathy persisting as long as 2 to 4 months. The most common severe complication is encephalopathy, which by various estimates occurs in 1% to 7% of cases and more commonly in adults and adolescents than in young children. The natural history of cat scratch disease and the full extent of its complications will be no doubt be defined more clearly with the availability of convenient serologic methods of diagnosis.

Treatment

The benefit of antibiotic therapy for "typical" cat scratch disease is unclear. If therapy is to be prescribed, a 5-day course of azithromycin is recommended. Additional agents that have been shown to be effective are ciprofloxacin, rifampin, trimethoprim-sulfamethoxazole (TMP/SMX), and gentamicin. Some patients benefit from incision and drainage of fluctuant nodes.

Expected Response

Azithromycin was shown to shorten the duration of typical cat scratch disease in a placebo-controlled study. Treatment of "atypical" cat scratch disease has not been standardized.

When to Refer

Referral is needed only for patients with "atypical" cat scratch disease manifested by such complications as encephalopathy, prolonged fever, granulomatous hepatitis, or neuroretinitis.

 KEY POINTS

CAT SCRATCH DISEASE
⤳ Cat scratch disease is a slowly progressive regional lymphadenitis caused by *B. henselae.*
⤳ Diagnosis can now be confirmed by measuring IgM and IgG antibodies to *B. henselae.*
⤳ The disease is usually self-limited. Encephalopathy occurs in 1% to 7% of cases. Other complications are neuroretinitis and granulomatous hepatitis.
⤳ Azithromycin may shorten the duration of "typical" cat scratch disease, but treatment is usually unnecessary.

SUGGESTED READING
Adal KA, Cockerell CJ, Petri WA. Cat scratch disease, bacillary angiomatosis, and other infections due to *Rochalimaea.* N Engl J Med 1994; 330: 1509-1515.

Arisoy EV, Correa AG, Wagner ML, et al. Hepatosplenic cat-scratch disease in children: selected clinical features and treatment. Clin Infect Dis 1999; 28: 778-784.

Bass JW, Freitas BD, Freiter AD, et al. Prospective randomized double blind placebo-controlled evaluation of azithromycin for treatment of cat-scratch disease. Pediatr Infect Dis J 1998; 17: 447-452.

Hulzebos CV, Koetse HA, Kimpen JL, et al. Vertebral osteomyelitis associated with cat-scratch disease. Clin Infect Dis 1999; 28: 1310-1312.

Margileth AM. Antibiotic therapy for cat scratch disease: clinical study of therapeutic outcome in 268 patients and a review of the literature. Pediatr Infect Dis J 1992; 11: 474-478.

Ormerod LD, Skolnick KA, Menosky MM, et al. Retinal and choroidal manifestations of cat-scratch disease. Ophthalmology 1998; 105: 1024-1031.

Smith DL. Cat-scratch disease and related clinical syndromes. Am Fam Physician 1997; 55: 1783-1789, 1793-1794.

Sexually Transmitted Diseases Manifested as Lymphadenopathy

Sexually transmitted diseases should be considered in the diagnosis when inguinal lymphadenopathy is present. In primary syphilis, lymphadenopathy is localized to the area near the chancre. Secondary syphilis occurs approximately 6 to 8 weeks after the initial lesion developed in the primary stage. Approximately half of patients untreated during the primary stage have fever, generalized lymphadenopathy (including the epitrochlear nodes), rash, and mucocutaneous lesions that are highly infectious. Lymphogranuloma venereum causes unilateral, tender inguinal and femoral lymphadenopathy. The inelastic inguinal (Poupart's) ligament runs between the femoral and inguinal nodal chains. When these nodes become infected and enlarged, the indentation resulting from the ligament is known as the groove sign. The nodes may also suppurate and drain spontaneously. Herpes simplex is now the most common cause of genital ulceration in the United States. The lesions are tender and initially appear as vesicles, grouped on an erythematous base. They subsequently erode and crust over. The associated lymphadenopathy may also be mildly tender. Chancroid lesions tend to be painful and friable with ragged undermined borders. Gray-yellow necrotic exudates typically cover the ulceration. The associated lymphadenopathy is suppurative, and spontaneous drainage can occur, leaving deep inguinal ulcers. Infection with *H. ducreyi* has been closely associated with coinfection of syphilis, and chancroid ulcers are considered a cofactor in HIV transmission.

Diagnosis and treatment are discussed in Chapter 16.

Bacterial and Mycobacterial Lymphadenitis

Both acute bacterial lymphadenitis and mycobacterial lymphadenitis are more common in children than in adults, but they should be considered as causes of regional lymphadenopathy in patients of all age groups.

Presentation and Progression
Causes

Acute bacterial lymphadenitis is usually related to a localized skin or soft tissue infection, most commonly caused by staphylococcal or streptococcal species. Mycobacterial species can cause either localized or generalized lymphadenopathy. Localized mycobacterial lymphadenitis is generally caused by *Mycobacterium tuberculosis* in adults and by mycobacteria other than *M. tuberculosis* ("atypical mycobacteria") in children. Mycobacteria of the *M. avium* complex now cause about 80% of cases of nontuberculous mycobacterial lymphadenitis in children in the United States. In recent years newly recognized and difficult-to-isolate mycobacterial species have been reported to cause cervical lymphadenitis in children.

Presentation

Acute bacterial lymphadenitis commonly manifests itself as fever associated with large (>3 cm), tender lymph nodes with or without fluctuance. Examination of the structures drained by the involved lymphatic chains often reveals the source of the infection (Table 8-2). Localized mycobacterial lymphadenitis occurs most commonly in the neck; this condition is known as scrofula. Examination often reveals a painless conglomerate of matted nodes, which may suppurate and drain superficially.

Diagnosis

For an uncomplicated presentation of localized adenopathy suggestive of bacterial infection (acute, unilateral, tender nodes), a presumptive course of antibiotic therapy can be initiated. Simple bacterial infections respond quickly. However, if the adenopathy follows an indolent course resembling tuberculous disease or does not respond to initial therapy, aspiration is indicated. With localized involvement, fine-needle aspiration can provide tissue for culture and sensitivity. Excision is indicated for significant lymph node involvement because it is both diagnostic and therapeutic. With a presentation of generalized lymphadenopathy, fever, night sweats, and possible weight loss, excisional biopsy is indicated rather than fine-needle aspiration. In this situation both tuberculosis and lymphoma are possible and nodal architecture must be examined for adequate diagnosis. Complications of sinus tract formation may occur with simple incisional biopsy. As with any case of suspected tuberculous disease, a tuberculin skin test and chest x-ray examination are indicated for diagnosis and to determine disease involvement.

Natural History
Expected Outcome

If untreated, acute bacterial lymphadenitis can lead to localized and systemic septic complications. Lymphadenitis in the axillary nodes can cause axillary and subclavian vein thrombosis. Cervical and supraclavicular lymphadenitis caused by *M. tuberculosis* in immunocompetent hosts may resolve spontaneously. Involvement of other lymph node groups by *M. tuberculosis* carries a worse prognosis without treatment. Cervical lymphadenitis caused by nontuberculous mycobacteria tends to be chronic and is sometimes associated with fistulas or draining sinuses.

Treatment
Methods

For lymphadenitis associated with a periodontal or oral infection, penicillin intramuscularly (procaine penicillin G) or orally (penicillin V) is adequate initial therapy. For lymphadenitis associated with skin and soft tissue infections, staphylococcal and streptococcal coverage with a penicillinase-resistant penicillin or other beta-lactam drug (dicloxacillin, nafcillin, cephalexin) is indicated. Macrolides are appropriate for penicillin-allergic patients. Failure to respond should prompt fine-needle aspiration to diagnose the disease and determine sensitivities of the organism.

When mycobacterial infection is suspected, isolation of the organism and susceptibility testing are highly desirable. Strains that are multidrug resistant require different therapeutic regimens than those used for susceptible strains. Treatment of nontuberculous mycobacteria such as *M. avium-intracellulare* is often problematic because chronic drainage and fistulas can occur.

Expected Results

Both acute bacterial lymphadenitis and mycobacterial lymphadenitis caused by *M. tuberculosis* usually respond well to therapy. Response to treatment of nontuberculous mycobacterial lymphadenitis is less predictable.

When to Refer

Patients with acute bacterial lymphadenitis require referral or hospitalization only when significant systemic toxicity or complications are present. Patients with suspected mycobacterial lymphadenitis should usually be referred for diagnosis and treatment.

KEY POINTS

BACTERIAL AND MYCOBACTERIAL LYMPHADENITIS

⊃ Both bacterial lymphadenitis and mycobacterial lymphadenitis are more common in children.

⊃ Acute bacterial lymphadenitis is usually caused by staphylococci or streptococci and manifested as fever and large (>3 cm), tender lymph nodes. Presumptive treatment, without diagnostic testing, is usually successful in uncomplicated cases.

⊃ Mycobacterial cervical lymphadenitis (scrofula) is commonly caused by *M. tuberculosis* in adults and by nontuberculous mycobacteria in children. *M. avium* complex now causes about 80% of cases in children in the United States. Newly recognized and difficult-to-isolate mycobacterial species have been reported to cause cervical lymphadenitis in children in recent years.

⊃ When mycobacterial lymphadenitis is suspected, fine-needle aspiration for culture and susceptibility testing is usually indicated.

SUGGESTED READING

Boyce JM. Severe streptococcal axillary lymphadenitis. N Engl J Med 1990; 323: 655-658.

Wallace RJ Jr, Cook JL, Glassroth J, et al. Diagnosis and treatment of disease caused by nontuberculous mycobacteria. American Thoracic Society Statement. Am J Respir Crit Care Med 1997; 156 (Suppl): S1-S25.

Wolinsky E. Mycobacterial lymphadenitis in children: a prospective study of 105 nontuberculous cases with long-term follow-up. Clin Infect Dis 1995; 20: 954-963.

Zoonoses Other Than Cat Scratch Disease That Cause Lymphadenopathy: Plague, Lyme Disease, and Tularemia

Cat scratch disease is now the most common cause of lymphadenopathy among the large group of diseases that are acquired by exposure to animals or transmitted from animals by vectors (zoonoses). Other important diseases in the United States are plague, Lyme disease, and tularemia.

Presentation and Progression

Causes

Yersinia pestis is the etiologic agent of bubonic plague and represents a serious yet treatable entity if diagnosed promptly. It is associated with rodent contact followed by a 10-day incubation period and is endemic in the southwestern United States. Lyme disease (see Chapter 7) is caused by the spirochete *Borrelia burgdorferi*. It is endemic in the northern Midwest and the northeastern regions of the United States and is transmitted by the bite of the *Ixodes* tick. Tularemia is caused by an intracellular gram-negative rod, *Francisella tularensis*. In the United States it is endemic in Arkansas, Missouri, and Oklahoma. Throughout the rest of the world it remains confined to the Northern Hemisphere. Infection may occur through numerous insect vectors, handling of contaminated animals or undercooked meat, or scratch- or bite-type injuries from infected animals. Disturbing animal carcasses by cutting brush or mowing has recently been described as another risk factor for tularemia.

Presentation

Bubonic plague is associated with a sudden onset of fever, chills, headache, and malaise. The patient experiences severe pain over the area of involved lymph nodes, and the symptom of pain can precede the actual enlargement of the nodes. The inguinal nodes are the most common chain involved; however, axillary and cervical node involvement has been described.

Patients with Lyme disease (see Chapter 7) typically have the distinctive rash of erythema migrans originating at the site of the tick bite (see Chapter 7). Regional lymphadenopathy may be present. Tularemia most commonly occurs as an ulceroglandular syndrome. After exposure, an ulcerative skin lesion develops at the site of inoculation in association with fever and tender lymphadenopathy (Figure 8-2). The lymphadenopathy occurs in the chains associated with the drainage of the ulcerative lesions, and involvement of the upper extremities is most typical; however, the ulcer itself may resolve before the development of lymphadenopathy. Oculoglandular tularemia is a less common presentation and involves exposure to the bacteria through contact with the eyes. Patients may have erythematous conjunctivae, periorbital erythema, and adenopathy of preauricular lymph nodes. Other clinical features suggestive of tularemia are high fever with relative bradycardia, patchy pulmonary infiltrates, and mild elevation of the aminotransferase levels.

Diagnosis

The diagnosis of plague should be considered with a presentation of fever, painful lymphadenopathy, and risks of exposure. Blood cultures, serologic tests, and aspirates of infected lymph nodes provide confirmation of the diagnosis. Communication with laboratory personnel should occur when plague is suspected so that they may exercise extra precaution in culturing the organism. Patients with suspected plague should also be placed under respiratory isolation until drug therapy has continued for 48 hours, sputum cultures are negative, and pneumonia is documented to be absent.

The diagnosis of Lyme disease can be made clinically based on the presentation and characteristic rash. IgG anti–*B. burgdorferi* antibodies are generally not detectable until 4 to 6 weeks after infection. ELISA testing can support the diagnosis, which can be further confirmed by Western blot

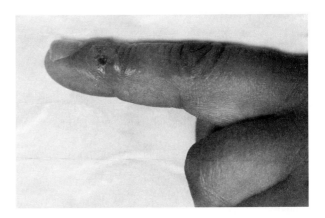

FIG. 8-2 Removal of a Band-Aid from a patient with high fever, relative bradycardia, massive epitrochlear lymphadenopathy, bilateral patchy pulmonary infiltrates, and abnormal liver function tests revealed a resolving ulcer, the portal of entry for ulceroglandular tularemia. (Courtesy of Dr. Charles S. Bryan.)

testing. Tularemia is diagnosed by combining the appropriate clinical presentation with serologic findings or ELISA. Because the antibody response appears about 2 weeks after the onset of the disease, treatment of suspected tularemia should not be postponed. Routine culturing of fluid and tissue is made difficult and is often negative in the presence of infection; moreover, attempts to isolate the highly infectious organism can be dangerous for laboratory personnel. PCR-based assays for *F. tularensis* DNA have been developed but are not widely available.

Natural History
Expected Outcome

Untreated, plague can lead to rapidly fatal illness with sepsis and pneumonia. Lyme disease may progress to chronicity (see Chapter 7). Complications of tularemia include draining lymphadenopathy and more severe forms of illness such as respiratory distress, pericarditis, and meningitis. Untreated tularemia also produces a protracted illness of fever, disabling malaise, recurrent lymphadenopathy, and weight loss.

Treatment
Methods

The drug of choice for *Yersinia pestis* is streptomycin (30 mg/kg/day up to 2 g per day in two divided doses for 10 days). Other agents that have been used successfully are tetracycline, doxycycline, chloramphenicol, and TMP/SMX. Antibiotic therapy is indicated at all stages of Lyme disease, although only early disease has been proved to respond (see Chapter 7). The traditional drug of choice for tularemia is streptomycin (10 mg/kg IM up to 2 g per day, q12h for a duration of 7 to 10 days); however, gentamicin, tetracycline, chloramphenicol, and erythromycin have been used with varying rates of success, and recent reports suggest that the fluoroquinolones may be effective.

Expected Response

All three of these infections usually respond well to treatment if begun early.

When to Refer

Hospitalization is required in severe cases of zoonotic illnesses.

 KEY POINTS

PLAGUE, LYME DISEASE, AND TULAREMIA

⊃ Plague is suggested by fever, lymphadenopathy, and sepsis in a person with exposure in an endemic area such as the southwestern United States.

⊃ Lyme disease should be considered when lymphadenopathy is associated with an annular skin lesion consistent with erythema migrans.

⊃ Tularemia should be considered when lymphadenopathy is accompanied by high fever, relative bradycardia, and systemic signs of illness such as patchy pulmonary infiltrates and elevated aminotransferases. A portal of entry is often apparent in ulceroglandular tularemia, the most common form of the disease. Diagnosis is supported by an appropriate exposure history, and treatment should be empiric because the antibody response usually occurs about 2 weeks after onset of the illness.

SUGGESTED READING

Johansson A, Berglund L, Gothefors L, et al. Ciprofloxacin for treatment of tularemia in children. Pediatr Infect Dis J 2000; 19: 449-453.

Limaye AP, Hooper CJ. Treatment of tularemia with fluoroquinolones: two cases and review. Clin Infect Dis 1999; 29: 922-924.

Medical Letter on Drugs and Therapeutics. Treatment of Lyme disease. Med Lett 2000; 42: 37-39.

Steinemann TL, Sheikholeslami MR, Brown HH, et al. Oculoglandular tularemia. Arch Ophthalmol 1999; 117: 132-133.

Nodular Lymphangitis: Sporotrichosis and Other Causes

The term "nodular lymphangitis" denotes nodular subcutaneous swellings along the path of lymphatic vessels, often with recognizable linear erythematous streaks (lymphangitis). Other terms for this syndrome are "chronic lymphangitis" and "lymphocutaneous syndrome." Sporotrichosis is the usual cause in the United States.

Presentation and Progression
Causes

Sporothrix schenckii is a dimorphic fungus found in soil and plant debris such as sphagnum moss. *M. marinum* is a nontuberculous mycobacterial organism found, as its name suggests, in water. *Nocardia brasiliensis,* like other *Nocardia* species, is a branching, filamentous, gram-positive bacterium found in soil, water, and organic matter. *Leishmania* species are endemic in developing countries, including rural areas of Central and South America. *F. tularensis* (the cause of tularemia, discussed previously) sometimes causes nodular lymphangitis. Occasional causes of nodular lymphangitis include other nontuberculous mycobacterial species such as *M. kansasii;* other fungi, including the agents of blastomycosis, coccidioidomycosis, cryptococcosis, and histoplasmosis; and pyogenic bacteria such as staphylococci and streptococci.

Presentation

Patients with sporotrichosis typically give a history of a skin break contaminated in some form by soil. Inoculation by thorny plants is common. The incubation period can be several weeks to 2 to 3 months. A shallow, painless ulcer or nodule develops at the site of injury, followed by characteristic erythematous nodules along the draining lymphatic channels (Figure 8-3). Pain over the lesions and nodes or nodules is usually very mild. Patients with *N. brasiliensis* may describe exposures similar to those of sporotrichosis, since the organisms are abundant in soil. *Nocardia* infection may be confused with cat scratch disease because trauma from a bite or scratch may be its route of inoculation. Acquisition of infection by *M. marinum* usually involves water exposure. The classic scenarios described include exposures in aquariums, in swimming pools, and to freshwater and saltwater fish. Following a 2- to 3-week incubation period after the injury, a papulonodular lesion appears on the extremity, progressively enlarges, and suppurates. Regional lymphadenitis and lymphangitis with characteristic satellite nodule formation may follow. The lesion is typically located on the distal extremities because *M. marinum* grows at a cooler temperature.

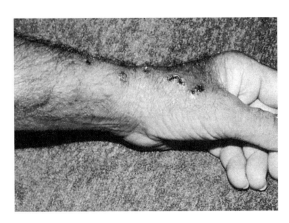

FIG. 8-3 Lymphonodular sporotrichosis. (Courtesy of Dr. Charles S. Bryan.)

Diagnosis

With the presentation of nodular lymphadenitis, aspiration of tissue or biopsy for culture is usually required for determining the causative organism and its sensitivities. The diagnosis of sporotrichosis is based on the clinical presentation along with detection of yeast in tissue by immunofluorescence or culture. Serologic tests for sporotrichosis are available, but their overall usefulness remains unclear. When mycobacteria, including *M. marinum,* are being considered in the differential diagnosis, laboratory personnel should be notified because acid-fast staining should be performed and cultures should be incubated at a lower-than-normal temperature, specifically 86° to 90° F (30° to 32° C). *Nocardia* species are slow-growing bacteria, and communication with the laboratory is necessary to ensure incubation periods long enough for maximal recovery of organisms. Acid-fast staining of specimens may reveal filamentous branching rods. A positive stain strongly supports the diagnosis and allows early presumptive therapy.

Natural History
Expected Outcome

Without treatment the infections causing nodular lymphangitis can progress to involve local lymph node chains and may also evoke systemic symptoms such as fever. A chronic destructive infection of the skin, soft tissue, and underlying supportive structures known as a mycetoma is sometimes associated with *Nocardia* infection.

Treatment
Methods

Itraconazole 200 mg/day for 3 to 6 months has become the drug of choice for sporotrichosis, replacing potassium iodide, which is also effective but less well tolerated. Amphotericin B is reserved for disseminated and life-threatening disease. Sulfonamides alone have been standard therapy for *Nocardia* infection. However, TMP/SMX (2.5 to 10 mg/kg of trimethoprim; 12.5 to 50 mg/kg of sulfamethoxazole) is now the most frequently used regimen to treat nocardiosis. Patients should be observed for evidence of myelosuppression during prolonged therapy with TMP/SMX. Other agents that have activity against *Nocardia* are sulfadiazine, minocycline, amikacin, imipenem, and certain third-generation cephalosporins. Antibiotic therapy should be continued for a minimum of 2 months because relapse is common. Treatment of *M. marinum* is based

on organism sensitivities but generally involves therapy with rifampin plus ethambutol, minocycline, or TMP/SMX. Duration of therapy should be 2 to 3 months or extend 4 to 6 weeks after resolution of skin lesions. With *M. marinum,* deep soft tissue infections of the hand or distal extremities may require surgical débridement.

Expected Response

Treatment of all the conditions described is usually successful eventually, but therapy must be prolonged and compliance ensured.

When to Refer

Referral for surgical débridement is sometimes required.

 KEY POINTS

NODULAR LYMPHANGITIS: SPOROTRICHOSIS AND OTHER CAUSES

- ⊃ Nodular lymphangitis consists of linear inflammation and nodule formation along the pathways of lymphatic vessels.
- ⊃ Sporotrichosis is the most common cause in the United States. Other important causes are *N. brasiliensis* and *M. marinum.*
- ⊃ Nodular lymphangitis caused by sporotrichosis and nocardiosis is usually associated with injury involving exposure to soil or organic matter. Nodular lymphangitis caused by *M. marinum* is usually associated with injuries involving freshwater exposure.
- ⊃ Drug therapy for nodular lymphangitis typically must exceed 2 months' duration.

SUGGESTED READING

Kauffman CA. Sporotrichosis. Clin Infect Dis 1999; 29: 231-236.
Kauffman CA, Hajjeh R, Chapman SW. Mycoses Study Group, Infectious Diseases Society of America. Practice guidelines for the management of patients with sporotrichosis. Clin Infect Dis 2000; 30: 684-687.
Kostman JR, DiNubile MJ. Nodular lymphangitis: a distinctive but often unrecognized syndrome. Ann Intern Med 1993; 118: 883-888.
Lerner, PI. Nocardiosis. Clin Infect Dis 1996; 22: 891-905.
Smego RA, Castiglia M, Asperilla MO. Lymphocutaneous syndrome: a review of non-*Sporothrix* causes. Medicine (Baltimore) 1999; 78: 38-63.
Tobin EH, Jih WH. Sporotrichoid lymphocutaneous infections: etiology, diagnosis and therapy. Am Fam Physician 2001; 63: 326-332.
Zaharopoulos P. Fine-needle aspiration cytologic diagnosis of lymphocutaneous sporotrichosis: a case report. Diagn Cytopathol 1999; 20: 74-77.

Noninfectious Causes of Lymphadenopathy: Autoimmune and Granulomatous Diseases and Diseases of Unknown Cause

Because many noninfectious etiologies of lymphadenopathy enter into the differential diagnosis, brief discussion is warranted. Several autoimmune and noninfectious granulomatous disorders have fever and lymphadenopathy as associated findings. Systemic lupus erythematosus (SLE) can cause a mild, generalized lymphadenopathy in as much as 50% of cases. Lymphadenopathy is more common in childhood-onset SLE than in adult-onset SLE (6% versus 0.5% in one series), and generalized lymphadenopathy is rare. The incidence of lymphadenopathy in rheumatoid arthritis has been reported to be as high as 50% to 70% of cases. The appearance of nodes tends to correlate with onset, disease exacerbation, or severe disease in general. Adult Still's disease (ASD), an inflammatory illness that resembles juvenile rheumatoid arthritis, occurs in adolescent and middle-aged individuals. The presentation of ASD can also closely mimic a mononucleosis syndrome, with lymphadenopathy that is typically cervical. On close examination of the lymphadenopathy in both rheumatoid arthritis and ASD, the nodes are soft, rarely tender, and nonfluctuant. Sarcoidosis, a granulomatous disease of unknown etiology, commonly features intrathoracic and peripheral lymphadenopathy. Peripheral lymph nodes are generally soft and nontender and occasionally cause symptoms if they become large enough to encroach on other structures.

Asymmetry of lymphadenopathy, acute enlargement (rapid progression), or acute tenderness is uncommon in any of these illnesses and should lead the physician toward a different diagnosis. Exceptions are acute vasculitis and severe SLE, in which severe lymphadenitis and some degree of tenderness may occur. Full node biopsy, allowing examination of node architecture, is indicated when the etiology of lymphadenopathy is unclear. Changes in baseline lymphadenopathy in patients with known autoimmune disease should prompt evaluation for superimposed infectious etiologies.

SUGGESTED READING

Belfer MH, Stevens RW. Sarcoidosis: a primary care review. Am Fam Physician 1998; 58: 2041-2050.

Dale DC. Lymphadenopathy and lymphoproliferative disorders. Immunol Allergy Clin North Am 1993; 13: 359-368.

Pai MR, Adhikari P, Coimbatore RV, et al. Fine needle aspiration cytology in systemic lupus erythematosus: a case report. Acta Cytol 2000; 44: 67-69.

Pouchot J, Sampalis JS, Beaudet F, et al. Adult Still's disease: manifestations, disease course, and outcome in 62 patients. Medicine (Baltimore) 1991; 70: 118-136.

Noninfectious Causes of Lymphadenopathy: Hypersensitivity Reactions

A number of drugs may induce fever and lymphadenopathy with long-term use in certain patients. (For a brief list, see Table 8-1.) On initial evaluation of the patient a thorough review of the current medications should take place and recent changes in medications should be noted. Drug reactions accompanied by fever and lymphadenopathy tend to be more severe than drug reactions without these features. Hypersensitivity to anticonvulsant drugs (notably phenytoin, phenobarbital, and carbamazepine) can cause a severe syndrome manifested as fever, lymphadenopathy, a pleomorphic skin eruption, eosinophilia, and hepatitis. Inquiry should be made about use of over-the-counter medications and illicit drugs, since lymphadenopathy may be a manifestation of hypersensitivity to any number of

agents. Injecting drug use has been associated with hypersensitivity-type syndromes, particularly if patients are injecting "contaminated" preparations. Their symptoms include fever, rash, myalgias, arthritis, and lymphadenopathy and typically resolve after the offending agent has been removed.

SUGGESTED READING

Morkunas AR, Miller MB. Anticonvulsant hypersensitivity syndrome. Crit Care Clin 1997; 13: 727-739.

Pastan, RS, Silverman SL, Goldenberg DL. A musculoskeletal syndrome in intravenous heroin users: association with brown heroin. Ann Intern Med 1977; 87: 22-29.

Noninfectious Causes of Lymphadenopathy: Neoplasms and Lymphomas

Malignant disease is always a concern in the evaluation of patients with fever and lymphadenopathy. Both lymphoma and leukemia can cause localized or generalized lymphadenopathy. Metastatic cancer can manifest itself in a similar manner. Clinical findings that should suggest malignancy on initial presentation include age beyond the fourth decade, a history of night sweats or weight loss, an abnormal chest radiograph, anemia, and node size >2 cm. The location of supraclavicular lymphadenopathy has a higher association with malignancy, and the finding of hard fixed nodes in any chain is also highly suggestive of malignancy.

Angioimmunoblastic lymphadenopathy is a rare lymphoproliferative disorder primarily affecting older persons and characterized by generalized lymphadenopathy, polyclonal hypergammaglobulinemia, hepatosplenomegaly, and hemolytic anemia. A characteristic histologic picture on lymph node biopsy supports the diagnosis. The clinical course is often aggressive. Malignant transformation has also been described in Castleman's disease, a lymphoproliferative disorder of unknown cause in which the presentation is occasionally fever, weight loss, and large nodes suggesting lymphoma.

When malignancy is suspected, obtaining a tissue diagnosis is necessary. Lymph node biopsy is indicated in most cases because the nodal architecture is needed to diagnose and classify lymphoma properly. An exception to this rule is the suspicion that head and neck cancer is present. Nodal biopsy in this case could interfere with future tissue dissection and adversely affect outcome. In this situation a fine-needle aspiration is an appropriate initial procedure.

SUGGESTED READING

Pangalis GA, Vassilakopoulos TP, Boussiotis VA, et al. Clinical approach to lymphadenopathy. Semin Oncol 1993; 20: 570-582.

Patt BS, Schaefer SD, Vuitch F. Role of fine-needle aspiration in the evaluation of neck masses. Med Clin North Am 1993; 77: 611-623.

Soldes OS, Younger JG, Hirschl RB. Predictors of malignancy in childhood peripheral lymphadenopathy. J Pediatr Surg 1999; 34: 1447-1452.

9

Eye Infections

CHARLES S. BRYAN, SANJEEV GREWAL

Ocular Emergencies
Blepharitis, Dermatoblepharitis, Hordeolum, and
    Chalazion
Infections of the Lacrimal System
Acute Conjunctivitis
Keratitis

The specialized vocabulary and instruments of ophthalmology and the danger of loss of vision make eye infections intimidating for the primary care clinician. Nevertheless, all primary care clinicians should be familiar with the anatomy of the eye (Figure 9-1), the basic vocabulary of eye infections (Table 9-1), the indications for urgent hospitalization or referral, the differential diagnosis of red eye (Table 9-2), the diagnosis and management of common periocular infections and acute conjunctivitis, and the dangers of using topical corticosteroids.

SUGGESTED READING

Seal DV, Bron AJ, Hay J. Ocular Infection: Investigation and Treatment in Practice. St. Louis: Mosby; 1998.
Tabbara RA, Hyndiuk RA, eds. Infections of the Eye. Boston: Little Brown and Company; 1986.

Ocular Emergencies

Situations requiring urgent referral include major trauma to the eye; minor trauma when the eye is contaminated with foreign bodies or vegetative matter; symptoms of keratitis or corneal ulcers; suspicion of uveitis, endophthalmitis, or retinitis; and preseptal cellulitis or orbital cellulitis.

Uveitis, Endophthalmitis, and Retinitis

Uveitis denotes inflammation of the pigmented tissues of the eye, or uvea, which includes the iris, ciliary body, and choroid. Anterior uveitis denotes inflammation of the iris (iritis), sometimes accompanied by inflammation of the adjacent ciliary body (iridocyclitis). Posterior uveitis denotes inflammation of the choroid and related structures. In either case the anatomic diagnosis is usually made by an ophthalmologist by slit lamp examination and other diagnostic techniques that are not generally available in primary care practices.

Common presenting symptoms of anterior uveitis are unilateral (or less commonly bilateral) inflammation of the eye with pain, redness, photophobia, tearing, and inflammation. Redness tends to be most prominent at the limbus (the outer margin of the cornea, or sclerocorneal junction), in contrast to conjunctivitis, in which the redness tends to be most prominent away from the cornea. Inflammation can be granulomatous or nongranulomatous. Often no specific cause is found. Infectious causes of anterior uveitis include herpes simplex and herpes zoster.

Posterior uveitis commonly manifests itself as vision loss. The eye is "externally quiet"; that is, redness is not a prominent clinical finding unless anterior uveitis is also present. Toxoplasmosis is a common cause of posterior uveitis in

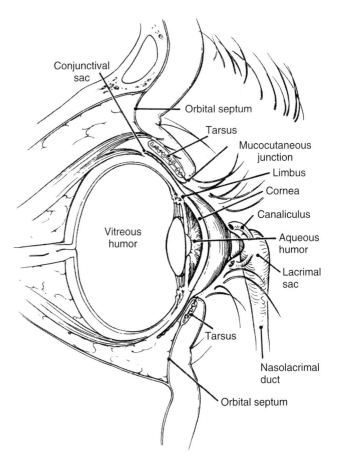

FIG. 9-1 Anatomy of the eye relevant to primary care. (From Kirk R, Wilhelmus MD. The red eye. Infect Dis Clin North Am 1988; 2: 99-116.)

TABLE 9-1
Some Terms Pertaining To Eye Infections

Term	Definition
Blepharitis	Inflammation of the margins of the eyelids
Blepharospasm	Spasm of the eyelids
Canaliculitis	Low-grade chronic inflammation of the canaliculi of the lacrimal apparatus
Chemosis	Excessive edema of the conjunctiva
Dacryoadenitis	Inflammation of the main lacrimal gland
Dacryocystitis	Inflammation of the lacrimal sac
Dermatoblepharitis	Inflammation of the eyelids and of the skin around the eyelids
Endophthalmitis	Inflammation (usually caused by infection) involving the vitreous humor and usually the retina and other tissues
Entropion	Inversion (in-turning) of the eyelid
Epiphora	Excessive tear formation
Episcleritis	Inflammation of tissues overlying the sclera or of the outer layers of the sclera
Hyphema	Hemorrhage within the anterior chamber of the eye
Hypopyon	Inflammation with layered white blood cells in the inferior aspect of the anterior chamber of the eye
Iritis	Inflammation of the iris (usually characterized by pain, photophobia, congestion in the region of the ciliary body, and contraction of the pupil)
Keratitis	Inflammation of the cornea
Madarosis	Loss of eyelashes
Scleritis	Inflammation of the sclera
Synechia	Adhesions between the iris and the cornea (anterior synechia) or between the iris and the lens (posterior synechia)
Trichiasis	In-turning of the eyelashes so that they scratch the surface of the eye
Uveitis	Inflammation of the uveal tissue of the eye in one or more areas; iritis refers to inflammation of the iris, cyclitis to inflammation of the ciliary body, and choroiditis to inflammation of the choroid

immunocompetent persons. Syphilis causes only about 1% of cases but should always be excluded by appropriate serologic tests because of the therapeutic implications. Other infectious causes include fungi (notably histoplasmosis and candidiasis); spirochetes, including *Borrelia burgdorferi* (Lyme disease; see Chapter 7); viruses; parasites (including *Toxocara canis*); and, in patients with advanced human immunodeficiency virus disease, cytomegalovirus. Numerous systemic inflammatory diseases are associated with uveitis. Uveitis provides an important clue to the diagnosis of sarcoidosis and juvenile rheumatoid arthritis and also occurs in other connective tissue disease, including the spondyloarthropathies (such as anky-

losing spondylitis and Reiter's syndrome), inflammatory bowel disease, psoriasis, and Behçet's disease. Tumors, notably lymphomas, sometimes masquerade as uveitis. Depending on the anatomy, posterior uveitis is described by various terms such as choroiditis, chorioretinitis, retinochoroiditis, retinitis, vitreitis, intermediate uveitis, and pars planitis.

Endophthalmitis denotes inflammation involving the vitreous and anterior chamber. It is most often of infectious origin but can also be caused by lens matter or toxic materials. Infectious endophthalmitis can be endogenous (in which case microorganisms gain access to the eye through the bloodstream) or exogenous (in which case microorganisms enter the eye

TABLE 9-2
Differential Diagnosis of the Red Eye

Feature	Bacterial conjunctivitis	Viral conjunctivitis	Allergic conjunctivitis	Bacterial keratitis	Viral keratitis	Iritis	Acute glaucoma
Blurred vision	0	0	0	+++	0 to ++	+ to ++	++ to +++
Pain	0	0	0	++	0 to +	++	++ to ++++
Photophobia	0	0	0	++	++	+++	− to ++
Discharge	Purulent + to +++	Watery + to ++	White, ropy +	Purulent +++	Watery +	0	0
Injection	+++	++	+	+++	+	0 to +	+ to ++
Corneal haze	0	0	0	+++	+ to ++	0	+ to +++
Ciliary flush	0	0	0	+++	+	++ to ++++	+ to ++
Pupil	Normal	Normal	Normal	Normal or miotic (iritis)	Normal	Miotic	Mid-dilated; nonreactive
Pressure	Normal	Normal	Normal	Normal	Normal	Normal, low, or high	High
Preauricular lymph nodes	Rare	Usual	0	0	0	0	0
Smear taken from conjunctiva	Bacteria; PMNs	Lymphocytes	Eosinophils	Bacteria; PMNs	0	0	0
Therapy	Antibiotics	Nonspecific	Nonspecific	Antibiotics	Antivirals	Cycloplegia; topical steroids	Medical or surgical

From Syed NA, Hyndiuk RA. Infectious conjunctivitis. Infect Dis Clin North Am 1992; 6: 789-805.
PMNs, Polymorphonuclear neutrophils.

because of trauma or surgery). Endogenous endophthalmitis is especially likely to occur in patients with endocarditis or infected central venous catheters. Common pathogens are staphylococci, streptococci, gram-negative bacilli, and *Candida* species. Exogenous endophthalmitis as a postoperative complication is most commonly caused by coagulase-negative staphylococci (notably *S. epidermidis*). More severe cases are often caused by *Staphylococcus aureus* or gram-negative bacilli, whereas more indolent cases are often caused by *Propionibacterium acnes*. Exogenous endophthalmitis related to trauma can be caused by a wide range of microorganisms, including common environmental contaminants such as *Bacillus* and *Clostridium* species and various fungi such as dematiaceous molds (see Chapter 21). Endophthalmitis is always an emergency and usually requires administration of antibiotics directly into the eye in addition to systemic therapy.

Retinitis can be caused by cytomegalovirus and various herpesviruses. Untreated, retinitis can be devastating to vision. Prompt referral is crucial.

Preseptal Cellulitis and Postseptal (Orbital) Cellulitis

In preseptal cellulitis, infection is confined to the tissues anterior to the orbital septum. The skin of the eyelids is edematous and inflamed. In postseptal (orbital) cellulitis, acute infection of the orbital contents poses a risk not only to vision but also of spread to the cavernous sinuses. Most cases of orbital cellulitis arise by spread of infection from contiguous structures, notably the paranasal sinuses. The orbit is separated from the ethmoid air cells by a thin piece of bone known as the lamina papyracea, which is easily injured by trauma. Hematogenous spread of bacteria to the orbit occurs but is rare. Preseptal cellulitis in children was often caused by *H. influenzae* type b before the introduction of the vaccine against that organism. Streptococci are now the major cause of preseptal cellulitis in children. *S. aureus* is the most common cause of orbital cellulitis in adults, but *Streptococcus pyogenes* and *Streptococcus pneumoniae* are also encountered.

The early symptoms of orbital cellulitis are typically fever, lid edema, and rhinorrhea. These are followed by orbital pain, tenderness on palpation of the lids, and headache. The lids become discolored and warm. Initially vision is usually normal. Later findings include conjunctival hyperemia, chemosis, and proptosis. Onset of postseptal cellulitis can be sudden in the form of the orbital apex syndrome, in which case vision loss and ophthalmoplegia are accompanied by minimal external signs of inflammation. The orbital apex syndrome results from spread of infection to the orbit from the ethmoid or sphenoid sinuses, and vision loss is probably due to vascular compromise.

Both preseptal and postseptal orbital cellulitis can spread to bone (subperiosteal abscess) and lead to cavernous sinus thrombosis. Orbital cellulitis carried a mortality rate of nearly 20% before the introduction of antibiotics. Suspicion of orbital cellulitis mandates urgent imaging of the orbits and paranasal sinuses. An ophthalmologist should be consulted, as well as an otolaryngologist if evidence of sinus disease is found.

 KEY POINTS

OCULAR EMERGENCIES

⊃ Loss of vision, sometimes with eye pain and conjunctival injection, may indicate uveitis or endophthalmitis.

⊃ Anterior uveitis commonly presents with red eye and vision symptoms. Posterior uveitis presents with vision symptoms; redness is absent unless anterior uveitis is also present.

⊃ Preseptal cellulitis and postseptal (orbital) cellulitis usually arise from sinusitis; complications include cavernous sinus thrombosis.

⊃ The orbital apex syndrome, a variant of orbital cellulitis, is manifested as vision loss and ophthalmoplegia, often with minimal external signs of inflammation.

SUGGESTED READING

Ambati BK, Ambati J, Azar N, et al. Periorbital and orbital cellulitis before and after the advent of *Haemophilus influenzae* type B vaccination. Ophthalmology 2000; 107: 1450-1453.

Barza M, Baum J, eds. Ocular infections. Infect Dis Clin North Am 1992; 6: 777-980.

Baum J. Infections of the eye. Clin Infect Dis 1995; 21: 479-488.

Donahue SP, Khoury JM, Kowalski RP. Common ocular infections: a prescriber's guide. Drugs 1996; 52: 526-540.

Donahue SP, Schwartz G. Preseptal and orbital cellulitis in childhood: a changing microbiologic spectrum. Ophthalmology 1998; 105: 1902-1905.

Gaynor BD, Margolis TP, Cunningham ET Jr. Advances in diagnosis and management of herpetic uveitis. Int Ophthalmol Clin 2000; 40: 85-109.

Uzcategui N, Warman R, Smith A, et al. Clinical practice guidelines for the management of orbital cellulitis. J Pediatr Ophthalmol Strabismus 1998; 35: 73-79.

Blepharitis, Dermatoblepharitis, Hordeolum, and Chalazion

Blepharitis, or inflammation of the eyelid margins, is usually chronic, bilateral, and difficult to treat. It is frequently associated with a localized infection (hordeolum) or a localized lipogranulomatous inflammation (chalazion).

Presentation and Progression
Cause

The cause of blepharitis remains controversial, and it is likely that no single cause applies to all patients. Staphylococci—both *S. aureus* and coagulase-negative staphylococci—are commonly implicated, but these bacteria are often found in cultures taken from normal eyelids. Many cases of blepharitis involve the skin around the eyelids (dermatoblepharitis), and in these cases dermatologic disease (e.g., seborrheic dermatitis or acne rosacea), specific infections (e.g., herpes simplex virus 1 or 2, varicella-zoster virus, and pyogenic bacteria), allergy, or connective tissue disease may be involved. Occasional cases are caused by infection with the pubic or "crab" louse, *Phthirus pubis*. Blepharitis involving the posterior lid margins is usually attributed to dysfunction of the meibomian glands.

Hordeolum is an acute, localized staphylococcal infection of one of the glands lining the eyelid. External hordeolum, the familiar "stye," is a microabscess involving the glands of Zeis (sebaceous glands connected with the follicles of the eyelashes) or the glands of Moll (apocrine sweat glands near the lid margin). Internal hordeolum is a staphylococcal infection of a meibomian gland. Chalazion is attributed to chronic inflammation of a meibomian gland.

Presentation

Blepharitis is nearly always chronic and bilateral. Staphylococcal blepharitis usually presents with inflamed eyelids accompanied by scaling and crusting around the cilia. Loss of eyelashes (madarosis) may occur. Seborrheic blepharitis, which is often associated with seborrheic dermatitis elsewhere, causes inflammation and oily or greasy scaling along the anterior border of the eyelid. Some patients with seborrheic blepharitis, however, have involvement mainly of the meibomian glands and inflammation of the posterior surface of the eyelid. Other patients with posterior blepharitis have primary inflammation of the meibomian glands (meibomianitis), and have dry eyes.

External hordeolum (stye) is a small, painful lesion of the anterior margin of the lid. The onset is acute. Internal hordeolum is also an acute, painful lesion and is frequently accompanied by diffuse swelling, tenderness, and edema of the lid. Chalazion is a lid nodule away from the lid margin. It may begin with inflammation and tenderness, is often accompanied by secondary infection, and usually points toward the conjunctival surface of the lid. Occasional chalazia are sufficiently large to distort vision by pressing on the globe.

Diagnosis

Diagnoses of blepharitis, hordeolum, and chalazion are made on clinical grounds. In patients with blepharitis the lids should be evaluated carefully for seborrhea and the eyelashes should be inspected for the small nits (0.5 to 1 mm) and adult lice (3 mm) of *Phthirus pubis*. Culture of the lid margins in anterior blepharitis may show a heavy growth of staphylococci. When patients with blepharitis complain of dry eyes, the possibility of keratoconjunctivitis sicca (which can be part of Sjögren's syndrome) should be suspected. When blepharitis is unilateral and chronic, the possibility of underlying malignancy should be considered.

External hordeolum, the familiar stye, presents little or no diagnostic problem. Internal hordeolum becomes apparent with the eyelid is inverted. There is often diffuse erythema of the lid, but the basic lesion can be identified as a yellowish nodule. Chalazion, especially if enlarging, must be distinguished from sebaceous gland carcinoma. This is a rare tumor (accounting for about 1% of malignancies of the eyelids) but carries a substantial mortality if diagnosis is delayed.

Natural History
Expected Outcome

Blepharitis seldom resolves spontaneously. In cases attributed to staphylococci, the lid margins commonly become thickened and irregular, often with thinning and misdirection of the eyelashes. External hordeolum (stye) usually ruptures spontaneously within several days. Internal hordeolum, however, is less likely to resolve spontaneously. Chalazia often resolve slowly but are prone to recurrence, especially in cases associated with severe blepharitis.

Treatment
Methods

Patients with blepharitis should be advised that the disease is chronic and that cure is unlikely. The mainstays of treatment are local hygiene and topical antibiotics. The eyelids should be scrubbed once or twice daily, as follows. First, a washcloth is soaked with hot water (as hot as the patient can tolerate) and applied to the closed eyelids for 5 to 10 minutes. As the washcloth cools, it should be replenished with more hot water. Next, the secretions and debris that are drawn out by the hot compress are removed by gentle scrubbing with a nonirritating baby shampoo, diluted 50% by water, using a clean moist washcloth, a cotton ball, or a cotton-tipped applicator. Care must be taken to keep the diluted shampoo from flowing into the eye. Finally, the eyelid should be thoroughly rinsed to remove all traces of the shampoo. In patients with obstructed meibomian glands it may be helpful to massage the lid margin against the globe with a small circular motion to express secretions. In patients with staphylococcal blepharitis the usual approach is to apply an antibiotic ointment to the lid margins one to four times daily, although the efficacy of topical antibiotics is not clearly established. Bacitracin or erythromycin ointment is most commonly prescribed for this purpose. Treatment should continue for a month after all signs of inflammation have subsided. Patients with acne rosacea, and occasional patients with seborrheic dermatitis who have secondary meibomianitis, may benefit from a course of tetracyclines (tetracycline HCl 250 mg q.i.d. or doxycycline 100 mg b.i.d.), given for 2 to 6 weeks with a warning to avoid ultraviolet light exposure. Topical metronidazole gel is effective in some patients with ocular rosacea. Patients with *P. pubis* infestation of the eyelids can be treated with a bland ointment in such a way as to smother the lice. A single application of lindane cream, 1%, is effective therapy, but care must be taken to avoid contact with the eyes.

External hordeolum usually ruptures spontaneously. Pricking the lesion with a fine, sterile needle hastens resolution. Warm compresses are also useful, but antibiotics are seldom required. Internal hordeolum, on the other hand, resolves much more slowly. Some patients with internal hordeolum benefit from an oral antistaphylococcal antibiotic (e.g., dicloxacillin).

Chalazia often need excision. Warm compresses can hasten resolution and may prevent obstruction of meibomian gland orifices. However, observation is a reasonable strategy, since most chalazia decrease in size.

Expected Response

Blepharitis is frustrating because of its tendency to chronicity and recurrence. Hordeolum and chalazion tend to recur. Some patients with hordeolum are chronic nasal carriers of *S. aureus*.

When to Refer

Patients with refractory blepharitis may benefit from referral to a dermatologist or ophthalmologist. Patients whose main complaint is dryness of the eyes should be evaluated for keratoconjunctivitis sicca. (The Schirmer test, which provides a crude measure of tear production, can be performed in the practitioner's office, but in general these patients should be evaluated by an ophthalmologist.) The possibility of underlying malignancy should be considered in patients with unilateral blepharitis, and sebaceous gland carcinoma should be considered in older patients with persistent or recurrent chalazion.

 KEY POINTS

BLEPHARITIS, HORDEOLUM, AND CHALAZION

- Blepharitis is nearly always bilateral; when it is persistent and unilateral, underlying malignancy should be suspected.
- Phthiriasis palpebrarum is blepharitis caused by the pubic or "crab" louse *(P. pubis)*, which can be transmitted sexually. Diagnosis is based on finding the nits or adult lice in the eyelashes.
- External hordeolum (stye) nearly always ruptures spontaneously within several days. Internal hordeolum sometimes requires systemic antibiotics.
- Chalazion usually occurs as a firm, localized nodule in the lid margin. Sebaceous gland carcinoma should be excluded by close observation and, when indicated, wide excision of the lesion.

SUGGESTED READING

Barnhorst DA Jr, Foster JA, Chern KC, et al. The efficacy of topical metronidazole in the treatment of ocular rosacea. Ophthalmology 1996; 103: 1880-1883.

Jackson TL, Beun L. A prospective study of cost, patient satisfaction, and outcome of treatment of chalazion by medical and nursing staff. Br J Ophthalmol 2000; 84: 782-785.

Lederman C, Miller M. Hordeola and chalazia. Pediatr Rev 1999; 20: 283-284.

McCulley JP, Shine WE. Meibomian secretions in chronic blepharitis. Adv Exp Med Biol 1998; 438: 319-326.

Infections of the Lacrimal System

Tears, essential to ocular health, form in the lacrimal gland, flow across the cornea, and drain into the nose by way of a series of tubes: the canaliculi, lacrimal sac, and lacrimal duct (Figure 9-1). Infections can occur at any of these sites and are usually best managed by an ophthalmologist.

Dacryoadenitis

Dacryoadenitis, or inflammation of the main lacrimal gland, is uncommonly encountered in primary care and can be acute or chronic.

Acute dacryoadenitis is characterized by localized tenderness and swelling of the outer margin of the upper eyelid, causing an S-curved deformity of the lid margin. Erythema and swelling of the lid may be present; the swelling can be so severe that the lid cannot be opened. *S. aureus* and streptococci are the most common pathogens, but *Chlamydia trachomatis* and *Neisseria gonorrhoeae* must also be considered. Some cases are caused by viruses, especially the mumps virus and the Epstein-Barr virus. Acute dacryoadenitis should be treated with parenteral antistaphylococcal antibiotics.

Chronic dacryoadenitis is usually painless and slowly progressive and is often bilateral. Mumps is a frequent cause in children. Other viruses that can cause chronic dacryoadenitis include the Epstein-Barr virus, varicella-zoster virus, cytomegalovirus, coxsackieviruses, and echoviruses. Chronic dacryoadenitis can also reflect granulomatous inflammation caused by tuberculosis; leprosy; syphilis; fungal diseases such as blastomycosis, histoplasmosis, and sporotrichosis; and parasitic diseases such as cysticercosis and schistosomiasis. However, most diseases that cause chronic swelling of the lacrimal gland are noninfectious. These include Sjögren's syndrome, sarcoidosis, tumors (both benign and malignant, which comprise about 25% of lacrimal gland swellings), and chronic dacryoadenitis of unknown cause, which occurs especially in older men.

Canaliculitis

Canaliculitis, or inflammation of the canaliculi, often causes low-grade symptoms that include itching and tearing of the eye with redness of the nasal conjunctiva. The origin of these symptoms often goes unrecognized for years. Swelling or pouting of the lacrimal punctum provides a clue to the diagnosis. Some cases of canaliculitis are caused by obstruction. Other cases are caused by infections. *Actinomyces israelii* is a frequent cause and is associated with "sulfur granules." Other infectious agents are *Propionibacterium propionicus*, *Malassezia pachydermatis*, and various fungi, chlamydiae, and viruses. When the diagnosis of canaliculitis is suspected, referral to an ophthalmologist is indicated to obtain material for Gram stain and culture, to remove by curettage material that has accumulated in the canaliculus, and to consider definitive surgery. Many ophthalmologists prefer to irrigate the canaliculus with an antibiotic solution (e.g., penicillin G 160,000 units/mL) or to prescribe antibiotic drops, but the value of antibiotics for canaliculitis is unclear.

Dacryocystitis

Dacryocystitis, or inflammation of the lacrimal sac, results from obstruction of the flow of tears from the lacrimal sac into the nose. The process can be acute or chronic.

Acute dacryocystitis is usually caused by bacteria. *Streptococcus pneumoniae* is the most common pathogen in neonates with congenital nasolacrimal obstruction; *S. aureus* is more common in acquired cases caused by trauma, tumors, and dacryoliths (stones that develop within the canaliculi or lacrimal sac). Acute dacryocystitis is characterized by pain and diffuse swelling over the lacrimal sac or just below the medial aspect of the eye. Gentle massage of the inflamed area beginning at the lower aspect and proceeding toward the lacrimal puncta produces pus. Acute dacryocystitis can progress to the formation of a significant localized abscess (dacryocystopyocele), orbital abscess, and orbital cellulitis; the latter condition can be life threatening. Other complications are involvement of the cornea and formation of a mucocele.

Acute dacryocystitis is treated with warm compresses and systemic antibiotics, ideally based on results of Gram stain and culture. An antistaphylococcal penicillin (such as dicloxacillin or a first-generation cephalosporin) is the drug of choice for empiric therapy in acquired cases. After the acute infection has resolved, the patient should be warned of the possibility of recurrence and taught to massage the lacrimal sac using gentle digital pressure. Topical antibiotic drops are often used after the acute infection has subsided.

Chronic dacryocystitis can result from prior episodes of acute dacryocystitis or can be caused by chronic diseases such as sarcoidosis. *Streptococcus pneumoniae* is often isolated, but a wide range of anaerobic bacteria, fungi, and even *Chlamydia trachomatis* are sometimes present. Pain and swelling over the lacrimal sac suggest the diagnosis, but epiphora is sometimes the only manifestation. Topical antibiotic drops and ointments are of limited usefulness in patients with chronic dacryocystitis.

Most patients with dacryocystitis should be evaluated at some point by an ophthalmologist. Surgical drainage is necessary for orbital abscess, and hospitalization is usually indicated for orbital cellulitis. Recurrent episodes of dacryocystitis or continued epiphora after treatment is an indication for dacryocystorhinostomy.

 KEY POINTS

INFECTIONS OF THE LACRIMAL SYSTEM

⊃ Acute dacryoadenitis (infection of the lacrimal gland) is rare but is usually caused by *S. aureus* or streptococci and associated with systemic toxicity.

⊃ Chronic dacryoadenitis can be caused by infections such as tuberculosis and syphilis but is frequently due to noninfectious conditions, including Sjögren's syndrome, sarcoidosis, and tumors (about 25% of cases). Chronic dacryoadenitis of unknown cause is especially likely to affect older men.

⊃ Canaliculitis, or inflammation of the canaliculi, often goes undiagnosed. Symptoms include itching and tearing of the eye and swelling in the area of the lacrimal punctum.

⊃ Acute dacryocystitis is manifested as painful swelling of the lacrimal sac that if untreated can lead to orbital cellulitis.

⊃ Chronic dacryocystitis is characterized by swelling of the lacrimal sac, which may or may not be painful.

⊃ Most infections involving the lacrimal system should be managed in consultation with an ophthalmologist.

SUGGESTED READING

Brook I, Frazier EH. Aerobic and anaerobic microbiology of dacryocystitis. Am J Ophthalmol 1998; 125: 522-524.

Campolattaro BN, Lueder GT, Tychsen L. Spectrum of pediatric dacryocystitis: medical and surgical management of 54 cases. J Pediatr Ophthalmol Strabismus 1997; 34: 143-153.

Janssen AG, Mansour K, Bos JJ, et al. Abscess of the lacrimal sac due to chronic or subacute dacryocystitis: treatment with temporary stent placement in the nasolacrimal duct. Radiology 2000; 215: 300-304.

McLean CJ, Rose GE. Postherpetic lacrimal obstruction. Ophthalmology 2000; 107: 496-499.

Acute Conjunctivitis

Acute conjunctivitis, defined by "red eye" of less than 3 weeks' duration, is a common problem in primary care that must be distinguished on clinical grounds from other, more serious illnesses (Table 9-2).

Presentation and Progression

Cause

Acute conjunctivitis is usually caused by bacteria, viruses, allergy, or nonspecific irritants. In pediatric practice the majority of cases (54% to 80%) are due to bacteria. In adult practice bacteria account for about 40% of cases and viruses for about 36%. *S. pneumoniae, H. influenzae,* and *Moraxella catarrhalis* are important causes of bacterial conjunctivitis in children. Some children have concurrent otitis media; this has been called the conjunctivitis-otitis syndrome and is usually due to *H. influenzae* or *S. pneumoniae.* In adults *S. aureus* is the most common cause of acute bacterial conjunctivitis. Other bacteria, including *Streptococcus mitis* and *Streptococcus pyogenes,* cause occasional cases. Adenoviruses are the most common agents of viral conjunctivitis and tend to be highly contagious. *Neisseria gonorrhoeae* and *Chlamydia trachomatis* can be transmitted to the eyes from patients with urethritis caused by these organisms.

Presentation

Presentation of acute conjunctivitis varies according to the pathogen.

Hyperacute bacterial conjunctivitis, which is usually caused by *N. gonorrhoeae,* is marked by rapidly progressive signs of inflammation: redness, tenderness, irritation, and purulent discharge. Findings include marked swelling of the lids, chemosis, and tender preauricular lymphadenopathy. This presentation is a medical emergency because of the potential for spread to the cornea.

Bacterial conjunctivitis caused by the more common pathogens, such as *S. aureus, S. pneumoniae, H. influenzae,* and *M. catarrhalis,* is characterized by redness and a purulent discharge at the lid margins and corners of the eye that is typically thick and globular. The process is usually but not always unilateral.

Viral conjunctivitis caused by adenoviruses or other agents usually causes injection, a "sandy" or "gritty" feeling in the eye, and a discharge that is predominantly watery or mucoserous. The process usually begins in one eye and then typically (but not always) spreads to the other eye within 24 to 48 hours. Tender preauricular lymphadenopathy is often present, and there may be other symptoms of viral infection such as sore throat or recent upper respiratory infection. Viral conjunctivitis is often highly contagious. Viruses can remain viable for several days outside of human hosts. Preventive measures include handwashing and thorough cleaning of medical equipment.

Epidemic viral keratoconjunctivis, caused by certain types of adenovirus (namely types 8, 19, and 37), has a more fulminant course than most cases of viral conjunctivitis and also—as the name implies—features corneal involvement. Patients have symptoms suggesting viral conjunctivitis and also have the sensation of a foreign body in the eye, indicating the keratitis component.

Allergic conjunctivitis, caused by various environmental allergens and often occurring in patients with a history of atopy or seasonal allergy, causes symptoms similar to those of viral conjunctivitis but is differentiated largely by itching as a prominent complaint. Chemosis is sometimes prominent and can be extreme, with the edematous conjunctiva bulging forward beyond the lid margins. Known as bullous chemosis, this finding is usually encountered in patients who are allergic to cats.

Nonspecific conjunctivitis can be caused by foreign bodies, such as dust, and by chemicals.

Conjunctivitis in contact lens wearers is often associated with keratitis (see later discussion).

Diagnosis

Conjunctivitis must be approached from the perspective of the differential diagnosis of the red eye (Table 9-2), since a firm diagnosis can be made only after other causes of red eye such as uveitis or angle-closure glaucoma have been excluded. In conjunctivitis the redness should be diffuse and should involve the inner surface of the lids (i.e., the palpebral and tarsal conjunctiva), as well as the conjunctiva covering the globe. The redness or injection of conjunctivitis tends to be more prominent away from the pupil, whereas the redness or injection of keratitis, iritis, and glaucoma spares the tarsal conjunctiva. When the patient has a history of recent trauma, the clinician should consider the possibilities of traumatic iritis and of corneal or conjunctival foreign body. In less-than-straightforward cases the eye should be examined systematically using a protocol as follows:

- Equipment. Disposable rubber or latex gloves (which should be worn from start to finish), visual acuity chart, penlight with cobalt blue filter, topical anesthetic drops, fluorescein strips, sterile solution for irrigation, cotton-tipped swabs, and direct ophthalmoscope set on +10 diopters.
- Visual acuity. Record for each eye (if possible, keeping the patient's lenses or eyeglasses in place).
- Examination for lymphadenopathy. Note whether palpable preauricular or submandibular lymph nodes are present (these are usually associated with viral conjunctivitis, especially adenovirus or herpes simplex virus, but are occasionally found in bacterial conjunctivitis).
- External examination of the eye. Note any changes in the eyelids, lid margins, and eyelashes, and look for ptosis and discharge.
- Initial examination of the eye with the ophthalmoscope, using an oblique approach. Examine the eyelids (vesicles or ulcers suggest primary herpes simplex virus conjunctivitis; follicles suggest a viral etiology), bulbar conjunctiva (i.e., the conjunctiva covering the globe), and cornea (keratitis is

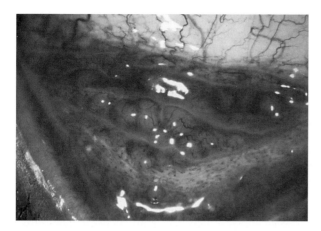

FIG. 9-2 Follicular conjunctivitis. The inferior eyelid has been everted. Numerous round, raised follicles are present in the tissue between the globe and the palpebral conjunctiva.

suggested by a poor light reflex, infiltrate, gray or white ulcer, or injection of the ciliary body or limbus).

- Examination of the inner surface of the lower lids. Pulling the lower lid down, examine for papillae, follicles, or membranes on the palpebral conjunctiva (i.e., the conjunctiva lining the inner surface of the lids).

- Examination of the cornea using fluorescein. Instill topical anesthetic drops into the eye, then place a fluorescein strip into the eye. Using the cobalt blue light, examine the cornea for areas of apple-green fluorescence, causes of which include herpes simplex keratitis, corneal ulcer, and abrasion.

- Clean-up. Discard gloves; wash hands; and disinfect equipment.

Examining both the bulbar conjunctiva (i.e., the conjunctiva covering the eyeball or globe) and the palpebral conjunctiva (the conjunctiva covering the inside surface of the lids) with magnification, the practitioner should look specifically for papillae, follicles, and membranes. Papillae are fine vascular tufts, each containing a central core <0.5 mm in diameter. The presence of numerous papillae causes the eye to appear diffusely red. Papillae are a nonspecific finding regarding etiology. Follicles are smooth, shiny elevations, usually 1 to 2 mm in diameter, on the conjunctival surface (Figure 9-2). Overlying blood vessels may be present, but, in contrast to papillae, no central vascular core exists. Follicles confer a "pebbly" or "cobblestone" appearance to the conjunctival surface. Follicles are highly characteristic of viral conjunctivitis but also occur in chlamydial conjunctivitis, and their formation can be induced by topical medications. Membranes and pseudomembranes, when present, are usually seen in the inferior fornix or on the palpebral conjunctiva. These are rarely seen in adenoviral conjunctivitis but are common in adenoviral epidemic keratoconjunctivitis and in herpetic keratoconjunctivitis. Corneal involvement is often barely visible when viewed with a penlight in cases of epidemic keratoconjunctivitis. Linear or dendritic ulcers are typical of keratoconjunctivitis caused by herpes simplex virus.

Gram stains and cultures should be obtained in cases of neonatal conjunctivitis, hyperacute conjunctivitis, and membranous conjunctivitis. Material can be obtained with a sterile cotton-tipped applicator moistened in thioglycollate medium. The patient is asked to look up. The lower lid is pulled down, and the lower conjunctival cul-de-sac is swabbed twice going from the temporal side to the nasal side in order to reduce the risk of touching the lid margin. Ideally the specimen is plated out promptly, using appropriate media. Alternatively a prepackaged applicator and transport medium system such as Culturette or CultureSwab Plus can be used.

When hyperacute conjunctivitis caused by *N. gonorrhoeae* is suspected, Gram staining of the exudate should be performed to look for the gram-negative, biscuit-shaped diplococci, and laboratory personnel should be asked to look specifically for this organism using modified Thayer-Martin media. When chlamydial infection is suspected, a conjunctival scraping should be sent for enzyme-linked immunosorbent assay or other assay for *Chlamydia*. In the interpretation of cultures it should be kept in mind that the normal flora of the eyelids and conjunctiva usually includes coagulase-negative staphylococci (up to 90% of normal persons), often includes *S. aureus* (about 25%), and occasionally includes other potential pathogens such as *S. pneumoniae*, *Pseudomonas* species and other gram-negative rods, and anaerobic bacteria.

Natural History
Expected Outcome

Hyperacute bacterial conjunctivitis caused by *N. gonorrhoeae* can spread quickly to the cornea, leading to keratitis and perforation. Bacterial conjunctivitis is usually but not always self-limited. Epidemic keratoconjunctivitis caused by certain adenoviruses and herpetic keratoconjunctivitis can permanently damage the cornea with loss of vision. Otherwise, viral conjunctivitis runs a self-limited course similar to that of the common cold, growing worse for several days and then gradually resolving over the next week or two, with 3 weeks sometimes required for complete resolution of the signs and symptoms.

Treatment
Methods

For patients who do not need immediate referral, the primary care clinician can use either of two strategies: treat for acute bacterial conjunctivitis, or tailor therapy depending on the likelihood of a bacterial, viral, or allergic etiology.

For acute bacterial conjunctivitis, topical antibiotic solutions or ointments are used, generally four times a day until response is obtained and then twice a day. Solutions are applied as 1 to 2 drops inside the lower lid. Ointments are applied as ½ inch (or 1.25 cm) inside the lower lid. Several appropriate alternatives are available (Table 9-3). Most adults prefer eye drops because they do not cause the short-lived but annoying blurring of vision that usually follows the application of ointments to the lower lids. Chloramphenicol eye drops should be used with care if at all because of the risk of aplastic anemia. Ointments are preferred for patients who may have trouble using eye drops and also for children. Children with the conjunctivitis-otitis syndrome should receive systemic antibiotics appropriate for acute otitis media (see Chapter 10). Because nearly 70% of *H. influenzae* strains now causing conjunctivitis produce β-lactamase, systemic treatment should probably consist of an oral

TABLE 9-3
Topical Ophthalmic Preparations Used in Treatment of Conjunctivitis

Class	Indications	Preparations	Dose
Lubricants	Nonspecific conjunctivitis	Eye lubricant drops (Hypotears, Refresh, Tears II)	1 or 2 gtts q1h, q.i.d, or prn
		Eye lubricant ointment (Lacrilube, Refresh PM)	½ inch (or 1.25 cm) h.s. or q.i.d., prn
Antibiotics	Nonspecific approach to treatment of conjunctivitis (see text) or treatment of acute bacterial conjunctivitis	Erythromycin ophthalmic ointment (Ilotycin)	½ inch q.i.d. for 5 to 7 days
		Sulfacetamide 10% ophthalmic drops (Bleph-10, Sulamyd, Sulf-10)	1 to 2 gtts q.i.d. for 5 to 7 days
		Fluoroquinolone ophthalmic drops (Ciloxan, Ocuflox, Quixin)	1 to 2 gtts q.i.d. for 5 to 7 days
Antihistamine/ decongestant combinations	Viral conjunctivitis and first-line therapy for allergic conjunctivitis	Naphcon-A, Ocuhist, Visine AC	1 to 2 gtts b.i.d.
Mast cell stabilizer/ antihistamine	Second-line therapy for allergic conjunctivitis (individually or with an antihistamine-decongestant combination)	Patanol, Zaditor, Optivar	1 to 2 gtts b.i.d.
Nonsteroidal antiinflammatory drug	Second-line therapy for allergic conjunctivitis (individually or with an antihistamine-decongestant combination)	Acular	1 to 2 gtts q.i.d. prn
Potent mast cell stabilizer/antihistamine	Third-line therapy for allergic conjunctivitis, for severe cases (used in conjunction with a first- and second-line agent)	Alomide, Crolom, cromolyn 4% ophthalmic solution (generic), Opticrom	1 to 2 gtts q.i.d.

third-generation cephalosporin or amoxicillin-clavulanate (Augmentin).

Patients with viral conjunctivitis are often treated with over-the-counter topical eye drops containing antihistamines or decongestants, since there is no specific therapy. Warm or cool compresses offer a measure of symptomatic relief.

Patients with allergic conjunctivitis are often treated by a step-wise approach, as follows. First-line therapy consists of over-the-counter combinations of antihistamines and decongestants (e.g., Naphcon-A or Ocuhist, for short-term use only). Second-line therapy consists of a drug with anti-histamine and mast cell–stabilizing properties (e.g., Patanol, Zaditor, or Optivar) or an NSAID (e.g., Acular), either of which can be added to the first-line agent. Third-line therapy for patients with clear-cut atopy or severe seasonal allergy can be a more potent drug with mast cell–stabilizing properties (e.g., Alomide, Crolom, or Opticrom). Systemic antihista-mines provide little additional benefit unless severe hyper-sensitivity reaction is present.

Patients with nonspecific conjunctivitis often benefit from lubricant drops (e.g., Hypotears, Refresh) or an eye lubricant ointment (e.g., Lacrilube, Refresh PM).

Topical corticosteroids should not be used in primary care for the treatment of conjunctivitis. Use of steroids in patients with keratitis caused by herpes simplex virus, bacte-ria, or fungi can lead to perforation, scarring, or melting of the cornea with permanent loss of vision. Topical cortico-steroids also promote cataract formation and glaucoma. These potent agents should be used only under the supervi-sion of an ophthalmologist.

Expected Response

Treatment probably shortens the duration of acute bacterial conjunctivitis and reduces the likelihood of person-to-person spread. Topical therapy with polymyxin-bacitracin ointment, for example, reduces the duration of symptoms by half and eradicates the causative bacteria by the tenth day in 79% of patients (versus 31% for placebo).

When to Refer

Patients with hyperacute bacterial conjunctivitis should be hospitalized and followed closely by an ophthalmologist. Referral to an ophthalmologist should also be considered for patients with acute bacterial conjunctivitis who do not respond to treatment within 1 to 2 days and for patients with chronic conjunctivitis (red eye lasting >3 weeks).

 KEY POINTS

ACUTE CONJUNCTIVITIS

⊃ Acute conjunctivitis is a diagnosis of exclusion, to be made after more serious disorders such as uveitis and angle-closure glaucoma have been considered.

⊃ Purulent discharge is the predominant complaint in patients with bacterial conjunctivitis, whereas burning, a "sandy" or "gritty" feeling, or itching is characteristic of viral conjunctivitis and allergic conjunctivitis.

⊃ Bacteria account for about 80% of cases of conjunctivitis in pediatric practice and for about 40% of cases in adults.

⊃ Some children with conjunctivitis also have otitis media (conjunctivitis-otitis syndrome).

⊃ Gram stains and cultures should be obtained in cases of neonatal conjunctivitis, hyperacute conjunctivitis, and membranous conjunctivitis. Cultures are unnecessary in most cases of conjunctivitis, which are managed clinically.

⊃ Hyperacute bacterial conjunctivitis, which is usually due to *N. gonorrhoeae,* is characterized by rapidly progressive, severe inflammation of the eye and requires prompt referral to an ophthalmologist.

⊃ Conjunctivitis in contact lens wearers should be referred to an ophthalmologist unless no evidence of keratitis is present and a prompt response to treatment occurs within 12 to 24 hours.

⊃ Patients with chronic conjunctivitis (red eye lasting >3 weeks) should usually be referred to an ophthalmologist.

⊃ For most patients with conjunctivitis there are two acceptable approaches to therapy: to treat all patients for bacterial conjunctivitis, or to tailor therapy based on the probability of bacterial, viral, or allergic conjunctivitis.

⊃ Topical corticosteroids should not be used to treat conjunctivitis in primary care because of the risk of corneal disease (severe keratitis, including perforation) and glaucoma.

SUGGESTED READING

Baratz KH, Hattenhauer MG. Indiscriminate use of corticosteroid-containing eyedrops. Mayo Clin Proc 1999; 74: 362-366.

Block SL, Hedrick J, Tyler R, et al. Increasing bacterial resistance in pediatric acute conjunctivitis (1997-1998). Antimicrob Agents Chemother 2000; 44: 1650-1654.

Leeming JP. Treatment of ocular infections with topical antibacterials. Clin Pharmacokinet 1999; 37: 351-360.

Morrow GL, Abbott RL. Conjunctivitis. Am Fam Physician 1998; 57: 735-746.

Thielen TL, Castle SS, Terry JE. Anterior ocular infections: an overview of pathophysiology and treatment. Ann Pharmacother 2000; 34: 235-246.

Wallace DK, Steinkuller PG. Ocular medications in children. Clin Pediatr 1998; 37: 645-652.

Weber CM, Eichenbaum JW. Acute red eye: differentiating viral conjunctivitis from other, less common causes. Postgrad Med 1997; 101: 185-186, 189-192, 195-196.

Keratitis

Keratitis, except in the mildest cases, should be managed by an ophthalmologist because of the potential that corneal inflammation will cause scarring or ulceration with permanent loss of vision. The primary care clinician's task is largely that of recognition. Primary care clinicians should also promote safe practices pertaining to contact lenses.

Presentation and Progression
Cause

Patients at increased risk of keratitis include contact lens users, elderly patients with preexisting eye problems, and seriously ill patients being treated in intensive care units.

Bacteria account for 80% to 90% of cases in which a causative agent is identified. Staphylococci, streptococci, and aerobic gram-negative rods are the most commonly isolated bacteria, with *S. aureus* being the most common microorganism at the present time. Various reports document regional differences within the United States; for example, *P. aeruginosa* and streptococci are relatively common in the South, *Moraxella* is relatively common in New York City, and marine vibrios have been recently reported from the Gulf Coast.

Herpes simplex viruses are the most common agents of viral keratitis, which can occur during the neonatal period (about 20% of infants born with herpes simplex infection), during childhood (often manifested mainly as follicular conjunctivitis), or during adulthood. Herpes simplex keratitis recurs within 12 months in about 25% of patients and within 24 months in about 33% of patients. These recurrences are explained by reactivation of latent virus particles in the trigeminal ganglion. Spread to the cornea by way of the trigeminal nerve also explains keratitis in cases of herpes zoster involving the ophthalmic branch of the fifth cranial nerve. Other viruses associated with keratitis include the measles virus and Epstein-Barr virus. Rabies and Creutzfeldt-Jakob disease have been transmitted by corneal transplantation.

Fungi cause about 16% of cases of keratitis. *Fusarium solanae* is the most common agent, but numerous filamentous fungi and yeasts have been implicated. There is often a history of penetrating trauma involving tree branches or other vegetative material. Use of soft contact lenses as a "bandage" for corneal disease also predisposes to fungal keratitis.

Parasites are commonly associated with keratitis in some areas of the world, the best-known example being river blindness caused by onchocerciasis (*Onchocerca volvulus;* see Chapter 23). Other parasites causing keratitis include *Leishmania* species, microsporidia, and trypanosomes (African trypanosomiasis). In recent years *Acanthamoeba* species have been widely recognized as causes of keratitis, and the major risk factors are exposure to contaminated water or use of contact lenses (Box 9-1).

Other causes of keratitis include trachoma (*Chlamydia trachomatis*), which is often said to be the most important cause of blindness worldwide; hypersensitivity reactions; syphilis, which causes interstitial keratitis, especially when the disease is congenital; and systemic vasculitis.

Presentation

The predominant symptom is usually intense pain caused by the cornea's rich supply of nerve endings. Most patients have loss of visual acuity. Excessive tear formation (epiphora), photophobia, and blepharospasm are common. Discharge is not a feature of keratitis unless conjunctivitis is also present (keratoconjunctivitis).

Diagnosis

The primary care clinician can confirm the diagnosis of keratitis by inspecting the eye with a penlight or direct ophthalmoscope with or without fluorescein (see "Examination of the Red Eye" earlier in the chapter). The normal cornea is a unique tissue in that it is clear and avascular. Loss of transparency, either local or generalized, is an early sign of keratitis. This finding is often subtle and is best appreciated by instilling fluorescein, then using a cobalt blue light. Corneal ulcers, including the dendritic ulcers of herpetic keratitis (Figure 9-3), are also best appreciated with this technique. Blood vessels invade the cornea in severe keratitis. Slit lamp examination allows localization of the inflammatory process and recognition of associated phenomena such as the presence

BOX 9-1
CONTACT LENS USE AND KERATITIS

- Bacterial keratitis, especially caused by *P. aeruginosa,* is a major risk of contact lens use.
- *Acanthamoeba* species are being recognized as a cause of keratitis related to contact lenses. Both diagnosis and treatment are difficult.
- Contact lenses should not be worn at night.
- Contact lenses should be rinsed regularly with special solutions made for this purpose. Saline solution does not suffice, and tap water is frequently contaminated.

of leukocytes and fibrin (hypopyon) in the lower portion of the anterior chamber (Figure 9-4) and synechiae.

Examination of the cornea using a cobalt blue light and fluorescein strips sometimes shows changes suggesting a specific diagnosis. Herpes simplex keratitis is classically manifested as dendritic ulcers, but other patterns of the disease include punctate ulcerations and maceration of the cornea in a geographic pattern.

Natural History
Expected Outcome

Herpes simplex keratitis heals spontaneously within 2 weeks in about 80% of cases. Many other forms of keratitis are often self-limited, but serious complications occur with sufficient frequency to make keratitis an urgent clinical problem.

Treatment
Methods

Patients with keratitis must be followed closely. In all but the mildest cases, consultation with an ophthalmologist is desirable. Hospitalization is frequently indicated.

The clinician must decide whether to treat keratitis empirically or to attempt a specific microbiologic diagnosis. For microbiologic diagnosis the procedure is as follows: (1) anesthetize the eye using an agent without antiseptic properties such as proparacaine HCl 0.5% (Ophthetic); (2) obtain corneal scrapings using a calcium alginate swab, a Kimura blunt platinum spatula, or a sterile surgical blade; (3) also obtain scrapings from the unaffected eye so that the patient's "normal ocular flora" can be compared with the results of studies on the diseased eye; and (4) submit the sample for multiple stains (Gram, Giemsa, acid-fast bacillus [AFB], calcofluor white, and methenamine silver stains) and cultures (routine, anaerobic, AFB, and fungal).

Empiric broad-spectrum topical antibiotic therapy for suspected bacterial keratitis includes such regimens as cefazolin plus gentamicin (or tobramycin) plus bacitracin (or polymyxin B) plus vancomycin. Empiric topical therapy for suspected herpes simplex keratitis includes trifluridine, vidarabine, or idoxuridine. Use of topical antibiotics should be avoided unless there is a strong risk of bacterial superinfection, since

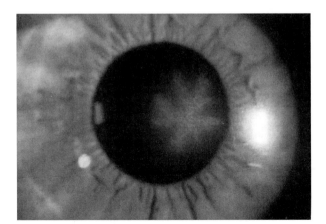

FIG. 9-3 Herpes simplex keratitis. A classic "dendritic" ulcer is demonstrated by fluorescein staining of the cornea.

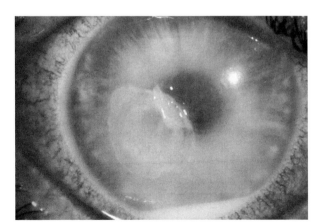

FIG. 9-4 Keratitis caused by *Pseudomonas aeruginosa* in a contact lens user. Note the opacity of the central cornea and also the layer of pus (hypopyon) in the inferior aspect of the anterior chamber.

antibiotics increase the risk of drug toxicity. Atropine ophthalmic drops are used if herpetic uveitis is also present. Long-term antiviral prophylaxis is recommended for patients with stromal keratitis caused by herpes simplex virus.

Expected Response

Most patients with keratitis respond to topical therapy. Patients with fungal keratitis usually require a corneal transplant.

When to Refer

All but the mildest cases of keratitis should be managed by an ophthalmologist.

 KEY POINTS

KERATITIS

⊃ The main symptoms of keratitis are pain and loss of vision. Tearing, photophobia, and blepharospasm are often present. Discharge is usually absent unless an associated conjunctivitis is present.

⊃ Bacteria, especially *S. aureus* and *P. aeruginosa,* are the most commonly identified causes of keratitis.

⊃ Fungi, especially filamentous fungi (molds), are relatively common causes of keratitis, especially when the predisposing factors are trauma involving tree branches or other vegetative matter or the use of soft contact lenses.

⊃ Herpes simplex keratitis is classically recognized because of dendritic corneal ulcers, but other forms of the disease exist and other diseases can cause dendritic ulcers.

⊃ *Acanthamoeba* is being recognized with increasing frequency as a cause of keratitis resulting from contaminated water or contact lens use.

SUGGESTED READING

Cruz CS, Cohen EJ, Rapuano CJ, et al. Microbial keratitis resulting in loss of the eye. Ophthalmic Surg Lasers 1998; 29: 803-807.

Forster RK. Conrad Berens Lecture. The management of infectious keratitis as we approach the 21st century. CLAO J 1998; 24: 175-180.

Garg P, Gopinathan U, Choudhary K, et al. Keratomycosis: clinical and microbiologic experience with dematiaceous fungi. Ophthalmology 2000; 107: 574-580.

Hart A, White S, Conboy P, et al. The management of corneal abrasions in accident and emergency. Injury 1997; 28: 527-529.

Herpetic Eye Disease Study Group. Acyclovir for the prevention of recurrent herpes simplex virus eye disease. N Engl J Med 1998; 339: 300-306.

McCulley JP, Alizadeh H, Niedreknorn JY. The diagnosis and management of *Acanthamoeba* keratitis. CLAO J 2000; 26: 47-51.

Micallef C, Cuschieri P, Bonnici MR. Contamination of contact-lens-related sources with *Pseudomonas aeruginosa.* Ophthalmologica 2000; 214: 324-331.

Penland RL, Boniuk M, Wilhelmus KR. *Vibrio* ocular infections on the U.S. Gulf Coast. Cornea 2000; 19: 26-29.

10 Upper Respiratory Tract Infections and Other Infections of the Head and Neck

CHARLES S. BRYAN, J. DAVID OSGUTHORPE

Upper respiratory tract infection (URI) causes at least of one half of all symptomatic illness in the community, exacting huge tolls that can be measured as morbidity, absenteeism from school and work, direct health care costs, and overuse of antibiotics leading to the emergence of drug-resistant bacteria. This disease burden is largely explained by anatomy (Figure 10-1). The nose, mouth, and pharynx are exposed to circulating viruses and are normally colonized by large numbers of bacteria, including potential pathogens such as *Staphylococcus aureus, Streptococcus pneumoniae, Haemophilus influenzae,* and group A streptococci. Mucosal injury caused by viral infection, allergy, or other factors compromises the mucociliary barriers designed to maintain sterility of the middle ears, paranasal sinuses, and lungs. Most URIs are self-limited, but progression to life-threatening acute illness occurs and progression to chronic disease is common.

During the first year of life infants have, on average, about eight URIs. Adults average three to four URIs per year, but the incidence is higher in young parents. Many people are unusually susceptible to URI for reasons that are poorly understood. When and now to prescribe antibiotics for such common conditions as acute otitis media in childhood (see Chapter 4) and acute sinusitis is highly problematic, and over-prescribing largely explains the emergence of β-lactamase–producing strains of *H. influenzae* and pneumococci with reduced susceptibility to penicillin. Primary care clinicians should have in place efficient, cost-effective protocols for management of URI symptoms. Newer imaging studies improve the understanding of conditions such as acute sinusitis but should be used on a selective basis. Patients with complicated problems should usually be referred to an otolaryngologist. Primary care clinicians must promote public awareness of the need for therapeutic restraint in the management of these common but usually self-limited disorders.

SUGGESTED READING

Carroll K, Reimer L. Microbiology and laboratory diagnosis of upper respiratory tract infections. Clin Infect Dis 1996; 23: 442-448.

Dolin R, Wright PF. Viral Infections of the Respiratory Tract. New York: Marcel-Dekker; 1999.

Dosh SA, Hickner JM, Mainous AG III, et al. Predictors of antibiotic prescribing for nonspecific upper respiratory infections, acute bronchitis, and acute sinusitis: an UPRNet study. J Fam Pract 2000; 49: 407-414.

Fagnan LJ. Prescribing antibiotics for upper respiratory infections. J Fam Pract 2000; 49: 415-417.

Johnson JT, Yu VL, eds. Infectious Diseases and Antimicrobial Therapy of the Ears, Nose and Throat. Philadelphia: W.B. Saunders Company; 1997.

The Common Cold

The common cold is an acute, self-limited catarrhal (Latin *catarrhus,* to flow down) syndrome limited to the mucosal membranes of the upper respiratory tract. Recently "viral rhinosinusitis" has been suggested as the technically correct term for this disorder because computed tomography (CT) shows abnormalities of the paranasal sinuses in most cases. However, "cold" is the preferred term for clinical use, since "rhinosinusitis" suggests to patients the need for antibiotics. The common cold accounts for up to three fourths of all illnesses in young infants and up to one half of illnesses in adults. Elimination of the common cold would also eliminate an estimated 27 million office visits, 23 million days of work absenteeism, 26 million days of school absenteeism, and nearly $2 billion worth of over-the-counter remedies in the United States each year.

Presentation and Progression
Cause

Rhinoviruses, of which more than 100 serotypes exist, cause an estimated 30% to 50% of colds. Coronaviruses account for perhaps 10% of cases. Respiratory syncytial virus (RSV) is an important cause of cold symptoms in young children and among the elderly. Influenza and parainfluenza viruses can cause colds but more often cause lower respiratory tract infection or systemic symptoms. Adenoviruses, of which at least 47 antigenic types exist, cause 5% to 10% of colds. Although echoviruses and coxsackieviruses have been associated with colds, they more commonly cause an undifferentiated flulike illness or distinctive syndromes such as aseptic meningitis or pharyngitis. Rhinoviruses and parainfluenza viruses cause outbreaks of cold symptoms during the fall and late spring; RSV, adenoviruses, and coronaviruses cause outbreaks during the winter and early spring. Viruses that remain to be discovered probably cause a substantial fraction of colds.

Rhinoviruses are transmitted most efficiently by direct contact. Hand contact with the eyes and nose is common in everyday life. Rhinoviruses remain viable on skin and also on objects (fomites) for at least 2 hours. Rhinoviruses can be recovered from the hands of 40% to 90% of persons with colds and from up to 15% of objects near persons with colds. However, brief exposure such as a handshake or even being around an infected person for 36 hours causes transmission in less than 10% of subjects and in one study transmission was only 38% between spouses. Rhinoviruses can also be transmitted by aerosolization, for example, by being in a crowded room where people are sneezing. Kissing does not seem to be a common mode of transmission, probably because only about 10% of persons with colds have demonstrable virus in their saliva. Studies carried out in Antarctica dispel the popular idea that cold weather increases susceptibility to rhinovirus infection.

The nasal epithelium of persons with colds is remarkably intact even when studied with the electron microscope. Symptoms are best explained by physiologic responses: the release of chemical mediators of inflammation and the sensitization and irritation of airway receptors, with stimulation of the parasympathetic nervous system (Figure 10-2).

Presentation

After an incubation period of 24 to 72 hours, usually a sore or scratchy throat develops, which is followed by nasal obstruction, rhinorrhea, and sneezing. A green or yellow nasal discharge should not be construed as evidence of secondary bacterial infection (neutrophils cause yellow-green discoloration because of their natural myeloperoxidase activity). By the second and third days of the illness, rhinitis with nasal congestion replaces sore throat as the major complaint. By the fourth and fifth days, nasal symptoms have usually decreased but in about 30% of cases are replaced by cough or "chest cold" (see "Acute Bronchitis" in Chapter 11).

Diagnosis

The common cold is a clinical diagnosis. Although the viral agents can sometimes be demonstrated by culture, antigen detection symptoms, or serologic tests, such studies are of little or no use in everyday clinical practice. The clinician's major obligation is to exclude bacterial sinusitis, otitis media, or more serious illness. High fever, myalgia, and chills should prompt a search for an alternative diagnosis.

In young children nasal foreign bodies, streptococcal nasopharyngitis, and congenital syphilis should be considered when symptoms are atypical. The key to early suspicion of a nasal foreign body is a unilateral discharge that may be bloody or foul smelling. The key to early diagnosis of streptococcal nasopharyngitis, which may be indistinguishable from the common cold in a child under the age of 3 years, is culture of the discharge; fever and excoriation of the nares are

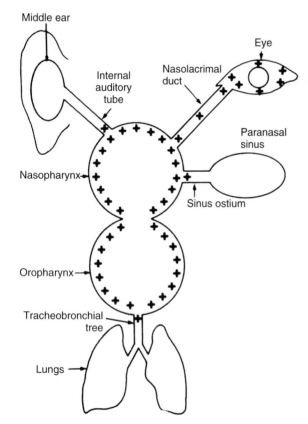

FIG. 10-1 Structures such as the middle ear, the paranasal sinuses, and the lungs are connected by various tubes to the oropharynx and nasopharynx, which normally carry a heavy microbial flora. Sterility is therefore difficult to maintain. (From Todd JK. Bacteriology and clinical relevance of nasopharyngeal and oropharyngeal cultures. Pediatr Infect Dis 1984; 3: 159-163.)

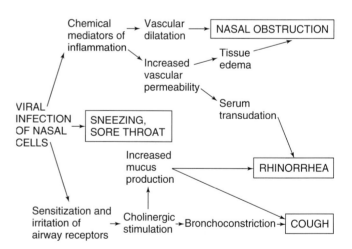

FIG. 10-2 Proposed pathogenesis of cold symptoms. This framework provides the rationale for various therapeutic interventions. For example, topical vasoconstrictors reverse the increased vascular permeability, and ipratropium bromide blocks cholinergic stimulation. New therapies are being developed to block viral attachment to nasal cells. (From Spector SL. The common cold: current therapy and natural history. J Allergy Clin Immunol 1995; 95: 1133-1138.)

found in some but not all of these children. The key to early diagnosis of congenital syphilis is the onset of a persistent clear rhinorrhea ("snuffles"), sometimes with excoriation, within the first 3 months (usually the first month) of life. In children, adolescents, and young adults, pertussis can be indistinguishable from the common cold during its early or "catarrhal" phase. Pertussis should be suspected when severe paroxysmal cough begins to dominate the illness or when pertussis is prevalent in the community.

Allergic rhinitis causes symptoms that can be almost indistinguishable from the common cold. Clinical clues to allergic rhinitis include seasonal occurrence, a personal or family history of asthma, itching of the eyes or palate, a watery nasal discharge (rather than the thick discharge of infection), and sneezing as the predominant complaint throughout the illness. A nasal smear for eosinophils can be useful. Finding more than 20% eosinophils has high specificity for allergic rhinitis; however, the sensitivity of this test is relatively low.

Acute severe bacterial sinusitis (see later discussion) is unlikely to be mistaken for a common cold, since this illness is characterized by facial pain, headache, and fever as well as by purulent rhinorrhea. However, less severe but persistent sinusitis can be difficult to distinguish from the common cold because the major symptoms are rhinorrhea and cough. The principal distinguishing feature is duration of the illness, since symptoms of the common cold usually begin to resolve within 5 to 7 days whereas symptoms of sinusitis persist or worsen. As compared with "colds," bacterial sinusitis is more commonly associated with unilateral aching of the cheek or maxillary molars, unilateral nasal discharge, forehead pain, or pain worsened by bending over or by the Valsalva maneuver.

KEY POINTS

THE COMMON COLD: DIAGNOSIS

⊃ The initial symptoms of the common cold are usually a sore or scratchy throat and sneezing.

⊃ Rhinitis with nasal congestion or obstruction is usually the most prominent symptom during the second and third days of the illness.

⊃ In about 30% of cases there is progression to cough ("chest cold") during the fourth to fifth days of the illness.

⊃ In young children the possibility of a nasal foreign body should be considered, especially if the nasal discharge is unilateral, bloody, or foul smelling.

⊃ Streptococcal nasopharyngitis in young children can be indistinguishable from the common cold; nasal excoriation is a valuable clue.

⊃ In children less than 3 months of age, clear rhinorrhea ("snuffles") should prompt suspicion of congenital syphilis.

⊃ Allergic rhinitis can resemble the common cold; distinguishing points include itchy eyes, >20% eosinophilia in nasal secretions, and seasonal occurrence.

⊃ Persistent, low-grade bacterial sinusitis is distinguished from the common cold on the basis of chronicity of symptoms.

⊃ Abnormalities of the paranasal sinuses can be seen on CT scan in up to 87% of patients with colds but are usually of little significance.

⊃ High fever, chills, myalgias, signs of meningeal irritation, or proptosis should prompt consideration of another diagnosis.

Natural History
Expected Outcome

The average duration of cold symptoms in immunologically normal persons is 3 to 7 days. Symptoms are usually worse during the second to fourth days of the illness. Symptoms persist for up to 2 weeks in about 25% of patients, and smokers tend to have a prolonged cough. Risk factors for more severe disease include prematurity, infancy, crowded living conditions, malnutrition, and the presence of chronic disease, including immunodeficiency disorders.

Sinusitis, presumed to be of viral etiology, can be demonstrated by plain x-ray examination of the sinuses in about 40% of patients and by CT scans in up to 87% of patients with colds, but it usually resolves without antibiotic therapy. About 0.5% to 2.5% of adults with common colds have clinical symptoms and signs of acute bacterial sinusitis (see later discussion). Other complications are acute otitis media (discussed later), exacerbations of chronic bronchitis (Chapter 11), and acute asthma. Colds have been associated with up to 40% of acute asthmatic attacks. Mounting evidence suggests that asthmatic symptoms are caused not only by the viral infection but also by the immune response to infection (Figure 10-3), which triggers airway hyperresponsiveness, leading to obstruction. By causing changes in the bacterial

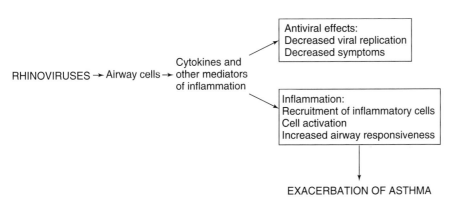

FIG. 10-3 Proposed mechanism for exacerbation of asthma by rhinovirus infection. The rationale for prednisone or inhaled corticosteroids is to block the inflammatory response. New therapies being developed include antiviral agents, inhibitors of signal transduction pathways in the airway cells, and specific cytokine inhibitors. (Modified from Gern JE, Busse WM. Association of rhinovirus infections with asthma. Clin Microbiol Rev 1999; 12: 9-18.)

flora of the upper respiratory tract, colds may predispose affected persons to invasive bacterial infections such as meningococcal disease and pneumococcal pneumonia. The frequency of these complications is unknown.

Treatment
Methods

Whether drugs help the common cold has been debated for many years. Osler is said to have remarked, "The only way to treat a cold is with contempt." Numerous remedies have been proposed (Table 10-1), but controlled trials have been

difficult to conduct because of the cost and because of the side effects of the illness. Aspirin, acetaminophen, and other nonsteroidal antiinflammatory drugs (NSAIDs) prolong symptomatic illness and the duration of viral shedding. At present, ipratropium bromide and zinc lozenges have the greatest support on the basis of critical reviews of available data (Table 10-1). Antihistamines are, in general, not recommended. On the basis of data from experimental rhinovirus colds, however, one authority recommends a first-generation antihistamine (brompheniramine 12 mg extended release) plus naproxen sodium 275 mg q12h.

TABLE 10-1
Drug Therapy for the Common Cold

Class	Dose	Theoretical basis	Evidence for efficacy	Consensus
Ipratropium bromide 0.06% nasal spray	Two 42-µg sprays per nostril t.i.d. to q.i.d. for 4 days	Parasympathetic nervous system reflexes are thought to mediate symptoms of rhinorrhea	Brought about a 31% reduction in rhinorrhea in a randomized, double-blinded, placebo-controlled trial	Approved by Food and Drug Administration; recommended but moderately expensive
Zinc lozenges	One lozenge of 13.3 mg of zinc q2h while awake	Zinc ions inhibit rhinovirus replication in vitro	Reduced the severity of cold symptoms in three of six studies, all of which were somewhat flawed	The data are inconclusive; however, the lozenges are inexpensive and the side effects are minor
Antihistamines	Brompheniramine (12 mg extended release) q12h; diphenhydramine; clemastine fumarate	Since there is little evidence that histamine is important in the pathogenesis of cold symptoms, the rationale is limited to the drying up of rhinorrhea	Reduced the severity of sneezing in a slight majority of studies, but otherwise caused little improvement; sedation can be an important side effect of older generation antihistamines	Not recommended by most authorities; however, recent work suggests first-generation antihistamines may be effective
Vitamin C	Variable doses	Suggested to be immunopotentiating drug by a Nobel laureate	In 23 studies, led to an average 23% decrease in symptom duration, but the studies were not well controlled	Not recommended
Echinacea extract	Variable doses	Suggested to be immunomodulating	Had no effect on the duration or severity of colds in a randomized, controlled trial	Not recommended
Antibiotics	Amoxicillin-clavulanate	May benefit patients who have pathogens in nasal discharge	In a controlled trial, hastened resolution of symptoms in patients whose nasal secretions showed *Haemophilus influenzae, Streptococcus pneumoniae,* or *Moraxella catarrhalis*	Not recommended; because of delay in receiving culture results, five patients would have to be treated for every patient who would respond
Nonsteroidal antiinflammatory drugs	Naproxen 220 mg q12h	Inhibits prostaglandin action	May be useful for cough and systemic symptoms such as headache; may also prolong viral shedding	Recommended by some authorities for symptomatic relief

When, if ever, are antibiotics indicated for the common cold? In one provocative study patients were randomly assigned to receive placebo or amoxicillin-clavulanate (Augmentin). The only patients who benefited from therapy were those who had nasal cultures positive for *H. influenzae, M. catarrhalis,* or *S. pneumoniae* (about one fifth of all patients). These patients were 10 times more likely to be asymptomatic at 5 days of the illness than control patients with positive nasal cultures who were not treated. However, use of antibiotics cannot be widely endorsed, especially since the disease is nearly always self-limited and the number of patients who would need to be treated to prevent one case of invasive bacterial disease is unknown.

Many researchers have sought a way to prevent colds. Interferon has been shown to be effective as prophylaxis against colds; however, it has local side effects. Use of virucidal-impregnated facial tissues has been shown to reduce transmission of the virus. Porous materials such as cotton handkerchiefs or paper tissues do not support survival of the virus. Decontamination of environmental tissues with virucidal disinfectants such as phenol-alcohol (Lysol) reduces the rate of transmission. Common courtesy requires that persons with cold symptoms minimize direct contact with other persons, such as handshaking.

Expected Response

The common cold is usually a self-limited condition.

When to Refer

Referral is indicated only for the most severe complications.

 ## KEY POINTS

TREATMENT OF THE COMMON COLD

- ⊃ Well-controlled trials are lacking for most of the agents reported to be beneficial.
- ⊃ Inhaled ipratropium bromide or zinc lozenges have the greatest support on the basis of the published literature.
- ⊃ Most of the literature provides little support for use of antihistamines, decongestants, antiinflammatory medicines, and herbal regimens, including *Echinacea*.
- ⊃ On the basis of experimental data in rhinovirus colds in adults, one authority recommends brompheniramine (12 mg extended release tablets) plus naproxen 275 mg q12h.
- ⊃ Antibiotics may benefit the one fifth of patients who have pathogens in their nasal secretions, but this approach is not practical at this time.
- ⊃ Preventive measures include frequent handwashing, use of disposable tissues by persons with colds, avoidance of hand contact with patients or fomites, and the vitamins supplied in a normal diet. Decontamination of surfaces with phenol-alcohol (Lysol) reduces the rate of transmission.

SUGGESTED READING

Barrett B, Vohmann M, Calabrese C. *Echinacea* for upper respiratory infection. J Fam Pract 1999; 48: 628-635.

Gern JE, Busse WW. Association of rhinovirus infections with asthma. Clin Microbiol Rev 1999; 12: 9-18.

Grimm W, Muller HH. A randomized controlled trial of the effect of fluid extract of *Echinacea purpurea* on the incidence and severity of colds and respiratory infections. Am J Med 1999; 106: 138-143.

Gwaltney JM Jr, Philips CD, Miller RD, et al. Computed tomographic study of the common cold. N Engl J Med 1994; 330: 25-30.

Hayden FG, Diamond L, Wood PB, et al. Effectiveness and safety of intranasal ipratropium bromide in common colds: a randomized, double-blind, placebo-controlled trial. Ann Intern Med 1996; 125: 89-97.

Jackson JL, Peterson C, Lesho E. A meta-analysis of zinc salts lozenges and the common cold. Arch Intern Med 1997; 157: 2373-2376.

Kaiser L, Lew D, Hirschel B, et al. Effects of antibiotic treatment in the subset of common-cold patients who have bacteria in nasopharyngeal secretions. Lancet 1996; 347: 1507-1510.

Luks D, Anderson MR. Antihistamines and the common cold: a review and critique of the literature. J Gen Intern Med 1996; 11: 240-244.

Winther B, Gwaltney JM Jr, Mygind N, et al. Viral-induced rhinitis. Am J Rhinol 1998; 12: 17-20.

Acute Bacterial Sinusitis

Few common problems in primary care are as confusing as sinusitis. Acute bacterial sinusitis is vastly overdiagnosed, but chronic sinusitis can be frustrating and disabling. The paranasal sinuses are accessible to direct examination only by sophisticated instruments. Adequate specimens for cultures can be obtained only by invasive procedures. Low-grade sinusitis is an intrinsic feature of the common cold. Clinicians must distinguish between self-limited viral rhinosinusitis and acute bacterial sinusitis, which usually calls for antibiotic therapy. It is therefore important to appreciate the spectrum of conditions that fall under the rubric "sinusitis" (Table 10-2). This section discusses acute bacterial sinusitis. Chronic sinusitis and fungal sinusitis are discussed separately later in the chapter, and acute, complicated frontal, ethmoid, or sphenoid sinusitis, which can be a life-threatening emergency, is discussed in Chapter 6.

Presentation and Progression
Cause

Sinusitis is usually caused by obstruction of the ostia, as from edema, damage to ciliated epithelial cells, and increased volume or viscosity of the mucous secretions. The pathogenesis of acute sinusitis can be discussed in three complementary ways: anatomy, physiology, and microbiology.

Anatomy. The outflow tract of the maxillary sinus sits in an awkward position high on the medial wall of the sinus cavity and is connected to the nasal cavity by a narrow tubular passage known as the infundibulum. Gravitational drainage of the maxillary sinus is therefore tenuous and easily disrupted. A small area between the middle and inferior nasal turbinates where drainage from the maxillary, ethmoid, and frontal sinuses converges is known as the ostiomeatal complex (Figure 10-4). Anatomic or physiologic compromise of the ostiomeatal complex predisposes not only to maxillary sinusitis, but also to infection of multiple sinuses (pansinusitis). Causes of mechanical obstruction of sinus drainage include deviated nasal septum, polyps, foreign bodies, tumors, concha bullosa (enlarged middle turbinates from pneumatization, present in 10% of the population), ethmoid bullae, choanal atresia, and—most commonly—mucosal swelling. Mucosal swelling is usually due to viral infection

TABLE 10-2
Categories of Community-Acquired Sinusitis According to Severity and Therapeutic Implications

Category of severity	Clinical features	Therapeutic implications
Trivial (viral rhinosinusitis)	The common cold or "rhinosinusitis," with symptoms of runny nose and nasal obstruction; CT scanning shows abnormalities of the paranasal sinuses (most often of the maxillary sinus) in a reported 87% of cases. The symptoms usually resolve within 1 week. The etiology is presumed to be viral.	Symptomatic therapy. Imaging studies, cultures, and antibiotic therapy are not indicated.
Nonurgent (elective) acute bacterial sinusitis	Symptoms of cold or flulike illness persist for ≥8 days with little or no improvement but little or no worsening. Imaging studies, if performed, usually show mucosal thickening. The etiology is presumed to be bacterial (see Table 10-3). Symptoms persist no longer than 4 weeks.	Oral antibiotic therapy plus supportive measures such as an oral decongestant, an antihistamine, and a mucoevacuant (see Table 10-6). Imaging studies are not indicated. Follow-up visits should be on an as-needed basis.
Urgent acute bacterial sinusitis	Fever (temperature ≥100.4° F [38° C]); facial pain sometimes with edema or erythema; maxillary toothache. Imaging studies often show a classic air-fluid level. The etiology is nearly always bacterial (see Table 10-3).	Same as above. Imaging studies are sometimes indicated based on the clinician's judgment. A follow-up visit should be scheduled.
Emergency acute sinusitis	Same as above *plus* symptoms and signs that point to extension into the orbit or brain. Imaging studies usually indicate involvement of the ethmoid, frontal, or sphenoid sinuses with intracranial or orbital extension. Complications include brain abscess, meningitis, and cavernous sinus thrombosis. The etiology is usually bacterial, with *Staphylococcus aureus* a frequent pathogen. Fungal disease (e.g., rhinocerebral mucormycosis) should also be considered.	Hospitalization on an emergency basis. Studies should include computed tomography and lumbar puncture, and otolaryngology consultation should be obtained. Initial intravenous antibiotic therapy should consist of vancomycin plus a third-generation (and cerebrospinal fluid–penetrating) cephalosporin.
Chronic sinusitis in children	Symptoms and signs of sinusitis persisting for ≥12 weeks *or* four or more episodes of sinusitis lasting ≥10 days occur each year. Imaging studies confirm mucosal thickening and other changes. The etiology varies and is poorly understood.	Referral to an otolaryngologist is usually indicated.
Chronic sinusitis in adults	Symptoms and signs of sinusitis persisting for ≥12 weeks *or* four or more episodes of sinusitis lasting ≥10 days occur each year. Imaging studies confirm mucosal thickening and other changes. The etiology varies and is poorly understood.	Referral to an otolaryngologist is usually indicated.
Fungal sinusitis	The clinical spectrum of disease includes simple colonization of the paranasal sinuses by fungi; mycetoma (fungus ball); allergic fungal sinusitis; and invasive fungal sinusitis. Invasive fungal sinusitis is potentially life threatening.	Referral to an otolaryngologist is usually indicated.
Sinusitis in patients with cystic fibrosis	Sinusitis is typically chronic and is often associated with nasal polyposis. Imaging studies typically show complete opacification of the maxillary and ethmoid sinuses. The frontal sinuses sometimes fail to develop, and the sphenoid sinuses are often small. Common bacterial isolates include *Pseudomonas aeruginosa* and *S. aureus* in addition to the pathogens that cause sinusitis in immunologically intact persons.	Referral to an otolaryngologist is usually indicated.

*Modified from Gwaltney JM Jr. Acute community-acquired sinusitis. Clin Infect Dis 1996; 23: 1209-1225.

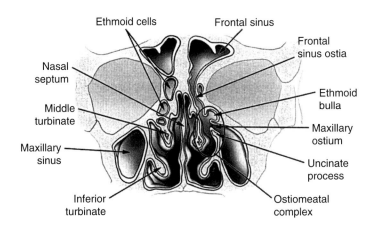

Ethmoid cells   Frontal sinus

Frontal
sinus ostia

Nasal
septum

Ethmoid
bulla

Middle
turbinate

Maxillary
ostium

Maxillary
sinus

Uncinate
process

Inferior
turbinate

Ostiomeatal
complex

FIG. 10-4   Anatomy of the nose and its relation to the maxillary, ethmoid, and frontal sinuses, showing the pivotal position of the ostiomeatal complex. (From Brook I, Gooch WM, Reiner SA, et al. Medical management of acute bacterial sinusitis: recommendations of a clinical advisory committee on pediatric and adult sinusitis. Ann Otol Rhinol Laryngol 2000; 109S [Suppl 182, May 2000]: 2-20.)

TABLE 10-3
Microbial Etiologies of Acute Sinusitis in Children and Adults

Agent	PERCENT OF CASES	
	Children	Adults
BACTERIA		
Streptococcus pneumoniae	31	36
Haemophilus influenzae	21	33
Both *S. pneumoniae* and *H. influenzae*	5	—
Anaerobic bacteria	6	—
Staphylococcus aureus	4	—
Streptococcus pyogenes (group A streptococci)	2	2
Moraxella catarrhalis	2	19
Gram-negative bacilli	9	2
VIRUSES		
Rhinoviruses	15	—
Influenza virus	5	—
Parainfluenza virus	3	—
Adenovirus	—	2

Modified from Carroll K, Reimer L. Microbiology and laboratory diagnosis of upper respiratory tract infection. Clin Infect Dis 1996; 23: 442-448.

or allergic inflammation but can also be caused by systemic disorders (e.g., cystic fibrosis and the dyskinetic cilia syndromes) or injury brought about by trauma, swimming or diving, or overuse of topical medication (rhinitis medicamentosa) or cocaine.

Physiology. The sinuses are kept sterile mainly by a mucociliary blanket that changes two to three times per hour, a rate sufficient to prevent mucus from accumulating in the sinuses. Sinusitis results when mucociliary drainage of the paranasal sinuses fails because of mucosal edema, dysfunction of the ciliated epithelial cells, or both. Viral rhinitis and allergic rhinitis disrupt the epithelium, as do cigarette smoking and intranasal cocaine use. Swimming predisposes to sinusitis for reasons that are somewhat unclear, although chlorine is known to irritate the mucosa. Other factors that may help to preserve the normal sterility of the paranasal sinuses include cellular and humoral immunity and nitric oxide.

Acute sinusitis typically starts with viral infection that paves the path for pathogenic bacteria. The major pathogens are *S. pneumoniae* and nontypeable strains of *H. influenzae.* Other bacteria associated with community-acquired sinusitis are group A streptococci, *Staphylococcus aureus, Moraxella catarrhalis,* and viridans streptococci (Table 10-3). Whether *Chlamydia pneumoniae* commonly causes sinusitis is currently being studied. Patients who have had nasogastric tubes in place are vulnerable to sinusitis caused by aerobic gram-negative rods such as *Pseudomonas aeruginosa* and *Klebsiella pneumoniae.* Anaerobic bacteria are associated with acute sinusitis mainly in the setting of dental disease. Anaerobic bacteria also play an important role in chronic sinusitis.

Presentation

Sinusitis usually begins with symptoms of the common cold such as runny nose, nasal obstruction, sore throat, cough, and the sensation of "pressure" or "tightness" in the face. Rhinosinusitis is divided into four subtypes based on patient history and limited physical examination (Table 10-4). The symptoms differ somewhat between children and adults. Symptoms are divided into "major" and "minor" groups (Box 10-1), and specific combinations of these allow the diagnosis based on patient history and the sole physical finding for diagnosis of uncomplicated acute sinusitis: nasal purulence, visualized by anterior rhinoscopy or as a postnasal discharge on examination of the pharynx.

Children with sinusitis can have either of two presentations. The more common presentation consists of *persistent* cold symptoms—that is, symptoms lasting more than 10 days. Children with persistent sinusitis seldom complain of head-

TABLE 10-4
Classification of Adult Rhinosinusitis

Classification	Duration	History and physical examination*	Special notes
Acute	<4 weeks	Two or more major factors; one major factor and two minor factors; or nasal or postnasal purulence on examination	Fever or facial pain and pressure does not constitute a suggestive history in the absence of other nasal symptoms or signs. Consider acute bacterial rhinosinusitis if symptoms worsen after 5 days, if symptoms persist for 10 days, or if symptoms are out of proportion to those typically associated with viral infection.
Subacute	4 to 11 weeks	Two or more major factors; one major factor and two minor factors; or nasal or postnasal purulence on examination	The condition resolves completely after effective medical therapy.
Recurrent acute	Four or more episodes per year with each episode lasting ≥7 days; absence of intervening symptoms and signs	Two or more major factors; one major factor and two minor factors; or nasal or postnasal purulence on examination	
Chronic	≥12 weeks	Two or more major factors; one major factor and two minor factors; or nasal or postnasal purulence on examination	Facial pain and pressure do not constitute a suggestive history in the absence of other nasal symptoms or signs.

Modified from Lanza D, Kennedy D. Adult rhinosinusitis defined. Otolaryngol Head Neck Surg 1997; 117: S1-S7.
*See Box 10-1 for definition of major and minor factors.

BOX 10-1
Factors Associated with the Diagnosis of Rhinosinusitis

MAJOR FACTORS
• Facial pain, pressure, congestion, fullness*
• Nasal obstruction, blockage
• Nasal or postnasal purulence by physical examination
• Hyposmia, anosmia
• Cough not caused by asthma (in children)

MINOR FACTORS
• Headaches
• Fever
• Halitosis
• Fatigue
• Dental pain
• Cough (in adults)
• Ear pain, pressure, fullness

Modified from Hadley J, Schaefer S. Clinical evaluation of rhinosinusitis. Otolaryngol Head Neck Surg 1997; 117: S8-S11.
*Facial pain and pressure alone do not constitute a suggestive history in the absence of another major factor.

ache or facial pain. Parents of young children often report malodorous breath. The less common presentation consists of *severe* cold symptoms—that is, cold symptoms accompanied by high fever (≥103° F [39° C]) and purulent nasal discharge. Some of these children have headaches, usu-

ally behind or around the eye and occasionally with periorbital edema.

Adults with sinusitis, compared with children, tend to have more prominent facial pain, sometimes with local tenderness, swelling, and erythema. Pain patterns and other findings vary according to which sinuses are involved:

■ Maxillary sinusitis (most common location). Pain is over the cheekbones or above the maxillary second molar teeth.
■ Ethmoid sinusitis (common). Pain is between the orbits and the nasal bridge.
■ Frontal sinusitis (uncommon). Pain is over the frontal bones.
■ Sphenoid sinusitis (least common, but dangerous—see Chapter 6). Pain can be frontal, temporal, orbital, or occipital. Facial pain resulting from fifth nerve involvement is characteristic. Pain is occasionally perceived over the vertex of the skull.

Low-grade fever is often present. Physical examination may reveal tenderness on percussion of the maxillary or frontal sinuses, and pinching the bridge of the nose may bring out tenderness if the ethmoid sinuses are involved. However, the sensitivity and specificity of these findings are unknown and the clinical findings are often subtle.

Diagnosis

Acute bacterial sinusitis is suggested in children by persistent or severe cold symptoms and in adults by fever, severe pain in a characteristic location, or the observation of pus coming from the nose (again, with the caveat that yellow or green discharge can be caused by uncomplicated colds). In maxillary,

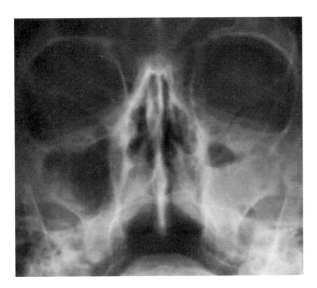

FIG. 10-5   Plain film (Waters' view) demonstrating an air-fluid level in one maxillary sinus.

anterior ethmoid, or frontal sinusitis, pus can often be observed in the middle meatus.

Sinus transillumination is a time-honored method for evaluating the maxillary and frontal sinuses. The procedure must be performed in a completely darkened room using a special device called a sinus transilluminator. Normal transillumination is considered evidence against sinusitis; complete opacification of the sinus correlates with active disease. Partial or reduced transillumination is a less helpful finding. This procedure is still considered worthwhile but has at least four limitations: inability to evaluate the ethmoid and sphenoid sinuses; relatively low sensitivity and specificity (73% and 54%, respectively, compared with radiographic evaluations); observer bias, since the technique requires experience for accurate interpretation; and technical difficulties in dark-skinned persons and those with unusually heavy bone structure or obesity.

Radiography (plain films or CT scans) has largely replaced sinus transillumination in many practices. The traditional series of plain films includes a Waters' view for the maxillary sinuses; a Caldwell's view for the frontal and ethmoid sinuses; a lateral view for information about all of the sinuses, including the sphenoid sinuses; and a submentovertical (base) view for the sphenoid and ethmoid sinuses. An air-fluid level on plain films (Figure 10-5) is 38% sensitive and 89% specific for acute maxillary sinusitis when compared with a positive culture obtained by antral puncture. CT scans provide much better detail, and the cost of a limited (or "mini") series of CT scans is now comparable to that of plain films in many areas. Axial images provide information about all of the sinuses, but most authorities prefer coronal images because they also provide information about the ostiomeatal complex. The key radiologic finding is complete opacification of the sinus or an air-fluid level. Mucosal thickening, common in chronic sinusitis, is not a specific feature of acute sinusitis. Magnetic resonance imaging, although useful for evaluation of suspected tumors of the sinuses, is not

generally applied to the evaluation of sinusitis because it is more expensive than CT and has a higher incidence of false-positive diagnoses.

Accurate microbiologic diagnosis can be made only by obtaining an uncontaminated specimen for microscopic examination and culture. Unfortunately, such a specimen can be obtained only by direct puncture of the involved sinus. Direct puncture of the maxillary sinus is feasible, but this procedure is seldom carried out in daily clinical practice. Specimens can also be obtained by microswab culture of the middle meatus as directed by sinus endoscopy. However, since the endoscope must pass through the nasal lumen, such specimens are inevitably contaminated unless a nasal speculum is used to hold the vibrissae away from the swab. For diagnosis of sinusitis in adults, clinical criteria have been developed based on the presence or absence of five findings: maxillary toothache, purulent secretions, poor response to decongestants, abnormal transillumination, and history of colored nasal discharge. On the basis of these five findings, the likelihood ratio of sinusitis was determined to be as follows: for four findings, 6.4; for three findings, 2.6; for two findings, 1.1; for one finding, 0.5; and for none of the findings, 0.1. These criteria (and others that have been developed) have not been fully validated by use of direct sinus puncture.

 KEY POINTS

DIAGNOSIS OF ACUTE BACTERIAL SINUSITIS

⊃ Acute bacterial sinusitis is overdiagnosed in clinical practice, in part because of the difficulty, morbidity, and expense of making an accurate diagnosis.

⊃ In a child, acute sinusitis should be suspected when cold symptoms are unusually severe or persist beyond 12 days.

⊃ In an adult, acute sinusitis should be suspected when cold symptoms are accompanied by fever or severe facial pain.

⊃ The certain diagnosis of acute sinusitis can be made only by obtaining an uncontaminated specimen of the sinus for microbiologic examination, but because of the expense (and morbidity if via antral puncture), this is not routinely done.

⊃ A strong presumptive diagnosis of acute sinusitis can be made on the basis of sinus opacification (sometimes with an air-fluid level) demonstrated by plain x-ray examination or CT scanning.

⊃ Some data suggest that the likelihood of acute bacterial sinusitis can be predicted on the basis of the presence or absence of five symptoms (Tables 10-4 and 10-5).

Natural History
Expected Outcome

Acute bacterial sinusitis is often self-limited, but the frequency with which this condition resolves spontaneously is unknown. Direct sinus puncture for accurate diagnosis has not been carried out in placebo-controlled clinical trials. Serious complications occur often enough to justify close follow-up, especially in the clinically more severe cases

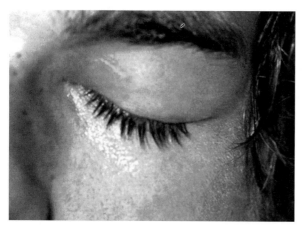

FIG. 10-6   Orbital cellulitis complicating ethmoid and frontal sinusitis.

(Table 10-2). The most common complication is progression to chronic sinusitis (see later discussion). Cavernous sinus thrombosis (see Chapter 6) can result from ethmoid, frontal, or sphenoid sinusitis. Ethmoid sinusitis can also cause orbital cellulitis (Figure 10-6). Frontal sinusitis can cause osteomyelitis of the frontal bone with swelling and edema of the forehead (Pott's puffy tumor) and subdural empyema. Sphenoid sinusitis can be a medical emergency (see Chapter 6).

Treatment
Methods

The standard approach consists of decongestants (especially phenylephrine nasal spray), with antibiotics reserved for the more severe cases (Table 10-2). Current consensus holds that for both children (Figure 10-7) and adults

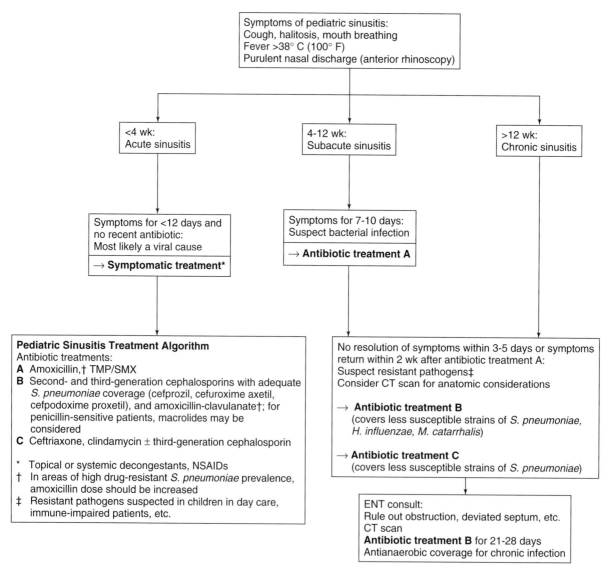

FIG. 10-7   Algorithm for diagnosis and antimicrobial therapy of acute sinusitis in children. (From Brook I, Gooch WM, Reiner SA, et al. Medical management of acute bacterial sinusitis: recommendations of a clinical advisory committee on pediatric and adult sinusitis. Ann Otol Rhinol Laryngol 2000; 109S [Suppl 182, May 2000]: 2-20.)

(Figure 10-8), antibiotics are generally recommended for patients whose symptoms have lasted at least 7 days. Phenylephrine (Neo-Synephrine) nasal spray often provides temporary relief but should be restricted to 3 or 4 days, since more prolonged use often leads to rebound rhinitis (rhinitis medicamentosa). Some data suggest that oxymetazoline (Afrin nasal spray) actually reduces nasal mucosal blood flow and may interfere with the healing of maxillary sinusitis. *Use of phenylpropanolamine-containing preparations is now contraindicated because of phenylpropanolamine's occasional association with stroke.* Although oral decongestants are often prescribed, no well-designed trial supports their use. Except for one study in HIV-positive patients, little direct evidence is available showing that mucolytic agents such as guaifenesin (e.g., Robitussin), antihistamines, or topical steroids are beneficial (Table 10-5).

Antibiotics recommended for sinusitis can be divided into first-line agents (amoxicillin and TMP/SMX), as recently recommended by the U.S. Agency for Healthcare Policy and Research, and second-line drugs, such as amoxicillin-clavulanate, cefaclor, cefuroxime, cefixime, clarithromycin, and doxycycline (Table 10-6). Some thoughtful reviewers conclude that amoxicillin remains the drug of choice, especially for patients likely to adhere to therapy and return for follow-up. The major reservations about amoxicillin are its lack of coverage of *S. aureus,* the possibility of β-lactamase–producing strains of *H. influenzae* and

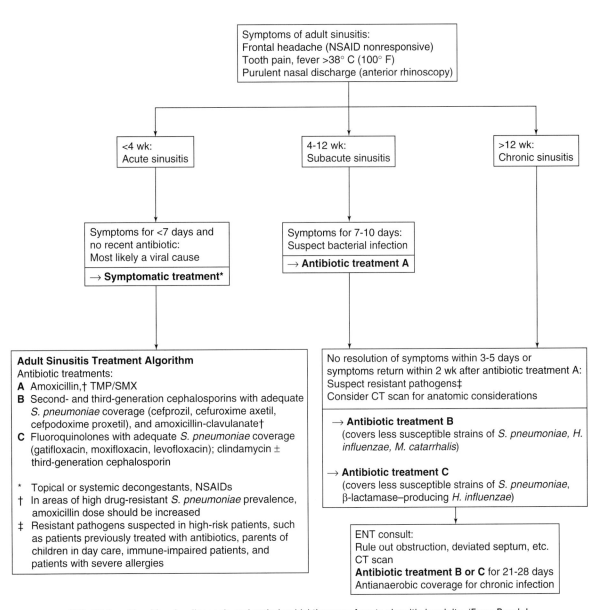

FIG. 10-8   Algorithm for diagnosis and antimicrobial therapy of acute sinusitis in adults. (From Brook I, Gooch WM, Reiner SA, et al. Medical management of acute bacterial sinusitis: recommendations of a clinical advisory committee on pediatric and adult sinusitis. Ann Otol Rhinol Laryngol 2000; 109S [Suppl 182, May 2000]: 2-20.)

TABLE 10-5
Adjunctive Therapy for Sinusitis

Class of drug	Examples	Action and duration	Dosage	Comments
Topical vasoconstrictors: sympathomimetic amines	Phenylephrine (Neo-Synephrine)	α_1-Adrenergic agonist; duration of action 1 to 4 hours	2 to 3 sprays in each nostril q3-4h	Use should be restricted to no more than 3 to 4 days because of the risk of rebound rhinitis.
Topical vasoconstrictors: imidazoline derivatives	Oxymetazoline (Afrin 12-hour)	α_2-Adrenergic agonists; duration of action 5 to 12 hours	2 to 3 sprays b.i.d.	Not recommended (see text).
Systemic vasoconstrictors	Phenylpropanolamine (Tavist-D timed release)	α_1- and α_2-adrenergic agonist; duration of action 8 to 12 hours	1 tablet q12h	These oral vasoconstrictors reduce nasal congestion; however, their systemic side effects can be significant and clinical trials do not document their efficacy for treating sinusitis.
	Pseudoephedrine (Sudafed; Novafed timed release)	α_1-, α_2-, β_1-, and β_2-adrenergic agonists; duration of action 4 to 8 hours (Sudafed); 8 to 12 hours (Novafed timed release)	60 mg q4-6h (Sudafed); 120 mg q12h (Novafed timed release)	These oral vasoconstrictors reduce nasal congestion; however, their systemic side effects can be significant and clinical trials do not document their efficacy for treating sinusitis.
Mucolytic agents	Guaifenesin (usually available in decongestant combinations, such as Entex L.A.)	Prescribed with the rationale that destruction of mucus will thin secretions		Little evidence has been shown that mucolytics are clinically effective.
Antihistamines				Little rationale exists for antihistamines; moreover, older generation antihistamines can thicken mucus and block the ostiomeatal complex.
Topical corticosteroids				Intranasal corticosteroids are of dubious benefit except in patients with inhalant allergies that complicate recovery from chronic sinusitis.

Moraxella catarrhalis, and the increasing resistance of *S. pneumoniae* to the penicillins. In geographic areas with a high prevalence of penicillin-resistant pneumococci, doubling the dose of amoxicillin (up to 80 to 90 mg/kg per day, or a maximum dose of 3 g per day) is recommended. Some authorities recommend TMP/SMX as the drug of first choice.

In a randomized trial a 3-day course of TMP/SMX was equivalent in results to a 7-day course.

Many newer antibiotics are, at least theoretically, effective for sinusitis but are not approved by the Food and Drug Administration (FDA) for this indication. Moreover, critical reviews suggest that newer, more expensive drugs

TABLE 10-6
Options for Oral Antibiotic Therapy for Acute Sinusitis

Antibiotic	FDA approved?	Dose for children	Dose for adults	Comments
Amoxicillin	Yes	40 mg/kg/day in divided doses (q8h)	500 mg t.i.d.	Despite rising prevalence of *Streptococcus pneumoniae* with reduced susceptibility to penicillin, amoxicillin is still considered the cost-effective drug of choice by many authorities.
Amoxicillin-clavulanate	Yes	40 mg/kg/day (based on amoxicillin component) in divided doses (q8h)	500/125 mg t.i.d.	Extends the spectrum of amoxicillin to include penicillin-resistant, methicillin-sensitive *Staphylococcus aureus* strains (and thus may be especially useful when frontal or sphenoid sinusitis is suspected) and β-lactamase–producing strains of *Haemophilus influenzae*.
TMP/SMX	No	8 mg/kg/day (TMP)/40 mg/kg/day (SMX) in divided doses (q12h)	One DS tablet (160 mg/800 mg) b.i.d.	Clinical efficacy of TMP/SMX (92% in one study) compares favorably with that of newer, more expensive agents.
Clarithromycin	Yes	7.5 mg/kg q12h	500 mg b.i.d.	Has been shown to be effective for treatment of sinusitis caused by sensitive pneumococcal strains. Little or no evidence for superiority over less expensive options.
Loracarbef	Yes	30 mg/kg/day in divided doses (q12h)	400 mg b.i.d.	Has been shown to be effective (93% in one study), but little or no evidence for superiority over less expensive options. May be less effective than alternatives against β-lactamase–producing organisms.
Cefaclor	No	40 mg/kg/day in divided doses (q8h)	500 mg t.i.d.	Effective, but probably overprescribed and with little or no evidence for superiority over less expensive options.
Cefuroxime	Yes	30 mg/kg/day in divided doses (q12h)	500 mg b.i.d.	Has been shown to be effective (95% in one study), but little or no evidence for superiority over less expensive options.
Azithromycin	No	12 mg/kg/day on days 1 through 5	500 mg on day 1, then 250 mg on days 2 through 5	Should be effective against susceptible organisms but has not undergone rigorous evaluation in studies using pretreatment and posttreatment sinus aspirates.
Cefpodoxime	Yes	5 mg/kg q12h	200 mg q12h	Should be effective against susceptible organisms but has not undergone rigorous evaluation in studies using pretreatment and posttreatment sinus aspirates.
Cefixime	No	8 mg/kg/day as a single dose or in divided doses (q12h)	400 mg/day as a single dose or in divided doses (q12h)	Has been shown to effective (91% in one study), but little or no evidence for superiority over less expensive options for most patients. Potentially useful for nosocomial sinusitis caused by gram-negative bacilli.
Levofloxacin	Yes	Contraindicated	500 mg/day	Like other "respiratory fluoroquinolones," effective against common pathogens; concern expressed that wide usage could promote resistance among *S. pneumoniae* strains.

FDA, Food and Drug Administration; *TMP/SMX,* trimethoprim-sulfamethoxazole.

are no more effective than older drugs for this purpose. Criteria for FDA approval have become more rigorous, causing some companies to be less inclined to sponsor the necessary studies. One approach is to use an older, less expensive regimen such as TMP/SMX or amoxicillin for 3 to 7 days. If the patient does not improve by the third day, a newer drug with broader coverage such as cefpodoxime or cefuroxime can be tried. Some authorities advise using amoxicillin-clavulanate (Augmentin) or a fluoroquinolone (in adults, not children) when there is a history of antibiotic therapy within the previous 2 weeks. When evidence clearly shows that the frontal sinuses are involved, we recommend a drug that covers *S. aureus,* such as amoxicillin-clavulanate (Augmentin), because extension of staphylococcal disease from the frontal sinuses into the brain can have tragic consequences.

Expected Response

Response to treatment of acute bacterial sinusitis is often disappointing. About 10% to 25% of patients continue to have symptoms. Whether these symptoms reflect unresolved bacterial infection or failure to restore mucociliary flow despite sterilization of the sinuses is unknown.

When to Refer

Referral should be considered for patients who fail to respond to treatment and continue to have severe symptoms. Referral is always indicated in cases with spread of infection beyond the bony confines of the sinuses (e.g., cheek, orbit, meninges) or bone involvement. Referral should also be considered in severe cases of frontal or sphenoid sinusitis. Functional endoscopic sinus surgery (FESS) has replaced older procedures such as the Caldwell-Luc (drainage of the maxillary sinuses via a buccal approach) or Lynch (medial orbital approach to the ethmoid or frontal sinuses) procedures except in complicated or life-threatening infections.

 KEY POINTS

TREATMENT OF ACUTE UNCOMPLICATED SINUSITIS

- ⊃ Standard therapy consists of decongestants (e.g., phenylephrine or oxymetazoline nasal spray), reserving antibiotics for the more severe or more prolonged cases (≥7 days).
- ⊃ At present, amoxicillin and TMP/SMX are considered the first-line antibiotics for acute bacterial sinusitises.
- ⊃ The dose of amoxicillin can be doubled (up to 80 to 90 mg/kg per day, with a maximum dose of 3 g/day) in areas where resistance of *S. pneumoniae* to penicillin G is high.
- ⊃ Newer antibiotics with better coverage against *S. aureus* and β-lactamase–producing strains of *H. influenzae* and *M. catarrhalis* should be considered if symptoms are unusually severe or the patient fails to respond within several days to TMP/SMX or amoxicillin.
- ⊃ Up to 25% of patients continue to have symptoms after resolution.
- ⊃ Referral should be considered for patients who fail to respond to therapy or who have severe disease involving the sphenoid, ethmoid, or frontal sinuses.

SUGGESTED READING

Benninger M, Sedory Holzer SE, Lau J. Diagnosis and treatment of uncomplicated acute bacterial rhinosinusitis: summary of the Agency for Health Care Policy and Research evidence-based report. Otolaryngol Head Neck Surg 2000; 122: 1-7.

Brooks I, Gooch WM III, Jenkins SG, et al. Medical management of acute bacterial sinusitis: recommendations of a clinical advisory committee on pediatric and adult sinusitis. Ann Otol Rhinol Laryngol 2000; 182 (Suppl 2000—May): 2-20.

Hamory BH, Sande MA, Sydnor A Jr, et al. Etiology and antimicrobial therapy of acute maxillary sinusitis. J Infect Dis 1979; 139: 197-202.

Osguthorpe JD. Adult rhinosinusitis: diagnosis and management. Am Fam Physician 2001; 63: 69-76.

Piccirillo JF, Mager DE, Frisse ME, et al. Impact of first-line vs second-line antibiotics for the treatment of acute uncomplicated sinusitis. JAMA 2001; 286: 1849-1856.

Sinus and Allergy Health Partnership. Antimicrobial treatment guidelines for acute bacterial rhinosinusitis. Otolaryngol Head Neck Surg 2000; 123: 5-31.

Snow V, Mottur-Pilson C, Hickner JM. Principles of appropriate antibiotic use for acute sinusitis in adults. Ann Intern Med 2001; 134: 495-497.

Vogan JC, Bolger WE, Keyes AS. Endoscopically guided sinonasal cultures: a direct comparison with maxillary sinus aspirate cultures. Otolaryngol Head Neck Surg 2000; 122: 370-373.

Williams JW Jr, Simel DL. Does this patient have sinusitis? Diagnosing acute sinusitis by history and physical examination. JAMA 1993; 270: 1242-1246.

Chronic Sinusitis

When acute sinusitis fails to resolve and becomes chronic, cultures may reveal a variety of opportunistic pathogens, including anaerobic bacteria. Some authorities believe that the problem is no longer mainly "infectious" but rather reflects permanent mucosal injury. Definitions of chronic sinusitis in children and adults are shown in Table 10-2. It has been estimated that chronic sinusitis causes morbidity, measured as absenteeism from school, work, or social activities, of the same magnitude as heart disease and arthritis.

Presentation and Progression
Cause

The prevailing view holds chronic sinusitis to be a disorder of abnormal anatomy and physiology of the paranasal sinuses with one or more causes: previous acute sinusitis, nasal polyposis (as in the triad of asthma, allergies, and aspirin sensitivity), previous sinus surgery, and cystic fibrosis. These processes lead to anatomic changes, including obstruction of the infundibula and ostia, mucosal edema and scarring, bone hypertrophy, polypoid degeneration, and mucosal fibrosis, rendering the mucociliary clearance mechanism defunct.

Numerous microorganisms can be isolated from patients with chronic sinusitis, but correlation between culture results and the disease process is often poor. Mixtures of aerobic and anaerobic organisms are common. In most patients no single microorganism can be assigned a pathogenic role. In some patients, however, *Pseudomonas aeruginosa* or *S. aureus* seems to be clearly pathogenic, and there are data suggesting roles for *H. influenzae* and *M. catarrhalis* (in children). Patients with chronic sinusitis often have exacerbations analogous to the acute exacerbations of chronic obstructive lung disease. In these instances, especially in children, *S. pneumoniae* and *H. influenzae* may be important. Numerous bacteria,

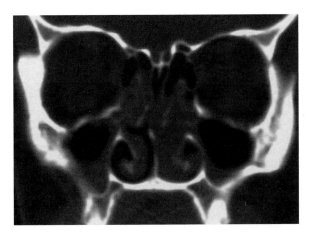

FIG. 10-9 Coronal computed tomogram of a patient with severe inhalant allergies and chronic sinusitis. Note mucosal thickening in the maxillary and ethmoid sinuses bilaterally, as well as the turbinate hypertrophy with compromise of mucous drainage from the ostiomeatal regions.

including gram-negative rods, have been isolated from patients with postoperative sinusitis. Some investigators believe that many patients with chronic sinusitis have allergic fungal sinusitis (discussed later in the chapter) in which the disease manifestations are caused by an immune response to extramucosal fungi.

Presentation

The typical history consists of nasal drainage, obstruction, and postnasal drip lasting for at least several months, often against a background of chronic "sinus trouble." Patients often complain of headache or "sinus pain," nocturnal cough, and bad breath. Loss of smell may also be a feature. Fever is unusual. A history of inhalant allergy is 4.5 times more common in patients with chronic sinusitis than in persons without this disease.

Diagnosis

Although physical examination can reveal such findings as nasal septal deviation or mucosal changes, imaging studies are necessary to make a correct diagnosis. The coronal CT scan represents the current "gold standard" (Figure 10-9), but axial CT scans are often useful, especially in children. Sinus endoscopy can also provide invaluable information.

Natural History
Expected Outcome

Chronic sinusitis may have a relapsing or remitting course, but without treatment patients seldom become entirely free of symptoms related to the paranasal sinuses. Complications include remodeling of the facial bones, osteomyelitis, and, occasionally, invasive disease of the central nervous system caused by bacteria or fungi.

Treatment
Methods

Antibiotics are usually prescribed, but their usefulness has not been convincingly demonstrated. A number of studies indicate, however, that 4- to 6-week courses of antibiotics

are superior to 10- to 14-day courses (80% rate of improvement versus 60%). Antibiotic selection is controversial. Many authorities favor amoxicillin-clavulanate or the newer fluoroquinolones.

Topical corticosteroids have been evaluated, but the results are unclear except in patients with inhalant allergies, in whom chronic mucosal edema compromises sinus drainage. Similarly, topical and systemic decongestants are commonly used. Decongestants and mucolytic agents are sometimes helpful. Referral to an allergist or an appropriately trained otolaryngologist for consideration of desensitization can be useful, especially for patients who give a history of seasonal allergy. Surgery is frequently useful, especially since advances in endoscopic surgery allow more precise approaches with less morbidity than with older procedures.

When to Refer

Patients in whom medical management of chronic sinusitis has failed and who have clear evidence of persistent disease by CT scan should be referred for consideration of endoscopic surgery.

 KEY POINTS

CHRONIC SINUSITIS

- ➲ Chronic sinusitis generally reflects permanent anatomic dysfunction and may not be cured by eradication of one or another microorganism.
- ➲ The microbiology of chronic sinusitis varies and includes both aerobic and anaerobic microorganisms.
- ➲ The role of specific antibiotic therapy for chronic sinusitis is unclear, but in general a 4- to 6-week course of a broad-spectrum agent (such as amoxicillin-clavulanate or a fluoroquinolone) is currently the therapy of choice.
- ➲ Some authors suggest the use of topical corticosteroids, decongestants, and mucolytic agents, but the role for these agents is unclear.
- ➲ Desensitization therapy should be considered, especially in patients who give a clear history of inhalant allergy.
- ➲ Surgery is often used in chronic sinusitis, but indications for surgery are unclear. Guidelines are under development.
- ➲ The possibility of fungal sinusitis should be considered in all patients.

SUGGESTED READING

Anand VK, Osguthorpe JD, Rice D. Surgical management of adult rhinosinusitis. Otolaryngol Head Neck Surg 1997; 117: S50-S52.

Ferguson BJ, Johnson JT. Allergic rhinitis and rhinosinusitis: is there a connection between allergy and infection? Postgrad Med 1999; 105: 55-58, 61, 64.

Kaliner MA, Osguthorpe JD, Fireman P, et al. Sinusitis: bench to bedside; current findings, future directions. Otolaryngol Head Neck Surg 1997; 116: S1-S20.

Osguthorpe JD. Surgical outcomes in rhinosinusitis: what we know. Otolaryngol Head Neck Surg 1999; 120: 451-453.

Fungal Sinusitis

Fungal sinusitis is relatively uncommon but should be considered in patients with chronic sinusitis because of its potentially serious complications.

Presentation and Progression

Cause

Aspergillus species are the most common causes of fungal sinusitis, and fungi of the order Mucorales are the most dangerous (see discussion of rhinocerebral mucormycosis in Chapter 21). Various widely distributed pigmented fungi that are collectively known as dematiaceous molds can cause a variety of syndromes that include life-threatening disease; examples of these organisms are *Alternaria, Bipolaris, Cladosporium, Curvularia,* and *Exserohilum.* Numerous other fungi sometimes cause sinusitis.

Presentation

Five syndromes are currently recognized, as follows:

- Simple colonization of the paranasal sinuses by fungi may be relatively common, although the incidence is unknown.
- Sinus mycetoma (fungus ball) occurs most often as a mass in the maxillary sinus. Underlying disease is usually absent, although some patients have nasal polyps and chronic bacterial sinusitis. Patients usually seek medical attention for nasal obstruction, facial pain, symptoms of chronic sinusitis, or fetid breath (cacosmia). Seizures have been reported as a presenting manifestation.
- Allergic fungal sinusitis usually manifests itself as intractable sinusitis with nasal polyposis in patients with atopy. Some patients also have allergic bronchopulmonary aspergillosis. In children with allergic sinusitis, hypertelorism or proptosis may develop when the frontal or ethmoid sinuses are involved. As mentioned previously, some investigators believe that allergic fungal sinusitis is present in a majority of patients who carry the diagnosis "chronic rhinosinusitis."
- Acute (fulminant) invasive fungal sinusitis is essentially synonymous with rhinocerebral mucormycosis (see Chapter 21), which usually occurs in patients with diabetes mellitus or severe immunosuppression from other causes. The sinuses have been called "way stations to the brain" in this medical emergency, which classically presents as a painless black eschar on the palate or a nasal turbinate followed by epistaxis, headache, changes in mental status, and focal neurologic symptoms and signs (e.g., diplopia). Other fungi, including *Aspergillus* species, *Fusarium* species, and *Pseudallescheria boydii,* can cause an identical syndrome, typically in patients who are severely immunosuppressed from disease (including acquired immunodeficiency syndrome) or chemotherapy for cancer or organ transplantation.
- Chronic invasive fungal sinusitis can occur not only in immunocompromised patients, but also in patients who are immunologically normal. Most of these latter patients have chronic sinusitis and nasal polyposis. Causative organisms include the dematiaceous molds noted previously; the condition is known as phaeohyphomycosis. Dense masses of fungal elements resembling mycetoma are found, but invasion into the mucosa and then into bone may also be seen. Patients initially have headache and localizing symptoms

such as decreased vision and loss of eye movement (orbital apex syndrome) or behavioral changes (mycetoma of the frontal lobe).

Diagnosis

CT scans showing small speckled calcifications within the sinuses or bowing of the bony margins suggest fungal sinusitis (Figure 10-10). True destruction of the bony walls or edema of adjacent soft tissues suggests an invasive fungal process (or a rapidly growing neoplasm such as a metastasis). Other radiologic signs of fungal sinusitis are nonspecific. Fungal culture of nasal mucus is unreliable and should not be performed. When fungal sinusitis is suspected, patients should be referred to an otolaryngologist to have culture specimens obtained directly from the affected sinuses or, when invasive fungal disease is suspected, to have biopsy specimens obtained for culture and histologic examination (including frozen section).

Criteria for the diagnosis of allergic fungal sinusitis include (1) symptoms and signs of chronic rhinosinusitis; (2) demonstration of eosinophils or their products (such as Charcot-Leyden crystals) in mucin obtained from the sinuses; and (3) demonstration of fungi by histology, culture, or both in mucin obtained from the sinuses. Investigators using a novel method for specimen collection recently found fungi in 96% of 210 patients with chronic rhinosinusitis. However, fungi were also isolated from 100% of normal, healthy volunteers. The key finding is the presence of both eosinophils and fungi in mucin; hence the proposed term "eosinophilic fungal rhinosinusitis."

Natural History

Untreated, sinus mycetoma causes symptoms of chronic sinusitis and facial pain that are unlikely to resolve spontaneously. The natural history of allergic fungal sinusitis is unclear, since this condition has been well described only within recent years. Acute (fulminant) invasive fungal sinusitis

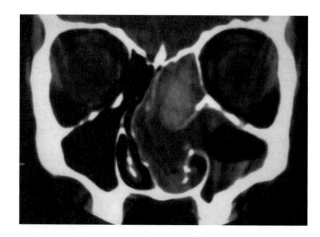

FIG. 10-10 Coronal computed tomogram of a patient with unilateral allergic fungal sinusitis. Note the characteristic calcium speckles in an obstructed ethmoid sinus, the air-fluid level in the adjacent and obstructed maxillary sinus, and the unilateral nasal airway blockage by polyps.

carries high mortality and substantial morbidity. Chronic invasive sinusitis can similarly cause death or serious disability.

Treatment
Methods

None of the syndromes of fungal sinusitis has been subjected to carefully designed randomized therapeutic trials. Treatment of mycetoma consists of débridement of the fungal elements and aeration of the sinuses. Treatment of allergic fungal sinusitis is similar but also includes short courses of oral antifungal agents and corticosteroids, long-term topical corticosteroids, and possibly the addition of desensitization therapy. Management of invasive fungal sinusitis requires aggressive surgery combined with antifungal drug therapy, usually amphotericin B.

Expected Response

The response of mycetoma to débridement is excellent. Allergic fungal sinusitis is prone to recur. Favorable outcome from acute or chronic invasive sinusitis hinges on prompt therapy; residual morbidity is common.

When to Refer

Most patients with fungal sinusitis should be referred to an otolaryngologist.

 KEY POINTS

FUNGAL SINUSITIS

⊃ Fungal sinusitis is a spectrum of conditions ranging from simple colonization to life-threatening invasive disease.

⊃ *Aspergillus* species are the most commonly encountered microorganisms. The agents of mucormycosis are the most dangerous. A large number of dematiaceous molds (the agents of phaeohyphomycosis) are now recognized as causes of invasive sinusitis in immunologically normal persons.

⊃ Patients with fungal sinusitis other than simple colonization should usually be referred to an otolaryngologist.

⊃ Allergic fungal sinusitis—also called eosinophilic fungal rhinosinusitis because the diagnosis depends on demonstrating eosinophils and fungi in mucin—may be a common condition in clinical practice. This entity is somewhat controversial at present.

SUGGESTED READING

deShazo RD, Chapin K, Swain RE. Fungal sinusitis. N Engl J Med 1997; 337: 254-259.

deShazo RD, O'Brien M, Chapin K, et al. Criteria for the diagnosis of sinus mycetoma. J Allergy Clin Immunol 1997; 99: 475-485.

Ferguson BJ. Definitions of fungal rhinosinusitis. Otolaryngol Clin North Am 2000; 33: 227-235.

Ferguson BJ. Mucormycosis of the nose and paranasal sinuses. Otolaryngol Clin North Am 2000; 33: 349-365.

Ponikau JU, Sherris DA, Kern EB, et al. The diagnosis and incidence of allergic fungal sinusitis. Mayo Clin Proc 1999; 74: 877-884.

Washburn RG, Kennedy DW, Begley MG, et al. Chronic fungal sinusitis in apparently normal hosts. Medicine (Baltimore) 1988; 67: 231-247.

Otitis Externa

Otitis externa, a spectrum of conditions caused by infection, allergy, or primary skin disease, affects up to 10% of all people during their lifetimes. Necrotizing (malignant) otitis externa is a medical emergency seen usually in patients with diabetes mellitus or a compromised immune system or in patients who have had prior irradiation of the head (see Chapter 6).

Presentation and Progression
Cause

Otitis externa begins with breakdown in the cerumen barrier. Cerumen, although commonly considered a nuisance, protects against infection by creating an acidic environment hostile to bacterial and fungal growth; promoting a dry environment through its hydrophobic properties; and trapping debris by its sticky nature. Excessive cleaning or scratching of the ear canal promotes breakdown of the cerumen barrier. Swimming notoriously predisposes to otitis externa, since it promotes a more alkaline pH, which in turn promotes bacterial growth. However, increased moisture of any origin leads to maceration of the skin and breakdown. Mechanical trauma from devices such as ear plugs (used for hearing conservation in many industries), headphones, hearing aids, and diving caps also predisposes to otitis externa.

P. aeruginosa and *S. aureus* are common causes of otitis externa. Group A streptococci and various gram-negative rods sometimes cause this condition, and anaerobic bacteria are involved in up to 25% of cases. About 10% of cases are caused by various fungi, with *Aspergillus* species the most common, followed by *Candida* species.

Presentation

Otitis media can be graded in severity from mild (minor pain and pruritus, minimal edema of the ear canal) to severe (severe pain and pruritus, complete occlusion of the ear canal, auricular and periauricular erythema, and frequently fever and lymphadenopathy). Syndromes include the following:

■ Acute localized otitis externa occurs as a single or several pustules or furuncles in the ear canal, usually caused by *S. aureus*. Initial symptoms include itching, pain, swelling, redness, and sometimes decreased hearing. A small furuncle that would be inconspicuous on most parts of the skin becomes intensely painful in the confines of the narrow ear canal.

■ Acute diffuse otitis externa (swimmer's ear) typically presents with pain (otalgia), itching, discharge, and hearing loss. The pain can become intolerable. There is often a history of recent exposure to water. Mobile redwood hot tub systems have been associated with a severe hemorrhagic form of the disease. *P. aeruginosa* is the most common pathogen. Other patients give a history of ear instrumentation, excessive cleaning, previous infection, otitis media, tinnitus, or vertigo. Examination reveals the ear canal to be diffusely red and edematous.

■ Erysipelas involving the concha and canal is caused by group A streptococci, with a pathogenesis similar to that of erysipelas elsewhere (see Chapter 15). When first seen, patients have a diffusely red and painful ear. Examination may reveal hemorrhagic bullae on the walls of the canal and on the tympanic membrane, and tender regional lymphadenopathy may be present.

■ Chronic otitis externa manifests itself with mild discomfort and flaking of the skin of long duration, often with a history of the use of numerous antibiotic and otic preparations. Eczematous otitis externa, a variant, indicates involvement of the ear by primary skin diseases such as contact dermatitis, seborrheic dermatitis, and atopic dermatitis. Severe itching is a cardinal symptom, and examination reveals a scaling skin surface with crusting, oozing, and erythema.

Diagnosis

Diagnosis of otitis externa is nearly always based on the history and physical examination (Figure 10-11). Pressure on the tragus or pulling the auricle superiorly causes pain; the latter maneuver is a valuable diagnostic aid. Examination of the ear canal shows erythema, edema, and in severe cases partial or complete occlusion of the canal. To exclude otitis media, the practitioner should demonstrate with pneumatic insufflation that the tympanic membrane is mobile. However, the tympanic membrane is often partially or totally obscured by edema in the ear canal.

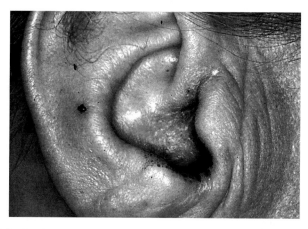

FIG. 10-11 Severe otitis externa with evidence of bleeding in the macerated canal lining. Note the preauricular swelling from spread of cellulitis into the parotid gland.

TABLE 10-7
Topical Preparations for Otitis Externa*

Drug or preparation	Trade name	pH
PREPARATIONS WITHOUT STEROIDS		
Acetic acid 2%	Otic Domeboro Solution, VO Sol Otic Solution, others	3.0
Methylrosaniline chloride 1% and 2%	Gentian violet solution	<6.1
Merthiolate 1:1000	Thimerosal solution	6.7
Phenol 1.5%, basic fuchsin, resorcinol, and acetone	Castellani paint	2.8-3.7
Sulfacetamide sodium 10%	Bleph-10 Ophthalmic Solution	7.4
Sulfisoxazole 4%	Gantrisin Ophthalmic Solution	7.2-7.9
Tobramycin 0.3%	Tobrex Ophthalmic Solution	7.0-8.0
Ofloxacin 0.3%	Floxin Otic Solution	—
Amphotericin B 3%	Fungizone Lotion	6.5-6.7
Nystatin 100,000 units/mL	Nystatin Suspension	—
Clotrimazole 1%	Lotrimin Solution Lotrimin Lotion Lotrimin Cream	4.5-8.0 — 5.0-7.0
m-Cresyl acetate 25%	Cresylate Solution	4.5
PREPARATIONS WITH STEROIDS		
Acetic acid 2% and hydrocortisone 1%	VO Sol HC Otic Solution	3.0
Acetic acid 2% and desonide 0.05%	Tridesilon Otic Solution	5.0-6.7

Natural History
Expected Outcome

Although otitis externa is usually considered a self-limited condition, serious complications can occur. Perforation of the tympanic membrane can be caused by extension of the disease process or by misguided attempts by patients or health care providers to relieve the condition through mechanical manipulation. Other complications include stenosis of the ear canal, auricular cellulitis, and chondritis.

Treatment
Methods

Cleaning the ear canal is the most important principle. Excessive cerumen should be removed along with desquamated skin and purulent material. The ear canal should be cleaned carefully through an otoscope using a cerumen wire loop or a cotton swab to gently remove the debris. If the tympanic membrane is visible and intact, the ear canal can be irrigated with half-strength hydrogen peroxide or 2% acetic acid (dilute vinegar). If the tympanic membrane is perforated, the clinician must keep in mind that all forms of topical therapy are potentially damaging to middle ear structures.

Topical antibiotics are usually prescribed (Table 10-7). The plethora of otic preparations can be confusing, and as with other classes of drugs, clinicians should become familiar with a small number of alternatives. Fluoroquinolones (e.g., ciprofloxacin and ofloxacin) are now available as otic solutions, but concern has been expressed about their ability to promote drug-resistant organisms. Systemic antibiotics have been used in severe cases and are appropriate for patients with erysipelas.

Patients with mild disease should be treated with an "aural toilet" (removing debris, with irrigation and suction as needed) and a topical agent and seen for follow-up examination in about 14 days. Simple acidifying agents can be used (e.g., acetic acid, hydrochloric acid, salicylic acid, boric acid, and citric acid). Topical steroids reduce inflammation. Cortisporin is commonly used for this purpose, but two potential dangers should be noted based on experimental studies: ototoxicity resulting from the neomycin component of Cortisporin, and damage to ear structures after daily introduction of Cortisporin into the middle ear. Ophthalmic preparations containing steroids or antibiotics are sometimes used, especially for patients who cannot tolerate the acidic otic preparations because of burning or stinging. The neutral or

TABLE 10-7—cont'd
Topical Preparations for Otitis Externa*

Drug or preparation	Trade name	pH
Neomycin sulfate 0.35%, colistin sulfate 0.3%, thonzonium bromide 0.05%, and hydrocortisone 1%	Cortisporin TC Otic Suspension	5.0
Neomycin sulfate 0.35%, polymyxin B sulfate 10,000 units, and hydrocortisone 1%	Cortisporin Otic Solution Cortisporin Otic Suspension PediOtic Suspension	2.9-4.0 3.0-5.5 >4.1
Polymyxin B sulfate 10,000 units and hydrocortisone 0.5%	Otobiotic Otic Solution; Pyocidin-Otic Solution	5.0-7.5
Sulfacetamide sodium 10%, prednisolone acetate 0.25%	Vasocidin Ophthalmic Solution Metimyd Ophthalmic Suspension	6.2-8.2 5.0-6.0
Tobramycin 0.3% and dexamethasone 0.1%	TobraDex Ophthalmic Suspension	6.0-8.0
Ciprofloxacin 10 mg/mL, hydrocortisone 10 mg/mL	Cipro HC Otic Solution	4.5-5.0
Clotrimazole 1% and betamethasone dipropionate 0.05%	Lotrisone Cream	5.0-7.0
Dexamethasone 0.1%	Decadron Solution	7.0-8.5
Prednisone sodium phosphate 1%	Inflamase Forte Ophthalmic Solution	6.2-8.2
Prednisolone sodium acetate 1%	Pred Forte Ophthalmic Suspension	5.0-6.0
Mometasone furoate 0.1%	Elocon Lotion	4.5

*In the presence of tympanic membrane perforation, all of the above agents should be used with caution if at all.
Note that ophthalmic preparations are, in general, more pH neutral than otic preparations and can therefore be useful in patients who cannot tolerate acidic preparations because of burning or stinging. Although ophthalmic preparations can be used in the ear, the reverse is not true—*otic preparations should not be used in the eye because of their acidic pH.*

slightly alkaline pH of ophthalmic solutions may limit their therapeutic efficacy; on other hand, the lower viscosity of ophthalmic preparations compared with otic preparations allows them to penetrate narrowed canal lumens. Another approach is to fill the ear canal with a single application of an ointment containing antibiotics and a steroid, using a syringe. The ear should be protected from water during recovery. This can be accomplished by using a cotton ball tipped with a thin coat of petroleum jelly during baths and showers. Most patients respond to topical therapy and need only NSAIDs for pain relief, but some require narcotic analgesics.

Patients should be advised to avoid any inciting factors. They should be told that the ear is self-cleaning and that they should not put objects into it. Swimmers should be told to shake the ear dry after swimming and to blow-dry the ear with the dryer held about 12 inches away from the ear. Ear drops containing alcohol or acetic acid can also be used to promote drying.

Expected Response

Acute otitis externa usually responds to appropriate therapy.

When to Refer

Patients with advanced or severe disease and complete occlusion of the ear canal should be referred to an otolaryngologist for placement of a stent. Stents (such as ribbon gauze or a small compressed cellulose wick) allow topical medication to reach the medial aspect of the ear canal and facilitate a longer contact time for topical solutions. Stents can be replaced every 1 to 3 days, usually in conjunction with ear canal cleaning to remove the desquamated epithelium characteristic of moderate or severe external otitis. Ear canal pruritus lasting for a month or so after external otitis results from the epithelial regeneration and is therefore not a reason for continued use of ototopical agents. Unfortunately, persistent pruritus prompts some patients to scratch the canal with a Q-tip or similar object, causing trauma that predisposes to new infection. In patients with severe disease, otolaryngologists can clean the infected ear under a dissecting microscope, which allows binocular magnified vision and frees both hands.

 KEY POINTS

OTITIS EXTERNA

⊃ Acute localized otitis externa usually begins as a pustule or furuncle caused by *S. aureus*.
⊃ Acute diffuse otitis externa (swimmer's ear) causes diffuse erythema and edema and is usually due to *P. aeruginosa*.
⊃ Erysipelas of the external ear is usually due to group A streptococci and can be associated with hemorrhagic bullae involving the ear canal and tympanic membrane.
⊃ An attempt should be made to exclude otitis media by examination of the tympanic membrane using pneumatic insufflation.
⊃ In most patients otitis externa can be managed conservatively with local care, including topical otic preparations, but patients with severe disease or complete occlusion of the ear canal should be referred to an otolaryngologist.

⊃ Ear canal pruritus lasting for a month or so after treatment of external otitis is due to epithelial regeneration and is not an indication for continued use of ototopical agents.

SUGGESTED READING

Hannley MT, Denneny JC III, Holzer SS. Use of ototopical antibiotics in treating 3 common ear diseases. Otolaryngol Head Neck Surg 2000; 122: 934-940.

La Rosa S. Primary care management of otitis externa. Nurse Pract 1998; 23: 125-128, 131-133.

Sander R. Otitis externa: a practical guide to treatment and prevention. Am Fam Physician 2001; 63: 927-936, 941-942.

Acute Otitis Media

The importance of otitis media in primary care cannot be overemphasized, especially in pediatric practice, where it accounts for about 25% of all office visits, 50% of office visits for illness, and 40% of antibiotic prescriptions. By age 5, between 75% and 95% of children have had at least one episode of otitis media. This disease is responsible for some 25 million office visits each year, with annual health care costs estimated to be between 3 and 5 billion dollars. Although 80% of patients with otitis media are less than 15 years of age, more than one fourth of all oral antibiotic prescriptions in the United States are written for this condition. Heavy prescribing of β-lactam antibiotics for otitis media is thought to be responsible in large measure for the decreasing drug susceptibility of *S. pneumoniae* strains.

Presentation and Progression
Cause

Acute otitis media is often preceded by viral URI that causes edema and obstruction of the eustachian tube, causing an ex vacuo serous transudate into the middle ear and paving the way for pathogenic bacteria (Figure 10-1). Children are predisposed because their eustachian tubes are shorter, wider, and straighter than those of adults. Recognition of otitis media requires knowledge of the relationship of the eustachian tube to the nasopharynx, the middle ear, and the mastoid air cells (Figure 10-12). The eustachian tube normally serves to regulate pressure in the middle ear, to protect against nasopharyngeal sound pressure and secretions, and to afford a pathway for the drainage of secretions produced within the middle ear into the nasopharynx. The latter function requires an intact mucociliary system. Factors predisposing to eustachian tube dysfunction and otitis media include allergy, cleft palate, ciliary dysmotility, immunodeficiency, exposure to tobacco smoke, exposure to frequent upper respiratory tract infections (notoriously, in day care centers), early age of first infection, and race. Native Americans are markedly predisposed to otitis media for reasons that are unclear. Adults can be predisposed to otitis media because of diabetes mellitus, cancer, immune deficiencies, and injection drug use. The adenoids have long been implicated in the pathogenesis of otitis media, for better or worse, since inflammation of the adenoids causes inflammatory obstruction of the adjacent eustachian tube orifices; colonization of the adenoids by pathogenic bacteria

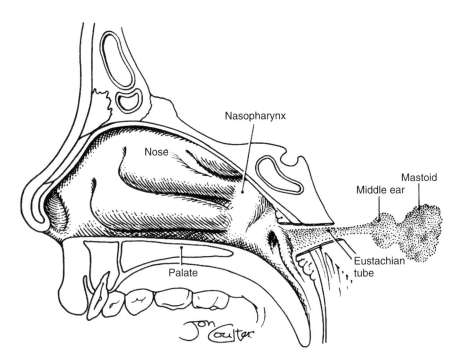

FIG. 10-12   Relationship of the eustachian tube to the nasopharynx, middle ear, and mastoid air cells. (From Johnson JT, Yu VL, eds. Infectious Diseases and Antimicrobial Therapy of the Ears, Nose, and Throat. Philadelphia: W.B. Saunders Company; 1997; 275.)

promotes invasion of the middle ear by these same bacteria; yet the adenoids provide local immunity in the form of secretory IgA secretion.

The microbiology in otitis media is similar in adults and children when tympanocentesis is carried out (Table 10-8). In about 40% of cases, culture of middle ear fluid fails to show a bacterial pathogen. This might reflect a viral etiology or sterile inflammation. RSV has been found relatively commonly, with a special tendency to cause the disease in children. Influenza viruses and parainfluenza viruses are also predisposing factors for otitis media. *S. pneumoniae* causes about 30% to 40% of cases, and the prevalence of strains with reduced susceptibility to penicillin is increasing. *H. influenzae* causes between 20% and 30% of cases, and *M. catarrhalis* between 10% and 15% of cases, especially in children. Group A streptococci cause less than 5% of cases but can cause up to 10% during the winter months.

Presentation

Acute otitis media in children usually presents with rapid onset of otalgia, fever, or irritability. Otalgia in young infants is manifest by pulling on the ear. Young children can also have anorexia, loose stools, and vomiting. Otalgia tends to be the major symptom in adults. A minority of patients experience spontaneous perforation of the tympanic membrane.

Diagnosis

The tympanic membrane is abnormal, often bulging, with loss of the usual landmarks. Erythema of the tympanic membrane alone is not diagnostic; it can be caused, for example, by crying. Purulent fluid is sometimes seen behind the tympanic membrane. The key procedures are pneumatic otoscopy and, when indicated, tympanocentesis (Box 10-2). Pneumatic otoscopy, which is performed by gently squeezing and then releasing a rubber bulb attached to the otoscope, provides information about the mobility of the tympanic membrane.

Normally the tympanic membrane moves rapidly inward when positive pressure is applied, then outward when the pressure is released. Reduced or absent mobility in response to pneumatic otoscopy indicates a middle ear effusion. When the diagnosis is in doubt, tympanometry can be carried out with a simple device that slowly changes the pressure in the external canal while directing a low-frequency tone at the eardrum to determine when the tone best passes through the eardrum. Negative middle ear pressure or fluid can be distinguished from normal middle ear aeration by tympanometry, even in a crying infant. Tympanocentesis provides fluid for culture, which is becoming more important because of the emergence of drug-resistant bacteria. Cultures of the nasopharynx correlate poorly with cultures of fluid obtained by tympanocentesis and are therefore of limited usefulness.

Acute otitis media must be distinguished from otitis media with effusion (serous otitis media). The latter consists of an asymptomatic or hyposymptomatic middle ear effusion, which can be acute (less than 3 weeks), subacute (3 weeks to 3 months), or chronic. Although hearing loss is frequently present in both acute otitis media and otitis media with effusion, patients with otitis media and effusion lack systemic signs and symptoms such as otalgia and fever.

Natural History
Expected Outcome

The natural history of untreated otitis media continues to prompt debate on whether most cases should be treated with antibiotics. A metaanalysis of the literature based on data obtained from 5400 children in 33 studies indicates that 81% percent of children have spontaneous resolution. Antimicrobial therapy accelerated resolution by only about 14%, which explains why some physicians (especially in Europe) choose not to treat the disease, since the overall benefit appears marginal. Others, however, believe that untreated patients are at

TABLE 10-8
Microbial Etiologies of Acute Otitis Media in Children and Adults and of Chronic Otitis Media

Mircoorganism	PERCENT OF CASES		
	Acute otitis media in children	Acute otitis media in adults	Chronic otitis media
BACTERIA			
Streptococcus pneumoniae	35	21	7
Haemophilus influenzae	23	26	5
Moraxella catarrhalis	14	3	10
Staphylococcus aureus	2	3	3
Group A streptococci *(Streptococcus pyogenes)*	3	3	1
Other bacteria	32	26	50
None	16	26	30
VIRUSES			
Respiratory syncytial virus	7		
Rhinovirus	3		
Influenza A	2		
Adenovirus	2		
Parainfluenza virus	1		
Enterovirus	1		

Modified from Carroll K, Reimer L. Microbiology and laboratory diagnosis of upper respiratory tract infections. Clin Infect Dis 1996; 23: 442-448.

BOX 10-2
Indications for Tympanocentesis in Acute Otitis Media

- Unusually severe otalgia or systemic toxicity
- Newborn infant or sick neonate (because of the possibility of an unusual organism)
- Onset of otitis media while receiving antibiotics
- Failure to respond to appropriate antibiotics
- Confirmed or suspected suppurative complication
- Immunodeficiency disorder

greater risk of mastoiditis and point out that the severe suppurative complications described in the preantibiotic era are now uncommon in the United States. Some data suggest that the incidence of acute mastoiditis in children with acute otitis media may now be increasing. In addition, hearing loss (20 to 30 decibels) from otitis media can impair speech development in young children and school performance in older ones if the hearing loss is present for more than 2 to 3 months. The rates of spontaneous resolution vary according

to the pathogen. Spontaneous resolution is most common with *M. catarrhalis* (about 80%), relatively common with *H. influenzae* (about 50%), and uncommon with *S. pneumoniae* (about 20%). However, whether an individual patient's disease will resolve spontaneously is difficult to predict on clinical grounds, and the current consensus in the United States is that all patients should be treated.

Treatment
Methods

Patients should be treated with antibiotics only after being seen and examined. Treatment over the telephone is to be discouraged. A strong case can be made for withholding antibiotics if the answer is yes to each of the following questions: Is the age greater than 2 years? Is the patient in a toxic condition? Are host defenses normal? Is the patient (or the patient's parents) likely to comply with recommendations and return for follow-up?

Amoxicillin continues to be the drug of choice for first-line therapy, but the literature should be watched because further reductions in antibiotic susceptibility of *S. pneumoniae* could cause the consensus recommendations to change.

It was recommended recently that the dose of amoxicillin in children be increased from 40 to 80 mg/kg/day because the higher dose provides sufficient drug levels in the middle ear to inhibit all but the most highly resistant pneumococcal strains (minimum inhibitory concentration ≥ 2 µg/mL), because no more than 16% of cases are likely to be caused by β-lactamase–producing strains of *H. influenzae* and *M. catarrhalis,* and because patients who fail to improve after several days of amoxicillin can be given an alternative drug. Alternative agents include amoxicillin-clavulanate (Augmentin), oral cephalosporins, TMP/SMX, erythromycin-sulfamethoxazole, and macrolides. Fluoroquinolones are theoretically excellent choices for acute otitis media but are currently contraindicated in patients under 17 years of age. A 10-day course of antibiotic therapy is currently recommended; longer courses offer little or no advantage. The efficacy of agents other than antibiotics has not been verified. Antihistamines, decongestants, and steroids should be used carefully if at all in young children because of the possible ill effects. Immune globulin therapy has been evaluated in children for prevention, but the results are unclear.

If one of the above regimens fails, tympanocentesis should be performed to define the microbiologic features and provide drainage to the ear.

Expected Response

Major complications of acute otitis media include persistent middle ear effusion and recurrent otitis media. Despite appropriate antibiotic therapy, middle ear effusions persist for 1 month in up to 40% of patients and 3 months or longer in about 10% of patients. These patients require close follow-up because of the risk of mild to moderate hearing loss. The effect of otitis media on speech development has not been clearly established.

Strategies for management of persistent middle ear infusion include (1) a second 10-day course of the same antibiotic used initially; (2) a 10-day course of a different antibiotic; (3) a topical or systemic nasal decongestant or antihistamine; (4) systemic corticosteroids; and (5) eustachian tube–middle ear inflation. Randomized, controlled trials do not support any of the above methods, making expectant observation a reasonable alternative strategy. Most effusions clear by 3 to 4 months, but patients with more persistent effusions may need to be approached differently.

Strategies for management of recurrent episodes of acute otitis media include (1) continuous chemoprophylaxis, for example, amoxicillin 20 mg/kg at bedtime, during the peak season for respiratory infections; (2) myringotomy with tube insertion; and (3) adenoidectomy. Patients receiving continuous antimicrobial prophylaxis should be examined frequently (every 6 to 8 weeks). The emergence of *S. pneumoniae* strains with reduced susceptibility to penicillin makes continuous prophylaxis with amoxicillin less attractive than was formerly the case. Myringotomy with tympanostomy tube insertion is a reasonable alternative to amoxicillin prophylaxis. Adenoidectomy, often advocated in the past, is supported to some extent by randomized trials and continues to be recommended for carefully selected patients. Pneumococcal vaccine should be considered for older children. Frequent recurrences of acute otitis media often prompt evaluation for

allergy, imaging studies of the paranasal sinuses, and screening tests for immunodeficiency, especially if frequent infections occur in other organs or if the patient is beyond early childhood.

Otitis media with effusion (serous otitis media), as mentioned previously, differs from acute otitis media primarily by the absence of otalgia and fever and by a usually benign course, tending to resolve within 2 to 3 months without therapy. However, this condition can be associated with hearing loss. Antibiotic therapy is often recommended because many of these patients have the same bacteria found in acute otitis media or, if a chronic condition, in chronic sinusitis. Analyses of the literature indicate that antibiotics have short-term efficacy but little or no long-term benefit for this condition. Corticosteroids can be helpful, but the contraindications must be carefully weighed. Middle ear insufflation, a time-honored procedure, is not recommended on the basis of current data, which show it to have no efficacy. In many patients serous otitis media is managed with combinations of topical nasal decongestants, immunotherapy, and control of allergy.

When to Refer

Referral to an otolaryngologist for consideration of tympanostomy tube insertion, sometimes in conjunction with adenoidectomy in children, should be considered in the scenarios indicated in Box 10-3. Randomized clinical trials fail to support tonsillectomy and adenoidectomy for recurrent otitis media in children not previously treated with tympanostomy tubes.

BOX 10-3
Indications for Tympanostomy Tube Insertion

- Recurrent otitis media with three or more episodes in 6 months or four or more episodes in 12 months, with one recent effusion, with failure of antimicrobial prophylaxis to reduce the frequency
- Chronic otitis media with effusion persistent for ≥ 3 months if bilateral or for ≥ 6 months if unilateral, especially when associated with hearing loss, speech, language delay, tinnitus, disequilibrium or vertigo, or severe retraction pocket
- Recurrent episodes of middle ear effusion not meeting criteria for chronic disease but with excessive cumulative duration (e.g., 6 of 12 months)
- Eustachian tube dysfunction (with or without effusion) when persistent, recurrent signs or symptoms (e.g., hearing loss, disequilibrium or vertigo, tinnitus, or severe retraction pocket) is not relieved by treatment
- Suspected presence of a suppurative complication

 KEY POINTS

ACUTE OTITIS MEDIA

⊃ Acute otitis media accounts for about 50% of office visits for illness in young children and for more than one fourth of all oral antibiotic prescriptions in the United States.

⊃ *S. pneumoniae* and *H. influenzae* are the most common bacterial pathogens isolated; *M. catarrhalis* (in children), group A streptococci, *S. aureus,* and other bacteria can also be found.

⊃ Pneumatic otoscopy is the key diagnostic procedure and shows reduced mobility of the tympanic membrane.

⊃ Tympanocentesis is required for accurate microbiologic diagnosis and should be considered in newborn infants, when the illness is unusually severe, when the patient fails to respond to antibiotics, or when a suppurative complication is confirmed or suspected.

⊃ Acute otitis media must be distinguished from otitis media with effusion (serous otitis media), which consists of an asymptomatic or hyposymptomatic middle ear effusion without fever or otalgia.

⊃ Amoxicillin in higher dose (80 mg/kg/day) remains the drug of choice for acute otitis media in children, but the literature should be closely watched in this regard.

⊃ The major complications of acute otitis media are persistent middle ear infusion and frequent recurrences of acute otitis media, both of which sometimes require referral to an otolaryngologist.

SUGGESTED READING

Bahadori RS, Schwartz RH, Ziai M. Acute mastoiditis in children: an increase in frequency in northern Virginia. Pediatr Infect Dis J 2000; 19: 212-215.

Bluestone CD, Klein JO, eds. Otitis Media in Infants and Children. 2nd ed. Philadelphia: W.B. Saunders Company; 1995.

Brook I, Yocum P, Shah K. Aerobic and anaerobic bacteriology of concurrent chronic otitis media with effusion and chronic sinusitis in children. Arch Otolaryngol Head Neck Surg 2000; 126: 174-176.

Craig WA, Andes D. Pharmacokinetics and pharmacodynamics of antibiotics in otitis media. Pediatr Infect Dis J 1996; 15: 255-259.

Dowell SF, Butler JC, Giebink GS, et al. Acute otitis media: management and surveillance in an era of pneumococcal resistance—a report from the Drug-Resistant *Streptococcus pneumoniae* Therapeutic Working Group. Pediatr Infect Dis J 1999; 18: 1-9.

Dowell SF, Marcy SM, Phillips WR, et al. Otitis media: principles of judicious use of antimicrobial agents. Pediatrics 1998; 101: 165-171.

Klein JO. Review of consensus reports on management of acute otitis media. Pediatr Infect Dis J 1999; 18: 1152-1155.

Paradise JL, Bluestone CD, Colborn DK, et al. Adenoidectomy and adenotonsillectomy for recurrent acute otitis media: parallel randomized clinical trials in children not previously treated with tympanostomy tubes. JAMA 1999; 282: 945-953.

Chronic Suppurative Otitis Media and Mastoiditis

Chronic suppurative otitis media is a complication of acute otitis media, usually occurring when a defect is present in the tympanic membrane, such as a "central" perforation or a tympanostomy tube. It is accompanied by purulent discharge (otorrhea). Mastoiditis is invariably present. The associated bacteria seem to vary depending on whether an infected cholesteatoma is present. Cholesteatoma is often associated with anaerobic bacteria and "skin flora" microorganisms, and the otorrhea often has a foul odor. When cholesteatoma is not present, gram-negative rods, including *P. aeruginosa* and *Escherichia coli,* are often found.

In the preantibiotic era, mastoiditis was often a dramatic and severe illness with retroauricular inflammation and serious intracranial complications. Today mastoiditis is more typically an indolent, low-grade, often painless infection of the temporal bone that tends to be clinically silent ("masked mastoiditis") unless a complication such as brain abscess develops. Patients at high risk of complications include newborn infants, persons with diabetes mellitus, the elderly, and the immunocompromised.

Spontaneous resolution is rare if it occurs at all. Local complications of chronic suppurative otitis media and mastoiditis include bone destruction, subperiosteal abscess (including Bezold's abscess, which may be manifested as a neck mass), facial paralysis, labyrinthitis, and petrositis. Intracranial complications include brain abscess, subdural abscess, epidural abscess, septic thrombosis of the lateral sinus, meningitis, and hydrocephalus. Patients with chronic suppurative otitis media or mastoiditis should be referred to an otolaryngologist, since effective treatment usually requires surgical intervention. Orally administered antibiotics may be effective for some patients, based on culture and susceptibility testing. Topical otic preparations are used in selected incidents, but caution is advised because of the potential ototoxicity, especially of drugs such as polymyxins B and E and neomycin (which are found in Cortisporin and Coly-Mycin preparations).

SUGGESTED READING

Nissen AJ, Bui H. Complications of chronic otitis media. Ear Nose Throat J 1996; 75: 284-292.

Acute Pharyngitis

Acute pharyngitis (sore throat) is one of the most common problems encountered in clinical practice. Viruses cause most cases as part of the common cold. However, about 15% of cases, and up to 50% of cases in children during some periods, are caused by group A β-hemolytic streptococci (*S. pyogenes*). Although usually self-limited, streptococcal pharyngitis demands respect as a cause of acute rheumatic fever and—less commonly—major suppurative complications, acute glomerulonephritis, and even the streptococcal toxic shock syndrome. The clinician's task is to determine in a cost-effective manner which patients need treatment and which do not.

Presentation and Progression
Cause

Acute pharyngitis has many known etiologies, and pathogens remain to be discovered for an estimated 30% of cases (Table 10-9). Viral infections are thought to cause sore throat by generating bradykinin and lysyl bradykinin, which stimulate nerve endings. Group A streptococci and certain other pathogens, including some of the respiratory viruses, cause pain by invading the mucosa.

Group A streptococci are carried in the human nasopharynx and transmitted from person to person usually by direct contact with saliva or nasal secretions. Acquisition is greatest in school-aged children, suggesting the gradual development of immunity over time. Children also serve as a reservoir for spread among family members. Asymptomatic pharyngeal carriage of group A streptococci is relatively common, and

TABLE 10-9
Microbial Etiologies of Acute Pharyngitis

Microorganism	Percent of cases (estimated)	Associations
Streptococcus pyogenes (group A β-hemolytic streptococci)	15-30	Pharyngitis, tonsillitis, scarlet fever, acute rheumatic fever, acute glomerulonephritis, toxic shock syndrome (rare)
Rhinoviruses	20	Common cold
Groups C and G β-hemolytic streptococci	5-10	Pharyngitis; tonsillitis; acute glomerulonephritis (rare)
Coronavirus	5	Common cold
Adenoviruses	5	Upper respiratory infection, pharyngoconjunctival fever
Herpes simplex viruses (1 and 2)	4	Gingivitis, stomatitis, pharyngitis
Parainfluenza viruses	2	Common cold, croup
Influenza viruses (A and B)	2	Influenza
Epstein-Barr virus	<1	Infectious mononucleosis
Cytomegalovirus	<1	Infectious mononucleosis
Human immunodeficiency virus (HIV-1)	<1	Acute retroviral syndrome (primary HIV infection)
Neisseria gonorrhoeae	<1	Pharyngitis
Corynebacterium ulcerans	<1	Pharyngitis; diphtheria
Corynebacterium diphtheriae	<1	Diphtheria
Arcanobacterium hemolyticum	<1	Pharyngitis, scarlatiniform rash
Yersinia enterocolitica	<1	Pharyngitis, enterocolitis
Yersinia pestis	<1	Plague
Francisella tularensis	<1	Tularemia
Treponema pallidum	<1	Secondary syphilis
Mycoplasma pneumoniae	<1	Pneumonia, bronchitis, pharyngitis
Chlamydia pneumoniae	Unknown	Pneumonia, bronchitis, pharyngitis
Chlamydia psittaci	<1	Pneumonia, "fever of unknown origin"
Mycoplasma hominis, type 1	Unknown	Pharyngitis in volunteers
Unknown	30	

Data from Bisno AL. Acute pharyngitis: etiology and diagnosis. Pediatrics 1996; 97 (6 part 2) (Suppl): 949-954; and Gwaltney JM, Bisno AL. Pharyngitis. In: Mandell GL, Bennett JE, Dolin R. Mandell, Douglas, and Bennett's Principles and Practice of Infectious Diseases. 5th ed., Philadelphia: Churchill Livingstone; 2000: 656-662.

the factors that cause the development of acute pharyngitis and other complications is some persons are poorly understood (for additional perspectives on *S. pyogenes,* see Chapters 1 and 6). Group C and group G streptococci cause a pharyngitis syndrome clinically indistinguishable from that caused by group A streptococci, sometimes recognized as outbreaks related to a common food source. Group C streptococci (*S. dysgalactiae* subspecies *equisimilis*) appear to be a frequent cause of pharyngitis in college-aged students.

Presentation

Pharyngitis caused by group A streptococci occurs most frequently in children between 5 and 15 years of age, usually during the winter and early spring. In its severe form the disease starts abruptly with fever, sore throat, and odynophagia. Chills, headache, and abdominal pain are sometimes present. Examination reveals diffuse erythema of the pharynx and tonsils accompanied by a patchy, purulent tonsillar and pharyngeal exudate, hypertrophy of the lymphoid nodules in the posterior pharyngeal mucosa, and tender cervical lymphadenopathy. Occasional strains of *S. pyogenes* elaborate the erythrogenic toxin of scarlet fever, resulting in a striking rash and "red strawberry tongue" with enlargement of the papillae. Rhinorrhea and cough may occur. However, these dramatic manifestations are absent in many, perhaps most, cases of streptococcal pharyngitis. Because the features of group A streptococcal pharyngitis blend imperceptibly with those of other causes of sore throat, numerous students of the disease have concluded that the diagnosis must be secured by laboratory methods before definitive treatment (see later discussion). Other syndromes include the following:

- Pharyngitis caused by the common cold is often accompanied by sore throat, which is frequently the first symptom but is usually not the main complaint when patients seek medical care. Rhinorrhea, postnasal drainage, and cough are usually more prominent symptoms than sore throat. Fever is seldom prominent, and severe sore throat with odynophagia is uncommon.

- Patients with influenza sometimes have sore throat as the chief complaint, but it is usually accompanied by other symptoms suggesting influenza, such as myalgia, headache, and cough. In pharyngitis caused by the common cold or by influenza, purulent pharyngeal or tonsillar exudates and tender cervical lymphadenopathy are absent. Tracheal tenderness may be present in influenza, indicating diffuse viral infection of the respiratory mucosa.

- In contrast to influenza, in adenoviral pharyngitis a sore throat is often the chief complaint. Fever, chills, headache, malaise, and myalgias can be prominent. About one third to one half of patients with adenoviral pharyngitis also have follicular conjunctivitis; this syndrome is known as pharyngoconjunctival fever. Patients with adenoviral pharyngitis often have a pharyngeal exudate, so the disease can mimic streptococcal pharyngitis. Epidemics of pharyngoconjunctival fever occur during the summer in civilian populations and during the winter in military recruits.

- Infectious mononucleosis caused by the Epstein-Barr virus produces exudative tonsillitis or pharyngitis in about one half of cases. Tonsillar and pharyngeal exudates can be prominent. If examined with Wright's stain, the exudates of mononucleosis consist mainly of mononuclear cells. In contrast the exudates of streptococcal pharyngitis consist mainly of polymorphonuclear neutrophils. Tender cervical lymphadenopathy is often prominent in the posterior triangles of the neck (spinal accessory chain of nodes), contrasting with the prominent anterior nodal enlargements (jugulodigastric chain) typical of bacterial pharyngitis. Patients with mononucleosis usually have headache, fatigue, and other features of the disease such as palpable splenomegaly (about one half of cases). Cytomegalovirus mononucleosis can also cause sore throat, but pharyngeal exudate is rare.

- Primary infection with HIV, known as the acute retroviral syndrome, sometimes presents with fever and pharyngitis. Pharyngeal erythema can be marked, but exudates do not seem to occur. This illness usually occurs within 3 to 6 weeks of the initial infection, during a phase of initial viral multiplication and before the appearance of HIV antibodies. Fever, lethargy, arthralgia, and myalgia are usually prominent, and many patients have a nonpruritic maculopapular rash. Lymphadenopathy, which can be in the anterior or posterior triangles of the neck, appears about 1 week after the onset of pharyngitis (see Chapter 8).

- Herpes simplex virus infection can cause pharyngitis, which sometimes resembles viral or streptococcal pharyngitis. Vesicles and shallow ulcers on the palate suggest the herpetic etiology. These can be extensive and confluent, causing severe oral pain (see "Mouth Ulcers" later in the chapter). Herpangina is an uncommon syndrome caused by coxsackieviruses and is seen mainly in children. It is characterized by small (1- to 2-mm) vesicles on the soft palate, uvula, and anterior tonsillar pillars, which rupture to form small white ulcers. Fever, sore throat, and dysphagia can be severe, and occasional patients have anorexia and abdominal pain suggesting acute appendicitis.

- *Chlamydia pneumoniae* can cause pharyngitis with or without infection of the lower respiratory tract. No distinctive features have been described. There is some epidemiologic evidence that *Mycoplasma pneumoniae* causes pharyngitis, usually mild and again without distinctive features.

- Diphtheria should be mentioned, since it still causes occasional cases of pharyngitis in the United States in patients who have not been vaccinated. Classic diphtheria (*Corynebacterium diphtheriae*) has a slow onset followed by marked systemic toxicity. Sore throat is usually not severe despite the finding of a gray "pseudomembrane" adherent to the tonsillar and pharyngeal mucosa. *Arcanobacterium hemolyticum* (formerly known as *Corynebacterium hemolyticum*) has been increasingly recognized as a cause of exudative pharyngitis in adolescents and young adults, associated with a diffuse and sometimes pruritic maculopapular rash on the trunk and extremities. Rarely, this disease mimics diphtheria. *Corynebacterium ulcerans* is a rare cause of pharyngitis associated with the ingestion of raw milk.

- Anaerobic pharyngitis (Vincent's angina) causes a purulent exudate and often a foul odor to the breath. This uncommon infection is caused by a mixture of anaerobic bacteria and spirochetes, with group A streptococci and *S. aureus* sometimes playing a role. The infection sometimes progresses to peritonsillar abscess (quinsy) or to septic thrombophlebitis of the internal jugular vein (Lemierre syndrome; see Chapter 6).

- *Yersinia enterocolitica* can cause exudative pharyngitis with a fulminant course associated with high mortality. Fever, tender cervical lymphadenopathy, and abdominal pain with or without diarrhea are prominent features. This illness can occur in outbreak form as the result of ingestion of contaminated food or beverages.
- The typhoidal form of tularemia can be manifested as pharyngitis because of inhalation of the organisms, which can occur, for example, while skinning an infected rabbit (see Chapter 8).
- Kawasaki disease (see Chapters 4 and 7), a systemic vasculitis affecting mainly infants and young children, can cause fever and sore throat. Diffuse oropharyngeal erythema without exudate is found during the acute febrile phase of the illness. Other features are bilateral, nonpurulent conjunctivitis; erythema with fissuring, cracking, and bleeding of the lips; strawberry tongue; edema of the hands and feet with erythema of the palms and soles; and an erythematous rash.
- Miscellaneous causes of sore throat include juvenile rheumatoid arthritis, systemic lupus erythematosus, bullous pemphigoid, Behçet's disease, paraquat ingestion, and drug reactions.

Diagnosis

Clinicians should keep in mind the many potential causes of pharyngitis (Box 10-4). However, the usual issue is whether streptococcal pharyngitis is present, warranting antimicrobial therapy.

The diagnosis of streptococcal pharyngitis is strongly suggested on clinical grounds when patients have fever, sore throat, and odynophagia accompanied by purulent tonsillar exudate, tender cervical lymphadenopathy, and leukocytosis (white blood cell count >12,000/mm³). Findings that point away from streptococcal pharyngitis are conjunctivitis, rhinitis, cough, hoarseness, anterior stomatitis, discrete ulcers, and diarrhea. A recent review determined that the most helpful findings pointing toward the diagnosis of streptococcal pharyngitis were tonsillar exudate, pharyngeal exudate, and

exposure to strep throat within the preceding 2 weeks (positive likelihood ratios were 3.4, 2.1, and 1.9, respectively). The most useful findings pointing away from the diagnosis of streptococcal pharyngitis were absence of tender cervical lymph nodes, tonsillar enlargement, or exudate (negative likelihood ratios were 0.60, 0.63, and 0.74, respectively). However, a wealth of experience suggests that clinicians' ability to predict which patients have streptococcal pharyngitis and which do not is poor. Pharyngeal exudates can also be caused by the Epstein-Barr virus, streptococci belonging to Lancefield groups C and G, adenoviruses, herpes simplex virus, and other agents. Thus, when treatment is being considered, an attempt to document group A streptococci should always be made. At present two complementary methods are used for diagnosis: the rapid streptococcal antigen detection test and throat culture.

The rapid streptococcal antigen test screens for the presence of group A streptococcal carbohydrate on a throat swab specimen. The several available tests of this type, when compared with the results of conventional throat culture, provide excellent specificity (≥95%) but only fair sensitivity (80% to 90% or lower). Throat culture, when properly performed, has a specificity of 100% and a sensitivity of 90% to 95% for the presence of *S. pyogenes* in the pharynx. For either method an adequate throat swab specimen is important and is obtained as follows. The swab is rubbed lightly against both tonsils (or tonsillar fossae in the absence of the tonsils) and against the posterior pharyngeal wall, taking care not to touch other areas of the mouth or oropharynx. It should then be processed by a laboratory with adequate quality control and should be reexamined at 48 hours if the initial result at 24 hours is negative.

What are the relative roles of the streptococcal antigen test and throat culture? A standard approach is to reserve throat cultures for patients whose rapid streptococcal antigen test results are negative (Figure 10-13). Some data suggest that throat culture is unnecessary when the results of a high-sensitivity rapid streptococcal antigen test are negative, since such patients seem to be at low risk for suppurative and non-suppurative complications of group A streptococcal infection irrespective of the results of cultures. Other authorities suggest that reliance on throat culture, rather than the rapid streptococcal antigen test, offers the most cost-effective strategy. Another approach is to use clinical findings, expressed

BOX 10-4
Differential Diagnosis of Sore Throat: Findings Pointing to Etiologies Other Than Streptococcal or Viral Pharyngitis

- Medial displacement of one tonsil or bulging of the ipsilateral soft palate suggests peritonsillar abscess, which should prompt referral.
- A gray pseudomembrane (which can be mistaken for an exudate) suggests diphtheria.
- A foul odor to the breath suggests anaerobic pharyngitis (Vincent's angina), which can cause serious complications such as peritonsillar abscess or the Lemierre syndrome.
- Fever with abdominal pain raises the possibility of *Yersinia enterocolitica,* which can have a fulminant course.
- Fever in a young child with conjunctivitis, erythema of the lips, strawberry tongue, edema of the hands and feet, and rash suggests Kawasaki disease.
- Fever with lethargy, arthralgia, myalgia, and maculopapular rash occurs in the acute retroviral syndrome (primary human immunodeficiency virus infection).

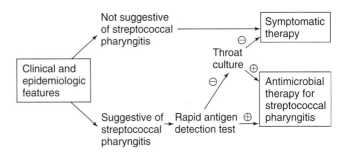

FIG. 10-13 Algorithm for diagnosis and treatment of streptococcal pharyngitis. (Modified from Bisno AL, Gerber MA, Gwaltney JM Jr, et al. Diagnosis and management of group A streptococcal pharyngitis. Clin Infect Dis 1997; 25: 574-578.)

TABLE 10-10
Use of a "Sore Throat Score" as a Guide to Diagnosis and Treatment of Pharyngitis

Step	Actions
Evaluation	1. Assign one point for each of the following: age <15 years; temperature ≥100.4° F (38° C) by history or physical examination; presence of tonsillar swelling or exudate; presence of tender anterior cervical lymphadenopathy; and absence of cough. 2. Subtract one point if age is ≥45 years. 3. Calculate the "sore throat score" on the basis of the number of points, as determined above.
Diagnosis and therapy	If score is ≤1, neither throat culture nor treatment is indicated. If score is 2 or 3, obtain a throat culture (or rapid streptococcal antigen test) as basis for treatment. If score is ≥4, either starting treatment or obtaining a throat culture is appropriate.
Validation in community practice	1. The sore throat score was found to be 85% sensitive and 92% specific for identifying group A streptococcal infection. 2. Use of the sore throat score would reduce prescriptions to patients without streptococcal pharyngitis by 64% and would reduce overall antibiotic prescriptions by 52%.

Modified from McIsaac WJ, Goel V, To T, et al. The validity of a sore throat score in family practice. CMAJ 2000; 163: 811-815.

as a "sore throat score," as the basis for diagnostic and therapeutic decisions (Table 10-10). Primary care clinicians should periodically review their strategies for diagnosis of streptococcal pharyngitis on the basis of new data and evolving opinion.

Serologic methods such as the Streptozyme test and the antistreptolysin O (ASO) titer are useful for retrospective diagnosis of streptococcal infection (as in cases of suspected acute rheumatic fever) but have no place in the differential diagnosis of acute pharyngitis.

Natural History
Expected Outcome
Group A streptococcal pharyngitis is usually a self-limited disease. Fever and other constitutional symptoms typically resolve within 3 to 4 days of onset. Suppurative complications are uncommon. Formerly it was said that 3% of cases of streptococcal pharyngitis were complicated by acute rheumatic fever; however, this observation was based on limited data in select populations, and the incidence of rheumatic fever now seems to be much lower. Streptococcal pharyngitis can also cause acute glomerulonephritis as an immunologic complication. Streptococcal toxic shock syndrome (see Chapter 6) as a complication of noninvasive streptococcal pharyngitis or from nasal packing (e.g., for control of epistaxis or after surgery on the sinuses or nasal septum) has now been reported.

Treatment
Methods
Antimicrobial therapy for streptococcal pharyngitis is recommended for patients with a positive rapid antigen detection test or positive throat culture (Figure 10-13). Postponing therapy for 24 to 48 hours while awaiting the results of throat culture does not reduce the efficacy of treatment. Indeed,

therapy has been shown to effectively prevent nonsuppurative sequelae such as acute rheumatic fever even if begun 9 days after onset of symptoms. When findings strongly suggest streptococcal pharyngitis despite a negative rapid antigen detection test or when patients insist on antibiotics, a reasonable strategy is to (1) obtain a throat culture, (2) provide a 2-day supply of antibiotics, and (3) discontinue antibiotics if the throat culture is negative for group A streptococci.

Standard treatment of streptococcal pharyngitis consists of a 10-day course of penicillin (Table 10-11) or, for young children, amoxicillin. Benzathine penicillin G as a single injection is recommended for patients who are likely to be noncompliant or who would prefer a painful buttock to 10 days of oral therapy. The controlled clinical trials that established the efficacy of penicillin for prevention of acute rheumatic fever used repository forms of the drug (procaine penicillin G in oil containing aluminum monostearate, a preparation now replaced by benzathine penicillin G). A large number of antibiotics (Table 10-11), if taken properly and for the recommended duration, are equally effective at eradicating *S. pyogenes,* and it is therefore assumed, although not proved, that these should be effective for the same purpose. Group A streptococci resistant to penicillin G have not yet been reported. Strains highly resistant to erythromycin have been reported elsewhere but are uncommon in the United States.

Follow-up throat cultures are not recommended in the absence of pharyngeal complaints.

Expected Response
Antimicrobial therapy effects a slight reduction in the severity and duration of streptococcal pharyngitis and, more important, prevents suppurative and nonsuppurative sequelae.

In occasional patients pharyngitis recurs as shown by positive throat cultures or rapid streptococcal antigen tests. These patients present a dilemma. Many are "streptococcal

TABLE 10-11
Some Recommended Antibiotic Regimens for Group A Streptococcal Pharyngitis*

Regimen	Dose (children)†	Dose (adults)
Benzathine penicillin G†	600,000 units IM (single dose)	1.2 million units IM (single dose)
Amoxicillin	250 mg PO b.i.d. for 10 days‡	
Penicillin V potassium	250 mg PO b.i.d. or t.i.d. for 10 days	250 mg t.i.d. or q.i.d. or 500 mg b.i.d. for 10 days
Erythromycin estolate (Ilosone)§	20-50 mg/kg/day in divided doses (q12h)	Not recommended
Erythromycin ethyl succinate (E.E.S., others)§	30-50 mg/kg/day in divided doses (q6h, q8h, or q12h)	400 mg q.i.d.
Cephalexin (Keflex)¶	50 mg/kg/day in divided doses (q12h)	500 mg q12h
Cefaclor (Ceclor)¶	20 mg/kg/day in divided doses (q8h)	250 mg q8h
Cefadroxil (Duricef)¶	30 mg/kg/day (one dose or in divided doses, q12h)	1 g daily or 500 mg b.i.d.
Cefuroxime(Ceftin)¶	20 mg/kg/day in divided doses (q12h)	250 mg q12h
Cefpodoxime (Vantin)¶	10 mg/kg/day in divided doses (q12h)	100 mg q12h
Cefprozil (Cefzil)¶	30 mg/kg/day in divided doses (q12h)	500 mg daily
Cefixime (Suprax)¶	8 mg/kg/day (one dose or in divided doses, q12h)	400 mg daily or 200 mg q12h
Cefdinir (Omnicef)¶	14 mg/kg/day (one dose or divided doses, q12h)	600 mg daily or 300 mg b.i.d.
Clarithromycin (Biaxin)¶	15 mg/kg/day in divided doses (q12h)	250 mg b.i.d.
Azithromycin (Zithromax)¶	12 mg/kg/day on days 1 through 5	500 mg on first day, then 250 mg daily for 4 days

*All regimens are oral except for benzathine penicillin G. Repository penicillin G is the only treatment shown in clinical trials to prevent acute rheumatic fever. The other regimens are approved for treatment of streptococcal pharyngitis and in theory should also prevent acute rheumatic fever. However, this has not been established.
†In general, the doses listed here are for children well beyond the neonatal period.
‡Amoxicillin suspension is recommended for young children because it is more palatable than the alternatives.
§Erythromycin is recommended by most authorities for patients who are allergic to β-lactam antibiotics.
¶All of these regimens are more expensive than amoxicillin, penicillin, and erythromycin but have not been shown to be more effective. Some data suggest that failures of penicillin or amoxicillin are caused by destruction of the drugs by β-lactamase–producing bacteria in the oropharyngeal flora. On this basis cephalosporins and other agents have been recommended especially for "treatment failures."

carriers" whose individual episodes of pharyngitis are often due to other etiologies, notably cold viruses. Throat cultures during asymptomatic intervals may be worthwhile to establish the diagnosis of a streptococcal carrier state. However, no compelling evidence in favor of treating asymptomatic carriers has been presented, since they are unlikely to transmit the organism to others and they have not been shown to be at risk for suppurative complications or acute rheumatic fever. There is some evidence that patients with frequent recurrences of streptococcal pharyn-

gitis may respond more favorably to clindamycin or to amoxicillin-clavulanate than to penicillin, a theoretical rationale being that "penicillin resistance" might actually reflect the presence of β-lactamase–producing bacteria in the oropharynx (Box 10-5).

When to Refer

Referral is indicated for the occasional patient with major suppurative complications, such as peritonsillar abscess, and for those with multiple recurrent infections.

BOX 10-5
Management of the Patient with Frequent Recurrences of Streptococcal Pharyngitis, Proven by Culture or by the Rapid Antigen Detection Test

- Current opinion holds that most patients with frequent recurrences of streptococcal pharyngitis are actually streptococcal carriers whose sore throats are usually due to viral pharyngitis. Thus a measure of reassurance should be offered.
- Throat cultures may be useful during asymptomatic intervals to establish the diagnosis of "streptococcal carrier state," which, however, does not mandate an attempt to eradicate the organism.
- Throat cultures for all family members and treatment of those with positive cultures may be useful (no good evidence has been presented that pets are reservoirs for the disease or contribute to spread within a family). However, affected individuals should minimize the chances of reintroduction of the streptococcus by treating any item they use orally (toothbrush, orthodontic retainers) in dilute bleach or hydrogen peroxide (rinsing thoroughly thereafter) on a daily basis during the period of oral antibiotic therapy.
- Individual episodes of pharyngitis can be treated with benzathine penicillin G or other standard regimens.
- Some evidence suggests that individual episodes may respond more favorably in this circumstance to a 10-day course of therapy with clindamycin (for children, 20 to 30 mg/kg/day in divided doses; for adults, 600 mg/day in two to four divided doses) or amoxicillin-clavulanate [Augmentin] 40 mg/kg/day in three divided doses).
- Selected patients may benefit from tonsillectomy, although the benefit is often short lived.

KEY POINTS

ACUTE PHARYNGITIS

⊃ Sore throat has numerous potential etiologies and is most commonly caused by the common cold. There is a wide consensus that antibiotics are overused.

⊃ Group A β-hemolytic streptococci cause about 15% to 30% of cases of acute pharyngitis and are more commonly isolated from children than from adults. Streptococcal pharyngitis is usually a self-limited disease but can cause major suppurative complications and acute rheumatic fever.

⊃ Rapid antigen detection tests or throat cultures should be obtained for patients with suspected streptococcal pharyngitis.

⊃ When streptococcal pharyngitis is strongly suspected, antibiotics can be prescribed while the results of throat cultures are awaited. However, antibiotics should be discontinued if throat cultures are negative for group A streptococci.

⊃ Primary care clinicians should have in place a strategy for cost-effective management of suspected streptococcal pharyngitis.

⊃ Follow-up throat cultures are not recommended after treatment of streptococcal pharyngitis.

⊃ Patients with frequent recurrences of pharyngitis and positive cultures for group A streptococci or positive rapid antigen detection tests are often streptococcal carriers whose sore throats are due to acute, self-limited viral illness.

SUGGESTED READING

Bass JW, Person DA, Chan DS. Twice-daily oral penicillin for treatment of streptococcal pharyngitis: less is best. Pediatrics 2000; 105: 423-424.

Bisno AL, Gerber MA, Gwaltney JM Jr, et al. Diagnosis and management of group A streptococcal pharyngitis: a practice guideline. Clin Infect Dis 1997; 25: 574-583.

Brook I. Microbial factors leading to recurrent upper respiratory tract infections. Pediatr Infect Dis J 1998; 17: S62-S67.

Ebell MH, Smith MA, Barry HC, et al. Does this patient have strep throat? JAMA 2000; 284: 2912-2918.

Hayes CS, Williamson H. Management of group A beta-hemolytic streptococcal pharyngitis. Am Family Physician 2001; 63: 1557-1564, 1565.

Linder JA, Stafford RS. Antibiotic treatment of adults with sore throat by community primary care physicians: a national survey, 1989-1999. JAMA 201; 286: 1181-1186.

McIsaac WJ, Goel V, To T, et al. The validity of a sore throat score in family practice. CMAJ 2000; 163: 811-815.

Snow V, Mottur-Pilson C, Cooper RJ, et al. Principles of appropriate antibiotic use for acute pharyngitis in adults. Ann Intern Med 2001; 134: 506-508.

Tsevat J, Kotagal UR. Management of sore throats in children: a cost-effectiveness analysis. Arch Pediatr Adolesc Med 1999; 153: 681-688.

Turner JC, Hayden FG, Lobo MC, et al. Epidemiologic evidence for Lancefield group C beta-hemolytic streptococci as a cause of exudative pharyngitis in college students. J Clin Microbiol 1997; 35: 1-4.

Webb KH, Needham CA, Kurtz SR. Use of a high-sensitivity rapid strep test without culture confirmation of negative results: 2 years' experience. J Fam Pract 2000; 49: 34-38.

Acute Laryngitis

Acute laryngitis is extremely common, usually occurring as part of upper respiratory tract infection. Treatment is symptomatic, but prolonged hoarseness mandates the search for other etiologies.

Presentation and Progression
Cause

Acute laryngitis is most often caused by respiratory viruses, but vocal abuse or gastroesophageal reflux must also be considered. Parainfluenza viruses are the usual cause in patients between ages 5 and 15. Hoarseness complicates up to 29% of rhinovirus infections, 35% of influenza virus and adenovirus infections, and 63% of coronavirus infections according to various studies. Hoarseness can also complicate acute streptococcal pharyngitis. *H. influenzae* and *Moraxella catarrhalis* are often isolated, but their pathogenic roles are unclear. Rarely, fungi such as *Candida* species, *Cryptococcus neoformans,* and *Coccidioides immitis* cause laryngitis. Uncommonly, laryngitis is also caused by tuberculosis and blastomycosis.

Presentation

Acute laryngitis is manifested as hoarseness. Speech and swallowing may be painful. The voice is hoarse, harsh, broken, or nearly absent. The patient often has concomitant symptoms of the common cold, including sore throat.

Diagnosis

Diagnosis of acute laryngitis is made on clinical grounds, typically by the history. Direct or indirect laryngoscopy shows erythema and edema of the vocal folds, sometimes with submucosal bruising or microhemorrhages (if the patient continues heavy use of the voice or has a bad cough). Viral cultures and special studies are seldom indicated.

Natural History
Expected Outcome

Median duration of hoarseness is about 3 days, but hoarseness lasts 8 days or longer in about 25% of cases and hoarseness lasting 2 to 3 weeks is not uncommon. A longer duration of hoarseness should prompt consideration of an etiology other than acute infection. Benign conditions include gastroesophageal reflux disease and continued voice abuse, but the serious possibilities are cancer, tuberculosis (laryngeal tuberculosis is highly infectious), blastomycosis, and histoplasmosis.

Treatment
Methods

Treatment is entirely symptomatic. Voice rest and humidification are often prescribed. Antibiotics are of no proven benefit. Oral steroids can temporarily alleviate the hoarseness of an infection or vocal abuse but are inappropriate.

Expected Response

Acute laryngitis is self-limited.

When to Refer

Persistent hoarseness requires referral for laryngoscopy. The primary care physician should keep in mind that sometimes a false diagnosis of cancer is returned on biopsy of the larynx in cases of histoplasmosis, blastomycosis, or (occasionally) tuberculosis because of overlying pseudoepitheliomatous hyperplasia.

  KEY POINTS

ACUTE LARYNGITIS
- Acute laryngitis is usually a self-limited illness of viral etiology.
- The median duration of hoarseness is about 3 days, but hoarseness lasts for 8 days in about 25% of patients and can last for several weeks.
- Patients with more prolonged hoarseness should be referred for laryngoscopy.

SUGGESTED READING

Hol C, Schalén C, Verduin CM, et al. *Moraxella catarrhalis* in acute laryngitis: infection or colonization? J Infect Dis 1996; 174: 636-638.

Ormseth EJ, Wong RK. Reflux laryngitis: pathophysiology, diagnosis and management. Am J Gastroenterol 1999; 94: 2812-2817.

Spiegel JR, Hawkshaw M, Markiewicz A, et al. Acute laryngitis. Ear Nose Throat J 2000; 79; 488-495.

Vrabec JT, Molina CP, West B. Herpes simplex viral laryngitis. Ann Otol Rhinol Laryngol 2000; 109: 611-614.

Odontogenic Infections

Odontogenic infections, the most common infections of the oral cavity, begin in and around the teeth and can spread to cause life-threatening local or systemic complications.

Presentation and Progression
Cause

The normal oral cavity contains dense masses of bacteria, of which 80% or more are anaerobic. Viridans streptococci (such as *S. mitis, S. sanguis, S. salivarius,* and *S. mutans*) preferentially colonize one or another anatomic site. *Streptococcus mutans* is the major cause of dental caries (cavities). As is well known, poor oral hygiene facilitates development of dental plaque, composed mainly of anaerobic bacteria. Diet high in simple sugars and carbohydrates predisposes to plaque. Periodontal disease, on the other hand, is unrelated to diet but is associated with poor oral hygiene, increasing age, various congenital immunodeficiency diseases, and juvenile diabetes mellitus. Gingivitis and periodontitis are caused mainly by anaerobic bacteria. Once established, suppuration arising in and around the teeth can spread along fascial planes, invade bone, or enter the bloodstream. Deeper infections requiring surgical drainage, such as periapical abscesses and deep fascial space infections (see Chapter 6), are associated with numerous anaerobic bacterial species.

Presentation

Odontogenic infections develop as one of several syndromes:
- Periapical abscess and acute alveolar abscess represent infection of the tooth pulp. In the early stages the tooth is sensitive to touch and also to both hot and cold. In the later stages the tooth is extremely painful when exposed to heat; the pain is relieved by cold.
- Gingivitis is often first manifest as friability and bleeding of the gums. A more severe form, acute necrotizing gingivitis (Vincent's angina or trench mouth), is characterized by a sudden onset of severe pain and necrosis of the gingiva, typically with a grayish pseudomembrane, halitosis, and systemic symptoms including fever, malaise, and generalized lymphadenopathy.
- Periodontitis, broadly defined as infections of the periodontium (the supporting structures of the teeth, which include alveolar bone, cementum, and the periodontal ligament, as well as the gingiva) begins gradually, usually in early adulthood, and is associated with plaque below the gingival margin. Patients sometimes complain of itchy sensations of the gums in between the teeth, bad taste in the mouth, vague jaw pains, and sensitivity to both hot and cold. Pus can sometimes be expressed by pressure on the gingival margin. Periodontal abscess can cause a red, fluctuant swelling of the gingival margin. Pus can readily be expressed after probing.
- Pericoronitis consists of acute localized pain over a partially erupted or impacted wisdom tooth. The gums are red and swollen, and a small amount of pus can usually be expressed by pressing on the gum flap overlying the partially erupted tooth. Trismus caused by irritation of the masseter or medial pterygoid muscle is often marked.

Diagnosis

Diagnosis of dentoalveolar infections, gingivitis, and periodontal infections is based on symptoms, examination, and, when indicated, dental radiographs. Radiographs are especially valuable for visualizing periapical abscess and acute alveolar abscess.

Natural History
Expected Outcome

Spontaneous cure without loss of tooth or tissue is uncommon.

Treatment

Apical abscess, dentoalveolar abscess, and periodontal abscess generally require surgical drainage. Pericoronitis often responds to gentle débridement with irrigation, but incision and drainage combined with antibiotic therapy are required for more severe cases. Gingivitis is usually treated with local débridement and lavage using oxidizing agents. Antibiotic treatment with penicillin or metronidazole is often useful. Periodontitis sometimes responds to tetracycline and metronidazole along with root débridement and surgical resection.

Expected Response

Response to definitive surgical treatment is usually excellent. Progressive periodontal disease, however, is the most frequent cause of gum loss in adults.

When to Refer

Serious odontogenic disease should usually be treated by a dentist. Deep fascial space infections (see Chapter 6) require hospitalization.

 KEY POINTS

ODONTOGENIC INFECTIONS
- Periapical abscess and acute alveolar abscess represent infection of the tooth pulp; the tooth is sensitive to touch and to hot stimuli.
- Pericoronitis represents localized pain over a partially erupted or impacted wisdom tooth.
- Periodontal abscess can develop as a red, fluctuant swelling of the gingival margin.
- Dental infections can have serious complications such as osteomyelitis, maxillary sinusitis, brain abscess, and deep soft tissue infections of the head and neck.
- Primary care clinicians should promote good oral hygiene, especially to prevent periodontal disease.

SUGGESTED READING

Heimdahl A. Culturing the exudate of an odontogenic infection—a useful procedure? Oral Surg 2000; 90: 2-4.

Kureishi A, Chow AW. The tender tooth: dentoalveolar, pericoronal, and periodontal infections. Infect Dis Clin North Am 1988; 2: 163-182.

Li X, Kolltveit KM, Tronstad L, et al. Systemic diseases caused by oral infection. Clin Microbiol Rev 2000; 13: 547-558.

Loesche WJ, Grossman NS. Periodontal disease as a specific, albeit chronic, infection: diagnosis and treatment. Clin Mircobiol Rev 2001; 14: 727-752.

Slavkin HC, Baum BJ. Relationship of dental and oral pathology to systemic illness. JAMA 2000; 284: 1215-1217.

Mouth Ulcers

Careful examination of the oral cavity often provides evidence of important systemic and local disease. Candidiasis, hairy leukoplakia, or the hyperpigmented lesions of Kaposi's sarcoma can be the first clues to advanced HIV disease (see Chapter 17). Mucositis—manifested as marked erythema with extensive ulceration—is a disabling complication of chemotherapy and radiation therapy in patients with malignancies. Oral lesions also occur in connective tissue disorders, Behçet's disease, systemic fungal infection, secondary syphilis (mucous patches), and primary dermatologic conditions such as lichen planus, pemphigoid, and pemphigus vulgaris. Persistent white lesions of the oral mucosa raise the possibility of squamous cell carcinoma, and pigmented lesions occasionally reflect melanoma. More commonly, primary care clinicians evaluate patients with self-limited diseases such as stomatitis caused by the herpes simplex viruses and aphthous stomatitis (canker sores). Here we briefly review these latter conditions and their differential diagnosis.

Presentation and Progression
Cause

Herpes simplex viruses 1 and 2 cause fever blisters and less commonly lesions elsewhere in the mouth, including the palate. The cause of aphthous stomatitis is unknown. Current opinion favors an immunopathogenesis involving T-cell immunity, possibly a delayed-type hypersensitivity reaction to an antigen residing within the epithelium. Some cases of aphthous stomatitis have been attributed to drugs. Stress, smoking, hormonal factors, and food allergy have also been invoked, but the evidence is unconvincing.

Presentation

Herpes simplex stomatitis begins with 1- to 2-mm vesicles that rupture, leading to ulceration. Confluent lesions can give rise to large areas of ulceration (Figure 10-14). Lesions typically occur on keratinized or attached oral mucosal surfaces such as the lips, the gingiva, the lateral surfaces of the tongue, or the palate. Aphthous stomatitis begins with ulcers of various size, usually from several millimeters to 1 cm or more in diameter. Lesions typically occur on nonkeratinized, unattached mucosal surfaces (Figure 10-15). Both types of lesions are painful.

Diagnosis

Diagnosis of both herpes simplex stomatitis and aphthous stomatitis is usually made on clinical grounds. In cases of extensive herpes simplex stomatitis (as shown in Figure 10-14), viral culture may be indicated. Differential diagnosis assumes importance when individual lesions fail to resolve within 7 to 14 days. Evidence of disease elsewhere may suggest a systemic disease such as lupus erythematosus, Sjögren's syndrome, Behçet's disease, pemphigus, pemphigoid, and the mouth and genital ulcers with inflamed cartilage (MAGIC) syndrome. Disseminated fungal infection such as histoplasmosis or blastomy-

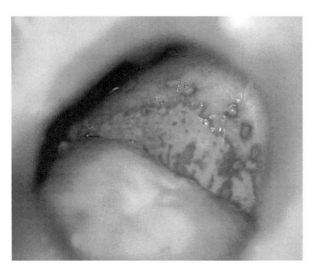

FIG. 10-14   Herpes simplex stomatitis with extensive confluent ulceration of the mucosal surface of the palate. The individual "unit" lesions are small ulcerations with erythematous halos.

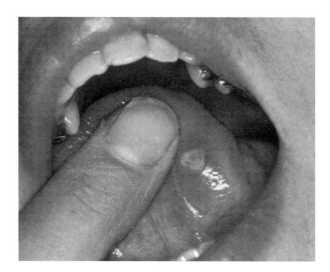

FIG. 10-15   Lesion consistent with aphthous stomatitis on the undersurface of the tongue.

cosis can cause indurated, "punched-out" ulcers. The margins of these ulcers often show pseudoepitheliomatous hyperplasia on biopsy, which can be misinterpreted as squamous cell carcinoma. Occasional patients with recurrent mouth ulcers have cyclic neutropenia, which can be diagnosed by serial complete blood counts (spontaneous resolution of granulocytopenia, mouth ulcers, and other symptoms such as fever). In 1987 a new syndrome known as PFADA (periodic fever, aphthous stomatitis, pharyngitis, and cervical adenitis) or Marshall's syndrome was described in children.

Natural History
Expected Outcome

In immunocompetent patients the lesions of both herpes simplex stomatitis and aphthous stomatitis usually resolve within 7 to 14 days. Both lesions tend to recur. Occasional patients with recurrent aphthous stomatitis experience disabling disease characterized by severe mouth pain leading to malnutrition ("complex aphthosis"). Patients with cyclic neutropenia or the PFADA syndrome (Marshall's syndrome) remain well between episodes.

Treatment
Methods

Oral-labial herpes simplex stomatitis can be treated with topical antiviral therapy such as pencilovir cream. Severe cases of herpes simplex stomatitis can be treated with systemic antiviral drugs such as acyclovir or famciclovir. Apthous stomatitis usually responds to topical corticosteroids. Severe cases of aphthous stomatitis (including "complex aphthosis") usually respond to high-dose oral corticosteroid therapy (e.g., prednisone 40 mg b.i.d. for 4 days). Short-course therapy and careful monitoring are advised, since patients may be tempted to self-medicate, leading to iatrogenic Cushing's syndrome. Thalidomide is useful for severe aphthous stomatitis and can be obtained for this purpose on an investigational basis.

Expected Response

Topical penciclovir cream has been shown to reduce pain and shorten the duration of recurrent oral-labial herpes simplex virus.

When to Refer

Patients with chronic mouth ulcers should usually be referred, for example, to a knowledgeable dentist or oral surgeon, for consideration of biopsy.

 KEY POINTS

MOUTH ULCERS

- ⊃ The most common causes of self-limited mouth ulcers in the United States are herpes simplex stomatitis and aphthous stomatitis (canker sores).
- ⊃ Oral-labial herpes simplex virus infection usually involves keratinized or attached mucosal surfaces such as the lips, gingiva, lateral surfaces of the tongue, and palate.
- ⊃ Aphthous stomatitis usually involves unkeratinized, unattached mucosal surfaces.
- ⊃ Recurrent aphthous stomatitis can be extremely disabling ("complex aphthosis").
- ⊃ Oral-labial herpes simplex virus infection can be treated with topical or systemic antiviral drugs.
- ⊃ Aphthous stomatitis usually responds to topical or systemic corticosteroids, but these agents should be used sparingly because patients may be tempted to self-medicate, leading to Cushing's syndrome.
- ⊃ Patients with persistent mouth ulcers should be referred to a dentist or oral surgeon for biopsy.

SUGGESTED READING

Callen JP. Oral manifestations of collagen vascular disease. Semin Cutan Med Surg 1997; 16: 323-327.

Cohen DM, Bhattacharyya I, Lydiatt WM. Recalcitrant oral ulcers caused by calcium channel blockers: diagnosis and treatment considerations. J Am Dent Assoc 1999; 130: 1611-1618.

Epstein JB. The painful mouth: mucositis, gingivitis, and stomatitis. Infect Dis Clin North Am 1988; 2: 183-202.

Eversole LR. Immunopathogenesis of oral lichen planus and recurrent aphthous stomatitis. Semin Cutan Med Surg 1997; 16: 284-294.

Feder HM Jr. Periodic fever, aphthous stomatitis, pharyngitis, adenitis: a clinical review of a new syndrome. Curr Opin Pediatr 2000; 12: 253-256.

Rogers RS III. Recurrent aphthous stomatitis: clinical characteristics and associated systemic disorders. Semin Cutan Med Surg 1997; 16: 278-283.

Schneider LC, Schneider AE. Diagnosis of oral ulcers. Mt Sinai J Med 1998; 65: 383-387.

11 Lower Respiratory Tract Infections

CHARLES S. BRYAN

Lower respiratory tract infections challenge primary care physicians on an almost daily basis. Otherwise healthy persons with acute bronchitis expect and often receive prescriptions for antibiotics despite the knowledge in medicine that the benefits are marginal at best. Elderly and immunocompromised persons often have symptoms and signs of pneumonia, raising the issue of whether hospitalization is indicated. Pneumonia and influenza are largely to blame for the increased mortality rates during winter months. Precise diagnosis of lower respiratory tract infection is desirable but difficult to obtain. Old pathogens such as the pneumococcus (*Streptococcus pneumoniae*) are becoming difficult to treat, and new pathogens continue to be discovered. The chapter covers the clinical spectrum of airways infection, the clinical spectrum of pneumonia, the more common causes of "typical" and "atypical" pneumonia, and influenza. Bronchiolitis and other respiratory infections in children are discussed in Chapter 4.

SUGGESTED READING

Mandell LA, Niederman MS, eds. Lower respiratory tract infections. Infect Dis Clin North Am 1998; 12: 535-825.

Marrie TJ, ed. Community-Acquired Pneumonia. New York: Plenum Publishing; 2000.

Pennington JE, ed. Respiratory Infections: Diagnosis and Management. New York: Raven Press; 1994.

Reimer LG, Carroll KC. Role of the microbiology laboratory in the diagnosis of lower respiratory tract infections. Clin Infect Dis 1998; 26: 742-748.

Acute Bronchitis ("Chest Cold")

Tracheobronchial infections without pneumonia comprise a spectrum of disorders with different clinical implications: acute bronchitis, chronic bronchitis, and bronchiectasis. Acute bronchitis or "acute simple bronchitis" in otherwise healthy persons is extremely common, usually of viral etiology, and a common reason for overuse of antibiotics. The term "acute infectious bronchitis" is sometimes used to distinguish this entity from other causes of cough, and the term "tracheobronchitis" is sometimes used for accuracy, since the trachea is also inflamed. However, "chest cold" is probably the best term for daily practice, since it implies that antibiotics are seldom necessary. *Bordetella pertussis,* the agent of whooping cough, is now recognized as a cause of acute bronchitis in adults. Infection by either *Mycoplasma pneumoniae* or *Chlamydia pneumoniae* accounts for many of the stubborn cases in which symptoms fail to resolve or recur soon after treatment has been discontinued.

Presentation and Progression
Cause

Infection of the tracheobronchial mucosa causes local inflammation, increased secretion of mucus, and damage to ciliary cells. Symptoms result both from the inflammatory response and from the interruption of the mucociliary blanket that normally cleanses the lower respiratory tract. Most cases of acute bronchitis (95% by some estimates) are caused by viruses. All the common viruses affecting the upper respiratory tract have been implicated: rhinoviruses, coronavirus, respiratory syncytial virus, adenoviruses, coxsackieviruses, influenza viruses A and B, and parainfluenza virus. In two studies in which attempts were made to establish a precise diagnosis, the etiology was established in only 16% and 29% of cases and viruses were the most common cause.

M. pneumoniae and *C. pneumoniae* probably play minor roles in acute bronchitis, at least in most populations. However, *M. pneumoniae* probably causes more cases of bronchitis than pneumonia, and *C. pneumoniae* may be an important cause of acute bronchitis in college-aged students. Whether *S. pneumoniae, Haemophilus influenzae,* and *Moraxella catarrhalis* cause chest cold in otherwise healthy persons is unclear, but the concept of "acute bacterial bronchitis" as a community-acquired disease has little support. Recently it has been emphasized that *B. pertussis* can infect adults, even when vaccinated, providing a reservoir for whooping cough among infants. *Bordetella parapertussis* causes a protracted illness similar to whooping cough but without systemic toxicity. Whether these observations can be generalized to other populations is undetermined.

Presentation

The incidence of acute bronchitis is highest in children <5 years of age, with another peak among the elderly. The disease is seasonal and is most common in midwinter and least common in midsummer. Most cases occur without obvious predisposing factors.

The onset is typically preceded by a prodrome of at least 24 hours with symptoms of coryza and pharyngitis. A dry cough, signifying early inflammation of the upper airway, often evolves into a cough productive of moderate amounts of mucopurulent sputum. Fever, headache, myalgias, and retrosternal chest pain or discomfort may be present. Fever is most common when an influenza virus or *M. pneumoniae* is the causative agent. The patient rarely looks toxic. Tracheal tenderness is often present. Auscultation may reveal a few coarse crackles with occasional wheezes in the chest, but signs of consolidation are absent.

Diagnosis

Acute bronchitis is a clinical diagnosis supported by the typical symptoms, the finding of tracheal tenderness, and the absence of pneumonia. Rigorous diagnosis requires a normal chest x-ray examination, but in most cases this is not indicated on the initial visit. Any attempt to identify specific viruses, *M. pneumoniae,* or *C. pneumoniae* is usually unrealistic, and microscopic examination of sputum is seldom performed. The usual indications for further studies or therapeutic trials are uncertainty about the diagnosis or duration of symptoms >3 weeks.

More than 90% of patients with cough lasting >3 weeks have the postnasal drip syndrome, asthma, gastroesophageal reflux, or drug-induced cough (of which angiotensin-converting enzyme [ACE] inhibitors are now the most common cause). Postnasal drip should be suspected when patients report having to clear the throat frequently. Postnasal drip is usually due to postinfectious rhinitis (often caused by the common cold), allergic rhinitis, vasomotor rhinitis, sinusitis, or irritants. Asthma usually causes wheezing, but wheezing is sometimes absent and, moreover, tests for reversible airway obstruction can have false-positive results. The best way to confirm asthma as the cause of chronic cough may be a therapeutic trial of an inhaled β-agonist. Gastroesophageal reflux can be confirmed by 24-hour esophageal pH monitoring, but a more practical approach may be a therapeutic trial of antacids, an H_2-receptor antagonist, or a proton pump inhibitor such as omeprazole (Prilosec).

Isolation of *B. pertussis* requires special media and 5 to 7 days of incubation. The organism can be identified more rapidly by a direct fluorescein-labeled antibody method. Newer strategies to identify *B. pertussis* are not yet widely available, and current criteria for serologic diagnosis are imprecise. *B. parapertussis* resembles *Haemophilus* species on agar and is often incorrectly assumed to be normal flora.

Natural History
Expected Outcome

Acute bronchitis of viral etiology resolves within 2 weeks in about 75% of cases. Cough caused by *M. pneumoniae* or *C. pneumoniae* can persist for 6 weeks or possibly longer. There is some evidence that recurrent attacks of acute bronchitis contribute to the pathogenesis of chronic obstructive pulmonary disease (COPD).

Treatment
Methods

Antibiotics are unnecessary in most cases. Numerous trials suggest that antibiotics confer only modest benefit. Antibiotics should be reserved for patients at high risk of complications: the elderly, those with chronic lung disease, and those with compromised host defenses.

Symptomatic therapy includes nonsteroidal antiinflammatory drugs (NSAIDs), aspirin (for adults but not for children because of the risk of Reye's syndrome), acetaminophen, ipratropium bromide (Atrovent), or a nasal decongestant. The most effective symptomatic therapy may be the combination of an NSAID (e.g., naproxen 250 to 350 mg t.i.d. or ibuprofen 400 mg q12h) and a first-generation antihistamine (e.g., brompheniramine 12 mg q12h). Placebo-controlled trials fail to support the use of narcotic-containing cough suppressants, even though these are widely prescribed. Intranasal corticosteroids or antihistamines may be appropriate for patients with symptoms of allergic rhinitis. The use of inhaled steroids has not yet been validated by well-controlled studies.

M. pneumoniae and *C. pneumoniae* respond to antibiotic therapy with a tetracycline or macrolide antibiotic. Clinical experience suggests that *C. pneumoniae* infections often recur, requiring additional courses of therapy. Erythromycin is the drug of choice for pertussis and is most effective if given early in the illness. When pertussis is diagnosed later in the illness, erythromycin is still indicated to eliminate pharyngeal carriage and thus reduce transmission of the agent. Neuraminidase inhibitors shorten the duration of symptoms in patients with influenza A or B.

Acute bronchitis provides an excellent opportunity to counsel patients about smoking.

When to Refer

Referral is seldom if ever indicated in patients with acute uncomplicated bronchitis. Chronic cough, on the other hand, should be evaluated further because of the possibility not only of treatable benign disease but also of lung cancer.

 KEY POINTS

ACUTE BRONCHITIS

⊃ Acute bronchitis is usually a self-limited disease of viral etiology. "Chest cold" may be a better term than "bronchitis," since the former implies that antibiotics are usually unnecessary.

⊃ Chest x-ray examination and laboratory studies are not indicated in straightforward cases.

⊃ At presentation, antibiotics are seldom if ever indicated except in elderly patients and those with severe underlying diseases.

⊃ *M. pneumoniae* and *C. pneumoniae* cause protracted cases of bronchitis. However, these agents seem to play a minor etiologic role in acute bronchitis as encountered in most ambulatory care practices.

⊃ In patients with cough lasting more than 3 weeks, acute bronchitis should be distinguished from other causes of chronic cough, notably postnasal drip syndrome, asthma, gastroesophageal reflux, and use of ACE inhibitors.

⊃ In recent studies *B. pertussis* (the agent of whooping cough) was found in 10% to 20% of adults with chronic cough lasting more than 3 weeks despite a history of prior immunization *B. pertussis* may be a more common cause of cough in adolescents and adults than has been generally thought to be the case. However, isolation of the organism can be difficult and current serologic criteria for diagnosis are imprecise.

⊃ The most effective therapy may be the combination of an NSAID (e.g., naproxen or ibuprofen) and a first-generation antihistamine (e.g., brompheniramine).

⊃ Acute bronchitis provides an opportunity for counseling about smoking cessation.

SUGGESTED READING

Bent S, Saint S, Vittinghoff E, et al. Antibiotics in acute bronchitis: a meta-analysis. Am J Med 1999; 107: 62-67.

Freestone C, Eccles R. Assessment of the antitussive efficacy of codeine on cough associated with the common cold. J Pharm Pharmacol 1997; 49: 1045-1049.

Gonzales R, Sande MA. Uncomplicated acute bronchitis. Ann Intern Med 2000; 133: 981-991.

Gonzales R, Steiner JF, Lunn A, et al. Decreasing antibiotic use in ambulatory practice: impact of a multidimensional intervention on the treatment of uncomplicated acute bronchitis in adults. JAMA 1999; 281: 1512-1519.

Gonzales R, Wilson A, Crane LA, et al. What's in a name? Public knowledge, attitudes, and experiences with antibiotic use for acute bronchitis. Am J Med 2000; 108: 83-85.

Gwaltney JM Jr, Druce HM. Efficacy of brompheniramine maleate treatment for rhinovirus colds. Clin Infect Dis 1997; 25: 1188-1194.

Hueston WJ, Mainous AG III. Acute bronchitis. Am Fam Physician 1998; 57: 1270-1276, 1281-1282.

Hueston WJ. Does acute bronchitis really exist? A reconceptualization of acute viral respiratory infections. J Fam Pract 2000; 49: 401-406.

Leiner S. Acute bronchitis in adults: commonly diagnosed but poorly defined. Nurse Pract 1997; 22: 104, 107-108, 113-117.

MacKay DN. Treatment of acute bronchitis in adults without underlying lung disease. J Gen Intern Med 1996; 11: 557-562.

Nennig ME, Shinefield HR, Edwards KM, et al. Prevalence and incidence of adult pertussis in an urban population. JAMA 1996; 275: 1672-1674.

Strebel P, Nordin J, Edwards K. Population-based incidence of pertussis among adolescents and adults, Minnesota, 1995-1996. J Infect Dis 2001; 183: 1353-1359.

Acute Infectious Exacerbations of Chronic Bronchitis

Chronic bronchitis is defined by the American Thoracic Society (ATS) as excessive sputum production with cough, present on most days for at least 3 months a year and not less than 2 successive years, without an underlying etiology such as tuberculosis or bronchiectasis. This common disorder, affecting up to 25% of the adult population, can lead to full-blown COPD, the fourth-leading cause of death in the United States. The extent to which acute exacerbations are due to treatable infections remains controversial.

Presentation and Progression
Cause

Chronic bronchitis is caused mainly by cigarette smoking. Air pollution, cold and damp climates, heredity, frequent lower respiratory tract infections, and immunodeficiency disorders (e.g., common variable hypogammaglobulinemia or isolated IgA deficiency) play a role in some patients. The essential feature is anatomic change in the larger airways, including an increased number of mucus-producing goblet cells and mucosal gland hypertrophy in the bronchial walls. Increased bronchial secretions and impaired ability to handle them lead to chronic cough and disabling complications.

Current opinion holds that most acute exacerbations of chronic bronchitis are caused by viruses or by noninfectious agents. Viruses have been found in as few as 7% to as many as 64% of cases in which they were sought. By conservative estimate viruses cause about one third of cases, the more common ones being influenza viruses A and B, parainfluenza virus, coronaviruses, and rhinoviruses.

Cultures of sputum often show nontypeable strains of *H. influenzae, S. pneumoniae,* or *M. catarrhalis.* However, the extent to which these bacteria explain exacerbations in a given patient is hard to determine, since they often colonize the damaged lower respiratory tract on a more or less permanent basis. Evidence suggests that repeated episodes of bacterial infections—especially when caused by *H. influenzae*—contribute to deterioration of pulmonary function. *Staphylococcus aureus* and aerobic gram-negative rods occasionally cause exacerbations of chronic bronchitis. The pathogens associated with "atypical pneumonia" such as *M. pneumoniae, C. pneumoniae,* and *Legionella pneumophila* probably cause <10% of exacerbations. Evidence to date suggests that *C. pneumoniae* is more strongly associated with the underlying chronic bronchitis than with its acute exacerbations. However, *C. pneumoniae* can cause a stubborn respiratory illness lasting several weeks or longer and tending to relapse after each course of antibiotics.

Diagnosis

The clinical diagnosis of chronic bronchitis is based on a daily productive cough, which is worse in the morning. When chronic bronchitis begins at an early age, the possibility of cystic fibrosis, immunoglobulin deficiency, or other underlying disease should be considered (see Chapters 3 and 4). Exacerbations are characterized by increased severity of cough, dyspnea, and sputum production. The appearance of sputum may change from mucoid to purulent. Some observers believe that the "sputum wet prep" can be useful, as follows. The patient is asked to bring a fresh morning sputum sample for microscopic examination using the oil immersion lens. The presence of numerous polymorphonuclear neutrophils and ciliated epithelial cells indicates disease activity, and the presence of eosinophils or their derivatives suggests the possibility of an "allergic" component. However, critical studies have not confirmed the presence of increased numbers of leukocytes in expectorated samples. The more significant change is in pulmonary function. Peak expiratory flow rate is usually markedly reduced, and hypoxemia is common.

A chest radiograph should be obtained to exclude pneumonia. Distortion of the pulmonary architecture in COPD renders pulmonary infiltrates less impressive than they would be in healthy persons. Most authorities believe that routine sputum cultures are not indicated during exacerbations. The two most common bacterial isolates—nontypeable strains of *H. influenzae* and *S. pneumoniae*—are relatively difficult to isolate; moreover, their isolation does not establish a causal role in the exacerbation, since these organisms are often merely colonizers. Sputum culture results during exacerbation and during remission tend to be similar. However, increasing resistance of *S. pneumoniae* to antibiotics could prompt a reappraisal of this issue in the future.

Natural History
Expected Outcome

Early in the history of COPD most exacerbations are self-limited. When COPD is more advanced, exacerbations often lead to respiratory failure requiring hospitalization.

Treatment
Methods

The role and choice of antibiotics for exacerbations of chronic bronchitis continue to be controversial subjects, with a wide variety of therapeutic options (Table 11-1). Antibiotic therapy usually leads to only modest improvement in airflow. Some authorities maintain that antibiotics should be reserved for patients with more severe COPD as defined by a scoring system that takes into account age, smoking status, other diseases, the frequency of acute exacerbations, and the results of baseline pulmonary function tests. However, most clinicians give antibiotics that will cover *S. pneumoniae, H. influenzae,* and *M. catarrhalis* because of the consequences of deteriorating pulmonary function in these patients. In practice, antibiotic therapy in this setting is usually empiric; indeed, results of culture and sensitivity testing can be misleading because multiple strains of organisms such as nontypeable *H. influenzae* are sometimes present.

Historically, the recommended drugs have been doxycycline, trimethoprim-sulfamethoxazole (TMP/SMX), and amoxicillin. Some authorities prefer amoxicillin–clavulanic acid (Augmentin), which is superior to amoxicillin alone because up to 15% of nontypeable *H. influenzae* and 75% of *M. catarrhalis* now produce β-lactamase. Also, amoxicillin–clavulanic acid has compared favorably with newer agents in clinical trials. Others prefer the newer "respiratory quinolones" (e.g., levofloxacin, moxifloxacin, gatifloxacin) for elderly patients and those with coexisting morbid disease such as heart failure, since the quinolones cover a broader spectrum of potential pathogens (see "Acute Community-Acquired Pneumonia" later in the chapter). When antibiotics are given, they are usually continued for 7 to 10 days. However, studies suggest that 5- to 7-day courses often suffice.

Adjunctive therapy, which is probably more important than antibiotic therapy in most cases, often consists of bronchodilators and judicious use of oxygen. Alternative drugs such as mucolytics, antiproteases, antioxidants, and immunostimulants are being investigated. All patients with chronic bronchitis should receive the pneumococcal vaccine and annual influenza immunization. Pneumococcal vaccine has not been shown to reduce the frequency of exacerbations of chronic bronchitis, but it clearly reduces the frequency and severity of invasive pneumococcal dis-

TABLE 11-1
Drug Regimens for Acute Exacerbations of Chronic Bronchitis*

Regimen	Cost ($)†
Doxycyline 100 mg b.i.d.‡	8
TMP/SMX one DS tablet b.i.d.‡	4
Amoxicillin-clavulanate (Augmentin) 500 mg/125 mg t.i.d. or 875 mg/125 mg b.i.d.	106 to 120
Azithromycin (Zithromax as Z-pack) 500 mg on first day, then 250 mg per day for 4 days	36
Cefepime (Suprax) 400 mg daily	82
Cefpodoxime proxetil (Vantin) 200 mg b.i.d.	80
Cefprozil (Cefzil) 500 mg b.i.d.	145
Cefuroxime axetil (Ceftin) 250 to 500 mg b.i.d.	77 to 146
Cefibuten (Cedax) 400 mg daily	75
Clarithromycin (Biaxin) 500 mg b.i.d.	80
Loracarbef (Lorabid) 400 mg b.i.d.	120
Levofloxacin (Levaquin) 500 mg daily	85
Ciprofloxacin (Cipro) 500 to 750 mg b.i.d.§	83 to 86
Ofloxacin (Floxin) 400 mg b.i.d.	99

*A 10-day course is recommended for all regimens except azithromycin (5 days).
†Data from 2001 Redbook. Montvale, NJ: Medical Economics Data Production Company; 2001.
‡Least expensive agents.
§I do not recommend for treatment of lower respiratory infections because of inferior activity against *S. pneumoniae* compared with other quinolones.

ease. Similarly, the influenza vaccine reduces the frequency and severity of influenza, a major cause of death in these patients. Enthusiasm for continuous use of amoxicillin or doxycycline during the winter months remains unsupported by clinical trials. Indeed, this practice should be discouraged because it fosters the emergence of drug-resistant strains.

Expected Response

Patients with advanced underlying COPD need close follow-up because of the variable course of exacerbations.

When to Refer

Patients with deteriorating pulmonary function should be hospitalized.

KEY POINTS

ACUTE EXACERBATIONS OF CHRONIC BRONCHITIS
⊃ Most exacerbations of chronic bronchitis are probably caused by viruses or noninfectious causes.

⊃ *S. pneumoniae* and nontypeable strains of *H. influenzae* are the most common bacterial isolates from sputum cultures, but a pathogenic role is usually unclear because these bacteria are frequent colonizers.

⊃ Antibiotics bring about only modest improvement in airflow but are usually given to patients with markedly impaired baseline pulmonary function because of the serious consequences of respiratory failure.

⊃ Antibiotic courses of 5 to 7 days are, in general, as effective as longer courses.

⊃ Amoxicillin-clavulanate (Augmentin) and the newer "respiratory quinolones" (e.g., levofloxacin, moxifloxacin, and gatifloxacin) are now preferred by some authorities over older drugs such as doxycycline, TMP/SMX, and amoxicillin.

⊃ The practice of giving prophylactic antibiotics through the winter months is not supported by rigorous trials and should be discouraged.

⊃ Patients with chronic bronchitis should receive the pneumococcal vaccine and yearly immunization against influenza.

SUGGESTED READING

Adams SG, Melo J, Luther M, et al. Antibiotics are associated with lower relapse rates in outpatients with acute exacerbations of COPD. Chest 2000; 117: 1345-1352.

Grossman RF. Guidelines for the treatment of acute exacerbations of chronic bronchitis. Chest 1997; 112 (6 Suppl): 310S-313S.

Heath JM, Mongia R. Chronic bronchitis: primary care management. Am Fam Phys 1998; 57: 2365-2372, 2376-2378.

Hill AT, Campbell EJ, Hill SL, et al. Association between airway bacterial load and markers of airway inflammation in patients with stable chronic bronchitis. Am J Med 2000; 109: 288-295.

Legnani D. Role of oral antibiotics in treatment of community-acquired lower respiratory tract infections. Diagn Microbiol Infect Dis 1997; 27: 41-47.

Murphy TF, Sethi S, Niederman MS. The role of bacteria in exacerbations of COPD: a constructive view. Chest 2000; 118: 204-209.

Sethi S, Muscarella K, Evans N, et al. Airway inflammation and etiology of acute exacerbations of chronic bronchitis. Chest 2000; 118: 1557-1565.

Snow V, Lascher S, Mottur-Pilson C. Evidence base for management of acute exacerbations of chronic obstructive pulmonary disease. Ann Intern Med 2001; 134: 595-599.

Wilson R, Wilson CB. Defining subsets of patients with chronic bronchitis. Chest 1997; 112 (6 Suppl): 303S-309S.

Bronchiectasis

Bronchiectasis is an acquired disorder characterized anatomically by abnormal dilatation of bronchi and bronchioles and clinically by chronic productive cough and frequent lower respiratory tract infections. Its prevalence fell dramatically after the introduction of broad-spectrum antibiotics and widespread immunization against measles and pertussis. Although bronchiectasis is now uncommon, it often goes undiagnosed until far advanced. Newer imaging studies now enable earlier diagnosis, and understanding of its causes continues to improve.

Presentation and Progression
Cause

Cigarette smoking, the major cause of chronic bronchitis, plays little role in bronchiectasis except for predisposing to recurrent infections. The basic problem in bronchiectasis is permanent structural damage to the walls of bronchi and bronchioles brought about by the concerted action of (1) infection and (2) impairment of the pulmonary toilet, airway obstruction, or a defect in host defenses.

In the past, bronchiectasis was associated especially with frequent or severe lower respiratory infections during childhood. Bronchiectasis continues to be associated with such infections—especially necrotizing pneumonias in which treatment is delayed—but the list of known causes has expanded. Bronchiectasis can be the earliest clue to cystic fibrosis manifesting itself during adolescence or early adulthood. *Mycobacterium avium-intracellulare* complex (MAC) infection is not infrequently associated with bronchiectasis, especially in older women and thin women. Allergic bronchopulmonary aspergillosis often leads to bronchiectasis, which might be prevented by early recognition of this syndrome. Immunodeficiency disorders, both congenital (hypogammaglobulinemia) and acquired (acquired immunodeficiency syndrome), predispose to bronchiectasis. The dyskinetic cilia syndromes are sufficiently common (about 1 in every 20,000 to 60,000 persons) that a case is likely to occur in every medium-sized city. Recent interest centers on a possible association with *Helicobacter pylori,* since patients with bronchiectasis are more likely to be seropositive for this agent than control subjects.

Presentation

Patients with advanced bronchiectasis experience daily cough productive of large amounts of mucopurulent, thick, tenacious sputum. However, most patients produce lesser amounts of sputum, at least during the early stages, and cough may be nonproductive ("dry bronchiectasis") or even absent. Dyspnea and hemoptysis are common. Patients often give a history of repeated respiratory infections and sometimes of recurrent pleuritic chest pain. Hard crackles are heard locally over the lung fields in about 70% of patients. Rhonchi and widespread expiratory wheezes are also common. Clubbing is present in only about 3% of patients. Plain chest radiographs (posteroanterior and lateral views) are usually abnormal.

Diagnosis

In some patients the history, physical findings, and plain chest radiographs are a sufficient basis for a diagnosis of bronchiectasis. In the past, bronchography was used to prove the diagnosis and to classify the disease as cylindrical, cystic, or varicose, depending on the pattern of airway destruction. Ultrasensitive computed tomographic (CT) scanning (either high-resolution or spiral volumetric) is now the procedure of choice for demonstrating bronchial wall thickening and luminal dilatation. When the diagnosis of bronchiectasis has been established, an effort should be made to establish its etiology if the cause remains unclear after close attention to the medical history and the radiographic findings.

Chronic sinus disease and upper airway obstruction should be sought in every case. Routine sputum culture and cultures for fungi and mycobacteria (acid-fast bacillus [AFB] culture) should be obtained. Screening for cystic fibrosis and hypogammaglobulinemia is appropriate if the patient is a child, adolescent, or young adult. Cystic fibrosis is usually diagnosed by means of the sweat chloride test. Some patients, however, have normal sweat chloride levels; in these, screening for mutations in the cystic fibrosis transmembrane conductance regulator gene may be necessary. Young's syndrome exhibits clinical features similar to those of cystic fibrosis but with normal sweat chloride levels. Immunoglobulin levels should probably be measured in most patients. Screening for IgG subclass deficiency is recommended for persons with early onset of diffuse bronchiectasis or those with recurrent infections outside the lung. Diagnosis of IgG subclass deficiency, however, is controversial because the range of IgG subclass levels varies widely among persons who do not have frequent infections. To help decide whether a low level is important, the clinician can (1) measure baseline antibody titers of *H. influenzae* type b and pneumococcal polysaccharide types; (2) give *H. influenzae* and pneumococcal vaccine; and (3) measure the titers 6 weeks later (persons with immunodeficiency will not generate an immune response).

The dyskinetic cilia syndromes can be diagnosed by specialized examination of epithelial samples obtained by nasal or bronchial brush or biopsy. The best-known example is Kartagener's syndrome (bronchiectasis, sinusitis, and situs inversus with dextrocardia), but more subtle variants are now being recognized. Allergic bronchopulmonary aspergillosis can be diagnosed by finding peripheral eosinophilia, high plasma IgE levels, and precipitating and specific antibodies to *Aspergillus*. Isolation of *Aspergillus* species from sputum helps but is not specific.

Natural History
Expected Outcome

Bronchiectasis is a serious disease often associated with deterioration of pulmonary function and complications similar to those of chronic obstructive lung disease. Even before the advanced stages the chronic productive cough greatly interferes with quality of life.

Treatment
Methods

There is no curative treatment other than resection of the diseased portion of the lung. Antibiotics are appropriate during episodes of fever with increased sputum production. Antibiotics should be given in high dose. Bacteria colonizing the airways can produce high levels of β-lactamases (enzymes that destroy β-lactam antibiotics). Although high-dose amoxicillin (e.g., 3 g b.i.d.) has been used in the past, amoxicillin–clavulanic acid (Augmentin) is now a better choice because of its β-lactamase inhibitor component. Treatment should usually be continued for 7 to 14 days. In patients with cystic fibrosis, treatment should be based on results of sputum cultures. Initially sputum cultures of patients with cystic fibrosis usually show *S. aureus* or mucoid strains of *Pseudomonas* species; later these patients tend to acquire *Burkholderia* (formerly *Pseudomonas*) *cepacia,* which is a poor prognostic sign. All patients should receive pneumococcal, *H. influenzae* type b, and yearly influenza vaccines.

When to Refer

Bronchiectasis tends to be a chronic, incurable, and unusually frustrating disease. Most patients benefit from referral to a pulmonary medicine specialist if only for a one-time opinion.

 KEY POINTS

BRONCHIECTASIS

⊃ Bronchiectasis should be suspected in patients with unusually severe, protracted, productive cough. Delayed diagnosis is common.

⊃ High-resolution or spiral volumetric CT scanning allows earlier, noninvasive diagnosis in most cases. Workup should usually include a complete blood count with differential, quantitative immunoglobulin levels (IgG, IgM, and IgA), routine sputum smear and culture, and sputum culture for mycobacteria (AFB culture) and fungi.

⊃ Cystic fibrosis and immunodeficiency should be suspected, especially when bronchiectasis begins in young patients.

⊃ Allergic bronchopulmonary aspergillosis, which commonly leads to bronchiectasis, is manifested as peripheral eosinophilia, elevated plasma IgE levels, and precipitating antibodies to *Aspergillus* species.

SUGGESTED READING

Cockrill BA, Hales CA. Allergic bronchopulmonary aspergillosis. Annu Rev Med 1999; 50: 303-316.

Conlan AA, Kopec SE. Indications for pneumonectomy: pneumonectomy for benign disease. Chest Surgery Clin North Am 1999; 9: 311-326.

De Gracia J, Rodrigo JM, Morell F, et al. IgG subclass deficiencies associated with bronchiectasis. Am J Respir Crit Care Med 1996; 153: 650-655.

Lynch DA. Imaging of asthma and allergic bronchopulmonary mycosis. Radiol Clin North Am 1998; 36: 129-142.

Mysliwiec V, Pina JS. Bronchiectasis: the "other" obstructive lung disease. Postgrad Med 1999; 106: 123-126, 128-131.

Bronchiolitis ("Wheezy Bronchitis"; "Asthmatic Bronchitis")

Bronchiolitis, a common disease of early childhood, is characterized by wheezing (hence the synonyms "wheezy bronchitis" and "asthmatic bronchitis"). It is nearly always caused by a virus, notably the respiratory syncytial virus (RSV). The diagnosis is usually based on clinical findings and observation of the self-limited course, with improvement beginning between the third and seventh days of illness. Antibiotics are not indicated except for the rare patient with bacterial superinfection. Bronchodilators, although often used, are of unclear benefit and may cause complications. Chest radiology, if performed, shows hyperinflation of the lungs and sometimes coexisting pneumonia, especially when RSV is the pathogen. Patients should be observed closely until improvement occurs. Increased work of breathing and hypoxemia are the indications for hospitalization (see Chapter 4 for further discussion).

Acute Community-Acquired Pneumonia: Overview of Diagnosis and Treatment

Pneumonia is an acute infection of the lung parenchyma confirmed by the presence of an infiltrate, detected on a chest radiograph or by physical examination. Lower respiratory symptoms usually predominate, but the majority of patients have other nonspecific symptoms such as headache, fatigue, anorexia, myalgias, or abdominal pain. Primary care physicians must determine whether the problem is pneumonia or something else, whether hospitalization or referral is necessary, what etiology is most likely, whether unusual causes might be present, and what therapy is appropriate. These issues are often far from straightforward.

Pneumonia accounts for an estimated 45,000 deaths in the United States each year. It is the sixth most common cause of death and the most common infectious cause of death. Since it is not a reportable disease, the precise incidence is unknown. Estimates suggest that 4 million cases occur each year, prompting 10 million physician visits and 600,000 to 1.2 million hospitalizations and adding $23 billion to health care costs. Data suggest a 28-fold increased cost for managing the disease on an inpatient basis ($7517 versus $264 for outpatient therapy). However, the mortality rate is 1% or less for outpatients versus 14% to 25% for those admitted to the hospital. Physicians often overestimate the short-term mortality risk, but erring toward hospitalization is understandable given the potentially fatal nature of the disease.

More than any other infectious disease, pneumonia has been the focus for clinical guidelines and algorithms. At least 14 major studies since 1987 have addressed predictors of adverse outcome. Major guidelines have been developed by the ATS, the British Thoracic Society, the Canadian Infectious Diseases Society, and the Infectious Diseases Society of America (IDSA). The IDSA guidelines, unlike the ATS guidelines, attempt to identify low-risk patients for whom outpatient therapy might be appropriate by use of the pneumonia severity index (PSI) prediction rule. Driving the development of these guidelines, at least in part, is the difficulty of making a precise etiologic diagnosis at the time of initial physician contact. The purpose of this section is to develop a framework for diagnosis and management.

Presentation and Progression
Cause

Microorganisms can enter the lungs by aspiration, by inhalation, or by way of the bloodstream (hematogenous pneumonia). Aspiration of bacteria that have colonized the oropharynx is by far the most common mechanism. Most humans aspirate small amounts of oropharyngeal secretions on a nightly basis. Microorganisms that are not removed by the mucociliary blanket are taken up and killed by pulmonary alveolar macrophages, the last line of defense. This process, called pulmonary clearance, is impaired by viral respiratory infections, tobacco smoke, chronic lung disease, alcohol, and many other factors associated with debilitating diseases. One or more chronic diseases are present in the majority of adult patients with pneumonia (58% to 89% of patients in various studies). Alcoholism predisposes to aspiration, but cigarette smoking is the main avoidable risk factor for community-acquired pneumonia in adults.

Inhalation of aerosolized particles is an important route of entry for many viruses, including the influenza viruses and, most recently, the Hantaviruses. Bacteria that cause pneumonia by airborne transmission are *M. tuberculosis, Yersinia pestis* (plague), *Bacillus anthracis* (anthrax), and probably *L. pneumophila* (legionnaire's disease) and *Francisella tularensis* (tularemia). Spore-producing fungi such as *Histoplasma capsulatum, Blastomyces dermatitidis,* and *Coccidioides immitis* also cause inhalation pneumonia.

Hematogenous pneumonia classically develops from septic pulmonary emboli, frequently resulting in patchy or nodular bilateral pulmonary infiltrates sometimes accompanied by pleural effusions. In inner-city populations, a familiar scenario consists of bilateral pneumonia associated with *S. aureus* endocarditis on the tricuspid or pulmonic valves of injecting drug users (see Chapter 3). Another scenario consists of emboli from septic thrombophlebitis, for example, of the pelvic veins (pelvic inflammatory disease, septic abortion; see Chapters 5 and 16), internal jugular vein (Lemierre syndrome; see Chapter 10), or any large vein where a catheter has been inserted (see Chapter 27). Hematogenous seeding of the lungs may explain some pneumonias caused by gram-negative bacteria and by unusually virulent organisms such as *F. tularensis* (tularemia).

The microbial cause of community-acquired pneumonia is usually difficult to determine. In prospective studies of patients requiring hospitalization, a cause is found in only 40% to 70% of cases. In primary care practice a far greater fraction of cases are never diagnosed. Most of these cases respond to empiric therapy. Published data concerning the causes of pneumonia vary among regions, but some generalizations are possible. *M. pneumoniae* is the most common cause in some communities, when presumptive diagnoses were taken into account, followed by *S. pneumoniae* and *C. pneumoniae.* Adults with compromised host defenses are likely to have pneumococcal pneumonia but can also have pneumonia caused by *H. influenzae, M. catarrhalis, S. aureus,* or aerobic gram-negative rods. *S. pneumoniae* is widely agreed to be the most common cause of community-acquired pneumonia requiring hospitalization. An emerging and controversial area concerns the frequency of pneumonia caused by more than one microorganism. In one study a second pathogen was found in about 10% of patients with pneumonia caused by a conventional bacterial pathogen but in 55% of patients in whom an "atypical" pathogen was found.

Presentation

Attack rates are highest at the extremes of life: <4 years or >65 years of age. Symptoms and signs of illness are subtle in the elderly (see Chapter 3). The incidence of pneumonia is greatest in the winter months, largely because of the seasonal increase in viral respiratory tract infections caused by confinement of people indoors.

Before the widespread use of radiology, the term "pneumonia" most often referred to a dramatic illness with high fever, chills, purulent sputum production, and lobar consolidation on physical examination. In 1938 the term "atypical pneumonia" was introduced to describe "an unusual form of tracheobronchopneumonia with severe constitutional symptoms." Later a differentiation between "classic bacterial pneumonia" and "atypical pneumonia" became customary. This distinction was challenged during the 1990s when researchers found these illnesses difficult if not impossible to differentiate on clinical grounds. Some authorities now suggest abandoning the term "atypical pneumonia." Others would keep the term, since it enriches the appreciation of the disease, forces physicians to consider unusual etiologies, and serves as a reminder that the "atypical pneumonias" do not respond to β-lactam antibiotics. For these latter reasons and for the sake of clarity, the terms are used here with the knowledge that in some cases "classic bacterial pneumonia" cannot be distinguished from "atypical pneumonia" in clinical practice (Figure 11-1).

PATIENTS 1 AND 2

A 35-year-old woman sought medical attention for fever and minimally productive cough of several days' duration. Questioning brought out that she had not felt well for about 2 weeks and that two of her four children had upper respiratory symptoms before the onset of her own symptoms. Physical examination revealed her to be in no acute distress with a temperature of 103.2° F (39.6° C), slight erythema of the right tympanic membrane, and a few fine crackles at the left lung base. Her white blood cell (WBC) count was 7800/mm³ with a normal differential. Chest x-ray examination showed an impressive left lower lobe infiltrate (Figure 11-2). She was treated with erythromycin and steadily improved over the next several days. Acute and convalescent serologic tests confirmed *M. pneumoniae* infection.

A 58-year-old man was brought to the hospital by relatives because of fever, confusion, and vague left-sided chest pain. His past medical history was remarkable for alcoholism and moderately heavy smoking. Physical examination revealed him to be confused and dyspneic with a temperature of 102.8° F (102.3° C) and hard crackles over the left lung base. Laboratory findings included a WBC count of 8320/mm3 with a marked shift to the left, arterial Po_2 on room air 52 mm Hg, Pco_2 48 mm Hg, pH 7.31, and mild azotemia. Chest x-ray examination showed an impressive left lower lobe infiltrate (Figure 11-3). The patient was treated initially with vancomycin and ceftriaxone. *S. pneumoniae* was isolated from both blood cultures. He required mechanical ventilation for 33 days and a secondary infection with methicillin-resistant *S. aureus* developed, but eventually he made a full recovery.

Classic bacterial pneumonia begins with sudden onset of fever, chills, pleuritic chest pain, and productive cough. In the absence of impaired consciousness or inebriation, patients usually seek medical care within 6 hours of the onset of symptoms. Chills occur in about 50% and chest pain in about 30% of patients. Most patients are febrile, although some, especially the elderly, have normal or subnormal temperatures. The respiratory rate is usually increased. Physical examination often reveals signs of consolidation such as dullness to percussion, pectoriloquy, and egophony (*e→a* change). Lobar consolidation is present on chest x-ray examination in about one third of patients. The WBC count is usually elevated with a shift to the left. However, leukopenia rather than leukocytosis may be present and portends a poor prognosis.

Atypical pneumonia, in contrast, usually begins gradually. The insidious onset is often brought out when the physician asks, "When was the last time you were in your usual good health?" Constitutional symptoms are usually more prominent than pulmonary symptoms. Chest pain is experienced as substernal discomfort. Cough is nonproductive or produces only scanty amounts of sputum. Relative bradycardia is frequently present. The trachea may be tender, but the lung fields are essentially clear on auscultation, causing the physician to be surprised by the extent of infiltrate visible on the chest radiograph. The WBC count is often normal or near normal. Modest elevation of liver enzyme levels (specifically the aminotransferases—aspartate aminotransferase [AST] and alanine aminotransferase [ALT])—is often present. Atypical pneumonia, in summary, seldom manifests itself as an acute, life-threatening medical problem but forces the physician to expand the differential diagnosis (Table 11-2).

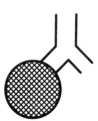

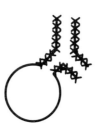

Alveolar inflammation
Peripheral (pleuritic) pain
Copious, purulent sputum
Elevated WBC count with
 shift to the left

Tracheobronchial-interstitial
 inflammation
Central (substernal) pain
Scanty, nonpurulent sputum
Normal WBC count

FIG. 11-1 Classic bacterial pneumonia, best exemplified by *Streptococcus pneumoniae*, primarily involves inflammation of the alveoli. Atypical pneumonia, best exemplified by *Mycoplasma pneumoniae*, primarily involves inflammation of the tracheobronchial mucosa and the interstitium of the lungs. *WBC*, white blood cell.

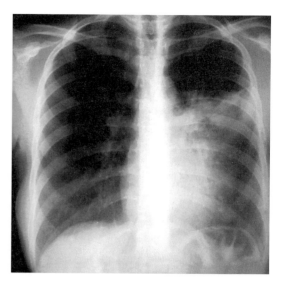

FIG. 11-2 Left lower lobe pneumonia caused by *Mycoplasma pneumoniae* in a 25-year-old woman.

Diagnosis

The diagnosis of acute pneumonia is usually based on the history, physical findings, and chest x-ray examination. Acute pneumonia is distinguished from chronic pneumonia (see later discussion) largely on the basis of the history. The three essential questions are: Is the problem pneumonia or something else? Is the pneumonia severe enough to warrant hospitalization? What is the likely etiology?

Is the Problem Acute Pneumonia or Something Else?

None of the symptoms and signs of pneumonia are specific for the disease. Nonspecific symptoms such as headache, anorexia, nausea, vomiting, myalgias, abdominal pain, and

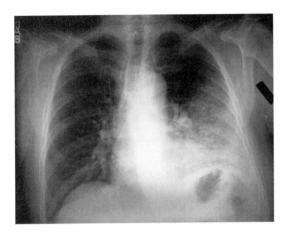

FIG. 11-3 Left lower lobe pneumonia caused by *Streptococcus pneumoniae* in a 58-year-old man.

diarrhea can dominate the clinical picture, suggesting that the primary problem lies elsewhere than in the chest. Signs of pulmonary consolidation are present in less than one third of cases. An abnormal chest radiograph is a *sine qua non* for confident diagnosis of pneumonia. Rarely the initial chest radiograph is normal, but "repeating the chest x-ray after adequate hydration" is not recommended unless new symptoms or physical signs develop. CT using newer methods (e.g., the high-resolution spiral CT method) increases the diagnostic precision but is seldom necessary. The clinician should always keep open the possibility of other disease processes (Box 11-1).

Pulmonary embolism often masquerades as "atypical pneumonia." Sudden onset of dyspnea and pleuritic chest pain in a patient at risk suggests pulmonary embolism, but this condition—like pneumonia—can be exceedingly subtle. Pulmonary embolism sometimes causes significant fever (Allen's sign). When pulmonary embolism is suspected, the patient should be referred for appropriate studies such as spiral CT scanning of the chest (which is sensitive for large, centrally located emboli) or ventilation-perfusion lung scanning (which is sensitive for peripherally located emboli).

Hypersensitivity pneumonitis can be caused by a wide variety of drugs. Nitrofurantoin, which can cause a pleural effusion in addition to pneumonia, is perhaps the most notorious, but other drugs that cause pulmonary reactions include aspirin, phenytoin (Dilantin), and gold salts. These reactions can be either abrupt or gradual in onset and may progress to pulmonary fibrosis if the drug is not discontinued. Many pneumonias are attributed to hypersensitivity pneumonitis caused by thermophilic actinomycetes. Recurrent pneumonia caused by thermophilic actinomycetes, attributed to contaminated air conditioners, has been observed in office workers.

TABLE 11-2
Some Causes of Typical and Atypical Pneumonias in Adults

Frequency	"Typical" pneumonias	"Atypical" pneumonias
Usual	*Streptococcus pneumoniae, Haemophilus influenzae*	*Mycoplasma pneumoniae, Chlamydia pneumoniae*
Less common	*Staphylococcus aureus;* mouth flora bacteria, predominantly anaerobes; aerobic gram-negative rods	*Legionella pneumophila,** influenza A and B viruses,† adenoviruses types 4 and 7,‡ *Pneumocystis carinii* (see Chapter 17),§ *Mycobacterium tuberculosis* (see Chapter 22)
Uncommon or rare	Moraxella catarrhalis,¶ *Streptococcus pyogenes* (group A streptococcus), *Neisseria meningitidis,*‡ enterococci	*Francisella tularensis* (tularemia; see Chapter 9); *Chlamydia psittaci* (psittacosis); *Yersinia pestis* (plague, see Chapter 6); fungi, including regional mycoses (see Chapter 21); rickettsiae (see Chapter 8); parasites (see Chapter 23); miscellaneous viruses (see Chapter 26); Hantavirus pulmonary syndrome (see Chapter 6)

*Legionnaire's disease, which has features of both classic bacterial pneumonia and atypical pneumonia, is common in some but not most geographic areas in the United States.

†Influenza A pneumonia is common during epidemics and pandemics.

‡Adenovirus pneumonia and meningococcal pneumonia are more common in military recruits.

§*Pneumocystis carinii* pneumonia is a common cause of pneumonia in human immunodeficiency virus–positive persons and a classic presenting manifestation of acquired immunodeficiency syndrome.

¶*Moraxella catarrhalis* more commonly causes bronchitis than pneumonia.

BOX 11-1

Conditions That Can Mimic Pneumonia Caused by a Treatable Infection

- Pulmonary thromboembolism—perhaps the most frequent cause of "atypical pneumonia"
- Foreign body aspiration—should be considered in children, the frail elderly, and those with impaired levels of consciousness
- Acute heart failure—can be mistaken for pneumonia, especially when caused by endocarditis or mitral valve disease
- Acute eosinophilic pneumonia—uncommon but, in contrast to chronic eosinophilic pneumonia (Carrington's syndrome), often associated with a normal peripheral eosinophil count
- Hypersensitivity pneumonias caused by a wide variety of drugs and antigens (notably the thermophilic actinomycetes)—can be manifested as chills, fever, cough, dyspnea, and patchy infiltrates
- Connective tissue diseases, especially systemic lupus erythematosus and variants of polyarteritis nodosa—frequently cause pulmonary symptoms with infiltrates
- Pulmonary alveolar proteinosis
- Allergic bronchopulmonary aspergillosis
- Tumors, primary and metastatic—especially choriocarcinoma
- Pulmonary hemorrhage—for example, Goodpasture's syndrome or mitral stenosis

BOX 11-2

Poor Prognostic Factors in Community-Acquired Pneumonia That Should Prompt Consideration of Hospitalization

- Age >65 years
- Chronic underlying diseases such as heart failure, chronic obstructive lung disease, diabetes mellitus, renal failure, malignancy, or a disease requiring immunosuppressive therapy
- Hospitalization within the previous year
- Vital signs suggesting severe sepsis: respiratory rate ≥30 breaths/min, systolic blood pressure <90 mm Hg, diastolic blood pressure <60 mm Hg, or temperature >101° F (38.3° C)
- Altered mental status
- Identified extrapulmonary site of infection
- Multilobar involvement on chest x-ray examination
- Presence of a large pleural effusion on chest x-ray examination
- Presence of a cavitary lesion on chest x-ray examination
- Severe hypoxemia (arterial Pao_2 <60 mm Hg or <90% saturation on pulse oximetry)
- White blood count <4000/mm^3 or >30,000/mm^3
- Renal failure or elevated blood urea nitrogen level
- Hematocrit value <30%
- Infection caused by *Streptococcus pneumoniae*, *Staphylococcus aureus*, or *Legionella pneumophila*

Bronchiolitis obliterans organizing pneumonia should be considered in the differential diagnosis of a subacute interstitial pneumonia with cough, dyspnea, fever, malaise, weight loss, and failure to respond to antibiotics. Diagnosis generally requires open lung biopsy. When this syndrome is suspected, patients should usually be referred to a specialist in pulmonary medicine.

Idiopathic acute eosinophilic pneumonia is an uncommon problem characterized by abrupt onset, high fever, and bilateral pulmonary infiltrates. Respiratory failure with severe hypoxemia is common. In contrast to chronic eosinophilic pneumonia (Carrington's syndrome), peripheral blood eosinophilia is usually absent. The diagnosis is usually made by demonstrating eosinophilia in fluid obtained by bronchoalveolar lavage or in transbronchial lung biopsy specimens. Treatment with corticosteroids usually results in dramatic recovery.

Chronic pneumonia is discussed more fully later in the chapter.

Is the Pneumonia Severe?

At the time of initial presentation, determining the severity of pneumonia is more important to management than making an accurate etiologic diagnosis. About 10% of cases of acute community-acquired pneumonia are sufficiently severe to warrant hospitalization (Box 11-2). In recent years the definition of "severe" community-acquired pneumonia has attracted a great deal of interest. Less emphasis has been placed on the definition of "mild" community-acquired pneumonia. Advanced age and underlying diseases greatly enhance the severity of the infection. Leukopenia is a poor prognostic sign in bacterial pneumonia. The combination of alcoholism, leukopenia, and pneumococcal sepsis is known as the ALPS syndrome, but this finding is not specific for pneumococcal disease. Fingertip pulse oximetry will probably prove to be a useful adjunct for assessing the severity of pneumonia in ambulatory settings.

What Is the Etiology?

In many cases the history, physical examination, sputum Gram stain, chest radiograph, and other laboratory studies point toward one or another specific etiology (Tables 11-3 to 11-5). In clinical practice the etiology is unclear more often than not. Newer diagnostic tests using molecular techniques could improve this unfortunate situation. In one study, for example, evaluating a single throat swab specimen by the polymerase chain reaction (PCR) was 88% sensitive and 100% specific for diagnosing causative agents later established by another method. In the meantime most cases of pneumonia are managed on a presumptive basis.

Researchers propose that the etiology of pneumonia is "definite" when a pathogen is isolated from a sterile site (blood, pleural fluid, or cerebrospinal fluid [CSF]) or if a pathogen that is not ordinarily a colonizer of the respiratory tract is identified in sputum specimens (e.g., *M. tuberculosis*, *L. pneumophila*, and *Pneumocystis carinii*). The etiology is "probable" if sputum culture showing a heavy or predominant growth of a pathogen correlates with findings on Gram stain. Serologic studies have varying degrees of specificity depending on the organism, the test, and the diagnostic criteria.

The value of the sputum Gram stain and culture has been debated for many years. The ATS guidelines downplay sputum evaluation, whereas the IDSA guidelines hold examination of the Gram stain to be "desirable" for outpatients and essential for seriously ill patients. Up to 30% of patients cannot produce sputum. Another 15% to 30% of patients have received antibiotics before evaluation, and in 35% to 65% the sputum Gram stain is unhelpful. However, Gram stains can be useful in at least three ways. First, Gram stains can suggest a specific etiology such as *S. pneumoniae* (Figure 11-4) or *H. influenzae* (Figure 11-5). When evaluated by an experienced practitioner, Gram stains are up to 85% specific for *S. pneumoniae* (although only 62% sensi-

TABLE 11-3
Clues to the Etiology of Pneumonia from the History and Physical Examination

Finding	Suggested pathogens
HISTORY	
Onset sudden or gradual	Sudden onset suggests acute bacterial pneumonia; gradual onset suggests "atypical" pneumonia (see text)
Family history of respiratory illness	*Mycoplasma pneumoniae;* respiratory syncytial virus; influenza
Chronic obstructive lung disease	*Streptococcus pneumoniae; Haemophilus influenzae; Moraxella catarrhalis*
Nursing home resident or recent hospitalization	*S. pneumoniae; H. influenzae;* aerobic gram-negative rods; respiratory syncytial virus
Alcoholism	*S. pneumoniae;* gram-negative rods (notably *Klebsiella pneumoniae);* mixed anaerobes ("mouth flora"); *Mycobacterium tuberculosis*
Altered mental status; seizures; alcoholism; recent dental manipulation	"Mouth flora aspiration pneumonia" (mixed anaerobic and aerobic bacteria); *S. pneumoniae*
Homelessness or incarceration	*S. pneumoniae; M. tuberculosis*
Injecting drug use	*Staphylococcus aureus; S. pneumoniae;* consider septic emboli from right-sided endocarditis
Home use of small-volume nebulizers	*Pseudomonas aeruginosa;* other aerobic gram-negative rods
Recent influenza A or B	*S. pneumoniae; S. aureus; Streptococcus pyogenes*
Diabetic ketoacidosis	*S. pneumoniae; S. aureus*
Exposure to small children	*M. pneumoniae*
Exposure to contaminated aerosols (showers, air coolers, water supplies)	*Legionella pneumophila* (legionnaire's disease)
Cystic fibrosis	*P. aeruginosa; S. aureus; Burkholderia cepacia*
History of splenectomy	*S. pneumoniae; H. influenzae* (see Chapters 3 and 6)
B-lymphocyte disorder (multiple myeloma, agammaglobulinemia, chronic lymphocytic leukemia)	*S. pneumoniae*
Sickle cell anemia	*S. pneumoniae*
Exposure to birds (parakeets, cockatoos, budgerigars)	*Chlamydia psittaci* (psittacosis)
Exposure to cats, cows, sheep, goats	*Coxiella burnettii* (Q fever)
Exposure to tissues or body fluids of rabbits, foxes, or squirrels	*Francisella tularensis* (tularemia; see Chapter 8)
Exposure to raw wool, goat hair, animal hides, cattle, pigs, horses	*Bacillus anthracis* (anthrax; see Chapter 6)
Exposure to ground squirrels, rats, chipmunks, prairie dogs	*Yersinia pestis* (plague; see Chapter 6)
Exposure to rodent droppings, urine, or saliva; exploring in the "Four Corners" area of the southwestern United States	Hantavirus pulmonary syndrome (see Chapter 6)

Continued

TABLE 11-3—cont'd
Clues to the Etiology of Pneumonia from the History and Physical Examination

Finding	Suggested pathogens
Exposure to water contaminated with animal urine, or to wild rodents, dogs, cattle, pigs, or horses	Leptospirosis (see Chapter 7)
Military recruit	*Neisseria meningitidis;* adenovirus type 4 or 7
Travel to southwestern United States or southern California, especially if exposed to a windstorm	*Coccidioides immitis* (coccidioidomycosis; see Chapter 21)
Travel to Ohio or Mississippi river valleys; exposure to bat droppings or dust from soil enriched by bird droppings; exploration of a cave	*Histoplasma capsulatum* (histoplasmosis; see Chapter 21)
Travel to Southeast Asia, West Indies, Australia, Guam, or South or Central America	*Burkholderia pseudomallei* (melioidosis)
Weight loss	Tuberculosis (see Chapter 22); postobstructive pneumonia behind endobronchial carcinoma
Associated acute arthritis	Drug reaction or connective tissue disease
Pulmonary alveolar proteinosis	*Nocardia* species (nocardiosis)
PHYSICAL EXAMINATION	
Altered mental status	Associated meningitis; tuberculosis; fungal disease; legionnaire's disease; endocarditis
Poor oral hygiene with foul odor to breath	"Mouth flora" aspiration pneumonia (mixed anaerobic/aerobic bacteria)
Bullous myringitis	*M. pneumoniae*
Relative bradycardia	Viral infection, tularemia, *M. pneumoniae;* legionnaire's disease
Skin lesions	Atypical measles, varicella-zoster, fungal pneumonia, nocardiosis, staphylococcal pneumonia with bacteremia
Furuncles	*S. aureus*
Erythema multiforme	*M. pneumoniae*
Erythema nodosum	Histoplasmosis, coccidioidomycosis, tuberculosis
Ecthyma gangrenosum	*P. aeruginosa; S. aureus*
Relatively clear lung fields on physical examination despite impressive infiltrates on chest x-ray examination	Agents of "atypical" pneumonia (Table 11-2)
Splenomegaly	Psittacosis, typhoid fever, brucellosis, endocarditis

TABLE 11-4
Implications of Some Chest X-Ray Findings in Pneumonia

Finding	Implications
X-ray film more impressive than physical examination would suggest	Atypical pneumonia (especially *Mycoplasma pneumoniae* pneumonia); pulmonary embolism
Patchy bilateral infiltrates	Right-sided endocarditis; septic embolism; atypical pneumonia (especially tularemia)
Multilobar consolidation	Hospitalization should be strongly considered
Bilateral lower lobe involvement	Thromboembolism or septic embolism; chronic aspiration; *M. pneumoniae* pneumonia
Volume loss	Tuberculosis; carcinoma
Miliary pattern	Tuberculosis; histoplasmosis; coccidioidomycosis; bacterial sepsis
Pulmonary nodules	Fungal infection (especially cryptococcosis); septic pulmonary embolism; *Legionella micdadei* pneumonia
Cavitary lesions	Aspiration pneumonia*; gram-negative pneumonia; rarely, tuberculosis, cavitary carcinoma
Massive pleural effusion	*Streptococcus pyogenes* (group A streptococcus)
Hilar lymphadenopathy	Tuberculosis; pertussis; inhalational anthrax; tularemia; pneumonic plague; carcinoma
Clear chest x-ray film despite suspicion of pneumonia	Experimental work and anecdotal reports support the notion that occasional patients with pneumonia have normal chest radiographs because of dehydration

*Aspiration pneumonia typically occurs in the superior (or apical) segment of the lower lobe if the patient aspirates while lying on the back, or in the posterior segment of the upper lobe if the patient aspirates while lying on one side.

tive) and are sometimes virtually diagnostic of *H. influenzae* (although only 40% to 80% sensitive). Second, Gram stains help exclude possible etiologies that might require unique therapies: for example, *S. aureus* (Figure 11-6) and aerobic gram-negative rods (Figure 11-7). Finally, the presence of purulent sputum—defined as the presence of >25 leukocytes and <10 epithelial cells per low-power field—indicates that a culture should be performed.

Blood cultures are recommended for patients who are sufficiently ill to require hospitalization. Overall, blood cultures are positive in up to 20% of patients with bacterial pneumonias and up to 11% of all severe community-acquired pneumonias. A new test for pneumococcal antigen in urine (Binax, Portland, Maine) is sensitive (up to 89% according to the manufacturer; in a recent study the sensitivity and specificity were both >95%) for patients with bacteremic pneumococcal pneumonia, but its utility in milder cases is not well defined. Soluble *L. pneumophila* antigen can be found in the urine in up to 80% of patients with *Legionella* infections caused by serogroup 1 (which accounts for about 80% of *Legionella* infections) and is probably 100% specific for this entity. Newer serologic methods have been developed for diagnosis of *Legionella* species, *M. pneumoniae*, *C. pneumoniae*, and

Coxiella burnettii. Unfortunately, these tests are not completely standardized.

For patients with severe pneumonia, several methods of diagnosis can be used in the hospital setting. Transtracheal (or translaryngeal) aspiration is no longer used because of the risk of uncontrollable hemorrhage. Direct lung puncture is occasionally used but carries the obvious risk of pneumothorax. Fiberoptic bronchoscopy to obtain samples using bronchoalveolar lavage or a protected specimen brush is a promising although invasive way to make a precise etiologic diagnosis. Open lung biopsy is sometimes used, especially in cases of chronic pneumonia or when unusual pathogens are suspected, as in severely immunocompromised patients.

Natural History
Expected Outcome
Patients who are well enough to be treated on an outpatient basis (a condition often called "walking pneumonia" by laypersons) generally recover (<1% mortality rate in some series). Hospitalized patients have a more serious prognosis. In the preantibiotic era, pneumonia and tuberculosis were commonly known as "captains of the men of death."

TABLE 11-5
Some Noninvasive Tests for the Diagnosis of Community-Acquired Pneumonia

Test	Merits	Drawbacks
Chest x-ray examination	Helps distinguish pneumonia from bronchitis; useful in determining severity and may point to one or another etiology (Table 11-4)	Unavailable in many offices; cost
Sputum Gram stain	Provides quick assessment of whether sputum is purulent and may point to one or another etiology; absence of gram-positive cocci in clumps and gram-negative rods has therapeutic implications	Many patients cannot produce sputum or have been previously treated with antibiotics; specimens often unsatisfactory; some microorganisms stain poorly if at all; interpretation subject to observer variability and bias
Sputum culture	Suggests one or another etiology and enables susceptibility testing to be carried out	Requires 24 to 48 hours to interpret, which can be difficult because of contaminating oropharyngeal flora
Blood culture	Isolation of *Streptococcus pneumoniae, Haemophilus influenzae, Staphylococcus aureus,* and gram-negative rods such as *Klebsiella pneumoniae* has high specificity	Low sensitivity (about 11% overall and ≤20% in patients with purulent sputum)
Streptococcus pneumoniae urinary antigen	High specificity	Unknown sensitivity for nonbacteremic disease
Legionella pneumophila urinary antigen	High specificity	Identifies only *Legionella pneumophila* serogroup 1 (which causes about 80% of cases of legionnaire's disease)
IgM serologic tests	Sometimes helpful in the diagnosis of *Legionella, Mycoplasma pneumoniae,* and *Chlamydia pneumoniae* pneumonias	Specificity largely unknown
IgG serologic tests	Provide a retrospective diagnosis in many cases; sensitivity and specificity better defined than with IgM serologic tests	Results usually not available for several weeks; nontuberculous mycobacteria (which may be contaminants) are being isolated more frequently than *M. tuberculosis* at many centers
Cold agglutinins	When present in high titer, heighten suspicion of *M. pneumoniae* and suggest severe disease caused by this pathogen	Nonspecific
Acid-fast stain	Offers rapid way to recognize mycobacteria, including *Mycobacterium tuberculosis*	Results usually not available for several weeks; nontuberculous mycobacteria (which may be contaminants) are being isolated more frequently than *M. tuberculosis* in some centers
Influenza antigen detection	Offers rapid way to diagnose influenza with high specificity, which is useful in deciding on isolation precautions	Test not universally available; positive result does not exclude possibility of a secondary pathogen
Respiratory syncytial virus antigen	Rapid, with high specificity	Test not universally available; pretest probability low except in children and the frail elderly
Cryptococcal antigen	High specificity	Low pretest probability except in immunocompromised persons with diffuse infiltrates

TABLE 11-5—cont'd
Some Noninvasive Tests for the Diagnosis of Community-Acquired Pneumonia

Test	Merits	Drawbacks
Histoplasma urinary antigen	High specificity	Low pretest probability except in highly endemic areas
Polymerase chain reaction for *M. pneumoniae, C. pneumoniae, S. pneumoniae,* and *Legionella* species	Potentially a rapid and accurate method of diagnosis	Sensitivity and specificity unknown at this time; minuscule amounts of contaminating DNA can cause false-positive result

Modified from Plouffe JE, McNally C, File TM Jr. Value of noninvasive studies in community-acquired pneumonia. Infect Dis Clin North Am 1998; 12: 689-699.

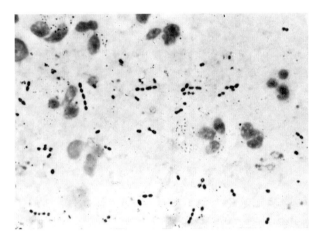

FIG. 11-4 Sputum Gram stain from a patient with bacteremic pneumococcal pneumonia. Note the presence not only of diplococci but also of short chains of gram-positive cocci. A rule of thumb is that the chains formed by *Streptococcus pneumoniae* rarely contain more than six individual cells.

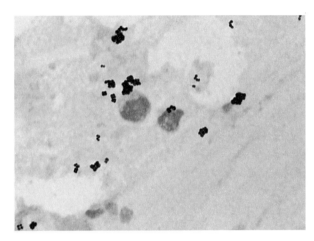

FIG. 11-6 Gram-positive cocci in clumps associated with polymorphonuclear leukocytes in a sputum Gram stain suggests *Staphylococcus aureus* as the cause of pneumonia.

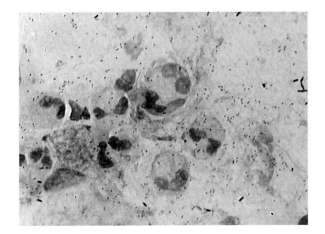

FIG. 11-5 The finding in a sputum Gram stain of tiny, pleomorphic gram-negative coccobacilli associated with polymorphonuclear neutrophils is virtually diagnostic of *Haemophilus influenzae* infection.

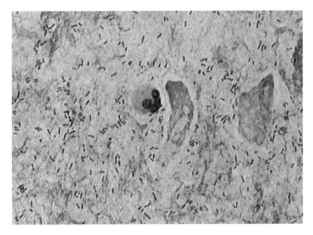

FIG. 11-7 Swarms of gram-negative bacilli in a sputum Gram stain in a patient with pneumonia caused by *Pseudomonas aeruginosa.*

TABLE 11-6
Activity of Antibiotics Against the More Common Causes of Community-Acquired Pneumonia

Antibiotic	Streptococcus pneumoniae*	Haemophilus influenzae	Moraxella catarrhalis	Mycoplasma pneumoniae	Chlamydia pneumoniae	Legionella pneumophila
β-LACTAMS						
Amoxicillin-clavulanate	+	+	+	−	−	−
Ampicillin-sulbactam	+	+	+	−	−	−
Cefotaxime or ceftriaxone	+	+	+	−	−	−
Macrolides						
Erythromycin	+	±	+	+	+	+
Clarithromycin	+	±	+	+	+	+
Azithromycin	+	+	+	+	+	+
"RESPIRATORY QUINOLONES"						
Levofloxacin	+	+	+	+	+	+
Moxifloxacin	+	+	+	+	+	+
Gatifloxacin	+	+	+	+	+	+
Gemifloxacin	+	+	+	+	+	+
OTHER AGENTS						
Doxycycline	−	±	−	+	+	+
TMP/SMX	±	+	+	−	−	−
Linezolid	+	−	−	−	−	−

TMP/SMX, Trimethoprim-sulfamethoxazole.
*The most active agents against *S. pneumoniae* strains with markedly reduced susceptibility to penicillin G (minimum inhibitory concentration >2 μg/mL) are vancomycin and the "respiratory quinolones." TMP/SMX, imipenem, and the first- and second-generation cephalosporins are unreliable against such strains, and the activity of third-generation cephalosporins (such as ceftriaxone and cefotaxime) may be marginal. The role of linezolid in the treatment of community-acquired pneumonia remains to be determined.

Treatment
Methods

The clinician must address three issues: where to treat, how to treat, and how long to treat. Indications for hospitalization are discussed later in this section ("When to Refer").

Guidelines for antibiotic therapy of pneumonia continue to evolve. The relative roles of the newer "respiratory quinolones" (e.g., levofloxacin, moxifloxacin, gatifloxacin, and gemifloxacin), the macrolides, and the traditional β-lactam antibiotics (e.g., cefotaxime or ceftriaxone) are much debated. In my opinion the "respiratory quinolones" are entirely appropriate for mild to moderately severe pneumonia treated on an outpatient basis. The advantage of the quinolones is their coverage not only of the classic bacterial pathogens, but also of the atypical pathogens causing pneumonia (Table 11-6). The macro-lides are, in general, also broadly active against atypical pathogens. However, the newer "respiratory quinolones" are superior to the macrolides against *S. pneumoniae* strains with reduced susceptibility to penicillin, and *S. pneumoniae* strains resistant to the macrolides are increasing in prevalence. For patients with pneumonia not requiring hospitalization, optimum choice of antibiotics depends to some extent on modifying circumstances (Table 11-7). For a patient with severe community-acquired pneumonia requiring hospitalization (Box 11-3), a current approach is to use both a β-lactam antibiotic and a second drug to cover the "atypical" pathogens. Whether the second drug should be a macrolide or a quinolone is much debated. A current consensus favors the macrolides for this purpose, partly to help slow the emergence of resistance of *S. pneumoniae* to the quinolones.

TABLE 11-7
Some Recommendations for Empiric Therapy for Adult Patients with Community-Acquired Pneumonia in Whom Initial Studies Are Nondiagnostic and in Whom Hospitalization Is Not Considered Indicated*

Host condition	Likely pathogens	Therapy (in order of preference)†
Healthy adult <60 years of age	*Streptococcus pneumoniae, Mycoplasma pneumoniae, Chlamydia pneumoniae, Haemophilus influenzae*	1 and 2. Macrolide (erythromycin, azithromycin, or clarithromycin) *or* respiratory quinolone (e.g., levofloxacin, moxifloxacin, or gatifloxacin)‡ 3. Doxycycline
Underlying disease (e.g., chronic obstructive lung disease, heart failure, neoplasm); no risk factors for penicillin-resistant *S. pneumoniae*	*S. pneumoniae, M. pneumoniae, C. pneumoniae, H. influenzae, Moraxella catarrhalis*	As above; consider an initial dose of ceftriaxone
Underlying disease; risk factors for penicillin-resistant *S. pneumoniae*	*S. pneumoniae, M. pneumoniae, C. pneumoniae, H. influenzae, M. catarrhalis*	Respiratory quinolone (e.g., levofloxacin, moxifloxacin, or gatifloxacin); consider an initial dose of ceftriaxone
Underlying disease; aspiration considered likely	*S. pneumoniae, M. pneumoniae, C. pneumoniae, H. influenzae, M. catarrhalis,* "mouth flora" (mixed aerobic and anaerobic bacteria)	Amoxicillin-clavulanate

*When hospitalization is indicated (see text), the initial drug therapy varies somewhat according to the pathogens suspected. Either ceftriaxone 2 g IV or levofloxacin 500 mg IV is appropriate for most patients. Combining ceftriaxone with either a macrolide or a respiratory quinolone is often appropriate to cover both "typical" and "atypical" pathogens. If "mouth flora" aspiration pneumonia is suspected, clindamycin 600 to 900 mg IV or ampicillin-sulbactam (Unasyn) would be appropriate. If penicillin-resistant *S. pneumoniae* or oxacillin-resistant *Staphylococcus aureus* is suspected, vancomycin 1 g should be given initially.

†Representative doses for oral regimens for adult patients: erythromycin 500 mg q.i.d.; azithromycin 500 mg on first day, then 250 mg daily for 4 days; clarithromycin 500 mg b.i.d.; levofloxacin 500 mg daily; doxycycline 100 mg b.i.d.; amoxicillin-clavulanate 875 mg/125 mg b.i.d. or 500 mg/125 mg t.i.d.

‡Whether a macrolide or a "respiratory quinolone" should be the drug of first choice for community-acquired pneumonia in healthy adults is controversial. The literature should be watched.

BOX 11-3
Consensus Definition of Severe Community-Acquired Pneumonia (American Thoracic Society)

Respiratory rate >30 breaths/min
Severe respiratory failure defined by PAO_2/FIO_2 ratio <250 mm Hg or by PO_2 <60 mm Hg
Requirement for mechanical ventilation
Chest x-ray film showing bilateral involvement or involvement of multiple lobes; in addition, a ≥50% increase in the size of the opacity within 48 hours of admission indicates severe pneumonia
Shock (systolic blood pressure <90 mm Hg or diastolic blood pressure <60 mm Hg)
Requirement for vasopressors for >4 hours
Urine output <20 mL/hr or total urine output <80 mL in 4 hours unless another explanation is available, or acute renal failure requiring dialysis
Altered mental status

Modified from American Thoracic Society. Guidelines for the initial management of adults with community-acquired pneumonia: diagnosis, assessment of severity and initial antimicrobial therapy. Am Rev Respir Dis 1993; 148: 1418-1426.

Historically, pneumococcal pneumonia has been treated with penicillin G or other β-lactam antibiotics. The usual causes of "atypical" pneumonia—*M. pneumoniae, C. pneumoniae,* and *L. pneumophila*—do not respond to β-lactam antibiotic therapy but generally respond to tetracyclines, macrolides, or quinolones. Whether these drugs shorten the duration of illness in pneumonia caused by *M. pneumoniae* or *C. pneumoniae* is controversial. In some studies patients with such atypical pneumonias usually made full recoveries even when they did not receive an "appropriate" drug.

A relatively new approach to management of pneumonia is to stratify patients according to the severity of illness. To this end a pneumonia severity index has been developed (Tables 11-8 and 11-9 and Figure 11-8) based on a multicenter study of 14,199 adults who were hospitalized for pneumonia. Points are assigned on the basis of age, underlying diseases, and clinical findings at the time of diagnosis. On the basis of the total number of points (from Table 11-8), patients are assigned to one of five risk classes and the place of treatment is chosen accordingly (Table 11-9). Studies designed to validate this approach to the management of pneumonia are now being carried out and reported in the literature. Many moderately ill patients (especially in class III) seem to benefit

TABLE 11-8
Pneumonia Severity Index: Risk Factors and Assigned Points

Category	Risk factors	Assigned points
Demography	Age for men Age for women Nursing home resident	Age (years) Age (years) − 10 +10
Coexisting illnesses	Neoplastic disease (active) Chronic liver disease Congestive heart failure Cerebrovascular disease Chronic renal disease	+30 +20 +10 +10 +10
Physical examination	Altered mental status* Respiratory rate ≥30 breaths/min Systolic blood pressure <90 mm Hg Temperature <95° F (35° C) or ≥104° F (40° C) Pulse ≥125 beats/min	+20 +20 +20 +15 +10
Laboratory	Arterial pH <7.35 Blood urea nitrogen ≥30 mg/dL Serum sodium <130 mmol/L Glucose ≥250 mg/dL Hematocrit <30% Arterial Pao_2 <60 mm Hg or oxygen saturation <90% on pulse oximetry Pleural effusion on chest x-ray film	+30 +20 +20 +10 +10 +10 +10
Total points		Sum of the above

Modified from Fine MJ, Auble TE, Yealy DM, et al. A prediction rule to identify low-risk patients with community-acquired pneumonia. N Engl J Med 1997; 336: 243-250.

*In patients with altered mental status, coexisting meningitis should be considered (see Chapter 6).

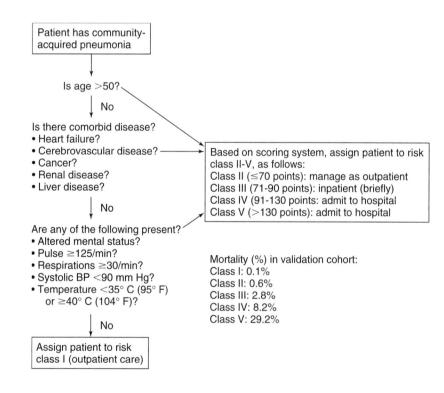

FIG. 11-8 Use of the pneumonia severity index (Tables 11-8 and 11-9) as a guide to management strategies. Note the correlation of mortality with the severity index. (Modified from Fine MJ, Auble TE, Yealy DM, et al. A prediction rule to identify low-risk patients with community-acquired pneumonia. N Engl J Med 1997; 336: 243-250.)

TABLE 11-9
Application of the Pneumonia Severity Index

Risk class	Number of points	Mortality (%)	Implications
I	See footnote*	0.1	Treat on outpatient basis, usually without seeking to determine the etiology.
II	≤70	0.6	Consider treating on an outpatient basis, usually without seeking to determine the etiology.
III	71-90	0.9	A brief period of inpatient observation is usually warranted.
IV	91-130	9.3	The patient should be admitted to the hospital.
V	>130	27.0	The patient should be admitted to the hospital and often to an intensive care unit.

Modified from Fine MJ, Auble TE, Yealy DM, et al. A prediction rule to identify low-risk patients with community-acquired pneumonia. N Engl J Med 1997; 336: 243-250.
*Patients in class I were defined by age <40 years and none of the risk factors shown in Table 11-8.

from a brief hospitalization. Determination of the pneumonia severity index is admittedly cumbersome and probably unnecessary in most instances provided the underlying principles are well understood (Figure 11-8).

For uncomplicated pneumonia in a patient under age 60 who does not have underlying disease, options for treatment include a macrolide (erythromycin, clarithromycin, or azithromycin), a "respiratory quinolone," or a β-lactam antibiotic. Recent data suggest decreasing susceptibility of *S. pneumoniae* not only to penicillin G but also to the macrolides. The "respiratory quinolones" have become popular agents for treating community-acquired pneumonia, but opinions vary about their appropriateness for most patients. Whether quinolones give adequate tissue penetration has been questioned, and the emerging resistance of *S. pneumoniae* to the quinolones is also a concern. A Therapeutic Working Group on the problem of drug-resistant *S. pneumoniae* recommended that the quinolones be limited to adult patients who (1) have failed to respond to treatment with another agent; (2) are allergic to other agents; or (3) have documented infection caused by *S. pneumoniae* strains that are highly resistant to penicillin G (minimum inhibitory concentration [MIC] ≥4 μg/mL). Primary care clinicians should strive to stay abreast of changing opinions on the relative role of the quinolones versus other agents for primary treatment of community-acquired pneumonia. For uncomplicated pneumonia in a patient over age 60 or with underlying disease, a penicillin or cephalosporin is recommended, with quinolones and macrolides reserved for penicillin-allergic patients. The duration of treatment, as in most infectious diseases, is arbitrary. Most authorities advise 10 to 14 days of antibiotic therapy.

Expected Response

With a few exceptions (e.g., bacteremic pneumococcal pneumonia; see later discussion), appropriate antibiotic therapy brings clinical improvement within 48 to 72 hours. The chest radiograph usually returns to normal within 4 weeks. In elderly patients and those with underlying lung disease, complete radiographic resolution may take 10 weeks or longer.

BOX 11-4
Steps to Take if the Patient Fails to Improve Within 48 to 72 Hours

- Review the diagnosis. Could the problem be something other than pneumonia?
- Review the history and physical findings. Has a clue to a specific cause been overlooked? Is evidence of extrapulmonary infection such as empyema present?
- Consider pathogens that are not being covered by the initial drug regimen, especially those associated with "atypical" pneumonia (e.g., *Pneumocystis carinii, Mycobacterium tuberculosis*), viruses, or drug-resistant microorganisms.
- Consider bronchoscopy to evaluate the possibility of airway obstruction and to obtain samples for microbiologic and cytologic diagnosis.

Failure of the host's defense mechanisms, rather than failure of antibiotics, is the most common reason for failure to improve. However, a number of specific steps should be undertaken if the patient fails to improve within 72 hours (Box 11-4). Bronchoscopy may provide useful information in about 40% of cases. Drug fever is always a possibility, but drug reaction is unlikely to account for the failure of fever to resolve within this time frame. Repeating the sputum culture is usually unhelpful after antibiotics have been started.

The diagnosis and treatment of acute community-acquired pneumonia are summarized in Box 11-5.

When to Refer

Patients with severe illness (Box 11-3 and Tables 11-8 and 11-9) should usually be hospitalized. Primary care physicians face mounting pressure to treat more cases of pneumonia on an outpatient basis. However, pneumonia is always a potentially life-threatening disease. When in doubt, admission to the hospital is usually the best course.

BOX 11-5
Diagnosis and Treatment of Acute Community-Acquired Pneumonia

- Diagnosis of acute community-acquired pneumonia is based on the history, physical examination, and chest x-ray examination.
- Other diagnostic possibilities such as pulmonary embolism, endocarditis, and causes of chronic pulmonary infiltrates should be considered.
- The decision whether to admit the patient to the hospital should be based on whether the patient's host defenses are compromised and on whether the pneumonia is severe.
- Classifying pneumonia as "severe" or "nonsevere" is more useful than trying to determine the precise cause.
- Differentiation between "classic bacterial pneumonia" and "atypical pneumonia" is frequently difficult or impossible on clinical grounds. Retaining these concepts is useful, if only for a reminder that the "atypical" pathogens do not respond to β-lactam antibiotics. Clinical findings that sometimes suggest "atypical" pathogens include headache, myalgias, relative bradycardia, and abnormal liver function tests.
- In community practice, atypical pneumonia is caused mainly by *Mycoplasma pneumoniae, Chlamydia pneumoniae,* and (in some but not all localities) *Legionella* species. Unfortunately, there are no rapid, widely available, and accurate tests for diagnosis.
- Mixed infections may be relatively common, hence the rationale for providing antimicrobial coverage for both "classic bacterial" and "atypical" pathogens in severe cases. Such broad coverage consists of a cell wall–active agent (penicillin, cephalosporin, or vancomycin) plus an agent such as a macrolide, quinolone, or tetracycline.
- PCR is a promising test for diagnosis of the agents of atypical pneumonia: *M. pneumoniae, C. pneumoniae,* and *Legionella pneumophila.*
- Efficacy of drug treatment for *M. pneumoniae* is arguable.
- Overuse of quinolones as monotherapy may promote the emergence of resistance.

SUGGESTED READING

Bartlett JG, Dowell SF, Mandell LA, et al. Practice guidelines for the management of community-acquired pneumonia in adults. Clin Infect Dis 2000; 31: 347-382.

Fang GD, Fine M, Orloff J. New and emerging etiologies for community-acquired pneumonia with implications for therapy: a prospective multicenter study of 359 cases. Medicine 1990; 69: 307-316.

Farr BM, Woodhead MA, Macfarlane JT, et al. Risk factors for community-acquired pneumonia diagnosed by general practitioners in the community. Respir Med 2000; 94: 422-427.

Fine MJ, Auble TE, Yealy DM, et al. A prediction rule to identify low-risk patients with community-acquired pneumonia. N Engl J Med 1997; 336: 243-250.

Fine MJ, Stone RA, Singer DE, et al. Processes and outcomes of care for patients with community-acquired pneumonia: results from the Pneumonia Patient Outcomes Research Team (PORT) cohort study. Arch Intern Med 1999; 159: 970-980.

Gleckman R, DeVita J, Hibert D, et al. Sputum Gram stain assessment in community-acquired bacteremic pneumonia. J Clin Microbiol 1988; 26: 846-849.

Heffelfinger JD, Dowell SF, Jorgensen JH, et al. Management of community-acquired pneumonia in the era of pneumococcal resistance: a report from the Drug-Resistant *Streptococcus pneumoniae* Therapeutic Working Group. Arch Intern Med 2000; 160: 1399-1408.

Hyde TB, Gay K, Stephens DS, et al. Macrolide resistance among invasive *Streptococcus pneumoniae* isolates. JAMA 2001; 286: 1857-1862.

Kelley MA, Weber DJ, Gilligan P, et al. Breakthrough pneumococcal bacteremia in patients being treated with azithromycin and clarithromycin. Clin Infect Dis 2000; 31: 1008-1111.

Marrie TJ, Lau CY, Wheeler SL, et al. CAPITAL Study Investigators. Community-Acquired Pneumonia Intervention Trial Assessing Levofloxacin: a controlled trial of a critical pathway for treatment of community-acquired pneumonia. JAMA 2000; 283: 749-755.

Mundy LM, Oldach D, Auwaerter PG, et al. Hopkins CAP Team. Implications for macrolide treatment in community-acquired pneumonia. Chest 1998; 113: 1201-1206.

Nathwani D, Rubinstein E, Barlow G, et al. Do guidelines for community-acquired pneumonia improve the cost-effectiveness of hospital care? Clin Infect Dis 2001; 32: 728-741.

Pope-Harman AL, Davis WD, Allen ED, et al. Acute eosinophilic pneumonia: a summary of 15 cases and review of the literature. Medicine 1996; 75: 334-342.

Ramirez JA, Ahkee S, Tolentino A, et al. Diagnosis of *Legionella pneumophila, Mycoplasma pneumoniae,* or *Chlamydia pneumoniae* lower respiratory infection using the polymerase chain reaction on a single throat swab specimen. Diagn Microbiol Infect Dis 1996; 24: 7-14.

Rosón B, Carratalà J, Verdaguer R, et al. Prospective study of the usefulness of sputum Gram stain in the initial approach to community-acquired pneumonia requiring hospitalization. Clin Infect Dis 2000; 31: 869-874.

Ruiz M, Ewig S, Torres A, et al. Severe community-acquired pneumonia: risk factors and follow-up epidemiology. Am J Respir Crit Care Med 1999; 160: 923-929.

Stahl JE, Barza M, DesJardin J, et al. Effect of macrolides as part of initial empiric therapy on length of stay in patients hospitalized with community-acquired pneumonia. Arch Intern Med 1999; 159: 2576-2580.

Vourlekis JS, Brown KK, Cool CD, et al. Acute interstitial pneumonitis: case series and review of the literature. Medicine (Baltimore) 2000; 79: 369-378.

Pneumonia in Nursing Home Residents

Pneumonia is a common problem in nursing home residents. In one study, for example, the incidence was 33 per 1000 patients per year, versus 1.4 per 1000 per year for ambulatory persons between 65 and 74 years of age and 12 per 1000 per year for ambulatory patients over age 75. This section briefly reviews ways in which pneumonia acquired in the nursing home differs from other cases of community-acquired pneumonias.

Presentation and Progression
Cause

Nursing home residents are especially vulnerable to pneumonia because of problems with swallowing, nasopharyngeal colonization by gram-negative bacilli, and the closed environment. The frequent finding of aspirated vegetable matter in their lungs at autopsy ("asylum pneumonitis") indicates how difficult it is for them to chew and swallow their meals. Patients with stroke are at especially high risk. Videofluorographic studies indicate that about 50% of stroke patients aspirate, especially those who have suffered multiple strokes, brainstem stroke, or subcortical stroke. The closed environment facilitates airborne transmission of respiratory pathogens (notably viruses and *M. tuberculosis*) and contact transmission of bacteria and fungi.

Aerobic gram-negative rods account for a substantial fraction of pneumonias among nursing home patients, especially in the more severely debilitated. Pneumococcal pneumonia is also common, and drug-resistant pneumococci may be especially frequent in this environment (see below). Pneumonia caused by *H. influenzae* is not uncommon, and pneumonia caused by *S. aureus* should be considered especially during influenza epidemics. The toll exacted by epidemic influenza A in nursing homes is well known, but in one study RSV was isolated as often as the influenza A virus and was associated with an even greater mortality.

Diagnosis

In general, diagnostic strategies are as outlined previously. Serologic tests are not useful. As discussed earlier, blood cultures are recommended for seriously ill patients.

Natural History
Expected Outcome

Death is more likely in patients who have cognitive or functional decline. The most important predictor of short-term mortality is severe dependency in activities of daily living.

Treatment

Antibiotic therapy is reviewed in the previous section (Table 11-7). In recent years the use of quinolone antibiotics has attracted enthusiasm, since the newer agents in this class provide coverage against aerobic gram-negative rods as well as against gram-positive cocci. However, potential resistance of *S. pneumoniae* to the quinolones should be kept in mind. Ribavirin is currently the treatment of choice for RSV infection.

Expected Response

The mortality rate for nursing home–acquired pneumonia is about twice that of community-acquired pneumonia (32% versus 14% in one study) but not substantially higher than the mortality for nursing home patients admitted to the hospital for other reasons. The extent of self-sufficiency before onset of pneumonia correlates with survival. The notion that pneumonia in nursing home patients leads to long-term decline in function is being challenged.

When to Refer

A substantial literature documents that many nursing home patients can be treated with oral antimicrobial agents without hospitalization. Recent data suggest that erring toward hospitalization does not improve the short-term mortality rate.

 KEY POINTS

PNEUMONIA IN NURSING HOME RESIDENTS
- ⊃ Mortality for pneumonia acquired in the nursing home is about twice that of pneumonia acquired in the community.
- ⊃ Modifiable risk factors include swallowing difficulties and lack of influenza and pneumococcal vaccination.
- ⊃ Outbreaks of pneumonia in nursing home patients are likely to be caused by influenza, RSV, and tuberculosis.
- ⊃ Aerobic gram-negative rods frequently cause pneumonia in nursing home patients after first colonizing the nasopharyngeal mucosa.

SUGGESTED READING

Ding R, Logemann JA. Pneumonia in stroke patients: a retrospective study. Dysphagia 2000; 15: 51-57.

Loeb M, McGeer A, McArthur M, et al. Risk factors for pneumonia and other lower respiratory tract infections in elderly residents of long-term care facilities. Arch Intern Med 1999; 159: 2058-2064.

Marrie TJ. Community-acquired pneumonia in the elderly. Clin Infect Dis 2000; 31: 1066-1078.

Medina-Walpole AM, McCormick WC. Provider practice patterns in nursing home–acquired pneumonia. J Am Geriatr Soc 1998; 46: 187-192.

Muder RR. Pneumonia in residents of long-term care facilities: epidemiology, etiology, management, and prevention. Am J Med 1998; 105: 319-330.

Nuorti JP, Butler JC, Crutcher JM, et al. An outbreak of multidrug-resistant pneumococcal pneumonia and bacteremia among unvaccinated nursing home residents. N Engl J Med 1998; 338: 1861-1868.

Thompson RS, Hall NK, Szpiech M, et al. Treatment and outcomes of nursing-home-acquired pneumonia. J Am Board Fam Pract 1997; 10: 82-87.

Thompson RS, Hall NK, Szpiech M. Hospitalization and mortality rates for nursing home-acquired pneumonia. J Fam Pract 1999; 48: 291-293.

Wald TG, Miller BA, Shult P, et al. Can respiratory syncytial virus and influenza A be distinguished clinically in institutionalized older persons? J Am Geriatr Soc 1995; 43: 170-174.

Pneumococcal Pneumonia

S. pneumoniae (see also Chapter 1) remains the major cause of severe community-acquired pneumonia and, worldwide, a leading cause of death. It accounts for about two thirds of cases of bacteremic pneumonia and is the most common cause of pneumonia leading to hospitalization in all age groups. Although *S. pneumoniae* is isolated in only 5% to 18% of all cases of community-acquired pneumonias, the following lines of evidence suggest that it is more common: (1) sputum cultures fail to show *S. pneumoniae* in about 50% of patients with pneumonia and positive blood cultures for this organism, suggesting that sputum culture is insensitive; (2) when transtracheal aspiration is performed to avoid upper airway contamination, the yield on culture is higher; and (3) a majority of pneumonias of unknown etiology respond to penicillin G therapy. Some authorities believe that *S. pneumoniae* may cause up to one half of all community-acquired pneumonias. There is concern that the incidence of pneumococcal disease may be increasing at the same time that drug resistance is becoming much more common. Primary care clinicians should strive to make pneumococcal vaccination an imperative for patients at increased risk.

Presentation and Progression
Cause

S. pneumoniae is a common colonizer of the nasopharynx. Invasive pneumococcal disease occurs most often after a new serotype has been acquired, typically after an incubation of 1 to 3 days. Viral illness increases the incidence of disease, presumably by interfering with normal host defenses. Risk factors for invasive pneumococcal disease include extremes of age, alcoholism, human immunodeficiency virus (HIV) disease, end-stage renal disease, sickle cell disease, diabetes mellitus, dementia, malnutrition, malignancies, diseases affecting B-lymphocyte function (notably multiple myeloma and hypogammaglobulinemia), and immunosuppressive disorders. The problem of pneumococcal disease in asplenic persons is discussed in Chapter 6. The pneumococcus does not invade cells as readily as do some of the other streptococci. However, once in the lungs it passes easily from one alveolus to another through the pores of Kohn until stopped by the dense connective tissue of a fissure; this is the basis for lobar consolidation.

In recent years an alarming spread in the incidence of penicillin-resistant strains has occurred in the United States and elsewhere. Technically the term "strains with reduced susceptibility to penicillin" is more appropriate, since high doses of penicillin G often remain effective. Strains with intermediate-level resistance (MICs between 0.1 and 1.0 μg/mL) now comprise about 30% of all pneumococcal isolates in some communities in the United States. High-level resistance (MIC ≥4 μg/mL) is uncommon, but such resistance is expected to become more common because of wide use of cephalosporins. Penicillin-resistant strains are fully virulent and can exhibit resistance to the newer cephalosporins (e.g., cefotaxime and ceftriaxone). Vancomycin is the most reliable drug for treatment of strains with high-level resistance, but—disturbingly—tolerance to vancomycin has now been reported.

Presentation

As classically described by previous generations of clinicians, *S. pneumoniae* causes a lobar pneumonia with the sudden onset of fever and a single, hard-shaking chill, cough productive of rusty-colored mucopurulent sputum, and pleuritic chest pain. Systemic toxicity, including tachypnea, is present. Physical examination reveals crepitant rales, tubular breath sounds, and signs of lobar consolidation (dullness to percussion, egophony with *e*→*a* change, and pectoriloquy). Today, however, pneumococcal disease is often a more subtle illness. Patchy infiltrates and bronchopneumonia are relatively common.

Diagnosis

A firm diagnosis is established most frequently by positive blood cultures. Bacteremia accompanies an estimated 20% to 30% of severe cases. Sputum cultures, as already noted, are relatively insensitive. A "probable" diagnosis of pneumococcal pneumonia is warranted if sputum culture reveals *S. pneumoniae* and the patient responds to a drug (usually a β-lactam antibiotic) that would not be effective against the causes of "atypical" pneumonia. When the patient is first seen, a "probable" diagnosis can be based on sputum Gram stain supported by a positive quellung reaction (capsular swelling of *S. pneumoniae* in the presence of type-specific antibody). Unfortunately, the quellung reaction is labor intensive and is not performed in most clinical laboratories. There is a great deal of interest in the development of rapid diagnostic tests, such as the demonstration of pneumococcal antigen in urine.

Natural History
Expected Outcome

The mortality rate for bacteremic pneumococcal pneumonia was more than 80% before the introduction of type-specific serum therapy. Patients recovered either gradually (called

"lysis") or abruptly (called "crisis"). Complications of pneumococcal pneumonia include parapneumonic effusion, empyema, necrotizing pneumonia with or without lung abscess, meningitis, pericarditis, septic arthritis, and endocarditis.

Treatment
Methods

These questions should be asked: Is the patient asplenic (see Chapter 6)? Is the pneumonia severe (see earlier discussion in this chapter)? Is meningitis a possibility (see Chapter 6)? Are there risk factors for pneumococcal strains with reduced susceptibility to penicillin G? Is penicillin allergy likely to be present?

Risk factors for *S. pneumoniae* strains with reduced susceptibility to penicillin G include the following:
- Extremes of age (≤2 years or ≥70 years)
- Prolonged hospitalization
- Recent β-lactam antibiotic therapy
- Attendance at a day care center (either as a child or as a staff person)
- Residence in a nursing home
- Chronic disease, such as cirrhosis, chronic obstructive lung disease, or HIV disease (according to some but not all studies)

Therapeutic options for patients with none of these risk factors include β-lactam antibiotics (Box 11-6), newer quinolones, macrolides, and cephalosporins. Treatment of drug-resistant pneumococcal infection is not well standardized. Newer cephalosporins (notably ceftriaxone or cefotaxime) are commonly used with the caveat that vancomycin should be added if meningitis is suspected. In most cases of uncomplicated pneumococcal pneumonia, treatment need be continued no more than 7 days, or no more than 3 days after the patient becomes afebrile.

BOX 11-6
Antibiotic Therapy for Pneumococcal Pneumonia

- Risk factors for intermediate resistance to penicillin G include extremes of age (≤2 years or ≥70 years), prolonged hospitalization, prior β-lactam antibiotic therapy, attendance in a day care center (either as a child or as a staff person), and—at least in some studies—human immunodeficiency virus disease.
- If none of these risk factors are present, pneumococcal pneumonia can be treated with a β-lactam antibiotic (e.g., penicillin G, ampicillin, or a cephalosporin), a macrolide, or a quinolone.
- If no risk factors to high-level resistance are present, high-dose aqueous penicillin G is appropriate therapy.
- Ceftriaxone 2 g q24h or cefotaxime 2 g q8h is also effective and is probably the most frequently used regimen in the United States.
- Vancomycin (1 g IV q12h for a 70-kg adult with normal renal function) should be used along with a third-generation cephalosporin if high-level resistance is suspected (minimum inhibitory concentration ≥4 μg/mL), if meningitis is suspected (see Chapter 6), or if type I allergy (anaphylaxis, urticaria, angioedema, or bronchospasm) to penicillins and cephalosporins is present.
- If concomitant meningitis is suspected, ceftriaxone plus vancomycin is appropriate initial therapy. Some authorities would add rifampin 300 mg PO b.i.d.

Expected Response

Severe pneumococcal disease remains a formidable problem. In recent series, mortality in bacteremic cases has been as high as 43%. Risk factors for a complicated course include older age; underlying lung disease; immunodeficiency, including HIV disease; and nosocomial acquisition. Clearing of the chest radiograph may take up to 6 weeks even in healthy persons. Elderly persons and those with chronic obstructive lung disease tend to have delayed resolution. Workup for malignancy is indicated only if infiltrates persist beyond 6 weeks. Occasionally, necrotizing pneumonia or lung abscess develops.

When to Refer

When having strong reason to suspect pneumococcal disease, and especially in a person with compromised host defenses, the clinician should be liberal about the need to hospitalize the patient. An emerging strategy might be intravenous administration of antibiotics and monitoring of vital signs in a holding area for 12 hours, but such an approach has not yet been validated by careful trials.

 KEY POINTS

PNEUMOCOCCAL PNEUMONIA

⊃ *S. pneumoniae* remains the leading cause of severe community-acquired pneumonia and a major cause of death.

⊃ Risk factors for invasive pneumococcal disease include extremes of age, alcoholism, HIV disease, end-stage renal disease, sickle cell disease, diabetes mellitus, dementia, malnutrition, malignancies, diseases affecting B-lymphocyte function (notably multiple myeloma and hypogammaglobulinemia), and immunosuppressive disorders.

⊃ The physician should consider these key clinical questions: Is the patient asplenic? Is the pneumonia severe? Is meningitis a possibility? Are there risk factors for pneumococcal strains with reduced susceptibility to penicillin G? Is penicillin allergy likely to be present?

⊃ Primary care clinicians should make pneumococcal vaccination a priority in their practices.

SUGGESTED READING

Chen DK, McGeer A, de Azavedo JC, et al. Canadian Bacterial Surveillance Network. Decreased susceptibility of *Streptococcus pneumoniae* to fluoroquinolones in Canada. N Engl J Med 1999; 341: 233-239.

Ho PL, Tse WS, Tsang KWT, et al. Risk factors for acquisition of levofloxacin-resistant *Streptococcus pneumoniae*: a case-control study. Clin Infect Dis 2001; 32: 701-707.

Marfin AA, Sporrer J, Moore PS, et al. Risk factors for adverse outcome in persons with pneumococcal pneumonia. Chest 1995; 107: 457-462.

Metersky ML, Fine JM, Tu GS, et al. Lack of effect of a pneumonia clinical pathway on hospital-based pneumococcal vaccination rates. Am J Med 2001; 110: 141-143.

Novak R, Henriques B, Charpentier E, et al. Emergence of vancomycin tolerance in *Streptococcus pneumoniae*. Nature 1999; 399: 590-593.

Whitney CG, Farley MM, Hadler J, et al. Increasing prevalence of multidrug-resistant *Streptococcus pneumoniae* in the United States. N Engl J Med 2000; 343: 1917-1924.

Bacterial Pneumonia Caused by Agents Other Than Streptococcus Pneumoniae

Among the numerous bacteria other than *S. pneumoniae* that sometimes cause acute community-acquired pneumonia (Table 11-2), the most common are *H. influenzae*, *S. aureus*, *Streptococcus pyogenes*, miscellaneous aerobic gram-negative rods, and anaerobic "mouth flora" bacteria. Patients with these pneumonias often have significant underlying disease, severe pneumonia, or both. Therefore hospitalization is usually indicated.

H. influenzae is a frequent cause of pneumonia in elderly patients and in patients with serious underlying diseases, including chronic obstructive lung disease. The pneumonia usually has a patchy or segmental distribution, which is characteristic of bronchopneumonia rather than lobar pneumonia. A sputum Gram stain showing small, pleomorphic gram-negative coccobacilli can be virtually diagnostic.

S. aureus pneumonia, when community acquired, tends to be an acute, fulminant process. *S. aureus* is an uncommon cause of community-acquired pneumonia, explaining 1% of cases, except during influenza epidemics. Influenza virus infection markedly predisposes to staphylococcal colonization of the respiratory mucosa. Staphylococcal pneumonia tends to be a necrotizing process with abscess formation. The chest radiograph sometimes shows air pockets known as pneumatoceles, especially in children.

S. pyogenes (group A streptococcal) pneumonia is uncommon except during influenza epidemics. This pneumonia is often accompanied by the rapid development of large empyemas. Chest tube drainage is often necessary, resulting in prolonged hospitalization.

Klebsiella pneumoniae is a relatively common cause of pneumonia in patients suffering from alcoholism. The pneumonia often assumes a lobar distribution. Classically this pneumonia affects the upper lobes and causes a "bulging fissure" on radiography. *E. coli* and other aerobic gram-negative rods are relatively common causes of pneumonia in the frail elderly. *Pseudomonas aeruginosa*, although a common cause of nosocomial pneumonia, is rarely associated with community-acquired pneumonia in patients without underlying lung disease or severe debility.

Pneumonia caused by "mouth flora" bacteria—by which is meant a combination of anaerobic and aerobic bacteria with the anaerobes usually predominating—occurs most frequently in patients with alcoholism and poor oral hygiene. "Mouth flora" pneumonia in an edentulous patient should prompt suspicion of underlying lung cancer. A foul odor of the breath is present in many but not all of these patients. This form of pneumonia is often associated with lung abscess and with empyema caused by bronchopleural fistula.

Pneumonias caused by *F. tularensis* (tularemia; see Chapter 8), *Y. pestis* (plague; see Chapter 6), *B. anthracis* (anthrax; see Chapter 6), and Hantavirus pulmonary syndrome (see Chapter 6) are discussed elsewhere.

Mycoplasma Pneumoniae Pneumonia

Formerly known as the "Eaton agent," *M. pneumoniae* is the most commonly identified cause of atypical pneumonia, although its precise incidence is unknown. Various investigators have determined this microorganism to be the cause of 13% to 27% of community-acquired pneumonias. It can also cause hospital-acquired pneumonias, and it has caused as many as 50% of pneumonias during epidemics in closed populations. *M. pneumoniae* pneumonia becomes less common after age 40, but older persons may have more severe manifestations.

Presentation and Progression
Cause

M. pneumoniae is a cell wall–deficient organism with particular affinity for the respiratory tract epithelium. Many of the disease manifestations are now thought to be immune mediated. Close, prolonged contact promotes transmission by respiratory secretions. The extent to which *M. pneumoniae* accompanies other agents as a concurrent pathogen has attracted interest. In one study an additional pathogen was found in about two thirds of patients with *M. pneumoniae* pneumonia who required hospitalization; *S. pneumoniae* was most commonly found, but *Legionella* species and *C. pneumoniae* were also identified.

Presentation

Of persons infected with *M. pneumoniae,* an estimated 20% or so are symptomatic. A mild respiratory illness (pharyngitis or tracheobronchitis) develops in about 70%, and pneumonia in >10%. The disease occurs in all age groups, including toddlers and the elderly, but peaks between ages 5 and 15 years.

After an incubation period of about 3 weeks, symptoms begin gradually with fever, headache, malaise, chills, sore throat, and substernal productive cough. The cough is initially nonproductive, paroxysmal, and worse at night. It commonly becomes productive later in the illness. Physical examination is usually unimpressive. Bullous myringitis is uncommon, occurring at most in about 5% of patients, but has a high positive predictive value for *M. pneumoniae* infection. More commonly the patient has mild tenderness over the paranasal sinuses, mild erythema of the posterior pharyngeal mucosa, soft cervical lymphadenopathy, and tracheal tenderness. Scattered rales and wheezes may be present but are usually unimpressive.

The WBC count is normal in 75% or more of cases. Thrombocytosis can occur as an acute-phase response. Levels of liver enzymes, notably the aminotransferases (AST and ALT), are often mildly elevated. The chest radiograph commonly shows infiltrates that are much more extensive than physical examination would suggest. The most common pattern is a peribronchial pneumonia in which thickened bronchial shadows are surrounded by streaky interstitial infiltrates and patchy atelectasis. Other patterns are nodular infiltrates and hilar lymphadenopathy. The lower lobes are most commonly involved, and pleural effusions—which can be especially severe in patients with sickle cell disease—occur in up to 20% of patients when carefully sought.

Extrapulmonary manifestations of *M. pneumoniae* pneumonia sometimes dominate the clinical picture and include the following:

- Hemolytic anemia, usually mild but sometimes life threatening, attributed to IgM antibodies to the I antigen on red blood cell membranes and suggested by a high reticulocyte count
- Rashes, ranging from mild erythematous, maculopapular or vesicular rashes to life-threatening Stevens-Johnson syndrome (of which *M. pneumoniae* may be the most common infectious cause, responsible for about 16% of cases)
- Central nervous system complications (in about 0.1% of patients, most often children), including aseptic meningitis, meningoencephalitis, transverse myelitis, cerebellar ataxia, cranial nerve palsies, and peripheral neuropathy; the CSF usually shows a lymphocytic pleocytosis with elevated protein and normal glucose levels, and morbidity can be significant
- Cardiac complications, including myocarditis, pericarditis, rhythm disturbances, and heart failure
- Polyarthralgia and rarely polyarthritis

Digestive disturbances are relatively common. Glomerulonephritis and pancreatitis have been described.

Diagnosis

M. pneumoniae pneumonia is usually diagnosed on clinical grounds. The disease often travels through young families, causing pharyngitis or tracheobronchitis in the children and pneumonia in one or both parents. Distinguishing features include gradual onset, absence of systemic toxicity, and presence of nasopharyngeal and constitutional symptoms that often dominate the patient's history. On the basis of clinical findings, *M. pneumoniae* cannot be distinguished from viral upper respiratory infections as a cause of ear pain (2% to 35% of patients), rhinorrhea (2% to 40%), or pharyngitis (6% to 59%), nor can it be distinguished reliably from most other causes of pneumonia, including pneumococcal pneumonia.

Most laboratories do not attempt to isolate *M. pneumoniae,* since isolation requires 2 to 3 months of incubation and a special medium (SP-4 medium). In the past, cold agglutinin titers were often used to make this diagnosis. However, cold agglutinin levels are elevated mainly in patients with severe disease and are nonspecific. Measurement of IgM antibodies with either a complement fixation assay or enzyme-linked immunosorbent assay (ELISA) is often used for diagnosis at present. However, the IgM antibody test can be negative during the first 10 days, and moreover, false-positive results occur. Demonstration of a four-fold or greater increase or decrease in either IgM or IgG titers in paired sera is also used for diagnosis. Antibody titers rise 7 to 9 days after infection and peak at 3 to 4 weeks. Newer methods for diagnosis are antigen detection systems, PCR, and gene probes.

Natural History
Expected Outcome

M. pneumoniae pneumonia is usually self-limited. Some patients have a persistent nonproductive or minimally productive cough. The need for and efficacy of antibiotic therapy has been debated. However, *M. pneumoniae* pneumonia can be a severe illness; a 1.4% mortality rate was determined by a metaanalysis of the literature. This illness tends to be more severe in patients with sickle cell disease, in whom pleural effusions often develop. According to recent reports, *M. pneumoniae* can cause an acute inflammatory bronchiolitis in adults, with normal chest x-ray findings, which can progress to bronchiolitis obliterans organizing pneumonia. Also, a case has been reported in which recurrent chest pain and intermittent constitutional symptoms resulted from pericarditis caused by *M. pneumoniae.*

Treatment
Methods

β-Lactam antibiotics are ineffective, since *M. pneumoniae* lacks a cell wall. Macrolides, tetracyclines, and fluoroquinolones are all effective therapy. The mainstays of drug therapy have been doxycycline (100 mg PO b.i.d.) or erythromycin (333 mg PO t.i.d.). Newer drugs such as azithromycin, clarithromycin, and the newer quinolones are commonly used in office practice, but their superiority over the older and less expensive agents is not clearly established. In severe cases requiring hospitalization, coverage should be given against the pneumococcus.

When to Refer

Clear indications for hospitalization include severe pneumonia in older patients, Stevens-Johnson syndrome, and marked hemolytic anemia.

 KEY POINTS

BACTERIAL PNEUMONIA CAUSED BY AGENTS OTHER THAN STREPTOCOCCUS PNEUMONIAE

➲ *M. pneumoniae* is the most commonly identified cause of atypical pneumonia, especially in adolescents and younger adults. The disease usually has a gradual onset of respiratory and constitutional symptoms.

➲ There is a wide spectrum of extrapulmonary manifestations.

➲ In adults *M. pneumoniae* occasionally causes acute inflammatory bronchiolitis that can lead to severe restrictive defects.

➲ Cold agglutinin titers are not specific for this diagnosis and should not be ordered routinely.

➲ Measurement of IgM and IgG antibodies to *M. pneumoniae* by complement fixation tests or ELISA is now the most common way to make the diagnosis, but patients should be treated empirically before the results are available. The IgM antibody test can be negative for 10 days, and false-positive results also occur.

➲ PCR is promising as a way to establish the diagnosis of pneumonia caused by *M. pneumoniae.*

SUGGESTED READING
Chan ED, Kalayanamit T, Lynch DA, et al. *Mycoplasma pneumoniae*–associated bronchiolitis causing severe restrictive lung disease in adults: report of three cases and literature review. Chest 1999; 115: 1188-1194.

Clyde WA Jr. Clinical overview of typical *Mycoplasma pneumoniae* infections. Clin Infect Dis 1993; 17 (Suppl 1): S32-S36.

Farraj RS, McCully RB, Oh JK, et al. *Mycoplasma*-associated pericarditis. Mayo Clin Proc 1997; 72: 33-36.

Lieberman D, Schlaeffer F, Lieberman D, et al. *Mycoplasma pneumoniae* community-acquired pneumonia: a review of 101 hospitalized adult patients. Respiration 1996; 63: 261-266.

Marrie TJ, Peeling RW, Fine MJ, et al. Ambulatory patients with community-acquired pneumonia: the frequency of atypical agents and clinical course. Am J Med 1996; 101: 508-515.

Tay YK, Huff JC, Weston WL. *Mycoplasma pneumoniae* infection is associated with Stevens-Johnson syndrome, not erythema multiforme (von Hebra). J Am Acad Dermatol 1996; 35: 757-760.

Chlamydia Pneumoniae Pneumonia

C. pneumoniae, described in 1986 as the TWAR agent, has been determined by some researchers to be the third or fourth most common cause of community-acquired pneumonia, explaining perhaps 10% to 14% of cases (up to 28% in some series). Pneumonia is recognized most frequently among the elderly, in whom it can be severe.

Presentation and Progression
Cause

C. pneumoniae is classified as a bacterium on the basis of its cell wall and growth properties. Unlike most bacteria, however, it grows only as an intracellular parasite. Serologic studies suggest that most humans gain experience with *C. pneumoniae* at some point in their lives, although immunity is short lived. About 50% of all persons have antibodies by age 20, and up to 75% of elderly persons are seropositive. It is also thought that most infections (up to 90%) are asymptomatic. Transmission is probably from person to person by respiratory secretions. In patients requiring hospitalization, *C. pneumoniae* can be a concurrent pathogen with *S. pneumoniae, M. pneumoniae,* or *L. pneumophila.*

Presentation

After an incubation period of several weeks, most patients experience gradual onset of nonspecific upper and lower respiratory symptoms, including those of sinusitis, otitis, and pharyngitis. Sore throat with hoarseness is often prominent among the initial symptoms and tends to be the dominant symptom in college-aged persons. Symptoms of pneumonia tend to develop slowly. Often patients have had symptoms for several weeks before seeking medical care. The history sometimes suggests a biphasic illness: an upper respiratory infection with sore throat that resolved, followed by lower respiratory infection with cough.

The severity is age dependent. Children under age 5 seldom have evidence of significant disease. University students often have a 10-day history of sore throat or hoarseness with minimal fever. The mean age of patients with pneumonia is about 56 years. Rhonchi and rales are present on physical examination more frequently than in *M. pneumoniae* pneumonia, even among patients who do not complain of cough. The WBC count is usually normal. Chest radiographs may show one or more infiltrates, most commonly a single, patchy, subsegmental infiltrate.

Wheezing is sometimes present. Accumulating evidence suggests that *C. pneumoniae* sometimes precipitates adult-onset asthma. Reported extrapulmonary manifestations of *C. pneumoniae* infection are meningoencephalitis, cerebellar dysfunction, Guillain-Barré syndrome, reactive arthritis, and myocarditis. The possibility that *C. pneumoniae* might cause coronary artery disease has received much attention. High levels of antibodies to *C. pneumoniae* have been observed in patients with chronic obstructive lung disease, sarcoidosis, and lung cancer, but an etiologic link is unclear.

Diagnosis

No "gold standard" for diagnosis has been established. The presentation is nonspecific, and *C. pneumoniae* infection cannot be distinguished from other causes of community-acquired pneumonia. Suggestive features include the unusually gradual onset and the frequent symptoms of sinusitis and pharyngitis with hoarseness. *C. pneumoniae* can be isolated from nasopharyngeal swabs by cell culture techniques, but most laboratories are not equipped for this cumbersome procedure. Specific serologic tests are not generally available. Tests available in reference laboratories or under development include antibody measurements (complement fixation and microimmunofluorescence), antigen detection systems (direct fluorescent antibody [DFA] and enzyme immunoassay [EIA]), and PCR.

Natural History
Expected Outcome

Symptomatic *C. pneumoniae* infection is usually a mild illness characterized by slow recovery. Cough can persist for weeks, prompting numerous physician visits. The illness is more severe and can be life threatening, especially when there is coinfection by another pathogen in the presence of an underlying disease in an older patient.

Treatment
Methods

Doxycycline (100 mg b.i.d.) or erythromycin (500 mg q.i.d.) for 10 to 14 days has been the treatment of choice. Treatment with newer macrolides, such as azithromycin and clarithromycin, both of which are highly active in vitro against the organism, has been the subject of considerable interest.

Expected Response

Treatment is often extremely frustrating because relapse frequently occurs after the course of antibiotics has been completed. *C. pneumoniae* infection provides a plausible explanation for at least a portion of the thousands of stubborn, slow-to-resolve respiratory infections that primary care practitioners see each year.

 KEY POINTS

CHLAMYDIA PNEUMONIAE PNEUMONIA
- *C. pneumoniae* pneumonia cannot be distinguished from other pneumonias on clinical grounds but tends to have gradual onset, hoarseness as a prominent complaint, and a single patchy subsegmental infiltrate.
- Young patients have mainly pharyngitis. Pneumonia occurs typically in elderly patients and can be severe.
- *C. pneumoniae* pneumonia can manifest itself as acute onset of asthma.
- Extrapulmonary manifestations have been described.
- Serologic tests are available in reference laboratories, but their value is uncertain. PCR offers promise as diagnostic test.

- The idea that *C. pneumoniae* plays a role in coronary artery disease is provocative, but the implications for primary care are unclear.
- Doxycycline is the treatment of choice.

SUGGESTED READING

Korman TM, Turnidge JD, Grayson ML. Neurological complications of chlamydial infections: case report and review. Clin Infect Dis 1997; 25: 847-851.

Kuo CC, Jackson LA, Campbell LA, et al. *Chlamydia pneumoniae* (TWAR). Clin Microbiol Rev 1995; 8: 451-461.

Lieberman D, Ben-Yaakov M, Lazarovich Z, et al. *Chlamydia pneumoniae* community-acquired pneumonia: a review of 62 hospitalized adult patients. Infection 1996; 24: 109-114.

Chlamydia Psittaci (Psittacosis; Ornithosis)

About 100 to 200 cases of psittacosis are reported in the United States each year, but the true incidence is thought to be much higher. Mortality can be high if the diagnosis is not suspected.

Presentation and Progression
Cause

Chlamydia psittaci infects many and perhaps all species of birds, which may remain asymptomatic or show symptoms and signs of illness such as anorexia, dyspnea, and ruffled feathers. Strains of *C. psittaci* that are most virulent for humans tend to be those associated with psittacine birds (from the Latin *psittacus,* or parrot), such as parrots, parakeets, macaws, cockatoos, and budgerigars, as well as with turkeys. Humans with psittacosis are commonly bird fanciers or work in poultry farms (notably turkey farms), abattoirs, processing plans, pet shops, or veterinarians' offices. The organism is usually acquired by inhalation, but human-to-human transmission occurs on rare occasions.

Presentation

After an incubation period of 5 to 15 days, symptoms and signs of illness ranging in severity from mild to life threatening develop. The major presenting features include the following:
- Atypical pneumonia manifested as headache, fever, and nonproductive cough (the most characteristic form of the disease; chest x-ray abnormalities, most commonly consolidation of one lower lobe, are seen in 75% of cases, and the radiographic findings are usually much more striking than the findings on auscultation of the chest)
- A typhoidal illness with fever, malaise, relative bradycardia, and hepatosplenomegaly
- A mononucleosis-like syndrome with fever, sore throat, lymphadenopathy, and hepatosplenomegaly
- Fever of unknown origin
- A nonspecific flulike "viral syndrome"

Occasional patients have severe complications. These include endocarditis (sometimes with embolic occlusion of large vessels), disseminated intravascular coagulation, and neurologic abnormalities, including encephalitis and transverse myelitis.

Diagnosis

Diagnosis depends largely on demonstration of complement-fixing or microimmunofluorescent antibodies. PCR, ELISA, and DFA tests are being developed. Culture is not recommended because it is dangerous to laboratory personnel.

Natural History

Expected Outcome

Untreated, the mortality from psittacosis is as high as 20%. Psittacosis can be a severe disease during pregnancy.

Treatment

Methods

Doxycycline (100 mg PO b.i.d. for 10 to 21 days) or tetracycline HCl (500 mg PO q.i.d. for 10 to 21 days) is currently the treatment of choice.

Expected Response

Effective treatment usually brings about clinical improvement within 24 hours and lowers mortality to 1%.

When to Refer

Patients with severe manifestations of psittacosis should be admitted to the hospital.

 KEY POINTS

CHLAMYDIA PSITTACI (PSITTACOSIS; ORNITHOSIS)

- ◯ *C. psittaci* possibly infects all avian species, but the most virulent strains for humans are associated with psittacine birds and turkeys.
- ◯ Psittacosis is a hazard to pet bird fanciers, veterinarians, pet shop owners, poultry farmers (especially turkey farmers), and workers in abattoirs and processing plans.
- ◯ The syndromes of psittacosis include pneumonia, a typhoidal illness, a mononucleosis-like syndrome, fever of unknown origin, and a minimally symptomatic illness.
- ◯ Diagnosis is often suspected on the basis of failure of pneumonia to respond to β-lactam antibiotics. The diagnosis is confirmed by serology.
- ◯ Treatment with doxycycline or tetracycline lowers mortality from about 20% to 1%.

SUGGESTED READING

Centers for Disease Control and Prevention. Compendium of measures to control *Chlamydia psittaci* infection among humans (psittacosis) and pet birds (avian chlamydiosis), 2000. MMWR 2000; 49 (RR-8): 1-17.

Gregory DW, Schaffner W. Psittacosis. Semin Respir Med 1997; 12: 7-11.

Hyde SR, Benirschke K. Gestational psittacosis: case report and literature review. Mod Pathol 1997; 10: 602-607.

Kirchner JT. Psittacosis: is contact with birds causing your patient's pneumonia? Postgrad Med 1997; 102: 181-182, 198-188, 193-194.

Legionnaire's Disease

First identified in 1976 during an outbreak at an American Legion convention in Philadelphia, legionnaire's disease is now recognized as a relatively common cause of both community- and hospital-acquired pneumonia. The incidence exhibits wide geographic variation—from <1% to >16% of community-acquired pneumonias—reflecting to a large extent the degree of contamination of water reservoirs by the causative organisms. Unlike pneumonias caused by *M. pneumoniae* and *C. pneumoniae,* cases that can be treated on an outpatient basis tend to be the exception rather than the rule.

Presentation and Progression

Cause

Legionella species are gram-negative bacteria that stain poorly and survive intracellularly. More than 40 species and more than 60 serogroups of *Legionella* are now recognized. *L. pneumophila* is the most commonly encountered species, causing at least 80% of clinical infections.

Legionellosis seems to be a disease of human progress, brought about by devices that maintain water at warm temperatures and produce aerosols. In water the organisms multiply within amebas; in humans they multiply within alveolar macrophages. The disease is spread by water rather than by person-to-person contact. Contamination of water sources has been associated with numerous outbreaks in settings ranging from inner-city hospitals to industrial plants to luxury cruise liners.

Clinically severe cases of legionnaire's disease tend to occur in persons with compromised host defenses, most often in the setting of COPD, immunosuppression, or advanced age. As discussed previously, coinfection is relatively common. In a study done in Israel, only 38% of patients with legionnaire's disease were infected solely by this pathogen; *S. pneumoniae* was the most common concurrent pathogen (about one half of cases), followed by *M. pneumoniae* and *C. pneumoniae.*

Presentation

A mild form of legionellosis, known as Pontiac fever, is a self-limited disease with fever, malaise, headaches, and chills without pneumonia. Pontiac fever resolves within a few days without antibiotic therapy. Legionnaire's disease, the more familiar and more severe form of legionellosis, affects persons of all ages and causes symptoms that overlap those of "classic bacterial" and "atypical" pneumonia.

After an incubation period of 2 to 10 days, fever, headache, anorexia, malaise, and myalgia occur. At this point, respiratory symptoms are usually not prominent, and the cough is only minimally productive. Some patients have chest pain, and if the sputum is blood tinged, pulmonary embolism is often suspected. Gastrointestinal symptoms with nausea, vomiting, diarrhea, and abdominal pain can also dominate the clinical picture. Alternatively, neurologic symptoms can be the presenting complaint, variably manifested as headache, lethargy, and change in mental status.

Fever is usually present. Relative bradycardia is found more often in older patients and those with severe pneumonia. Examination of the chest usually shows rales and, later in the illness, signs of consolidation. The peripheral blood commonly shows leukocytosis and thrombocytopenia. Hyponatremia (serum sodium level <130 mEq/L) is more common in legionnaire's disease than in most other pneumonias. Hypophosphatemia also occurs. Evidence of liver and renal dysfunction is frequently found. Hematuria and proteinuria are common. There is no characteristic radiologic feature. The most common pattern is a patchy infiltrate involving one lobe, which progresses to consolidation. Infiltrates can assume a diffuse or interstitial pattern, and pleural effusions are common.

Diagnosis

In geographic areas where legionnaire's disease is not well publicized, early diagnosis requires a high index of suspicion. The possibility of legionnaire's disease is suggested by the combination of extrapulmonary symptoms, signs, and laboratory abnormalities and by pneumonia that progresses during therapy with a β-lactam antibiotic. However, some experts hold that legionnaire's disease is difficult if not impossible to distinguish from other pneumonias on clinical grounds. Unfortunately, no laboratory test is entirely satisfactory.

The urinary antigen test for *L. pneumophila* serogroup 1 is at least 80% sensitive and 99.5% specific if performed within the first week of the illness. Since serogroup 1 accounts for about 80% of cases of legionnaire's disease, this test should allow a diagnosis in more than 60% of cases. The sensitivity of the urinary antigen test gradually declines over the next 6 months. DFA staining of sputum or lung biopsy tissue has a sensitivity of up to 70% but requires experienced laboratory personnel. Sputum culture using specialized media (typically, buffered charcoal yeast extract media) is up to 60% sensitive; a higher yield (about 80%) can be obtained in specialized laboratories with use of several media. Growth of the organism usually requires incubation of cultures for 3 to 5 days. Serologic studies usually do not help clinical decision making, since they require convalescent serum. Application of the PCR to clinical practice has not been especially promising to date.

Natural History
Expected Outcome

The mortality of untreated legionnaire's disease ranges from 16% to 30%. The prognosis depends mainly on the presence of chronic underlying disease. In a metaanalysis of the literature, the mortality rate for community-acquired pneumonia caused by *L. pneumophila* was 15%.

Treatment
Methods

To be effective against the intracellular *Legionella* bacteria, antibiotics must penetrate cells, including macrophages, in therapeutic concentrations. Erythromycin, with or without rifampin, has been the mainstay of therapy. Erythromycin is now being replaced by the newer macrolides, especially azithromycin. Compared with erythromycin, the newer agents have less gastrointestinal toxicity, superior pharmacokinetics that permits once- or twice-daily doses, better penetration into lung tissue and macrophages, and more potent intracellular activity. The newer quinolones such as ciprofloxacin and levofloxacin are also highly active.

For patients without underlying disease and with relatively mild infections, a 7- to 10-day course of azithromycin may suffice because of the long intracellular half-life and slow release of this agent. Combined therapy with a macrolide and a quinolone (e.g., azithromycin and levofloxacin) is now

being recommended for seriously ill patients. Rifampin remains a useful adjunct for some patients. Doxycycline and TMP/SMX are also useful for some patients.

Expected Response

Patients with legionnaire's disease, especially younger patients without underlying disease, generally improve and feel well within 3 to 5 days if treated early. Delay in the initiation of treatment affects prognosis. Some patients have residual fatigue for several months. The infection seems to confer immunity, since second cases are uncommon.

When to Refer

Older and immunocompromised patients with suspected legionnaire's disease should usually be hospitalized.

 KEY POINTS

DIAGNOSIS OF LEGIONNAIRE'S DISEASE

- ⤷ Features common to "atypical pneumonia" include gradual onset and extrapulmonary symptoms and signs of disease.
- ⤷ Features typical of "classic bacterial pneumonia" include frequent lobar consolidation and severity of illness.
- ⤷ Specific diagnostic clues include prominent gastrointestinal symptoms (notably diarrhea), failure to find a predominant organism on Gram stain of a purulent sputum specimen, hyponatremia, and failure to respond to β-lactam antibiotics.
- ⤷ The urine antigen test for *L. pneumophila* serogroup 1 has a sensitivity of about 80% and a specificity approaching 100%; this serogroup accounts for about 80% of cases of legionnaire's disease.
- ⤷ The organism can be isolated in about 60% to 80% of cases by use of specialized media.

SUGGESTED READING

Edelstein PH. Antimicrobial chemotherapy for Legionnaires disease: time for a change. Ann Intern Med 1998; 129: 328-330.

Kazandjian D, Chiew R, Gilbert GL. Rapid diagnosis of *Legionella pneumophila* serogroup 1 infection with the Binax enzyme immunoassay urinary antigen test. J Clin Microbiol 1997; 35: 954-956.

Lieberman D, Porath A, Schlaeffer F, et al. *Legionella* species community-acquired pneumonia: a review of 56 hospitalized adult patients. Chest 1996; 109: 1243-1249.

Stout JE, Yu VL. Legionellosis. N Engl J Med 1997; 337: 682-687.

Waterer GW, Baselski VS, Wunderink RG. *Legionella* and community-acquired pneumonia: a review of current diagnostic tests from a clinician's viewpoint. Am J Med 2001; 110: 41-48.

Influenza

The importance of influenza to primary care physicians cannot be overemphasized. Primary care practitioners form the front line of defense against this highly contagious infection of the upper and lower respiratory tract. The three influenza pandemics of the 20th century—the "Spanish flu" of 1918-1919, the "Asian flu" of 1957-1958, and the "Hong Kong flu" of 1968-1969—caused an estimated 654,000 deaths in the United States alone.

Yearly epidemics commonly cause at least 10,000 deaths in the United States, and death rates exceeding 40,000 are not uncommon. The annual cost of influenza in the United States is estimated to be $14.6 billion, of which 10% reflects direct costs for medical care and 90% represents the costs of lost productivity and employee absenteeism.

There is now concern that a major pandemic, perhaps caused by an H5N1 virus, will strike during the early years of the third millennium. Development, manufacture, and distribution of an inactivated strain-specific influenza vaccine take about 9 months. Pandemic influenza can cause huge increases in the demand for medical services. New advancements—the development of rapid office tests for diagnosis and of new drugs for treatment—will increase the demand for medical services. Appropriate recognition, diagnosis, treatment, and prevention of influenza will continue to be a major challenge in primary care.

Presentation and Progression
Cause

Influenza viruses that infect humans are classified as influenza A, the cause of epidemic and pandemic influenza, and influenza B, which is usually a milder illness that occurs throughout the year (Box 11-7).

Influenza A virus is classified on the basis of changes in the antigenic characteristics of the envelope glycoproteins known as hemagglutinin (H) and neuraminidase (N). The RNA genome of influenza viruses is constantly undergoing rearrangement. Antigenic shifts reflect major changes in these glycoproteins, designated by a change in type, for example, a change from HxNx to HyNy. Antigenic shifts in the virus set the stage for epidemics and pandemics. Pandemics take place when an antigenic shift occurs in such a way that few members of the world's population have naturally occurring antibodies to the virus. Antigenic drifts are minor changes associated with more localized outbreaks of disease. The influenza B virus is less inclined to mutate; antigenic drifts in its H antigen have been reported, but antigenic shifts do not seem to occur.

The Centers for Disease Control and Prevention (CDC) monitors influenza viruses in collaboration with the World Health Organization. Much of the story of circulating influenza

BOX 11-7
Epidemiology of Influenza

- Epidemics and pandemics of influenza A occur because of major changes in the antigenic structure of hemagglutinin and neuraminidase glycoproteins. These changes are called "antigenic shifts," to distinguish them from minor changes ("antigenic drifts") that occur between epidemics.
- Influenza B virus usually causes a milder disease than influenza A. Outbreaks of influenza B are less extensive and pandemics do not occur, probably because the influenza B virus, unlike the influenza A virus, does not undergo major antigenic shifts.
- Weekly information about influenza can be obtained from the CDC, either on the worldwide web at http://www.cdc.gov/ncidod/diseases/flu/weekly.htm or by telephone at 888-232-3228.
- Epidemics and pandemics of influenza can occur with devastating rapidity. Attack rates are generally 10% to 20% of the general population during epidemics and can exceed 50% during pandemics.

viruses is summarized in their names. For example, the designation "A (H1N1)/Sydney/5/93" identifies the strain as an influenza A virus with hemagglutinin type 1 and neuraminidase type 1 (thus H1N1) first isolated in Sydney, Australia, in 1993 as the fifth strain in a sequence. Influenza B viruses have only one recognized type of the H antigen and one of the N antigen, and hence their designations are shorter. Thus "B/Beijing/184/93" identifies an influenza B virus first isolated in Beijing during 1993 as the 184th strain of a sequence. Since 1977, H1N1 and H3N2 subtypes of influenza A have concurrently circulated around the globe along with influenza B viruses. Each year the composition of the influenza vaccine is changed to reflect the current viruses.

Influenza A is highly infectious. Most outbreaks have attack rates of 10% to 20% in the general population. Attack rates are especially high among children in day care centers, who usually escape the brunt of the disease but transmit it to others. Attack rates are also high in institutions and in semiclosed populations. During pandemics, attack rates can exceed 50% in the general population. Outbreaks of influenza B viruses, which are usually less extensive, have been reported especially in schools and military camps; occasionally such outbreaks occur in chronic care facilities and nursing homes.

Presentation

The clinical spectrum ranges from a self-limited illness resembling the common cold to fulminant disease with death from overwhelming viral pneumonia within a few hours. Symptoms usually begin abruptly. A common chief complaint is, "I feel like I've been hit by a truck." Although the disease requires a 2- to 4-day incubation period, adult patients can often date to the hour the onset of symptoms such as fever, throbbing headache, photophobia, myalgia, sore throat, substernal soreness, nonproductive cough, and persistent malaise. In preschool children the major symptoms tend to be fever, rhinitis, pharyngitis, vomiting, and diarrhea. In elderly patients the course is often dominated by high fever, nasal obstruction, lassitude, and confusion. In all age groups the constitutional symptoms may be more impressive initially than the respiratory symptoms.

Physical findings are likewise nonspecific. The patient may appear febrile and exhausted. The skin is often hot and moist, the face is flushed, and the eyes are red and watery. More than 50% of patients have physical evidence of upper respiratory tract infection such as nasal obstruction, nasal discharge, and pharyngeal injection. Younger patients often have nontender cervical lymphadenopathy. The trachea is often tender. In the absence of complications the chest is usually clear on auscultation.

Diagnosis

Recognizing an epidemic of influenza is easier than making a precise diagnosis in an individual case. Isolated or sporadic cases cannot be distinguished from infections caused by other viral respiratory infections. When influenza has been confirmed in a community, acute respiratory illness should be considered to be influenza until proved otherwise. However, the physician should be alert for alternative diagnoses, since other life-threatening diseases such as severe sepsis caused by *S. aureus* are often manifested as undifferentiated "flulike" illness. Recent, well-publicized cases make inhalational anthrax (see Chapter 6) another consideration in the differential diagnosis.

Influenza viruses can be isolated from sputum samples, nasal washes, nasal swabs, throat swabs, or combined nose-and-throat swab specimens. Isolation usually takes 3 to 7 days, which is too late to benefit the individual patient. Antigen detection systems have recently been introduced and are now available commercially. Methods include EIA, optical immunoassay, time-resolved immunofluorescence, and an assay that detects neuraminidase activity. Several office laboratory tests have been approved by the Food and Drug Administration and are now available for diagnosis of both influenza A and influenza B. The sensitivity of these tests for influenza A ranges from 65% to 81% and the specificity from 93% to 100% in various studies; the sensitivity for influenza B is not reported. Of the three tests Flu OIA, Quickvue, and Zstatflu, Quickvue was concluded by *Medical Letter* consultants to be the easiest and fastest. However, it was noted that no direct comparisons had been made. These tests are especially useful for making treatment decisions about patients with flulike symptoms in the absence of reported influenza in a community. The methodology in this area is changing rapidly, and primary care clinicians should consult their local laboratories concerning the optimum available test.

Natural History
Expected Outcome

In the absence of complications, symptoms gradually improve over 2 to 5 days. The total illness may last somewhat longer than a week. Some patients feel "washed out" for several weeks, a state called postinfluenza asthenia.

The major complication of influenza is pneumonia (Box 11-8). Primary influenza pneumonia should be suspected when symptoms of influenza fail to resolve within several days. It is characterized by high fever and dyspnea. It is the least common but most severe of the pulmonary complications of influenza. Patients with elevated left ventricular pressures seem to be especially predisposed. Patients in high-risk groups for influenza are at risk for pneumonia. Rarely it occurs in otherwise healthy young adults. Secondary bacterial pneumonia is brought about by damage to the tracheobronchial epithelium, which impairs mucociliary clearance and leads to infection of the lung parenchyma. Often it appears after initial improvement and is characterized by high fever, cough, purulent sputum, and pulmonary infiltrates. *S. pneumoniae* is the most common cause (nearly one half of cases), but *S. aureus* explains about 20% of cases. *H. influenzae* is also a cause. Frequently patients have features of both primary influenza pneumonia and secondary bacterial pneumonia.

Extrapulmonary complications of influenza include the following:

■ Reye's syndrome, characterized by nausea and vomiting followed by cerebral edema, liver failure, and hypoglycemia. Reye's syndrome typically occurs between the ages of 2 and 16 years and has been associated with influenza A more often than with influenza B. The incidence has declined since warnings were issued against the use of aspirin for children with viral illnesses.

■ Acute myositis and rhabdomyolysis, with extreme muscle tenderness, most prominently in the legs. This complication occurs most often in children, and myoglobulinuria sometimes results in renal failure. The serum creatinine phosphokinase (CPK) concentration is markedly elevated.

■ Complications of *S. aureus* superinfection, including not only pneumonia but also complications of bacteremia such

---

BOX 11-8
Primary Influenza Pneumonia and Secondary Bacterial Pneumonia Complicating Influenza

• Primary influenza pneumonia should be suspected when, instead of improving within several days, symptoms persist with high fever and dyspnea.
• Secondary bacterial pneumonia should be suspected when, after a period of initial improvement from influenza, fever returns with productive cough.
• Secondary bacterial pneumonia is most often caused by *Streptococcus pneumoniae* (up to one half of cases), but *Staphylococcus aureus* is a common cause of pneumonia in this setting.
• Primary influenza pneumonia and secondary bacterial pneumonia often coexist.
• Mortality is highest in persons with chronic underlying diseases and in the elderly. However, during pandemics, about 50% of deaths occur in people <65 years of age.
• Much of the mortality occurs in people with heart, lung, or renal disease. Extrapulmonary complications occasionally occur and can be severe.

---

as endocarditis or epidural abscess. Toxic shock syndrome has been associated with influenza (especially influenza B) and *S. aureus* infection.

■ Myocarditis and pericarditis. These were associated with the 1918 pandemic but have been reported infrequently since that time.

■ Central nervous system complications. Reported complications include instances of encephalitis, transverse myelitis, and Guillain-Barré syndrome, but a clear causal relationship has not been established.

Treatment and Prevention
Methods

Symptomatic therapy for influenza consists mainly of rest, hydration, and acetaminophen. Especially in persons <18 years of age, use of aspirin should be avoided because of its association with Reye's syndrome. Empiric initial therapy for suspected bacterial superinfection, in the absence of clear evidence pointing to one or another pathogen, should provide adequate coverage against *S. pneumoniae*, *S. aureus*, and *H. influenzae*.

Drug therapy against influenza now consists of three classes of agents: tricyclic amines (amantadine and rimantadine), ribavirin, and recently introduced neuraminidase inhibitors (zanamivir and oseltamivir) (Table 11-10). Amantadine and rimantadine have been effective for prevention of influenza, especially in institutional settings such as nursing homes. Both are associated with central nervous system effects. Ribavirin given by aerosol has been shown to be somewhat effective. The recently introduced neuraminidase inhibitors, zanamivir (Relenza) and oseltamivir (Tamiflu), shorten the duration of the illness by about 1½ days if given within the first 48 hours of symptoms. These new agents are less likely to induce resistance and seem thus far to have fewer side effects than amantadine and rimantadine. Recent studies indicate that both zanamivir and oseltamivir are effective in preventing influenza of household contacts, when combined with treatment of index cases. However, use of these agents has also been shown to promote drug-resistant mutants of the influenza virus.

TABLE 11-10
Drugs For Treatment and Prevention of Influenza

Class	Drugs and usual adult dosage	Efficacy and safety
Antiparkinson drugs with antiviral activity (tricyclic amines)	Amantadine (Symmetrel) 200 mg daily or 100 mg PO b.i.d.; rimantadine (Flumadine) 200 mg daily or 100 mg PO b.i.d.	Amantadine and rimantadine are at least 70% effective as prophylaxis against influenza A in institutional settings and reduce the duration of the symptoms and signs of influenza A by about 50% if given within the first 48 hours. Neither is effective against influenza B. The major side effects are on the central nervous system: jitteriness, insomnia, anxiety, confusion, and, rarely, seizures. Dosage should be reduced in patients with impaired renal function.
Nucleoside analog	Ribavirin (Virazole) 1.1 g daily by inhalation	Ribavirin may be active against influenza A and B when given by aerosol. It is not currently a drug of choice for this indication.
Neuraminidase inhibitors	Zanamivir (Relenza) 10 mg by inhalation b.i.d.; oseltamivir (Tamiflu) 75 mg PO b.i.d.	Both drugs reduce the average duration of symptoms in influenza A and B by about 36 hours. Whether they will prevent serious complications, including death, has not yet been determined.

BOX 11-9
Causes of Pulmonary Infiltrates with Eosinophilia (PIE Syndrome)

- Allergic bronchopulmonary aspergillosis should be suspected when patients seek treatment for asthma. This entity, which is discussed earlier in the chapter (see "Bronchiectasis"), responds to corticosteroid therapy.
- Chronic eosinophilic pneumonia (Carrington's syndrome) often is manifested as cough, fever, weight loss, and peripherally located pulmonary infiltrates. The chest x-ray appearance has been called a "photographic negative of pulmonary edema," since, in contrast to pulmonary edema, the perihilar regions are relatively spared. This entity, which may have diverse causes, often responds to corticosteroid therapy.
- Acute eosinophilic pneumonia, discussed previously in the differential diagnosis of acute community-acquired pneumonia, is a dramatic illness characterized by fever, dyspnea, hypoxia, and bilateral diffuse pulmonary infiltrates in a previously healthy young adult. Because eosinophilia is usually not present in the peripheral blood, a high index of suspicion is required. The diagnosis is made by documenting pulmonary eosinophilia through the use of bronchoscopy with bronchoalveolar lavage.
- Various parasitic infections can cause transient or prolonged pulmonary infiltrates (see Chapter 23).
- *Pneumocystis carinii* pneumonia occasionally manifests itself as the PIE syndrome in human immunodeficiency virus–positive patients.
- Hypersensitivity pneumonitis from diverse causes (e.g., pigeon breeder's disease) can cause acute pulmonary infiltrates with dyspnea.
- Chronic infections, including tuberculosis, psittacosis, brucellosis, and regional mycoses (e.g., histoplasmosis, coccidioidomycosis), occasionally cause eosinophilia.
- Tropical eosinophilia, now thought to be a hypersensitivity reaction to microfilariae in most cases, is manifested as cough, wheezing, dyspnea, and constitutional symptoms such as fatigue, weight loss, and anorexia in persons who have been to the tropics. The characteristic x-ray finding consists of interstitial infiltrates with scattered 2- to 4-mm nodules, concentrated at the bases of the lungs.
- Noninfectious causes of the PIE syndrome include numerous entities such as the Churg-Strauss syndrome (asthma, diffuse infiltrates, and allergic angiitis with granulomatosis), eosinophilic leukemia, sarcoidosis, Hodgkin's disease, and drug allergy.

Expected Response

Amantadine, rimantadine, and probably the neuraminidase inhibitors are moderately effective at preventing influenza and have some effect on the course of the disease. Whether these drugs will prevent overwhelming influenza, however, remains to be determined. The best strategy for influenza is clearly immunization (see Chapters 3 and 25). Recent studies document the effectiveness of influenza immunization of children in day care centers and also of working adults, suggesting that wider use of the vaccine may be worthwhile.

When to Refer

Patients with suspected primary influenza pneumonia or severe secondary bacterial pneumonia should be hospitalized.

SUGGESTED READING
Bridges CB, Thompson WW, Meltzer MI, et al. Effectiveness and cost-benefit of influenza vaccination of healthy working adults: a randomized controlled trial. JAMA 2000; 284: 1655-1663.

Couch RB. Prevention and treatment of influenza. N Engl J Med 2000; 343: 1778-1787.

Gubareva LV, Kaiser L, Matrosovich MN, et al. Selection of influenza virus mutants in experimentally infected volunteers treated with oseltamivir. J Infect Dis 2001; 183: 523-531.

Hayden FG, Gubareva LV, Monto AS, et al. Inhaled zanamivir for the prevention of influenza in families. N Engl J Med 2000; 343: 1282-1289.

Horimoto T, Kawaoka Y. Pandemic threat posed by avian influenza A viruses. Clin Microbiol Rev 2001; 14: 129-149.

Hurwitz ES, Haber M, Chang A, et al. Effectiveness of influenza vaccination of day care children in reducing influenza-related morbidity among household contacts. JAMA 2000; 284: 1677-1682.

Monto AS. Preventing influenza in healthy adults: the evolving story (editorial). JAMA 2000; 284: 1699-1700.

Rapid diagnostic tests for influenza. Med Lett 1999; 41: 121-122.

Stamboulian D, Bonvehi PE, Nacinovich FM, et al. Influenza. Infect Dis Clin North Am 2000; 14: 141-166.

Welliver R, Monto AS, Carewicz O, et al. Effectiveness of oseltamivir in preventing influenza in household contacts: a randomized controlled trial. JAMA 2001; 285: 748-754.

Pulmonary Infiltrates with Eosinophilia (PIE Syndrome)

Rarely the primary care clinician encounters a patient with pulmonary infiltrates associated with eosinophilia in the peripheral blood. This presentation, commonly known as the PIE syndrome, poses a wide range of diagnostic possibilities (Box 11-9). Occasionally the diagnosis is straightforward, but in many cases referral is indicated.

SUGGESTED READING

Kim Y, Soo Lee K, Choi DL, et al. The spectrum of eosinophilic lung disease: radiologic findings. J Comput Assist Tomogr 1997; 21: 920-930.

Marchand E, Reynaud-Gaubert M, Lauque D, et al. Idiopathic chronic eosinophilic pneumonia: a clinical and follow-up study of 62 cases. Medicine 1998; 77: 299-312.

Marshall BG, Wilkinson RJ, Davidson RN. Pathogenesis of tropical pulmonary eosinophilia, parasitic alveolitis, and parallels with asthma. Respir Med 1998; 92: 1-3.

Chronic Pneumonias

Sometimes a primary care clinician encounters a patient with an unexpected, chronic, or persistent infiltrate on chest x-ray examination. Most such patients require referral to a pulmonary specialist for consideration of bronchoscopy and other specialized studies. The primary care clinician should carefully evaluate these patients for clues to the possible etiology (Box 11-10).

In a nonimmunocompromised patient the usual causes of chronic pneumonia are mycobacterial infection (see Chapter 22), fungal infection (see Chapter 21), cancer (often with post-

---

BOX 11-10
Some Clues to the Etiology of Chronic Pneumonia

- Age and sex. In elderly patients tuberculosis and aspiration pneumonia are the primary considerations. The incidence of pulmonary disease caused by *Mycobacterium avium-intracellulare* is increasing in middle-aged women. Young and middle-aged women are also susceptible to pulmonary lymphangioleiomyomatosis.
- Geography. Histoplasmosis and coccidioidomycosis have unique geographic distributions within the United States (see Chapter 21). International residence or travel correlates with paracoccidioidomycosis (Latin America), melioidosis (Southeast Asia), and paragonimiasis (Asian rim).
- Occupation. Diseases acquired through work or hobbies include pneumoconioses such as silicosis and asbestosis (sandblasters, shipyard workers), hypersensitivity pneumonitis, berylliosis, and injury from noxious gases.
- Alcoholism. Alcoholism predisposes to tuberculosis, aspiration pneumonia, chronic pneumonia caused by gram-negative bacteria, and pulmonary sporotrichosis.
- Esophageal disease. Persons with esophageal disease (e.g., achalasia) are prone to chronic aspiration, which can cause lower lobe pulmonary infiltrates. Lipoid pneumonia (mineral oil pneumonia) sometimes occurs, as does superinfection with saprophytic mycobacteria.
- Drugs. Nitrofurantoin (Macrodantin), amiodarone, gold salts, penicillamine, and a wide variety of drugs used in cancer chemotherapy can cause chronic pneumonia or pulmonary fibrosis.

---

obstructive pneumonia), chronic aspiration, connective tissue diseases, and primary lung diseases. Evaluation of these patients must be individualized based on the history and radiographic findings. Except when an etiology such as *M. tuberculosis* is readily established, most patients undergo further imaging studies (e.g., CT) followed by invasive procedures (e.g., bronchoscopy, transthoracic lung biopsy, or surgical exploration).

SUGGESTED READING

Marik PE. Aspiration pneumonitis and aspiration pneumonia. N Engl J Med 2001; 344: 665-671.

Ost D, Fein A. Evaluation and management of the solitary pulmonary nodule. Am J Respir Crit Care Med 2000; 162: 782-787.

12 Gastrointestinal and Intraabdominal Infections

RADU CLINCEA, CHARLES S. BRYAN, NATHAN M. THIELMAN, J. ROBERT CANTEY

Acute gastroenteritis (mainly infectious diarrhea) is second only to cardiovascular disease as a cause of death worldwide. In the United States, acute gastroenteritis is second only to viral respiratory disease as a cause of acute illness, prompting an estimated 73 million physician consultations each year. Most episodes are self-limited, but infectious diarrhea and various foodborne illnesses account annually for more than 5000 deaths. Other intraabdominal infections are also relatively common and present dilemmas in diagnosis and management. Pitfalls for primary care physicians include the following:

- Acute bacterial meningitis is sometimes misdiagnosed as "gastroenteritis" because of prominent nausea and vomiting. Headache is a valuable clue, and the "jolt test" may be useful in deciding whether lumbar puncture is indicated (see Chapter 6).
- Intrathoracic disorders such as pneumonia, pulmonary thromboembolism, and acute myocardial infarction sometimes cause pain in the upper abdomen. Conversely, pain in the lower chest sometimes indicates an intraabdominal pathologic condition.
- Unrecognized esophageal disease with reflux can cause asthma, persistent sore throat, and chronic aspiration pneu-

monia, leading to such complications as bronchiectasis and atypical mycobacterial infection.
- Fever with right lower quadrant pain suggesting acute appendicitis (pseudoappendicitis syndrome) can be caused by *Yersinia enterocolitica* (the usual cause), *Salmonella enteritidis,* or *Campylobacter jejuni.* A high index of suspicion can avert the need for surgery.
- Abdominal pain in a person with diabetes mellitus can indicate a life-threatening syndrome such as emphysematous pyelonephritis or emphysematous cholecystitis. Appropriate imaging procedures usually lead to the correct diagnosis (see Chapter 3).
- Abdominal pain, fever, or evidence of sepsis in a person with cirrhosis and ascites should suggest the possibilities of spontaneous bacterial peritonitis or spontaneous bacteremia (see Chapter 3). Paracentesis is usually indicated.
- Abdominal pain and evidence of sepsis in an elderly person should raise the possibility of an "acute abdomen" caused by such disorders as acute cholecystitis, diverticulitis, perforation of the colon, acute appendicitis, or ruptured aortic aneurysm. When in doubt, the physician should err toward requesting imaging procedures (see Chapter 3).
- Abdominal pain and fever in a patient who has recently had diverticulitis, cholecystitis, or pancreatitis should suggest the possibility of intraabdominal abscess.

All clinicians should know the salient features of acute cholecystitis, appendicitis, and diverticulitis, since these are common diseases. Fever and abdominal pain can also be caused by infections of the urinary tract or reproductive organs (see Chapters 5, 14, and 16).

SUGGESTED READING
Blaser MJ, Smith PD, Ravdin JI, et al., eds. Infections of the Gastrointestinal Tract. New York: Raven Press; 1995.

Helicobacter Pylori

Recognition of the role of *Helicobacter pylori* in peptic ulcer disease and gastric carcinoma has spawned an enormous body of research and numerous ongoing controversies. Here, current aspects of *H. pylori* infection are summarized as they pertain to primary care.

Presentation and Progression

H. pylori is a spiral-shaped, microaerophilic, gram-negative rod that attaches to epithelial cells in the stomach, especially in the antrum, where it resides in the mucous layer. *H. pylori* damages mucus-secreting cells and also promotes an acute and chronic inflammatory response that may lead to a sequence of events: acute gastritis followed by chronic superficial gastritis, then atrophic gastritis, intestinal metaplasia, dysplasia, and adenocarcinoma. The stomach infected with *H. pylori* also develops lymphoid follicles (lymphoid tissue is not normally present in the stomach), which can evolve into a low-grade malignancy known as MALT (mucosa-associated lymphoid tissue) lymphoma. Why these various manifestations of *H. pylori* infection develop in some persons and not others remains unclear.

H. pylori colonizes at least one half of the world's population, with high colonization rates in developing countries where the infection is usually acquired during childhood. About 35% of persons in the United States are colonized, and since the frequency of colonization is approximately 0.5% per year, about 50% of persons >60 years of age in the United States and other developed countries may be infected. Fecal-oral transmission occurs, and lower prevalence rates correlate with higher standards of living and sanitation.

H. pylori is associated with about 70% to 90% of duodenal ulcers, about 70% of gastric ulcers, and about 60% to 80% of gastric carcinomas. The prevalence of *H. pylori* in the United States appears to be declining, and this may explain, at least in part, the declining incidence of peptic ulcer disease and adenocarcinoma of the stomach. However, the incidence of reflux esophagitis, Barrett's esophagus, and adenocarcinoma of the esophagus in the United States has been increasing, leading to the provocative suggestion that certain strains of *H. pylori* may be protective against the serious consequences of gastroesophageal reflux disease (GERD).

Presentation

H. pylori infection does not manifest itself as an infectious disease in the usual sense; rather, the manifestations are those of gastritis, duodenal ulcer, gastric ulcer, adenocarcinoma of the stomach, or MALT lymphoma. Whether *H. pylori* contributes substantially to "dyspepsia" is a matter of ongoing controversy.

Diagnosis

Several alternative methods for diagnosis are available, each with >95% accuracy when properly performed but varying considerably in cost and inconvenience. Serologic tests for IgG antibody are currently the most practical and cost-effective approach to diagnosis in primary care (in large studies, sensitivity 90% to 100% and specificity 76% to 96%). Other relatively noninvasive approaches to diagnose are the urea breath test (sensitivity 88% to 95%, specificity 95% to 100%), which requires expensive instrumentation; a stool antigen test (sensitivity 94%, specificity 86% to 92%); and the newly approved 13C-bicarbonate assay (sensitivity 91%, specificity 86%). Identification of the organism in mucosal biopsy specimens obtained during endoscopy remains the "gold standard" for diagnosis. The organism can be isolated by culture, but this is not optimally sensitive. The urease test on samples obtained at endoscopy can also be performed.

The availability of diagnostic tests for *H. pylori* infection raises an important issue: who should be tested? In 1998 the American College of Gastroenterology, American Gastroenterological Association, American Society for Gastrointestinal Endoscopy, and American Association for the Study of Liver Diseases endorsed the following guidelines:

- Testing for *H. pylori* should be carried out only if treatment is intended.
- Testing for *H. pylori* is indicated for patients with active peptic ulcer disease, past history of documented peptic ulcer, or gastric MALT lymphoma.
- Testing for *H. pylori* is not indicated for patients without a past history of peptic ulcer disease.
- Testing for *H. pylori* is not indicated as part of the evaluation of patients with gastroesophageal reflux disease.
- Testing for *H. pylori* may be considered for patients with nonulcer dyspepsia on a case by case basis.

Testing might also be considered for patients with a strong family history of carcinoma of the stomach, but testing for *H. pylori* as a preventive method for carcinoma of the stomach should not be considered a standard of care.

Natural History
Expected Outcome

Peptic ulcer disease occurs in about one in six persons (17%) with *H. pylori* infection. Carcinoma of the stomach eventually develops in about 1% to 3% of patients with *H. pylori* infection. It has been suggested that each year about 1% to 2% of persons infected with *H. pylori* have a major complication. Rarely, low-grade T cell–dependent B-cell lymphoma (MALT lymphoma) develops. Suggested but unproven associations with *H. pylori* infection include coronary artery disease, gallstones, thyroid disease, chronic urticaria, diabetes mellitus, Raynaud's phenomenon, and short stature.

Treatment
Methods

Three broad categories of drugs are useful: antacids, notably bismuth subsalicylate; antisecretory agents, notably proton pump inhibitors (PPIs) such as omeprazole or lansoprazole; and antibiotics, notably amoxicillin, clarithromycin, metronidazole, and tetracycline. Trials to define the optimum regimen are ongoing, especially since the organism develops resistance to various antibiotics. Currently recommended regimens associated with >90% rates of eradication generally include at least three drugs:

- A PPI (omeprazole 20 mg b.i.d. or lansoprazole 30 mg b.i.d.), amoxicillin 1 g b.i.d., and clarithromycin 500 mg b.i.d., for 2 weeks. For penicillin-allergic patients, metronidazole 500 mg b.i.d. can be substituted for amoxicillin, with the notation that resistance of *H. pylori* to metronidazole (up to 50% in some areas) is more common than resistance to amoxicillin.
- A PPI (as above), bismuth subsalicylate 525 mg q.i.d., and two antibiotics (e.g., metronidazole 250 mg q.i.d. and tetracycline 500 mg q.i.d.) for 2 weeks.

Two-drug regimens (such as a PPI or bismuth plus either amoxicillin or clarithromycin) have been approved but are not generally recommended because of lower eradication rates.

Patients with peptic ulcer disease should not be treated empirically for *H. pylori* infection without confirmation because treatment requires compliance with a complicated regimen and produces side effects and because up to 40% of persons with gastric ulcer and up to 27% of persons with duodenal ulcer lack evidence of *H. pylori* infection.

Little or no evidence supports therapy for *H. pylori* infection in patients with nonulcer dyspepsia. However, a recent study suggests that eradication of *H. pylori* infection in patients with atrophic gastritis improves intestinal metaplasia and may therefore help prevent stomach cancer.

Expected Results

Treatment as outlined previously eradicates *H. pylori* in about 90% of cases, which usually correlates with healing of duodenal or gastric ulcer. Eradication of *H. pylori* causes regression of MALT lymphoma. Treatment of *H. pylori* infection has not been shown to benefit gastric carcinoma.

When to Refer

Patients with disease manifestations attributable in part to *H. pylori* infection are commonly referred to gastroenterologists.

 KEY POINTS

HELICOBACTER PYLORI

⊃ *H. pylori* has strong associations with duodenal ulcer, gastric ulcer, gastric carcinoma, and MALT lymphoma. The possible association with nonulcer dyspepsia is controversial.

⊃ Serologic testing for IgG antibodies to *H. pylori* is the most convenient method of diagnosis in primary care. Serologic testing should be performed only if treatment is planned. Testing is therefore recommended mainly for patients with peptic ulcer disease.

⊃ Treatment of asymptomatic persons for *H. pylori* is not recommended. Some strains of *H. pylori* are thought to be protective against GERD and its complications, notably adenocarcinoma of the esophagus.

SUGGESTED READING

Blaser MJ. Hypothesis: the changing relationships of *Helicobacter pylori* and humans; implications for health and disease. J Infect Dis 1999; 179: 1523-1530.

Childs S, Roberts A, Meineche-Schmidt V, et al. The management of *Helicobacter pylori* infection in primary care: a systematic review of the literature. Fam Pract 2000; 17 (Suppl 2): S6-S11.

Howden CW, Hunt RH. Ad Hoc Committee on Practice Parameters of the American College of Gastroenterology. Guidelines for the management of *Helicobacter pylori* infection. Am J Gastroenterol 1998; 93: 2330-2338.

Laine L, Schoenfeld P, Fennerty MB, et al. Therapy for *Helicobacter pylori* in patients with nonulcer dyspepsia: a meta-analysis of randomized, controlled trials. Ann Intern Med 2001; 134: 361-369.

Ohkusa T, Fujiki K, Takashimizu I, et al. Improvement in atrophic gastritis and intestinal metaplasia in patients in whom *Helicobacter pylori* was eradicated. Ann Intern Med 2001; 134: 380-386.

Solnick JV, Schauer DB. Emergence of diverse *Helicobacter* species in the pathogenesis of gastric and enterohepatic diseases. Clin Microbiol Rev 2001; 14: 59-97.

Uemura N, Okamoto S, Yamamoto S, et al. *Helicobacter pylori* infection and the development of gastric cancer. *N Engl J Med* 2001; 345: 784-789.

Food Poisoning

Centralized food processing and distribution combined with the growing trend toward meals away from home make food poisoning an increasingly important problem in the United States and elsewhere. About 5000 outbreaks of foodborne disease are reported to the Centers for Disease Control and Prevention (CDC) each year, but the magnitude of the problem is thought to be far greater. By various estimates 6 to 81 million cases of food poisoning occur in the United States annually, causing 323,000 hospitalizations, 5000 deaths, and expenditures exceeding $5 billion. Symptoms range from mild facial flushing (Chinese restaurant syndrome) or gastroenteritis to life-threatening paralysis or colitis. Emerging problems include the hemolytic-uremic syndrome caused by Shiga toxin–producing strains of *Escherichia coli* (notably *E. coli* O157:H7 but also others) and increasing drug resistance among *Salmonella, Shigella,* and other relatively common bacteria. In this section we review briefly the major syndromes of food poisoning (Table 12-1). Many of the specific pathogens are discussed elsewhere in this chapter or in other chapters.

Presentation and Progression
Cause

Food poisoning is due in part to risky food handling or food consumption practices. A recent survey of more than 19,000 adults in the United States indicated that 19% did not wash their hands or cutting boards adequately after contact with raw meat or chicken. During the previous year 50% of respondents had eaten undercooked eggs, 20% of respondents had eaten pink hamburgers, 8% had eaten raw oysters, and 1% had drunk raw milk. Risky practices were more common among men and among persons of higher socioeconomic status.

An outbreak of food poisoning is defined by the CDC as the occurrence of two cases with identical or nearly identical symptoms and signs traced to a single exposure. The cause of food poisoning is determined in only about one third of outbreaks. About 75% of outbreaks of determined cause are due to bacteria, 17% to chemical agents, about 6% to viruses, and about 2% to parasites.

Bacterial food poisoning can result from one of four mechanisms:

- Ingestion of food containing preformed toxin is characteristic of food poisoning caused by *Staphylococcus aureus, Bacillus cereus* (short incubation type), and *Clostridium botulinum* (other than infant botulism). Symptoms of *S. aureus* and short-incubation *B. cereus* food poisoning typically begin within 1 to 6 hours, since the organism need not multiply in the host to cause disease. Symptoms of botulism are delayed because the toxin must be absorbed and then fixed to neural tissue.

- Toxin production within the patient's gastrointestinal tract after ingestion of the organism is characteristic of food poisoning caused by *B. cereus* (long incubation type), infant botulism, *Clostridium perfringens,* enterotoxigenic *E. coli,* Shiga toxin–producing *E. coli,* and *Vibrio cholerae* infection (O1, O139, and non-O1). Symptoms typically begin 8 hours or more after ingestion.

- Tissue invasion by the microorganism is characteristic of foodborne disease caused by *Salmonella* species, *Shigella* species, *C. jejuni,* and invasive *E. coli.* Symptoms typically begin 16 hours or more after ingestion, since the organism must multiply and then invade tissue.

TABLE 12-1
Food Poisoning Syndromes

Syndrome	Nature of cause	Specific causes	Mechanism	Comments
Nausea and vomiting within 1 to 6 hours	Infectious	*Staphylococcus aureus*	Preformed enterotoxin	Symptoms usually last <12 hours
		Bacillus cereus	Heat-stable toxin	Symptoms usually last <12 hours
	Noninfectious	Heavy metals	Most important: copper, zinc, tin, cadmium	Symptoms (including cramps) typically begin within 15 minutes and resolve within 3 hours
Paresthesias within 1 hour	Noninfectious	Histamine fish poisoning (scromboid)	Release of histamine and inhibitors of histamine degradation	Burning of mouth and throat; flushing, headache, dizziness; abdominal cramps, nausea, and vomiting; urticaria and bronchospasm
		Paralytic shellfish poisoning	Neurotoxins produced by dinoflagellates (e.g., saxitoxin)	Paresthesias of mouth, lips, face, and extremities; in severe paralysis, ataxia, respiratory failure
		Neurotoxic shellfish poisoning	Neurotoxins produced by dinoflagellates	Similar to paralytic shellfish poisoning, except that paralysis does not occur
		Amnesic shellfish poisoning	Domoic acid (a toxin produced by a dinoflagellate)	Permanent antegrade amnesia (25% of patients) caused by destruction of hippocampi
		Chinese restaurant syndrome	Monosodium L-glutamate	Burning sensation in upper body; headache, flushing, diaphoresis; cramps; resolves within several hours
		Niacin		Facial erythema, which rapidly resolves
Paresthesias within 1 to 6 hours	Noninfectious	Paralytic shellfish poisoning	Neurotoxins produced by dinoflagellates (e.g., saxitoxin)	Paresthesias of mouth, lips, face, and extremities; in severe cases, paralysis, ataxia, respiratory failure
		Ciguatera	Ciguatoxin, produced by dinoflagellates	Numbness and paresthesias of lips, tongue, and throat; abdominal cramps, nausea, vomiting, and diarrhea; shooting pains in the legs; may last several months
Syndrome resembling alcohol intoxication or disulfiram (Antabuse)-like reaction within 2 hours	Noninfectious	Various mushrooms	Various toxins: ibotenic acid, muscarine, muscimol, psilocybin, psilocin, disulfiram-like substance	Symptoms include confusion, restlessness, visual disturbances, evidence of parasympathetic hyperactivity (e.g., salivation, blurred vision, abdominal cramps), psychotic reactions, and disulfiram-like reactions.

■ Toxin production and tissue invasion are characteristic of infection caused by *Vibrio parahaemolyticus* and *Y. entero-colitica,* which thus seem to cause disease by more than one mechanism.

Some microorganisms, for example, *B. cereus,* cause disease by more than one mechanism.

Salmonella species are the most frequently reported cause of foodborne outbreaks and are sometimes associated with severe disease. *Shigella* species, the classic agents of bacillary dysentery, currently cause <2% of outbreaks in the United States, while *C. jejuni,* although responsible for >200,000 cases of diarrhea each year, causes <1% of reported foodborne outbreaks. Shiga toxin–producing *E. coli* strains assume importance disproportionate to their frequency because of the severe complications (discussed later in the chapter). *Listeria monocytogenes* causes occasional outbreaks of foodborne illness in the United States, which can result in life-threatening disease,

TABLE 12-1—cont'd
Food Poisoning Syndromes

Syndrome	Nature of cause	Specific causes	Mechanism	Comments
Abdominal cramps and diarrhea within 8 to 16 hours	Infectious	*Clostridium perfringens*	Five types of *C. perfringens* toxin produced in vivo (notably, toxin A)	Nausea; vomiting (less frequently); symptoms usually resolve within 24 hours
		Bacillus cereus	Heat-labile enterotoxin produced in vivo	Nausea; vomiting (less frequently); symptoms usually resolve within 24 hours
Abdominal cramps and diarrhea within 6 to 24 hours, followed by hepatic and renal failure	Noninfectious	Mushrooms (notably *Amanita phalloides, Amanita virosa,* and *Amanita verna*)	Amatoxins; phallotoxins	Abdominal cramps and diarrhea, which usually resolve within 24 hours, followed 1 or 2 days later by hepatic and renal failure
Fever, abdominal cramps, and diarrhea within 16 to 48 hours	Infectious	*Campylobacter jejuni, Salmonella* species, *Shigella* species, *Vibrio parahaemolyticus,* invasive *Escherichia coli*	See "Infectious Diarrhea: Overview" and specific pathogens in text	See "Infectious Diarrhea: Overview" and specific pathogens in text
Fever and abdominal cramps within 16 to 48 hours	Infectious	*Yersinia enterocolitica*	Enterotoxin or tissue invasion	Diarrhea occurs especially in younger children; can mimic acute appendicitis (pseudoappendicitis syndrome)
Abdominal cramps and watery diarrhea within 16 to 72 hours	Infectious	Enterotoxigenic *E. coli, Vibrio parahaemolyticus, Vibrio cholerae* (O1 and non-O1), *Campylobacter jejuni, Salmonella* species, *Shigella* species	Various enterotoxins and cytotoxins	See "Infectious Diarrhea: Overview" and specific pathogens; headache and vomiting are prominent features of disease caused by Norwalk virus ("winter vomiting disease")
Nausea, vomiting, diarrhea, and paralysis within 18 to 36 hours	Infectious	*Clostridium botulinum*	Neurotoxins (A, B, and E) produced by *C. botulinum*	Gastrointestinal symptoms are followed by descending weakness or paralysis.
		Campylobacter jejuni	? Cross-reactivity with myelin (see text)	Guillain-Barré syndrome
Bloody diarrhea without fever within 72 to 120 hours	Infectious	Shiga toxin–producing strains of *E. coli* (notably *E. coli* O157:H7)	Shiga toxin (verotoxins)	Hemorrhagic colitis; hemolytic-uremic syndrome; thrombotic thrombocytopenic purpura
Persistent diarrhea within 1 to 3 weeks	Infectious	*Cyclospora cayatanensis*	Damage to intestinal epithelial cells by parasite	Diarrhea (often intermittent and relapsing) with anorexia, nausea, fatigue, and weight loss
	Noninfectious	Raw milk (? component)	Unknown	Watery diarrhea

especially in young children and among the elderly. *Brucella* species cause occasional outbreaks of disease (brucellosis) in the United States and are usually acquired from cheese made from unpasteurized milk, raw milk, or raw meat. Parasites associated with outbreaks of foodborne disease in the United States in recent years include *Cyclospora cayetanensis, Cryptosporidium parvum,* and *Listeria monocytogenes.*

Presentation

The syndromes of food poisoning vary according to the organism, the organ(s) affected, and the time of onset after ingestion:

- Onset within 1 hour suggests ingestion of a chemical.
- Onset between 1 and 6 hours suggests ingestion of a preformed toxin, usually in food contaminated with *S. aureus* or *B. cereus.*

- Onset within 8 to 16 hours raises a number of possibilities (Table 12-1), especially bacteria such as *C. perfringens* and enterotoxin-producing strains of *B. cereus* that must multiply in the gastrointestinal tract before causing disease.
- Onset beyond 16 hours also raises a number of possibilities, including various bacteria and viruses.

Staphylococcal food poisoning and short-incubation *B. cereus* food poisoning are characterized by vomiting and crampy abdominal pain. Diarrhea occurs in about one third of cases. A later onset of crampy abdominal pain with diarrhea is characteristic of *C. perfringens* and long-incubation *B. cereus* food poisoning, but these same symptoms can be caused by many other enteric pathogens. The usual presentations of infectious diarrhea caused by *E. coli, Salmonella* and *Shigella* species, and *C. jejuni* are discussed more fully later in the chapter.

Diagnosis

When food poisoning is suspected, diagnosis has two purposes: to take proper care of the individual patient, and to uncover a possible outbreak that may pose special danger to persons at risk, such as the elderly and the immunocompromised. Because most cases of food poisoning are self-limited, extensive studies are unnecessary for care of the individual patient. When an outbreak is suspected, however, the aid of local health authorities should usually be enlisted. Investigation may include evaluation not only of the stools, vomitus, and blood of affected patients, but also of leftover food, the environment in which the food was prepared, and in some instances the food handlers. Laboratories should be asked to save bacterial isolates for possible special studies such as serotyping or pulsed-field gel electrophoresis. When botulism or mushroom poisoning is suspected, every effort should be made to secure the incriminated source.

Natural History
Expected Outcome

The outcome of food poisoning depends on the specific cause and the general health of the patient (Table 12-1).

Treatment and Prevention
Methods

Treatment depends on the specific cause.

When to Refer

A suspected foodborne outbreak should be brought to the attention of local health authorities.

 KEY POINTS

FOOD POISONING

- Although a specific cause is found in only about one third of foodborne outbreaks in the United States at present, the most likely causes are usually suggested by the nature of the symptoms and the time of onset in relation to ingestion of the suspected vehicle.
- When a foodborne outbreak is suspected, local health authorities should be notified, since the diagnosis may prove important to persons at increased risk of serious complications.

- Preventive measures include properly storing and preparing food, washing hands and cutting boards after contact with raw meat or chicken, and avoiding ingestion of undercooked eggs, pink hamburgers, raw oysters, and raw milk.

SUGGESTED READING

Centers for Disease Control and Prevention. Diagnosis and management of foodborne illnesses: a primer for physicians. MMWR 2001 (RR-2): 1-69.

Mead PS, Slutsker L, Dietz V, et al. Food-related illness and death in the United States. Emerg Infect Dis 1999; 5: 607-625.

Olsen J, MacKinnon LC, Goulding JS, et al. Surveillance for foodborne diseases—United States, 1993-1997. MMWR 2000; 49: 1-62.

Slutzer L, Altekruse SF, Swerdlow DL. Foodborne diseases: emerging pathogens and trends. Infect Dis Clin North Am 1998; 12: 199-216.

Infectious Diarrhea: Overview

Infectious diarrhea is the second most common cause of death worldwide and the leading cause of death in early childhood. In the United States infectious diarrhea causes death mainly in older and debilitated persons. However, disastrous consequences can occur in previously healthy persons. Pathogen-associated complications from infectious diarrhea include mycotic aneurysm of the aorta with *Salmonella* species (see Chapter 6), the hemolytic-uremic syndrome and renal failure with Shiga toxin–producing strains of *E. coli,* and Guillain-Barré syndrome with *C. jejuni.* The clinician's primary task is to discern which patients need further investigation, including stool cultures; which need empiric antimicrobial therapy; and which need only "tincture of time." According to various estimates, >200 million episodes of diarrhea occur in the United States each year (by one estimate, 1.4 episodes per person), resulting in >73 million physician consultations, 28 million office visits, 1.8 million hospitalizations, and 5000 deaths. Answers to a series of questions usually determine the optimum approach to diagnosis and therapy (Figure 12-1).

Questions to Ask When Patients Seek Treatment for Diarrhea

The clinician must determine whether diarrhea is "medically important."

- Is the problem best classified as diarrhea? Diarrhea is usually defined as three or more loose stools per day, two loose stools with abdominal symptoms, or >250 g of stool per day for 7 days. "Loose stools" not meeting one of these criteria may be part of another illness or may fall within the range of normal bowel functioning. However, it is acceptable to consider any increased frequency or decreased consistency of bowel movements as "diarrhea."
- Is the problem more likely infectious or noninfectious? Most cases of community-acquired diarrhea are probably caused by infection. Noninfectious causes include drugs, primary gastrointestinal diseases such as inflammatory bowel disease, food allergies, endocrine disorders (e.g., thyrotoxicosis), carcinoid syndrome, and paraneoplastic syndromes. Ischemic colitis caused by cocaine should be considered in the differential diagnosis of abdominal pain and bloody diarrhea in a young or middle-aged adult.

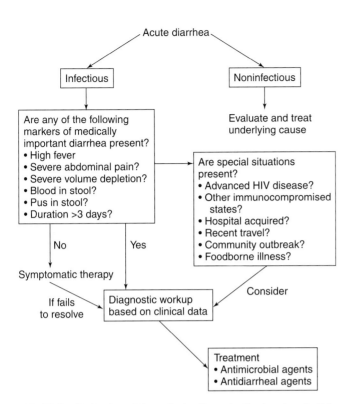

FIG. 12-1 Evaluation of the patient with acute diarrhea (see text) is based on the answers to a series of structured questions. (Modified from Aranda-Michel J, Giannella RA. Acute diarrhea: a practical review. Am J Med 1999; 106: 670-676.)

- What is the duration of the illness, and did it begin suddenly or gradually? Sudden onset of diarrhea can be caused by a preformed toxin or by a specific enteric pathogen usually associated with an acute diarrheal syndrome. Diarrhea of gradual onset is often caused by pathogens that tend to cause prolonged diarrheal illness, such as *Giardia lamblia.*
- What is the epidemiologic setting? Has the patient recently traveled to a developing country (see Chapter 24)? Has the patient recently taken antibiotics (raising the possibility of *C. difficile* colitis)? Has the patient been exposed to persons who have diarrhea or are at high risk for diarrhea (such as children in day care centers)? Is there a history of ingestion of unsafe foods (such as unpasteurized milk or cheese, raw shellfish, raw eggs, or raw meat) or water (such as from lakes or streams)? Has there been contact with animals or pets, including reptiles (which are notoriously associated with *Salmonella* species)?
- How is the patient's general health and immunocompetence? Dehydration caused by acute diarrheal illness carries an increased risk of morbidity and mortality at the extremes of life: infants and the elderly. Persons who are taking immunosuppressive medication or who have advanced HIV disease are at high risk of diarrhea caused by opportunistic pathogens, including parasites.
- Is the diarrhea likely to involve mainly the small bowel or the large bowel? About 90% of cases of acute, community-acquired infectious diarrhea in the United States represent "small bowel diarrhea" characterized by infrequent watery

stools. About 5% to 10% of cases represent "large bowel diarrhea" or the dysentery syndrome, characterized by frequent, small-volume stools that often contain mucus or blood (Table 12-2). Frequently, however, the pattern of diarrhea does not fit neatly into one or the other of these categories.
- Is the diarrhea medically important? Diarrhea is a common experience and usually runs a benign course, even in persons with underlying medical conditions. Most patients do not require stool cultures and other studies. The character and duration of the diarrhea, the associated symptoms and signs, and the epidemiologic features usually determine whether further investigation is warranted (Box 12-1 and Figure 14-1).

The distinction between noninflammatory and inflammatory diarrhea (Table 12-2) has clinical relevance even though considerable overlap is often present. Inflammatory diarrhea is commonly caused by *Shigella* species, *Salmonella* species, and *C. jejuni.* Shiga toxin–producing strains of *E. coli* (enterohemorrhagic *E. coli,* and especially *E. coli* O157:H7), although causing <1% of all cases of acute diarrheal illness in the United States, are important to recognize because of the serious complications. The many causes of noninflammatory diarrhea can be divided into those that typically cause short-lived diarrhea and those that typically cause persistent diarrhea (>10 to 14 days). In the United States acute, self-limited watery diarrhea is usually of viral etiology (rotavirus, the Norwalk agent, and other viruses). Other causes are enterotoxigenic *E. coli,* enteropathogenic *E. coli,* and *C. jejuni.* Prolonged diarrheal illness is often caused by protozoal pathogens such as *G. lamblia, C. parvum, Cyclospora cayatenensis,* and *Isospora belli.* In patients with advanced HIV disease, microsporidial organisms become another consideration.

Examination of Stool

Routine stool cultures for patients with infectious diarrhea are not cost effective, since the expenditure would exceed $1000 for each positive culture result. However, examination of the stool is helpful in most cases of severe acute infectious diarrhea and need not be expensive. Cultures and other studies can be selected on the basis of clinical and epidemiologic features (Table 12-3).

Gross inspection of stool is worthwhile. Patients should be asked to bring a specimen to the office in a convenient container, such as a large, sealed glass jar. Watery and nonbloody stool suggests noninflammatory diarrhea. The presence of mucus or blood suggests dysentery. Examination of stool for fecal leukocytes provides a rapid, inexpensive clue to the presence of inflammation. The technique is as follows: (1) a drop of stool is placed on a glass slide, (2) a drop of methylene blue is added (reticulocyte stain, available in most clinical laboratories, can be substituted for methylene blue), (3) a coverslip is applied, and (4) the preparation is examined using the high-dry or oil-immersion lens of the microscope. Fecal polymorphonuclear leukocytes are found in cases of inflammatory diarrhea caused by *Salmonella, Shigella, Campylobacter,* and *Yersinia* species, Shiga toxin–producing *E. coli* strains (notably *E. coli* O157:H7), and noninfectious inflammatory diseases such as ulcerative colitis and ischemic colitis. Fecal mononuclear leukocytes predominate in enteric fever (*Salmonella typhi*). Degenerating fecal leukocytes are sometimes found in

TABLE 12-2
Comparison of Small Bowel Diarrhea and Large Bowel Diarrhea

	Small bowel diarrhea	Large bowel diarrhea
Medical synonym	Noninflammatory diarrhea	Inflammatory diarrhea (dysentery)
Vernacular synonym	"The runs"	"The squirts"
Character of stools	Watery	Semiformed, typically with mucus and blood
Frequency of stools	Infrequent	Frequent
Pain on defecation	Usually absent	Often present
Pathophysiology	The small bowel secretes excessive fluid or fails to absorb fluids; the large bowel functions normally as a reservoir and therefore stores a large volume of fluid until overdistention prompts a bowel movement	The colon is inflamed and therefore fails in its normal function as a reservoir, prompting frequent, small-volume bowel movements, which are often painful because of inflammation involving the rectum
Polymorphonuclear leukocytes in stool*	Seldom present	Usually present
Fever	Usually absent	Often present
Associated symptoms	Abdominal cramping, bloating, and gas; symptoms of volume depletion (dehydration) if severe	Systemic toxicity; pain and tenderness in the left lower quadrant of the abdomen

*Fecal lactoferrin test can be a substitute for examination for polymorphonuclear leukocytes in stool.

BOX 12-1
Medically Important Diarrhea (Investigation Warranted)

- High fever (≥101.3° F [38.5° C])
- Profuse watery diarrhea with severe volume depletion
- Severe abdominal pain, especially in a person >50 years of age
- Bloody diarrhea
- Diarrhea in a patient with hemolytic anemia or renal failure
- Dysentery syndrome (small-volume stools with blood and mucus)
- Duration >3 days
- Advanced age (≥70 years)
- Immunocompromised state (including advanced human immuno-deficiency virus disease)
- Many similar cases, suggesting a community outbreak

---

dysentery caused by *Entamoeba histolytica* (amebiasis; see Chapter 23). The experience needed to identify fecal leukocytes can be gained with a modicum of practice. In recent years the lactoferrin test (Leukotest, TechLab) has been introduced as a surrogate marker for fecal polymorphonuclear neutrophils. The test is based on an immunoassay for this leukocyte product.

Stool cultures or toxin assays are indicated on a selective basis (Table 12-3). In a study carried out in the United States during 1997, the frequency of pathogens in stool cultures was estimated to be 2.3% for *Campylobacter*, 1.8% for *Salmonella* species, 1.1% for *Shigella* species, and 0.4% for *E. coli* O157:H7. However, the frequency of *E. coli* O157:H7 was nearly 8% if the stool was visibly contaminated with blood. Obtaining "stools for ova and parasites" from immunocompetent patients with diarrhea of less than 7 days' duration is not cost effective.

Therapy for Patients with Diarrhea

Supportive treatment of diarrhea consists of close attention to fluid and electrolyte replacement and judicious use of antimotility drugs. Patients with mild diarrhea are advised to focus on adequate fluid intake, including soups and juices for nutrition. Patients with more severe diarrhea who have signs of volume depletion such as lightheaded-ness require more aggressive hydration that includes electrolyte solutions. The recognition that sodium and glucose absorption from the intestines is "coupled" ranks high among the medical discoveries of the 20th century and is responsible for saving countless lives. The coupled absorption of sodium and glucose provides the rationale for the many commercially available replacement solutions, such

TABLE 12-3
Tests to Be Performed on Diarrheal Stools on a Selective Basis

Clinical setting	Modifying circumstances	Culture or test	Comments
Acute community-acquired diarrhea or traveler's diarrhea that has not responded to empiric therapy with a fluoroquinolone or TMP/SMX	None	Culture for *Salmonella* species, *Shigella* species, and *Campylobacter jejuni*	Routine stool cultures have a relatively low yield unless blood or mucus is present. Most laboratories now include selective media for *Campylobacter* in routine stool cultures.
	Acute bloody diarrhea, or hemolytic-uremic syndrome	Culture for *Escherichia coli* O157:H7*	SMAC agar is used for this purpose and is now suggested by the CDC for all cases of acute, bloody diarrhea.
		Assay for Shiga toxin†	This assay is necessary as a screen for Shiga toxin–producing strains of *E. coli* other than O157:H7.†
	Shellfish ingestion or seacoast exposure within 3 days of onset of diarrhea	Culture for *Vibrio* species*	Selective thiosulfate–citrate–bile salts–sucrose (TCBS) agar is used for this purpose.‡
	Fall or winter months in at-risk populations, or persistent abdominal pain or fever	Culture for *Yersinia* species	Cefsulodin-irgasan-novobiocin agar, incubated at room temperature, is used for this purpose.
	Recent antibiotics, chemotherapy, or hospitalization	Assay for *Clostridium difficile* toxins A ± B	Toxin assay rather than culture is preferred for routine use.
	Outbreak of diarrhea during summer months; severe diarrhea without other explanation	Culture for *Aeromonas hydrophila*	Cefsulodin-irgasan-novobiocin agar is incubated at 95° F (37° C).‡
Persistent diarrhea lasting more than 7 days	None	Evaluation for ova and parasites§	"Stool for ova and parasites" has a low yield in diarrhea of short duration.
	Advanced HIV disease	Evaluation for ova and parasites, as above, and also for *Microsporidia* species and *Mycobacterium avium* complex	Stool should also be processed for the same pathogens associated with acute, community-acquired diarrhea in immunocompetent persons.

CDC, Centers for Disease Control and Prevention; *HIV,* human immunodeficiency virus; *SMAC,* Sorbitol-MacConkey; *TCBS,* thiosulfate–citrate–bile salts–sucrose; *TMP/SMX,* trimethoprim-sulfamethoxazole.
*These cultures require selective media.
†Assay for Shiga toxin is necessary because strains of *E. coli* other than O157:H7 sometimes produce this toxin and will not be identified with standard culture media. Such strains (that is, Shiga toxin positive but O157:H7 negative) should be sent to a reference laboratory for further identification.
‡Alternatively, colonies isolated on blood agar can be screened for a positive oxidase reaction.
§Evaluation for parasites now includes not only a standard microscopic examination of stool but also immunologic tests (immunofluorescence, enzyme immunoassay) for *Giardia lamblia* and *Cryptosporidium parvum* and acid-fast stains for *Cryptosporidium, Cyclospora, Isospora,* and *Mycobacterium* species.

as Pedialyte and Ceralyte (see Chapter 4). Patients become less thirsty as they become rehydrated, which helps protect against overhydration. Replacement of vitamin A and zinc is recommended for persons with likely deficiency of either.

Antimotility drugs provide symptomatic relief, with the caveat that they can make dysentery syndromes much worse. Some authorities believe, however, that the risk of antimotility drugs may have been overestimated. Use of antimotility drugs should be avoided in patients with bloody diarrhea,

patients who might have colitis caused by *Clostridium difficile,* and patients with bloody diarrhea or proven infection with Shiga toxin–producing *E. coli.*

Specific antimicrobial therapy for diarrhea is recommended for at least five situations commonly encountered in primary care in the United States: traveler's diarrhea, shigellosis, *C. difficile* colitis, *C. jejuni* infection, and *Salmonella* gastroenteritis in persons >50 years of age. Rationales and treatment regimens are discussed more fully later in the chapter.

KEY POINTS

INFECTIOUS DIARRHEA: OVERVIEW

⊃ Diarrhea should be considered "medically important" if any of the following features are present: high fever; severe volume depletion; severe abdominal pain, especially in a person >50 years of age; dysentery syndrome; bloody diarrhea; renal failure; hemolytic anemia; or immunocompromised state.

⊃ Patients with diarrhea sufficiently severe to prompt an office visit should be instructed to bring with them a stool specimen (most conveniently, in a clean container such as a cup or glass jar placed in a brown paper bag). Stool containing blood or mucus can be examined for fecal leukocytes. Stool cultures and toxin assays are indicated on a selective basis.

⊃ Small bowel diarrhea (noninflammatory diarrhea) accounts for most episodes (about 90%) of infectious diarrhea in community practice. It is characterized by infrequent, large, watery bowel movements with little or no fever.

⊃ Large bowel diarrhea (inflammatory diarrhea, dysentery) is characterized by frequent small bowel movements accompanied by pain on defecation (tenesmus), blood or mucus in the stool, and frequently fever.

⊃ Symptomatic treatment of infectious diarrhea includes rehydration, preferably by the oral route, and judicious use of antimotility drugs. The latter should be avoided in patients with severe inflammatory diarrhea and especially in children with hemorrhagic colitis.

⊃ Specific antimicrobial therapy is recommended for several diarrheal diseases, notably traveler's diarrhea, shigellosis, *C. difficile* colitis, salmonellosis in persons with risk factors including age >50 years, and various parasitic infections.

SUGGESTED READING

Aranda-Michel J, Giannella RA. Acute diarrhea: a practical review. Am J Med 1999; 106: 670-676.

DuPont HL The Practice Parameters Committee of the American College of Gastroenterology. Guidelines on acute infectious diarrhea in adults. Am J Gastroenterol 1997; 92: 1962-1975.

Guerrant RL, Van Gilder T, Steiner TS, et al. Practice guidelines for the management of infectious diarrhea. Clin Infect Dis 2001; 32: 331-350.

Hennessy TW, Hedberg CW, Slutsker L, et al. The Investigation Team. A national outbreak of *Salmonella enteritidis* infections from ice cream. N Engl J Med 1996; 334: 1281-1286.

Linder JD, Monkemuller KE, Raijman I, et al. Cocaine-associated ischemic colitis. South Med J 2000; 93: 909-913.

Slutsker L, Ries AA, Greene KD, et al. *Escherichia coli* O157:H7 diarrhea in the United States: clinical and epidemiologic features. Ann Intern Med 1997; 126: 505-513.

Surawicz CM, ed. Infectious diarrhea. Gastroenterol Clin North Am 2001; 30: 599-861.

Shiga Toxin–Producing Escherichia Coli (Escherichia Coli O157:H7 and Other Serotypes)

Strains of *E. coli* that produce Shiga toxin, also known as enterohemorrhagic *E. coli* strains, were recognized in the United States in 1982 and now cause an estimated 20,000 cases of diarrheal disease each year. Although uncommon in primary care (<1% of all cases of infectious diarrhea), these strains can cause severe hemorrhagic colitis, the hemolytic-uremic syndrome, and thrombotic thrombocytopenic purpura.

Presentation and Progression
Cause

E. coli O157:H7 differs from most *E. coli* strains by its production of one or more Shiga toxins and by its inability to ferment sorbitol. Other serotypes of *E. coli* sometimes produce Shiga toxins, but these are uncommon in the United States. These *E. coli* strains adhere tightly to mucosal cells, especially in the ascending and transverse colon. The toxin molecule damages mucosal cells and also enters the systemic circulation, where it causes vascular and endothelial damage that can lead to capillary leak syndrome, thrombosis, hemolysis, and renal failure.

Most human infections have been transmitted by beef and are thought to result from fecal contamination of meat during slaughter. Undercooked hamburger meat has been famously associated with *E. coli* O157:H7 outbreaks. It has been estimated that a hamburger purchased at a fast food restaurant in the United States contains meat from as many as 1000 cows. Outbreaks have also been associated with the ingestion of unchlorinated drinking water, unpasteurized apple cider, alfalfa sprouts, leaf lettuce, mesclun lettuce, radish sprouts, milk, and other foods and beverages. New standards for food processing have been introduced in the United States with the aim of reducing the prevalence of this pathogen. However, the infectious dose is low, possibly as low as 100 bacteria. Therefore prevention is difficult and person-to-person spread may occur.

Presentation

After an incubation period of 3 to 4 days (range 1 to 8 days), the classic onset of crampy abdominal pain and bloody stools occurs. The pain is often severe and out of proportion to the findings on physical examination of the abdomen. About one third of patients have fever, which characteristically follows the appearance of blood in the stool. Some persons infected with *E. coli* O157:H7 remain asymptomatic, and others experience crampy abdominal pain with little or no diarrhea. Most patients, however, have bloody diarrhea caused by hemorrhagic colitis. Data from large series suggest that up to 90% of patients have bloody diarrhea at some point during the illness and about 60% of patients have blood in their stools at the time of presentation. Severe abdominal pain before the onset of fever often suggests acute appendicitis, and pain combined with bloody stools suggests inflammatory colitis.

Diagnosis

Acute bloody diarrhea is an urgent medical problem. Baseline studies include urinalysis and measurement of hemoglobin, serum albumin, and serum creatinine, since results of these studies may become abnormal later in the illness. Plain films of the abdomen may show imprinting of the bowel mucosa like that seen in ischemic colitis. *E. coli* O157:H7 can be distinguished from other *E. coli* strains by its translucent colonies on sorbitol-MacConkey agar. After such colonies are confirmed as *E. coli* by the usual biochemical reactions, they can be tested with antisera to the O157 antigen. The CDC recommends that all stools from patients with bloody diarrhea be screened for this *E. coli* serotype. Screening for serotypes other than *E. coli* O157:H7 that produce Shiga toxin is currently based on testing for the toxin by enzyme immunoassay (EIA), since selective culture media for such serotypes have not yet been developed. An EIA kit is available for this purpose. *E. coli* isolates that have been presumptively identified as O157:H7 or that test positive for the Shiga toxin should be sent to a reference laboratory for confirmation or further identification.

Natural History
Expected Outcome

Hemorrhagic colitis from *E. coli* O157:H7 is a severe disease, necessitating hospitalization in about one quarter to one half of patients and carrying a 1% to 2% mortality rate. Mortality is higher in the very young and the elderly. In the absence of complications the illness usually resolves in about 1 week. Serious complications occur most commonly in children <10 years of age. The hemolytic-uremic syndrome develops in up to 9% of children with *E. coli* O157:H7 and is manifested as the triad of hemolytic anemia, thrombocytopenia, and acute renal failure. The illness is called thrombotic thrombocytopenic purpura when further complicated by fever and neurologic symptoms and signs. About 50% of patients with the hemolytic-uremic syndrome require dialysis, about 3% to 5% die of the disease, and up to 10% have permanent residua. The hemolytic-uremic syndrome is now the most common cause of acute renal failure in children in the United States and is associated with *E. coli* in over half of all cases.

Treatment
Methods

Treatment is supportive. However, use of antimotility drugs should be avoided because they tend to increase the duration of exposure to toxin. In a recent study, treatment with trimethoprim-sulfamethoxazole (TMP/SMX) or a β-lactam antibiotic was associated with a 17-fold increase in the incidence of hemolytic-uremic syndrome. Antibiotic treatment of children <10 years of age is therefore strongly discouraged. Therapeutic strategies designed to prevent absorption of the toxin or to neutralize its systemic effect are under active investigation. Prompt and adequate hydration is the cornerstone of therapy and may ameliorate the effects of diffuse endothelial damage such as capillary leak syndrome, thrombosis, hemolytic anemia, and renal failure.

Expected Results

Most patients recover with supportive therapy.

When to Refer

Patients with severe abdominal pain and bloody diarrhea, especially young children and elderly persons, should be hospitalized.

 KEY POINTS

SHIGA TOXIN–PRODUCING ESCHERICHIA COLI (ESCHERICHIA COLI O157:H7 AND OTHER SEROTYPES)

⊃ Stool cultures are positive for *E. coli* O157:H7 in up to 8% of patients with infectious diarrhea whose stools are visibly bloody.

⊃ Hemorrhagic colitis suspected to be caused by *E. coli* O157:H7 requires hospitalization because of the potential for severe complications such as hemolytic-uremic syndrome.
⊃ Use of antimotility drugs should be avoided in children, since they increase the duration and extent of exposure to the toxin.
⊃ Use of TMP/SMX or β-lactam antibiotics carries a 17-fold increased risk of hemolytic-uremic syndrome. Antibiotic therapy should therefore be discouraged.

SUGGESTED READING
Jackson LA, Keene WA, McAnulty JM, et al. Where's the beef? The role of cross-contamination in 4 chain restaurant–associated outbreaks of *Escherichia coli* O157:H7 in the Pacific Northwest. Arch Intern Med 2000; 160: 2380-2385.
Mead PS, Griffin PM. *Escherichia coli* O157:H7. Lancet 1998; 352: 1207-1212.
Su C, Brandt LJ. *Escherichia coli* O157:H7 infection in humans. Ann Intern Med 1995; 123: 698-714.
Tarr PI, Neill MA. *Escherichia coli* O157:H7. Gastroenterol Clin North Am 2001; 30: 735-751.
Wong CS, Jelacic S, Habeeb RL, et al. The risk of the hemolytic-uremic syndrome after antibiotic treatment of *Escherichia coli* O157:H7 infections. N Engl J Med 2000; 342: 1930-1936.

Salmonella Species Other Than Salmonella Typhi (Salmonellosis)

Gastroenteritis caused by nontyphoidal *Salmonella* strains is extremely common in the United States, with an estimated 0.8 to 3.7 million cases each year. Many cases, and probably the vast majority of sporadic cases, go unrecognized. Outbreaks are usually associated with food products. Between 1985 and 1994, *S. enteritidis* was identified with 582 outbreaks that accounted for 28,058 cases of disease, 2290 hospitalizations, and 70 deaths. Typhoid fever (discussed separately later in the chapter) is usually associated with international travel.

Presentation and Progression
Cause

Salmonellae are aerobic gram-negative rods. Recent studies showing high levels of DNA similarity among *Salmonella* isolates have led to the reclassification of all clinically important salmonellae into a single species, *Salmonella choleraesuis*. This species has seven subgroups, and more than 2300 serovars are recognized based on three major antigens (the somatic O, surface Vi, flagellar H antigens). Most clinical laboratory reports continue to identify isolates by their familiar names, for example, *Salmonella typhimurium* rather than *Salmonella choleraesuis* serotype *typhimurium*.

Although *S. typhi* and *S. paratyphi* colonize only humans, nontyphoidal *Salmonella* strains are widespread throughout the animal kingdom. Human disease is usually associated with food products, most commonly poultry and eggs. Infection of poultry flocks is widespread. Ingestion of uncooked or lightly cooked eggs is therefore a risk factor for disease. However, outbreaks and cases have been linked to numerous foods, including tomatoes, alfalfa sprouts, cantaloupe, and freshly squeezed orange juice. Some patients with salmonellosis give a history of keeping exotic pets, especially reptiles, of which up to 90% harbor *Salmonella* organisms.

Salmonella infection is frequently asymptomatic. No reliable serologic test has been developed, and a single negative stool culture does not exclude the possibility that a food handler might be an intermittent shedder of *Salmonella* organisms. Given both the wide distribution of *Salmonella* in foodstuffs and the frequency of asymptomatic *Salmonella* carriage, it is difficult to envision how any restaurant might prevent the occasional case of *Salmonella* transmission despite emphasis on hygienic practices. *Salmonella* infection is a risk of everyday life, especially for persons who dine out frequently.

Salmonella infection nearly always arises because of ingestion of the bacteria. Gastric acidity is the first line of host defense, since *Salmonella* survives poorly if at all at the normal gastric pH (<1.5). On the basis of previous data, it has been accepted that ingestion of $>10^5$ *Salmonella* organisms is necessary to cause disease. However, more recent data indicate that a lower inoculum ($>10^3$ organisms) can cause disease. Because *Salmonella* survives well at pH values of 4.0 or higher, persons who have atrophic gastritis (which is common among the elderly) or are taking gastric pH–raising medications (antacids, H_2-blockers, or proton pump inhibitors) are at increased risk of salmonellosis. Containment of *Salmonella* infection depends on an intact T-lymphocyte system, including macrophage function. Persons at risk for serious consequences of *Salmonella* infection include those with impaired T-cell function because of lympho-proliferative disorders, other malignancies, HIV disease, or immunosuppressive medication and those with disorders that cause "macrophage blockade," such as hemoglobinopathies (notably sickle cell disease), bartonellosis, malaria, schistosomiasis, and disseminated histoplasmosis.

Presentation

The five recognized syndromes of salmonellosis are gastroenteritis, enteric fever (discussed separately later in the chapter), bacteremia and endovascular infection, localized metastatic infections, and the asymptomatic carrier state.

Gastroenteritis caused by nontyphoidal *Salmonella* is usually manifested as nausea, vomiting, and diarrhea 6 to 48 hours after the ingestion of contaminated food or water. A high inoculum of *Salmonella* correlates with increased severity and duration of the illness. The stools are usually loose, of moderate volume, and without blood. Occasionally the presentation is the classic "small bowel diarrhea" with large-volume, watery stools or the classic "large bowel diarrhea" with small-volume stools accompanied by tenesmus (Table 12-2). Fever, chills, nausea, vomiting, and abdominal cramps are common. Occasionally, right lower quadrant pain suggesting acute appendicitis dominates the clinical picture (pseudoappendicitis).

Bacteremia is documented, when sought, in up to 4% of immunocompetent persons with *Salmonella* gastroenteritis. Unrecognized episodes of transient bacteremia are probably common. More prolonged bacteremia correlates with immunosuppression. Multiple positive blood cultures for *Salmonella* should raise the possibility of intravascular infection, including mycotic aneurysm (see Chapter 6) or endocarditis.

Localized metastatic infection occurs in up to 10% of patients. The major syndromes are as follows:

- Endocarditis occurs in up to 0.4% (or 1 in 250) patients with *Salmonella* bacteremia, usually in persons with pre-existing heart disease.
- Central nervous system infections, including meningitis, ventriculitis, and brain abscess, are more common in infants, especially neonates.
- Osteomyelitis and septic arthritis are encountered most frequently in persons with sickle cell disease, bone disease, or immunosuppression. Osteomyelitis caused by *Salmonella* species most commonly affects the femur, tibia, humerus, or lumbar vertebrae. Septic arthritis caused by *Salmonella* species most commonly affects the knee, hip, or shoulder. Reactive arthritis affecting multiple joints occurs most often in persons who have the HLA-B27 histocompatibility antigen (see Chapter 15).
- Soft tissue infections usually occur in the setting of local trauma and immunosuppression.
- Urinary tract infection usually occurs in the setting of ureteral or bladder stones, malignancy, renal transplants, or, in some parts of the world, schistosomiasis. Successful treatment often requires attention to structural abnormalities.
- Other complications are pneumonia, hepatobiliary infection, splenic infection, and genital infections.

The asymptomatic carrier state develops in 0.2% to 0.6% of persons with nontyphoidal salmonellosis and is more common in women and in persons with abnormalities of the biliary tract. The long-term carrier state is defined by persistence of *Salmonella* in stool or urine cultures for >1 year.

Diagnosis

Salmonella is readily isolated from stool cultures, although at least 48 hours of incubation is generally required. The role of serologic tests in diagnosis is negligible.

Natural History
Expected Outcome

Salmonella gastroenteritis is usually a self-limited illness, lasting 3 to 7 days. Fever generally resolves within 47 to 72 hours. Diarrhea lasting >10 days should suggest another diagnosis. The mean duration of carriage, as determined by follow-up stool cultures, is about 4 to 5 weeks but varies according to the serotype. The mortality for *Salmonella* gastroenteritis is <0.5%, with most deaths occurring in severely debilitated persons. Bacteremia with metastatic infection, however, carries high mortality in some situations (see earlier discussion).

Treatment
Methods

There is wide agreement that antimicrobial therapy is not indicated for *Salmonella* gastroenteritis unless disease is severe, with high fever and frequent stools (more than nine per day), or unless specific risk factors are present, including age <1 year or >50 years, vascular grafts, or the presence of a disorder affecting T lymphocytes or phagocytes (Table 12-4). The disease is usually self-limited. All antimicrobials, including the fluoroquinolones, seem to prolong the carriage state. Relapse may follow discontinuation of antibiotics.

Treatment of major systemic complications of *Salmonella* infection currently relies mainly on the fluoroquinolones or

TABLE 12-4
Recommended Drug Therapy for Specific Pathogens Causing Diarrhea

Pathogen	Drug of choice	Alternative drugs	Comments
Enterotoxigenic *Escherichia coli* (traveler's diarrhea)	Fluoroquinolone (e.g., ciprofloxacin 500 mg b.i.d., norfloxacin 400 mg b.i.d., or ofloxacin 300 mg b.i.d.) for 3 days*	TMP/SMX 160 mg/800 mg (one double-strength tablet) b.i.d. for 3 days	Drug therapy reduces the duration of traveler's diarrhea from 3 to 5 days to <1 to 2 days.
Shigella species	Fluoroquinolone (e.g., ciprofloxacin 500 mg b.i.d., norfloxacin 400 mg b.i.d., or ofloxacin 300 mg b.i.d.) for 3 days*	TMP/SMX 160 mg/800 mg (one double-strength tablet) b.i.d. for 3 days; ceftriaxone; azithromycin	Many *Shigella* strains are now resistant to TMP/SMX and also to ampicillin, a former drug of choice.
Clostridium difficile	Metronidazole 250 mg q.i.d. for 10 days	Vancomycin 125 mg PO q.i.d. for 10 days	Some gastroenterologists prefer vancomycin for more severely ill patients.
Salmonella species in a patient with risk factors†	Fluoroquinolone (e.g., ciprofloxacin 500 mg b.i.d., norfloxacin 400 mg b.i.d., or ofloxacin 300 mg b.i.d.) for 5 to 7 days*	TMP/SMX 160 mg/800 mg (one double-strength tablet) b.i.d. for 5 to 7 days	Treatment is not generally recommended for patients without risk factors.
Campylobacter jejuni, severe disease	Erythromycin, 500 mg PO b.i.d. for 5 days	Fluoroquinolone (same drugs and doses as above) for 5 days*	Antibiotic therapy is recommended only for severe cases. Resistance to fluoroquinolones is being reported.
Yersinia species, severe disease	Fluoroquinolone (e.g., ciprofloxacin 500 mg b.i.d., norfloxacin 400 mg b.i.d., or ofloxacin 300 mg b.i.d.) for 5 to 7 days*	TMP/SMX 160 mg/800 mg (one double-strength tablet) b.i.d. for 5 to 7 days or doxycycline	For immunocompromised patients, severe infections, or bacteremia, hospitalization and combination therapy with doxycycline or an aminoglycoside can be used. Septicemia caused by *Yersinia* species is associated with a high case-fatality rate.
Vibrio cholerae O1 or O39	Fluoroquinolone (one dose)*	Doxycycline 300 mg (one dose), tetracycline 500 mg q.i.d. for 3 days, or TMP/SMX 160 mg/800 mg (one double-strength tablet) b.i.d. for 3 days	Antibiotic therapy is secondary to aggressive rehydration.
Aeromonas or *Plesiomonas*	Fluoroquinolone (e.g., ciprofloxacin 500 mg b.i.d., norfloxacin 400 mg b.i.d., or ofloxacin 300 mg b.i.d.) for 3 days	TMP/SMX (if susceptible) 160 mg/800 mg (one double-strength tablet) b.i.d. for 3 days	Anecdotal experience and small studies suggest that antimicrobial therapy may be of value for diarrhea caused by *Aeromonas* and *Plesiomonas* species, but controlled trials are lacking.
Giardia lamblia	Metronidazole 250 to 750 mg t.i.d. for 7 to 10 days	Tinidazole, quinacrine HCl, or furazolidone	Relapses may occur after treatment.
Entamoeba histolytica	Metronidazole (750 mg t.i.d. for 5 to 10 days) plus either iodoquinol (650 mg t.i.d. for 20 days) or paromomycin	Dehydroemetine 1 to 1.5 mg/kg/day IM for 5 days (rarely used; available only through CDC)	Iodoquinol and paromomycin are used to treat invasive intestinal infection and liver abscess. Asymptomatic cyst passers (500 mg t.i.d. for 7 days) can be treated with a luminal agent only (i.e., metronidazole).
Cryptosporidium species, severe case	Paromomycin 500 mg t.i.d. (see comments)	Azithromycin; hyperimmune bovine colostrums; consider nitazoxanide (compassionate use)	Optimum duration of treatment is not established; suggested treatment is 7 days for severe cases or indefinitely (at b.i.d. rather than t.i.d. dose) for patients with advanced HIV disease.

Continued

TABLE 12-4—cont'd
Recommended Drug Therapy for Specific Pathogens Causing Diarrhea

Pathogen	Drug of choice	Alternative drugs	Comments
Isospora species	TMP/SMX 160 mg/800 mg (one double-strength tablet), q.i.d. for 10 days, then b.i.d. for 3 weeks	Pyrimethamine plus folinic acid	Patients with severe HIV disease may require indefinite maintenance therapy.
Cyclospora species	TMP/SMX 160 mg/800 mg (one double-strength tablet), b.i.d. for 7 days		
Microsporidia species, immunocompromised patient	Albendazole 200 to 400 mg PO b.i.d. for 3 weeks or longer		Available for compassionate use only. Albendazole is more effective against *Encephalitozoon intestinalis* than against *Enterocytozoon bieneusi*.

CDC, Centers for Disease Control and Prevention; *HIV*, human immunodeficiency virus; *TMP/SMX*, trimethoprim-sulfamethoxazole.
*Fluoroquinolones are contraindicated in persons <16 years of age (see Chapter 19).
†Risk factors for severe *Salmonella* infection, including metastatic infection occurring during transient bacteremia: age <6 months or >50 years (older persons are at risk of mycotic aneurysm of the aorta; see Chapter 6), sickle cell disease (risk of osteomyelitis; see Chapter 15), prosthetic device, malignancy, uremia, HIV disease.

third-generation cephalosporins (notably ceftriaxone). Emerging resistance of *Salmonella* to these and other antimicrobials continues to be a source of great concern.

The long-term carrier state can be treated with TMP/SMX (one double-strength tablet for 3 months) or ampicillin. Both have been associated with cure rates >80%, which seems paradoxic in view of their apparent inability to eradicate the organism during active disease.

Expected Results

Treatment of *Salmonella* gastroenteritis, according to most studies, achieves only a modest clinical benefit. Antimicrobial therapy may reduce the number of bacteria in stools (even while prolonging the carriage state) and may therefore be useful in limiting epidemics in closed settings. Follow-up stool cultures are not generally recommended for patients with *Salmonella* gastroenteritis, especially since excretion of the organisms can be intermittent.

When to Refer

Patients with high fever, severe diarrhea, or dehydration should be hospitalized. Laboratories are required by law to report *Salmonella* isolates to state health departments.

 KEY POINTS

SALMONELLA SPECIES OTHER THAN SALMONELLA TYPHI (SALMONELLOSIS)

⊃ *Salmonella* species are widespread in food products. Because many cases of *Salmonella* gastroenteritis are asymptomatic and intermittent fecal shedding is common, occasional transmission through food handling is inevitable.

⊃ The five syndromes of *Salmonella* infection are gastroenteritis, enteric fever, bacteremia with endovascular infection, localized metastatic infections, and the asymptomatic carrier state.

⊃ *Salmonella* gastroenteritis usually begins with nausea, vomiting, and diarrhea within 6 to 48 hours after ingestion of contaminated food or water. Stools are usually loose, of moderate volume, and without blood. Occasional patients show classic features of "small bowel diarrhea" or "large bowel diarrhea" (Table 12-2), but most patients do not clearly fit into one or the other pattern.

⊃ Treatment of *Salmonella* gastroenteritis is recommended for two groups of patients: those with severe disease, manifested as high fever, frequent stools (more than nine per day), or dehydration, and those predisposed to complications, such as persons <2 years of age or >50 years of age, those with impaired T-cell function, those with disorders that cause "phagocyte blockade," and those with vascular grafts.

SUGGESTED READING

Baumler AJ, Hargis BM, Tsolis RM. Tracing the origins of *Salmonella* outbreaks. Science 2000; 287: 50-52.

Dunne EF, Fey PD, Kludt P, et al. Emergence of domestically acquired ceftriaxone-resistant *Salmonella* infections associated with ampC β-lactamase. JAMA 2000; 284: 3151-3156.

Hohmann EL. Nontyphoidal salmonellosis. Clin Infect Dis 2001; 32: 263-269.

Shimoni Z, Pitlik S, Leibovici L, et al. Nontyphoid *Salmonella* bacteremia: age-related differences in clinical presentation, bacteriology, and outcome. Clin Infect Dis 1999; 28: 822-827.

Shigella Species (Shigellosis)

Shigella species are the classic agents of dysentery (Table 12-2) and are highly communicable. Shigellosis remains an important cause of morbidity and mortality in developing countries, mainly in children. At least 19,000 cases occur in the United States each year.

Presentation and Progression
Cause

Shigella are gram-negative bacilli with four recognized serogroups: group A (*S. dysenteriae*), group B (*S. flexneri*), group C (*S. boydii*), and group D (*S. sonnei*). Within these four serogroups are about 40 serotypes, of which *S. dysenteriae* serotype 1 (also known as the Shiga bacillus) causes the most severe disease. *S. sonnei* now accounts for about 60% to 80% of cases of shigellosis in the United States.

Like *Salmonella*, *Shigella* can contaminate food and water, causing occasional common source outbreaks. However, person-to-person transmission is the dominant mode of transmission. As few as 10 to 100 *Shigella* organisms can cause disease; therefore shigellosis is highly communicable. After exposure to a case of shigellosis in a household, the disease develops in about 40% of persons between 1 and 4 years of age and about 20% of persons of all ages. Outbreaks of shigellosis occur in crowded, closed environments such as nurseries, day care centers, institutions, and cruise ships.

After ingestion, *Shigella* organisms multiply in the small intestine, resulting in concentrations of 10^7 to 10^9 bacteria per milliliter of intestinal fluid. Symptoms commonly result from small intestinal involvement, but the hallmark symptoms of shigellosis result from mucosal invasion and toxin production in the colon. Inflammation is severe but relatively superficial, and bacteremia is therefore uncommon.

Presentation

Shigellosis occurs most often during the summer months and in children between 1 and 4 years of age. The usual incubation period is 1 to 7 days (average, 3 days). Initial symptoms of small bowel involvement are fever and crampy abdominal pain. Within a few days pain and tenderness become localized to the lower quadrants of the abdomen and are accompanied by urgency, tenesmus, and small stools that usually contain mucus and blood. Overall, fever occurs in about 30% to 40% of patients, vomiting in about 35%, abdominal pain in 70% to 90%, and diarrhea in most. Patients usually pass 8 to 10 stools per day but can have as many as 100 stools per day. Significant fluid loss leading to dehydration seldom occurs. *S. sonnei*, the dominant serogroup in the United States, usually causes milder disease than the other serogroups and in some cases the diarrhea remains watery.

Diagnosis

Shigellosis should be suspected in all cases of dysentery (Table 12-2). Findings on physical examination, which may include tenderness over the lower abdominal quadrants, are nonspecific. Fecal leukocytes are present and provide an important clue to the nature of the process (Table 12-2). Diagnosis is established by isolation of *Shigella* species on stool culture, but these bacteria are relatively fastidious. Culture of a stool specimen provides a higher yield than culture based on a rectal swab specimen, and the highest yield comes from the mucoid portion of the stool.

Natural History
Expected Outcome

Untreated, shigellosis is usually a self-limited disease, typically lasting 1 to 30 days (average, 7 days). Deaths occur mainly in malnourished young children and in the elderly. However, epidemics caused by the Shiga bacillus can cause mortality rates of up to 20%. Complications of shigellosis are more common with serogroups other than *S. sonnei* and include proctitis or rectal prolapse (in infants and young children), toxic megacolon, intestinal obstruction, perforation of the colon, leukemoid reaction, bacteremia, seizures, hemolytic-uremic syndrome, thrombotic thrombocytopenic purpura, and reactive arthritis, including Reiter's syndrome (see Chapter 15).

Malnutrition sometimes complicates shigellosis and is due in part to protein-losing enteropathy.

Treatment
Methods

Although most cases of shigellosis are self-limited, antibiotics such as ampicillin and tetracycline shorten the duration of the illness. Some authorities believe that antibiotics should be reserved for the most severely ill patients, especially since drug-resistant *Shigella* strains continue to pose a major problem. TMP/SMX is generally the drug of choice when the sensitivity pattern of the infecting microorganism is unknown. However, resistance to TMP/SMX is increasing (59% of 430 recent isolates from Oregon were resistant to TMP/SMX; none were resistant to ciprofloxacin). Azithromycin has been used recently to treat shigellosis caused by strains resistant to multiple drugs.

Expected Results

Successful treatment typically shortens the duration of the illness, but the disease is usually self-limited.

When to Refer

Patients with shigellosis who have severe systemic toxicity should be admitted to the hospital.

 KEY POINTS

SHIGELLA SPECIES (SHIGELLOSIS)

⊃ *Shigella* species are the classic cause of dysentery and are highly communicable, since only a few organisms (<200) are necessary to cause disease.

⊃ *S. dysenteriae* serogroup 1 (the Shiga bacillus) is the most virulent of the *Shigella* species and worldwide is an important cause of morbidity and mortality in young children. *S. sonnei*, which causes relatively mild disease, accounts for 60% to 80% of shigellosis in the United States

⊃ The highest attack rates occur in children between 1 and 4 years of age.

⊃ Shigellosis should be suspected when acute diarrhea is characterized by systemic toxicity and frequent, small-volume, bloody stools with tenesmus. Fecal leukocytes are present and provide a clue to the diagnosis. Milder cases do not require antimicrobial therapy.

SUGGESTED READING

Khan WA, Dhar U, Salam MA, et al. Central nervous system manifestations of childhood shigellosis: prevalence, risk factors, and outcome. Pediatrics 1999; 103: E18.

Khan WA, Seas C, Dhar U, et al. Treatment of shigellosis. V. Comparison of azithromycin and ciprofloxacin: a double blind, randomized, controlled trial. Ann Intern Med 1997; 126: 697-703.

Kotloff KL, Winickoff JP, Ivanoff B, et al. Global burden of *Shigella* infections: implications for vaccine development and implementation of control strategies. Bull World Health Org 1999; 77: 651-666.

Martin JM, Pitetti R, Maffei F, et al. Treatment of shigellosis with cefixime: two days vs. five days. Pediatr Infect Dis J 2000; 19: 522-526.

Replogle ML, Fleming DW, Cieslak PR. Emergence of antimicrobial-resistant *Shigella* in Oregon. Clin Infect Dis 2000; 30: 515-519.

Campylobacter Species

Diarrhea caused by *C. jejuni* is one of the most common infectious diseases worldwide. More than 1 million cases occur each year in the United States, where *Campylobacter* is isolated from stool cultures more frequently than either *Salmonella* or *Shigella* species. *C. jejuni* is therefore an important pathogen in primary care. *Campylobacter fetus* is encountered much less frequently and causes a bacteremic illness.

Presentation and Progression
Cause

Campylobacter species are small, comma-shaped or curved, gram-negative bacilli, of which *C. jejuni* and *C. fetus* are of medical importance. *C. jejuni* causes an intestinal infection manifested as acute gastroenteritis and colitis. *C. fetus* is more likely to cause a systemic infection with bacteremia, meningitis, intravascular infections including endocarditis, and metastatic abscesses. Human disease is predominantly foodborne but can result from direct contact with animals, including household pets (notably puppies or kittens with diarrhea). Fecal-oral transmission occurs, and men who have sex with men are at increased risk. However, transmission from food handlers appears to be uncommon. Some studies suggest that disease can result from ingestion of as few as 500 bacilli. Like *Salmonella*, *Campylobacter* is inhibited by hydrochloric acid in the stomach and might therefore occur more commonly when gastric pH is raised because of gastritis or medications. *Campylobacter* species invade the intestinal mucosa and also elaborate various extracellular toxins with cytopathic activities.

Presentation

C. jejuni causes disease throughout the year in the United States, but sharp peaks of *Campylobacter* disease occur during the summer and early fall. The disease especially affects children <1 year of age and persons between 15 and 29 years of age. This pattern in the United States contrasts sharply with the pattern in developing countries, where *Campylobacter* affects persons of all ages and especially those in the first 5 years of life. Mishandling of raw poultry and consumption of undercooked poultry are now considered the major risk factors for *Campylobacter* infection.

The incubation period of *C. jejuni* gastroenteritis is usually between 1 and 7 days (average, 2 to 4 days). In about two thirds of cases the disease begins with abdominal pain and diarrhea. The remaining patients have a prodrome that suggests a flulike illness (see later discussion). Pain is often severe and can be the predominant symptom. In other patients fever is the predominant manifestation of the disease. The diarrhea can consist of frequent loose stools, massive watery stools, or grossly bloody stools. Most patients (at least 50% in one study) have 10 or more bowel movements on the worst day of the illness. Gross blood is commonly present in bowel movement during the second and third days of the illness. Mild leukocytosis is often present.

Three presentations of *C. jejuni* gastroenteritis merit special comment:

■ A flulike prodrome occurs in about one third of patients and is characterized by high fever, chills, myalgias, dizziness, and delirium. These patients tend to have severe disease.

■ A pseudoappendicitis syndrome, manifested as pain and tenderness in the right lower quadrant, occurs most often in children between 6 and 15 years of age. True rebound tenderness is absent, and ultrasound examination suggests enteritis involving the enterocecal region rather than appendicitis. *C. jejuni* has been isolated in up to 3% of persons undergoing surgery for acute appendicitis.

■ Acute colitis, with bloody diarrhea as the disease manifestation, can raise the possibility of ulcerative colitis or Crohn's disease. *C. jejuni* infection should therefore be considered as a cause of acute inflammatory bowel disease, especially since this infection tends to occur in the same age groups as ulcerative colitis and Crohn's disease.

Other complications of *Campylobacter* infection are cholecystitis, pancreatitis, hepatitis, peritonitis, hemolytic-uremic syndrome, and exacerbation of preexisting inflammatory bowel disease.

C. fetus infection less commonly causes diarrhea, although nonspecific abdominal pain may be the initial manifestation. *C. fetus* infection can cause a prolonged relapsing illness with fever, chills, and myalgias. This microorganism exhibits a marked predilection for vascular sites. Endocarditis, pericarditis, and thrombophlebitis all occur.

Diagnosis

Fecal leukocytes are often present. Isolation of *Campylobacter* species from stool specimens requires selective media (generally, blood-based, antibiotic-containing media) and an atmosphere with 5% to 10% oxygen, 1% to 10% carbon dioxide, and ideally some hydrogen as well. Stool samples should be kept cool before culture. Microscopic examination of Gram stain of stool is useful if comma-shaped, gram-negative bacilli are present, a finding with high specificity but relatively low sensitivity (50% to 75%). *C. jejuni* is occasionally isolated from blood cultures. Blood cultures are customarily used to isolate *C. fetus*, with the caveat that the organism is usually slow growing.

Natural History
Expected Outcome

Gastroenteritis caused by *C. jejuni* is often self-limited, with gradual resolution occurring over several days. However, about 10% to 20% of persons who seek medical attention for *Campylobacter* gastroenteritis have significant symptoms for >1 week. Diarrhea typically lasts 4 to 5 days (although in one study the mean duration of diarrhea was 11 days). Weight loss of ≥10 pounds is common. Children usually tolerate *Campylobacter* gastroenteritis relatively well. Some patients with gastroenteritis or colitis caused by *C. jejuni* have severe disease, occasionally progressing to toxic megacolon.

Reactive arthritis occurs in about 1% of persons with *C. jejuni* gastroenteritis and is similar to reactive arthritis caused by other microorganisms (see Chapter 15). Guillain-Barré syndrome complicates about 1 in 2000 cases of *C. jejuni* gastroenteritis. However, about 20% to 50% of cases of Guillain-Barré syndrome follow *C. jejuni* infection. A Guillain-Barré variant known as the Miller Fisher syndrome, in which cranial nerves are affected in addition to the ascending polyneuritis, is also associated with *C. jejuni* infection. Current opinion holds that Guillain-Barré syndrome may result from cross-reactivity between a *C. jejuni* epitope and a ganglioside (GM1) present in nerve sheath myelin.

Excretion of *C. jejuni* in stool continues for an average of 2 to 3 months after clinical resolution of infection. Relapse occurs in 5% to 10% of persons after apparently successful eradication of their infections.

Treatment
Methods

As in other cases of diarrheal disease, aggressive fluid and electrolyte replacement is probably more important than antimicrobial therapy. *C. jejuni* is generally sensitive in vitro to macrolides, fluoroquinolones, aminoglycosides, tetracycline, and chloramphenicol. Erythromycin is still considered the drug of first choice when the diagnosis is confirmed, even though about 5% of *C. jejuni* isolates are now resistant to erythromycin. The dose is 500 mg PO b.i.d. for 5 days. For children the dose is 40 mg/kg/day for 5 days. Fluoroquinolones, including ciprofloxacin, have been quite effective therapies for *C. jejuni* infection. However, resistance occurs rapidly.

Treatment of gastroenteritis caused by *C. jejuni* can be problematic because isolation from stool cultures may take several days; the disease is usually self-limited; and the drug of choice, erythromycin, is not the drug of choice for the other common enteric pathogens (Table 12-4). Several courses of action are available:

- Observation with supportive care is appropriate for some patients.
- In patients with severe illness or debilitation, initiation of therapy with a fluoroquinolone may be appropriate, since this will provide broad coverage against various enteric pathogens.
- Erythromycin, the drug of choice, can be given after bacteriologic confirmation of *Campylobacter* infection or when *Campylobacter* infection is a strong likelihood, as in persons who are part of a known outbreak.

C. fetus generally requires intravenous antimicrobial therapy in the hospital setting.

Expected Results

The effect of treatment on the course of *Campylobacter* infection is difficult to evaluate, since many, perhaps most, patients arc improving when treatment is initiated.

When to Refer

Most patients with severe gastroenteritis caused by *C. jejuni* and nearly all patients with *C. fetus* gastroenteritis should be hospitalized.

 KEY POINTS

CAMPYLOBACTER SPECIES

- ⊃ *C. jejuni* is now the most common bacterial pathogen isolated from stool cultures in the United States. An estimated 1 million cases of *Campylobacter* gastroenteritis occur in the United States each year. The disease affects mainly children <1 year of age and adults 15 to 29 years of age.
- ⊃ Abdominal pain and fever can be the dominant clinical features of *C. jejuni* gastroenteritis. Atypical presentations include a severe flulike illness (about one third of patients), a pseudoappendicitis syndrome, and acute colitis suggesting inflammatory bowel disease (ulcerative colitis or Crohn's disease).
- ⊃ *C. fetus* usually causes a bacteremic illness, sometimes with endocarditis.

SUGGESTED READING

Allos BM. *Campylobacter jejuni* infections: update on emerging issues and trends. Clin Infect Dis 2001; 32: 1201-1206.

Altekruse SF, Stern NJ, Fields PI, et al. *Campylobacter jejuni*—an emerging foodborne pathogen. Emerg Infect Dis 1999; 5: 28-35.

Nachamkin I, Allos BM, Ho T. *Campylobacter* species and Guillain-Barré syndrome. Clin Microbiol Rev 1998; 11: 555-567.

Clostridum Difficile and Antibiotic-Associated Colitis

Diarrhea is a relatively common complication of antimicrobial therapy and is associated with *C. difficile* in about 10% to 30% of cases. Pseudomembranous colitis caused by *C. difficile,* the most severe form of antibiotic-associated diarrhea, occurs in about 1 in 10,000 courses of antibiotic therapy in ambulatory patients. Primary care clinicians are likely to encounter *C. difficile* colitis in three groups of patients: patients given broad-spectrum antibiotics, including some of the newer oral cephalosporins; patients recently released from the hospital; and patients in long-term care facilities, such as nursing homes, where *C. difficile* has become a major problem.

Presentation and Progression
Cause

Antibiotics alter the colonic microflora, causing diarrhea by at least two mechanisms: osmotic diarrhea, caused by depletion of bacteria that normally ferment carbohydrates in the gut, and toxin-mediated diarrhea caused by overgrowth of *C. difficile. C. difficile* elaborates two large toxin molecules, an enterotoxin known as toxin A and a cytotoxin known as toxin B. About 60% of adults in the United States have serum antibodies to *C. difficile,* suggesting that asymptomatic colonization is relatively common. Prevalence surveys indicate colonization of the colon by *C. difficile* in about 3% or less of healthy adults, 2% to 8% of elderly persons in nursing homes, and up to 20% of persons who are hospitalized. Person-to-person transmission of *C. difficile* occurs and can be reduced by handwashing before and after patient encounters and by use of disposable gloves (followed by handwashing) during direct contact with patients.

Various antibiotics are associated with *C. difficile* colitis in roughly the following frequencies:

- Frequently associated antibiotics: ampicillin, amoxicillin, cephalosporins, clindamycin
- Occasionally associated antibiotics: penicillins other than ampicillin, including β-lactamase–stable penicillins (antistaphylococcal penicillins); erythromycin and other macrolides; tetracyclines; TMP/SMX; sulfonamides; and fluoroquinolones
- Rarely or never associated antibiotics: metronidazole, vancomycin, chloramphenicol, parenteral aminoglycosides

Third-generation cephalosporins are more likely than the penicillins to predispose to *C. difficile* colitis. The extent to which fluoroquinolones promote *C. difficile* colitis is unclear, but a case-control study suggests an association.

Presentation

Symptoms typically begin 5 to 10 days after a course of antimicrobial therapy but can start as early as the first day of treatment and as late as 10 weeks after treatment has been discontinued. A common presentation consists of acute onset of watery diarrhea with low-grade fever and abdominal pain. The disease ranges in severity from mild to fulminant. Overall, about 30% to 50% of patients have fever and 20% to 33% have abdominal pain. Despite prominent involvement of the rectosigmoid area in most cases, gross blood is seldom present in the stool. Variants of the presentation include the following:

- Antibiotic-associated colitis without pseudomembranes, associated with 5 to 15 or more watery bowel movements a day, leading to dehydration
- Fulminant colitis (2% to 3% of cases) with diarrhea and complications that include perforation, megacolon, and ileus along with high fever, chills, and marked leukocytosis (up to 40,000 white blood cells [WBCs]/mm^3).
- "Acute abdomen" with toxic megacolon but without diarrhea
- Pseudomembranous colitis with protein-losing enteropathy, causing hypoalbuminemia.

  C. difficile colitis can complicate the course of ulcerative colitis or Crohn's disease.

Diagnosis

Fecal polymorphonuclear leukocytes are demonstrated in about 50% of cases of *C. difficile* colitis and are usually present in severe cases. At present, diagnosis is based largely on demonstration of toxins in stool specimens. Various assay methods are available, including eight commercial enzyme-linked immunosorbent assay (ELISA) kits for determining the presence of toxin A and toxin B. In most laboratories these newer assay methods have replaced the cytotoxicity assay, which, however, remains the "gold standard." The newer toxin assays are 63% to 94% sensitive and 75% to 100% specific. Rare strains of *C. difficile* produce toxin B without producing toxin A. Stool culture for *C. difficile* is seldom used in clinical practice, since the organism is a frequent colonizer and up to 25% of *C. difficile* isolates do not produce toxin. Newer methods for diagnosis, such as the polymerase chain reaction (PCR), continue to be developed.

Proctoscopy, sigmoidoscopy, and colonoscopy are generally reserved for cases in which the diagnosis is in doubt. Findings are usually most pronounced in the rectosigmoid area. Colonoscopy is required in about 10% of cases. Overall, endoscopy has a sensitivity of about 45% but a specificity of 100% for *C. difficile* colitis. The finding of raised, yellowish, 2- to 10-mm plaques or pseudomembranes interspersed with "skip" areas of normal mucosa is considered pathognomonic. In severe cases the lesions coalesce, giving an appearance of diffuse colitis. Radiographic findings in severe cases include marked thickening of the colonic wall on CT scan; dilatation of the colon (>6 cm) in cases of toxic megacolon, often with a "thumb sign" of submucosal edema and air-fluid levels suggesting obstruction; and free air under the diaphragm in cases of perforation.

Natural History
Expected Outcome

Most patients recover, but morbidity and mortality occur in elderly patients and patients with severe disease. Toxic megacolon carries a mortality of up to 64%. Rare extraintestinal complications include bacteremia, splenic abscess, osteomyelitis, and reactive arthritis.

Treatment
Methods

Current recommendations of the American College of Gastroenterology and the Society for Healthcare Epidemiology of America include the following:

- Discontinue the offending antibiotic if possible. If continuation of antimicrobial therapy is necessary, choose an agent less frequently associated with *C. difficile* colitis, such as fluoroquinolone.
- Replace fluid and electrolyte losses.
- Avoid use of antimotility drugs.
- If the above measures do not suffice, or if the disease is moderately severe, prescribe metronidazole 250 mg q.i.d. for 10 days.

  Vancomycin is reserved for patients who fail to respond to metronidazole, who cannot tolerate vancomycin, or who are critically ill. Treatment of asymptomatic carriers of *C. difficile* is not recommended. Two drugs not available in the United States, oral teicoplanin and fusidic acid, have been shown to be as effective as oral vancomycin and oral metronidazole in controlled studies.

Expected Results

Metronidazole and vancomycin are both associated with cure rates of about 94% to 95%. However, relapses occur in 5% to 20% of treated patients. Recurrences should be treated as for first episodes. Attempts to eradicate the carrier state have been disappointing. Occasional patients have persistent symptoms and signs of disease. Numerous remedies, none of which has gained general acceptance, have been tried in such cases.

When to Refer

Patients with severe disease should be hospitalized. Patients with toxic megacolon may require colectomy. The overall mortality rate in patients requiring surgery is about 30% to 50%. Patients with relapses should be referred to specialists to rule out inflammatory bowel disease.

KEY POINTS

CLOSTRIDIUM DIFFICILE AND ANTIBIOTIC-ASSOCIATED COLITIS

⊃ Antibiotics cause diarrhea by altering the colonic microflora. Osmotic diarrhea results from impairment of carbohydrate fermentation. About 10% to 30% of cases of antibiotic-related diarrhea are caused by *C. difficile,* which elaborates two toxins.

⊃ The antibiotics most frequently associated with *C. difficile* colitis are ampicillin, amoxicillin, cephalosporins (especially third-generation cephalosporins), and clindamycin.

⊃ The usual presentation of *C. difficile* colitis is watery diarrhea (bloody diarrhea is rare), crampy lower abdominal pain, and fever. Fecal leukocytes are often present. Diagnosis is confirmed by demonstrating *C. difficile* cytotoxins in stool. Sigmoidoscopy or colonoscopy is indicated when the diagnosis is in doubt. Treatment consists of discontinuing the offending antimicrobial agent, correcting fluid and electrolyte losses, and in severe cases prescribing oral metronidazole. Vancomycin is reserved for special circumstances. Use of agents that alter the normal intestinal motility should be avoided.

SUGGESTED READING

Hogenauer C, Hammer HF, Krejs GJ, et al. Mechanisms and management of antibiotic-associated diarrhea. Clin Infect Dis 1998; 27: 702-710.

Johnson S, Gerding DN. *Clostridium difficile*–associated diarrhea. Clin Infect Dis 1998; 26: 1027-1034.

Kyne L, Warny M, Quamar A, et al. Asymptomatic carriage of *Clostridium difficile* and serum levels of IgG antibody against toxin A. N Engl J Med 2000; 342: 390-397.

Mylonakis E, Ryan ET, Calderwood SB. *Clostridium difficile*–associated diarrhea: a review. Arch Intern Med 2001; 161: 525-533.

Thielman NM. Antibiotic-associated colitis. In: Mandell GL, Bennett JE, Dolin R, eds. Mandell, Douglas, and Bennett's Principles and Practice of Infectious Diseases. 5th ed., Philadelphia: Churchill Livingstone; 2000: 1111-1126.

Miscellaneous Gastrointestinal Pathogens

Gastroenteritis of presumed viral origin is extremely common in primary care. Diarrhea caused by *E. coli, V. cholerae,* and noncholera vibrios is discussed briefly. Parasitic diarrhea is discussed in Chapter 23.

Viruses

One of the most common human infections, viral gastroenteritis causes an estimated 3 to 5 billion cases of diarrhea each year worldwide, with some 5 to 10 million deaths.

Rotaviruses *(see Chapter 4)*

Rotaviruses, so named because they resemble a wheel with spokes under the electron microscope (*rota* is Latin for "wheel"), cause about one third of diarrhea-related hospitalizations worldwide and about 800,000 deaths each year. Nearly all children are infected by age 3 years. In the United States diarrhea caused by rotaviruses accounts for an esti-

mated 500,000 physician visits, 50,000 hospitalizations, and 20 to 40 deaths, at an annual cost >$1 billion.

Of the three recognized groups of rotaviruses (A, B, and C), group A accounts for most outbreaks. The disease is presumably spread mainly by fecal-oral transmission, which explains in part its high frequency in child care centers. Rotaviruses infect villous epithelial cells in the jejunum and ileum. Children with rotavirus infection typically have fever, vomiting, and diarrhea. Dehydration can be significant. Adults remain susceptible to rotavirus infection, but serious morbidity and mortality are rare except among the elderly. Outbreaks of rotavirus diarrhea can occur in nursing homes, sometimes with dehydration and death.

Diagnosis of rotavirus diarrhea is usually based on enzyme-linked immunosorbent assay of stool. Several kits are commercially available, with sensitivity 63% to 100%, specificity 100%, positive predictive value 100%, and negative predictive value 91% to 100%. Other methods of diagnosis are PCR of stool and virus isolation using cell culture.

Oral rehydration therapy is nearly always effective for rotavirus diarrhea, but hospitalization for intravenous therapy may be required. Although the Food and Drug Administration approved a tetravalent rotavirus vaccine in August 1998, it was voluntarily withdrawn from the market in 1999 because of a strong association between the vaccine and intussusception in some infants.

Norwalk Virus and Other Caliciviruses

Caliciviruses, so named because of cuplike indentations on their surfaces (*calix* is Latin for "cup" or "goblet"), cause vomiting, diarrhea, or both. Norwalk virus and similar agents cause more than one third of outbreaks of nonbacterial gastroenteritis in the United States, affecting persons of all age groups. Some studies suggest that up to 90% of persons are eventually infected. Like rotaviruses, caliciviruses are spread mainly by fecal-oral transmission and infect villous cells in the small intestine, causing diarrhea as a result of malabsorption. Onset of illness can be gradual or abrupt, with crampy abdominal pain as the usual first symptom. Most patients have both vomiting and diarrhea, but either of these symptoms can predominate. Some patients experience only mild watery diarrhea, whereas others have a more severe illness with vomiting, headache, and constitutional symptoms. Caliciviruses have been difficult to isolate by culture. No convenient diagnostic test is available, although numerous tests are in various stages of development. Treatment is supportive, and recovery within 48 to 72 hours is the rule.

Astroviruses and Other Agents of Viral Gastroenteritis

Astroviruses and enteric (group F) adenoviruses have been firmly established as causes of diarrhea. Astroviruses cause diarrhea primarily in young children. Serologic studies indicate that the majority of children are infected by 6 years of age. Illness is usually manifested as headache, malaise, and diarrhea, and less commonly as nausea. The illness tends to be milder than rotavirus diarrhea, although occasional patients require hospitalization. Secondary cases in adult contacts are less common, and experimental studies indicate that astroviruses usually do not produce symptoms in adults. Both astroviruses and enteric adenoviruses have been isolated by culture. A commercially available test is available for detection of enteric adenoviruses, which also cause diarrheal disease in children.

Other viruses that may sometimes cause diarrhea but in which the etiologic or causal relationship has not yet been firmly established are coronaviruses, echoviruses, coxsackie A and B viruses, non–group F adenoviruses, picobirnaviruses, picotrirnaviruses, pestiviruses, and toroviruses.

Escherichia Coli Other Than Shiga Toxin–Producing Strains

Escherichia coli, a major component of the normal intestinal flora and the most carefully studied of all living organisms, causes diarrhea by at least six mechanisms, identified by the adjectives used to describe the respective strains:

- Shiga toxin–producing strains (STEC; also called entero-hemorrhagic *E. coli* [EHEC]) are discussed previously in the chapter.
- Enterotoxigenic strains (ETEC) are the usual cause of traveler's diarrhea (see Chapter 24).
- Enteroinvasive strains (EIEC) cause dysentery with high fever and bloody diarrhea that contains polymorphonuclear leukocytes. These strains belong to certain serogroups (e.g., O28, O52, and O112) that are rare in the United States
- Enteropathogenic strains (EPEC) cause disease by adhering tightly to epithelial cells and effacing their brush borders. These strains, also called "enteroaggressive," have been associated with nursery outbreaks and with persistent diarrhea in young children.
- Enteroaggregative strains (EAEC, also known as EaggED) adhere to cells and seem to cause diarrhea by several mechanisms, including both stimulation of the guanylate cyclase system and cytotoxicity. These strains have been associated with diarrhea mainly in developing countries but also cause persistent diarrhea in persons with advanced HIV disease.
- Diffusely adherent *E. coli* (DAEC) may cause disease by massive attachment to the gut mucosa, thereby diminishing the absorptive surface.

Most clinical laboratories cannot diagnose *E. coli* as the cause of diarrhea in these latter syndromes. Therefore consultation with a state health department may be advisable when an outbreak of severe diarrhea occurs and cultures for the usual pathogens are unrevealing.

Cholera and Noncholera Vibrios

V. cholerae causes a life-threatening secretory diarrhea by stimulating the adenylate cyclase system of the gastrointestinal tract. The disease has an abrupt onset with watery diarrhea. Fever and abdominal pain are seldom prominent, if they occur at all. Death results from dehydration. Treatment requires aggressive fluid replacement, with antibiotics (notably tetracyclines, ciprofloxacin, or for children TMP/SMX or erythromycin) having a secondary role. Cholera is rare in the United States and is seen almost exclusively in travelers, but an eighth pandemic of the disease remains a real possibility.

Vibrio parahaemolyticus is an important cause of gastroenteritis associated with the ingestion of inadequately cooked seafood or food that has been contaminated with seawater. Raw oysters are incriminated in about one half of cases in the Gulf Coast states, where the disease is most common in the United States, but outbreaks are associated with other types of shellfish. Between 1973 and 1998, 40 outbreaks of *V. parahaemolyticus* infection were reported to the CDC,

accounted for >1000 illnesses. Explosive watery diarrhea is usually the first symptom and is often accompanied by crampy abdominal pain. The organism can be isolated on thiosulfate–citrate–bile salts–sucrose (TCBS) agar (Table 12-3). The disease is usually mild and self-limited, but occasional deaths occur in young children, elderly persons, or severely debilitated persons.

 KEY POINTS

OTHER PATHOGENS THAT CAUSE GASTROENTERITIS AND DIARRHEA

- Rotaviruses, the most common agents of nonbacterial gastroenteritis in children, cause an estimated 500,000 office visits and 20 to 40 deaths in the United States each year. A tetravalent vaccine is now available.
- Norwalk virus and other caliciviruses cause vomiting and diarrhea throughout the year in persons of all ages, often as outbreaks. Patients seldom become acutely ill and generally make a full recovery within 48 to 72 hours.
- *V. cholerae* causes life-threatening secretory diarrhea by stimulation of the adenylate cyclase system in the gastrointestinal mucosa.
- *V. parahaemolyticus* gastroenteritis, usually manifested as a self-limited diarrheal illness, is associated mainly with the ingestion of undercooked seafood or food that has been contaminated with seawater.

SUGGESTED READING

Atmar RL, Estes MK. Diagnosis of noncultivatable gastroenteritis viruses, the human caliciviruses. Clin Microbiol Rev 2001; 14: 15-37.

Belhorn T. Rotavirus diarrhea. Curr Probl Pediatr 1999; 29: 198-207.

Daniels NA, MacKinnon L, Bishop R, et al. *Vibrio parahaemolyticus* infections in the United States, 1973-1998. J Infect Dis 2000; 181: 1661-1666.

Kaper JB. Enterohemorrhagic *Escherichia coli.* Curr Opin Microbiol 1998; 1: 103-108.

Nataro JP, Steiner T, Guerrant RL. Enteroaggregative *Escherichia coli.* Emerg Infect Dis 1998; 4: 251-261.

Offit PA, Clark HF. The rotavirus vaccine. Curr Opin Pediatr 1999; 11: 9-13.

Parashar UD, Bresee JS, Gentsch JR. Rotavirus. Emerg Infect Dis 1998; 4: 561-570.

Raufman JP. Cholera. Am J Med 1998; 104: 386-394.

Walter JE, Mitchell DK. Role of astroviruses in childhood diarrhea. Curr Opin Pediatr 2000; 12: 275-279.

Wanke CA. To know *Escherichia coli* is to know bacterial diarrheal disease. Clin Infect Dis 2001; 32: 1710-1712.

Enteric Fever (Typhoid and Paratyphoid Fevers)

The elimination of typhoid as a major public health problem in the United States is due largely to improved sanitation rather than to antibiotics or to the vaccine, which is only partially effective. Occasional outbreaks of typhoid fever still occur, but about three fourths of cases are acquired abroad, especially in Mexico, the Philippines, and India. The risk of typhoid among U.S. travelers is greatest among those who visit the Indian subcontinent. Paratyphoid fever is an enteric fever syndrome caused by *Salmonella* species other than *S. typhi.*

Presentation and Progression
Cause

Typhoid fever is caused by *Salmonella choleraesuis* subspecies *choleraesuis* serotype *typhi,* commonly known as *S. typhi.* A similar illness is caused by *S. paratyphi* A, *S. schottmülleri* (formerly *S. paratyphi* B), and *S. hirschfeldii* (formerly *S. paratyphi* C), and occasionally by other *Salmonella* species. Enteric fever is a "penetrating" intestinal infection in the sense that the bacteria penetrate the small bowel mucosa, where they multiply in intestinal lymphoid tissue and especially in the large aggregates of lymphocytes in the ileum known as Peyer's patches. Lymphohematogenous dissemination results in high fever and other disease manifestations. The organisms grow within reticuloendothelial cells, and satisfactory host defenses require intact cell-mediated (T-lymphocyte) immunity.

Presentation

Typhoid fever usually affects persons <30 years of age (children, adolescents, and young adults). After an incubation period of 5 to 21 days, abdominal pain, fever, chills, and constitutional symptoms develop. Diarrhea is seldom the presenting complaint, and about 30% of patients, especially adults, have constipation rather than diarrhea.

The illness characteristically evolves over several weeks:
- First week: stepwise fever that becomes sustained (that is, the temperature does not return to the baseline), often with relative bradycardia. Blood cultures are usually positive.
- Second week: abdominal pain. In some cases (<50%) a rash consisting of faint salmon-colored macules is seen on the trunk and abdomen (rose spots).
- Third week: hepatosplenomegaly with, in severe cases, intestinal bleeding or perforation caused by erosions of Peyer's patches. Complications include shock, stupor, delirium, seizures, psychosis, myelitis, and pneumonia.

Diagnosis

Typhoid should be included in the differential diagnosis of fever in a returning traveler. Microscopic examination of stool stained with methylene blue may reveal fecal mononuclear leukocytes. Other laboratory findings include anemia and either leukopenia or leukocytosis. Eosinophils are frequently decreased or absent on peripheral blood smear, which suggests the diagnosis in geographic areas where parasites are common. Abnormal results of liver function tests are common and sometimes suggest acute viral hepatitis. Urinalysis may reveal pyuria, proteinuria, and casts; the presence of red blood cells suggests an immune complex glomerulonephritis. Chest radiographs are abnormal in about 10% of patients.

Diagnosis is most conveniently made on the basis of blood cultures, which are positive in 40% to 80% of patients. *S. typhi* may require longer than the usual 24 to 48 hours to become apparent in blood cultures. Stool cultures are positive in 30% to 40% of patients. When typhoid fever is suspected and blood and stool cultures are negative, bone marrow should be aspirated for culture. In one study 98% of bone marrow cultures were positive, versus 70% of blood cultures. Serologic tests, although widely available, are of limited diagnostic usefulness.

Typhoid and paratyphoid fevers have a broad differential diagnosis. Diseases that sometimes mimic typhoid can be divided into those that are relatively common in the United States and those that are relatively uncommon:

- Diseases that are relatively common in the United States and that occasionally mimic typhoid fever include acute bacterial pneumonia (e.g., *Streptococcus pneumoniae*), *Chlamydia pneumoniae* infection, Crohn's disease, ehrlichiosis, granulomatous hepatitis, hepatitis B, infectious mononucleosis, influenza, intraabdominal abscess, legionnaire's disease, malignancy, *Mycoplasma pneumoniae* infection, sarcoidosis, tuberculosis, ulcerative colitis, and vasculitis (e.g., polyarteritis nodosa).
- Diseases that are uncommon in the United States and that can mimic typhoid fever include abdominal actinomycosis, acute bartonellosis (Oroya fever), acute schistosomiasis (Katayama fever), amebiasis, babesiosis, Brill-Zinsser disease, brucellosis, *C. fetus* infection, dengue, epidemic typhus, intestinal anthrax, leptospirosis, malaria, relapsing fever caused by *Borrelia hermsii,* melioidosis, rat bite fever, scrub typhus, septicemic plague, trichinosis, typhoidal tularemia, Q fever, scrub typhus, and visceral larva migrans.

Natural History
Expected Outcome

Mortality of typhoid fever was >12% before the introduction of antibiotics, with many deaths caused by perforation of the intestines or hemorrhage. Intestinal perforation is more common in adults than in children.

Treatment
Methods

Current treatment of typhoid fever consists of a fluoroquinolone (such as ciprofloxacin) or ceftriaxone. Occasional resistance to both of these agents occurs.

Expected Response

Current mortality from typhoid fever in immunocompetent persons, with treatment, is <1.5%.

When to Refer

Patients with suspected typhoid fever should be admitted to the hospital.

 KEY POINTS

ENTERIC FEVER (TYPHOID AND PARATYPHOID FEVER)
- Typhoid fever usually occurs in persons <30 years of age. Classically it begins as a stepwise fever that becomes sustained (i.e., the temperature does not return to the baseline), often with relative bradycardia (in adults but not in children). Abdominal pain, sometimes with "rose spots" on the trunk and abdomen, develops during the second week, and serious complications, including perforation of the bowel or hemorrhage, occur during the third week.

⊃ Blood cultures are positive in 40% to 80% of cases, stool cultures in 30% to 40%, and bone marrow cultures in up to 98%.

⊃ Most cases of typhoid fever in the United States are seen in returning travelers. However, occasional outbreaks still occur in the United States, so typhoid fever should be considered in the broad differential diagnosis of fever with abdominal pain.

SUGGESTED READING

Cobelens FG, Kooij S, Warris-Versteegan A, et al. Typhoid fever in group travelers: opportunity for studying vaccine efficacy. J Travel Med 2000; 7: 19-24.

Davis TM, Makepeace AE, Dallimore EA. Relative bradycardia is not a feature of enteric fever in children. Clin Infect Dis 1999; 28: 582-586.

Kamath PS, Jalihal A, Chakraborty A. Differentiation of typhoid fever from fulminant hepatic failure in patients presenting with jaundice and encephalopathy. Mayo Clin Proc 2000; 75: 462-466.

Memon LA, Billoo AG, Memon HI. Cefixime: an oral option for the treatment of multidrug-resistant enteric fever in children. South Med J 1997; 90: 1204-1207.

Mermin JH, Townes JM, Gerber M, et al. Typhoid fever in the United States, 1985-1994: changing risks of international travel and increasing antimicrobial resistance. Arch Intern Med 1998; 158: 633-638.

Misra S, Diaz PS, Rowley AH. Characteristics of typhoid fever in children and adolescents in a major metropolitan area in the United States. Clin Infect Dis 1997; 24: 998-1000.

Rowe B, Ward LR, Threfall EJ. Multidrug-resistant *Salmonella typhi*: a worldwide epidemic. Clin Infect Dis 1997; 24 (Suppl 1): S106-S109.

Biliary Tract Infections

Cholecystitis and cholangitis are relatively common causes of acute, recurrent, and chronic abdominal pain. Occasional complications of biliary tract disease include acute pancreatitis caused by gallstones and liver abscess.

Presentation and Progression

Cause

Cholecystitis usually results from obstruction of the cystic duct with subsequent bacterial invasion of the gallbladder. In the United States cholelithiasis is the cause of cystic duct obstruction in >90% of cases, and women are affected twice as frequently as men. Cholecystitis can be acute or chronic. More often than not, both types of inflammation are present, and evidence of chronic inflammation, including fibrosis, is found in about 95% of gallbladders removed for presumed acute cholecystitis.

Bile is normally sterile. Bacterial contamination of the gallbladder (bactobilia) occurs when gallstone impaction of the cystic duct or the common bile duct alters the local environment, allowing bacterial overgrowth to occur in the duodenum with subsequent invasion of the biliary tree through the ampulla of Vater. Endoscopic or surgical manipulation of the biliary tract can lead to polymicrobial contamination of the gallbladder by anaerobic or aerobic bacteria. Infection and inflammation often involve the full thickness of the gallbladder wall, causing ischemia with transmural necrosis, empyema, gangrenous cholecystitis, emphysematous cholecystitis, perforation with pericholecystic or intraperitoneal abscess, or frank peritonitis. Common pathogens in biliary infections are aerobic gram-negative bacilli (e.g., *E. coli, Klebsiella* species, *Enterobacter* species, *Proteus* species, and *Pseudomonas aeruginosa*), aerobic gram-positive cocci (enterococci, streptococci, and staphylococci), and anaerobic bacteria (e.g., *Bacteroides* species, *Clostridium* species, *Fusobacterium* species, and peptostreptococci).

About 2% to 12% of cases of acute cholecystitis are not associated with gallstones (acalculous cholecystitis). These cases sometimes result from infection of the gallbladder by *Salmonella* or *Campylobacter* species. Acalculous cholecystitis tends to occur in seriously ill patients. Predisposing factors include recent surgery, extensive burns, systemic sepsis or trauma, and total parenteral nutrition for >3 weeks with no oral intake. The pathogenesis of acalculous cholecystitis is poorly understood but may involve transmural ischemia of the gallbladder with subsequent necrosis.

Acute ascending cholangitis (also called toxic or suppurative cholangitis) occurs in the setting of common bile duct obstruction, most commonly from gallstones (choledocholithiasis). Other causes of common bile duct obstruction are benign or malignant strictures, extrinsic compression, and parasitic infestation (usually *Ascaris lumbricoides* in the United States; others include *Strongyloides stercoralis* and various trematodes and cestodes; see Chapter 23). Reflux of infected bile leads to inflammation in the extrahepatic and intrahepatic bile ducts, which often becomes complicated by multiple liver abscesses. Bacteremia, frequently polymicrobial, occurs in about 30% to 50% of patients with bacterial cholangitis. Bacteria isolated from bile are the same as those associated with acute cholecystitis (see earlier discussion) and are most commonly enteric gram-negative bacilli and various anaerobic bacteria. *E. coli, B. fragilis,* and *C. perfringens* are the most common blood isolates in patients with acute ascending cholangitis. *Pseudomonas aeruginosa* is encountered in patients with biliary stents or with a history of previous endoscopic or surgical procedures involving the bile ducts.

Emphysematous cholecystitis, characterized by gas within the gallbladder wall or lumen, is most often encountered in elderly diabetic men (see Chapter 3). The pathogenesis is unclear but may involve obstruction of the cystic duct. *C. perfringens* is found in about 45% of these cases.

Presentation

Acute cholecystitis, with or without gallstones, typically causes pain in the right upper quadrant of the abdomen, fever, nausea, and vomiting. Acute ascending cholangitis has a similar presentation, but fever is likely to be accompanied by signs of severe sepsis (see Chapters 1 and 6) and jaundice is frequently present. About 50% to 60% of patients with acute ascending cholangitis manifest Charcot's triad (fever, jaundice, and right upper quadrant abdominal pain). Patients with acute emphysematous cholecystitis are usually seriously ill.

Diagnosis

Suspicion of acute cholecystitis or cholangitis usually prompts evaluation in the hospital setting. Leukocytosis and abnormal liver function tests are frequently present, especially in patients with cholangitis. Abdominal ultrasound has an overall accuracy of 95% for diagnosis of gallstones and is usually the initial procedure of choice. In acute cholecystitis, gallstones are sometimes seen impacted in the cystic duct or the neck of the gallbladder, which often has a thickened wall and may contain intraluminal sludge. Maximum tenderness over a stone-containing gallbladder (Murphy's sign) localized by ultrasound may have a positive predictive value of >90% for acute cholecystitis. In patients with jaundice, CT scanning, although less sensitive than ultrasound for identification of gallstones, usually provides more useful information. CT scanning may also be more accurate than ultrasound for diagnosis of emphysematous cholecystitis (in which gas bubbles outlining the biliary tract can sometimes be seen on plain x-ray films).

Natural History
Expected Outcome

Perforation of the gallbladder occurs in up to 15% of cases of acute cholecystitis. Infection and inflammation are usually contained by the omentum and serosal surfaces of adjacent viscera, but rupture into an adjacent viscus sometimes occurs. Mortality from acute cholecystitis is increased in elderly persons, and high mortality is associated with acalculous cholecystitis (in large part because of the underlying conditions), acute ascending cholangitis, and acute emphysematous cholecystitis.

Treatment
Methods

Patients with acute biliary tract infection are generally admitted to the hospital for treatment with broad-spectrum intravenous antibiotics and consultation with a surgeon or gastroenterologist.

When to Refer

Patients with acute cholecystitis should usually be admitted to the hospital. Patients with suspected acute ascending cholangitis, acalculous cholecystitis, emphysematous cholecystitis, or gallstone pancreatitis should be hospitalized.

 KEY POINTS

BILIARY TRACT INFECTIONS

⊃ Acute cholecystitis is usually associated with gallstones and in the United States occurs more frequently in women than in men. Acalculous cholecystitis (about 2% to 12% of cases) generally occurs in patients with significant underlying diseases. Acute emphysematous cholecystitis occurs most commonly in elderly men with diabetes mellitus.

⊃ Ultrasound is usually the initial imaging procedure of choice for patients with suspected biliary tract infection.

⊃ Most patients with acute cholecystitis and all patients with suspected acute ascending cholangitis, acalculous cholecystitis, or emphysematous cholecystitis should be admitted to the hospital for intravenous antibiotic therapy and surgical consultation.

SUGGESTED READING

Carpenter HA. Bacterial and parasitic cholangitis. Mayo Clin Proc 1998; 73: 473-478.

Hashizume M, Sugimachi K, MacFadyen BV. The clinical management and results of surgery for acute cholecystitis. Semin Laparosc Surg 1998; 5: 69-80.

Ko CW, Sekijima JH, Lee SP. Biliary sludge. Ann Intern Med 1999; 130: 301-311.

Lillemoe KD. Surgical treatment of biliary tract infections. Am Surg 2000; 66: 138-144.

Paulson EK. Acute cholecystitis: CT findings. Semin Ultrasound CT MR 2000; 21: 56-63.

Raraty MG, Finch M, Neoptolemos JP. Acute cholangitis and pancreatitis secondary to common duct stones: management update. World J Surg 1998; 22: 1155-1161.

Acute Appendicitis and Mesenteric Lymphadenitis (Pseudoappendicitis Syndrome)

The possibility of acute appendicitis should be considered for all patients with fever, right lower quadrant abdominal pain, anorexia, and vomiting. However, these findings are nonspecific and the clinical presentation of acute appendicitis can be atypical. Several diseases closely mimic acute appendicitis, including mesenteric lymphadenitis. Studies suggest that 8% of all persons and up to 20% of those admitted to the hospital for suspected acute appendicitis may have mesenteric lymphadenitis instead. Newer imaging studies hold the potential for more accurate diagnosis, but when doubt exists, surgical exploration is nearly always the best course.

Presentation and Progression
Cause

Acute appendicitis is usually caused by obstruction of the organ's narrow lumen by fecaliths, foreign bodies, enlarged lymphatic follicles, or tumors. The mucosa and wall become ischemic, promoting bacterial invasion. Unchecked, the inflammatory process progresses to gangrene (infarction) and then perforation, allowing aerobic and anaerobic bacteria to enter the peritoneal cavity. Peritonitis can be localized as a right lower quadrant mass or abscess or can be generalized. In either case sepsis usually develops.

Mesenteric lymphadenitis (pseudoappendicitis) is most commonly caused by *Y. enterocolitica* and *Yersinia pseudotuberculosis*. Nontyphoid *Salmonella* species and *C. jejuni* have also been associated with this syndrome. Streptococci were sometimes associated with the syndrome in the preantibiotic era. Unusual etiologies reported in recent years include infectious mononucleosis (Epstein-Barr virus) and intestinal anthrax.

Presentation

The classic presentation of acute appendicitis is fever, anorexia, nausea, and abdominal pain with maximal tenderness, including rebound tenderness, over McBurney's point. McBurney's point was described by Charles McBurney in 1889 as "very exactly between an inch and a half and two inches from the anterior spinous process of the ilium on a straight line drawn from that process to the umbilicus." Atypical locations of pain and tenderness correlate with atypical locations of the appendix. Maximum pain in the flank or back correlates with retrocecal location of the appendix, and maximum pain in the suprapubic area correlates with pelvic location. Nausea is prominent in acute appendicitis, and its absence militates against the diagnosis. Acute appendicitis can occur at any age.

The incidence of acute appendicitis in the United States has declined in recent decades.

Mesenteric lymphadenitis also manifests itself as fever, vomiting, and abdominal pain. Diarrhea can be present as well. This disorder typically occurs in children or young adults, especially boys between ages 5 and 14. The disease is more common during the winter and spring months, and outbreaks occur.

Diagnosis

The broad differential diagnosis of fever and lower abdominal pain includes acute salpingitis (or pelvic inflammatory disease; see Chapter 16), ectopic pregnancy, gastroenteritis and enteric fever (discussed previously), diverticulitis (discussed later in the chapter), typhlitis (neutropenic enterocolitis, typically involving the cecum and occurring in severely immunocompromised patients), mesenteric arterial or venous thrombosis, and many other disease entities. Leukocytosis is usually present in patients with acute appendicitis but is also common in patients with mesenteric lymphadenitis and other conditions that can mimic acute appendicitis. In patients with mesenteric lymphadenitis, fecal leukocytes are sometimes present and stool cultures are sometimes positive for an enteric pathogen.

The diagnosis of acute appendicitis is established in only about one half of patients admitted to the hospital for this possibility. Recent interest has been directed toward the use of imaging procedures, notably ultrasound and CT examination, to distinguish between acute appendicitis, mesenteric lymphadenitis, and other conditions that can cause fever with right lower quadrant abdominal pain. Ultrasound examination reveals an inflamed appendix in up to 86% of patients with acute appendicitis and can also reveal enlargement of the mesenteric lymph nodes with mural thickening of the ileum suggestive of "pseudoappendicitis" caused by *Y. enterocolitica, C. jejuni,* or other microorganisms. Helical CT scanning in acute appendicitis shows an inflamed appendix with periappendiceal fat stranding in 93% of cases (Figure 12-2). Less common but more specific changes include the presence of one or more appendicoliths (fecaliths). CT scanning of the appendix after instillation of contrast material into the colon

has been shown to be an effective, cost-saving means of avoiding unnecessary appendectomy. At this time, however, the consensus holds that results of imaging studies should not form the basis for postponing surgical exploration, especially in high-risk groups (see below).

Natural History
Expected Outcome

Acute mesenteric lymphadenitis (pseudoappendicitis syndrome) is a self-limited illness. Acute appendicitis with rupture, however, is extremely serious with a high degree of systemic toxicity. Morbidity and mortality from acute appendicitis are substantially higher in infants, children, and the elderly compared with adolescents and young adults. In infants and children the presentations tend to be nonspecific, yet the disease progresses rapidly with a high rate of rupture. In elderly patients symptoms tend to be blunted and rupture of the appendix is found in 60% to 90% of patients at surgery (compared with overall rates of rupture of 15% to 30% in patients undergoing surgery for acute appendicitis).

Treatment

When reason exists to suspect acute appendicitis and the diagnosis cannot be excluded with reasonable certainty, surgery should not be postponed. Whether laparoscopic surgery is a valid alternative to open appendectomy remains controversial. The appendix should be removed even if found to be normal.

Appropriate antimicrobial therapy for mesenteric lymphadenitis caused by *Yersinia* species includes TMP/SMX, a third-generation cephalosporin, or ciprofloxacin (which is contraindicated, however, in children).

Expected Response

Prognosis for acute appendicitis is generally good, provided extensive peritonitis with sepsis has not occurred before surgery. About 50% of deaths from acute appendicitis occur in persons >60 years of age, who comprise <10% of patients undergoing surgery for this condition. Acute mesenteric lymphadenitis is self-limited.

When to Refer

Patients in whom acute appendicitis figures prominently in the differential diagnosis should nearly always be admitted to the hospital.

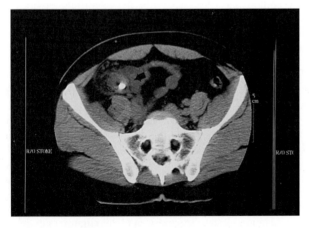

FIG. 12-2 Computed tomographic scan of a patient with acute appendicitis, showing an inflammatory mass surrounding the appendix, which contains an appendicolith (fecalith).

▶ KEY POINTS

ACUTE APPENDICITIS AND MESENTERIC LYMPHADENITIS (PSEUDOAPPENDICITIS SYNDROME)

⊃ The classic presentation of acute appendicitis is fever, nausea, vomiting, right lower abdominal pain, and leukocytosis. However, only about one half of patients admitted to the hospital for suspected acute appendicitis prove to have this diagnosis.

⊃ Morbidity and mortality from acute appendicitis are highest in infants, children, and the elderly.

⊃ Acute mesenteric lymphadenitis, caused by *Y. enterocolitica, C. jejuni,* nontyphoidal *Salmonella* species, and other microorganisms, can mimic acute appendicitis (hence "pseudoappendicitis syndrome").

⊃ Imaging studies, notably ultrasound and CT scanning, can help to distinguish between acute appendicitis and mesenteric lymphadenitis preoperatively. However, because of the potential seriousness of acute appendicitis, exploratory surgery should be carried out whenever acute appendicitis is a serious diagnostic possibility.

SUGGESTED READING

García-Corbeira P, Ramos JM, Aguado JM, et al. Six cases in which mesenteric lymphadenitis due to non-typhi *Salmonella* caused an appendicitis-like syndrome. Clin Infect Dis 1995; 21: 231-232.

Hardin DM Jr. Acute appendicitis: review and update. Am Fam Physician 1999; 60: 2027-2034.

Lane MJ, Mindelzun RE. Appendicitis and its mimickers. Semin Ultrasound CT MR 1999; 20: 77-85.

Rao PM, Rhea JT, Novelline RA, et al. Effect of computed tomography of the appendix on treatment of patients and use of hospital resources. N Engl J Med 1998; 338: 141-146.

Rothrock SG, Pagane J. Acute appendicitis in children: emergency department diagnosis and management. Ann Emerg Med 2000; 36: 39-51.

Acute Diverticulitis

Acute diverticulitis is a common problem in primary care because of the high prevalence of diverticulosis of the colon in developed nations. Acute diverticulosis is often self-limited but can lead to serious complications, including sepsis, intraabdominal abscess formation, and death.

Presentation and Progression
Cause

Diverticulosis has been linked to the low fiber content in diets of highly urbanized, industrialized nations. It may therefore be a deficiency disorder, preventable by changing from diets rich in refined carbohydrates to diets containing more fruit and vegetable fiber. The prevalence of diverticulosis increases with age. Recent data indicate an equal gender distribution. In persons of European ancestry, diverticulosis affects predominantly the distal colon in about 85% of cases. In persons of Asian ancestry, involvement of the right side (ascending colon) predominates in about 70% of cases. Diverticulitis develops in about 25% of persons with colonic diverticula.

Acute diverticulitis is actually a "peridiverticulitis" in that the inflammatory reaction is almost entirely extrinsic to the colon. Microperforations of diverticula cause contamination of the peritoneal cavity by the aerobic and anaerobic flora resident in the normal colon (see Chapter 1). The result is often a small abscess within the pericolonic fat (stage 1) that if not contained may expand and spread (stage 2) and then rupture, causing generalized suppurative peritonitis (stage 3). If the bowel lumen communicates with the inflammatory process, more colonic contents enter the peritoneal cavity, leading to extensive fecal contamination of the peritoneal cavity (stage 4). The inflammatory process can compress the bowel lumen, resulting in obstruction. The obstruction, however, is rarely complete.

Presentation

Since acute diverticulitis, as encountered in the United States, affects predominantly the sigmoid colon and descending colon, most patients have lower abdominal pain, usually maximal in the left lower quadrant. The presence of a redundant sigmoid colon can displace the symptoms from the left lower quadrant to the suprapubic region and even to the right lower quadrant. Right lower quadrant pain is common in Asian-American patients with acute diverticulitis. The patient often has a history of diarrhea, constipation, or both. Fever is generally present. Physical examination usually reveals marked tenderness, sometimes with guarding and rebound tenderness. Tenderness may also be present on rectal examination. In some patients a palpable abdominal mass is detected. Bowel sounds are diminished in the majority of patients. Hyperactive bowel sounds can be heard when intestinal obstruction is present.

Increased frequency of urination, urgency, or dysuria can result from contiguity of the inflammatory process with the urinary bladder. Pain is sometimes referred to the genital or suprapubic area. Recurrent urinary tract infections with a polymicrobial flora or with anaerobic bacteria, in the absence of an indwelling Foley catheter, suggest colovesicular fistula. Pneumaturia or fecaluria virtually establishes the diagnosis of this complication. Frank rectal bleeding is not a feature of acute diverticulitis and suggests an alternative diagnosis.

Diagnosis

Clinical diagnosis of acute diverticulitis is often based on the triad of fever, left lower quadrant abdominal pain and tenderness, and leukocytosis in a patient with known colonic diverticulosis. However, the nonspecificity of the symptoms, the frequent occurrence of diverticulitis in persons <50 years of age (about 20% of cases), the occasional presentation as right lower quadrant pain (hence, mimicking acute appendicitis), and the range of alternative possibilities make diagnosis a difficult challenge in many instances. The differential diagnosis includes acute appendicitis, pancreatitis, inflammatory bowel disease, urinary tract infection with or without ureteral stone, penetrating peptic ulcer, volvulus, carcinoma of the colon, ischemic colitis, mesenteric arterial or venous thrombosis, pseudomembranous colitis, amebic colitis, and, in women, pelvic inflammatory disease, torsion of the ovary, and ectopic pregnancy. Initial laboratory studies generally include a complete blood count with differential and plain radiographs of the chest and abdomen. Erect and supine abdominal films are abnormal in about 50% of cases; findings include pneumoperitoneum (about 11% of cases), ileus, obstruction, pericolonic tissue densities suggesting abscesses (mass effect), and air within the bowel wall (suggesting cecal necrosis).

CT scanning has become the imaging procedure of choice for patients in whom the diagnosis is unclear or who are at high risk of complications, such as those who are elderly, debilitated, or immunocompromised. Criteria for diverticulitis include thickening of the bowel wall (>5 mm), inflammation of the pericolonic soft tissue (stranding, increased attenuation, poor margination), and evidence of an intramural or peridiverticular abscess. CT scanning may suggest an alternative diagnosis and complications of diverticulitis, such as formation of fistulous tracts. Some authorities now consider ultrasonography of the abdomen and pelvis to be the second-line imaging procedure of choice (after CT scanning), and it is especially useful in women for exclusion of tubo-ovarian pathology. Abnormalities on ultrasound examination include hypoechoic thickening of the colonic wall, increased echogenicity of the pericolonic soft tissue, and the presence of an abscess. Ultrasonography tends, however, to be observer dependent. Both CT and ultrasonography can be falsely negative. Neither procedure is recommended on a routine basis for patients who can be managed without hospitalization.

Contrast enema and endoscopy (sigmoidoscopy or colonoscopy) should be performed with caution, if at all, in patients with acute diverticulitis, since insufflation of the colon with air during these procedures can cause bowel perforation. Contrast enemas have been widely used in the past and are now used mainly to provide additional information when CT scans are inconclusive. Use of barium should be avoided in favor of water-soluble contrast media because barium might leak into the peritoneal cavity, causing a foreign body reaction. Most authorities recommend colonoscopy 6 to 8 weeks after an episode of acute diverticulitis to exclude carcinoma of the colon.

Natural History
Expected Outcome

Acute diverticulitis is often a self-limited disease but tends to recur. Complications include life-threatening sepsis, abscesses, and fistulas.

Treatment
Methods

First episodes of acute diverticulitis or mild recurrences in generally healthy persons can often be managed on an outpatient basis with a clear liquid diet and an oral antimicrobial regimen designed to provide broad-spectrum coverage against the colonic flora. TMP/SMX or ciprofloxacin can be used to cover the aerobic component of the colonic flora, and metronidazole or clindamycin can be used to cover the anaerobic component. Although many patients make apparent full recoveries when only aerobic coverage is provided, anaerobic coverage is advisable, especially because of the strong correlation between *B. fragilis* contamination of the peritoneal cavity and abscess formation. Appropriate regimens include ciprofloxacin (500 to 750 mg PO b.i.d.) plus metronidazole (500 to 750 mg PO t.i.d.); TMP/SMX (one double-strength tablet PO b.i.d.) plus metronidazole; or either ciprofloxacin or TMP/SMX plus clindamycin (300 to 450 mg q6-8h). Patients receiving metronidazole should be told to avoid use of alcohol, including alcohol-containing medication.

Expected Results

Clinical improvement, indicated by a decrease in abdominal pain, fever, and WBC count, should occur within 48 to 72 hours.

When to Refer

Admission to the hospital for intravenous antibiotic therapy and surgical consultation is indicated in the following settings: (1) high fever, intense abdominal pain requiring narcotic analgesics, and marked leukocytosis at the outset of the illness; (2) nausea and vomiting that preclude oral antibiotic therapy; (3) elderly and immunocompromised patients; (4) right-sided diverticulitis and other instances in which the diagnosis may be in doubt; (5) acute diverticulitis in younger patients (<50 years

of age) because these patients tend to have more severe disease with higher rates of complication and often require surgery; and (6) failure to improve after 48 to 72 hours of an oral regimen.

KEY POINTS

ACUTE DIVERTICULTIS

⊃ Classic manifestations are left lower quadrant abdominal pain, fever, and leukocytosis. In about 15% of patients of European ancestry and about 70% of patients of Asian ancestry the disease involves primarily the right side of the colon (ascending colon), in which case the symptoms and signs can resemble those of acute appendicitis.

⊃ CT scanning of the abdomen and pelvis is now the imaging procedure of choice but is unnecessary (and may give false-negative results) in mild cases of acute diverticulitis.

⊃ Indications for hospitalization, IV antibiotics, and surgical consultation include severe disease; advanced age; comorbid conditions, including immunosuppression; age <50 years (in which case the complications tend to be more severe); and failure to improve within 48 to 72 hours.

⊃ Severe recurrent attacks often respond poorly to medical therapy alone and carry higher rates of complications and increased mortality.

SUGGESTED READING

Elsakr R, Johnson DA, Younes Z, et al. Antimicrobial treatment of intra-abdominal infections. Dig Dis 1998; 16: 47-60.

Ferzoco LB, Raptopoulous V, Silen W. Acute diverticulitis. N Engl J Med 1998; 21: 1521-1526.

Urban BA, Fishman EK. Targeted helical CT of the acute abdomen: appendicitis, diverticulitis, and small bowel obstruction. Semin Ultrasound CT MR 2000; 21: 20-39.

Wolff BG, Devine RM. Surgical management of diverticulitis. Am Surg 2000; 66: 153-156.

Young-Fadok TM, Roberts PL, Spencer MP. Colonic diverticular disease. Curr Probl Surg 2000; 37: 457-514.

Peritonitis and Intraabdominal Abscesses

Intraabdominal infections can be confined to the peritoneal cavity or to one or another organ: more commonly both are involved. Infectious peritonitis can be diffuse or localized. Examples of localized peritonitis caused by acute cholecystitis, acute appendicitis, and acute diverticulitis have already been discussed. Diffuse (generalized) peritonitis and intraabdominal abscess nearly always mandate admission to the hospital. An appreciation of the anatomy and pathophysiology of these life-threatening infections enhances the primary care clinician's index of suspicion that one of them might be present.

Presentation and Progression
Cause

In this section the anatomy of intraabdominal infections, the nature of abdominal pain, the microbiology of peritonitis, and the immediate causes of primary and secondary peritonitis are reviewed.

The anatomy of the abdomen determines the routes of spread of infection from the primary site. Organs that either protrude into or are suspended in the cavity include the stomach, jejunum, cecum, appendix, transverse colon, sigmoid colon, liver, gallbladder, and spleen. The remaining organs and parts of the intestine are retroperitoneal. The various omenta and organs divide the abdominal cavity into upper and lower halves, with pockets, pouches, and gutters dividing the remainder of the cavity. Fluid typically moves between the upper and lower compartments by way of the right and left paracolic gutters. As an oversimplification, the abdominal cavity may be considered to be divided into quarters, with good communication between the right upper and lower quarters and the left upper and lower quarters. Physicians are taught to report their abdominal examination by quarters (or quadrants), and these quarters coincide roughly with the anatomic quarters. More detailed accounts of the anatomy are available in standard textbooks of anatomy and surgery.

Abdominal pain accompanying infection is of two principal types: parietal and visceral. Parietal pain is by far the more severe and is also better localized. Anterior parietal pain is sharper and better localized than posterior parietal pain. Visceral pain is usually vague and poorly localized. The evolution of acute appendicitis illustrates the interplay of the different mechanisms of sensing abdominal pain. Initially the pain is visceral and is felt in the periumbilical and epigastric regions, with accompanying nausea. Later, when the parietal peritoneum becomes involved, the pain is felt more in the right lower quadrant and with greater intensity.

Structures that are covered by the visceral peritoneum have their origin in the embryonic foregut, which is innervated by the vagus nerve. Pain, usually a dull discomfort, is produced only by stretching of the visceral peritoneum and is referred to the dermatome of the organ or structure as follows: central portion of the diaphragm, C4 to C8; stomach, T5 to T7; liver and gallbladder, T6 to T8; intestines and colon, T8 to L1; kidneys and uterus, T10 to L1; and urinary bladder, S2 to S4. Nausea may also result from stretching of the visceral peritoneum. For example, pain from the gallbladder is referred to the right upper back between the shoulder and epigastrium. The nerve supply of the parietal peritoneum arises from branches of the cutaneous nerves in the anterior abdominal wall. These nerves are exquisitely sensitive in the same way as the cutaneous nerves. Pain can be localized with some precision, and this is the basis for the so-called peritoneal signs. Pain from inflammation of the peripheral portion of the diaphragm is referred to the adjacent body wall, whereas pain arising from the central portion of the diaphragm is referred to the right shoulder (because of the embryologic origin of the central tendon of the diaphragm in the neck).

Primary peritonitis (spontaneous bacterial peritonitis) occurs in up to 10% of patients with alcoholic cirrhosis (see Chapter 3) and occurs rarely in patients with ascites caused by congestive heart failure, nephritic syndrome, metastatic tumors, systemic lupus erythematosus, or other disorders. Anaerobic bacteria are rare in primary peritonitis.

Peritonitis can also be caused by tuberculosis (see Chapter 22) and by *Neisseria gonorrhoeae* and *Chlamydia trachomatis* infections (see Chapter 16). Secondary peritonitis usually results from spillage of bacteria from the gastrointestinal tract, as occurs in acute appendicitis with rupture, acute diverticulitis, ischemic bowel disease, intestinal obstruction caused by neoplasm, and penetrating injuries. Other causes of secondary peritonitis include acute suppurative cholecystitis (see earlier discussion), chronic ambulatory peritoneal dialysis, complicated genitourinary tract infections, and ruptured abscess from an intraabdominal organ such as the liver, pancreas, kidney, or fallopian tube. Secondary peritonitis typically involves both aerobic and anaerobic bacteria. *Candida* species are often present in patients who have recently received antibiotics. Intraabdominal abscesses arise from one of several mechanisms: local spread of infection within the peritoneal cavity, hematogenous seeding of an organ, and necrosis of an organ followed by bacterial colonization and superinfection.

Presentation

Primary peritonitis in a patient with cirrhosis and ascites generally manifests itself with fever (50% to 80% of patients) or abdominal pain, often accompanied by encephalopathy or by abdominal symptoms such as anorexia, nausea, vomiting, or diarrhea. Physical findings include ascites, diffuse abdominal tenderness with rebound, and hypoactive or absent bowel sounds (see Chapter 3).

Secondary peritonitis most commonly causes moderate to severe abdominal pain that is made worse by motion. Anorexia, nausea, and vomiting are also common, and some patients complain of abdominal distention. The evolution of the pain depends on the source. Peritonitis caused by cholecystitis, diverticulitis, or appendicitis usually spreads slowly, whereas peritonitis caused by a ruptured liver abscess or perforated peptic ulcer spreads rapidly and even catastrophically. Reduction in the intensity of pain and the extent of tenderness suggests that localization may be occurring. Physical findings in secondary peritonitis are more dramatic than in primary peritonitis. The patient typically lies quietly in bed with the knees flexed. There is marked tenderness to palpation. Rebound tenderness, when present, signifies inflammation of the parietal peritoneum and may accurately localize the source of the peritonitis (as in acute appendicitis or diverticulitis). Rigidity of the abdominal muscles can be voluntary (guarding) or reflex. The abdomen may be distended because of an ileus, and bowel sounds may be absent. Examination of the abdomen can be deceptively benign in patients with lax abdominal musculature, including postpartum women, and also in patients who have been receiving corticosteroids. In these patients absence of bowel sounds may be the only significant finding. Rectal and, in female patients, pelvic examination should be performed because the findings may help to localize the pain and also the source (e.g., rectal pain in a patient with ruptured retrocecal appendix).

Tertiary peritonitis is defined as recurrent peritonitis after surgery for secondary bacterial peritonitis and usually occurs in the setting of severe illness.

Intraabdominal abscesses usually are manifested as fever accompanied by pain that may point to one or another location. Thus appendiceal abscess typically causes right lower quadrant pain; diverticulitis causes left lower quadrant pain (for exceptions, see the previous section); liver abscess causes right upper quadrant pain; splenic abscess causes left upper quadrant pain; and pancreatic abscess causes midabdominal pain. Patients with subphrenic abscess, which frequently follows a subacute course, often have symptoms and signs related to the chest, including pleuritic pain and rib tenderness.

Diagnosis

Diagnosis of primary peritonitis in the patient with ascites is based largely on paracentesis. Peritonitis is suggested by an ascitic fluid WBC count $>300/\text{mm}^3$, and 85% of patients have an ascitic fluid WBC count $>1000/\text{mm}^3$ with a predominance of neutrophils. Ascitic fluid pH <7.35 and lactate concentration >25 mg/dL are more specific but less sensitive than the cell count. Ascitic fluid cultures may be negative in up to 35% of patients believed to have primary peritonitis on the basis of other criteria. Of those, one third have positive blood cultures. Ascitic fluid cultures have a better yield if the fluid is inoculated into blood culture bottles at the bedside. Diagnosis of tuberculous peritonitis is discussed in Chapter 22.

Secondary peritonitis is often more difficult to diagnose, since ascites, when present, is usually less marked than in primary peritonitis. Most patients have peripheral blood leukocytosis, in contrast to primary peritonitis in which the peripheral blood WBC count can be normal. Blood cultures are sometimes positive. Chest radiography should be performed to exclude a pulmonary source. Supine, upright, and lateral decubitus x-ray films of the abdomen may reveal distended bowel and a possible cause of the distention. Free air under the diaphragm suggests a ruptured viscus or gas-producing microorganisms. Ultrasound examination is often the initial imaging procedure, although abdominal tenderness or dilated loops of bowel may hinder optimum examination. Ultrasound is especially useful for examination of the right upper quadrant, retroperitoneum, and pelvis. CT examination of the abdomen with contrast usually provides more information than ultrasound and should be the initial imaging procedure when possible. If fluid is identified by ultrasound or abdominal CT scan, it should be tapped.

Diagnosis of intraabdominal abscesses is now frequently suspected on the basis of the CT scan. Plain x-ray films are sometimes helpful, especially for patients with subphrenic abscess. Ultrasound is useful in many instances, although in general it is less sensitive than CT scanning for intraabdominal abscess. Radionuclide scans, especially those using labeled leukocytes, are sometimes used to resolve difficult cases.

Needle aspiration using CT or ultrasound guidance can be extremely helpful, but some patients still require open surgical exploration for diagnosis.

Natural History
Expected Outcome

Peritonitis from any source carries substantial mortality without treatment.

Treatment
Methods

Antibiotics are the mainstay of treatment of primary and secondary peritonitis. Empiric regimens should provide coverage against the common Enterobacteriaceae, *Pseudomonas aeruginosa,* and anaerobic bacteria. Typical choices are piperacillin-tazobactam or imipenem.

When to Refer

Patients with suspected peritonitis should be admitted promptly to the hospital and usually to the intensive care unit. Patients with secondary peritonitis should be under the care of either a surgeon or a medical subspecialist, depending on the likely source.

 KEY POINTS

PERITONITIS

⊃ Patients with suspected peritonitis should be admitted promptly to the hospital, preferably to the intensive care unit.
⊃ Intraabdominal abscesses may present characteristic symptoms and signs, but diagnosis usually requires CT scanning followed by needle aspiration or open surgery.

SUGGESTED READING

Johnson CC, Baldessare J, Levison ME. Peritonitis: update on pathophysiology, clinical manifestations, and management. Clin Infect Dis 1997; 26: 1035-1045.

Levison ME, Bush LM. Peritonitis and other intra-abdominal infections. In Mandell GE, Bennett JE, Dolin R, eds. Mandell, Douglass, and Bennett's Principles and Practice of Infectious Diseases. 5th ed., Philadelphia: Churchill Livingstone; 2000; 821-856.

Solomkin JS, Wittman DW, West MA, et al. Intraabdominal infections. In: Schwartz SI, Shires GT, Spencer FT, et al., eds. Principles of Surgery. 7th ed., New York: McGraw-Hill; 1999: 1515-1550.

13 Viral Hepatitis

ROBERT L. SWORDS, EDWIN A. BROWN

Viral hepatitis is a common and potentially serious infection of the liver that results in significant morbidity and mortality. At least five distinct hepatotropic viruses cause viral hepatitis: hepatitis A virus (HAV); hepatitis B virus (HBV); hepatitis C virus (HCV), formerly known as non-A, non-B hepatitis; hepatitis D virus (HDV); and hepatitis E virus (HEV). These viruses cause liver inflammation and necrosis without significant involvement of other organs. Because the acute illness caused by these viruses is clinically similar, exposure history and specific diagnostic tests are necessary to make an etiologic diagnosis. In addition to the morbidity and mortality of the acute illness, HBV, HCV, and HDV can progress to a chronic infectious state and result in serious sequelae such as cirrhosis, hepatocellular carcinoma, polyarteritis nodosa, cryoglobulinemia, glomerulonephritis, and aplastic anemia. Although progress has been made in the identification and diagnosis of the etiologic agents of this disease, effective strategies for the treatment of chronic infection and prevention of long term complications are still limited.

Differential Diagnosis of Abnormal Liver Function Tests

Patients with mildly abnormal liver function tests and no risk factors by history or physical examination are at low risk for significant liver pathology. However, if the abnormalities persist, the patient should undergo further testing. Initial laboratory studies should include the evaluation of hepatic enzymes, excretory products, and synthetic products.

The hepatic enzymes include aminotransferases (aspartate aminotransferase [AST], alanine aminotransferase [ALT]), alkaline phosphatase (AP), and γ-glutamyl transpeptidase (GGT). Markedly elevated aminotransferase levels (>500 U/L) typically occur with acute hepatocellular injury as seen in

acute viral hepatitis, drug-induced hepatitis, and shock liver. Modest elevation of AST and ALT (<300 U/L) may be seen in chronic hepatitis, infiltrative diseases, and biliary obstruction. An AST/ALT ratio greater than 1.5 suggests the possibility of alcohol-induced liver damage. AP is found primarily in the liver, bones, and intestines. Serum AP levels are often elevated in cholestasis, biliary obstruction, and infiltrative liver disease; heat fractionation may be performed to establish a source of an elevated AP level. GGT is also present in a variety of tissues, but elevated levels in the presence of an elevated AP level strongly suggests a hepatic source. A GGT/AP value greater than 2.5 should evoke a strong suspicion of alcohol abuse.

Abnormalities in excretory products such as bilirubin and ammonia are often associated with liver disease. Bilirubin levels may be elevated because of increased production or impaired excretion. Overproduction of unconjugated bilirubin is seen in hemolysis and cases of ineffective erythropoiesis. Conjugated bilirubin elevations usually result from hepatocellular dysfunction or biliary tract obstruction. Serum ammonia levels may be elevated in hepatic dysfunction, affecting the urea cycle as seen in cirrhosis of various causes, although the usefulness of ammonia levels in the management of hepatic disease is questionable.

Synthetic products of the liver can also be helpful markers of hepatic injury. Decreased levels of albumin are most often seen in chronic liver disease. Prothrombin time is prolonged as a consequence of impaired coagulation factor synthesis (liver disease), consumption (disseminated intravascular coagulation), or vitamin K deficiency. Normalization of prothrombin time with the administration of vitamin K supports vitamin deficiency. The liver synthesizes cholesterol and its hormone derivatives. As a result, chronic liver disease may result in decreased levels of cholesterol or of hormones such as testosterone.

 KEY POINTS

DIFFERENTIAL DIAGNOSIS OF ABNORMAL LIVER FUNCTION TESTS

⊃ Marked elevation (>500 U/L) of levels of the aminotransferases (AST, ALT; also known as transaminases) typically occurs in acute viral hepatitis, drug-induced hepatitis, and shock liver.

⊃ Modest elevation of AST and ALT levels (<300 U/L) is seen in chronic liver disease, infiltrative diseases, and biliary obstruction.

⊃ An AST/ALT ratio greater than 1.5 or a GGT/AP ratio greater than 2.5 suggests alcohol-related liver disease.

Acute Viral Hepatitis

Acute viral hepatitis is a self-limited illness characterized by inflammation and necrosis of the liver. Over the past 20 years five distinct hepatitis viruses have been identified: HAV, HBV, HCV, HDV, and HEV. Hepatitis F virus, hepatitis GB virus, hepatitis G virus, and TT virus are thought to be potential liver pathogens, but their significance is still uncertain. Other viruses that cause a hepatitis-like syndrome but are not specifically hepatotropic are Epstein-Barr, cytomegalovirus, herpes simplex, varicella-zoster, rubeola, rubella, coxsackie B, adenovirus, and yellow fever virus.

The diagnosis of acute viral hepatitis is based on the combination of clinical and laboratory findings (Figure 13-1). The disorder is separated into four stages: incubation, preicteric, icteric, and convalescent, with the spectrum of disease ranging from inapparent, to anicteric with symptoms, to icteric, to fulminant. The incubation period may last from a few weeks to several months, during which time the patient is asymptomatic. During the preicteric phase, lasting 3 to 14 days, the patient has nonspecific symptoms such as malaise and weakness, followed by anorexia, nausea, vomiting, and right upper quadrant pain. Malaise occurs in approximately 95% of patients and is often the first symptom to appear and the last to resolve. About 5% to 15% of patients have a serum sickness–like illness with fever, rash (often urticarial), and migratory arthritis. These symptoms generally resolve with the onset of jaundice or dark urine, characteristic of the icteric phase, which lasts from several days to several weeks. The convalescent period follows, during which symptoms resolve and aminotransferase and bilirubin levels become normal by 3 to 6 months. Although this sequence represents the "typical" case, the course can vary considerably depending on the virus involved. For example, hepatitis A is more likely to have a sudden onset with jaundice, whereas hepatitis B and C are often more insidious and anicteric.

The physical findings of acute viral hepatitis are few. Vital signs are usually normal except for occasional fever. Icterus may be noted when bilirubin levels exceed 2.5 to 3 mg/dL and is most readily detected in the conjunctivae or under the tongue. Examination of the abdomen often reveals an enlarged and tender liver and occasionally splenomegaly. Skin findings include vascular spiders, hemangiomas, excoriation resulting from pruritus, and exacerbation of preexisting acne. Patients with serum sickness–like syndrome may exhibit fever, urticaria, and arthritis.

Although the physical findings of acute viral hepatitis are nonspecific, the laboratory findings are characteristic. Concentrations of the aminotransferases (AST, ALT) are usually five or more times normal at the onset of jaundice. The AST/ALT ratio is usually less than 1, whereas it often exceeds 1.5 in alcohol-induced hepatitis. AP, GGT, and lactic dehydrogenase concentrations can be mildly increased. The bilirubin level is variably elevated in icteric hepatitis, involving both direct and indirect fractions.

A rare but serious manifestation of acute viral hepatitis is fulminant disease. This is characterized by increasing jaundice, worsening coagulopathy, persistence of abnormally high aminotransferase levels, and hepatic encephalopathy. Symptoms and signs include lethargy, somnolence, personality change, asterixis, fetor hepaticus, ecchymoses, and petechiae. Fulminant hepatitis develops less than 2 weeks after the onset of jaundice and occurs more commonly in hepatitis B and D than in the other forms of acute viral hepatitis. Hepatitis E also has an increased incidence of fulminant disease and a high mortality rate, particularly in pregnant women during the third trimester. Clinical findings may include varying degrees of confusion and the presence of asterixis, spider nevi, ascites, splenomegaly, and occasionally varices. These complications seem to occur most frequently in those >40 years of age, injecting drug users, and persons with underlying illness.

FIG. 13-1 Approach to the diagnosis of acute viral hepatitis.

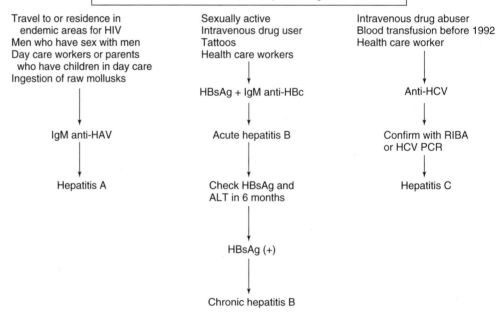

Suspicion of viral hepatitis based on history, physical examination, elevated transaminase levels, or epidemiologic risk factors

Travel to or residence in endemic areas for HIV
Men who have sex with men
Day care workers or parents who have children in day care
Ingestion of raw mollusks
↓
IgM anti-HAV
↓
Hepatitis A

Sexually active
Intravenous drug user
Tattoos
Health care workers
↓
HBsAg + IgM anti-HBc
↓
Acute hepatitis B
↓
Check HBsAg and ALT in 6 months
↓
HBsAg (+)
↓
Chronic hepatitis B

Intravenous drug abuser
Blood transfusion before 1992
Health care worker
↓
Anti-HCV
↓
Confirm with RIBA or HCV PCR
↓
Hepatitis C

KEY POINTS

ACUTE VIRAL HEPATITIS

⊃ The spectrum ranges from inapparent, to anicteric with symptoms, to icteric, to fulminant.

⊃ A serum sickness–like prodrome with fever, rash (often urticarial), and migratory arthritis occurs in 5% to 15% of patients.

⊃ Physical findings are usually few and nonspecific.

⊃ Aminotransferase levels are usually five or more times normal at the onset of jaundice, with the AST/ALT ratio usually less than 1.

⊃ Fulminant disease, which is rare, is characterized by increasing jaundice, worsening coagulopathy, persistence of abnormal aminotransferase elevations, and hepatic encephalopathy.

SUGGESTED READING

Specter S. Viral Hepatitis: Diagnosis, Therapy, and Prevention. Totowa, NJ: Humana Press; 1999.

Zuckerman AJ, Thomas HC, eds. Viral Hepatitis. 2nd ed., London: Churchill Livingstone; 1998.

Chronic Viral Hepatitis

Chronic viral hepatitis has traditionally been defined as the persistence of aminotransferase abnormalities or clinical evidence of liver disease for >6 months. However, a new classification system has been adopted to predict more accurately the long-term risk of developing cirrhosis. Prospective studies have shown that HBV and HCV are rarely if ever completely cleared from the liver when treatment has resulted in normalization of serum aminotransferase levels. Also, it appears that the previous emphasis on piecemeal necrosis was misguided, since other forms of cellular damage such as bridging necrosis are equally, if not more, important in determining prognosis. Therefore the term "chronic hepatitis" should not be applied solely on the basis of disease duration or the presence or absence of abnormalities on liver biopsy but rather on what has been identified as the most likely cause. This should help to predict outcome and dictate appropriate therapeutic interventions.

Together HBV and HCV are the leading cause of chronic hepatitis worldwide. Chronic disease is not known to follow HAV or HEV infection, although infection with HAV may lead to a form of autoimmune hepatitis. Other possible causes include autoimmune hepatitis, hemochromatosis, Wilson's disease, drug-induced liver disease, fatty liver disease, α-antitrypsin deficiency, granulomatous hepatitis, alcoholic liver disease, and nonalcoholic steatohepatitis.

KEY POINTS

CHRONIC VIRAL HEPATITIS

⊃ A new classification system emphasizes the most likely cause of liver abnormalities rather than disease duration or histologic findings on liver biopsy.

⊃ HBV and HCV are the leading causes of chronic hepatitis worldwide.

⊃ Noninfectious diseases such as hemochromatosis and Wilson's disease should be included in the differential diagnosis.

Hepatitis A

The incidence of hepatitis A in the United States has decreased because of improvements in water quality, sewage disposal, and food sanitation. However, hepatitis A still accounts for 26% to 28% of all acute hepatitis cases reported to the Centers for Disease Control and Prevention (CDC) each year, and the incidence tends to increase in a cyclic fashion approximately every 10 years. Hepatitis A is typically a self-limited illness that rarely results in death. It is characterized by an acute onset of a flulike illness with a predominance of constitutional symptoms such as fever, headache, malaise, and myalgias. The severity of clinical disease and risk of death increase with age. Children are more likely to be asymptomatic and anicteric, whereas older adults usually have clinically apparent disease with a greater risk of acute liver failure. HAV is not associated with chronic liver disease and does not result in persistent viremia or an intestinal carrier state.

Presentation and Progression
Cause

HAV is a nonenveloped, thermostable, acid-resistant RNA virus that is now classified into a unique genus hepatovirus. After oral ingestion HAV crosses the intestinal epithelium, enters the bloodstream, and is taken up by hepatocytes where it replicates in the cytoplasm. New infectious particles pass through the biliary system into the intestines, forming the basis for fecal-oral transmission.

The incubation period of HAV is 15 to 50 days (average 28 days). HAV is excreted into the feces for 1 to 2 weeks before onset of illness and for at least 1 week afterward. Virus concentrations in feces are highest during the late incubation period, after the onset of symptoms, and then rapidly decline.

Oral ingestion of HAV is the major route of transmission. HAV has, albeit rarely, also been isolated from saliva and serum, but other than infected feces, only serum has been implicated in the transmission of the virus. Person-to-person contact is the most common mode of fecal-oral transmission as demonstrated by the high rates of infection among household contacts of people with hepatitis A and among children in day care centers. Household crowding, poor education, and inadequate human waste disposal systems contribute to community outbreaks.

Foodborne outbreaks occur with the distribution of contaminated food that is uncooked or undercooked and when food is prepared by HAV-infected individuals with poor personal hygiene. Consuming mollusks poses a significant risk because they are commonly served raw and, as bivalve organisms, they filter and concentrate HAV, which can survive for months in water at room temperature. Salads, cold meats, hamburgers, orange juice, pastries, and raw milk have all been reported as sources of HAV.

In the United States about 33% of the population has serologic evidence of previous infection. Nonetheless, from 1992 to 1994 hepatitis A ranked as the third most common reportable infectious disease among children, and fifth and sixth among adult men and woman, respectively. It is the low seroprevalence rate that makes travel to developing countries where HAV is endemic a well-defined risk.

Other risk factors for HAV infection include homosexuality and intravenous drug use. The increased risk in homosexuals is thought to be related to oral-anal sexual practices. Intravenous drug users are at risk from the presence of HAV in serum, fecal contamination of injection equipment because of poor hygiene, and possible contamination of the illicit drug during transport in the intestines after being swallowed or during carriage in the rectum.

Presentation

Hepatitis A typically begins with the abrupt onset of constitutional and gastrointestinal symptoms. These include fever, malaise, anorexia, nausea, abdominal discomfort, itching, myalgias, and headache. The prodromal symptoms usually abate with the onset of jaundice, although the anorexia and malaise may persist for weeks. Dark urine also commonly precedes the onset of jaundice and occurs in >80% of patients. In the rare event of acute liver failure, patients may have mental status changes and coagulopathy. Possible findings on physical examination include an enlarged and tender liver, a palpable spleen tip, low-grade fever, posterior cervical lymphadenopathy, and scleral icterus if the bilirubin level exceeds 2.5 to 3 mg/dL. The most distinctive biochemical feature is the dramatic increase in serum aminotransferase levels, which may reach a maximum of 500 to 5000 U/L. The bilirubin level is variably elevated, and AP and lactic dehydrogenase levels are usually normal to mildly elevated. The prothrombin time is generally normal and, when prolonged, should raise the suspicion of fulminant hepatic failure. Hepatitis A is unique among the forms of viral hepatitis in causing a nonspecific elevation of serum immunoglobulin levels, with IgM levels doubling during the course of the disease.

Diagnosis

Diagnosis depends on finding IgM antibody to HAV during the acute phase of illness (Figure 13-2). IgM antibody is present 5 to 10 days before the onset of symptoms and persists for 3 to 6 months. Patients with asymptomatic illness may have detectable IgM for a shorter period than those with symptomatic disease. IgG anti-HAV is often present early in infection, persists for decades, and when detected without the presence of IgM, indicates recovery and protection from reinfection. Commercial diagnostic tests are available for the detection of IgM and total (IgM and IgG) anti-HAV in serum.

Natural History
Expected Outcome

Most patients have complete resolution of their symptoms within 2 months. Disease morbidity and mortality correlate with age. The case-fatality rate in infants and children up to 14 years of age is 0.1%; for adults requiring hospitalization it is 3%. However, 10% to 15% of symptomatic persons have an atypical course of prolonged or relapsing disease that falls into one of three major categories:

- Acute liver failure heralded by increasing aminotransferase levels and bilirubin, change in mental status, and profound coagulopathy.

- Cholestatic hepatitis, defined as persistent marked elevation of the serum bilirubin level (>10 mg/dL for >12 weeks) in the absence of hemolysis or renal failure. The prognosis for recovery is excellent.
- A relapsing or biphasic form, seen in 6% to 10% of patients and typically occurring 4 to 15 weeks after the initial onset. The relapse may be more or less severe than the initial episode with recurrence of symptoms and liver test abnormalities and the presence of HAV in the stool. Despite the protracted course characteristic of this variant, the prognosis for complete recovery is excellent.

Treatment and Prevention
Methods

Management consists of supportive measures, relief of symptoms, and prevention of further injury. Symptomatic therapy for nausea and pain is commonly required, but otherwise medications are best avoided. Sedatives should not be given because their elimination is delayed in patients with hepatic disease. A reduction in physical activity may be necessitated by fatigue, although studies have not shown bed rest to affect the duration of symptoms. No dietary restrictions are required except that alcohol is prohibited during the acute phase of illness.

Because hepatitis A remains a major public health problem, the importance of prevention is enhanced. Two important tools in the prevention of HAV infection are vaccines and immune globulin. Before the development of the HAV vaccines, passive immunization with human immune globulin containing IgG anti-HAV was the mainstay of prophylaxis. Human serum immune globulin (IG) is of greatest value when used before or within 2 weeks of exposure to HAV. It is not indicated for people who already have clinical manifestations of hepatitis A. When used for preexposure prophylaxis, as before travel to endemic areas, a dose of 0.02 mL/kg of IG administered intramuscularly confers protection for <3 months, and a dose of 0.06 mL/kg confers protection for 4 to 6 months. If administered within 2 weeks after exposure to HAV, 0.02 mL/kg of IG is >85% effective in preventing hepatitis A.

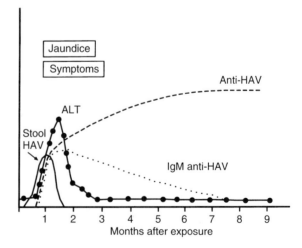

FIG. 13-2 Clinical course and serologic markers of hepatitis A. Note the diagnostic value of IgM anti-HAV in the acute illness, whereas total anti-HAV (measured as IgM and IgG but consisting mainly of IgG after the first several months) can persist for decades.

The goals of hepatitis A immunization are to protect persons from infection and reduce disease incidence by preventing transmission. Several inactivated and attenuated hepatitis A vaccines have been developed. The vaccines currently licensed in the United States are Havrix by SmithKline Beecham Biologicals and Vaqta by Merck & Company. Both of these vaccines are inactivated. The vaccine is recommended for children living in areas where rates of hepatitis A are at least twice the national average (which is 10 cases per 100,000 population), travelers to endemic areas, homosexuals, illegal drug users, persons working with nonhuman primates, and susceptible persons who have chronic liver disease (hepatitis C in particular). The pediatric dose is 0.5 mL followed by a booster dose of 0.5 mL 6 to 18 months later. Adults age 18 or older should receive a 1-mL dose followed by a 1-mL booster dose 6 to 12 months later. Protective antibody levels develop in 94% to 100% of adults 1 month after the first dose, and almost all persons have protective levels after the second dose. Immunity against HAV with two doses of the current vaccines is estimated to last 15 to 20 years.

Complications

Serious adverse events from immune globulin are rare. Anaphylaxis has been reported after repeated administration to patients who have immunoglobulin A deficiency, and thus IG should not be given to these persons. Since IG can interfere with the response to live-attenuated vaccines, the administration of such vaccines should be delayed for 3 to 6 months after use of IG. If IG must be used within 2 to 4 weeks after administration of a live-attenuated vaccine, the patient must be revaccinated.

The most frequently reported side effect of hepatitis A vaccines, occurring within 3 days after administration, were soreness at the injection site, headache, and malaise. Review of data from multiple sources for >5 years did not identify any *serious* adverse events among children or adults that could be definitively attributed to the vaccine.

When to Refer

Referral of a patient with HAV infection to a subspecialist is rarely needed. Situations in which this may be indicated are the development of encephalopathy or other signs of liver failure, when the patient has chronic liver disease, or clinical deterioration for unclear reasons.

 KEY POINTS

HEPATITIS A

⊃ An incubation period of 15 to 50 days is followed by an acute onset of hepatitis.

⊃ Transmission is fecal-oral.

⊃ Diagnosis is made by finding anti-HAV IgM antibodies.

⊃ The course is self-limited. A relapsing or biphasic course is seen in 6% to 10% of patients, but the disease does not lead to cirrhosis.

⊃ Occasionally hepatitis A leads to fulminant hepatitis.

⊃ Therapy is supportive.

⊃ Prevention is with inactivated HAV vaccine or prophylaxis with IG.

SUGGESTED READING

Centers for Disease Control and Prevention. Demographic differences in notifiable infectious disease morbidity—United States, 1992-1994. MMWR 1997; 46: 637-641.

Centers for Disease Control and Prevention. Prevention of hepatitis A through active or passive immunization: recommendations of the Advisory Committee on Immunization Practices (ACIP). MMWR 1999; 48 (RR-12).

Cuthbert JA. Hepatitis A: old and new. Clin Microbiol Rev 2001; 14: 38-58.

Glikson M, Galun E, Oren R, et al. Relapsing hepatitis A: review of 14 cases and literature survey. Medicine (Baltimore) 1992; 71: 14-23.

Lemon SM, Thomas DL. Vaccines to prevent viral hepatitis. N Engl J Med 1997; 336: 196-204.

Willner IR, Uhl MD, Howard SC, et al. Serious hepatitis A: an analysis of patients hospitalized during an urban epidemic in the United States. Ann Intern Med 1998; 128: 111-114.

Hepatitis B

Hepatitis B is a major cause of acute and chronic hepatitis, cirrhosis, and hepatocellular carcinoma worldwide. In the United States each year approximately 300,000 individuals contract hepatitis B and an estimated 1 to 1.25 million people have chronic HBV infection. These persons are the major reservoir of HBV and are at high risk for the serious long-term sequelae of chronic infection. The risk of chronic infection is inversely proportional to age. It occurs in 90% of infants infected at birth, 25% to 50% of children infected at 1 to 5 years of age, and 5% to 10% of people infected as older children or adults. In addition, immunosuppressed patients or individuals with comorbid conditions are at greater risk for chronic hepatitis B infection.

Because more than 90% of childhood HBV infections are asymptomatic, the true incidence of childhood illness is unclear. The incidence of acute hepatitis B reached a peak in 1985 but by 1991 had declined by 40%. The rate of acute hepatitis B has continued to decline, probably from changes in disease transmission patterns and use of hepatitis B vaccine.

Presentation and Progression
Cause

HBV is a small, enveloped DNA virus of the Hepadnaviridae family. HBV replicates in the liver and causes hepatic dysfunction. It is transmitted by percutaneous or mucosal exposure to infectious blood or other body fluids, blood products, or contaminated instruments; by sexual contact with an infected person; and perinatally from an infected mother to her infant. Sexual contact in both heterosexual and homosexual populations is the most commonly recognized mode of transmission. The highest prevalence of HBV infection is among injecting drug users, male homosexuals, and persons born in areas of high HBV endemicity and their descendants. Other groups at substantial risk include heterosexuals with multiple sexual partners, household contacts of HBV carriers, and health care workers. Practices that involve percutaneous exposure to blood products, such as acupuncture, body piercing, and tattooing, are documented but less common causes of transmission.

The incubation period of hepatitis B ranges from 45 to 160 days (average 120 days). After inoculation, HBV replication begins with binding of the virus to the hepatocyte cell surface. The virus is transported unprocessed into the nucleus where it undergoes replication without integration into the host genome. The mature viral particles are packed into the virus envelope along with HBV surface antigen (HBsAg) and then exported from the cell. Although HBsAg has been detected in a wide variety of body fluids, only serum, semen, and saliva have been demonstrated to be infectious. The presence of hepatitis Be antigen (HBeAg) in serum correlates with greater infectivity.

Presentation

The clinical manifestations of acute hepatitis B are highly variable and age dependent. In the majority of cases acute infection is clinically silent, particularly when acquired early in life. Neonates generally do not develop signs or symptoms and infection produces typical illness in only 5% to 15% of children 1 to 5 years of age. Older children and adults are symptomatic in 33% to 50% of cases. Symptoms are usually self-limited and last less than 4 to 6 months in most immunocompetent adults. Prodromal symptoms include malaise, anorexia, low-grade fever, nausea, vomiting, dark urine, pale stools, and abdominal discomfort. After approximately 2 weeks these symptoms resolve and jaundice may develop. Jaundice is typically mild and lasts no longer than 1 month. Occasionally, a serum sickness–like syndrome occurs with skin rash (often urticarial), arthralgias, and arthritis.

Physical examination during the acute illness is often unrevealing. Low-grade fever and right upper quadrant tenderness may be present, and, less commonly, there may be hepatomegaly and splenomegaly. Skin abnormalities, when found, are usually a nonspecific rash or icterus.

As a result of its tendency to be a clinically silent disease, hepatitis B is often diagnosed in its chronic form. Chronic infection with HBV is defined as the presence of HBsAg in serum for at least 6 months or the presence of HBsAg and the absence of IgM anti-HBc. Hepatitis B often comes to medical attention when serum liver enzyme tests are performed during routine examination or during screening for insurance eligibility. In chronic infection symptoms are frequently nonspecific and the most common complaints are anorexia, malaise, and fatigue. Physical findings in patients with chronic infection are variable and are related to the severity of liver disease. Chronic

stigmata of liver disease, including spider angiomas, palmar erythema, peripheral edema, ascites, splenomegaly, and gynecomastia, are commonly present in patients with decompensated liver disease.

Diagnosis

Hepatitis B is associated with both virus-specific and nonspecific laboratory features. The aminotransferase levels are usually elevated as in other forms of viral hepatitis, but the degree is variable. The earliest nonspecific abnormality tends to be elevation of the AST and ALT, which reflect hepatic inflammation during the prodrome. During the acute infection the ALT levels are usually greater than the AST levels and peak ALT values can be greater than 1000 IU/L. Following these elevations the serum bilirubin level rises gradually. Jaundice becomes apparent when the level exceeds 2.5 mg/dL. In severe hepatitis, hepatic synthesis function may be impaired, resulting in reduced serum albumin levels and prolonged prothrombin time.

Although the laboratory features may be suggestive of HBV infection, the diagnosis depends on serologic markers (Table 13-1). Acute HBV infection is characterized by the presence of HBsAg in serum and the development of IgM anti-HBc. HBsAg is the earliest serologic evidence of infection and precedes all other biochemical features by several weeks (Figures 13-3 and 13-4). In a typical case of acute hepatitis B the disappearance of HBsAg and the appearance of antibody to HBsAg (anti-HBs) herald resolution of infection (Figure 13-3). Anti-HBs is a long-lived antibody that can wane with time. During the "window period" that sometimes occurs between the disappearance of HBsAg and the appearance of anti-HBs, the only indication of infection is the presence of antibody to the viral core protein (IgM anti-HBc). This marker becomes detectable approximately 2 weeks after the appearance of HBsAg. As the infection evolves, IgM anti-HBc is replaced by IgG anti-HBc, which remains detectable for years. IgM anti-HBc can be helpful in differentiating between acute (IgM anti-HBc–positive) and chronic (IgM anti-HBc–negative) infections. Also, acute HBV infection without detectable HbsAg has been reported. In such a case the presence of IgM anti-HBc supports the diagnosis.

TABLE 13-1
Interpretation of Results of Serologic Tests for Hepatitis B*

HBsAg	IgM anti-HBc	Total anti-HBc	Anti-HBs	Interpretation
+	−	−	−	Early HBV infection before anti-HBc response
+	+	−	−	Early HBV infection, onset within past 6 months
−	+	+	±	Recent HBV infection with resolution
+	−	+	−	Probable chronic HBV infection*
−	−		+	Response to hepatitis B vaccine; no evidence of infection
−	−	+	+	Past HBV infection, recovered

*The presence of HbeAg in the absence of anti-HBe indicates high infectivity.

Hepatitis B early antigen (HBeAg) is detectable at the onset of illness and usually disappears after ALT levels peak. Its detection in serum implies active viral replication and high infectivity. The presence of HBeAg >8 to 10 weeks after acute illness is predictive of chronic infection. Anti-HBe appears in the serum after the resolution of HbeAg, although these markers may overlap for a short time. As patients respond to treatment or spontaneously improve, HBeAg disappears from serum and anti-HBe becomes detectable, suggesting a quiescent state.

Diagnosis of chronic hepatitis B depends on documentation of persistence of HBsAg for >6 months (Figures 13-4 and 13-5). Chronic infection can be divided into three phases:

- An early high replication phase characterized by elevated aminotransferase levels, high infectivity, and markers of HBV replication such as HBeAg
- A low-replication or latent phase after seroconversion of HBeAg to anti-Hbe, characterized by normalizing aminotransferase levels, reduced infectivity, and loss of markers of viral replication
- A nonreplicative or convalescent phase characterized by loss of HBsAg with development of anti-HBs

The infection may periodically be "reactivated" from the latent or convalescent phase to the high-replication phase.

Natural History
Expected Outcome

Hepatitis B is often asymptomatic, and when symptoms do occur, they are usually transient and resolve over 4 to 6 months. However, acute hepatitis B has unusual variants. Occasionally, unique phenomena such as polyarteritis nodosa, cryoglobulinemia, glomerulonephritis, and serum sickness–like syndrome are seen. Fulminant hepatitis occurs in about 1% to 2% of persons with acute disease and has a case-fatality ratio of 63% to 93%. It is characterized by sudden and progressive liver dysfunction and massive necrosis of liver tissue. Occurrence of encephalopathy within 8 weeks of the onset of symptoms defines fulminant hepatitis.

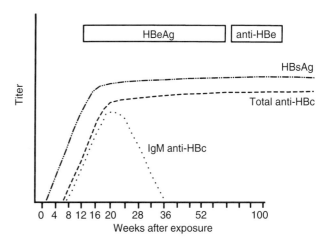

FIG. 13-4 Clinical course and serologic markers of hepatitis B in patients with an unfavorable response leading to chronic hepatitis B, as defined by the persistence of hepatitis B viral particles (measured as HBsAg) and the absence of protective antibodies (anti-HBs). The subset of patients with chronic hepatitis B who have the worst prognosis and the greatest infectivity are those who have persistence of HBeAg and do not develop anti-HBe antibodies.

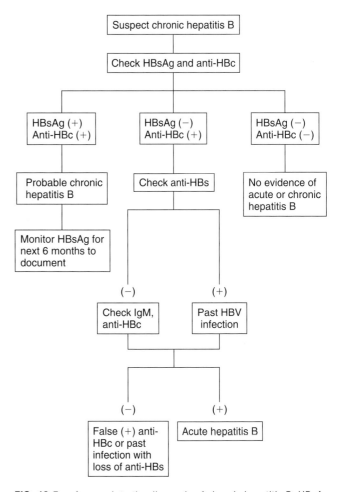

FIG. 13-5 Approach to the diagnosis of chronic hepatitis B. HBeAg and anti-HBe should be measured in patients with confirmed cases of chronic hepatitis B.

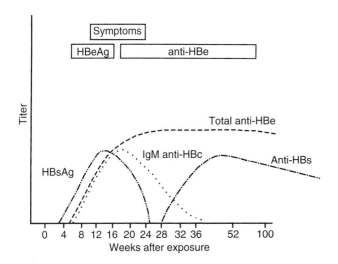

FIG. 13-3 Clinical course and serologic markers of hepatitis B in patients with a favorable response, as defined by the disappearance of hepatitis B viral particles (measured as HBsAg) and the appearance of protective antibodies (anti-HBs).

Chronic hepatitis B develops in about 5% to 10% of infected adults. The majority of these individuals (75%) have chronic persistent hepatitis B, whereas the remaining 25% have chronic active hepatitis B. Persons with persistent hepatitis remain clinically well but are potentially infectious. Their aminotransferase levels may be slightly elevated, and their disease can progress to terminal liver failure. Those with chronic active hepatitis are more likely to have persistently elevated aminotransferase concentrations and tend to be symptomatic with frequent flare-ups of disease. A serious complication of chronic infection is the development of cirrhosis with decompensated liver disease that occurs in up to 25% of these patients. The clinical signs of cirrhosis typically develop 10 to 30 years after the onset of hepatitis B, and the 5-year survival rate in these patients is about 50%. Another serious complication of chronic infection is hepatocellular carcinoma (HCC). Patients with chronic hepatitis B have a 50- to 200-fold greater risk of HCC. Risk factors for the development of HCC include infection early in life, preexisting immunocompromised condition, and male gender.

Treatment and Prevention
Methods

No specific treatment is available for acute HBV infection; care is supportive and symptomatic. Management consists of maintaining adequate nutrition, managing symptoms, and avoiding others to limit the spread of infection. Exercise can be continued as tolerated, although most patients prefer bed rest. Use of potentially hepatotoxic drugs such as acetaminophen and alcohol should be avoided. Most individuals can be managed on an outpatient basis with regular assessment of symptoms and serum aminotransferase levels. Tests for HBsAg should be repeated after clinical improvement and until seroconversion to anti-HBs. Patients with persistent HBsAg and sustained elevation of aminotransferase levels should be evaluated for possible antiviral therapy.

Treatment of chronic hepatitis B is justified by the severity of the long-term sequelae and the high infectivity of the disease. Currently, alpha-2b interferon is first-line therapy for chronic hepatitis B. Treatment with interferon-α is recommended for patients with persistent elevations of aminotransferase levels; detectable levels of HBsAg, HBeAg, and HBV DNA in serum; and chronic hepatitis as confirmed by liver biopsy. Approved regimens include either 5 million units administered intramuscularly five times a week or 10 million units three times a week for 16 weeks. Treatment response, defined as the loss of HBeAg from serum, is achieved in approximately 30% of patients. Patient characteristics associated with a favorable response to therapy include low pretherapy HBV DNA levels, high pretherapy aminotransferase levels, short duration of infection, female gender, absence of cirrhosis, and acquisition of disease in adulthood. Elimination of HBsAg from the serum and appearance of anti-HBs have occurred in approximately 65% of the responders at 5 years after treatment. This response seems to reflect immune clearance of infected hepatocytes and may predict long-term remission.

Because relatively few patients respond to interferon therapy, considerable research on other antiviral agents has been conducted. Although originally studied as an antiretroviral agent, lamivudine (3TC) has been found clinically useful against HBV. Lamivudine is the first nucleoside analog to be approved by the Food and Drug Administration (FDA) for use in chronic HBV infection and is the only nucleoside analog that has been studied in long-term clinical trials. Preliminary data suggest that long-term therapy with lamivudine is well tolerated but development of resistance is common, and further studies are needed to assess the effect of suppressive therapy. Other nucleoside analogs under investigation for use in chronic hepatitis B are famciclovir, lobucavir, and adefovir.

Liver transplantation should be considered if medical treatment has failed to prevent the progression to end-stage liver disease or in cases of fulminant acute hepatitis B. Patients receiving liver transplants for hepatitis B have lower 1-year survival rates than patients receiving transplants for other liver diseases because of the morbidity and mortality associated with reinfection of the graft by HBV, which occurs in 80% to 100% of cases if prophylaxis is not given.

At present the two forms of immunization against HBV infection are hepatitis B vaccine, which provides long-term protection and is recommended for preexposure and postexposure prophylaxis, and hepatitis B immune globulin, which provides temporary protection (3 to 6 months) and is indicated only in certain postexposure situations.

Currently available vaccines (Recombivax HB and Engerix-B) are preparations of HBsAg produced by recombinant DNA technology. Standard vaccination involves three intramuscular injections of HBV vaccine, at 0, 1, and 6 months. The CDC's strategy to eliminate hepatitis B transmission includes prenatal testing of pregnant women for HBsAg to identify newborns who require immunoprophylaxis, routine vaccination of children born to HBsAg-negative mothers, and vaccination of certain adolescents and adults at high risk of infection. High-risk groups for whom vaccination is recommended include persons with occupational risk, clients and staff of institutions for the developmentally disabled, patients receiving hemodialysis, recipients of clotting factor concentrates, household contacts and sex partners of HBV carriers, international travelers, injecting drug users, sexually active homosexual and bisexual men, sexually active heterosexual men and women, and inmates of long-term correctional facilities.

Hepatitis B immune globulin (HBIG) is recommended for nonimmune individuals who are exposed to HBV-contaminated fluids or material. In these situations HBIG 0.06 mL/kg IM for adults is given along with the complete course of HBV vaccine. The first dose of vaccine administered concurrently with HBIG should be given at a different site. The guidelines for HBIG administration apply in cases of perinatal exposure of an infant born to an HBsAg-positive mother; percutaneous or mucous membrane exposure to HBsAg-positive blood; and sexual exposure to an HBsAg-positive person. Data are limited, but HBIG is estimated to be 75% to 95% effective in preventing such infections if administered within 14 days of exposure. HBIG may also be used to protect patients from severe recurrent HBV infection after liver transplantation.

Complications

Side effects from interferon-α treatment are common and appear to be dose related. The most common adverse effect is a flulike syndrome, which generally occurs within the first several hours to days and has been reported in up to 98% of patients receiving the drug. Administering acetaminophen before each dose of interferon may attenuate this syndrome. Other side effects are diarrhea, lethargy, depression, alopecia, nausea, anorexia, and irritability. In addition, interferon can cause induce autoimmune thyroiditis. Therefore thyroid function tests should be obtained before and at the midpoint of treatment. Because granulocytopenia, anemia, and thrombocytopenia can occur during therapy, a complete blood count should be obtained on a regular basis. The interferon dose may need to be decreased or discontinued altogether if blood counts decline to unacceptable levels.

Hepatitis B vaccines have been shown to be safe when administered to adults and children. The most frequently reported side effects are pain at the injection site (3% to 29%) and temperature $\geq$99.8° F (37.7° C) (1% to 6%). In the United States, surveillance of severe adverse reactions has shown a possible association between Guillain-Barré syndrome and receipt of the first dose of plasma-derived hepatitis B vaccine in adults. Data from reporting systems for adverse events, however, do not indicate an association between recombinant hepatitis B vaccine and Guillain-Barré syndrome. Surveillance for vaccine-associated adverse events will continue to be an important part of public health. Any adverse event suspected to be associated with hepatitis B vaccination should be reported to the Vaccine Adverse Event Reporting System (VAERS) at 1-800-822-7967.

When to Refer

Referral for acute hepatitis B is limited to patients with severe cases characterized by marked prolongation of the prothrombin time, encephalopathy, ascites, edema, or inability to maintain adequate hydration. Chronically infected patients with new symptoms or signs of jaundice, weight loss, increasing ascites, or abdominal pain should be evaluated for hepatocellular carcinoma. In addition, patients with comorbid illness or an immunocompromised state may require referral to a subspecialist. Patients with chronic hepatitis B should be referred for possible treatment with interferon-α or other agents such as lamivudine.

 KEY POINTS

HEPATITIS B

- The incubation period is 30 to 150 days. The onset can be insidious or acute.
- Transmission is by blood, sexual, or perinatal exposure.
- The disease can lead to chronic illness with such sequelae as cirrhosis and hepatocellular carcinoma.
- Diagnosis is based on serologic markers.
- Therapy is supportive for acute infection, interferon-α or lamivudine for chronic infection.
- Prevention is via recombinant vaccine with or without HBIG.

SUGGESTED READING

Alter MJ, Mast EE. The epidemiology of viral hepatitis in the United States. Gastroenterol Clin North Am 1994; 23: 437-455.

Dienstag JL, Schiff ER, Wright TL, et al. Lamivudine as initial treatment for chronic hepatitis B in the United States. N Engl J Med 1999; 341: 1256-1263.

Mahoney FJ. Update on diagnosis, management, and prevention of hepatitis b virus infection. Clin Microbiol Rev 1999; 12: 351-366.

Malik AH, Lee WM. Chronic hepatitis B virus infection: treatment strategies for the next millennium. Ann Intern Med 2000; 132: 723-731.

Rogers S, Liang T. Acute and Chronic Hepatitis B and D. In: Wu G, Israel J, eds. Diseases of the Liver and Bile Ducts: Diagnosis and Treatment. Totowa, NJ: Humana Press Inc.; 1998: 121-129.

Hepatitis C

Hepatitis C virus (HCV) is the most important cause of chronic liver disease and the most common chronic blood-borne infection in the United States. Formerly known as non-A, non-B hepatitis, HCV infection accounts for about 20% of acute viral hepatitis, 60% to 70% of chronic hepatitis, and 30% of cirrhosis and liver cancer. The incidence of acute hepatitis C remained stable through much of the 1980s but declined dramatically between 1989 and 1995. Most of the decline in transfusion-associated hepatitis C occurred before testing of blood donors for anti-HCV began and was temporally associated with changes in the donor population resulting from exclusion of HIV-antibody positive donors. However, additional reduction in incidence has been noted since the introduction of surrogate testing. An estimated 4 million Americans (1.8%) have antibody to HCV (anti-HCV). Most of these persons are chronically infected and are unaware of their infection because they are not clinically ill. These individuals serve as a source of transmission to others and are at risk for chronic liver disease or other HCV-related chronic diseases during the years after primary infection.

A distinct characteristic of hepatitis C is its tendency to cause chronic liver disease. Chronic infection will develop in >75% of patients with acute HCV infection; of these, 60% to 70% will have fluctuating or persistently elevated ALT levels. Cirrhosis will develop in an estimated 20% to 50% of chronically infected persons. Population-based studies indicate that 40% of chronic liver disease is HCV related, resulting in an estimated 8000 to 10,000 deaths each year. HCV-associated end-stage liver disease is the most frequent indication for liver transplantation in adults.

Presentation and Progression
Cause

HCV is an enveloped RNA virus of which there are least six genetically distinct genotypes and more than 50 subtypes. Little difference in the severity of disease has been observed among the various genotypes, but data suggest that genotype 1, which is the most common in the United States, is less likely to respond to treatment with interferon-α. Like other RNA viruses, the HCV genome exhibits substantial heterogeneity as a result of mutations that occur during viral replication. Therefore an individual patient with HCV infection may have multiple heterogeneous variants called quasi-species. This characteristic is thought to contribute to HCV's tendency to cause chronic infection by avoiding the host immune response.

The incubation period for acute HCV infection ranges from 2 weeks to 6 months with an average of 6 to 7 weeks. Viral replication can, however, be detected as early as 1 week after exposure. The pathogenic mechanisms responsible for liver injury in acute and chronic HCV infection are unclear. It is thought that cellular immunity, specifically CD8+ and

CD4$^+$ lymphocytes and the proinflammatory cytokines they produce, plays a significant role in the liver damage associated with chronic infection.

HCV is spread primarily by contact with blood and blood products. Blood transfusions before 1992 and the use of shared, unsterilized needles and syringes have been the main source of HCV infections in the United States. Anyone, including persons without signs and symptoms of hepatitis C, who received blood products before 1992 or who has used intravenous drugs should be offered HCV testing. Another major risk group is people who have frequent exposure to blood products such as patients with hemophilia, solid-organ transplants, chronic renal failure, or malignancy requiring chemotherapy. Health care workers who suffer needle stick injuries are at significant risk, with transmission rates ranging from 0.1% from random needle sticks to 5% to 10% from a needle stick associated with an HCV RNA–positive index case. Groups thought to be at a slightly increased risk for hepatitis C are infants born to HCV-infected mothers, people with high-risk sexual behavior, and people who use cocaine. Intranasal cocaine use can cause ulceration and bleeding, potentiating the transmission of HCV between individuals who share drug paraphernalia. Transmission through nonsexual household contact has not been reported.

Presentation

Of patients with acute HCV infection, 60% to 70% have no symptoms, 20% to 30% have jaundice, and 10% to 20% have nonspecific symptoms such as malaise, anorexia, and abdominal discomfort. Fulminant hepatitis is unusual, but occasional patients have severe infection resembling severe cases of hepatitis A or B. The course of hepatitis C is variable, but elevations in serum ALT levels, often in a fluctuating pattern, are its most characteristic feature. The majority of patients seeking medical care for acute HCV infection have ALT levels greater than 600 U/L.

As a result of its insidious course, hepatitis C often manifests itself late in the disease process. The presence of infection may come to medical attention through routine physical examination and laboratory studies, blood donor screening, or clinical features of chronic liver disease such as hepatomegaly, splenomegaly, jaundice, ascites, and peripheral edema. The diagnosis of hepatitis C may also be suspected because of the presence of extrahepatic manifestations such as cryoglobulinemia, membranoproliferative glomerulonephritis, and porphyria cutanea tarda.

Diagnosis

The diagnosis of HCV infection can be made by detecting antibody to HCV (anti-HCV) or by the presence of HCV RNA (Figure 13-6). Anti-HCV is detected by enzyme immunoassay (EIA) with a sensitivity of ≥97%, but this will not distinguish among acute, chronic, and resolved infection. The majority (90%) of patients with hepatitis C infection have detectable anti-HCV by 12 weeks. Therefore anti-HCV testing should be repeated if acute hepatitis C is suspected and the initial test result is negative. As with other screening tests, the positive predictive value of anti-HCV varies depending on the prevalence of the infection in the population (Bayes' theorem, Chapter 1). Therefore a positive anti-HCV test should be confirmed either with a recombinant immunoblot assay (RIBA) or by nu-

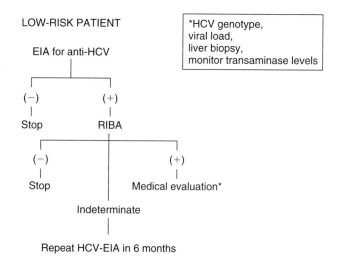

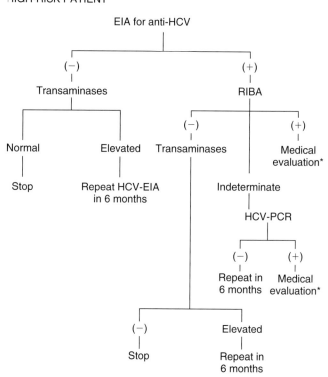

FIG. 13-6 Approach to the diagnosis of hepatitis C. Demonstration of hepatitis C virus DNA by the polymerase chain reaction can be useful in problem cases.

cleic acid detection with reverse transcriptase polymerase chain reaction (RT-PCR). RT-PCR may be particularly useful when ALT levels are normal or only slightly elevated or when anti-HCV is not present, as may occur in immunocompromised patients unable to produce antibodies for detection by EIA. Although RT-PCR assays are available from several commercial laboratories, the results may vary considerably among laboratories and at this time no such assays are approved by the FDA. In addition to variability resulting from lack of standardization among laboratories, HCV RNA levels may fluctuate during the course of infection and therefore a single negative test is not conclusive.

Several methods are available for measuring the titer of HCV in serum, which is an indirect assessment of viral load. These methods include a branched-chain DNA assay and quantitative PCR. These quantitative assays are less sensitive than the standard RT-PCR and so should not be used as a primary test to confirm or exclude the diagnosis of hepatitis C. The viral load does not correlate with the severity of the hepatitis or with a poor prognosis, but a low viral titer may indicate a greater likelihood of response to antiviral therapy. Sequential measurement of HCV RNA levels has not thus far proved useful in managing patients with hepatitis C.

Liver biopsy is not necessary for the diagnosis of HCV infection but is useful for grading the severity of disease and staging the degree of liver fibrosis. Biopsy will also determine the presence of other causes of liver disease, such as alcoholic injury and iron overload. Information gained from liver biopsy is most helpful in deciding when to initiate therapy. Patients found to have fibrosis or moderate to severe inflammation should be offered treatment if they do not have signs of decompensation such as ascites, persistent jaundice, variceal hemorrhage, or hepatic encephalopathy.

Natural History
Expected Outcome

The course of hepatitis C is variable, but its most characteristic feature is fluctuating, polyphasic ALT patterns. As stated earlier, chronic infection develops in most patients (>75%) with acute HCV infection. No clinical features of the acute disease or risk factors for infection have been found to be predictive of chronicity.

The majority of those chronically infected will have chronic hepatitis and are at increased risk for cirrhosis and hepatocellular carcinoma. Cirrhosis develops in 10% to 20% of persons with HCV over a period of 20 to 30 years. When cirrhosis is established, the rate of hepatocellular carcinoma may be as high as 1% to 4% per year. Factors implicated in the progression from chronic hepatitis to cirrhosis include age at exposure, duration of infection, and level of liver damage on liver biopsy. Host immunity, alcohol intake, and concomitant infection with HBV or HDV and HIV may also influence the progression of HCV infection. Although factors predicting the severity of liver disease have not been well defined, data suggest that increased alcohol intake, age greater than 40 years at the time of infection, and male gender are associated with more severe liver disease. Chronic alcohol use increases the risk of cirrhosis three-fold and hepatocellular cancer five-fold compared with the risk in nondrinkers.

Treatment and Prevention
Methods

Once identified as HCV positive, patients should be evaluated for the presence and severity of chronic liver disease. Therapy is recommended for patients with persistently elevated ALT levels, detectable HCV RNA, and a liver biopsy that reveals moderate inflammation and necrosis. Those who do not meet these criteria should be managed on an individual basis with regular monitoring of ALT levels if no treatment has been initiated. The decision to treat should not be based on the presence or absence of symptoms, viral genotype, or serum HCV RNA levels.

Patients with advanced cirrhosis that might be at risk for decompensation with therapy should not be treated. Those with compensated cirrhosis (without jaundice, ascites, variceal bleeding, or encephalopathy) might not benefit from therapy. Interferon treatment is not FDA approved for patients aged <18 years, and its use in children, patients >60 years, and pregnant women is relatively contraindicated. Contraindications to interferon therapy include severe depression, active substance or alcohol abuse, autoimmune disease, and cytopenias.

The appropriate management of HCV infection in patients with persistently normal serum ALT levels has not been resolved. The National Institutes of Health Consensus Conference did not recommend liver biopsy, but an emerging consensus is that a liver biopsy should be performed in most if not all infected individuals. Studies of these patients have shown markedly different results, but in 10% to 20% of individuals with persistently normal ALT levels, liver biopsy reveals cirrhosis or active necroinflammatory changes. Treatment of these individuals is even more controversial but should be considered for those with significant histologic findings.

Patients coinfected with HCV and HIV pose a significant problem. Studies thus far have been inconclusive regarding the benefits of HCV treatment in this population. The decision to treat people coinfected with HIV should be made with consideration of the patient's immune status (CD4 count) and concurrent medications. Response rates to interferon therapy appear to be similar for patients with HIV having near-normal CD4 counts and those without HIV. The efficacy of combination therapy has not been documented in patients with HIV, and ribavirin may have significant interactions with other antiretroviral medications.

In the United States the FDA has approved two regimens for hepatitis C therapy:

- Monotherapy with interferon-α, given subcutaneously three times weekly in doses of 3 million units for 12 months. This results in normalization of ALT levels in approximately 50% of patients and the loss of detectable HCV RNA in serum in 33%. Unfortunately, ≥50% of these responders will relapse when treatment is stopped. Thus, only 15% to 25% have a sustained response based on ALT and HCV RNA levels. Patients who have not responded to therapy by 3 months or who have only partially responded at the end of therapy are unlikely to respond, and a decision to discontinue treatment should be considered.

- Combination therapy with interferon-α and ribavirin, an oral antiviral agent given twice a day in 200-mg capsules for a total daily dose of 1000 to 1200 mg. Combination therapy leads to loss of HCV RNA after treatment in 50% to 55% and a sustained response in 35% to 45%. Patients with genotypes 2 and 3 tend to have a higher rate of response (60% to 70%), and a 24-week course yields results equivalent to those of a 48-week course. Patients with genotype 1 tend to have a lower response rate (25% to 35%), and a 48-week course yields a more sustained response.

Combination therapy may be attempted in patients who have had a relapse after monotherapy or in patients with an incomplete response to monotherapy. In either case therapy requires close monitoring and should probably be undertaken only by physicians experienced in the use of interferon-α and ribavirin and committed to keeping up with the rapidly evolving literature in this area.

As stated earlier, chronic hepatitis C is the most common indication for liver transplantation in the United States. The recurrence rate of HCV infection after liver transplantation approaches 100%. Recurrent HCV infection, however, in contrast to recurrent hepatitis B infection, tends to be less aggressive. The 5-year survival of approximately 60% among patients with HCV-related transplants supports the continued use of liver transplantation in these patients.

The currently available therapy for hepatitis C is obviously inadequate. New medications and approaches to treatment are sorely needed. At this time the only means of preventing HCV infection are screening the blood supply, using caution when handling blood and body fluids, and avoiding high-risk behavior. Studies have been inconsistent with respect to sexual transmission. Some studies have suggested that sexual intercourse with multiple partners is associated with HCV infection, but unrevealed percutaneous exposures may confound these results. In contrast, studies of monogamous, stable sexual partners have failed to document efficient transmission of HCV. Although a definitive answer to the risk of sexual transmission is not available, the overall risk of sexual transmission is estimated to be ≤5%. Since sexual intercourse is a potential risk factor for HCV transmission, the CDC now recommends the use of a barrier method of protection during sexual intercourse. The data do not support advising HCV-positive individuals against pregnancy, but couples should be informed of the small but finite (approximately 5%) risk of vertical transmission. This risk is increased if the mother is also HIV infected. In addition, no evidence for HCV transmission through breastfeeding has been presented. Available data regarding the prevention of HCV infection with immune globulin (IG) indicates that IG is not effective for postexposure prophylaxis of hepatitis C. Postexposure use of interferon to prevent HCV infection has not been assessed. A recent study suggests that treatment of acute hepatitis C prevents chronic infection, but the indications for treatment of acute HCV infection are unclear at the time of this writing. No vaccine is currently available, and the development of one will probably take many years because it will require protection against multiple genotypes of HCV. Since patients with hepatitis C are at increased risk of fulminant hepatitis if they contract HAV or HBV, they should be vaccinated against these viruses.

Complications

Side effects of interferon occur in more than 10% of patients and include flulike symptoms, severe fatigue, depression, thyroid dysfunction, arrhythmias, and bone marrow suppression. Ribavirin also causes significant side effects, including hemolytic anemia, bone marrow failure, and renal failure. Ribavirin is teratogenic, and female patients should avoid becoming pregnant during therapy.

When to Refer

Patients with chronic hepatitis C should be referred for liver biopsy at the time of diagnosis. If they do not meet the criteria for treatment, follow-up with routine measurement of ALT levels and assessment for signs of progressive liver disease may be needed. The presence of extrahepatic manifestations may also warrant referral, since these patients may not meet the criteria for hepatitis therapy, yet still require input from various subspecialists. Hepatitis C should be treated by a physician experienced in the use of interferon-α and ribavirin.

 KEY POINTS

HEPATITIS C

⊃ The incubation period is 15 to 120 days.
⊃ Insidious hepatocellular damage occurs.
⊃ Transmission is primarily bloodborne; uncommonly, it is perinatal.
⊃ The majority of patients have chronic infection with increased risk of cirrhosis and hepatocellular carcinoma. The risk of complications is increased by alcoholism.
⊃ Diagnosis is based on measurement of anti-HCV with confirmation by RIBA or RT-PCR.
⊃ Chronic infection may be treated with interferon-α alone or in combination with ribavirin.
⊃ A recent study suggests that treatment of acute hepatitis C with interferon-α prevents chronic infection. However, the indications for treating acute hepatitis C are at present unclear.
⊃ No vaccine is available.

SUGGESTED READING

Alter MJ, Kruszon-M D, Nainan OV, et al. The prevalence of hepatitis C virus infection in the United States, 1988 through 1994. N Engl J Med 1999; 341: 556-562.

Centers for Disease Control and Prevention. Recommendations for prevention and control of hepatitis C virus (HCV) infection and HCV-related chronic disease. MMWR 1998; 47 (RR-19): 1-39.

Hirsch KR, Wright TL. The dilemma of disease progression in hepatitis C patients with normal serum aminotransferase levels. Am J Med 2000; 109: 66-67.

Hoofnagle JH. Therapy for acute hepatitis C. N Engl J Med 2001; 345: 1495-1497.

Jaeckel E, Cornberg M, Wedemeyer H, et al. Treatment of acute hepatitis C with interferon alfa-2b. N Engl J Med 2001; 345: 1452-1457.

Lauer GM, Walker BD. Hepatitis C virus infection. N Engl J Med 2001; 345: 41-52.

Liang T, Rehermann B, Seeff L, et al. Pathogenesis, natural history, treatment, and prevention of hepatitis C. Ann Intern Med 2000; 132: 296-305.

McHutchison JG, Gordon SC, Schiff ER, et al. Interferon alfa-2b alone or in combination with ribavirin as initial treatment for chronic hepatitis C. N Engl J Med 1998; 339: 1485-1492.

Hepatitis D

Hepatitis D virus (HDV) is a defective RNA virus that can be acquired as a coinfection with HBV or as a superinfection of chronic HBV carriers. HDV requires the presence of HBsAg within its lipoprotein viral coat to be infective. The prevalence of HDV among HBsAg-positive individuals is low (1.4% to 8%) and, as might be expected, is highest among injecting drug users and hemophiliacs. Interestingly, infection with HDV is virtually absent from populations with high rates of HBV infection resulting from transmission during infancy and childhood. Uncommon in the United States, HDV has its highest prevalence in areas of moderate HBV endemicity such as the Mediterranean countries and the Middle East.

HDV is transmitted most efficiently by blood and blood products. However, in countries where HDV is endemic, infection is thought to be spread by sexual contact and close living arrangements. Perinatal infection is rare and has not been documented in the United States.

The clinical course and serologic changes are different for the two patterns of HDV infection. In either case hepatitis D may be difficult to diagnose. Two tests for antibody to HDV (anti-HDV) are commercially available. High titers of anti-HDV are present in most infected individuals, but the antibody response is quite variable. Acute coinfection with HBV may result in a severe biphasic hepatitis or even fulminant disease. Chronic hepatitis rarely develops. In contrast, superinfection in patients with chronic hepatitis B commonly results in chronic HDV infection. Superinfection often manifests itself as a sudden, unexplained clinical and biochemical deterioration in a previously stable patient. As with coinfection, the likelihood of severe hepatitis and fulminant disease are increased with superinfection. More commonly, though, superinfection results in a particularly aggressive, chronic course of liver disease. The role of HDV in the development of cirrhosis and hepatocellular cancer is unclear, but its effect on the severity and chronicity of disease may have an effect on these sequelae.

The only therapeutic agent that has proved effective in patients with hepatitis D superinfection is interferon-α. The same regimen used for the treatment of hepatitis B has been shown to lower serum aminotransferase levels in approximately 30% to 70% of patients infected with HDV. Histologic improvement has also been noted in these individuals, but loss of viral replication is uncommon and relapse after treatment occurs in the majority of patients. Because of the aggressive and chronic nature of superinfection, prolonged or even continuous treatment with high-dose interferon-α may be warranted. Since HDV depends on HBV for replication, HBV-HDV coinfection can be prevented with either preexposure or postexposure prophylaxis for HBV; however, no existing vaccine prevents HDV superinfection of HBsAg carriers. Therefore prevention of HDV superinfection depends on education to reduce risk behaviors among HBsAg carriers.

 KEY POINTS

HEPATITIS D

⊃ Hepatitis D occurs with hepatitis B as a coinfection or superinfection.

⊃ Coinfection with hepatitis B increases the risk of fulminant hepatitis.

⊃ Superinfection with hepatitis B tends to be chronic and aggressive.

⊃ Transmission occurs through blood and blood products, through sexual contact, and possibly perinatally.

SUGGESTED READING

Fattovich G, Giustina G, Christensen E, et al. The European Concerted Action on Viral Hepatitis. Influence of hepatitis delta virus infection on morbidity and mortality in compensated cirrhosis type B. Gut 2000; 46: 420-426.

Hoofnagel J. Type D (delta) hepatitis. JAMA 1989; 261: 1321-1325.

Katelaris PH, Jones DB. Fulminant hepatic failure. Med Clin North Am 1989; 73: 1989.

Lettau LA, McCarthy JG, Smith MH, et al. Outbreak of severe hepatitis due to delta and hepatitis B viruses in parenteral drug abusers and their contacts. N Engl J Med 1987; 317: 1256-1262.

Taylor J. Hepatitis delta virus. Intervirology 1999; 42: 173-178.

Hepatitis E

Hepatitis E virus (HEV), formerly called enterically transmitted non-A, non-B hepatitis, is an RNA virus related to the calicivirus family. It is transmitted by the fecal-oral route, and fecally contaminated drinking water has been the most commonly documented source of transmission. This often occurs in areas of poor socioeconomic and hygienic conditions, typically during rainy seasons or after floods. HEV is endemic in Asia, India, Pakistan, Mexico, the Middle East, and the former Soviet Union but is rare in the United States. The majority of documented cases in North America have been in individuals who originated from or had traveled to regions of known endemicity.

The typical incubation period has been reported to range from 2 to 9 weeks, with an average of 40 days. Overt disease predominantly occurs between the ages of 15 and 40 years, with an approximately equal gender distribution. Clinical hepatitis E is usually a mild, self-limited disease with no known tendency for chronicity. As with hepatitis A, the severity of hepatitis E seems to increase with age. A characteristic feature of hepatitis E infection is the high mortality rate (approaching 20%) among pregnant women infected during the third trimester.

Clinical hepatitis E occurs in two phases. The first, or prodromal phase, is preicteric and characterized by fever and nausea. The second, or icteric phase, is characterized by jaundice and dark urine. Other symptoms are anorexia, abdominal pain, arthralgias, clay-colored stools, diarrhea, and pruritus. Findings on physical examination may include hepatosplenomegaly, abdominal tenderness, rash, and jaundice.

A number of diagnostic tests for HEV have been developed, but none are yet commercially available in the United States. In practice the diagnosis is one of exclusion. Patients with symptoms and clinical findings consistent with viral hepatitis should have serologic tests for the other hepatotropic viruses. They should also be asked about travel to areas of HEV endemicity. The difficulty in using exclusion to diagnose HEV is that simultaneous infection with HEV and another hepatotropic virus may prevent the recognition of hepatitis E infection.

In the majority of cases hepatitis E can be managed supportively in the outpatient setting. Careful follow-up with evaluation of liver biochemistry findings will identify the patients at risk for fulminant hepatitis. Because of the high mortality rate in pregnant women, observation in a hospital environment should be considered for these individuals. Prophylaxis is an important issue for travelers to endemic countries. At this time no vaccine is available, and immune globulin has proved ineffective in preventing HEV transmission. Hepatitis E antibodies in affected individuals, however, are protective against repeat exposure. Currently the best prophylaxis is to advise travelers to drink water only from safe sources, avoid uncooked fruits and vegetables, and wash the hands frequently.

When to Refer

Because of the high mortality, pregnant women with suspected hepatitis E should be placed in a hospital capable of handling high-risk pregnancy. Any patient who exhibits signs of liver decompensation should be referred to a subspecialist.

KEY POINTS

HEPATITIS E

⊃ Hepatitis E is rare in the United States; most cases are imported.

⊃ After an acute onset the disease is usually self-limited, but fulminant hepatitis occurs in 1% to 2%.

⊃ The mortality rate is higher in pregnant women.

⊃ The disease is diagnosed by exclusion and travel history.

⊃ Preventive measures include use of a safe water supply, proper food handling, and handwashing.

SUGGESTED READING

Aggarwal R, Krawczynski K. Hepatitis E: an overview and recent advances in clinical and laboratory research. J Gastroenterol Hepatol 2000; 15: 9-20.

Harrison TJ. Hepatitis E virus—an update. Liver 1999; 19: 171-176.

Kwo PY, Schlauder GG, Carpenter HA, et al. Acute hepatitis E by a new isolate acquired in the United States. Mayo Clin Proc 1997; 72: 1133-1136.

Mast EE, Kuramoto IK, Favorov MO, et al. Prevalence of and risk factors for antibody to hepatitis E virus seroreactivity among blood donors in Northern California. J Infect Dis 1997; 176: 34-40.

Hepatitis G and TT Virus

Search continues for causes of viral hepatitis that cannot be attributed to hepatitis viruses A, B, C, D, or E. Two such candidate viruses are hepatitis G virus and transfusion-transmitted virus (TT virus; TTV).

Hepatitis G virus (HGV) is a single-stranded RNA virus that belongs to the family Flaviviridae. It has a global distribution but is predominantly found in West Africa where the seroprevalence has been estimated at 15%. HGV is present in 1% to 2% of blood donors in the United States and in 3% to 6% of cases of hepatitis that cannot be attributed to the known hepatitis viruses. However, whether infection with HGV leads to disease is still controversial. A majority of patients who become HGV positive after blood transfusion have normal serum aminotransferase levels and are not found to develop liver disease during prolonged follow-up. Furthermore, when aminotransferase levels are elevated, they rarely correlate with levels of viremia. Interestingly, infection with one type (type C) of HGV seems to have a protective effect on the course of infection caused by the human immunodeficiency virus (HIV), as evidenced by a slower progression to AIDS. No sensitive and reliable serologic assays are commercially available for the detection of HGV infection. Whether blood banks should screen for hepatitis B remains unclear. It seems unlikely that excluding a significant proportion of blood donors would be beneficial at this time.

TT virus (TTV), a nonenveloped DNA virus, was first isolated from a Japanese patient with posttransfusion hepatitis. About 12% of Japanese and 3% to 7.5% of U.S. blood donors have TTV DNA in their bloodstreams. As with HGV, the role of TTV as an independent cause of hepatitis remains to be defined. A strong argument against the role of TTV in hepatitis is that although its prevalence in blood donors is significant, the incidence of transfusion-associated hepatitis continues to decline. In addition, the presence of TTV in serum does not appear to correlate with abnormal serum aminotransferase levels. Favoring the role of TTV as a primary agent of hepatitis is that TTV DNA titers in the liver are 10 to 100 times those of the corresponding serum. Clearly, further studies are needed before TTV can be identified as the next hepatitis virus.

SUGGESTED READING

Alter HJ. The cloning and clinical implications of HGV and HGBV-C. N Engl J Med 1996; 334: 1356-1357.

Bendinelli M, Pistello M, Maggi F, et al. Molecular properties, biology, and clinical implications of TT virus, a recently identified widespread infectious agent of humans. Clin Microbiol Rev 2001; 14: 98-113.

Lefrere JJ, Roudot-Thoraval F, Lefrere F, et al. Natural history of the TT virus infection through follow-up of TTV DNA-positive multiple-transfused patients. Blood 2000; 95: 347-351.

Mphahlele MJ, Lau GK, Carman WF. HGV: the identification, biology, and prevalence of an orphan virus. Liver 1998; 18: 143-155.

Stosor V, Wolinsky S. GB virus C and mortality from HIV infection. N Engl J Med 2001; 345: 761-762.

TABLE 14-2
Some Microorganisms Causing Urinary Tract Infection and Their Clinical Correlates

Microorganism	Clinical correlates
Escherichia coli	Causes 75% to 80% of uncomplicated UTIs and is often found in complicated UTIs. Some strains are notoriously more "uropathogenic" than others.
Staphylococcus saprophyticus	Causes up to 15% of uncomplicated UTIs in women and is more common during the spring and summer. Since it is a coagulase-negative staphylococcus and often grows to a low concentration in urine (10^2 to 10^4 CFUs/mL), it can be dismissed as a contaminant by unsuspecting laboratory personnel. It can be distinguished from other coagulase-negative staphylococci by its resistance to novobiocin.
Proteus mirabilis	A urea-splitting gram-negative rod that causes the urine to be alkaline (pH ≥ 7), which promotes the formation of struvite calculi capable of becoming large "staghorn calculi" that can completely obstruct the renal pelvis.
Aerobic gram-negative rods other than *E. coli* and *P. mirabilis*	*Klebsiella* species sometimes cause uncomplicated community-acquired UTI, but the presence of other gram-negative species usually signifies complicated infection. Enterobacteriaceae such as *Enterobacter, Serratia,* and *Providencia* species are typically encountered in patients who have received multiple courses of antibiotics or have indwelling bladder catheters. Most patients with UTI caused by *Pseudomonas aeruginosa* have obstructive uropathy and have been seen by a urologist.
Enterococci	Enterococci are the most common gram-positive bacteria causing UTI. Their presence in the urine usually correlates with some combination of prior antibiotic therapy, urologic instrumentation, or obstructive uropathy. Enterococcal UTI is a risk factor for enterococcal endocarditis, which occurs mainly in younger women and older men. Enterococci resistant to vancomycin are becoming a major epidemiologic problem in the United States and elsewhere.
Staphylococcus aureus	The presence of coagulase-positive staphylococci (*S. aureus*) in urine often represents a "spill-over" from bacteremia rather than infection of the urinary tract per se. However, *S. aureus* bacteriuria can also signify the presence of an intrarenal abscess (renal carbuncle).
Staphylococcus epidermidis	This coagulase-negative staphylococcus is most often seen as a hospital-acquired pathogen related to indwelling urinary catheters. *S. epidermidis* is also a frequent contaminant of urine cultures due to its heavy presence in the normal skin flora.
Anaerobic bacteria and fastidious aerobic bacteria	These microorganisms are seldom encountered in urine cultures because the urinary tract is a hostile environment to their growth. Because anaerobic bacteria can be part of the normal periurethral flora, proof of an etiologic role in UTI generally requires aspiration of urine by suprapubic puncture.
Candida albicans and other yeasts	Yeasts are usually encountered in catheterized patients who have received multiple courses of antibiotics. Patients are often asymptomatic, and specific therapy is often not required. However, yeasts can infect the kidneys and can give rise to "fungus balls" that can completely obstruct the ureters.
Adenoviruses	Adenoviruses occasionally cause acute hemorrhagic cystitis, mainly in children and young adults.
Lactobacillus, Gardnerella vaginalis, and *Mycoplasma*	These microorganisms have been implicated as causes of UTI, but their relative importance is unclear.

CFU, Colony-forming unit; *UTI,* urinary tract infection.

mainly a disease of females until the sixth decade. During the reproductive years women have a 50-fold increased incidence of UTI compared with men. After the fifth decade the sex distribution of UTI is approximately equal between the sexes, since problems with voiding develop in both men and women and prostatism occurs in men. In the past, all UTIs in males were considered "complicated." It is now thought that UTI results from sexual activity in some men without predisposing anatomic or functional abnormalities.

Over 90% of UTIs are caused by a single microorganism. Most uncomplicated UTIs are caused by *Escherichia coli* (Table 14-2), which frequently colonizes the periurethral tissues. *Staphylococcus saprophyticus,* one of the coagulasenegative staphylococci, accounts for 10% to 15% of uncomplicated UTI, mainly during the summer months. Complicated UTI is caused by a more diverse group of microorganisms that, compared with *E. coli,* are more difficult to treat.

Laboratory Diagnosis

The ease of obtaining urine specimens from most patients and the availability of dipsticks, microscopes, and facilities for culture in most clinics make the laboratory diagnosis of urinary tract infection a relatively straightforward matter. Key findings pointing toward UTI are pyuria (which can, however, have other causes), hematuria (a finding helpful mainly in excluding alternative diagnoses such as urethritis and vaginitis), and significant bacteriuria (as defined previously, again with the caveat that $\geq 10^5$ bacteria per milliliter can sometimes be significant). Recent studies have focused on the extent to which dipsticks can replace traditional microscopy and urine culture for patients with uncomplicated UTI. Patients with complicated UTI, however, should have cultures because therapy tends to be more prolonged and difficult.

Obtaining Urine Specimens

Especially in women, the bacterial flora of the distal urethra, vagina, and perineum often contaminates urine cultures. Specimens should be collected carefully and processed or refrigerated promptly. They should not be allowed to sit out on countertops, since aerobic bacteria double about every 20 minutes at room temperature, causing false-positive results on microscopy, dipstick urinalysis, and culture.

Clean-catch midstream urine specimens usually suffice for diagnosis of UTI in older children, nonmenstruating women, and men. Female patients should be instructed to wash their hands, squat over the toilet, and spread the labia with the nondominant hand. Using sterile gauze pads soaked in sterile water or a sponge soaked with a mild nonhexachlorophene soap, they should then swab the vulva three times, front to back, using the dominant hand. The first 10 mL of urine should be discarded unless the diagnosis of urethritis is being considered. Male patients should be instructed to retract the foreskin if present, clean the glans, and similarly discard the first 10 mL of urine (the importance of cleaning the glans before obtaining a midstream specimen in a male is debatable, but this ritual is harmless).

Catheterized specimens are indicated in certain situations, such as patients who are unable to provide clean-catch specimens because of urologic or neurologic problems, including impaired consciousness. Suprapubic aspiration of the urinary bladder can be performed safely provided the bladder is distended, but it is seldom used in current practice.

Gross Inspection of Urine

Although the days are long past when clinicians determined urine to be "good" or "evil" based on gross inspection, this simple procedure remains valuable. Urine can be cloudy because of the presence of WBCs (≥ 200/mL), red blood cells (RBCs) (≥ 500/mL), bacteria ($> 10^6$/mL), fat, chyle, or sediment such as crystals. Crystals are more prominent in alkaline specimens. The urine of patients with clinical UTI is typically cloudy, but cloudy urine is not synonymous with UTI. The finding of grossly clear urine has a 91% to 99% negative predictive value for UTI. An important caveat is that urine can be clear (and urinalysis entirely normal) in patients with perinephric abscess or obstructed ureter.

Dipstick Analysis of Urine

Rapid dipstick techniques are increasingly used as a supplement to or substitute for traditional methods of diagnosis based on microscopy and culture. Chemical reagents on separate test pads of the dipstick evaluate different properties of urine, such as pH, glucose and protein content, and the presence or absence of WBCs (pyuria), RBCs (hematuria), and significant bacteriuria. The procedure is to dip the stick into fresh, uncentrifuged urine, covering all of the test pads. The strip is then withdrawn immediately along the edge of the container in such a way as to remove any excess urine. It should be held horizontally before being read to prevent mixing of the reagents in adjacent pads. Dipsticks should be stored and read according to the manufacturer's recommendations.

The leukocyte esterase test is used to screen for WBCs in urine. The dipstick should be read at 1 minute. Some experts suggest that it be read again at 5 minutes to increase the sensitivity of the test, which detects the presence of the enzyme leukocyte esterase contained in WBCs. This test has a reported 75% to 96% sensitivity and a 94% to 98% specificity for detecting pyuria. False-positive tests are usually caused by contamination, often by vaginal secretions. False-negative specimens can be caused by hypertonic urine (as determined by high specific gravity), glycosuria, and urobilinogen. Noninfectious causes of pyuria (sterile pyuria) are discussed below.

The nitrite test is used to screen for significant bacteriuria. It is based on two observations: normal urine contains nitrates but not nitrites, and about 90% of bacterial species causing UTI can convert urinary nitrates to nitrites. The nitrite test has a 92% to 100% sensitivity for UTI but only a 35% to 85% specificity. It is most useful for detecting $\geq 10^5$ CFUs/mL of aerobic gram-negative rods. The nitrite test is especially useful to determine whether or not patients with indwelling urinary catheters are infected. In children the sensitivity of the nitrite test is high (up to 98%) but specificity is lower (29% to 44%) than in adults. False-positive tests can result from substances that cause red urine such as the ingestion of beets in susceptible subjects or the bladder analgesic phenazopyridine. False-negative nitrite tests can occur in "low-count" UTI ($\leq 10^5$ CFUs of bacteria per milliliter of urine), infections caused by bacteria that do not produce nitrites (such as enterococci), short bladder dwell time, dilute urine specimens, or acid urine.

Dipstick reagents for hematuria screen for the presence of RBCs, free hemoglobin, and myoglobin. The test is reported to be 91% to 100% sensitive and 65% to 99% specific for microscopic hematuria as defined in the following section. False-positive tests result most often from contamination with menstrual blood. Other causes of false-positive results are exercise and dehydration. Because WBCs produce a peroxidase that interferes with the peroxidase reaction of the test, dense pyuria can cause a false-positive test result. Ascorbic acid and certain antibiotics inhibit the peroxidase color change of the dipstick, resulting in a false-negative test result. The finding of hematuria is helpful in the differential diagnosis of dysuria in women, since hematuria is found in 40% to 60% of patients with cystitis but is seldom caused by urethritis or vaginitis.

Microscopic Examination of Urine

Although some authorities hold that dipstick analysis of urine is highly reliable and that microscopic examination changes the management in less than 10% of cases, microscopy of both "unspun" and "spun" samples can be extremely rewarding.

Examination of "unspun" (uncentrifuged) urine begins by placing a drop of urine on a glass slide, adding a coverslip, and using the high, dry objective of the microscope. Bacteria, recognizable as rod- or brick-shaped structures, are usually visible in patients whose urine contains gram-negative rods in an amount $\geq 10^5$ CFUs/mL. Finding one or more such bacterial structures in each high, dry magnification field carries high positive predictive value for significant bacteriuria caused by gram-negative bacilli. Round or irregularly shaped structures, on the other hand, may represent nonspecific debris or amorphous phosphates in the urine rather than gram-positive cocci. Observing WBCs in unspun urine indicates pyuria. These observations on unspun urine can be made without the application of a stain but require some experience for interpretation. The most accurate method for detecting pyuria is to look at an unspun midstream urine sample with a hemocytometer; 10 or more leukocytes per milliliter is abnormal.

Examination of "spun" (centrifuged) urine entails centrifuging at 2000 rpm for 5 minutes, discarding the supernatant, and placing a drop of the sediment on a glass slide. A coverslip is added, and the specimen is examined with the high, dry objective of the microscope as described previously. Alternatively, the drop of sediment is allowed to dry and is then stained with the Gram method (see Chapter 2). These two methods can be complementary. The presence of >5 leukocytes per high-power field indicates pyuria. This finding is 90% to 95% sensitive for detecting significant bacteriuria. However, it is not specific, since sterile pyuria can be caused by other types of infections (genitourinary tuberculosis is a classic cause; others include endocarditis, gonorrhea, and vaginitis) and also by noninfectious conditions such as glomerulonephritis, drugs (notably steroids and cyclophosphamide), trauma, and inflammation of structures abutting the urinary tract (e.g., diverticulitis or appendicitis). The absence of bacteria on Gram stain of spun urine sediment has a high negative predictive value for significant bacteriuria.

Urine Culture

Urine cultures add enormous specificity to the diagnosis of UTI and continue to be the "gold standard" for diagnosis. Unfortunately, urine culture by commercial laboratories adds significantly to the cost of managing this common infection. In uncomplicated UTI, and more specifically in the absence of fever or back pain, a case can be made for empiric treatment of UTI without culture. Treatment can be based on any combination of bacteriuria, pyuria, or hematuria. Indications for culture include suspected upper UTI, failure to respond to therapy, and frequent recurrences. A case can also be made for culture when dipstick analysis shows the urine to have a highly alkaline pH, since urea-splitting bacteria (notably *Proteus mirabilis*) can foreshadow the development of large struvite calculi.

Determining the number of bacteria in urine is accomplished by plating out cultures using a calibrated loop. A number of alternative methods have been developed such as dipslides and pipettes coated with culture media. The definition of "significant bacteriuria" as the finding of >10^5 CFUs/mL of urine (see earlier discussion) derives in part from the bimodal frequency distribution of colony counts in urine cultures. Patients with symptomatic infection usually have counts significantly $<10^5$ CFUs/mL (e.g., 10^6 or 10^7 CFUs/mL), while contaminated cultures usually show >10^3 CFUs/mL of urine. In other words, most urine cultures show $<10^3$ CFUs/mL or >10^5 CFUs/mL, with relatively few cultures falling in the gray zone between (i.e., 10^4 CFUs/mL of urine).

Colony counts $<10^5$ CFUs/mL of urine can be significant in at least four situations. First, patients with pyelonephritis—in whom the bacteria are multiplying mainly in the kidneys rather than in the urinary bladder—not infrequently have $<10^4$ CFUs/mL. Second, some patients with symptoms of lower urinary tract infection have low colony counts, which may indicate the "urethral syndrome" discussed later. Third, low colony counts can be important in patients with prostatitis and epididymitis. Fourth, low colony counts can be important in patients with fungal urinary tract infection (as discussed later).

Perspectives on Laboratory Diagnosis

Primary care clinicians should develop one or more strategies for laboratory diagnosis of UTI. There is now growing enthusiasm for use of dipsticks for diagnosis of uncomplicated UTI. A combined leukocyte esterase nitrite test, for example, has a reported sensitivity of 70% to 90% for suspected symptomatic UTI, and a Uriscreen test based on the detection of catalase (an enzyme present in leukocytes), WBCs, and RBCs has a reported sensitivity of 87%, specificity of 78%, positive predictive value of 35%, and—perhaps most important—a negative predictive value of 98% for significant bacteriuria. Microscopic examination of urine remains useful and rewarding but requires interested and experienced personnel. From the behavioral perspective, studies of urine do not seem to have much effect on the actual management of UTI by many, perhaps most, primary care clinicians. Nearly all patients with symptoms of dysuria, frequency, and urgency receive antibiotics irrespective of the results of urinalysis and culture. For more rigorous diagnosis, as in the conduct of clinical trials of antimicrobial efficacy, it is reasonable to insist on a urine culture showing >10^5 CFUs/mL for diagnosis of lower UTI (sensitivity 80%, specificity 90%) and $\geq 10^4$ CFUs/mL for diagnosis of pyelonephritis (sensitivity 90%, specificity 95%).

 KEY POINTS

LABORATORY DIAGNOSIS

⊃ Urine culture remains the "gold standard" for diagnosis but is unnecessary in most cases of uncomplicated lower UTI.

⊃ The term "significant bacteriuria" traditionally refers to >10^5 CFUs/mL of urine. This criterion should be used to diagnose UTI in asymptomatic patients.

⊃ Fewer than 10^5 CFUs/mL of urine often signifies infection in acutely symptomatic patients (especially those with pyelonephritis) and in patients whose specimens are obtained directly from an indwelling catheter.

⊃ Grossly clear urine has a negative predictive value of 91% to 99% for bacteriuria. However, the urine can be clear and the urinalysis normal in patients with perinephric abscess or obstructed ureter. The physician should therefore consider these possibilities in patients with symptoms of upper UTI and a normal urinalysis.

⊃ The combined leukocyte esterase–nitrite test has a sensitivity of between 70% and 90% for suspected symptomatic UTI. Patients whose test results are negative but who have symptoms of UTI should have a microscopic examination of the urine, a urine culture, or both.

⊃ Nearly all (nongranulocytopenic) patients with symptomatic UTI have pyuria.

⊃ Urine culture should be obtained for patients with complicated UTI, as well as patients with recurrent uncomplicated UTI if the recurrences are not clearly related to sexual activity.

- ⊃ Because the bacteria that typically cause UTI multiply rapidly at room temperature, false-positive urine cultures can occur when specimens are not plated out or refrigerated promptly.
- ⊃ The presence of bacteria on microscopic examination of unspun urine (either unstained or stained with the Gram method) predicts significant bacteriuria on culture. The absence of bacteria on microscopic examination of a Gram stain of spun urine predicts the absence of significant bacteriuria on culture.
- ⊃ Pretest probability of a positive urine culture is increased by history of UTI symptoms, back pain, pyuria, hematuria, or bacteriuria (by dipstick analysis). The presence of two or more of these findings indicates a 73% chance of a positive urine culture.

SUGGESTED READING

Jou WW, Powers RD. Utility of dipstick urinalysis as a guide to management of adults with suspected infection or hematuria. South Med J 1998; 91: 266-269.

McLeod D, Kljakovic M. What do general practitioners do when patients present with symptoms indicative of urinary tract infections? NZ Med J 1998; 111: 189-191.

Phillips G, Fleming LW, Khan I, et al. Urine transparency as an index of absence of infection. Br J Urol 1992; 70: 191-195.

Rubin RH, Shapiro ED, Andriole VT, et al. Evaluation of new anti-infective drugs for the treatment of urinary tract infection. Clin Infect Dis 1992; 15: S216-S227.

Wigton RS, Hoellerich VL, Omato JP, et al. Use of clinical findings in the diagnosis of urinary tract infection in women. Arch Intern Med 1985; 145: 2222-2227.

Winkens RAG, Leffers P, Trienekens TAM, et al. The validity of urine examination for urinary tract infections in daily practice. Fam Pract 1995; 12: 290-293.

Imaging of the Urinary Tract

Imaging studies of the urinary tract are seldom indicated in patients whose infections are limited to the lower urinary tract and are not indicated in the majority of patients who have typical signs and symptoms of pyelonephritis and respond to therapy. The traditional methods of intravenous pyelography (IVP; also known as excretory urography) and retrograde pyelography (which requires cystoscopy) have been largely replaced by CT scanning, ultrasound, and nuclear medicine studies. The newer methods are considerably safer. Risks of IVP include not only allergic reactions to iodides but also acute renal failure, to which certain patients—such as those with underlying renal disease, multiple myeloma, or diabetes mellitus—are particularly vulnerable.

Helical CT scanning is probably the most useful currently available imaging procedure for evaluation of patients with suspected acute complicated UTI. Noncontrast helical CT scanning is especially useful for patients with flank pain and suspected renal colic. About one half of these patients are found to have an obstructing calculus, for which the procedure is 97% accurate. Some are found to have acute pyelonephritis. In other patients the procedure may disclose an alternative diagnosis such as appendicitis, cholecystitis, or pelvic mass. Helical CT scanning with contrast media provides excellent detail that can point to such diagnoses as acute pyelonephritis, intrarenal abscess (renal carbuncle), perinephric abscess, renal cell carcinoma, and dilatation of the ureter (ureterectasia).

Ultrasound examination of the kidney has two advantages over CT scanning: no radiation exposure and greater accessibility. However, tissue contrast is less than with CT scanning. Ultrasound examination is less sensitive than CT scanning for diagnosis of pyelonephritis but usually shows renal swelling. Ultrasound provides an excellent way to diagnose renal abscess. A common use of ultrasound is to exclude ureterectasia resulting from obstruction. Ultrasound is also useful in excluding malformations of the urinary tract in children.

Nuclear medicine procedures for evaluation of UTI continue to evolve. Among the most popular in recent years has been DMSA scanning, that is, scintigraphy using dimercaptosuccinic acid, a compound that binds to sulfhydryl groups in the proximal renal tubules and thereby localizes to the renal cortex.

Plain x-ray examination of the lower abdomen (commonly known as the KUB, for kidney-ureter-bladder) remains useful, especially when the newer methods are unavailable. Findings of great diagnostic value include radiopaque stones in patients with renal colic or complicated upper UTI and gas in or around the kidneys in patients with emphysematous pyelonephritis, a life-threatening infection usually encountered in patients with diabetes mellitus and discussed more fully later in the chapter.

Voiding cystourethrography is commonly used for diagnosis of vesicoureteral reflux.

 KEY POINTS

IMAGING OF THE URINARY TRACT

- ⊃ Noncontrast helical CT scanning has a 97% diagnostic accuracy for detection of renal calculi and is especially useful for patients with flank pain and renal colic.
- ⊃ Contrast-enhanced helical CT scanning is, overall, the most useful imaging procedure for patients with acute UTI.
- ⊃ Ultrasound examination of the kidney is a rapid way to exclude obstructive uropathy and is sensitive for diagnosis of renal abscess and other conditions.
- ⊃ Plain x-ray examination of the lower abdomen (KUB) is helpful in the diagnosis of calculus and emphysematous pyelonephritis.

SUGGESTED READING

Baumgarten DA, Baumgartner BR. Imaging and radiologic management of upper urinary tract infections. Urol Clin North Am 1997; 24: 545-569.

Johnson JR, Vincent LM, Wang K, et al. Renal ultrasonographic correlates of acute pyelonephritis. Clin Infect Dis 1992; 14: 15-22.

Asymptomatic Bacteriuria

Asymptomatic bacteriuria is a relatively common finding. It is present in up to 5% of unselected medical outpatients, 10% of pregnant patients at term, 14% of hypertensive patients, and 20% of patients with diabetes mellitus. Anatomic obstruction of any kind markedly increases the incidence of asymptomatic bacteriuria. Thus asymptomatic bacteriuria has been found in 23% of women with cystocele, 57% of patients with congenital urologic disease, 85% of patients with hydronephrosis and nephrolithiasis, and nearly all patients in whom an indwelling retention catheter has been left in place with open drainage for more than 48 hours. Issues in primary care include when and how to diagnose asymptomatic bacteriuria and treat affected patients.

Presentation and Progression
Cause

Asymptomatic bacteriuria affects mainly women until the age when prostatism develops in men. Bacteria colonize the vaginal introitus and then invade the urinary bladder. The mechanism of colonization by *E. coli* has been studied extensively. The organism adheres to uroepithelial cells by specific binding of bacterial surface molecules (adhesins) to complementary receptors on the host's epithelial cells. The ability of *E. coli* strains to adhere to uroepithelial cells correlates with the presence of pili or fimbriae. Many studies indicate a genetic susceptibility to colonization in some women. Estrogens increase the likelihood of colonization, and oral contraceptives increase the risk of bacteriuria, apparently by causing physiologic changes in the urinary tract.

Presentation

By definition, patients are asymptomatic when bacteriuria is discovered.

Diagnosis

The diagnosis is often suggested by urinalysis (dipstick or microscopic examination) and is confirmed by urine culture. If treatment is being considered, many authorities recommend a second urine culture to exclude contamination or improper processing of the first specimen.

Natural History
Expected Outcome

Most patients remain asymptomatic. In patients without anatomic factors predisposing to UTI, bacteriuria often resolves through normal host defense mechanisms, including the mechanical flushing of the urinary stream. Complications such as pyelonephritis and sepsis are likely to occur in pregnant women, patients undergoing genitourinary surgery, and patients undergoing urethral catheterization in the presence of complicating disease.

Treatment
Methods

Treatment is indicated during pregnancy, in young children with gross vesicoureteral reflux, and in selected patients with urologic problems or ureteral obstruction (Table 14-3). Treatment is also indicated in renal transplant recipients during the early posttransplant period and in patients with severe granulocytopenia. Regimens for asymptomatic bacteriuria are the

TABLE 14-3
Efficacy of Treating Asymptomatic Bacteriuria in Different Populations

Patient group	Efficacy of treatment based on current evidence
PATIENTS FOR WHOM TREATMENT IS NOT RECOMMENDED	
School-aged girls	Treatment reduces the incidence of bacteriuria at 2 years, but there is no difference in the eventual outcome measured as symptomatic UTI or loss of renal function.
Nonpregnant adult women	Treatment does not reduce the incidence of symptomatic UTI, and bacteriuria recurs in about one half of treated patients within 12 months.
Adult men	Bacteriuria is difficult to eradicate because anatomic abnormalities are present or the prostate is infected. Persistent bacteriuria does not appear to impair renal function.
Patients with diabetes mellitus	Treatment is often followed by reinfection. Moreover, treatment does not reduce the incidence of symptomatic UTI or affect the long-term prognosis.
Elderly patients	Treatment is often followed by reinfection. Treatment does not improve overall morbidity and mortality. Treatment does not reduce the incidence of urinary incontinence.
PATIENTS FOR WHOM TREATMENT IS RECOMMENDED	
Pregnant women	Treatment reduces the incidence of symptomatic pyelonephritis.
Patients scheduled for urologic surgery	Treatment reduces the risk of complications of surgery, including urosepsis.
Some patients who have just had an indwelling bladder catheter removed	Treatment should not be attempted while the catheter is in place. Treatment is not mandatory in this patient group but may be advisable if asymptomatic bacteriuria was not documented before catheterization.
Preschool children with gross vesicoureteral reflux	Treatment may reduce the risk of complications such as renal failure and hypertension.
Some patients with struvite stones	Patients with struvite stones associated with urea-splitting organisms such as *Proteus mirabilis* should be treated aggressively in consultation with a urologist.

UTI, Urinary tract infection.

same as those for symptomatic UTI (discussed later). During pregnancy the least toxic drugs (such as β-lactam antibiotics) should be used to minimize drug exposure of the fetus (see Chapter 5). Current opinion holds that treatment of asymptomatic bacteriuria in other patient groups can actually be harmful because it poses a risk of drug toxicity that outweighs the therapeutic benefit and because it selects for resistant microorganisms.

Expected Response

Bacteriuria nearly always resolves with appropriate therapy. However, it nearly always recurs in patients who are predisposed to colonization and infection by either hereditary or anatomic factors. Frequent treatment of such patients predisposes to new infections by microorganisms that are becoming increasingly difficult to treat, such as enterococci, *Pseudomonas aeruginosa,* and yeasts. For this reason asymptomatic bacteriuria is generally best left untreated except in well-defined patient groups (Table 14-3).

When to Refer

Referral of patients for management of asymptomatic bacteriuria alone is seldom necessary.

 KEY POINTS

ASYMPTOMATIC BACTERIURIA

⊃ Asymptomatic bacteriuria is a relatively common finding in certain patient groups.

⊃ Treatment is indicated during pregnancy, in young children with gross vesicoureteral reflux, in selected patients with urologic problems or ureteral obstruction, in renal transplant recipients during the early postoperative period, and in patients with severe granulocytopenia.

⊃ In other patient groups treatment of asymptomatic bacteriuria can actually be harmful. Therefore it is usually best left alone.

SUGGESTED READING

Hooton TM, Scholes D, Stapleton AE, et al. A prospective study of asymptomatic bacteriuria in sexually active young women. N Engl J Med 2000; 343: 992-997.

Nicolle LE. Asymptomatic bacteriuria—important or not? N Engl J Med 2000; 343: 1037-1039.

Urinary Tract Infection in Children (see also Chapter 4)

During the neonatal period UTI affects mainly boys. Thereafter childhood UTI mainly affects girls. About 30% to 50% of children with UTI have vesicoureteral reflux, which can lead to permanent renal damage. Ultrasonography and voiding cystourethrography are generally recommended for boys who have had one episode of UTI and for preschool girls who have had two episodes. Children with frequent recurrent UTIs and those with severe vesicoureteral reflux should be evaluated by a urologist.

TABLE 14-4
Syndromes of Infections Causing Acute Dysuria in Women

Syndrome	Typical presentation	Pyuria	Hematuria	Urine culture (CFUs/mL)	Usual pathogens
Cystitis	Acute onset with multiple and severe symptoms (dysuria, frequency, urgency), suprapubic or low back pain, suprapubic tenderness on examination	Usually	Sometimes	10^2 to $\geq 10^5$	*Escherichia coli, Staphylococcus saprophyticus, Proteus* species, *Klebsiella* species
Urethritis	Gradual onset, milder symptoms, vaginal discharge or bleeding (caused by concomitant cervicitis), lower abdominal pain, new sex partner, cervicitis or vulvovaginal herpetic lesions on examination	Usually	Rarely	$<10^2$	*Chlamydia trachomatis, Neisseria gonorrhoeae,* herpes simplex virus
Vaginitis	Vaginal discharge or odor, pruritus, dyspareunia, external dysuria, no increased frequency or urgency, vulvovaginitis on examination	Rarely	Rarely	$<10^2$	*Candida* species, *Trichomonas vaginalis, Gardnerella vaginalis* (bacterial vaginosis)

Modified from Stamm WE, Hooton TM. The management of urinary tract infections in adults. N Engl J Med 1993; 329: 1328-1334.
CFUs, Colony-forming units.

Uncomplicated Lower Urinary Tract Infection (Cystitis) in Nonpregnant Adult Women

Acute dysuria affects millions of women in the United States each year and usually reflects one of three conditions: acute bacterial cystitis, urethritis, or vaginitis (Table 14-4). At the time of the initial evaluation a determination of whether acute cystitis is complicated or uncomplicated may not be possible. Subclinical involvement of the kidney (pyelonephritis) is present in up to 30% to 50% of these cases. This observation may be one reason that single-dose regimens are not as effective as multidose regimens (discussed later in the chapter).

Presentation and Progression
Cause

Why symptomatic inflammation of the bladder (acute cystitis) develops in some patients and not others (asymptomatic bacteriuria) is unclear. Experimentally, 99.9% of a bladder inoculum of bacteria is promptly eliminated by voiding. Thus establishment of infection is the exception rather than the rule.

UTI in women is facilitated by sexual intercourse, during which the urethra often becomes intravaginal and bacteria are literally massaged from the periurethral mucosa into the bladder. Daily intercourse for 1 week increases the likelihood of cystitis by nine-fold. The risk is increased by the use of a diaphragm and by spermicidal contraceptives, which increase the vaginal pH, alter the microbial environment, and enhance the ability of *E. coli* to adhere to the mucosa.

E. coli causes 70% to 90% of episodes of acute cystitis in sexually active younger women. *S. saprophyticus* causes most other episodes, especially during the spring and summer months. Enterococci and various gram-negative rods explain most of the remainder of the cases.

Postmenopausal women with recurrent UTI often have urologic problems such as incontinence (41% of women in

a recent study), cystocele (about 41% of patients in a recent study), cystocele (19%), or increased postvoiding residual volume (28% of patients; defined as "mild" if <50 mL of urine, "moderate" if 50 to 100 mL, and "severe" if >100 mL).

Patients with uncomplicated lower UTI ("cystitis") usually report a recent onset of dysuria, frequency, and urgency, sometimes with suprapubic pain or discomfort. Distinguishing between external dysuria and internal dysuria by careful history helps clarify the diagnosis (Table 14-5). Internal dysuria is the typical symptom in acute cystitis, whereas external dysuria, in which the pain is experienced mainly during or after urination, usually indicates a nonurinary condition such as a sexually transmitted disease. Also, the acute onset of dysuria helps distinguish acute cystitis from other causes of dysuria, which tend to have a subacute or gradual onset.

Diagnosis (Box 14-1)

Pyuria as identified by dipstick or microscopic examination of a midstream urine specimen is present in nearly all women with acute cystitis; its absence suggests another cause.

The dipstick leukocyte esterase test is often used for screening. When this test is negative, microscopic examination for pyuria or a urine culture is indicated. Microscopic evaluation of urine for bacteriuria is generally not recommended for acute cystitis because bacteria can be present in low quantities ($\leq 10^4$ CFUs/mL) and these are difficult to find on a wet mount or Gram stain, even on a spun specimen. Urine cultures are usually not indicated in uncomplicated cystitis because causative organisms and their antimicrobial susceptibility profiles are predictable. Culture results become available only after the patient's symptoms have greatly improved or resolved. However, if the presence of a complicated infection is suspected or if symptoms are not typical for cystitis, culture of midstream urine is indicated. Many women with low colony counts ($<10^5$ CFUs/mL of urine) have the acute urethral syndrome.

TABLE 14-5
Internal Versus External Dysuria

Variable	Internal dysuria	External dysuria
Clinical history	A dull, visceral pain that may be either constant or experienced only with urination, often accompanied by a sense of bladder fullness and urgency	A sharp, burning sensation experienced during or after urination, often relieved by sitting in warm water
Pathophysiology	Inflammation of the urethra or urinary bladder	Passage of urine over inflamed introital or periurethral tissues
Causes	Most often caused by cystitis or urethritis. Urethritis (the so-called urethral syndrome) can be caused by *Escherichia coli* and other bacteria and also by *Chlamydia trachomatis, Neisseria gonorrhoeae, Trichomonas vaginalis,* and (rarely) *Mycobacterium tuberculosis.*	Most often caused by nonurinary pathologic conditions; infectious causes: genital herpes simplex virus infection, vaginitis, condyloma acuminatum, *Candida* infection, and periurethral infection such as abscess; noninfectious causes: sexual trauma, atrophic vaginitis (in patients with estrogen deficiency), foreign body, manipulation, allergies, irritants, cancer, and dysplasia
Diagnosis	Urine culture; urethral cultures or screens for *Chlamydia* and gonococci when sexually transmitted disease is suspected	Pelvic examination with appropriate studies based on clinical findings

BOX 14-1
Diagnosis of Acute Uncomplicated Urinary Tract Infection in Women

- Consider urethritis caused by *Neisseria gonorrhoeae* or *Chlamydia trachomatis* if the patient has a past history of sexually transmitted disease, a new sex partner, a sex partner with urethral symptoms, or gradual onset of symptoms over several weeks rather than an acute onset of dysuria.
- Consider vaginitis if the patient has a history of vaginal discharge or odor, pruritus, dyspareunia, external dysuria, and absence of frequency or urgency.
- Evaluate for fever, flank pain, adnexal area tenderness, and the presence of nausea or vomiting.
- Carry out pelvic examination if any of the features point to urethritis or vaginitis. Evaluate for vaginitis, urethral discharge, herpetic ulcerations, and cervicitis, and obtain cervical and urethral cultures (or other tests, such as urine ligase chain reaction tests) for *N. gonorrhoeae* and *C. trachomatis.*
- Urinalysis shows pyuria in nearly all cases of acute cystitis.
- Hematuria is a helpful finding, since it is not present in urethritis or vaginitis. However, it is not a predictor for complicated infection.
- For women with acute symptoms and pyuria, a culture showing $\geq 10^2$ CFUs/mL of the same microorganism is significant; most such women have urinary tract infection.
- The leukocyte esterase test can be used for screening. Patients with a negative leukocyte esterase test should have a microscopic evaluation for pyuria or a culture performed.
- Postmenopausal women with recurrent urinary tract infection often have a specific urologic problem such as incontinence, cystocele, or postvoiding residual urine.

Natural History
Expected Outcome

Acute cystitis, even when uncomplicated, causes substantial morbidity. In one study it was determined that each episode of UTI in young women was associated with 6.1 days of symptoms, 2.4 days of restricted activity, 1.2 days of being unable to attend classes or work, and 0.4 day in bed.

Treatment
Methods

A wealth of data supports empiric treatment without culture when an otherwise healthy woman with UTI shows signs of dysuria but no signs of pyelonephritis, such as fever or flank pain. Numerous treatment regimens can be endorsed (Table 14-6). Knowledge of antimicrobial susceptibility profiles in the community can be useful. Trimethoprim-sulfamethoxazole (TMP/SMX; Bactrim, Septra, and other brands) has been widely used, but bacteria resistant to trimethoprim or to the combination now cause up to 20% of UTIs in some communities. β-Lactam antibiotics are less effective than TMP/SMX for 3-day regimens but are safer during pregnancy. The most important predictor of high-cost effectiveness of various regimens for uncomplicated UTI seems to be efficacy against *E. coli*. Less potent regimens may promote recurrent UTI and progression to pyelonephritis. For all of the preceding reasons, fluoroquinolones are being used with increasing frequency for primary treatment of UTI, especially when the prevalence of resistance to TMP/SMX

exceeds 20% in a community. However, the quinolones are generally contraindicated during pregnancy (see Chapter 5).

The optimum duration of treatment has been debated for many years. A consensus opinion holds that 3-day regimens are more effective than single-dose regimens and more practical than longer regimens. Although some trials have shown equivalent efficacy between single-dose and 3-day treatment regimens, it should again be pointed out that many of these patients have subclinical pyelonephritis. Also, 3-day regimens are associated with better compliance, lower risk of adverse drug reaction, and lower cost than 7- to 10-day courses of treatment.

Self-start therapy is a growing trend. This can be based on telephone consultation (Figure 14-1) or, in selected patients with recurrent UTI, on self-diagnosis and treatment. Women with recurrent UTI are given a dipslide urine culture kit and a supply of medication (e.g., six norfloxacin or ciprofloxacin tablets). This practice should be discouraged for patients thought to be at substantial risk of sexually transmitted disease.

There is no proven basis for the common practice of "forcing fluids." Although overhydration might help flush bacteria out of the urine, it might also reduce the urinary concentration of antibiotics. The use of cranberry juice is also widely recommended but is unsupported by rigorous studies. Large volumes of cranberry juice can provide hippuric acid levels in the bladder sufficient to have some bacteriostatic activity. Patients with severe dysuria—present in about 10% of cases—may benefit from bladder analgesia with phenazopyridine (Pyridium) 200 mg PO t.i.d. Most patients, however, respond rapidly to therapy and therefore do not need bladder analgesia.

Expected Response

Acute cystitis nearly always responds to appropriate therapy. However, 20% to 25% of young women with acute cystitis have two or more infections per year, most commonly from reinfection with a new *E. coli* strain. Several strategies are available for prevention of recurrences (Table 14-7). One or more of these strategies may be tried for women with frequent episodes of uncomplicated lower UTI, especially when such episodes are accompanied by significant morbidity necessitating absence from school or work.

When to Refer

Referral of otherwise healthy women with acute uncomplicated cystitis is seldom necessary. In the past, there was overemphasis on referral for cystoscopy, which was usually unhelpful to long-term clinical management. Women with recurrent symptoms should undergo a thorough pelvic examination. Referral to a urologist should be considered for postmenopausal women with frequent recurrences.

 KEY POINTS

UNCOMPLICATED LOWER URINARY TRACT INFECTION (CYSTITIS) IN NONPREGNANT ADULT WOMEN

⊃ A 3-day course of an appropriate antibiotic is often recommended. TMP/SMX has been widely used in recent years, but resistance is emerging. The fluoroquinolones are one alternative. Alternative agents, notably the fluoroquinolones, are now recommended when the prevalence of resistance of *E. coli* to TMP/SMX exceeds 20% in a community (with the caveat that quinolones are generally contraindicated during pregnancy).

TABLE 14-6
Some Oral Regimens for Acute Uncomplicated Lower Urinary Tract Infection in Women

Regimen	Duration of therapy (days)	Approximate cost* ($)
NEWER QUINOLONES		
Ciprofloxacin 100 to 250 mg q12h	3†	23 to 17
Enoxacin 200 mg q12h	3	20
Levofloxacin 250 mg q24h	3†	22
Norfloxacin 400 mg q12h	3†	23
Ofloxacin 200 mg q12h	3	24
TRIMETHOPRIM-BASED REGIMENS		
Trimethoprim 100 mg q12h	3†	1.35
TMP/SMX 160 mg/800 mg (one double-strength tablet) q12h	3†	1.20
NEWER CEPHALOSPORINS		
Cefixime 400 mg q24h	3†	23
Cefpodoxime proxetil 100 mg q12h	3†	18
OTHER AGENTS		
Amoxicillin-clavulanate 500 mg q12h	7	55
Nitrofurantoin macrocrystals (Furadantin) 50 mg q6h	7	20
Nitrofurantoin monohydrate macrocrystals (Macrodantin) 100 mg q12h	7	24

TMP/SMX, Trimethoprim-sulfamethoxazole.
*Based on average wholesale price, 2001. From 2001 Redbook. Montvale, NJ: Medical Economics Data Production Co.; 2001.
†A 7-day regimen rather than a 3-day regimen is advisable when any of the following are present: symptoms >7 days' duration, recent urinary tract infection, use of a diaphragm for contraception, diabetes mellitus, or age >65 years.

⊃ Patients with severe dysuria (about 10% of cases) can be given phenazopyridine (Pyridium) for symptomatic relief. Most patients respond rapidly and do not need bladder analgesia. Forcing fluids has not been proved beneficial, and cranberry juice is probably unhelpful unless given in unusually large quantities.

⊃ Several strategies are available for prevention and treatment of recurrent UTI. These include patient-initiated self-treatment of symptomatic episodes, continuous low-dose prophylaxis, and postcoital prophylaxis.

⊃ Referral for studies such as cystoscopy or CT scanning of the kidney are seldom necessary for healthy women with recurrent acute uncomplicated lower UTI.

SUGGESTED READING

Barry HC, Ebell MH, Hickner J. Evaluation of suspected urinary tract infection in ambulatory women: a cost-utility analysis of office-based strategies. J Fam Pract 1997; 44: 49-60.
Gupta K, Hooton TM, Roberts PL, et al. Patient-initiated treatment of uncomplicated recurrent urinary tract infections in young women. Ann Intern Med 2001; 135: 9-16.
Gupta K, Hooton TM, Stamm WE. Increasing antimicrobial resistance and the management of uncomplicated community-acquired urinary tract infections. Ann Intern Med 2001; 135: 41-50.
Engel JD, Schaeffer AJ. Evaluation of and antimicrobial therapy for recurrent urinary tract infections in women. Urol Clin North Am 1998; 25: 685-701.
Raz R, Gennesin Y, Wasser J, et al. Recurrent urinary tract infections in postmenopausal women. Clin Infect Dis 2000; 30: 152-156.
Rosenberg M. Pharmacoeconomics of treating uncomplicated urinary tract infections. Int J Antimicrob Agents 1999; 11: 247-251.
Scholes D, Hooton TM, Roberts PL, et al. Risk factors for recurrent urinary tract infection in young women. J Infect Dis 2000; 182: 1177-1182.

Acute Upper Urinary Tract Infection (Pyelonephritis) in Adult Women

Acute pyelonephritis is a relatively common problem in adult women, accounting for >250,000 hospitalizations per year by some estimates. Many of these patients can be managed as outpatients, sometimes after brief observation in an acute-care facility.

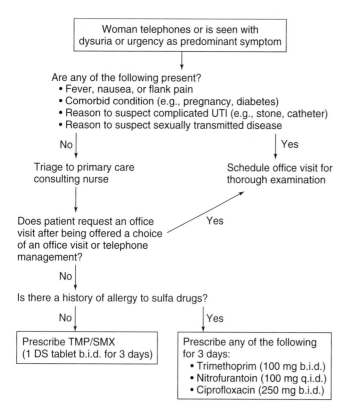

FIG. 14-1 Algorithm for management of presumptive lower urinary tract infection in otherwise healthy, sexually active women. (Modified from Saint S, Scholes D, Fihn SD, et al. The effectiveness of a clinical practice guideline for the management of presumed uncomplicated urinary tract infection in women. Am J Med 1999; 106: 636-641.)

Presentation and Progression

Cause

Bacteria are generally believed to ascend from the bladder to the renal pelvis by way of the ureters. Some researchers suggest that bacteria first enter the bloodstream from the renal pelvis through pyelovenous communications and then recirculate to the kidney. Be that as it may, it is easiest to consider most cases of pyelonephritis to be the result of "ascending UTI" as defined previously. The renal medulla has been called an "immunologic desert," since host defenses are rendered relatively helpless by the low pH and high osmolality. Multiplying bacteria can enter the bloodstream, causing the sepsis syndrome.

Pyelonephritis in patients with structurally normal urinary tracts is usually caused by so-called uropathogenic strains of *E. coli.* Other aerobic gram-negative rods sometimes cause acute pyelonephritis, especially in patients with complicated urologic histories. *S. saprophyticus,* although a common cause of acute cystitis, seldom causes pyelonephritis. Whether atypical microorganisms such as *Ureaplasma urealyticum* and *Mycoplasma hominis* cause acute uncomplicated pyelonephritis is unclear.

Presentation

Acute pyelonephritis occurs both with and without symptoms of lower UTI, such as frequency, urgency, and dysuria. The hallmark symptoms are fever and flank pain. However, nausea and generalized abdominal pain often dominate the clinical picture. Acute disease of the gastrointestinal tract (such as acute appendicitis, cholecystitis, or pancreatitis) and pelvis (pelvic inflammatory disease, ectopic pregnancy) must be considered in the differential diagnosis.

Physical examination should focus on the vital signs, the abdomen, and the costovertebral angle (CVA). Careful

TABLE 14-7
Strategies for Prevention of Recurrent, Uncomplicated Urinary Tract Infection in Premenopausal Women

Strategy	Appropriate patient group	Comments
Patient-initiated self-treatment (e.g., TMP/SMX as a single dose or as a 3-day course)*	Relatively well-educated women who have had relatively low recurrence rates of UTI	With single-dose TMP/SMX, an 85% success rate has been reported. Even higher rates would be expected with a 3-day course.
Continuous low-dose prophylaxis†	Patients with three or more infections per year	This strategy seems to be safe and highly effective. Emergence of drug-resistant bacteria is a potential complication.
Postcoital prophylaxis‡	Patients who have three or more infections per year and relate their recurrences to coitus.	This strategy also seems to be safe and highly effective.

TMP/SMX, Trimethoprim-sulfamethoxazole.

*The most commonly used single-dose regimens have been one or two double-strength tablets of TMP/SMX and 3 g of amoxicillin. Any of the 3-day regimens shown in Table 14-6 could be substituted.

†Regimens recommended for this purpose include TMP/SMX, trimethoprim alone (100 mg/day), norfloxacin, nitrofurantoin, sulfonamides, cephalexin, cefaclor, and cephradine.

‡One-dose postcoital regimens that have been studied include TMP/SMX (one regular-strength tablet), cephalexin 250 mg, cinoxacin 250 mg, and nitrofurantoin 50 mg. Both cinoxacin and nitrofurantoin have been shown to be effective during pregnancy.

measurement of temperature is important, since fever with UTI strongly suggests pyelonephritis. An increased respiratory rate can indicate respiratory compensation for metabolic acidosis. The abdomen should be examined especially for adnexal tenderness, which may suggest that the correct diagnosis is actually pelvic inflammatory disease. CVA tenderness is the classic physical finding in pyelonephritis.

Pyuria is nearly always present. As already mentioned, it can be absent if the site of infection is excluded from the normal flow of urine, as is the case with complete ureteral obstruction or perinephric abscess. Hematuria may be present but does not help differentiate pyelonephritis from cystitis. Urine culture reveals $>10^5$ CFUs/mL in 80% to 95% of cases. Some patients, as discussed previously, have lower colony counts. Between 10% and 20% of patients have positive blood cultures. However, no evidence has shown that patients with positive blood cultures do worse than patients whose blood cultures are sterile, and therefore blood cultures can be limited to patients who require hospitalization.

Diagnosis (Box 14-2)

Diagnosis of acute pyelonephritis hinges on the presence of typical findings (fever, flank pain, CVA tenderness, and pyuria) and the absence of findings pointing to alternative diagnoses as discussed earlier. WBC casts in the urine are, in the appropriate setting, nearly pathognomonic (Figure 14-2). When doubt exists or when findings are severe, pelvic examination should be performed. CT scans can be useful for confirming the diagnosis of acute pyelonephritis when the clinical picture is confusing or pain patterns are atypical.

Many researchers have sought ways to differentiate between upper and lower UTI. These include ureteral catheterization (accurate but invasive), Fairley's bladder washout test (helpful but labor intensive), the antibody-coated bacteria test (generally out of favor because of questions about its accuracy), measurement of urinary concentrating ability, serum antibody levels, and urinary levels of various enzymes and β_2-microglobulin. To date, none of these tests or procedures can be recommended for management of UTI in daily office practice. Patients with UTI and any combination of fever, flank pain, or CVA tenderness should be treated appropriately for pyelonephritis.

BOX 14-2
DIAGNOSIS OF ACUTE PYELONEPHRITIS

- Fever, flank pain, nausea, and vomiting—with or without symptoms of lower urinary tract infection (dysuria, frequency, urgency)—suggest the diagnosis of acute pyelonephritis.
- Pelvic inflammatory disease is often misdiagnosed as acute uncomplicated pyelonephritis. Pelvic examination should therefore be undertaken when risk factors for sexually transmitted disease are present.
- Pyuria is nearly always present. White blood cell casts have diagnostic value.
- Urine culture should be performed, since the nitrite test lacks sensitivity and will not provide the information about the causative organism that will be needed if initial treatment fails.
- Blood cultures should be performed in patients who require hospitalization, but they are not needed in most cases.
- A pregnancy test should be performed if the reliability of contraception is in doubt or menses are irregular.

Natural History
Expected Outcome

In healthy younger persons, life-threatening infection is rare. Even in the preantibiotic era most such patients survived.

Treatment
Methods

A variety of antibiotic regimens are effective in acute uncomplicated pyelonephritis (Table 14-8). Oral regimens are effective for milder cases unaccompanied by nausea and vomiting. The newer quinolone antibiotics and TMP/SMX are well absorbed. Because resistance to TMP/SMX is increasing (nearly 20% of uropathic *E. coli* strains in some localities), some authorities recommend quinolones as first-line therapy. Patients with severe symptoms, including nausea and vomiting, should be started on parenteral antibiotic therapy. Ceftriaxone (Rocephin) is an excellent choice unless a strong reason exists to suspect *P. aeruginosa* (which occurs almost exclusively in patients with a complicated urologic history). Once-daily aminoglycoside therapy (2.5 to 5 mg/kg/day) results in marked, sustained drug levels in renal tissue and is also cost-effective therapy for difficult cases (see Chapter 19).

In most cases parenteral antibiotic therapy can be replaced by oral therapy within 24 to 48 hours. The typically excellent response of uncomplicated pyelonephritis to antibiotic therapy has stimulated efforts to manage the disease on a strictly outpatient basis. One strategy involves the administration of parenteral antibiotics and fluids in a holding area. In one study 43 of 44 patients with pyelonephritis managed in this way could be sent home with oral antibiotics after 12 hours of observation, without adverse consequences.

In the past, antibiotics were continued for 6 weeks or longer. It is now known that prolonged therapy, compared with a 2-week regimen, carries greater risk of side effects and reinfection with drug-resistant bacteria. Recent data suggest that 7 days of therapy may suffice if a newer quinolone antibiotic (e.g., ciprofloxacin, ofloxacin, or levofloxacin) is used, presumably because these agents reach high concentrations within the infected kidney. When β-lactam antibiotics or TMP/SMX is used, the drug should be given for 14 days because shorter regimens are likely to result in therapeutic failure. Nitrofurantoin should not be

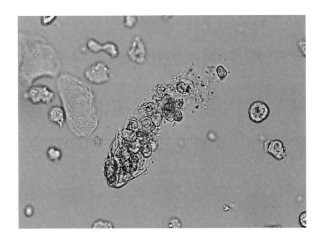

FIG. 14-2 White blood cell (leukocyte) cast. In the setting of pyuria, fever, and flank pain, this observation is essentially pathognomonic of pyelonephritis.

TABLE 14-8
Some Treatment Regimens for Empiric Therapy of Acute Pyelonephritis*

Regimen	Cost† ($)
ORAL REGIMENS	
Ciprofloxacin 500 mg q12h	90
Enoxacin 400 mg q12h	96
Levofloxacin 250 to 500 mg q24h	73 to 85
Norfloxacin 400 mg q12h	76
Ofloxacin 200 to 300 mg q12h	82 to 98
TMP/SMX 160 mg/800 mg (one double-strength tablet) q12h	6
Cefixime 400 mg q24h	77
Cefpodoxime proxetil 200 mg q12h	80
Amoxicillin-clavulanate 500 mg/125 mg q8h	80
PARENTERAL REGIMENS	
Ciprofloxacin 400 mg q12h	600
Levofloxacin 500 mg q24h	396
Ofloxacin 400 mg q12h	740
Ceftriaxone 1 g q24h	400
Aztreonam 1 g q8h to q12h	540 to 360
Cefepime 1 g q12h	340
Gentamicin 1 mg/kg q8h or 3-5 mg/kg q24h ± ampicillin 2 g q6h	66 or 121
TMP/SMX 160 mg/800 mg q12h	260
Imipenem-cilastatin 20 mg/500 mg q6h to q8h	1200 to 960
Piperacillin-tazobactam 3.375 g q6h to q8h	660 to 495
Ticarcillin-clavulanate 3.1 g q6h	616

TMP/SMX, Trimethoprim-sulfamethoxazole.
*See text. Oral regimens can be endorsed for patients who have mild to moderate illness and do not have nausea and vomiting. Hospitalization should be considered for patients with severe illness and those with nausea and vomiting. Some patients with moderately severe illness can be given a short course of intravenous antibiotics as outpatients and then—if response is rapid and nausea subsides—treated with oral regimens. Regimens with antipseudomonal activity (e.g., ciprofloxacin, cefepime, imipenem-cilastatin, piperacillin-tazobactam, and ticarcillin-clavulanate) are recommended for initial therapy when the patient has a history of urinary tract infection caused by *Pseudomonas aeruginosa*.
†Cost for regimen is based on 2000 Redbook. Montvale, NJ: Medical Economics Data Production Co.; 2000.

used for treatment of pyelonephritis, since tissue levels are inadequate.

Expected Response

Marked improvement within 72 hours of the start of antibiotic therapy usually distinguishes acute uncomplicated pyelonephritis from infection associated with obstruction, renal or perinephric abscess, or other serious complications. Routine posttreatment follow-up is not indicated for patients who respond promptly to therapy.

Failure to respond within 72 hours should prompt evaluation of the urinary tract with a contrast CT scan or ultrasound examination. Imaging studies are also indicated if recurrent acute pyelonephritis develops within 2 weeks of completion of therapy. For these patients retreatment with a different agent should be considered. For patients who have a relapse after 2 weeks, the approach should be the same as with initial episodes.

When to Refer

Patients with evidence of severe sepsis should be hospitalized. Other indications include uncertainty about the diagnosis, concerns about compliance, and inability to keep down oral medications. Urologic evaluation is not needed in most cases. In one study only 1 of 25 young women had a predisposing anatomic abnormality.

 KEY POINTS

ACUTE UPPER URINARY TRACT INFECTION (PYELONEPHRITIS) IN ADULT WOMEN

- ⟳ Outpatient therapy suffices for most nonpregnant women who have mild to moderately severe disease and are compliant with treatment.
- ⟳ Some authorities prefer quinolones to TMP/SMX for oral therapy, since resistance of uropathic *E. coli* to TMP/SMX now approaches 20% in some areas.
- ⟳ Indications for hospitalization include severe sepsis, uncertainty about the diagnosis, and inability to maintain oral hydration.
- ⟳ A growing trend is the treatment of selected patients as outpatients with a brief course of parenteral fluids and intravenous antibiotics followed by oral antibiotics when nausea and vomiting have subsided.
- ⟳ Factors that complicate the treatment of pyelonephritis include obstruction, vesicoureteral reflux, complicated urologic disease, pregnancy, diabetes mellitus, renal failure, renal transplantation, immunosuppression, and multiresistant organisms.
- ⟳ Imaging of the upper urinary tract (CT scan or ultrasound) should be performed if the patient does not show significant improvement within 72 hours. Imaging of the upper urinary tract can be performed if a patient has had two recurrences of pyelonephritis.
- ⟳ Duration of treatment depends on the antibiotic used. Some studies indicate that quinolones may be useful for 7 days, whereas β-lactam antibiotics need to be given for 14 days.

SUGGESTED READING

Behr MA, Drummond R, Libman MD, et al. Fever duration in hospitalized acute pyelonephritis patients. Am J Med 1996; 101: 277-280.

Talan DA, Stamm WE, Hooton TM, et al. Comparison of ciprofloxacin (7 days) and trimethoprim-sulfamethoxazole (14 days) for acute uncomplicated pyelonephritis in women: a randomized trial. JAMA 2000; 283: 1583-1590.

Ward G, Jorden RC, Severance HW. Treatment of pyelonephritis in an observation unit. Ann Emerg Med 1991; 20: 258-261.

Urinary Tract Infection During Pregnancy
(see also Chapter 5)

Pregnancy markedly predisposes to pyelonephritis, which can harm both the mother and the fetus. Bacteriuria during pregnancy is associated with prematurity and low birth weight, although a cause-and-effect relationship is unclear.

Urine culture should be obtained at the first prenatal visit. Dipstick methods are insufficiently sensitive to screen for bacteriuria in pregnancy. Patients with asymptomatic bacteriuria should be treated with a 3-day course of antibiotics and close follow-up.

Complicated Urinary Tract Infection in Adults

A minority of women with acute pyelonephritis have complications that can lead to chronic pyelonephritis and renal failure. UTI in men is often complicated and is discussed more fully later in the chapter.

Presentation and Progression
Cause

Complicated UTI occurs in specific clinical settings (Table 14-1). Renal abscess can result from hematogenous seeding of the renal cortex (most often caused by *Staphylococcus aureus*) or from ascending infection leading to severe pyelonephritis (most often caused by gram-negative rods). Perinephric abscess usually occurs in the setting of structural or functional abnormalities of the urinary tract. Vesicoureteral reflux, although less common than in children, sometimes occurs in adults (generally women). Struvite or infection stones result from UTI caused by urease-producing bacteria, most often *Proteus* species. The range of causative bacteria is much more diverse than in uncomplicated UTI. Aerobic gram-negative rods, such as *Klebsiella, Enterobacter, Serratia,* or *Providencia* species, enterococci, and fungi are commonly encountered. Complicated UTI is often polymicrobial (i.e., urine culture reveals two or more species of microorganisms). Fungal UTI presents special problems (Box 14-3).

Presentation

Symptoms of complicated UTI generally begin more insidiously and less dramatically than is the case with acute UTI. Gradually worsening symptoms sometimes antedate the diagnosis by weeks to months, as opposed to less than 3 days in most causes of acute uncomplicated pyelonephritis. Complicated UTI should also be suspected when standard therapy for upper UTI fails to bring about clinical improvement (return of temperature and WBC count to normal) within 5 days.

Perinephric abscess is often associated with urinary calculi or diabetes mellitus. Symptoms often begin insidiously but may

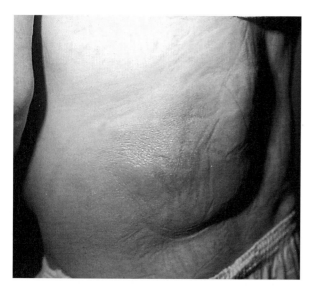

FIG. 14-3 Large perinephric abscess in a patient with diabetes mellitus, showing swelling with erythema over the left flank. At surgery 1500 mL of creamy pus was obtained, from which *Staphylococcus aureus* was isolated.

suggest acute pyelonephritis. A palpable mass is occasionally present (Figure 14-3). The urinalysis is normal in about 30% of patients, and the urine culture sterile in about 40%. Patients with renal abscess (renal carbuncle) may have symptoms suggesting acute pyelonephritis but responding poorly to therapy.

Xanthogranulomatous pyelonephritis is an unusual variant of chronic pyelonephritis that occurs most often in middle-aged women with a history of recurrent UTI. This lesion is unilateral, and presenting symptoms are some combination of fever, malaise, anorexia, weight loss, and flank pain. Imaging studies show a large, nonfunctioning kidney, usually containing several stones or a staghorn calculus. CT scan suggests the diagnosis. Xanthogranulomatous pyelonephritis is often confused with malignancy, which, however, can occasionally occur in this setting.

Diagnosis

Pyuria and bacteriuria are usually present, but they may be absent if the infection does not communicate with the collecting system (e.g., infected cyst, renal carbuncle, or perinephric abscess) or if the collecting system is obstructed. Urine cultures reveal bacteriuria. A colony count of $\geq 10^3$ CFUs/mL is significant unless the specimen was obtained through a newly inserted catheter, in which case a colony count of $\geq 10^2$ CFUs/mL of urine may be significant.

Imaging studies should always be performed in cases of complicated UTI. For diagnosis of renal abscess or perinephric abscess, CT scan has been found to be 96% sensitive and ultrasound 92% sensitive. Vesicoureteral reflux in adults, although uncommon, merits consideration in some cases (Box 14-4).

Natural History

The course varies according to the specific complication. Renal abscess caused by *S. aureus,* fortunately uncommon, can cause fulminant staphylococcal septicemia. Similarly, perinephric abscess can be a fatal disease if appropriate therapy, including drainage, is not carried out.

BOX 14-4
Vesicoureteral Reflux in Adults

- Vesicoureteral reflux is more common in women than in men (ratio about 5:1), is usually associated with urinary tract infections, and classically causes reflux nephropathy resulting in chronic pyelonephritis.
- Women with vesicoureteral reflux are 12 times more likely than men to have lower urinary tract infections and 7 times more likely to have upper urinary tract infections. However, men are more likely to have impaired renal function and proteinuria.
- Hypertension occurs in about one third of patients with ureterovesical reflux, but malignant hypertension is uncommon.
- Back pain occurs in about 40% of patients with vesicoureteral reflux, and renal calculi occur in about 20% of patients.
- Diagnosis can be confirmed by micturating cystography.

Treatment
Methods

Successful treatment includes not only antibiotics but also restoration of urine flow, usually by relief of obstruction. Empiric antibiotic regimens should include agents with some activity against *P. aeruginosa*. Use of certain antibiotics, such as nitrofurantoin, should be avoided in cases of renal failure. Long-term success of treatment of complicated UTI hinges on correction of the underlying abnormality. If it cannot be corrected, a failure rate of 50% at 4 to 6 weeks after therapy can be expected. Percutaneous drainage is being substituted for open surgical drainage in many cases of renal and perinephric abscess.

Expected Response

The outcome of complicated UTI is generally favorable provided there is a prompt diagnosis and institution of appropriate therapy.

When to Refer

Patients with complicated UTI should usually be hospitalized and managed in consultation with a urologist.

 KEY POINTS

COMPLICATED URINARY TRACT INFECTION IN ADULTS

- ⊃ Complicated UTI should be suspected when UTI occurs in any patient other than a nonpregnant young woman, when symptoms and signs of UTI are present with a normal urinalysis, when fever and leukocytosis fail to resolve within 5 days of appropriate therapy for pyelonephritis, and when urine culture shows an unusual organism (e.g., *P. aeruginosa* or a yeast) or more than one organism.
- ⊃ In a nonpregnant young woman, complicated UTI should be suspected when response to therapy is poor or when upper UTI caused by the same microorganism occurs within 2 weeks.
- ⊃ Imaging of the urinary tract should usually begin with a CT scan or ultrasound examination. These studies are especially useful for diagnosis of renal cortical abscess and perinephric abscess.
- ⊃ Struvite stones should be suspected in patients with alkaline urine and infection by a urease-producing organism, especially *P. mirabilis.*

⊃ The etiologic spectrum of organisms in complicated UTI is more diverse than that in uncomplicated UTI and includes such bacteria as *P. aeruginosa* and enterococci.

⊃ Symptoms of complicated UTI often begin insidiously. Patients with stones, however, may respond with renal colic and gross hematuria.

⊃ Patients with complicated UTI should generally be managed as inpatients.

⊃ Empiric antibiotic therapy should include agents with activity against *P. aeruginosa*.

SUGGESTED READING

Cohen TD, Preminger GM. Struvite calculi. Semin Nephrol 1996; 16: 425-434.

Fowler JE Jr, Perkins T. Presentation, diagnosis and treatment of renal abscesses, 1972-1988. J Urol 1994; 151: 847-851.

Hutchinson FN, Kaysen GA. Perinephric abscess: the missed diagnosis. Med Clin North Am 1998; 72: 993-1014.

Kohler J, Tencer J, Thysell H, et al. Vesicoureteral reflux diagnosed in adulthood: incidence of urinary tract infections, hypertension, proteinuria, back pain and renal calculi. Nephrol Dial Transplant 1997; 12: 2580-2587.

Nicolle LE. A practical guide to the management of complicated urinary tract infection. Drugs 1997; 53: 583-592.

Cystitis and Pyelonephritis in Men

At some time about one half of all men seek medical attention for UTI, a disease burden similar to that of women. Men, like women, have urethritis, cystitis, and pyelonephritis. Isolated urethritis (i.e., urethritis without cystitis or prostatitis) usually implies sexually transmitted disease (see Chapter 16). UTI in men is most commonly manifested as prostatitis, which is actually a spectrum of incompletely understood disorders. Most UTIs in men are complicated, and most patients eventually require evaluation by a urologist.

Presentation and Progression
Cause

Men are less prone to UTIs because of a longer urethra, a drier periurethral environment (causing less frequent colonization around the urethra), and the presence of antibacterial substances in prostatic fluid. Isolated cystitis in men, in contrast to women, nearly always indicates an abnormality such as hypospadias, prostatic hypertrophy, or prior instrumentation. Bacteria usually enter the prostate gland by way of reflux of urine into the prostatic ducts. Microorganisms can then spread from the prostate into the seminal vesicles and epididymis. Some data suggest that smoking increases the frequency of urinary tract symptoms in men. The notion that sexual abstinence, trauma, or dehydration predisposes men to UTI has not been proved.

E. coli is the most common cause of cystitis and pyelonephritis in women, as in men. Other gram-negative organisms causing UTI, such as *Klebsiella, Enterobacter, Proteus,* and *Pseudomonas* species, assume relatively greater importance in men who have undergone urologic instrumentation. Similarly, enterococcal UTI is usually seen in men with complicating factors. *S. aureus,* when isolated from urine, usually implies a hematogenous source (as discussed previously).

Presentation

Acute cystitis occurs occasionally in middle-aged men; the incidence is about five to eight UTIs per 10,000 such men per year. Cystitis is less common in healthy older men. Lower urinary tract symptoms, including incontinence, are relatively common in men and increase with advancing age. Incontinence is experienced by about 4% of men by age 50 and by 28% of men by age 90, but less than one half of these men seek medical advice. The symptoms and signs of cystitis and pyelonephritis in men are similar to those in women.

Diagnosis

Diagnosis of cystitis and pyelonephritis in men follows the same principles as in women, with the addition that men should usually undergo imaging procedures to exclude obstructive uropathy. Up to 80% of men with UTI who have no history of prior instrumentation or trauma are found to have abnormalities of the genitourinary tract, most commonly prostatic hypertrophy.

Natural History

Because of the high incidence of associated anatomic abnormalities, UTI resolves more slowly and is more prone to recur in men. The natural history of prostatitis, which often accompanies cystitis in men, is discussed later in the chapter.

Treatment
Methods

The choice of antibiotics is similar to that for women (Tables 14-6 and 14-8). Short-course regimens are seldom if ever appropriate for men, who should be treated for 10 to 14 days. Men with lower urinary tract symptoms of uncertain cause should be encouraged to stop smoking.

Expected Response

The response to treatment of UTI in men depends largely on successful resolution or palliation of the underlying urologic condition.

When to Refer

UTI in men usually warrants referral to a urologist. Men with UTI associated with hypertension, renal calculi, back pain, or proteinuria should probably be evaluated for the possibility of vesicoureteral reflux.

 KEY POINTS

CYSTITIS AND PYELONEPHRITIS IN MEN

⊃ About one half of adult men seek medical attention for UTI during their lifetimes.

⊃ The prevalence of urinary incontinence and lower urogenital tract symptoms, including voiding problems and symptoms of UTI, increases linearly with age.

⊃ Symptoms, signs, and diagnostic principles of UTI in men are similar to those in women.

⊃ Men with UTI should usually undergo imaging procedures to exclude obstructive uropathy.

SUGGESTED READING

Koskimaki J, Hakama M, Huhtala H, et al. Association of smoking with lower urinary tract symptoms. J Urol 1998; 159: 1580-1582.

Acute Bacterial Prostatitis

The term "prostatitis" encompasses a spectrum of disorders, some of which are infections and some of which are probably not (Table 14-9). Among these disorders, acute bacterial prostatitis is by far the most serious but also the least common. For reasons that are unclear, acute bacterial prostatitis is more common in patients infected with human immunodeficiency virus.

Presentation and Progression
Cause

Bacteria usually enter the prostate by reflux of urine from the urethra into the prostatic ducts. *E. coli* and *Proteus* species are the most commonly isolated bacteria.

Presentation

Patients with acute bacterial prostatitis usually have dramatic systemic and local symptoms. Fever, chills, malaise, and myalgia suggest acute infection. Dysuria, pelvic or perineal pain, and difficulty voiding suggest the site of infection. Laboratory findings include leukocytosis and pyuria. When all of these findings are present and the diagnosis seems straightforward, rectal examination should be avoided because it will be painful and may cause bacteremia.

Diagnosis

In doubtful cases, gentle rectal examination confirms the presence of a swollen, tender prostate. Prostatic massage should never be performed in this setting. Urine cultures are typically positive, and blood cultures are often positive. The serum prostate specific antigen (PSA) test should not be performed in patients with acute prostatitis, since the result is often abnormal in the absence of prostate cancer.

Natural History
Expected Outcome

Complications of acute bacterial prostatitis include spread of infection to other genitourinary structures (epididymides, bladder, kidneys), bacteremia (with the potential for metastatic infection elsewhere), and prostatic abscess. Prostatic abscess occurs most commonly in patients who have diabetes mellitus, are immunocompromised, or were inadequately treated for acute prostatitis.

Treatment
Methods

Acute bacterial prostatitis is a serious order that requires aggressive treatment. Empiric antibiotic regimens before the availability of culture results should include broad-spectrum activity against aerobic gram-negative rods, including *P. aeruginosa* and gram-positive cocci (see discussion of empiric treatment of sepsis in Chapter 6, as well as Appendix 2). Gram stain of centrifuged urine can be extremely helpful in this setting:

■ If only gram-negative rods are present, treatment can be started with ciprofloxacin, cefepime, or an aminoglycoside.

TABLE 14-9
Clinical Features of the Major Syndromes of Prostatitis

Feature	Acute bacterial prostatitis	Chronic bacterial prostatitis	Chronic nonbacterial (noninflammatory) prostatitis	Chronic pelvic pain (prostatodynia)
Approximate percentage of patients	1 to 5	5 to 10	40 to 65	20 to 40
Typical age at onset (years)	40 to 60	50 to 80	30 to 50	30 to 40
Typical presentation	Acute illness with tender, warm prostate	Recurrent urinary tract infections with large, "boggy" prostate	Genitourinary and voiding discomfort; prostate findings highly variable	Pain; voiding problems; prostate usually normal on examination
Prostatic fluid white blood cells*	Contraindicated†	Always present	Always present	Rarely present
Bacterial cultures	Positive	Positive four- or two-cup test‡	Negative	Negative
Response to antibiotic therapy	Predictable and usually satisfactory	Usual but slow	Occasional	None

*Presence of at least 10 white blood cells per high-power field on microscopic examination.
†Prostatic massage is contraindicated in acute bacterial prostatitis.
‡Data from Lipsky BA. Prostatitis and urinary tract infection in men: what's new; what's true? Am J Med 1999; 106: 327-334.

- If only gram-positive cocci in clusters are present, treatment should be appropriate for staphylococcal disease (nafcillin or, if oxacillin-resistant strains [methicillin-resistant *S. aureus*] are suspected, vancomycin).
- If only gram-positive cocci in chains are identified, treatment should be appropriate for enterococcal infection (high-dose ampicillin with or without gentamicin).

Many patients with acute bacterial prostatitis require hospitalization for parenteral antibiotic therapy, intravenous fluids, and relief of urinary tract obstruction. Adjunctive measures include use of nonsteroidal antiinflammatory drugs (NSAIDs) for management of pain and resolution of the inflammatory response. Urethral catheters can obstruct drainage of the prostate and should therefore not be used. Suprapubic cystostomy is the preferred treatment for acute urinary retention.

Expected Response

Symptomatic improvement with clearing of fever usually occurs within 2 to 6 days after the start of therapy. Treatment should be continued for 4 to 6 weeks. Urine culture should be repeated 7 days after treatment has been initiated. If the urine culture remains positive, an alternative drug regimen should be considered. Some data indicate that a negative urine culture at 7 days predicts cure after 4 to 6 weeks, at least when a quinolone antibiotic is used. Failure of the infection to resolve raises the possibility of prostatic abscess, which can be confirmed by transrectal ultrasound examination or by CT scan.

When to Refer

Any combination of severe sepsis, inability to void, or failure of the infection to respond to therapy warrants urologic referral.

 KEY POINTS

ACUTE BACTERIAL PROSTATITIS

- ↻ Acute bacterial prostatitis is usually manifested as some combination of fever, dysuria, pelvic or perineal pain, and pyuria.
- ↻ Rectal examination, which is painful and can cause bacteremia, should be avoided when the diagnosis seems straightforward.
- ↻ Initial empiric antibiotic coverage, unless guided by Gram stain of spun urine sediment, should include drugs with broad-spectrum activity against aerobic gram-negative rods and gram-positive cocci.
- ↻ Complications include bacteremia, urinary obstruction, and prostatic abscess.
- ↻ Urologic consultation is often warranted.

SUGGESTED READING

Lipsky BA. Prostatitis and urinary tract infection in men: what's new; what's true? Am J Med 1999; 106: 327-334.

Weidner W, Madsen PO, Schiefer HG, eds. Prostatitis: Etiopathology, Diagnosis and Therapy. Berlin: Springer-Verlag; 1994.

Chronic Bacterial Prostatitis

Compared with acute bacterial prostatitis, chronic bacterial prostatitis is a more common and more subtle illness, with recurrent UTIs accompanied by a large, "boggy" prostate (Table 14-9). A somewhat cumbersome procedure known as the four-cup test is the cornerstone of accurate diagnosis.

Presentation and Progression

Cause

Chronic bacterial prostatitis, by definition, results from acute bacterial prostatitis whether or not the initial infection was clinically apparent. Gram-negative rods such as *E. coli* are the most common causes. *E. coli* strains causing prostatitis have virulence factors similar to those that cause pyelonephritis in women. The disease can be caused by enterococci and perhaps by *S. saprophyticus*. A few cases are polymicrobial. Evidence that *Chlamydia trachomatis* causes chronic prostatitis is inconclusive.

Presentation

Some patients have asymptomatic bacteriuria. Others have recurrent symptoms typical of lower UTI, including dysuria, frequency, urgency, and pain that may be experienced in the perineum, suprapubic area, lower back, or testicles. Systemic symptoms such as fever are usually absent.

Diagnosis

Classically, rectal examination discloses a tender, boggy prostate. However, examination usually shows no abnormalities. The key to diagnosis is microscopic examination and culture of voided urine (and also of prostatic secretions, if obtained) after prostatic massage. This office procedure, sometimes called the four-cup test, begins with four specimen cups labeled VB1, VB2, EPS (for "expressed prostatic secretions"), and VB3. After the periurethral area is cleansed, the patient is instructed to void. The initial 5 to 10 mL of urine is placed in the first container (VB1), the next 100 to 200 mL of urine is discarded, and a midstream specimen of 5 to 10 mL is voided into the second container (VB2). The patient should be instructed to stop voiding ("hold your urine"). The prostate is then massaged, and any expressed secretions are placed in the third container (VB3). The first 5 to 10 mL of the remaining urine is then placed in the fourth container (VB4). Microscopic examination is carried out for leukocytes, and quantitative cultures are performed.

The four-cup test is interpreted as follows. Urethritis is inferred to be the principal diagnosis if the first specimen (VB1) contains the highest concentration of WBCs and bacteria (some authorities would omit the VB1 specimen, since—as noted previously—isolated urethritis in men is unusual apart from sexually transmitted diseases). Chronic prostatitis is inferred when the EPS specimen is strikingly positive for leukocytes or when the third specimen (VB3) contains more than 12 leukocytes per high-power field. The presence of $\geq 10^3$ CFUs/mL in the second specimen (VB2) renders the test uninterpretable for diagnosis of prostatitis, since bacteriuria of bladder origin will mask the typically small number of bacteria from the prostate.

Unfortunately, the true diagnostic accuracy of the four-cup test is unclear because no "gold standard" exists for excluding the diagnosis short of autopsy. Prostate tissue can contain microorganisms even when culture of the EPS specimen is sterile.

Occasionally prostatitis is the sole manifestation of tuberculosis or fungal disease (notably blastomycosis, coccidioidomycosis, and cryptococcosis and rarely histoplasmosis). These patients have granulomatous prostatitis, and the prostate is often indurated, firm, or nodular on rectal examination. Diagnosis is usually based on prostate biopsy, although urine cultures for mycobacteria and fungi are also helpful.

Natural History
Expected Outcome

Chronic bacterial prostatitis is prone to remissions and relapses.

Treatment
Methods

Quinolones (e.g., ciprofloxacin or ofloxacin) have become the drugs of choice because of their superior penetration into the non–acutely inflamed prostate. Quinolones have now been shown to be superior to TMP/SMX, the previous drug of choice. The optimum duration of treatment is unknown, but most authorities advise treatment for 4 to 12 weeks. For patients with frequent relapses, long-term, low-dose suppressive therapy with regimens similar to those for women with frequent recurrences of UTI (Table 14-7) is often effective.

Expected Response

A cure rate, at least on short-term follow-up, of about 70% has been achieved with quinolone therapy for chronic bacterial prostatitis.

When to Refer

Although chronic bacterial prostatitis, unlike acute bacterial prostatitis, is seldom a severe illness, many patients ultimately require referral to a urologist. When granulomatous prostatitis (including tuberculous and fungal prostatitis) is suspected because of the clinical course or the finding of an indurated, firm, or nodular prostate, biopsy should be considered.

 KEY POINTS

CHRONIC BACTERIAL PROSTATITIS

- ⊃ The diagnosis is usually made in the course of investigating the cause of recurrent UTI or asymptomatic bacteriuria.
- ⊃ Rectal examination classically shows a tender and boggy prostate but is frequently normal.
- ⊃ The four-cup test of urine is the cornerstone of accurate diagnosis. Unfortunately, there is no "gold standard" short of autopsy for excluding the diagnosis.
- ⊃ The treatment of choice is generally a quinolone antibiotic given for 4 to 12 weeks.
- ⊃ Although 70% cure rates have been achieved with quinolones, relapse is common.
- ⊃ Occasional patients have granulomatous prostatitis (tuberculous or fungal), which is suggested by failure to respond to antibiotics and by the finding of an indurated, firm, or nodular prostate.

SUGGESTED READING

Andreu A, Stapleton AE, Fennell C, et al. Urovirulence determinants in *Escherichia coli* strains causing prostatitis. J Infect Dis 1997; 176: 464-469.

Chronic Nonbacterial (Noninflammatory) Prostatitis and Chronic Pelvic Pain in Men (Prostatodynia)

Most men evaluated for prostatitis (>90% by some estimates) are given the diagnosis of chronic nonbacterial prostatitis or chronic pelvic pain syndrome. These overlapping syndromes are extremely common, poorly understood, and differentiated from each other mainly on the basis of examination of the prostate and microscopic examination of prostatic secretions (Table 14-9).

Presentation and Progression
Cause

The cause of neither syndrome is known. The presence of leukocytes in the prostatic secretions of patients with chronic nonbacterial prostatitis suggests an infectious etiology, but little or no convincing evidence has shown a role for such microbial candidates as *C. trachomatis, U. urealyticum,* and *Trichomonas vaginalis.* A wide variety of noninfectious etiologies have been proposed over the years. "Prostatodynia" has long been considered a diagnosis of exclusion. Recent data suggest that some of these patients have bladder outlet obstruction localized mainly to the vesical neck.

Presentation

Patients with nonbacterial prostatitis complain of dysuria, frequency, and pain. Patients with prostatodynia, who are often young and middle-aged men, sometimes complain mainly of voiding difficulties. Pain is often vague, described as a dull ache and variably localized to the perineum, suprapubic area, inguinal area, or scrotum. Patients sometimes complain of erectile dysfunction or pain on ejaculation.

Diagnosis

Operational criteria for the diagnosis of nonbacterial prostatitis include the presence of leukocytes (>20 per high-power field) in prostatic secretions, sterile cultures of prostatic secretions, and failure to respond to antibiotic therapy that would be appropriate for chronic bacterial prostatitis (namely a quinolone antibiotic given for 4 to 12 weeks).

Operational criteria for the diagnosis of prostatodynia include a normal urinalysis, the absence of significant numbers of leukocytes in prostatic secretions, and sterile cultures of prostatic secretions. In many of these patients urodynamic studies show various disorders such as bladder neck obstruction or dysfunction, urethral spasm, or abnormal tension in the pelvic floor.

Natural History
Expected Outcome

Both nonbacterial prostatitis and pelvic pain syndrome can, in the absence of specific treatment, be expected to be chronic with a fluctuating course.

Treatment
Methods

Sitz baths and NSAIDs may provide symptomatic relief in both of these syndromes. Psychotherapy is often useful for patients with associated sexual dysfunction.

For patients who meet the criteria for chronic nonbacterial prostatitis, a 2- to 4-week trial of doxycycline or erythromycin can be given because of the possible role of chlamydial or mycoplasmal infection. To date, however, clinical trials do not provide a clear rational basis to support this common practice.

Specialized urologic treatments help some patients. Those with chronic nonbacterial prostatitis may achieve some relief with transurethral microwave thermotherapy. Those with prostatodynia may benefit from treatment based on urodynamic findings: α-adrenergic blocking agents may help those with bladder neck and urethral spasm, surgical incision in the bladder neck may help those with bladder neck obstruction, and benzodiazepines (such as diazepam) may help those with pelvic floor dysfunction.

Expected Response

Both syndromes are frustrating to patients and physicians alike.

When to Refer

Although neither condition is life threatening, referral to a urologist may be helpful.

SUGGESTED READING

Egan KJ, Krieger JL. Chronic abacterial prostatitis—a urological chronic pain syndrome. Pain 1997; 69: 213-218.

Mayo ME, Ross SO, Krieger JN. Few patients with "chronic prostatitis" have significant bladder outlet obstruction. Urology 1998; 52: 417-421.

Epididymitis

Epididymitis, which is usually but not always an infectious disease, accounts for >600,000 physician visits in the United States each year according to one estimate. In younger men it is usually caused by sexually transmitted pathogens. In older men it is usually a bacterial disease associated with prostatic enlargement. Epididymitis must be distinguished from testicular torsion, a urologic emergency.

Presentation and Progression
Cause

Microorganisms can enter the epididymis from the prostate by way of the ejaculatory duct. Healthy younger men with sexually transmitted disease usually have no predisposing factors. The usual pathogens, in order of frequency, are *C. trachomatis*, *Neisseria gonorrhoeae*, and *U. urealyticum*. In older men the usual causes are aerobic gram-negative rods such as *E. coli*, other Enterobacteriaceae, and *Pseudomonas* species, but gram-positive cocci are also common. Tuberculous epididymitis was formerly a common condition, and epididymitis continues to be the most common manifestation of genitourinary tuberculosis in men. Predisposing factors to epididymitis include acute or chronic bacterial prostatitis, neurogenic bladder, indwelling urinary catheters, recent urologic surgery, and recent or remote prostatectomy or vasectomy.

Diagnosis

Early in the course of epididymitis, inflammation is localized to the epididymis, which is in its usual anatomic location. The inflammation may spread to involve the adjacent testis to the extent that the two organs are indistinguishable. In testicular torsion—the major entity to exclude—the epididymis is often high riding or rotated. When scrotal swelling complicates either condition, however, the exact anatomic location of the epididymis can be unclear. Other entities in the differential diagnosis are testicular cancer, trauma, orchitis, and spermatocele (Box 14-5).

Urinalysis sometimes shows pyuria. Urethral discharge should be examined microscopically, cultured, or in young men, tested for *C. trachomatis* and *N. gonorrhoeae* by culture or the enzyme-linked assays.

BOX 14-5
Differential Diagnosis of Epididymitis

- Both epididymitis and testicular torsion cause unilateral scrotal swelling and pain. Isolated epididymal tenderness in the organ's normal anatomic location, especially when accompanied by fever and pyuria, suggests epididymitis.
- Testicular torsion usually occurs in adolescents (peak age 12 to 14 years) but can occur in early adulthood. The epididymis is often high riding or rotated.
- Prepubescent and adolescent males should be presumed to have testicular torsion, prompting urgent urologic consultation.
- About 15% of patients with testicular cancer have symptoms and signs of epididymitis.

Natural History
Expected Outcome

Complications of acute epididymitis include abscess formation, progression to chronic disease, obliteration of the vas deferens, infertility, and testicular atrophy. The latter complication results from occlusion of the testicular blood flow by the epididymal swelling.

Treatment
Methods

Patients with sexually transmitted epididymitis should be treated with regimens appropriate for gonococcal and chlamydial infection (see Chapter 16). Patients with bacterial epididymitis can usually be treated with oral antibiotics (TMP/SMX or a quinolone in doses appropriate for treatment of pyelonephritis; see Table 14-8). Symptomatic relief can be obtained with NSAIDs (which may also shorten the clinical course) and bed rest, with the scrotum elevated with an athletic supporter. Patients with either complicated genitourinary disease or severe sepsis should be hospitalized and treated with intravenous antibiotics.

Expected Response

Patients usually respond to effective therapy for epididymitis within 3 days. Failure to respond indicates the need for reevaluation.

When to Refer

Patients with sepsis or toxicity should be hospitalized. Urologic follow-up should be carried out, since epididymitis is the presenting symptom in about 15% of patients with testicular cancer. When testicular torsion is a possible diagnosis, surgical consultation should be considered because delay in diagnosis can result in loss of the organ.

 KEY POINTS

EPIDIDYMITIS

⊃ Epididymitis in younger adults is most often the result of sexually transmitted disease; epididymitis in older adults is usually caused by gram-negative or gram-positive bacteria and associated with prostatic disease.

⊃ Epididymitis usually responds to appropriate therapy within 3 days.

⊃ Occasional patients with epididymitis require hospitalization because of sepsis.

SUGGESTED READING
Mittemeyer BT, Lennox KW, Borski AA. Epididymitis: review of 610 cases. J Urol 1966; 95: 390-392.

Seminal Vesiculitis

Seminal vesiculitis is a generally benign disease that usually causes painful ejaculation with blood (hematospermia). Semen should be cultured because it may contain the causative microorganism. Diagnostic evaluation proceeds along the same lines as the workup for acute prostatitis. TMP/SMX or a quinolone (such as ciprofloxacin) is currently the preferred drug for treatment. The alarming symptoms usually cause considerable anxiety, and patients should be reassured that the disease process is self-limited and benign.

Orchitis

The classic infectious cause of orchitis (inflammation of the testicle) is mumps, a vaccine-preventable disease. The incidence is highest in males infected with mumps after puberty; the disease may develop in nearly one third of this group. The process is manifested as severe pain in the scrotum with redness, erythema, and tenderness, developing toward the end of the first week of the illness. It is unilateral in the majority of cases. Parotitis may or may not be clinically apparent. Sterility can result. Other causes of orchitis include prostatitis, seminal vesiculitis, gonorrhea, and such systemic infections as tuberculosis, leptospirosis, brucellosis, and chickenpox. Orchitis must be distinguished from tumor, trauma, and testicular torsion.

Urinary Tract Infection in Frail Elderly Patients

Both asymptomatic and symptomatic UTIs are common in elderly patients. Complications are relatively common, but in general UTI serves as a marker for underlying disease. Attempting to eradicate asymptomatic bacteriuria is not recommended.

Presentation and Progression
Cause

The spectrum of microorganisms is the same as in younger patients. However, patients with obstructive uropathy or previous instrumentation, including indwelling catheters, often have difficult-to-treat pathogens such as *Enterobacter, Serratia,* and *Providencia* species, *P. aeruginosa,* enterococci, and yeasts. Fungal UTI is becoming increasingly common in elderly patients who have received multiple courses of antibiotics. Common predisposing factors for UTI are prostatism in men, bladder prolapse in women, neurologic disease, and inability to maintain good hygiene.

Presentation

Asymptomatic bacteriuria is common, affecting about 10% of men and 20% of women over 65 years of age. Careful studies have failed to establish a relationship between asymptomatic bacteriuria and general well-being or urinary continence in the elderly. However, symptoms of UTI can be subtle because both the febrile response to infection and the experience of pain and other symptoms may be blunted in the frail elderly.

Diagnosis

Diagnosis is made according to the same principles outlined above. In-and-out bladder catheterization is sometimes necessary to obtain a valid urine specimen.

Natural History
Expected Outcome

UTI in the elderly is in many ways a marker of general debility. Data suggesting that UTI reduces quality of life and increases mortality are unconvincing. However, urosepsis (UTI with positive blood cultures) in elderly people has been associated with an in-hospital mortality of about 16%. Risk factors for death include chronic urinary catheters, admission from a nursing home, and identification of a gram-positive microorganism as the source. Most of the fatalities occur in extremely debilitated patients.

Treatment
Methods

Treatment, when indicated, follows the principles outlined previously (Tables 14-6 and 14-8). Longer treatment may be necessary in older women. Attention should be paid to predisposing factors, especially impaired bladder emptying, genital prolapse, estrogen deficiency, perineal hygiene, and urolithiasis. When prescribing potentially toxic drugs, the physician should remember that renal function is reduced in elderly patients even when the serum creatinine level is normal.

Expected Response

In general, the elderly respond less well than younger patients to treatment of UTI. The poor response seems to be related to obstructive uropathy and to the severity of underlying disease rather than to age.

When to Refer

Older patients with symptomatic UTI that does not respond to antibiotic therapy should usually be referred for urologic evaluation.

SUGGESTED READING
Ackermann RJ, Monroe PW. Bacteremic urinary tract infection in older people. J Am Geriatr Soc 1996; 44: 927-933.

Matsumoto T, Kumazawa J. Urinary tract infection in geriatric patients. Int J Antimicrob Agents 1999; 11: 269-273.

Nygaard IE, Johnson JM. Urinary tract infections in elderly women. Am Fam Physician 1996; 53: 175-182.

Urinary Tract Infection in Patients with Diabetes Mellitus (see also Chapter 4)

Factors that potentially promote UTI in patients with diabetes mellitus include glycosuria, age, structural abnormalities of the urinary tract, recurrent episodes of vaginitis, generalized vascular disease, and—most important—autonomic neuropathy. Autonomic neuropathy impairs bladder function and sensation, causing a "diabetic cystopathy" that promotes vesicoureteral reflux. Patients with diabetes mellitus have up to a four-fold increase in the incidence of acute pyelonephritis compared with patients without diabetes mellitus. Unusual complications of UTI in diabetes mellitus include renal corticomedullary abscess (two-fold increase compared with nondiabetic patients), renal carbuncle (increased incidence), and emphysematous pyelonephritis and cystitis. Plain x-ray examination of the kidneys (KUB) or CT scanning should be strongly considered for diabetic patients with clinically severe UTI because of the possibility of emphysematous pyelonephritis or emphysematous pyelitis, both of which are potentially life threatening. Indications for hospitalization of patients with diabetes mellitus and UTI include high fever, nausea, vomiting, inability to take oral medications, advanced age, and debility.

Urinary Tract Infection in Patients with Polycystic Kidney Disease

Diagnosis and management of UTI in patients with polycystic kidney disease, a relatively common genetic disorder, pose several problems.

Presentation and Progression
Cause

Autosomal dominant polycystic kidney disease is a genetic disorder with a prevalence of 1:300 to 1:1000 in the general population. About 90% of cases are inherited, and about 10% arise from spontaneous mutations.

Presentation

Unlike the rare autosomal recessive form of polycystic kidney disease, which is usually diagnosed in the first year of life, symptoms of autosomal dominant polycystic kidney disease usually begin in the third or fourth decade. The presenting symptom is most often acute or chronic flank pain. Urinary tract infection is common and can involve cystitis, pyelonephritis, or infection of a cyst (pyocyst). In infected pyocyst the urine culture may be sterile because the cyst may not communicate with the collecting system. Pyuria is found in up to 45% of uninfected patients with polycystic kidney disease. Hematuria also occurs from the underlying disease.

Diagnosis

Diagnosis of polycystic disease is best made by ultrasound examination of the kidney, which reveals at least three to five cysts per kidney (the standard diagnostic criterion) in at least 80% of patients by age 20 and in nearly 100% by age 30. Radiologic studies offer relatively little help in the localization of UTI in these patients. CT scans may show evidence of pyelonephritis but in general are less helpful than in other patients. Indium scanning localizes only inflammation and is positive in only about one half of cases.

Natural History
Expected Outcome

In most patients with polycystic kidney disease, end-stage renal disease requiring dialysis or transplantation develops. Infected pyocysts seldom resolve spontaneously.

Treatment
Methods

Patients with parenchymal renal infection (pyelonephritis) should be treated similarly to patients without polycystic kidney disease. If pyocyst is suspected, however, treatment must be different. The aminoglycosides and β-lactam antibiotics do not penetrate well into cysts. TMP/SMX, ciprofloxacin, and chloramphenicol appear to provide the best penetration into

cysts among the currently available antibiotics. Prolonged therapy with TMP/SMX or ciprofloxacin is recommended for patients with pyocysts; 4 to 6 weeks of treatment is usually recommended, but 3 months or longer may be necessary.

Expected Response

Patients with pyelonephritis respond like other patients to therapy. Pyocyst should be strongly suspected if full recovery has not been achieved within 5 to 7 days. Most patients eventually respond. Percutaneous aspiration of the cyst has been performed but is difficult.

When to Refer

If fever, flank pain, and toxicity develop in a patient with polycystic kidney disease, hospitalization is usually needed.

 KEY POINTS

URINARY TRACT INFECTION IN PATIENTS WITH POLYCYSTIC KIDNEY DISEASE
- Cystitis, pyelonephritis, or infected cyst (pyocyst) can occur in patients with polycystic kidney disease.
- Pyuria and hematuria occur as part of the underlying disease and therefore lose diagnostic value.
- Distinguishing between pyelonephritis and pyocyst can be difficult because fever and flank pain are common to both.
- Infection of a cyst (pyocyst) is likely to be present if the patient has positive blood cultures, new renal pain, or failure to improve with a standard course of antibiotics.
- Antibiotics that penetrate well into cysts include TMP/SMX, ciprofloxacin, and chloramphenicol.

SUGGESTED READING

Gibson P, Watson ML. Cyst infection in polycystic kidney disease: a clinical challenge. Nephrol Dial Transplant 1998; 13: 2455-2457.

Urinary Tract Infection in Patients with Indwelling Catheters

Over 1 million catheter-associated UTIs occur in the United States each year. Risk factors including female sex, duration of catheterization, and disconnection of the junction between the catheter and the collecting tube. Microorganisms can gain access to the bladder either by migrating along the periurethral space on the outer surface of the catheter (especially in women) or by migrating up the catheter lumen after contamination of the collecting tube–drainage bag system (the main mechanism in men). Catheter-associated UTI is the most common factor predisposing to hospital-acquired gram-negative bacteremia in the United States. Males are predisposed to catheter-associated prostatitis, which can be difficult or impossible to cure.

Presentation and Progression
Cause

Microorganisms can gain access to the urinary tract through two routes: intraluminal (through the lumen of the catheter) and extraluminal (by way of the mucous film that forms between the external surface of the catheter and the patient's urethral epithelium). Intraluminal infections result from failure of the closed drainage system, contamination of the collecting bag, or disconnection of the urinary catheter from the drainage system. Recent studies suggest that about two thirds of these infections result from extraluminal infection; these infections are therefore not prevented even by the strictest adherence to closed-drainage technique. Extraluminal spread of bacteria is more likely to involve enterococci, staphylococci, and yeasts. Gram-negative bacilli cause intraluminal and extraluminal infections with approximately equal frequency. Each day asymptomatic bacteriuria develops in about 5% of catheterized patients despite good infection control practices.

Diagnosis

Diagnosis of UTI is easily made in catheterized patients by aspiration of urine from the catheter or from a port designed for that purpose. The catheter should not be disconnected from the collection tube unless absolutely necessary, since this predisposes to infection. Determining that bacteriuria or funguria explains clinical symptoms and signs in these patients requires interpretation of the urinalysis and urine culture findings in the context of an overall evaluation of the patient.

Natural History
Expected Outcome

Asymptomatic bacteriuria and funguria in catheterized patients are often well tolerated. However, pyelonephritis is probably underrecognized in these patients. In a study of autopsy findings among nursing home patients, the presence of a catheter at the time of death increased the likelihood of inflammation of the kidneys by seven-fold (38% versus 5% for patients without catheters). Bacteremia can occur. Yeast infection promotes the formation of "fungus balls" capable of obstructing the ureters. Whether the increased mortality in patients with catheter-associated UTI results from the infection per se or from debilities that led to catheterization has not been determined.

Treatment
Methods

Asymptomatic bacteriuria or funguria should not be treated while the catheter is in place. In general, routine urine cultures are not recommended for patients with long-term bladder catheters. For symptomatic patients with fever, it is best to obtain a urine for culture through the catheter and then remove the catheter while administering antibiotics. Urinary drainage can usually be managed by intermittent catheterization.

Expected Response

Provided the catheter is removed, treatment with standard regimens is probably as effective as in patients who have not been catheterized.

When to Refer

Patients who have frequent symptomatic catheter-associated UTIs and require long-term management of urinary drainage should be evaluated by a urologist.

SUGGESTED READING

Olsson ES, Cookson BD. Do antimicrobials have a role in preventing septicaemia following instrumentation of the urinary tract? J Hosp Infect 2000; 42: 85-97.

Saint S, Wiese J, Amory JK, et al. Are physicians aware of which of their patients have indwelling urinary catheters? Am J Med 2000; 109: 476-480.

Tambyah PA, Halvorson KT, Maki DG. A prospective study of pathogenesis of catheter-associated urinary tract infections. Mayo Clin Proc 1999; 74: 131-136.

Warren JW, Muncie HL, Hall-Craggs M. Acute pyelonephritis associated with bacteriuria during long-term catheterization: a prospective clinicopathological study. J Infect Dis 1988; 158: 1341-1346.

15 Infections of the Skin and Its Appendages, Muscle, Bones, and Joints

CHARLES S. BRYAN, STEPHEN J. HAWES

Infections of the skin and its appendages such as hair follicles and nails are common in primary care and must sometimes be distinguished from life-threatening conditions such as necrotizing fasciitis (see Chapter 6). Infections of muscle, bones, and joints are typically more serious than skin infections and usually require referral or hospitalization.

Overview of Skin Infections

Skin infections are best classified according to the nature of the lesion (e.g., macule, papule, vesicle, or pustule; see Chapter 7), the layer involved (Figure 15-1), and the microbial etiology (Table 15-1). Some of these infections, for example, uncomplicated impetigo, can be treated in the primary setting without resort to special studies such as Gram stains and cultures. The clinician should be alert to the possibility of rare but serious lesions, such as the membranous ulcers of cutaneous diphtheria or the malignant pustule of anthrax; of sexually transmitted diseases; and of the possibility that skin lesions signify underlying diseases (see Chapter 7).

SUGGESTED READING
Aly R, Maibach HI. Atlas of Infections of the Skin. New York: Churchill Livingstone; 1999.
Harahap M, ed. Diagnosis and Treatment of Skin Infections. Oxford: Blackwell Science; 1997.
Sanders CV, Nesbitt LT, eds. The Skin and Infection: A Color Atlas and Text. Philadelphia: Lippincott, Williams & Wilkins; 1995.
Suhonen R, Dawber RPR, Ellis DH. Fungal Infections of the Skin, Hair and Nails. London: Martin Dunitz; 1999.

Nonbullous Impetigo

Impetigo is a common superficial infection of the epidermis usually encountered in children, typically on the face and extremities.

Presentation and Progression
Cause

In the past most cases of impetigo have been attributed to *Streptococcus pyogenes* (group A streptococcus). Group A streptococcal strains causing impetigo are, in general, of different M serotypes from those causing pharyngitis. In recent years *Staphylococcus aureus* has emerged as the more common etiology, at least in some localities. Group A streptococci and *S. aureus* are often encountered together, and asymptomatic carriage of either or both of these bacteria is a predisposing factor for impetigo. Some data suggest that anaerobic bacteria play a prominent role in impetigo development. Group B streptococci can cause impetigo in newborns, but streptococci belonging to Lancefield groups C and G rarely cause this condition. Predisposing factors include warm, humid climates, poor personal hygiene, poverty, and minor skin trauma. Recent data suggest that impetigo occurs frequently in patients with atopic dermatitis.

Presentation

Impetigo typically involves exposed areas of the skin, especially the face, but also the extremities. The initial lesions are small vesicles that quickly become pustules and then rupture, leaving a purulent discharge on the skin that dries to form honey-colored or golden-brown "stuck-on" crust. The lesions are painless but often pruritic, prompting scratching that in turn

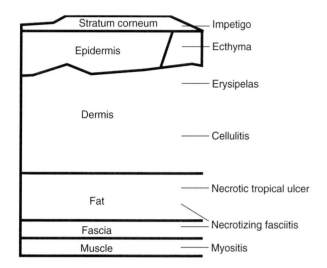

FIG. 15-1 Layers of the skin, showing tissue planes associated with various infectious syndromes. (From Wilhelmus KR. The red eye: infectious conjunctivitis, keratitis, endophthalmitis, and periocular cellulitis. Infect Dis Clin North Am 1998; 2: 99-116.)

spreads the infection to new areas. Mild lymphadenopathy is common, but high fever or other systemic symptoms should prompt a search for another diagnosis. The disease infects the most superficial layers of the epidermis (Figure 15-1).

Diagnosis

The thick, honey-colored crust of impetigo, once seen, becomes a familiar lesion that is seldom mistaken for other conditions. The grouped vesicles of herpes simplex, varicella, or herpes zoster can resemble the early lesions of impetigo. The crusts formed by a varicella-zoster viral infection are typically dark brown rather than honey colored and are harder than those caused by impetigo. Less common conditions that can be confused with impetigo include localized acute pustular psoriasis, acute palmoplantar pustulosis (a self-limited eruption of the palms and soles of unknown etiology), and primary cutaneous listeriosis (which is usually found on the forearms of farmers or veterinarians who have been involved in calving). The presumptive diagnosis of impetigo is strengthened by finding gram-positive cocci on Gram-stained smears of material obtained by unroofing the vesicles or the crust. *S. aureus*, group A streptococci, or both are isolated by culture. When a retrospective serologic diagnosis is desired, as in patients with acute glomerulonephritis, measurement of anti-DNase B antibodies to *S. pyogenes* gives a much higher yield than the antistreptolysin O (ASO) titer, which is usually unimpressive.

Natural History
Expected Outcome

Impetigo is nearly always a self-limited disease that heals without scarring. However, it is a common cause of acute poststreptococcal glomerulonephritis, which is life threatening.

Treatment
Methods

Oral cephalosporins (such as cephalexin and cefadroxil) or penicillinase-resistant penicillins (such as dicloxacillin) have replaced penicillin in recent years as the treatment of choice because of the emergence of *S. aureus* as a relatively common cause of nonbullous impetigo. In the past, penicillin G (often given as a single intramuscular injection) was considered the drug of choice. Erythromycin has traditionally been used as an alternative to penicillin, but the emergence of streptococci and staphylococci resistant to this agent has tempered enthusiasm.

Patients should be advised to remove the crusts gently after softening them with soap and water. Topical antibiotic ointments are usually prescribed. Mupirocin (Bactroban) is now the most popular agent; a cream formulation of mupirocin may be as effective or even superior to oral antibiotics, but further research is needed. Concern has been expressed that wide use of mupirocin will promote *S. aureus* resistance to this agent, thus negating the utility of mupirocin for treatment of the staphylococcal nasal carrier state.

Expected Response

Whether treatment reduces the incidence of poststreptococcal glomerulonephritis associated with impetigo has not been clearly established. This disease makes its presence known by dark urine and peripheral or facial edema and progresses to acute renal failure.

When to Refer

Impetigo seldom requires referral except for the infrequent complication of acute glomerulonephritis.

▶ KEY POINTS

NONBULLOUS IMPETIGO

- ⤴ Nonbullous impetigo is a superficial vesiculopustular infection of the stratum corneum.
- ⤴ The disease usually occurs in children during the summer months.
- ⤴ Vesicles quickly rupture to form golden-yellow or honey-colored, thick, "stuck-on" crusts.
- ⤴ Once the usual causative agent was group A streptococci, but *S. aureus* may be more common today, at least in some localities.
- ⤴ The disease is typically self-limited, although poststreptococcal glomerulonephritis develops in some patients.
- ⤴ Antibiotic therapy can be supplemented with removal of the crusts after soaking followed by application of a topical antibiotic ointment.

SUGGESTED READING

Bass JW, Chan DS, Creamer KM, et al. Comparison of oral cephalexin, topical mupirocin and topical bacitracin for treatment of impetigo. Pediatr Infect Dis J 1997; 16: 708-710.

Brook I, Frazier EH, Yeager JK. Microbiology of non-bullous impetigo. Pediatr Dermatol 1997; 14: 192-195.

Gisby J, Bryant J. Efficacy of a new cream formulation of mupirocin: comparison with oral and topical agents in experimental skin infections. Antimicrob Agents Chemother 2000; 44: 255-260.

Sadick NS. Current aspects of bacterial infections of the skin. Dermatol Clin 1997; 15: 341-349.

Ecthyma

Ecthyma resembles nonbullous impetigo in that it is usually caused by group A streptococci or staphylococci and begins with vesicles that become pustules and then rupture, leaving

TABLE 15-1
Descriptions and Usual Etiologies of Some Common Skin Infections

Infection	Description	Usual etiology
Impetigo (nonbullous)	Superficial vesiculopustular infection of the stratum corneum, featuring a thick, honey-colored, "stuck-on" crust	Group A streptococci and *Staphylococcus aureus* are the most common etiologies; anaerobic bacteria possibly have a role.
Bullous impetigo	Rupture of flaccid bullae, leaving an exposed skin surface that resembles a small burn; later, development of a thin, light-brown, "varnishlike" crust	*S. aureus* strains belonging to phage group II (usually type 71), which produces two extracellular exfoliative toxins, are the cause.
Ecthyma	Initial lesions resembling nonbullous impetigo; however, the process penetrates through the epidermis, leaving a "punched-out" ulcer with a raised, violaceous margin and covered by a greenish yellow crust	Group A streptococci are the cause. A similar-appearing lesion in the setting of systemic infection is known as ecthyma gangrenosum and is most commonly caused by *Pseudomonas aeruginosa* (see Chapter 7).
Folliculitis	Small (2- to 5-mm) erythematous papules that often contain small pustules at their apices; tend to be multiple and pruritic; associated with hair follicles	*S. aureus* is the usual cause in nonimmunocompromised persons. Other causes include *P. aeruginosa* (associated with water exposure), *Candida albicans*, *Malassezia furfur*, and *Pityrosporum ovale*.
Furuncle	The common "boil," an inflammatory nodule involving a hair follicle that usually begins as folliculitis	*S. aureus* is the cause.
Carbuncle	A group or series of abscesses in subcutaneous tissue that, compared with the common "boil," tend to be larger, deeper, and more irregular.	*S. aureus* is the cause.
Hidradenitis suppurativa	Chronic infection of the apocrine glands of the axillary, inguinal, and perianal areas	Secondary bacterial pathogens include *S. aureus*, aerobic gram-negative bacilli, and anaerobic bacteria.
Erysipelas	Fiery, bright red discoloration of the skin, sharply demarcated from the adjacent normal tissue and often with lymphangitis streaks and tender regional lymphadenopathy	Cause is usually group A streptococci (*S. pyogenes*), sometimes other streptococci (e.g., groups B, C, and G), and rarely staphylococci or other microorganisms.
Cellulitis (other than erysipelas)	Reddish discoloration of the skin in a diffuse pattern, with the involved skin often less clearly demarcated from the adjacent normal tissue than is the case in erysipelas	Group A streptococci and *S. aureus* are the usual pathogens. Unusual pathogens such as *Aeromonas hydrophila*, *Vibrio vulnificus*, *Erysipelothrix rhusiopathiae*, and *Cryptococcus neoformans* are usually suggested by the history.
Membranous ulcers (including cutaneous diphtheria)	Necrotic debris resembling a membrane and covering the base of a cutaneous ulcer	Various pyogenic bacteria can be the cause, but cutaneous diphtheria (*Corynebacterium diphtheriae*) should be considered in the differential diagnosis.
Erythrasma	Slowly spreading, pruritic, reddish brown macules in the genitocrural area	*Corynebacterium minutissimum* is the cause.

exudates on the skin surface. In ecthyma, however, the process does not remain confined to the stratum corneum but rather extends through the epidermis (Figure 15-1). The result is typically a "punched-out" ulcer with raised violaceous margins. The ulcer is covered with a greenish yellow crust. The lesions are most commonly located on the lower extremities. Ecthyma occurs most frequently in young children and in the elderly. Unusual causes of ecthyma include cutaneous diphtheria (see later discussion), gonococcal infection, mucormycosis, molluscum contagiosum, and herpes simplex virus infection.

"Uncomplicated ecthyma" must be distinguished from ecthyma resulting from systemic infection (ecthyma gangrenosum; see Chapter 7). Treatment is similar to that for impetigo, and systemic antibiotics are usually appropriate.

SUGGESTED READING

Hirschmann JV. Skin infections caused by staphylococci, streptococci, and the resident cutaneous flora. In: Arndt KA, LeBoit PE, Robinson JK, et al, eds. Cutaneous Medicine and Surgery. Philadelphia: W.B. Saunders Company; 1996: 919-930.

Kimyai-Asadi A, Tausk FA, Nousari HC. Ecthyma secondary to herpes simplex virus infection. Clin Infect Dis 1999; 29: 454-455.

Bullous Impetigo and the Staphylococcal Scalded Skin Syndrome

Bullous impetigo is a serious form of the disease that usually occurs in newborn infants and young children, is manifested as large, flaccid bullae, and is caused by strains of *S. aureus* capable of making exfoliative toxins. More extensive skin involvement caused by the same staphylococcal strains is known as the staphylococcal scalded skin syndrome or, when it affects neonates, pemphigus neonatorum (Ritter's disease).

Presentation and Progression
Cause

Bullous impetigo is attributed to *S. aureus* strains belonging to phage group II and capable of producing two extracellular exfoliative toxins (known as A and B) that separate the stratum corneum from the rest of the epidermis.

Presentation

The more common and milder form of the disease—representing about 10% of all cases of impetigo—differs from nonbullous impetigo in that the vesicles enlarge into flaccid bullae before rupturing. The exposed skin surface is at first moist and red, resembling a small burn. A thin, light brown, "varnishlike" crust then develops. The more severe form, which usually affects younger children, is known as the staphylococcal scalded skin syndrome. Widespread, flaccid bullae rupture, causing exfoliation of the skin that resembles an extensive third-degree burn. This form of the disease can occur in epidemic form in nurseries, where it is known as pemphigus neonatorum or Ritter's disease. Fever and other systemic symptoms are usually absent in the more localized forms of the disease but are invariably present in patients with the staphylococcal scalded skin syndrome. Staphylococcal

scalded skin syndrome in adults is rare and is usually associated with immunosuppression.

Diagnosis

Gram stain of material obtained by unroofing the bullae reveals gram-positive cocci in clumps, and cultures nearly always reveal *S. aureus*.

Natural History

Localized bullous impetigo is nearly always a self-limited disease. However, the staphylococcal scalded skin syndrome, which resembles a third-degree burn, is life threatening.

Treatment
Methods

Treatment of localized bullous impetigo is identical to that of nonbullous impetigo with the caveat that penicillin G, penicillin V, and amoxicillin are inappropriate therapy because nearly all *S. aureus* strains now produce β-lactamase. Patients with the staphylococcal scalded skin syndrome should be hospitalized and treated with parenteral antibiotic therapy and aggressive supportive care.

Expected Response

Localized bullous impetigo is self-limited, but the staphylococcal scalded skin syndrome carries a significant mortality rate.

When to Refer

Patients with the staphylococcal scalded skin syndrome should be hospitalized.

 KEY POINTS

BULLOUS IMPETIGO AND THE STAPHYLOCOCCAL SCALDED SKIN SYNDROME

⊃ Bullous impetigo and the staphylococcal scalded skin syndrome usually occur in infants and young children.

⊃ These diseases are caused by *S. aureus* belonging to phage group II, which produces exfoliative toxins.

⊃ Vesicles become large flaccid bullae that rupture, leaving exposed, moist, red skin before the formation of a thin, light brown, "varnishlike" crust.

⊃ The mild, localized form of bullous impetigo is self-limited.

⊃ The staphylococcal scalded skin syndrome (called pemphigus neonatorum when it occurs in neonates) is life threatening and requires aggressive treatment in the hospital.

SUGGESTED READING

Farrell AM. Staphylococcal scalded-skin syndrome. Lancet 1999; 354: 880-881.

Plano LR, Gutman DM, Woischnik M, et al. Recombinant *Staphylococcus aureus* exfoliative toxins are not bacterial superantigens. Infect Immun 2000; 68: 3048-3052.

Scales JW, Fleischer AB Jr, Krowchuk DP. Bullous impetigo. Arch Pediatr Adolesc Med 1997; 151: 1168-1169.

Shirin S, Gottlieb AB, Stahl EB. Staphylococcal scalded skin syndrome in an immunocompetent adult: possible implication of low-dosage prednisone. Cutis 1998; 62: 223-224.

Folliculitis

Folliculitis or pyoderma involving the hair follicles and apocrine glands affects nearly everyone at one time or another but is usually self-limited. Occasionally, folliculitis progresses to larger lesions known as furuncles and carbuncles.

Presentation and Progression

Cause

S. aureus is the usual cause of folliculitis in nonimmunocompromised patients. The infection probably arises from prior nasal colonization by this bacterium. *Pseudomonas aeruginosa* (usually of serogroup O:11) has emerged as an important cause of extensive folliculitis after exposure to contaminated hot tubs, whirlpools, heated swimming pools, or diving suits. *P. aeruginosa* can also cause extensive folliculitis in immunosuppressed patients. Other gram-negative bacilli typically cause folliculitis in patients who have undergone prolonged antibiotic therapy for acne or rosacea, but some recent data suggest that gram-negative folliculitis also occurs in persons without this predisposition. Fungi that cause folliculitis include *Candida albicans* (especially in hospitalized patients who have received corticosteroids and antibiotics) and *Malassezia furfur* (in patients who have diabetes mellitus or granulocytopenia or who have received corticosteroids). A condition known as eosinophilic folliculitis, of unknown origin, usually occurs in patients with advanced human immunodeficiency virus (HIV) disease.

Presentation

The characteristic unit lesion is a 2- to 5-mm erythematous papule that often contains a small pustule at its apex. The lesions are often multiple and tend to be pruritic. When multiple deep lesions appear on the bearded area of the face, the condition is known as sycosis barbae.

Folliculitis caused by *P. aeruginosa* following exposure to contaminated water is often widespread, affecting most commonly the axillae, hips, and buttocks. These lesions are pruritic and evolve into pustules. External otitis caused by the same bacterium is often present. Folliculitis caused by *C. albicans* in immunocompromised patients tends to occur as satellite lesions around areas of *Candida* infection involving the skin folds (intertriginous candidiasis). Folliculitis caused by *M. furfur* often involves the trunk, upper extremities, and face.

Variants of folliculitis include the following:

- Eosinophilic folliculitis ("itchy folliculitis") occurs mainly in HIV-infected patients, especially over the trunk but also over the face, is intensely pruritic, and is indistinguishable from other forms of folliculitis on clinical grounds.
- Pseudofolliculitis barbae ("razor bumps"; "ingrown hairs") is a papular or pustular inflammatory reaction affecting persons with curly hair (especially African-American males) who shave.
- "Steroid acne" is a folliculitis resulting from systemic or topical steroid therapy. It may be associated with fungal superinfection caused by *Pityrosporum ovale.*
- Viral folliculitis is caused most commonly by the herpesviruses (herpes simplex virus and varicella-zoster virus), especially in immunocompromised patients. Molluscum contagiosum can also cause folliculitis.
- Papular drug eruptions can mimic folliculitis. Sometimes called acneiform dermatoses, these eruptions tend to begin

suddenly, be widespread, occur in unusual locations such as the forearm and buttocks, and dissipate after the offending drug is discontinued.

Diagnosis

Folliculitis is a clinical diagnosis made by recognition of the typical unit lesion. Gram stains and cultures of unroofed lesions, when performed, usually reveal the causative microorganism. Eosinophilic pustular folliculitis in HIV-infected persons is best diagnosed by skin biopsy.

Natural History

Expected Outcome

Folliculitis is usually self-limited but can lead to the formation of furuncles or boils. Extensive folliculitis caused by *P. aeruginosa* often includes otitis externa as a manifestation. Rarely, folliculitis caused by *P. aeruginosa* progresses to ecthyma gangrenosum (see Chapter 7). The lesions of sycosis barbae, however, tend to be deeper and more chronic than those of other forms of folliculitis.

Treatment

Methods

Systemic antibiotics are seldom indicated for uncomplicated cellulitis. Appropriate treatment consists of application of warm saline compresses and topical antimicrobial agents (such as bacitracin ointment or, when fungal disease is suspected, an antifungal drug such as clotrimazole 1%). In immunosuppressed patients folliculitis caused by *M. furfur* that is refractory to clotrimazole usually responds to oral fluconazole therapy. Patients with severe, recurrent folliculitis or furunculosis (see later discussion) may benefit from nasal culture for *S. aureus.* Those with positive nasal cultures can then be treated with mupirocin ointment (Bactroban nasal, b.i.d. for 5 days each month).

Expected Response

Response is usually excellent.

When to Refer

Referral is seldom necessary.

 KEY POINTS

FOLLICULITIS

- Small (2- to 5-mm) erythematous papules often capped by a centrally located pustule.
- *S. aureus* is the usual pathogen.
- *P. aeruginosa* causes widespread folliculitis in patients exposed to contaminated hot tubs, whirlpools, or swimming pools.
- Other gram-negative bacilli sometimes cause folliculitis in patients who have received prolonged courses of antibiotic therapy for acne or rosacea.
- *C. albicans* and *M. furfur* can cause cellulitis in patients who are immunocompromised, who have diabetes mellitus, or who have received antibiotic or steroid therapy.
- Papular drug eruptions ("acneiform dermatoses") can cause folliculitis; they are often widespread and in unusual locations.
- Folliculitis is usually self-limited and responds to topical measures.

⊃ Sycosis barbae, a deep-seated folliculitis affecting bearded areas, often becomes chronic.
⊃ Local treatment usually suffices.

SUGGESTED READING

Crutchfield CE III. The causes and treatment of pseudofolliculitis barbae. Cutis 1998; 61: 351-356.

Jang KA, Kim SH, Choi JH, et al. Viral folliculitis on the face. Br J Dermatol 2000; 142: 555-559.

Neubert U, Jansen T, Plewig G. Bacteriologic and immunologic aspects of gram-negative folliculitis: a study of 46 patients. Int J Dermatol 1999; 38: 270-274.

Plewig G, Jansen T. Acneiform dermatoses. Dermatology 1998; 196: 102-107.

Weinberg JM, Mysiwiec A, Turiansky GW, et al. Viral folliculitis: atypical presentations of herpes simplex, herpes zoster, and molluscum contagiosum. Arch Dermatol 1997; 133: 983-986.

Yu HJ, Lee SK, Son SJ, et al. Steroid acne vs. *Pityrosporum* folliculitis: the incidence of *Pityrosporum ovale* and the effect of antifungal drugs in steroid acne. Int J Dermatol 1998; 37: 772-777.

Zichichi L, Asta G, Noto G. *Pseudomonas aeruginosa* folliculitis after shower/bath exposure. Int J Dermatol 2000; 39: 270-273.

Furuncles, Carbuncles, and Skin Abscesses

The familiar furuncle or "boil" is thought to arise from folliculitis. The term furunculosis refers to multiple boils or to frequent recurrences. Carbuncles are more extensive and difficult-to-treat lesions that often require surgical intervention. Skin abscesses, although similar to carbuncles histologically, are usually deeper infections that do not originate in hair follicles.

Presentation and Progression
Cause

S. aureus is the usual cause of both furuncles and carbuncles and is also the sole or predominant pathogen in about 50% of skin abscesses. Predisposing factors to recurrent furuncles (furunculosis) include obesity, corticosteroid therapy, disorders of neutrophil function, and possibly diabetes mellitus. Immunoglobulin levels are usually normal in patients with furunculosis. (Low IgM levels have been demonstrated in some patients, but this is of uncertain significance and, in contrast to IgG deficiency, replacement therapy is impractical.) However, most patients with recurrent furuncles have no obvious predisposing factors other than being nasal carriers of *S. aureus* (see Chapter 1). Outbreaks of furunculosis have been described in families, athletic teams, and village residents who took steam baths together. Repeated courses of omeprazole therapy were recently described as a possible risk factor; whether other drugs cause a predisposition to furunculosis is unclear. Skin abscesses can result from minor trauma, injection drug use (the practice of subcutaneous and intramuscular injection is known as "skin popping"), or bacteremia. Congenital immunodeficiency syndromes such as the hyperimmunoglobulin E–recurrent infection syndrome (Job's syndrome) are sometimes present in patients with recurrent skin abscesses. Rarely, skin abscesses are self-inflicted (factitious abscess), in which case Gram stain and culture may reveal "mouth flora" bacteria.

Presentation

Furuncles are commonly tender, firm, round subcutaneous nodules. The typical lesion is 1 to 2 cm in diameter, or about the size of a marble. The overlying skin is often erythematous, but fever and other systemic signs of illness are seldom present. Common sites for furuncles include the face, neck, axillae, and buttocks, but any area of the body that contains hair follicles can be affected.

Carbuncles differ from furuncles in that they are larger, deeper, irregular lesions that are usually associated with fever and malaise. Indeed, some patients with carbuncles are acutely ill and meet criteria for the sepsis syndrome. Common sites for carbuncles include the nape of the neck, the back, and the thighs.

Skin abscesses manifest themselves as local pain, swelling, and erythema. Systemic toxicity is usually absent unless cellulitis is present or unless the abscesses originated from bacteremia caused by a deep infection elsewhere. A majority of skin abscesses are located over the extremities, although any part of the body can be involved.

Diagnosis

Recognition of furuncles, carbuncles, and skin abscesses is usually straightforward. Lesions that sometimes resemble furuncles include infected cysts (such as epidermoid inclusion cysts and sebaceous cysts), nodular lesions caused by bloodstream infection in severely ill patients (causative organisms include *P. aeruginosa* and *Candida* species), and, rarely, metastatic cancer. Definitive diagnosis can be made by incision of the lesion and expression of purulent material from which *S. aureus* can usually be isolated. Incision, if carried out, must be done carefully to reduce the risk of causing bacteremia.

Natural History
Expected Outcome

Furuncles often break down and drain spontaneously, after which complete healing occurs. Carbuncles, if untreated, tend to become chronic. Lesions and particularly carbuncles can give rise to bacteremia, which can result in metastatic lesions such as endocarditis or osteomyelitis. Furuncles or carbuncles located in the "dangerous area" of the face—that is, the nose and medial aspects of the cheeks—can spread to the brain and cause cavernous sinus thrombosis (see Chapter 6). Most skin abscesses, if untreated, eventually "point" and drain spontaneously, but serious complications can result from bacteremia.

Treatment
Methods

Patients should be advised not to apply pressure to or squeeze carbuncles or furuncles because of the risk of causing bacteremia. The time-honored treatment of furuncles consists of the application of warm, wet compresses. The lesions usually "come to a head" and drain spontaneously, followed by complete resolution without residua. Surgical incision is indicated for unusually large lesions and is nearly always necessary for patients with carbuncles. Antibiotic therapy is indicated for furuncles when cellulitis or systemic toxicity is present, when the dangerous area of the face is involved, and when the patient has a condition that predisposes to life-threatening metastatic infection, such as a prosthetic heart valve. Long-term antibiotic therapy is often necessary for patients with carbuncles.

Skin abscesses are usually treated with antistaphylococcal antibiotics combined with surgical incision and drainage when fluctuance or "pointing" is present. Gram stain and culture of the lesion may help to clarify the etiology and occasionally suggest a factitious illness (see earlier discussion). Although data in the literature are conflicting regarding the frequency of bacteremia during incision and drainage of a skin abscess, patients with underlying heart lesions should be given prophylaxis against endocarditis with an antistaphylococcal drug (e.g., 1 or 2 g cefazolin IV just before incision of the abscess).

Patients with furunculosis (i.e., recurrent furuncles) present a therapeutic challenge, and no method has been uniformly effective (Table 15-2). Prolonged systemic antibiotic therapy (e.g., for 2 months) has, in general, not been successful. One study suggested that low-dose clindamycin (150 mg per day for 3 months) might be useful, but prolonged use of clindamycin exposes patients to the risk of pseudomembranous colitis.

Because many, perhaps most, patients with furunculosis are chronic nasal carriers of *S. aureus*, attempts to eradicate or suppress the carriage state are thought to be worthwhile. Topical antibiotic ointments (e.g., 2% mupirocin, applied to both nares twice daily for 5 days) are now recommended. A more aggressive approach is to combine topical antibiotic therapy with a 10- to 14-day course of oral antibiotic therapy (Table 15-2). A program designed to eradicate *S. aureus* nasal carriage should include follow-up cultures as a guide to retreatment, but the optimum frequency of such follow-up cultures has not been determined. Limited experience suggests that a strategy of repeating a 5-day course of mupirocin nasal ointment every month may be cost effective.

Vitamin C (1 g daily for 4 to 6 weeks) was shown to be effective for prevention of furunculosis in patients with impaired neutrophil function in a small study. Patients had no recurrences for 1 to 3 years after vitamin C was discontinued. Since this dose of vitamin C is seldom harmful, and since neutrophil function studies are expensive and available in only a few centers, a short course of vitamin C is not unreasonable for persons with severe furunculosis.

Individualized treatment is recommended. A flowchart for the patient might include columns for the date, results of nasal cultures, topical and systemic antibiotic therapy administered, new furuncles, and miscellaneous observations.

Expected Response

Furunculosis usually resolves spontaneously without scarring. Carbuncles are often chronic, and permanent scarring is the rule rather than the exception.

When to Refer

Patients with furunculosis are sometimes referred for a second opinion, but "cure" as defined by absence of recurrences over many years is the exception rather than the rule. Patients with carbuncles often need surgical drainage, since the lesions tend to be complicated and separated from one another by dense bands of connective tissue.

▶ KEY POINTS

FURUNCLES, CARBUNCLES, AND SKIN ABSCESSES
- ⊃ Furuncles, carbuncles, and skin abscesses rise from hair follicles and are nearly always caused by *S. aureus*.

- ⊃ Furuncles or "boils" are nodular lesions that usually resolve spontaneously.
- ⊃ Carbuncles are deeper, complex lesions that often require surgical drainage.
- ⊃ Skin abscesses are deeper than carbuncles, differ from furuncles and carbuncles in that they do not usually originate in hair follicles, and are caused by *S. aureus* in the majority of cases.
- ⊃ Applying pressure to carbuncles or furuncles or squeezing them can give rise to bacteremia and metastatic infection, such as endocarditis or osteomyelitis.
- ⊃ Furunculosis (recurrent formation of furuncles) is frustrating to manage; eradication of *S. aureus* nasal carriage may be worthwhile.

SUGGESTED READING

Binswanger IA, Kral AH, Bluthenthal RN, et al. High prevalence of abscesses and cellulitis among community-recruited injection drug users in San Francisco. Clin Infect Dis 2000; 30: 579-581.

Ellis AE. Immunization with bacterial antigens: furunculosis. Dev Biol Stand 1997; 90: 107-116.

Landen MG, McCumber BJ, Asam ED, et al. Outbreak of boils in an Alaskan village: a case-control study. West J Med 2000; 172: 235-239.

Levy R, Shriker O, Porath A, et al. Vitamin C for the treatment of recurrent furunculosis in patients with impaired neutrophil functions. J Infect Dis 1996; 173: 1502-1505.

Raz R, Miron D, Colodner R, et al. A 1-year trial of nasal mupirocin in the prevention of recurrent staphylococcal nasal colonization and skin infection. Arch Intern Med 1996; 156: 1109-1112.

von Eiff C, Becker K, Machka K, et al. Nasal carriage as a source of *Staphylococcus aureus* bacteremia. N Engl J Med 2001; 344: 11-16.

West BC, Agastya G, Sodeman W, et al. Furunculosis associated with repeated courses of omeprazole therapy. Clin Infect Dis 1998; 26: 1234-1235.

Hidradenitis Suppurativa

Hidradenitis suppurativa is a chronic disease of the apocrine glands of the axillae (hidradenitis suppurativa axillaris), inguinal region (hidradenitis suppurativa inguinalis), and perianal skin. The lesions become secondarily infected, leading to abscesses, fistulas, and scarring. Surgery rather than antimicrobial therapy is the usual cure for severe cases.

Presentation and Progression
Cause

Although the basic cause is unknown, the mechanism of disease appears to be the plugging of apocrine gland ducts by keratin. Pressure within the ducts causes them to dilate and rupture into surrounding tissues. The initial inflammatory lesions are sterile, but bacterial superinfection quickly occurs. Pathogens that have been isolated include *S. aureus*, streptococci (including *S. anginosus*), aerobic gram-negative rods (such as *Escherichia coli*, *Proteus mirabilis*, and *P. aeruginosa*), and anaerobic bacteria.

The disease especially affects young woman; the prevalence is 0.3% to 4% in developed countries. Familial occurrence and a possible association with cigarette smoking have been reported.

TABLE 15-2
Measures Used in the Management of Furunculosis

Measure	Methods	Comment
Antibiotic therapy	Antistaphylococcal penicillin, cephalosporin, clindamycin, or macrolide	Antibiotics are useful for acute episodes, but studies show that prolonged treatment (>2 weeks) does not help to prevent recurrences.
Bathing	Soap and water	Many authorities suggest use of an antimicrobial skin cleanser, including one with chlorhexidine (4%) or hexachlorophene.
Bath linens	Private (that is, reserved for the patient) towels and washcloths	The washcloth should be rinsed with hot water after each use and before the next use.
Bed linens and underwear	Laundering carried out at high temperatures	It may help to change bed linens on a daily basis.
Evaluation for immunodeficiency	Evaluation of neutrophil function (expensive and available in only a few areas)	Immunoglobulins are nearly always normal in patients with furunculosis or show isolated IgM deficiency, which, however, is not amenable to replacement therapy. Occasional patients have neutrophil disorders; vitamin C may benefit such patients (see later discussion).
Evaluation for the staphylococcal nasal carrier state	Nasal culture for *S. aureus* is performed by gently swabbing the anterior nasal mucosa	Although most patients with furunculosis are chronic nasal carriers, eradication or suppression of the carriage state may be worthwhile.
Topical treatment of the staphylococcal nasal carriage state	Mupirocin ointment (Bactroban nasal ointment) or less expensive alternatives such as bacitracin	Although mupirocin ointment eliminates the nasal carriage state in a substantial number of patients, repeat culturing is recommended because the carriage state nearly always recurs.
Systemic treatment of the staphylococcal nasal carriage state	Rifampin (600 mg per day) plus an amoxicillin-clavulanate or an antistaphylococcal penicillin (if the strain is methicillin susceptible) or TMP/SMX, ciprofloxacin, or minocycline (if the strain is methicillin resistant) or clindamycin alone	Rifampin should not be used alone, since *S. aureus* rapidly acquires resistance. Systemic therapy should be supplemented with topical therapy (we are aware of no evidence that these two methods are antagonistic).
Bacterial interference therapy	Colonization of the nose with "nonpathogenic" *S. aureus* after eradication of the nasal carriage state with a short course of aggressive antibiotic therapy	This approach is no longer recommended because the so-called nonpathogenic strain (known as 502A) was found to cause disease.
Vitamin C	1 g daily for 4 to 6 weeks	This approach was shown to be effective in a small group of patients with neutrophil disorders, with the benefit apparently lasting for 1 to 3 years after vitamin C was discontinued.
Vaccination	Staphylococcal vaccines	Trials of staphylococcal vaccines have, in general, failed to prevent recurrences.

Presentation

Early lesions consist of irregular reddish purple nodules, typically located in the axillae, groin, or perianal area. These lesions gradually enlarge and become fluctuant. Drainage results in sinus tracts. A foul odor to the drainage signifies anaerobic infection.

Diagnosis

Diagnosis is made clinically on the basis of the characteristic location and appearance of the lesions.

Natural History
Expected Outcome

In many patients the lesions remain generally stable. Spontaneous resolution is rare. In some patients the disease progresses relentlessly, resulting in extensive inflammation, undermining of the skin with sinus tracts, chronic drainage, and scarring. An associated spondyloarthropathy sometimes develops. Complications tend to be more severe in the perineal and perianal forms of the disease and include fistulas and squamous cell carcinomas.

Treatment
Methods

Early lesions of hidradenitis suppurativa should be treated aggressively with local moist heat followed by judicious incision and drainage. Topical clindamycin is apparently the only antimicrobial therapy shown to be effective by randomized clinical trial. Isotretinoin is possibly effective. In general, however, antimicrobial agents and retinoids have been disappointing. Smoking cessation should be encouraged. When material is obtained by incision and drainage, Gram stain and culture should be performed as a guide to antimicrobial therapy. Agents effective against anaerobic bacteria (e.g., metronidazole) should be used when a foul odor is present.

Many authorities recommend surgical intervention as the patient's best prospect for long-term cure.

Expected Response

In some patients hidradenitis suppurativa can be controlled for extended periods by conservative measures. In others, however, the disease progresses relentlessly, leading to chronic drainage and scarring. Surgical excision of the involved tissue with skin grafting is usually curative.

When to Refer

Patients with extensive disease require referral to a surgeon for radical excision of the involved tissue followed by skin grafting.

 KEY POINTS

HIDRADENITIS SUPPURATIVA

⊃ Hidradenitis suppurativa involves the apocrine glands in the axillary, inguinal, and perianal lesions.

⊃ The disease begins as a plugging of apocrine gland ducts by keratin; ductal obstruction leads to inflammation in the surrounding tissues.

⊃ Secondary bacterial pathogens include staphylococci, streptococci, aerobic gram-negative bacilli, and anaerobes.

⊃ Treatment of early lesions consists of the local application of moist heat followed by incision and drainage, combined with antimicrobial therapy directed at secondary pathogens determined to be present by Gram stain and culture. Topical clindamycin and isotretinoin are possibly effective. Medical therapy is, in general, disappointing.

⊃ Definitive treatment consists of excision of the involved tissue followed by skin grafting.

SUGGESTED READING

Brook I, Frazier EH. Aerobic and anaerobic microbiology of axillary hidradenitis suppurativa. J Med Microbiol 1999; 48: 103-105.

Brown TJ, Rosen T, Orengo IF. Hidradenitis suppurativa. South Med J 1998; 91: 1107-1114.

Endo Y, Tamura A, Ishikawa O, et al. Perianal hidradenitis suppurativa: early surgical treatment gives good results in chronic or recurrent cases. Br J Dermatol 1998; 139: 906-910.

Jemec GB, Wendelboe P. Topical clindamycin versus systemic tetracycline in the treatment of hidradenitis suppurativa. J Am Acad Dermatol 1998; 39: 971-974.

Konig A, Lehmann C, Rompel R, et al. Cigarette smoking as a triggering factor of hidradenitis suppurativa. Dermatology 1999; 198: 261-264.

Libow LF, Friar DA. Arthropathy associated with cystic acne, hidradenitis suppurativa, and perifolliculitis capitis abscedens et suffodiens: treatment with isotretinoin. Cutis 1999; 64: 87-90.

Erysipelas (Superficial Cellulitis)

The term "cellulitis" refers to spreading infection in the subcutaneous tissue. Erysipelas is a superficial form of cellulitis in which the involved skin assumes a fiery red color (hence the alternative name, "St. Anthony's fire"). Erysipelas is usually caused by group A streptococci and especially by *S. pyogenes.*

Presentation and Progression
Cause

Group A streptococci (*S. pyogenes*) cause most cases of erysipelas. Group B streptococci cause some cases of erysipelas in newborn infants, and streptococci belonging to groups C and G have caused erysipelas in adults. In one study more than 96% of cases of erysipelas were attributed to streptococci on the basis of extensive studies that included cultures of punch biopsy specimens. Rarely, *S. aureus* causes erysipelas.

Two notorious predisposing factors for erysipelas are breaks in the skin and lymphatic obstruction. Examples of the former are minor skin infections, including athlete's foot (tinea pedis), local trauma or abrasions, eczema, and cutaneous ulcers. Patients with lymphedema caused by congenital anomalies of the lymphatic system or with a history of surgery (e.g., radical mastectomy) or disease (e.g., filariasis or, quite commonly, previous episodes of cellulitis) are markedly predisposed to erysipelas. Erysipelas develops in about 50% of persons with severe lymphedema, compared with about 1 in 1000 persons in the general population. Other predisposing factors are the nephrotic syndrome, diabetes mellitus, alcoholism, and venous stasis of any etiology.

Presentation

Erysipelas is usually a rapidly progressive infection accompanied by fever and other signs of systemic toxicity. The involved skin is usually bright red, indurated, and edematous. A sharp demarcation divides involved and uninvolved skin (Figure 15-2). When the extremities are involved, frequently one or more bright red "lymphangitic streaks" connect the involved skin to one or more tender regional lymph nodes. Erysipelas most commonly occurs on the lower extremities. The upper extremities can be involved, especially in patients who have undergone radical mastectomy. The face, most often the nose and cheeks, is involved in about 20% of cases. A bullous form of erysipelas accounted for about 5% of cases in a recent series; patients with this form of the disease had a more prolonged clinical course.

Diagnosis

Erysipelas is a clinical diagnosis. A rapidly progressive erythema that is sharply demarcated from surrounding normal skin, one or more lymphangitic streaks, and tender regional lymphadenopathy constitute a virtually diagnostic triad. The following conditions can be confused with erysipelas: primary skin lesions such as giant urticaria or severe contact dermatitis

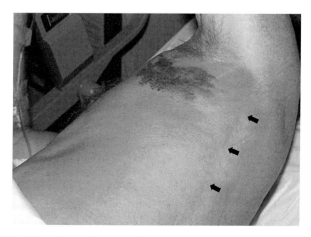

FIG. 15-2 Erysipelas caused by *Streptococcus pyogenes* involving the chest wall and flank, originating from pyoderma beneath the axilla. Note sharp demarcation from adjacent normal skin (*arrows*).

(in which fever is absent and itching is present), herpes zoster involving the face (in which localized pain precedes the skin lesions and vesicles soon appear), erythema chronica migrans (which progresses much less dramatically and with less fever), and diffuse inflammatory carcinoma of the breast (which also progresses less dramatically). Rarely, erysipelas-like lesions have been described in other conditions such as familial Mediterranean fever and hypogammaglobulinemia (with *Campylobacter jejuni* as the etiologic agent).

Attempts to confirm the streptococcal etiology are probably unnecessary in straightforward cases of erysipelas. Blood cultures are positive in only 2% to 5% of cases. Specimens for culture can be obtained by aspiration from the subcutaneous tissue after a small amount of sterile saline without preservative is injected (see Chapter 2). However, the yield is small from this procedure and it is not recommended for nonimmunocompromised patients.

Natural History
Expected Outcome

Untreated, erysipelas is often a self-limited disorder. However, it can progress to the deeper tissues, resulting in more severe cellulitis or even necrotizing fasciitis. In the preantibiotic era, protracted cases of erysipelas were probably a relatively common cause of group A streptococcal bacteremia, which carried an 80% mortality rate.

Treatment
Methods

Penicillin has traditionally been the treatment of choice. Oral penicillin (e.g., penicillin V, 250 to 500 mg q6h) or intramuscular procaine penicillin G (e.g., 600,000 units q12h) can be used in milder cases. When the clinical features are not clearly indicative of the "usual" erysipelas caused by streptococci, an agent with antistaphylococcal activity should be used. Many clinicians prefer to treat erysipelas with a cephalosporin or a macrolide antibiotic. Patients with more severe cases of erysipelas should receive intravenous antibiotic therapy. Small studies support the use of adjunctive corticosteroids, but this has yet to become a standard recommendation.

Patients who have had one or more episodes of erysipelas should be informed about the tendency of the disease to recur in the same location because of damage to the lymphatics. They should be advised to maintain scrupulous skin hygiene; treat any local skin diseases, including athlete's foot; and minimize their risk of cuts and abrasions. They should be advised that any sign of inflammation in the previously involved area should prompt medical attention. When travel to a remote area is planned (e.g., a camping trip in the wilderness), it may be prudent to prescribe an oral antibiotic (such as azithromycin or amoxicillin-clavulanate) with instructions to self-medicate when the earliest signs of inflammation occur.

Expected Response

Response to treatment is often slow. Fever usually subsides within 48 hours, but the skin lesion can actually progress during the first day or two after treatment is begun before the erythema and edema begin to subside (see the subsequent section "Cellulitis"). Complete resolution is usual, but some patients are left with residual lymphedema or worsening of preexisting edema. About 30% of patients, usually those with chronic lymphedema or venous insufficiency, have recurrent episodes years after an attack.

When to Refer

Hospitalization is recommended for patients with erysipelas accompanied by marked systemic toxicity, especially if they are elderly or have significant underlying diseases.

 KEY POINTS

ERYSIPELAS (SUPERFICIAL CELLULITIS)
- ⊃ Erysipelas is a superficial cellulitis in which the involved bright red skin is sharply demarcated from the adjacent normal skin.
- ⊃ Lymphangitic streaks and tender regional lymphadenopathy are often present and, with the skin lesions, form a triad that is virtually pathognomonic.
- ⊃ Rapid progression, fever, and systemic toxicity distinguish erysipelas from most of the conditions with which it might be confused.
- ⊃ Most cases are caused by group A streptococci (*S. pyogenes*).
- ⊃ Fever and local inflammation sometimes progress for a day or two after institution of adequate therapy.
- ⊃ Recurrence is common, especially in patients with lymphedema or venous insufficiency.
- ⊃ Patients should be advised about the potential for recurrence.

SUGGESTED READING

Bergkvist PI, Sjöbeck K. Antibiotic and prednisolone therapy of erysipelas: a randomized, double blind, placebo-controlled study. Scand J Infect Dis 1997; 29: 377-382.

el Tayeb SH, el Soliman AA, el Sehrawy AS. Role of *Streptococcus pyogenes* in the etiology of erysipelas. Adv Exp Med Biol 1997; 418: 95-97.

Guberman D, Gilead LT, Zlotogorski A, et al. Bullous erysipelas: a retrospective study of 26 patients. J Am Acad Dermatol 1999; 41: 733-737.

Roldan YB, Mata-Essayag S, Hartung C. Erysipelas and tinea pedis. Mycoses 2000; 43: 181-183.

Cellulitis (Other Than Erysipelas)

Cellulitis other than erysipelas is a deeper infection of the subcutaneous tissue usually caused by streptococci, staphylococci, or both. However, the etiologic spectrum is diverse. The primary care clinician should insist on close follow-up or hospitalization, especially because of the possibility that what initially appears to be a straightforward case of cellulitis might evolve into a life-threatening infection such as necrotizing fasciitis or clostridial myonecrosis (see Chapter 6).

Presentation and Progression
Cause

Cellulitis usually results from introduction of a pathogen into the skin by way of a wound or preexisting skin lesion. Examples of the former are cuts and punctures; examples of the latter are ulcers (such as stasis ulcers or decubiti), eczema, or furuncles. Predisposing factors include tinea pedis; peripheral vascular disease; peripheral edema, including lymphedema; prior history of cellulitis; and diabetes mellitus. *S. pyogenes* (group A streptococci) and *S. aureus* are the usual etiologies, but careful studies have established that cellulitis is often a mixed infection involving both of these microorganisms. A large and growing number of microorganisms have been associated with cellulitis, including the following, which have therapeutic implications:

- *Aeromonas hydrophila* cellulitis begins in wounds exposed to freshwater and can progress rapidly with marked systemic toxicity.
- *Vibrio vulnificus* and other marine vibrios cause cellulitis in wounds exposed to saltwater or brackish water. The infection progresses to necrosis of skin and subcutaneous tissue. This pathogen also causes sepsis in patients with liver disease after the ingestion of raw seafood (see Chapter 4).
- *Cryptococcus neoformans* causes cellulitis in immunosuppressed patients.
- *Haemophilus influenzae* was an important cause of cellulitis in children, often involving the face, before the introduction of the conjugated vaccine.
- Aerobic gram-negative rods (e.g., *E. coli, Proteus* species) sometimes cause cellulitis in immunocompromised persons or persons with diabetes mellitus.
- *Streptococcus pneumoniae* can cause severe cellulitis in immunocompromised persons and persons suffering from alcoholism.
- Non–group A β-hemolytic streptococci (e.g., groups B, C, or G) cause cellulitis in neonates, frail elderly persons, and persons with lymphedema of the lower extremities.
- *Erysipelothrix rhusiopathiae* causes erysipeloid ("fish-handler's disease"), which typically appears as a painful, violaceous, expanding lesion on an upper extremity on which an abrasion has been exposed to freshwater fish, shellfish, meat, hides, or poultry. "Seal finger," a cellulitis of unknown origin incurred while caring for seals, resembles erysipeloid but seems to respond best to tetracyclines.

Numerous microorganisms occasionally cause cellulitis, including non–serogroup O1 *Vibrio cholerae, Legionella* species, and even *Mycobacterium tuberculosis*.

Presentation

Cellulitis manifests itself by the classic signs of inflammation—redness, pain, warmth, and swelling—accompanied by fever, malaise, and other symptoms of toxicity. The line of demarcation

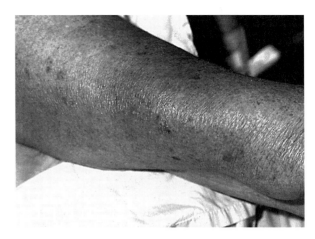

FIG. 15-3 Cellulitis in a patient with multiple myeloma. Note that demarcation from adjacent normal skin is less distinct than in erysipelas (Figure 15-2). *Staphylococcus aureus* was isolated from an aspirate of the lesion, following injection of a small amount of sterile saline without preservative. Cultures of aspirates from cellulitis have a higher yield in patients who are immunocompromised than in persons with normal host defenses.

between involved and uninvolved skin is often not as clear as is the case with erysipelas (Figure 15-3). Lymphangitic streaks are usually absent, but there may be tender regional lymphadenopathy. Depending to some extent on the pathogen, abscess formation or extension into fat or fascial layers may occur.

The clinical scenario may suggest the etiology and have therapeutic implications. In addition to the syndromes caused by the usual pathogens just summarized, the clinician should bear in mind the following:

- Cellulitis as a complication after surgery, including minor office procedures, can be a rapidly progressive and life-threatening infection in which hypotension and other features of sepsis dominate the clinical picture. Severe sepsis may be present even when signs of inflammation around the wound are minimal. This form of cellulitis is usually caused by group A streptococci.
- Perianal cellulitis occurs mainly in children and if untreated can become chronic. Clinical features include anal fissures, bloody stools, and pain on defecation. These infections can be caused by *S. pyogenes* but are often polymicrobial with mixtures of aerobic (e.g., *S. aureus* and *E. coli*) and anaerobic (e.g., *Bacteroides fragilis* and peptostreptococci) bacteria.
- Dissecting cellulitis of the scalp produces painful nodules, draining abscesses, and undermining of the skin; the highly descriptive Latin name for this condition is *perifolliculitis capitis abscedens et suffodiens*. *S. aureus* is the usual pathogen.
- Cellulitis related to saphenous vein harvest sites in patients who have undergone saphenous vein bypass surgery is often recurrent and of unclear microbial etiology. Non–group A β-hemolytic streptococci (e.g., streptococci belonging to groups B, C, or G) have been frequent causes in cases in which an etiology has been ascertained.
- The agent causing cellulitis of the vulvar or inguinal areas or lower abdominal wall in women who have undergone surgery or irradiation for gynecologic cancer is usually unclear, but most of the pathogens recovered have been

non–group A streptococci. Because these infections seem to be related to vaginal intercourse, the condition has been dubbed "streptococcal sex syndrome."

Diagnosis

The diagnosis of cellulitis is largely clinical. When features such as pain, hypotension, or other evidence of systemic toxicity seem disproportionate to the local signs of inflammation, imaging studies (such as magnetic resonance imaging [MRI]) may be advisable to exclude the possibility of a deeper and more serious process, such as necrotizing fasciitis or clostridial myonecrosis. Blood cultures should be obtained when marked systemic toxicity is present or when unusual pathogens are suspected (Figure 15-4), even though the yield is relatively low. For most patients with cellulitis, blood cultures are not cost effective. Aspiration of the lesion by the fine-needle technique, following injection through unbroken skin of a small amount of normal saline without preservative, has a higher yield than is the case with erysipelas; cultures from such aspirates reveal the causative organism in up to 30% of cases. Skin biopsy is occasionally worthwhile, especially when reason exists to suspect an unusual etiologic agent such as *C. neoformans.* When a primary site of infection is apparent, such as an ulcer or wound with surrounding erythema, culture of the lesion is often useful.

Natural History
Expected Outcome

Cellulitis often resolves spontaneously, but the high mortality (about 80%) exacted by streptococcal and staphylococcal bacteremia before the introduction of antibiotics should be remembered. Even today, group A streptococcal cellulitis complicating a trivial wound can cause life-threatening bacteremia or evolve into streptococcal toxic shock syndrome. As previously discussed (see discussion of erysipelas), episodes of cellulitis usually result in permanent local damage to the lymphatic system and thereby predispose the patient to recurrences. Recurrent cellulitis of the lower extremities or in the upper extremities of women who have undergone axillary lymph node dissection carries substantial morbidity.

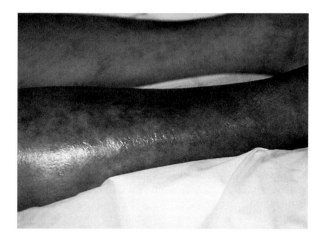

FIG. 15-4 Diffuse cellulitis of the lower extremity in a patient who had stepped on an oyster shell. Blood cultures revealed *Vibrio parahaemolyticus.*

Treatment
Methods

Presumptive antimicrobial therapy for patients without evidence of an unusual etiology should be directed mainly against group A streptococci and *S. aureus.* Appropriate choices for parenteral therapy are cefazolin (1 g IV q8h), nafcillin (2 g IV q4h), or oxacillin (2 g IV q4h). An appropriate oral regimen for mild cases consists of dicloxacillin (500 mg to 1 g q.i.d., taken 1 hour before meals and at bedtime, with no food intake in the previous 2 or 3 hours). Alternative regimens for parenteral therapy include ampicillin-sulbactam (Unasyn) and ticarcillin-clavulanate (Timentin); alternative regimens for oral therapy include azithromycin or clarithromycin.

Necrotizing fasciitis (see Chapter 6), although uncommon, is an important diagnostic consideration, since many cases are misdiagnosed as cellulitis. Clues to the presence of necrotizing fasciitis include pain disproportionate to the clinical findings, bullae, crepitance, and grayish or dusky discoloration of the skin. In patients with diabetes mellitus, aerobic gram-negative rods are sometimes involved, especially if crepitance is present. Antimicrobial coverage in these patients should therefore include an agent with broad-spectrum coverage against aerobic gram-negative rods, such as a third-generation cephalosporin, aztreonam, or an aminoglycoside. Note that in each of these instances a drug with broad activity against streptococci and staphylococci must be included. If reason exists to suspect methicillin-resistant *S. aureus,* initial therapy should include vancomycin.

Expected Response

Cellulitis sometimes becomes worse during the first day or two, even with effective antimicrobial therapy. The probable explanation for this phenomenon is the presence in the subcutaneous tissue of bacterial antigens that continue to evoke an intense inflammatory response even when the bacteria have become nonviable. Cellulitis may take several weeks to resolve completely. Patients who have recovered from cellulitis are typically vulnerable to recurrences in the same anatomic area caused by damage to lymphatic vessels.

When to Refer

Patients with severe cellulitis or in whom necrotizing fasciitis cannot be excluded with reasonable certainty on clinical grounds should be admitted to the hospital.

 KEY POINTS

CELLULITIS (OTHER THAN ERYSIPELAS)
⊃ Group A streptococci, *S. aureus,* or both are the usual pathogens.
⊃ The line of demarcation between involved and normal skin is not as sharp as is the case with erysipelas (superficial cellulitis).
⊃ Blood cultures are in general not cost effective for cellulitis and should probably be obtained only for patients who have marked systemic toxicity.
⊃ Necrotizing fasciitis should be considered as a possible alternative diagnosis when pain is disproportionate to the clinical findings or when unusual features, such as bullae, crepitance, or grayish discoloration of the skin, are present.

⊃ Group A streptococcal cellulitis complicating a wound can manifest itself as severe sepsis with hypotension before the skin lesion becomes obvious.

⊃ The history may suggest an unusual pathogen with therapeutic implications, such as wound exposure to freshwater (*A. hydrophila*) or saltwater (*V. vulnificus*), fish handling (*E. rhusiopathiae*), or immunosuppressive therapy (*C. neoformans*).

⊃ *S. pneumoniae* sometimes causes cellulitis in patients with underlying illnesses; it is often associated with systemic toxicity and positive blood cultures.

⊃ Cultures from aspirates yield the causative microorganism in up to 30% of cases and are more likely to be positive in immunocompromised patients.

⊃ Cellulitis may progress slightly during the first day or two of effective treatment before the patient begins to improve.

⊃ Recurrent cellulitis carries substantial morbidity.

SUGGESTED READING

Anderson DJ, Schmidt C, Goodman J, et al. Cryptococcal disease presenting as cellulitis. Clin Infect Dis 1992; 14: 666-672.

Barzilai A, Choen HA. Isolation of group A streptococci from children with perianal cellulites and from their siblings. Pediatr Infect Dis J 1998; 17: 358-360.

Cox NH, Colver GB, Paterson WD. Management and morbidity of cellulitis of the leg. J R Soc Med 1998; 91: 634-637.

Hook EW III, Hooton TM, Horton CA, et al. Microbiologic evaluation of cutaneous cellulitis in adults. Arch Intern Med 1986; 146: 295-297.

Koutkia P, Mylonakis E, Boyce J. Cellulitis: evaluation of possible predisposing factors in hospitalized patients. Diagn Microbiol Infect Dis 1999; 34: 325-327.

Markham RB, Polk BF. Seal finger. Rev Infect Dis 1979; 1: 567-569.

Parada JP, Maslow JN. Clinical syndromes associated with adult pneumococcal cellulitis. Scand J Infect Dis 2000; 32: 133-136.

Perl B, Gottehrer NP, Raveh D, et al. Cost-effectiveness of blood cultures for adult patients with cellulitis. Clin Infect Dis 1999; 29: 1483-1488.

Membranous Ulcers, Including Cutaneous Diphtheria

Cutaneous ulcers such as those associated with venous or arterial insufficiency in the lower extremities are relatively common in primary care. Occasionally, such an ulcer manifests at its base a layer of necrotic debris resembling a membrane. Analysis of the associated purulent drainage, which is often abundant, usually discloses a mixture of various aerobic and anaerobic bacteria. Rarely, such ulcers are caused by cutaneous diphtheria, which is now the most common form of diphtheria reported in the United States and which serves as a reservoir for transmission of the disease. A majority of confirmed cases in the United States in recent years have been imported from other countries, but vulnerable populations include homeless persons, Native Americans, and certain populations in the southeastern states and the Pacific Northwest. Primary cutaneous diphtheria occurs as an indolent, nonhealing, "punched-out" skin ulcer with a dirty gray or gray-brown membrane at its base. Wound diphtheria involves secondary infection of a preexisting wound, all or part of which becomes covered by a membrane. Cutaneous diphtheria can also occur as superinfection of an eczematoid skin lesion. Diagnosis in each of these syndromes is suspected on the basis of the characteristic membrane. Examination of a methylene blue–stained smear of material obtained from the edge of the membrane may reveal metachromatically staining, beaded bacilli consistent with *Corynebacterium diphtheriae.* Suspicion of cutaneous diphtheria should prompt attempts to make a definitive diagnosis by culture and to demonstrate the presence of the toxin by special methods. All cases of suspected or confirmed diphtheria should be reported promptly to the local health department.

Erythrasma

Erythrasma is a common skin disease that is usually found in the groin and is often asymptomatic. The etiology appears to be *Corynebacterium minutissimum,* which, as its name implies, is a small gram-positive bacillus. This same organism also seems to be the cause of pitted keratolysis, a process in which irregular craters or pits form on the pressure-bearing areas of the soles of the feet and toes and which is associated with increased sweating (hyperhidrosis) and an unpleasant odor. Erythrasma occurs most commonly in men, who are often obese, have diabetes mellitus, or both. The lesions begin insidiously as erythematous, reddish brown macules in the groin area. These spread and often coalesce until they cover a large portion of the genitocrural area. The diagnosis of erythrasma is made on clinical grounds. A Wood's lamp, if available, can be used for rapid diagnosis of erythrasma, since the lesions exhibit a coral red fluorescence. Gram stain of material obtained from the skin surface reveals myriad small, gram-positive bacilli. Erythrasma is often confused with tinea versicolor and tinea cruris. Tinea cruris tends to be a deeper infection of the skin with more inflammation and a more rapidly progressive course. Erythromycin is the drug of choice, generally given as 250 mg PO for 5 to 14 days. Success has been reported with a single dose of clarithromycin or with topical clindamycin HCl (2%). After treatment the lesions usually resolve within several weeks but may recur.

SUGGESTED READING

Wharton JR, Wilson PL, Kincannon JM. Erythrasma treated with single-dose clarithromycin. Arch Dermatol 1998; 134: 671-672.

Decubitus Ulcers

Primary care clinicians encounter decubitus ulcers in severely debilitated persons such as nursing home patients with neurologic deficits and persons with paraplegia. Between 7% and 23% of patients in nursing homes have pressure ulcers according to various surveys. Treatment is difficult, and prevention is therefore paramount.

Presentation and Progression

Cause

Decubitus ulcers result from the ischemic necrosis of tissue that is caused by prolonged pressure (hence the common name "pressure sores"). Risk factors include neurologic deficit, paraplegia, and immobilization for any reason, such as fracture, malnutrition, hypoalbuminemia, peripheral vascular disease, and urinary or fecal incontinence. Necrosis typically begins in either or both of two areas: the epidermis and the deep subcutaneous tissue adjacent to bony prominences.

Secondary bacterial colonization is inevitable and typically involves staphylococci, streptococci, aerobic gram-negative bacilli, and anaerobic bacteria, including *B. fragilis.*

Presentation

Early ulcers are usually recognized as breaks in the skin. Other presentations include unexplained fever or thromboembolism.

Diagnosis

Diagnosis is usually straightforward because of erosion with ulceration of the skin over bony prominences. Pressure sores are staged as follows:

- Stage 1: nonblanching erythema with intact skin
- Stage 2: partial-thickness skin loss (abrasion, blister, or shallow crater)
- Stage 3: full-thickness skin loss with damage or necrosis of subcutaneous tissue that may extend to, but not through, the underlying fascia
- Stage 4: full-thickness skin loss with extensive tissue destruction, necrosis, and damage to underlying muscle, bone, joints, or tendons

When necrosis of deep subcutaneous tissue predominates, the extent of the problem is often appreciated only at the time of surgical débridement or exploration.

Natural History
Expected Outcome

Neglected decubitus ulcers frequently become extensive and deep, leading to such complications as osteomyelitis of the adjacent bone, cellulitis, septic thrombophlebitis, and the sepsis syndrome. Sepsis from decubitus ulcers has been associated most clearly with *B. fragilis,* but other microorganisms causing sepsis from ulcers include *S. aureus* and aerobic gram-negative bacilli. Decubitus ulcers are an important reservoir for drug-resistant bacteria such as methicillin-resistant *S. aureus* and vancomycin-resistant enterococci. Colonization of decubitus ulcers occasionally leads to such complications as the toxic shock syndrome, tetanus, or wound botulism. The overall prognosis of patients with decubitus ulcers is poor, mainly because of underlying conditions. The 1-year mortality rate for patients admitted to nursing homes with decubitus ulcers is 50%, compared with a 27% mortality rate for persons admitted to nursing homes without decubitus ulcers.

Treatment and Prevention
Methods

Measures useful for both prevention and treatment of decubitus ulcers include frequent turning, special mattresses and beds designed to distribute pressure more evenly, and nutritional supplementation. When ulcers are first recognized, the essence of treatment is aggressive local wound care with débridement of dead tissue. Antimicrobial agents should generally be reserved for complications such as surrounding cellulitis. When sepsis occurs in patients with decubitus ulcers, blood cultures should be obtained and antimicrobial therapy initiated with agents that provide coverage against *S. aureus,* aerobic gram-negative rods, and *B. fragilis.*

Expected Results

Treatment of extensive decubitus ulcers is difficult, and recurrence is common. Emphasis should properly be placed on preventive measures.

When to Refer

Advanced decubitus ulcers generally require the assistance of a surgeon.

 KEY POINTS

DECUBITUS ULCERS
- Decubitus ulcers result from ischemic necrosis of tissue, typically over bony prominences.
- The extent of necrosis of deep subcutaneous tissue is often much greater than would be predicted from the appearance of the skin.
- Complications include cellulitis, osteomyelitis, thrombophlebitis, and sepsis. Sepsis is often due to *B. fragilis* in addition to aerobic pathogens, such as *S. aureus* and gram-negative bacilli.
- Decubitus ulcers are an important reservoir for drug-resistant organisms such as methicillin-resistant *S. aureus* and vancomycin-resistant enterococci.

SUGGESTED READING

Bergstrom NI. Strategies for preventing pressure ulcers. Clin Geriatr Med 1997; 13: 437-454.

Bryan CS, Dew CE, Reynolds KL. Bacteremia associated with decubitus ulcers. Arch Intern Med 1983; 143: 2093-2095.

Cervo FA, Cruz AC, Posillico JA. Pressure ulcers: analysis of guidelines for treatment and management. Geriatrics 2000; 55: 55-60.

Orlando PL. Pressure ulcer management in the geriatric patient. Ann Pharmacother 1998; 32: 1221-1227.

Smith DM. Pressure ulcers in the nursing home. Ann Intern Med 1995; 123: 433-442.

Smith PW, Black JM, Black SB. Infected pressure ulcers in the longterm-care facility. Infect Control Hosp Epidemiol 1999; 20: 358-361.

Pyomyositis

Pyomyositis, an acute pus-forming infection of skeletal muscle, was in the past usually called "tropical pyomyositis" to denote its geographic association. Recent reports indicate that pyomyositis is becoming more common in the United States and other developed countries. These reports also emphasize an association with HIV disease and with injection drug use, but some patients have no obvious predisposing condition. *S. aureus* causes about 95% of cases in tropical areas and about two thirds of cases in the United States. Streptococci (most often group A streptococci but also groups B, C, and G, *S. pneumoniae,* and *S. anginosus*) are as a group the second most common cause in the United States. Uncommon causes include the Enterobacteriaceae (*E. coli, Klebsiella* species, *Serratia marcescens, Salmonella* species, and others), *A. hydrophila, H. influenzae, Neisseria gonorrhoeae,* anaerobic bacteria (such as *Fusobacterium nucleatum* and *Clostridium septicum*), fungi (such as *Candida* and *Aspergillus* species), mycobacteria (not only *M. tuberculosis* but also, in HIV disease, *M. avium*), and other microorganisms. A history of recent blunt trauma or unusual exertion is obtained in up to one half of patients with pyomyositis, suggesting that local muscle injury created a "place of least resistance" (*locus minoris resistentiae*) that was subsequently infected during what would otherwise have been a transient, self-limited bloodstream infection. Whereas most

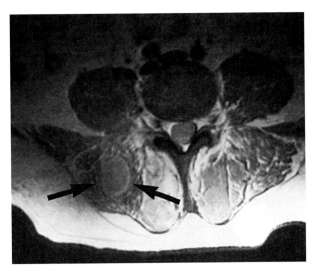

FIG. 15-5 Computed tomographic scan demonstrating a deep abscess of the lower back caused by *Staphylococcus aureus* in a 57-year-old man with persistent pain and low-grade fever.

patients with tropical pyomyositis have no underlying disease, about 60% of patients with pyomyositis in temperate climates have a defect in host defenses.

Pyomyositis usually affects the large muscles of the lower extremities or trunk. The illness typically unfolds over several weeks. The usual presenting symptoms are pain and tenderness localized to the body of a muscle, but an occasional patient has an acute illness with marked systemic toxicity. Unusual presentations include toxic shock syndrome and infection of the abdominal wall resembling the presentation of acute abdomen. Early diagnosis requires a high index of suspicion, especially since localized pain and swelling over a skeletal muscle after trauma are relatively common in primary care. When pyomyositis is suspected, imaging studies should be carried out. MRI may provide the most detail, typically showing a hyperintense rim on unenhanced T1-weighted images and peripheral enhancement after injection of gadolinium. Computed tomography (CT) and ultrasound examinations are also useful (Figure 15-5). Untreated, pyomyositis often progresses to severe sepsis with shock and death. Patients with pyomyositis should be hospitalized and treated with high-dose intravenous antibiotics combined with surgical drainage of any localized abscess.

SUGGESTED READING

Al-Tawfiq JA, Sarosi GA, Cushing HE. Pyomyositis in the acquired immunodeficiency syndrome. South Med J 2000; 93: 330-334.

Cone LA, Lamb RB, Graff-Radford A, et al. Pyomyositis of the anterior tibial compartment. Clin Infect Dis 1997; 25: 146-148.

Harbarth SJ, Lew DP. Pyomyositis as a nontropical disease. Curr Clin Top Infect Dis 1997; 17: 37-50.

Patel SR, Olenginski TP, Perruquet JL, et al. Pyomyositis: clinical features and predisposing conditions. J Rheumatol 1997; 24: 1734-1738.

Spiegel DA, Meyer JS, Dormans JP, et al. Pyomyositis in children and adolescents: report of 12 cases and review of the literature. J Pediatr Orthop 1999; 19: 143-150.

Wheeler DS, Vazquez WD, Vaux KK, et al. Streptococcal pyomyositis: case report and review. Pediatr Emerg Care 1998; 14: 411-412.

Infectious Arthritis and Bursitis: Overview

An infectious etiology must be considered in patients with pain and swelling in or around the joints, a common problem in office practice. Arthralgia (pain in the joints) must be distinguished from arthritis (pain accompanied by other signs of inflammation such as swelling, warmth, and erythema), since the latter process is often caused by pyogenic bacteria and can lead to a loss of joint function. It is often convenient to consider arthritis as monoarthritis (one joint) or polyarthritis (Tables 15-3 and 15-4). Joint involvement must be distinguished from involvement of a tendon sheath (tendonitis or tenosynovitis) or bursal sac (bursitis). Newer imaging studies are often helpful in making these and other distinctions. Aspiration of the affected joint or bursa is crucial to establishing the diagnosis of acute infectious arthritis or bursitis.

SUGGESTED READING

El-Gabalawy HS, Duray P, Goldbach-Mansky R. Evaluating patients with arthritis of recent onset: studies in pathogenesis and prognosis. JAMA 2000; 284: 2368-2373.

Mader JT, Mohan D, Calhoun J. A practical guide to the diagnosis and management of bone and joint infections. Drugs 1997; 54: 253-264.

Perry CR. Bone and Joint Infections. London: Martin Dunitz; 1996.

Acute Septic Arthritis (Acute Infectious Arthritis)

Here the term "septic arthritis" is used for acute infectious arthritis of bacterial etiology. This condition is uncommon in the general population (annual incidence 2 to 5 per 100,000 persons) but is more common in patients with rheumatoid arthritis (28 to 38 per 100,000) and in patients with a joint prosthesis (40 to 68 per 100,000). The disease usually affects a single joint, most commonly the knee. *S. aureus* is the most common pathogen, but special note should be taken of *N. gonorrhoeae* in sexually active young adults and of a wide range of bacteria under special circumstances (Table 15-3).

Presentation and Progression
Cause

Septic arthritis usually results from hematogenous seeding of the synovium, a highly vascular tissue that lacks a basement membrane. Especially vulnerable patients include young infants because of the rich vascularity surrounding their epiphyseal growth plates and patients with chronic arthritis, joint implants, recent trauma, or chronic debilitating diseases, including the frail elderly. Septic arthritis can also follow penetrating trauma. Septic arthritis of the hands and wrists is commonly caused by trauma, including animal and human bites.

In newborn infants the usual etiologies are group B streptococci, aerobic gram-negative rods, and *S. aureus*. *H. influenzae* type b was formerly the usual cause of septic arthritis in toddlers, but wide use of the conjugated vaccine has virtually eliminated this disease. *Kingella kingae*, a fastidious gram-negative rod, is emerging as an important joint pathogen in children. After age 2, *S. aureus* becomes the most common cause of septic arthritis in persons other than sexually active young adults, in whom gonococcal arthritis is common. Streptococci (not only group A but also groups B, C, and G) are relatively common causes. *Pasteurella multocida* causes par-

TABLE 15-3
Common and Uncommon Causes of Monoarticular Arthritis

Infectious or noninfectious	Frequency	Disease or pathogen	Comments, characteristics, and associations
Infectious (synovial fluid typically shows 50,000 to 100,000 white blood cells/mm³, of which >90% are polymorphonuclear cells; lower cell counts may represent tuberculous, fungal, or spirochetal arthritis)	Common	*Staphylococcus aureus*	Most frequent cause of monoarthritis, overall, in persons >2 years of age
		Neisseria gonorrhoeae	Most common cause of monoarthritis in sexually active adults <30 years of age
		Streptococci	Non–group A streptococci (groups B, C, and G) are being recognized with increasing frequency; cause about 13% to 27% of all cases
		Streptococcus pneumoniae	Infrequently encountered as a cause of suppurative arthritis; associated with sickle cell disease
		Enteric gram-negative bacilli	Usually associated with underlying disease, including urinary tract infection, decubitus ulcers, chronic arthritis, or advanced age; cause about 9% to 20% of all cases
	Uncommon	*Haemophilus influenzae*	Before the vaccine, an important cause of acute arthritis in young children
Noninfectious (synovial fluid typically shows between 3000 and 50,000 white blood cells/mm³ in gout, pseudogout, and rheumatoid arthritis)		*Pseudomonas aeruginosa*	Strongly associated with injecting drug use; often occurs in atypical locations (see text)
		Pasteurella multocida	Animal bite (typically, cat bite)
		Capnocytophaga canimorsus	Animal bite (typically, dog bite)
		Eikenella corrodens, "mouth flora" anaerobes	Human bite (including clenched-fist injury)
		Brucella species	Unpasteurized dairy products
		Mycobacterium tuberculosis	See Chapter 22; reactive tuberculin skin test; evidence of pulmonary tuberculosis in about 50% of cases

ticularly aggressive disease after a cat bite. Aerobic gram-negative rods cause up to one fifth of cases, usually in the setting of chronic underlying disease or injection drug use. *S. pneumoniae* occasionally causes septic arthritis, especially in children with sickle cell disease. A wide variety of bacteria cause occasional cases (Table 15-4). Septic arthritis caused by *P. aeruginosa* and occurring in unusual places (e.g., sternoclavicular joints, sacroiliac joints, or pubic symphysis) is well documented among injecting drug users.

Presentation

Presenting symptoms of acute septic arthritis are pain, swelling, and limitation of motion of the affected joint. Most patients are febrile. A single large joint is involved in about 90% of children and about 80% to 90% of adults. The knee is the most commonly involved joint, followed by the hip and shoulder. Patients with rheumatoid arthritis are more likely to have multiple joint involvement. Patients with gonococcal arthritis also have involvement of multiple large and small joints, but closer inspection often finds little or no joint effusion despite prominent inflammation of the adjacent tendons

(tenosynovitis). Associated vesiculopustules strongly suggest the gonococcal arthritis-dermatitis syndrome (see Chapter 7 and Figure 15-6). Rat-bite fever can also involve multiple joints distinct from the original bite. An associated palmar rash can be seen with rat-bite fever and gonococcal arthritis. *M. pneumoniae* can be associated with a painful polyarthritis.

Diagnosis

Acute septic arthritis must be distinguished from primary rheumatic conditions such as gout, chondrocalcinosis (pseudogout), and rheumatoid arthritis. All of these conditions can cause acute inflammation of a joint with a high synovial fluid leukocyte count consisting primarily of polymorphonuclear neutrophils.

Whenever possible, joint fluid should be collected for Gram stain and culture, as well as for synovial fluid leukocyte count. Since septic arthritis after hematogenous seeding usually involves large joints such as the knee, arthrocentesis is often easily accomplished. When gonococcal arthritis is suspected, inoculation of gonococcal media at the bedside is preferable because of the fastidious nature of the microorganism. Blood

TABLE 15-3—cont'd
Common and Uncommon Causes of Monoarticular Arthritis

Infectious or noninfectious	Frequency	Disease or pathogen	Comments, characteristics, and associations
		Nontuberculous mycobacteria	Trauma in an aquatic environment suggests *Mycobacterium marinum*
		Fungi	Especially *Sporothrix schenckii, Blastomyces dermatitidis,* and *Coccidiodes immitis;* occasionally *Cryptococcus neoformans*
		Spirochetes	*Borrelia burgdorferi* (Lyme disease; see Chapter 7); syphilis
	Common	Gout	Negatively birefringent urate crystals in joint fluid; response to antiinflammatory drugs
		Pseudogout	Positively birefringent calcium pyrophosphate crystals in joint fluid; chondrocalcinosis on x-ray examination
		Rheumatoid arthritis	More typically polyarticular; rheumatoid factor present in serum of 80% of patients; bacterial superinfection occurs especially in patients who have had steroid injections
		Trauma	History of trauma obtained, but be aware that trauma also predisposes to bacterial infection as a place of least resistance (*locus minoris resistentiae*)
		Osteoarthritis	Age of patient; history; characteristic radiographic changes
	Uncommon	Palindromic rheumatism	Suggested by a history of recurrent arthritis in the same joint; a poorly understood condition that sometimes evolves into rheumatoid arthritis
		Pigmented villonodular synovitis	Suggested by a persistently bloody joint effusion

cultures should be obtained for febrile patients. Cultures of the pharynx, rectum, and cervix or urethra are recommended when the patient is a sexually active young adult. Synovial fluid cultures are positive in about 90% of patients with non-gonococcal septic arthritis and in about 50% of patients with gonococcal arthritis. Attempts are being made to use the polymerase chain reaction (PCR) for early, specific diagnosis.

Natural History
Expected Outcome

Untreated, septic arthritis often leads to permanent damage to joints with loss of function.

Treatment
Methods

Attempts should be made to secure a diagnosis with Gram stain and culture before empiric parenteral antimicrobial therapy is initiated. If Gram stain is not available or the results are equivocal, appropriate empiric therapy for both children and adults consists of a penicillinase-resistant penicillin (e.g., nafcillin or oxacillin) combined with a third-generation cephalosporin (e.g., ceftriaxone or cefotaxime). If Gram stain reveals the unequivocal presence of gram-positive cocci, nafcillin or oxacillin

can be given as monotherapy. Vancomycin is the preferred alternative if methicillin-resistant *S. aureus* is suspected. If Gram stain reveals intracellular gram-negative diplococci or if the clinical scenario clearly points to gonococcal arthritis (e.g., characteristic skin lesions), ceftriaxone (1 g IV daily) or cefotaxime (1 g IV q8h) is appropriate initial therapy. In cases of septic arthritis caused by *S. aureus,* some infectious disease specialists would add rifampin (e.g., 300 mg PO t.i.d.) to take advantage of its activity against intracellular bacteria.

An orthopedic surgeon should be consulted for drainage of the joint. The literature supports either serial aspirations of the joint or arthrotomy. Most orthopedic surgeons prefer arthrotomy, which allows decompression of the joint and is especially useful when the joint space is filled with thick, loculated pus.

Expected Response

Complete recovery can usually be expected with prompt, aggressive therapy. However, staphylococcal arthritis is especially likely to leave some residual disability.

When to Refer

Patients with acute septic arthritis require parenteral antimicrobial therapy and should usually be admitted to the hospital.

TABLE 15-4
Common and Uncommon Causes of Polyarthritis

Infectious or noninfectious	Frequency	Disease or pathogen	Comments, characteristics, and associations
Infectious causes	Common	*Neisseria gonorrhoeae*	Disease is often polyarticular at onset and then "settles" in one or two joints; characteristic skin lesions (see Chapter 7).
		Infective endocarditis	Polyarthralgias and polyarthritis may be an immune complex phenomenon in some patients (see Chapter 6).
		Hepatitis prodrome	Migratory polyarthralgia, often with urticaria, can be part of the prodrome of hepatitis B (see Chapter 13).
		Reactive arthritis (in response to various infections)	An asymmetric oligoarthritis typically affecting the lower extremities; possibly the most common form of polyarthritis in young men; considered one of the spondyloarthropathies (see text).
	Uncommon	*Neisseria meningitidis*	Sepsis syndrome usually dominates over arthritis manifestations; arthritis can be a key feature of chronic meningococcemia (rare) (see Chapter 6).
		Streptobacillus moniliformis (rat-bite fever)	History of rat bite or ingestion of contaminated food. Polyarthritis may be accompanied by a macular or petechial rash, especially around involved joints.
		Spirillum minus (rat-bite fever)	Rat bite; joint involvement is usually less prominent than in rat-bite fever caused by *S. moniliformis.*
		Rubella	Rubella is rendered uncommon by the availability of rubella vaccine.
		Mumps	Mumps is rendered uncommon by the availability of mumps vaccine.
		Parvovirus B19	Parvovirus B19 is an important cause of arthritis and rash (see Chapter 7).
		Human immunodeficiency virus disease	Spectrum ranges from mild polyarthralgia to a severe, deforming pauciarticular arthritis.
		Secondary syphilis	Polyarthralgia or polyarthritis occasionally accompanies fever, rash, and other manifestations (see Chapter 7).
		Borrelia burgdorferi (Lyme disease)	Lyme disease is typically an asymmetric oligoarthritis with predilection for the knees (see Chapter 7). Occasionally resembles rheumatoid arthritis.
		Coccidioides immitis	Arthritis with erythema nodosum may complicate acute infection; chronic polyarthritis may complicate disseminated infection.
		Lymphogranuloma venereum	A history consistent with recent lymphogranuloma venereum including inguinal lymphadenopathy is usually present; serologic tests can be positive.
		Reiter's syndrome	The complete syndrome consists of arthritis, urethritis, and uveitis (see text); a form of reactive arthritis.
		Tropheryma whippelii	Whipple's disease; polyarthritis can precede other manifestations (diarrhea, abdominal pain, hyperpigmentation, lymphadenopathy) by many years.

TABLE 15-4—cont'd
Common and Uncommon Causes of Polyarthritis

Infectious or noninfectious	Frequency	Disease or pathogen	Comments, characteristics, and associations
		Acute rheumatic fever	The Jones criteria for diagnosis include arthritis, carditis, chorea, erythema marginatum, and subcutaneous nodules in a patient with antecedent group A streptococcal infection (see Chapter 7).
	Rare	Typhoid fever	High fever, abdominal pain, rose spots, and positive blood cultures suggest the diagnosis (see Chapter 12).
		Brucellosis	An important cause of arthritis in African, Middle Eastern, and Eastern European countries, often affecting the knee or the spine. Serologic tests are usually helpful.
		Cat scratch disease	Arthritis is an occasional manifestation of this important cause of lymphadenopathy (see Chapter 8).
		Viruses	Epstein-Barr virus; influenza; arboviruses; hepatitis A virus.
		Mycoplasma pneumoniae	Part of the diverse spectrum of extrapulmonary manifestations (see Chapter 11).
		Parasitic infections	Notably filariasis.
Noninfectious causes	Common	Systemic lupus erythematosus	Features include fever, anemia, leukopenia, polyarthritis, and polyserositis; fluorescent antinuclear antibodies are present in 95% of patients.
		Rheumatoid arthritis	Polyarthritis is classically symmetric and accompanied by morning stiffness. Periarticular swelling is also present. Bacterial arthritis (septic arthritis) can be superimposed.
		Juvenile rheumatoid arthritis	Usually begins before puberty but can occur in adults (Still's disease). An important cause of fever of unknown origin (see Chapter 1); clues include an evanescent salmon-colored rash, iritis, and elevated sedimentation rate.
		Gout	Classically a monoarticular arthritis involving the great toe, but can develop as polyarthritis; demonstration of sodium urate crystals in joint fluids is diagnostic.
		Pseudogout	Often involves the knees; chondrocalcinosis may be present on x-ray film; calcium pyrophosphate crystals in joint fluid.
	Uncommon	Sarcoidosis	Polyarthritis can be part of the clinical syndrome; pulmonary infiltrates and hilar or mediastinal lymphadenopathy are usually present. Other features include hypercalcemia, skin lesions, iritis, and heart block.
		Psoriasis	Characteristic rash; pitting of fingernails.
		Neoplasms	Especially leukemias and lymphomas.
		Serum sickness	Clinical features include polyarthritis, fever, urticaria, and nephritis. History of precipitating antigen is often obtained. Eosinophilia may be present, and the serum complement level is usually low.
		Miscellaneous	Inflammatory bowel disease, hemoglobinopathies, amyloidosis, ochronosis, Behçet's syndrome, familial Mediterranean fever, jejunoileal bypass, and palindromic rheumatism.

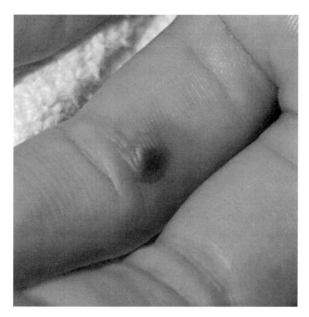

FIG. 15-6 Vesiculopustular lesion on the long finger of a patient with the gonococcal arthritis-dermatitis syndrome.

 KEY POINTS

ACUTE SEPTIC ARTHRITIS (ACUTE INFECTIOUS ARTHRITIS)

⊃ Infection should be considered in any patient with fever and acute arthritis, even (or especially) when underlying rheumatic disease is present.

⊃ *H. influenzae* was formerly the usual cause in childhood but has been rendered less common by the *H. influenzae* vaccine.

⊃ *S. aureus* is the most common cause after early childhood.

⊃ *N. gonorrhoeae* is the most common cause in sexually active young adults and can cause either arthritis or tenosynovitis.

⊃ The knee is the most commonly involved joint, followed by the hip and the shoulder.

⊃ Patients with rheumatoid arthritis are especially prone to multiple joint involvement.

SUGGESTED READING

Cucurull E, Espinoza LR. Gonococcal arthritis. Rheum Dis Clin North Am 1998; 24: 305-322.

Donatto KC. Orthopedic management of septic arthritis. Rheum Dis Clin North Am 1998; 24: 275-286.

Goldenberg DL. Septic arthritis. Lancet 1998; 351: 197-202.

Ike RW. Bacterial arthritis. Curr Opin Rheumatol 1998; 10: 330-334.

Louie JS, Liebling MR. The polymerase chain reaction in infectious and post-infectious arthritis: a review. Rheum Dis Clin North Am 1998; 24: 227-236.

Pioro MH, Mandell BF. Septic arthritis. Rheum Dis Clin North Am 1997; 23: 239-258.

Sack K. Monarthritis: different diagnosis. Am J Med 1997; 102 (Suppl 1A): 30S-34S.

Schattner A, Vosti KL. Bacterial arthritis due to beta-hemolytic streptococci of serogroups A, B, C, F, and G: analysis of 23 cases and a review of the literature. Medicine (Baltimore) 1998; 77: 122-139.

Shetty AK, Gedalia A. Septic arthritis in children. Rheum Dis Clin North Am 1998; 24: 287-304.

Smith JW, Piercy EA. Infectious arthritis. Clin Infect Dis 1995; 20: 225-231.

Septic Bursitis

Septic bursitis most commonly involves the olecranon or prepatellar bursae. *S. aureus* causes most cases of acute septic bursitis; chronic cases can be due to a wide range of microorganisms. Minor trauma is likely to be a precipitating factor, especially when bursae of the lower extremities are involved. Persons vulnerable to recurrent trauma, such as painters and brick masons, are at risk, and rheumatoid arthritis is sometimes present. Chronic infectious bursitis, which typically follows minor trauma, is associated with a wide variety of bacteria and fungi of low virulence. Examples include fungi that are soil contaminants (see discussion of phaeohyphomycosis in Chapter 21) and nontuberculous mycobacteria. Septic bursitis has its onset with some combination of pain, tenderness, erythema, warmth, and swelling over the affected bursa in a person vulnerable to recurrent trauma, such as a painter or brick mason. The presentation may be acute when the bursitis is caused by *S. aureus* or may be subacute or chronic when it is caused by an organism of lesser virulence. Absence of pain on movement of the joint helps distinguish septic bursitis from arthritis. Although septic bursitis is an uncommon lesion, the diagnosis is easily made on clinical grounds when suspected and is confirmed by aspiration or open exploration of the bursa. Appropriate therapy for acute septic bursitis consists of a penicillinase-resistant penicillin (nafcillin or oxacillin) combined with daily aspiration of the bursa. Patients with acute septic bursitis should usually be admitted to the hospital. Patients who respond to initial therapy can be treated with an oral agent such as dicloxacillin. Treatment of chronic septic bursitis should be based on identification of the infecting microorganism if possible. Surgical excision of the bursa is reserved for refractory or recurrent cases.

SUGGESTED READING

Stell IM. Management of acute bursitis: outcome study of a structured approach. J R Soc Med 1999; 92: 516-521.

Zimmermann B III, Mikolich DJ, Ho G Jr. Septic bursitis. Semin Arthritis Rheum 1995; 24: 391-410.

Viral Arthritis

Arthritis, usually symmetric and self-limited, is a prominent feature of several viral infections. Most cases result from viral invasion of the synovium or deposition of circulating immune complexes. The usual causes of viral arthritis in the United States are rubella, mumps, parvovirus B19, and hepatitis B. Arthritis caused by the rubella virus occurs in about one half of women with naturally occurring disease and in about 40% of susceptible women after vaccination. Arthritis caused by the mumps virus occurs in about 1 in 200 patients with the disease, most often men. Parvovirus B19 is now recognized as a cause of arthritis with skin lesions. Arthritis caused by hepatitis B occurs in about 20% of patients with the acute disease. Less common causes of viral arthritis in the United States are the lymphocytic choriomeningitis virus, hepatitis C virus, varicella virus, Epstein-Barr virus, cytomegalovirus, rubeola virus, influenza viruses, adenoviruses, and echoviruses. Arthritis is a relatively common manifestation of certain viral infections that are prevalent elsewhere in the world, such as the O'nyong-nyong (East Africa), Chikungunya (East Africa and India), Mayaro (South Africa and the Caribbean), and Ross River and Barmah Forest (Australia) viruses. Presentations vary according to the etiology:

- Rubella usually causes polyarthritis in adult women that most often affects the small joints of the hands. The knees, wrists, and ankles can also be involved. The arthritis usually begins simultaneously with the rash or within the next 72 hours. Effusions can be sufficiently large to permit aspiration for synovial fluid analysis, which usually discloses a predominance of mononuclear cells.
- Mumps typically causes a polyarthritis that involves multiple small and large joints. The arthritis usually begins shortly before the onset of parotitis or within the next 2 weeks. Effusions are uncommon.
- Parvovirus B19 causes arthritis that is usually symmetric and involves the joints of the upper or lower extremities. Carpal tunnel syndrome sometimes occurs. A rash that can be maculopapular, reticular, or hemorrhagic usually accompanies the arthritis. A history of exposure to a child with fifth disease (erythema infectiosum, which is manifested by a "slapped cheeks" facial rash) is often obtained.
- Acute hepatitis B causes, in about 20% of patients, a symmetric arthritis affecting (in order of frequency) the hands, knees, and ankles. The arthritis usually begins within 2 days before onset.

Most cases of viral arthritis are self-limited, but some patients have prolonged joint pain. The issue of whether viral arthritis precipitates chronic rheumatic diseases remains open.

SUGGESTED READING

Phillips PE. Viral arthritis. Curr Opin Rheumatol 1997; 9: 337-344.
Ytterberg SR. Viral arthritis. Curr Opin Rheumatol 1999; 11: 275-280.

Chronic Monoarticular Arthritis Caused by Infection

Chronic arthritis involving a single joint, when caused by infection, is usually caused by mycobacteria (including *M. tuberculosis*), fungi, nocardia, brucellosis, or Whipple's disease. Most cases of chronic monoarticular arthritis arise hematogenously. *Sporothrix schenckii* (sporotrichosis) is perhaps the most common fungal etiologic agent in nonimmunocompromised patients and most often involves the knee. Injection of a joint with corticosteroids can rarely introduce an opportunistic fungus such as *C. albicans*. *Brucella* species are notorious causes of chronic arthritis in parts of the world where brucellosis remains prevalent. Whipple's disease, recently attributed to a bacterium named *Tropheryma whippelii*, can also cause chronic monoarticular arthritis.

Onset of symptoms is insidious and slowly progressive, reflecting the granulomatous nature of these diseases. Patients sometimes note that abnormalities of the joint have been present for months or even years. Fever is seldom present, and the joints are seldom red or painful. Synovial thickening gives the joint a "boggy" feel, and the range of motion is reduced. In some patients the major symptoms are extraarticular and the presentation suggests bursitis or carpal tunnel syndrome. Imaging studies usually suggest the nature of the disease by revealing erosion of cartilage and bone. A tuberculin skin test and a serologic test for *Brucella* antibodies should be performed. However, synovial biopsy with simultaneous aspiration of fluid is the diagnostic procedure of choice. Open biopsy may be

required. The microbiology laboratory should be alerted to look for mycobacteria, including *M. marinum* (for which the optimum incubation temperature is 87.8° F [30° C] rather than the usual 95° F [35° C]), fungi including *S. schenckii*, and *Brucella* species (which may require special media). The histology laboratory should be asked to use special stains for mycobacterial and fungal pathogens.

SUGGESTED READING

Durand DV, Lecomte C, Cathébras P, et al. Whipple disease: clinical review of 52 cases. Medicine (Baltimore) 1997; 76: 170-184.
Harrington JT. Mycobacterial and fungal arthritis. Curr Opin Rheumatol 1998; 10: 335-338.
O'Duffy JD, Griffing WL, Li CY, et al. Whipple's arthritis: direct detection of *Tropheryma whippelii* in synovial fluid and tissue. Arthritis Rheum 1999; 42: 812-817.
Zacharias J, Crosby LA. Sporotrichal arthritis of the knee. Am J Knee Surg 1997; 10: 171-174.

Reactive Arthritis, Including Reiter's Syndrome

The term "reactive arthritis" denotes a systemic illness precipitated by infection and characterized by synovitis, but in which no viable microorganism can be isolated by culture. The term "Reiter's syndrome" should be reserved for the subset of patients who manifest the triad of arthritis, urethritis, and uveitis, as described in 1916 by Hans Reiter. Reactive arthritis and Reiter's syndrome belong to the spondyloarthropathy family of disorders, which also includes ankylosing spondylitis (both adult- and juvenile-onset varieties), spondyloarthropathy associated with systemic diseases (psoriasis, Crohn's disease, and ulcerative colitis), and undifferentiated spondyloarthropathy.

Urethritis caused by *Chlamydia trachomatis* is strongly associated with reactive arthritis, including Reiter's syndrome. For this reason reactive arthritis may be the most common form of arthritis in young men. Reactive arthritis is not uncommonly associated with infection by enteric pathogens (see Chapter 12), including *Salmonella*, *Shigella*, *Campylobacter*, *Yersinia*, and *Clostridium difficile*. Numerous investigators have found microbial DNA, RNA, and various antigens within joints of patients with reactive arthritis. Atypical elementary bodies consistent with *C. trachomatis* have been identified by electron microscopy. However, chlamydial elements have been also been found in patients with other forms of arthritis. Thus the precise etiology of reactive arthritis remains unknown.

A history of urethritis or gastroenteritis within the previous 4 weeks is often obtained, and, when combined with arthritis, suggests the diagnosis. Reactive arthritis is typically an asymmetric oligoarthritis affecting predominantly the joints of the lower extremities, especially the knees, ankles, and feet. Often only one to three joints are involved. The knees and ankles may be considerably swollen. Asymmetric oligoarthritis has a 44% sensitivity and 95% specificity for spondyloarthropathy. Patients with Reiter's syndrome may manifest several distinctive symptoms:

- Inflammation of the eye as conjunctivitis or, more typically, iritis. Iritis usually begins acutely in one eye with redness, pain, and photophobia.
- Painless, shallow ulcers on the glans penis or urethral meatus. These ulcers are known as circinate balanitis.
- Skin lesions on the palms and soles that begin as vesicles on an erythematous base and evolve into macules, papules,

and nodules. These lesions, which can resemble pustular psoriasis, are known as keratoderma blennorrhagicum.

Other manifestations of spondyloarthropathy include enthesopathy (inflammation around the insertions of ligaments, tendons, joint capsules, or fascia to bone) and pain in the cervical spine or lower back caused by inflammation (spondylitis). Patients with reactive arthritis and spondyloarthropathy usually benefit from consultation with a rheumatologist. Patients with iritis should be referred to an ophthalmologist for slit lamp examination.

SUGGESTED READING

Aviles RJ, Ramakrishna G, Mohr DN, et al. Poststreptococcal reactive arthritis in adults: a case series. Mayo Clin Proc 2000; 75: 144-147.

Barth WF, Segal K. Reactive arthritis (Reiter's syndrome). Am Fam Physician 1999; 60: 499-503, 507.

Ebringer A, Wilson C, Tiwana H. Is rheumatoid arthritis a form of reactive arthritis? J Rheumatol 2000; 27: 559-563.

Leirisalo-Repo M. Prognosis, course of disease, and treatment of the spondyloarthropathies. Rheum Dis Clin North Am 1998; 24: 737-751.

Sieper J, Braun J. Reactive arthritis. Curr Opin Rheumatol 1999; 11: 238-243.

Yli-Kerttula T, Luukkainen R, Yli-Kerttula U, et al. Effect of a three month course of ciprofloxacin on the outcome of reactive arthritis. Ann Rheum Dis 2000; 59: 565-570.

Erythema Nodosum

Erythema nodosum, classically defined by the presence of inflammatory nodules on the extensor surfaces of the lower extremities, is often accompanied by arthralgia and sometimes by swelling that suggests arthritis. Erythema nodosum is believed to be an immune response to a variety of antigens, including various infectious agents. These include group A streptococci, fungi associated with regional mycoses (histoplasmosis, blastomycosis, coccidioidomycosis), *M. tuberculosis,* and enteric pathogens, including *Yersinia* species. Some cases are associated with drugs, especially oral contraceptives. Sarcoidosis is a relatively common cause, and erythema nodosum occasionally complicates other diseases of unknown origin such as ulcerative colitis. In a large recent European study, the cause was undetermined in 55% of patients; 28% of patients had streptococcal infections and 11% had sarcoidosis. Occasional causes include mycoplasmal infection, cat scratch disease, psittacosis, brucellosis, and viral hepatitis.

Prodromal symptoms include fever and arthralgia. Periarticular ankle pain is common and often accompanied by slight swelling. The characteristic eruption consists of bilateral nodules over the anterior tibial surfaces (Figure 15-7). Löfgren's syndrome refers to the presence of erythema nodosum or periarticular ankle inflammation in patients with unilateral or bilateral hilar lymphadenopathy or right paratracheal lymphadenopathy caused by sarcoidosis. The diagnosis is usually made on clinical grounds, based on the typical nodules over the shins. Skin biopsy, if performed, reveals a trabecular panniculitis.

Erythema nodosum usually resolves within 3 to 5 weeks. Occasional patients, especially middle-aged women, may have a more protracted course (erythema nodosum migrans). Erythema nodosum associated with tuberculosis was once thought to por-

tend a poor prognosis; whether this observation remains valid in the chemotherapy era is unclear. Erythema nodosum occurring early in the course of sarcoidosis (Löfgren's syndrome) generally portends a favorable prognosis, especially if the serum angiotensin-converting enzyme level is normal at the time of diagnosis. Erythema nodosum is also thought to be a favorable sign in coccidioidomycosis, especially during pregnancy.

Treatment is usually symptomatic with nonsteroidal antiinflamatory drugs unless a specific microbial cause is identified. Corticosteroids are sometimes used for treatment of erythema nodosum in sarcoidosis. Referral may be indicated in severe cases or when the diagnosis is unclear.

SUGGESTED READING

Arsura EL, Kilgore WB, Ratnayake SN. Erythema nodosum in pregnant patients with coccidioidomycosis. Clin Infect Dis 1998; 27: 1201-1203.

Cribier B, Caille A, Heid E, et al. Erythema nodosum and associated diseases: a study of 129 cases. Int J Dermatol 1998; 37: 667-672.

García-Porrúa C, González-Gay MA, Vázquez-Caruncho M, et al. Erythema nodosum: etiologic and predictive factors in a defined population. Arthritis Rheum 2000; 43: 584-592.

Mañá J, Gómez-Vaquero C, Montero A, et al. Löfgren's syndrome revisited: a study of 186 patients. Am J Med 1999; 107: 240-245.

Overview of Osteomyelitis

Infections of bone require accurate diagnosis and precise antimicrobial therapy to achieve the optimum clinical result, which is defined as "arrest" rather than "cure," since osteomyelitis can recur decades after the acute infection. Thus the role of the primary care physician is to ensure accurate diagnosis and compliance with therapy and to follow up closely. Most patients require hospitalization and surgical consultation at some stage of their disease.

Two methods of classifying osteomyelitis are prevalent. The first, commonly known as the Waldvogel classification, groups osteomyelitis into three categories: (1) hematogenous osteomyelitis; (2) osteomyelitis secondary to a contiguous focus of infection; and (3) osteomyelitis secondary to vascular insufficiency, which is usually seen in the small bones

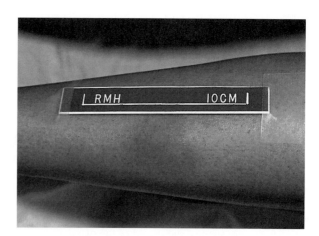

FIG. 15-7 Erythema nodosum. Note the relatively poor demarcation of erythema between the tender, slightly elevated nodule and the adjacent normal skin.

of the feet of persons with severe diabetes mellitus. The second method of classification, developed by Cierny and Mader, recognizes 12 stages of osteomyelitis based on four anatomic variations (medullary, superficial, localized, or diffuse osteomyelitis) and three categories of patients (otherwise healthy, compromised because of coexisting systemic or local disease, or severely disabled to the extent that treatment would be worse than the disease). Here the older Waldvogel classification is followed because it promotes appreciation of the syndromes of osteomyelitis as the primary care practitioner evaluates the patient.

SUGGESTED READING

Carek PJ, Dickerson LM, Sack JL. Diagnosis and management of osteomyelitis. Am Fam Physician 2001; 63: 2413-2420.

Lew DP, Waldvogel FA. Osteomyelitis. N Engl J Med 1997; 336: 999-1007.

Mader JT, Shirtliff M, Calhoun JH. Staging and staging application in osteomyelitis. Clin Infect Dis 1997; 25: 1303-1309.

Acute Hematogenous Osteomyelitis

Hematogenous osteomyelitis results when microorganisms enter the bloodstream from a distant source (such as a minor skin lesion), enter bone through a nutrient artery, and establish infection. The disease occurs most often in infants and children but can occur in any age group. Hematogenous osteomyelitis in adults most often involves the spine (vertebral osteomyelitis) and is discussed separately.

Presentation and Progression
Cause

Acute hematogenous osteomyelitis is nearly always caused by a single organism. *S. aureus* is common in all age groups and is the most frequent cause in adults. Group B streptococci and *E. coli* commonly cause the disease in infants, and group A streptococci often cause the disease in older children. *H. influenzae* was a common cause of osteomyelitis in young children before the wide use of the vaccine. *Salmonella* species frequently cause hematogenous osteomyelitis in patients with sickle cell disease or other hemoglobinopathies.

The occurrence of hematogenous osteomyelitis is best explained by the fragile nature of the arterial supply to the metaphyseal regions of bones, especially those of growing children. Minor trauma such as the "lumps and bumps" of childhood disrupts the delicate capillary loops of these regions, causing small areas of necrosis that provide safe harbor for any bacteria entering through the bloodstream. In infants <1 year of age the growth plates of bone have a rich blood supply; therefore hematogenous osteomyelitis often affects the epiphyses of long bones. Thereafter, the growth plates lose their blood supply, causing osteomyelitis to be confined to the metaphysis and diaphysis.

Presentation

Symptoms vary according to age but can be subtle in all age groups. In neonates symptoms often consist of localized swelling and decreased motion in an extremity, accompanied by an effusion in the adjacent joint in about 60% of cases.

About one half of children with osteomyelitis have an acute or subacute illness over several weeks with fever and other constitutional symptoms accompanied by signs of inflammation over the affected bone. In many children and in most adults the illness evolves over a month or longer with vague constitutional symptoms and nonspecific bone pain.

Diagnosis

The diagnosis of acute hematogenous osteomyelitis is usually based on imaging studies followed by aspiration or biopsy of material from the involved bone. Blood cultures sometimes yield the causative organism, obviating the need for bone biopsy.

Radionuclide, CT, and MRI scanning are now generally preferred to plain x-ray examination for early diagnosis because osteolytic changes become evident on x-ray films only after at least 50% of bone matrix is destroyed and usually after a lag period of 2 weeks or more. Scanning with technetium-99m polyphosphate can achieve positive results as early as 48 hours after onset of infection. False-negative results occasionally occur, possibly because of impaired circulation to the bone. The popularity of MRI scanning is increasing, especially because of the ability to distinguish between bone and soft tissue infection. Ultrasound and ultrasound-guided aspiration have been used successfully in children, who are often unable to cooperate with CT and MRI scanning.

Unless blood cultures are positive, specimens should nearly always be obtained by bone biopsy or open débridement to guide therapy (see later discussion). A tuberculin skin test should be performed on patients not known to be tuberculin positive.

Natural History
Expected Outcome

Observations made in the preantibiotic era indicate that acute hematogenous osteomyelitis often resolves spontaneously. However, the disease is notoriously prone to relapse, even decades later.

Treatment
Methods

Treatment usually consists of at least 4 to 6 weeks of appropriate antibiotic therapy based on identification of the causative microorganism. Patients should usually be hospitalized initially for appropriate studies and intravenous antibiotic therapy. Children usually respond more readily to therapy than do adults, and treatment of childhood osteomyelitis can often be completed with an oral regimen after an initial 2 weeks of intravenous therapy. Compliance must, however, be ensured. Adults often require débridement and other surgical procedures.

Expected Response

Response to treatment based on identification of the causative organism is usually gratifying. However, talk of a "cure" is inappropriate because osteomyelitis can relapse many years later.

When to Refer

Patients with acute hematogenous osteomyelitis should usually be hospitalized. Outpatient parenteral therapy is being used increasingly for good-risk patients.

KEY POINTS

ACUTE HEMATOGENOUS OSTEOMYELITIS

⊃ Hematogenous osteomyelitis is most common in childhood, but can occur at any age.

⊃ In adults the disease often involves the spine (discussed below as "vertebral osteomyelitis").

⊃ *S. aureus* is the most common cause.

⊃ Presentation is often subtle, with low-grade constitutional symptoms and poorly localized pain.

⊃ Bone changes are seen earlier on radionuclide, CT, and MRI scanning than on plain x-ray films, which usually lag well behind the clinical course.

⊃ Appropriate therapy requires isolation of the infecting microorganism by blood cultures or, more often, by cultures obtained through bone biopsy.

⊃ Hospitalization is usually indicated for appropriate studies followed by initiation of intravenous antibiotic therapy.

SUGGESTED READING

Boutin RD, Brossmann J, Sartoris DJ, et al. Update on imaging of orthopedic infections. Orthop Clin North Am 1998; 29: 41-66.

Fox IM, Brady K. Acute hematogenous osteomyelitis in intravenous drug users. J Foot Ankle Surg 1997; 36: 301-305.

Ma LD, Frassica FJ, Bluemke DA, et al. CT and MRI evaluation of musculoskeletal infection. Crit Rev Diagn Imaging 1997; 38: 535-568.

Mader JT, Shirtliff ME, Bergquist S, et al. Bone and joint infections in the elderly: practical treatment guidelines. Drugs Aging 2000; 16: 67-80.

Sammak B, Abd El Bagi M, Al Shahed M, et al. Osteomyelitis: a review of currently used imaging techniques. Eur Radiol 1999; 9: 894-900.

Tice AD. Outpatient parenteral antimicrobial therapy for osteomyelitis. Infect Dis Clin North Am 1998; 12: 903-919.

Wall EJ. Childhood osteomyelitis and septic arthritis. Curr Opin Pediatr 1998; 10: 73-76.

Vertebral Osteomyelitis and Diskitis

Vertebral osteomyelitis typically involves two adjacent vertebrae and the intervertebral disk; when the disk alone is involved, the process is called diskitis. Vertebral osteomyelitis is often a subacute or chronic illness with constitutional symptoms and localized back pain. Occasionally the presentation is acute fever with back pain. Fever is absent in about one half of patients. Complications include paraspinous abscess, epidural abscess (see Chapter 6), and spinal cord compression. Neurologic symptoms such as weakness in the lower extremities or impaired bladder or bowel function indicate spinal cord compression. The disease occurs mainly in adults. In children the initial complaint is usually refusal to walk, a limp, or back pain.

Most cases are of hematogenous origin, but occasional cases result from inoculation of bacteria during spinal surgery, lumbar puncture, myelography, or other medical procedures. *S. aureus* is the most common pathogen. Aerobic gram-negative rods are a relatively common cause, especially in patients with chronic urinary tract infections. Tuberculosis of the spine (Pott's disease) should always be considered. Occasional cases are caused by fungi or unusual pathogens.

Localized tenderness over the spine is an invaluable physical finding. The erythrocyte sedimentation rate is usually

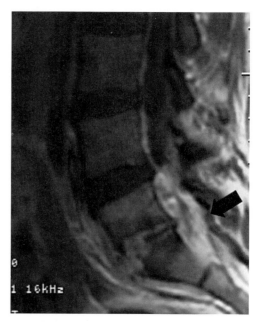

FIG. 15-8 T1-weighted, gadolinium-enhanced magnetic resonance image demonstrating vertebral osteomyelitis of L5-S1 with an associated epidural abscess. *Staphylococcus aureus* was isolated from cultures of blood and of the abscess.

elevated. The tuberculin skin test is usually but not always positive in Pott's disease. Blood cultures, although positive in a minority of cases (24% to 50% in recent series), should be obtained in all instances, since a positive blood culture for a pathogenic microorganism often obviates the need for invasive diagnostic procedures.

In well-established cases, plain x-ray films of the spine show bone destruction involving the anterior edges of two adjacent vertebral bodies with narrowing of the intervertebral disk. CT and MRI scans show evidence of bone destruction and soft tissue swelling before the changes become apparent on x-ray films (Figure 15-8). Bone biopsy is nearly always the diagnostic procedure of choice. The biopsy specimen should be obtained with CT or ultrasound guidance and should be taken promptly to the laboratory for aerobic and anaerobic culture, fungal culture, acid-fast bacillus (AFB) culture, and histologic examination. Gram stain and stains for AFB and fungi should be obtained especially when purulent material is obtained. Material obtained by closed aspiration or biopsy yields the causative microorganism in about one half of cases. If this approach is unsuccessful, open biopsy may be necessary. Establishing a definitive diagnosis is highly desirable, since directing aggressive, extended antimicrobial therapy simultaneously against bacterial, mycobacterial, and fungal pathogens is impractical.

Patients with vertebral osteomyelitis should usually be hospitalized, and consultation should be obtained with an orthopedic surgeon or neurosurgeon.

SUGGESTED READING

Babinchak TJ, Riley DK, Rotheram EB Jr. Pyogenic vertebral osteomyelitis of the posterior elements. Clin Infect Dis 1997; 25: 221-224.

Colmenero JD, Jíminez-Mejías ME, Sánchez-Lora FJ, et al. Pyogenic, tuberculous, and brucellar vertebral osteomyelitis: a descriptive and comparative study of 219 cases. Ann Rheum Dis 1997; 56: 709-715.

Fernandez M, Carrol CL, Baker CJ. Discitis and vertebral osteomyelitis in children: an 18-year review. Pediatrics 2000; 105: 1299-1304.

Frazier DD, Campbell DR, Garvey TA, et al. Fungal infections of the spine: report of eleven patients with long-term follow-up. J Bone Joint Surg 2001; 83-A: 560-565.

Shih TT, Huang KM, Hou SM. Early diagnosis of single segment vertebral osteomyelitis—MR pattern and its characteristics. Clin Imaging 1999; 23: 159-167.

Torda AJ, Gottlieb T, Bradbury R. Pyogenic vertebral osteomyelitis: analysis of 20 cases and review. Clin Infect Dis 1995; 20: 320-328.

Osteomyelitis Following Nail Puncture Wounds

Nail puncture wounds can result in various combinations of cellulitis, abscess, osteochondritis, septic arthritis, and osteomyelitis. Osteomyelitis complicates about 1% to 2% of nail puncture wounds in children. Most of these infections occur during the warm summer months. Osteomyelitis caused by *P. aeruginosa* is strongly associated with wearing tennis shoes at the time of the injury (up to 93% of cases). *S. aureus* is the other major pathogen, and in one series both *P. aeruginosa* and *S. aureus* were isolated in about one half of the cases. Rarely, other pathogens such as nontuberculous mycobacteria (e.g., *Mycobacterium fortuitum* and *M. chelonei*) have been reported. Patients with diabetes mellitus and neuropathy frequently have multiple pathogens.

Pain is usually the chief complaint. The patient may report that pain subsided after the initial injury, only to recur and progress over several days to weeks. Erythema, tenderness, and swelling are sometimes seen. An occasional patient has fever, leukocytosis, and elevation of the erythrocyte sedimentation rate. Plain x-ray films may be normal, especially early in the presentation. MRI scanning now provides more precise diagnosis and localization. Surgical débridement is strongly recommended to define the extent of the disease and obtain appropriate cultures. Parenteral ceftazidime is appropriate therapy for most patients. Ciprofloxacin (750 mg PO b.i.d.) has been used in adult patients. Optimum duration of therapy is unclear. In one series treatment with antimicrobial therapy for 7 days after surgery resulted in cure of all but 2 of 38 patients. Treatment of polymicrobial osteomyelitis in patients with diabetes mellitus is discussed later in the chapter.

SUGGESTED READING

Jacobs RF, McCarthy RE. *Pseudomonas* osteochondritis complicating puncture wounds of the foot in children: a 10-year evaluation. J Infect Dis 1989; 160: 657-661.

Lau LS, Bin G, Jaovisidua S, et al. Cost effectiveness of magnetic resonance imaging in diagnosing *Pseudomonas aeruginosa* infection after puncture wound. J Foot Ankle Surg 1997; 36: 36-43.

Laughlin RT, Reeve F, Wright DG, et al. Calcaneal osteomyelitis caused by nail puncture wounds. Foot Ankle Int 1997; 18: 575-577.

Miron D, El AL, Zuker M, et al. *Mycobacterium fortuitum* osteomyelitis of the cuboid after nail puncture wound. Pediatr Infect Dis J 2000; 19: 483-485.

Raz R, Miron D. Oral ciprofloxacin for treatment of infection following nail puncture wounds of the foot. Clin Infect Dis 1995; 21: 194-195.

Chronic Osteomyelitis

Chronic osteomyelitis, which can reflect persistence of infection from acute osteomyelitis or recurrence of prior infection, presents a difficult clinical problem that primary care clinicians will usually manage in concert with one or more consultants. The clinical presentation varies considerably. In some patients, local inflammation and draining sinus tracts make the diagnosis obvious. In others, symptoms and signs suggest acute osteomyelitis but a history of previous osteomyelitis at the same anatomic site is obtained. Chronic osteomyelitis often causes long-term disability. Life-threatening bacteremia caused by *S. aureus* or other pathogens can occur at any point in the disease. Carcinoma occasionally develops in chronically draining sinus tracts. Optimal treatment consists of surgical débridement of devitalized bone (e.g., sequestrectomy) combined with aggressive antimicrobial therapy based on isolation of the causative microorganism(s) from culture specimens that have not been contaminated by surface microorganisms. When the probability of successful surgical management is low, treatment usually consists of local wound management and suppressive antimicrobial therapy.

SUGGESTED READING

Ciampolini J, Harding KG. Pathophysiology of chronic bacterial osteomyelitis: why do antibiotics fail so often? Postgrad Med J 2000; 76: 479-483.

Mackowiak PA, Jones SR, Smith JW. Diagnostic value of sinus-tract cultures in chronic osteomyelitis. JAMA 1978; 239: 2772-2775.

Mader JT, Shirtliff ME, Bergquist SC, et al. Antimicrobial treatment of chronic osteomyelitis. Clin Orthop 1999; 360: 47-65.

Rissing JP. Antimicrobial therapy for chronic osteomyelitis in adults: role of the quinolones. Clin Infect Dis 1997; 25: 1327-1333.

Tetsworth K, Cierny G III. Osteomyelitis debridement techniques. Clin Orthop 1999; 360: 87-96.

Infections of the Hand

Infections of the hand are relatively common. About one third of these infections involve the fingertip region (paronychia, felon, and herpetic whitlow). These infections can often be managed successfully by the primary care clinician, but deeper infections usually warrant referral to an orthopedic surgeon.

Acute Paronychia

Acute paronychia, usually caused by *S. aureus,* is an infection involving the lateral fold of soft tissue surrounding the fingernail. Trauma to the nail, including nail biting, foreign bodies, manicures, or hangnail, is the usual predisposing cause. Injury to the seal between the nail plate and the nail fold allows bacteria to enter, causing cellulitis and the abscess. Mild infections are commonly treated with antistaphylococcal antibiotics, warm saline soaks, and split. Surgical drainage is required when the patient has fluctuance or an obvious abscess. Using digital nerve block anesthesia, the nail fold is carefully incised with a No. 11 or 15 scalpel blade, taking care to direct the blade away from the nail bed in order to avoid injury. In more severe cases part or all of the nail plate must be incised. The abscess is irrigated and then packed with plain gauze. Herpetic whitlow (see later discussion) should be considered as an alternative diagnosis before surgical drainage, since manipulation of a herpetic lesion can lead to serious consequences.

Herpetic Whitlow

Herpetic whitlow, caused by the herpes simplex virus (HSV-1 or HSV-2), usually involves the fingertip, including structures related to the nail bed. This lesion is an occupational hazard for health care workers and is frequently encountered among nurses, surgeons, and dentists. Patients with herpetic gingivostomatitis and genital herpes are also at risk. HSV-1 is the common cause in persons <20 years of age, and HSV-2 in persons >20 years of age. The lesions begin as fluid-filled vesicles that may rupture or progress to purpuric lesions. Pain is typically more severe and disproportionate to the appearance of the lesion. Tender lymphadenopathy, lymphangitis, and signs of systemic illness may occur, especially if the lesion is excised. Diagnosis is usually based on the patient's risk factors, the history of a vesicle as the first manifestation, the presence of considerable pain, and the clinical appearance of the lesion. Viral culture, fluorescent antibody staining, Tzanck preparation, or PCR could be used to confirm the diagnosis (see Chapter 20) but are seldom necessary. The lesion gradually resolves over 3 to 4 weeks. Acyclovir should be used in the occasional case in which surgical drainage is necessary to relieve pain because of direct involvement of the nail bed.

Chronic Paronychia

Chronic paronychia is usually associated with *C. albicans* (in about 95% of cases), but a wide range of bacterial, fungal, and mycobacterial pathogens have been recovered. A typical history is the frequent immersion of the hands in water. Persons at risk include housewives, dishwashers, swimmers, bartenders, and persons who have diabetes mellitus or are immunosuppressed. The condition most commonly affects women between the ages of 30 and 60 years. Recurrent episodes of pain, inflammation, and swelling eventually lead to chronic induration around the nail, often involving the eponychium (the thin membrane on the proximal aspect of the nail that serves as a seal between the nail wall and the nail plate). Treatment is often difficult and frustrating. Topical antifungal ointments with or without steroids are seldom successful. Definitive surgical treatment sometimes consists of marsupialization of the eponychium with excision of the nail plate.

Felon

Anatomic structures in the pulp of the fingertip include multiple vertical fibrous septa that run between the skin and the periosteum of the underlying bone. A felon is an abscess that begins in the closed space defined by two or more of these fibrous septa. *S. aureus* is the usual causative microorganism. Trauma is a frequent predisposing factor, and a history of multiple finger sticks for blood tests, splinters, abrasions, or minor cuts is often elicited. Patients usually have rapidly progressing, throbbing pain and swelling of the entire pulp. The pulp of the fingertip is exquisitely tender. The distal interphalangeal joint is not involved unless a complication such as cellulitis, septic arthritis, or infection of the flexor tendon sheath is present. Treatment consists of surgical incision and drainage using digital nerve block. The optimum surgical approach remains controversial. Most commonly a longitudinal incision is made over the area of maximal tenderness. Incision and drainage are supplemented with a 10- to 14-day course of an antistaphylococcal antibiotic unless cultures reveal a different microorganism. The association of felon with methicillin-resistant *S. aureus* has

been reported recently, and therefore culture and sensitivity testing is recommended.

Deep Subfascial Space Infections, Pyogenic Flexor Tenosynovitis, Septic Arthritis, and Osteomyelitis

Deep infections of the hand must be distinguished from noninfectious diseases such as gout, pseudogout, rheumatoid arthritis, foreign bodies, brown recluse spider bites, and the numerous other causes of localized pathologic conditions. Deep infection should always be suspected when hand infection complicates penetrating trauma. Deep subfascial space infections comprise about 5% to 15% of hand infections and are usually suspected on the basis of pain, swelling, tenderness, warmth, or limitation of motion. The spaces or potential spaces involved include the thenar space, the hypothenar space, the midpalmar space, the interdigital (web) space, the dorsal subaponeurotic space, and Parona's space (which is situated within the distal forearm but is contiguous with the midpalmar space and the radial and ulnar bursae of the wrist). These infections usually arise from a chronic lesion such as a fissure, blister, or callus or from penetrating trauma. Prompt surgical drainage is the cornerstone of management. Pyogenic flexor tenosynovitis involves the flexor tendon sheath of the finger or thumb or the radial or ulnar bursae. Patients report pain and swelling along the flexor tendon sheath and often give a history of penetrating trauma. The presence of pain on palpation of the flexor tendon sheath helps to distinguish this serious infection from other conditions such as herpetic whitlow, gout, and septic arthritis. Septic arthritis of the joints of the hand and wrist is uncommon but should be considered in the differential diagnosis of a painful joint even when another diagnosis such as gout or rheumatoid arthritis seems more likely. Appropriate management includes joint aspiration or surgical exploration to define the etiology as a guide to antimicrobial therapy. Osteomyelitis of the hand is often related to bite wounds or trauma. Although *S. aureus* is the most common pathogen, unusual etiologic agents, including *Eikenella corrodens* and *Pasteurella multocida,* must be considered (see Chapter 26).

 KEY POINTS

INFECTIONS OF THE HAND

- ⊃ Acute paronychia is usually caused by *S. aureus.* Mild infections are treated with antistaphylococcal antibiotics. More severe infections with abscess formation require surgical drainage using digital nerve block.
- ⊃ Herpetic whitlow must be distinguished from acute paronychia because attempts to incise and drain the lesion can cause severe local and systemic complications.
- ⊃ Chronic paronychia usually occurs in persons whose hands are frequently immersed in water, is most commonly associated with *C. albicans,* and is difficult to treat.
- ⊃ Felon is an abscess of the closed space between the vertical fibrous septa in the distal pulp of the fingertip. It is usually caused by *S. aureus.*
- ⊃ Deep subfascial space infections, pyogenic flexor tenosynovitis, septic arthritis, and osteomyelitis usually warrant surgical referral.

SUGGESTED READING

Boustred AM, Singer M, Hudson DA, et al. Septic arthritis of the metacarpophalangeal and interphalangeal joints of the hand. Ann Plast Surg 1999; 42: 623-628.

Connolly B, Johnstone F, Gerlinger T, et al. Methicillin-resistant *Staphylococcus aureus* in a finger felon. J Hand Surg [Am] 2000; 25: 173-175.

Jebson PJL, Louis DS, ed. Hand infections. Hand Clin 1998; 14: 511-725.

Mohler A. Herpetic whitlow of the toe. J Am Board Fam Pract 2000; 13: 213-215.

Tsai E, Failla JM. Hand infections in the trauma patient. Hand Clin 1999; 15: 373-386.

Infections of the Foot in Patients with Diabetes Mellitus, Including Polymicrobial Osteomyelitis

In the Waldvogel classification of osteomyelitis (see earlier discussion), osteomyelitis associated with vascular insufficiency is essentially synonymous with polymicrobial osteomyelitis of the small bones of the foot in patients with diabetes mellitus. Most of these patients have sensory neuropathy in addition to vascular insufficiency. In patients with diabetes mellitus, osteomyelitis must be distinguished from other types of foot infection. Foot ulcers and infections account for more hospitalizations than any other diabetic complication and for about two thirds of all nontraumatic amputations performed in the United States. Preventing these infections is an important challenge for primary care clinicians (see Chapter 3).

Presentation and Progression
Cause

Patients with diabetes mellitus often have small and large vessel arterial disease and peripheral neuropathy. Foot ulcers in patients with diabetes mellitus can result from ischemia, neuropathy, or, in an estimated one third of patients, both ischemia and neuropathy. Diabetic foot ulcers are also associated with long-term diabetes mellitus, advanced age, cigarette smoking, and microalbuminuria. Trauma is necessary, however, to initiate an ulcer. Superinfection results in ulcers and skin necrosis with or without gangrene. *S. aureus* or streptococci are commonly isolated from superficial infections such as cellulitis. Deep infections associated with penetrating ulcers are typically polymicrobial. Carefully obtained and processed cultures usually disclose a mixture of aerobic and anaerobic bacteria. The former include *S. aureus* (an increasing percentage of which is methicillin resistant, at least in some geographic areas), streptococci, enterococci (which are seldom primary pathogens in this setting), coagulase-negative staphylococci, *E. coli* and other enteric gram-negative bacilli, and occasionally *Pseudomonas* or *Acinetobacter* species. Anaerobic pathogens include peptostreptococci and *B. fragilis.*

Presentation

In many patients foot ulcers are the initial complaint. Pain, redness, and fever are often minimal. Cellulitis, deep ulcerations, and fistulous tracts suggest more extensive disease. Systemic symptoms including poor diabetic control (marked hyperglycemia) usually imply complications such as abscess, deep space infection, or gangrene. Osteomyelitis develops in 20% to 30% of patients, typically by extension of a plantar ulcer to bone. Some patients with osteomyelitis have no break in the skin; in these patients, osteomyelitis possibly results from hematogenous seeding of a previously damaged bone or joint (e.g., "Charcot foot" resulting from repetitive trauma in the presence of diabetic neuropathy).

Diagnosis

Cultures are probably unnecessary for patients with mild cellulitis. In patients with plantar ulcers, determining whether osteomyelitis is present can be difficult. Exposed bone at the base of an ulcer strongly suggests osteomyelitis. In recent years a "probe-to-bone test" has been used. A stainless steel probe is passed carefully to the base of the ulcer; contact with bone produces a characteristic resistance suggesting osteomyelitis. When performed by an experienced practitioner, the "probe-to-bone test" compares favorably with costly imaging procedures. Plain x-ray films can be difficult to interpret. An uninfected "Charcot foot" can cause heat, swelling, and radiographic changes typical of osteomyelitis. Gas in the tissues suggests a mixed infection with aerobic gram-negative rods and anaerobic pathogens. Gas gangrene caused by *Clostridium perfringens* is infrequent but should be considered in the differential diagnosis. MRI scans can be invaluable for managing the disease. However, differentiation on MRI between osteomyelitis and marrow edema resulting from peripheral neuropathy is not always possible; the sensitivity of MRI is much higher than the specificity (98% versus 81%). Indium-labeled leukocyte scintigraphy is sometimes useful, but the sensitivity (89%) and specificity (69%) are lower than with MRI.

Accurate bacteriologic diagnosis is desirable when osteomyelitis is suspected. Blood cultures are usually sterile even when fever is present. Superficial cultures of an ulcer are of limited if any value, since diverse colonizing bacteria are inevitably present. Cultures obtained by curettage of a foot ulcer are superior to those obtained by swabbing. Even better cultures can be obtained from a bullous lesion, if present, or from an abscess provided care is taken to decontaminate the skin. When osteomyelitis is suspected, the procedure of choice involves obtaining a deep culture through unbroken skin by aspiration, biopsy, or open surgical exploration.

Natural History

Untreated, most diabetic foot ulcers fail to heal and most cases of polymicrobial osteomyelitis cause significant disability and often result in amputation. Intactness of the arterial circulation to the foot is the best predictive factor for healing. Measurement of transcutaneous oxygen tension and toe blood pressure, available in specialized centers, correlates with a favorable outcome.

Treatment
Methods

Treatment is based on the extent of the wound and the probability of osteomyelitis. Patients with mild cellulitis can be treated empirically with an oral antibiotic with antistaphylococcal activity, such as dicloxacillin, amoxicillin-clavulanate, or cephalexin. Patients with infected foot ulcers without osteomyelitis are also treated empirically, in most instances, with antimicrobial agents that provide coverage against staphylococci and streptococci. Oral cephalexin 500 mg q.i.d. and clindamycin 300 mg t.i.d. for 2 weeks were shown to be equally effective in a clinical trial. Fluoroquinolones have also been used successfully. We prefer to avoid the use of fluoroquinolones, since *S. aureus* often acquires resistance, and to use a combination of cephalexin, dicloxacillin, or amoxicillin-clavulanate with metronidazole (Flagyl 500 to 750 mg t.i.d.). Therapy should be continued for at least 7 to 14 days and sometimes for extended periods. Prolonged use of metronidazole can aggravate a preexisting sensory neuropathy.

Local wound care is extremely important, and consultation with a surgeon is often desirable. Wound care consists of performing extensive débridement, the patient's cleansing the ulcer twice daily, covering the lesion with nonadherent dry dressing, keeping the foot elevated, and avoiding unnecessary walking. The use of human skin–equivalent material has recently been shown to be an effective adjunct.

When osteomyelitis is present, an effort should be made to secure an accurate microbiologic diagnosis if this can be done with reasonable safety. Most authorities recommend parenteral therapy. Appropriate regimens for initial empiric therapy include cefoxitin, cefotetan, ceftizoxime, ticarcillin—clavulanic acid, and ampicillin-sulbactam. For more severe infections an aminoglycoside can be added or imipenem (or meropenem) can be used as monotherapy. Osteomyelitis may require 6 to 12 weeks of parenteral therapy, especially if the quality of the débridement is uncertain. Some patients, however, can be given a short course of intravenous antibiotics and then treated for extended periods with an oral regimen as outlined previously. Most patients require close surgical follow-up. Patients with large vessel disease should be evaluated for revascularization. Surgical attention should also be given to corns, calluses, and bony prominences to prevent future wounds. Patients should be educated and reeducated about diabetic foot care.

Expected Results

In one study 75% of foot ulcers that were not associated with cellulitis, abscess formation, or osteomyelitis healed within 2 weeks with oral antibiotic therapy and aggressive local care. In other studies, however, less than one half of ulcers healed within 6 months despite appropriate care. On the other hand, studies carried out in multidisciplinary diabetic foot clinics indicated improved rates of foot salvage. In one study major amputation was avoided in 95% of all patients with diabetes and foot infection. In another study major amputation was avoided in 81% of patients with skin ulcer, 70% of patients with deep tissue infection or suspected osteomyelitis, and 7% of patients with gangrene. Risk factors for a poor result included fever, elevated serum creatinine level, prior hospitalization for a diabetic foot lesion, and presence of gangrene.

When to Refer

Although superficial lesions can often be managed successfully in primary care settings, patients with deep lesions or osteomyelitis usually benefit from referral to one or more specialists (e.g., infectious diseases or orthopedic surgery).

 KEY POINTS

INFECTIONS OF THE FOOT IN PATIENTS WITH DIABETES MELLITUS, INCLUDING POLYMICROBIAL OSTEOMYELITIS

⊃ Primary care clinicians play an essential role in the prevention of limb-threatening complications in diabetic patients.

⊃ Superficial infections involving foot ulcers are often due to staphylococci and streptococci. An increasing percentage of *S. aureus* strains in some areas are methicillin resistant.

⊃ Bone involvement (osteomyelitis) occurs in 20% to 30% of patients but can be difficult to diagnose. Deep infections, including osteomyelitis, are frequently polymicrobial with mixtures of aerobic and anaerobic bacteria.

⊃ When osteomyelitis is present, an effort should be made to secure an accurate bacteriologic diagnosis if this can be accomplished with reasonable safety.

⊃ Recent studies suggest improved rates of foot salvage (i.e., fewer major amputations) when patients are managed aggressively by a multidisciplinary team.

SUGGESTED READING

Armstrong DG, Lavery LA. Diabetic foot ulcers: prevention, diagnosis and classification. Am Fam Physician 1998; 57: 1325-1332, 1337-1338.

Boyko EJ, Ahroni JH, Stensel V, et al. The Seattle Diabetic Foot Study. A prospective study of risk factors for diabetic foot ulcer. Diabetes Care 1999; 22: 1036-1042.

Brem H, Balledux J, Bloom T, et al. Healing of diabetic foot ulcers with human skin equivalent: a new paradigm in wound healing. Arch Surg 2000; 135: 627-634.

Caputo GM, Cavanagh PR, Ulbrecht JS, et al. Assessment and management of foot disease in patients with diabetes. N Engl J Med 1994; 331: 854-860.

Caputo GM, Ulbrecht JS, Cavanagh PR, et al. The role of cultures in mild diabetic foot cellulitis. Infect Dis Clin Pract 2000; 9: 241-243.

Grayson ML, Gibbons GW, Balogh K, et al. Probing to bone in infected pedal ulcers: a clinical sign of underlying osteomyelitis in diabetic patients. JAMA 1995; 273: 721-723.

Hill SL, Holtzman GI, Buse R. The effects of peripheral vascular disease with osteomyelitis in the diabetic foot. Am J Surg 1999; 177: 282-286.

Holstein PE, Sørensen S. Limb salvage experience in a multidisciplinary diabetic foot clinic. Diabetes Care 1999; 22 (Suppl 2): B97-B103.

Lipsky BA, Pecoraro RE, Larson SA, et al. Outpatient management of uncomplicated lower-extremity infections in diabetic patients. Arch Intern Med 1990; 150: 790-797.

Lipsky BA. Osteomyelitis of the foot in diabetic patients. Clin Infect Dis 1997; 25: 1318-1326.

Pittet D, Wyssa B, Herter-Clavel C, et al. Outcome of diabetic foot infections treated conservatively: a retrospective cohort study with long-term follow-up. Arch Intern Med 1999; 159: 851-856.

Shea KW. Antimicrobial therapy for diabetic foot infections: a practical approach. Postgrad Med 1999; 106: 85-86, 89-94.

Sumpio BE. Foot ulcers. N Engl J Med 2000; 343: 787-793.

Temple ME, Nahata MC. Pharmacotherapy of lower limb diabetic ulcers. J Am Geriatr Soc 2000; 48: 822-828.

Tentolouris N, Jude EB, Smirnof I, et al. Methicillin-resistant *Staphylococcus aureus*: an increasing problem in a diabetic foot clinic. Diabet Med 1999; 16: 767-771.

16 Sexually Transmitted Diseases

SRI EDUPUGANTI, ARLENE C. SEÑA, MYRON S. COHEN

Sexually transmitted diseases (STDs) have been described as "hidden epidemics," comprising 5 of the 10 most frequently reported diseases in the United States. An estimated 12 million new cases of STDs occur each year in the United States, which has the highest rate among all developed countries. In the developing world STDs are an even greater public health problem and the second leading cause of healthy life lost among women between 15 and 44 years of age. The STD epidemic in the developing world, where atypical presentations, drug-resistant organisms, and coinfections (especially with human immunodeficiency virus [HIV]) are common, can have a potentially larger impact on the U.S. population because of increased international travel and migration. The health consequences of STDs have occurred primarily in women, children, and adolescents, especially among racial and ethnic minority groups. In the United States each year more than 1 million women are estimated to have an episode of pelvic inflammatory disease (PID). The number of ectopic pregnancies has been estimated as 1 in 50, and approximately 15% of infertile American women are thought to have tubal inflammation as a result of PID. Adverse outcomes of pregnancy resulting from untreated STDs include neonatal ophthalmia, neonatal pneumonia, physical and mental developmental disabilities, and fetal death from congenital

syphilis (see Chapter 5). Of all age groups, adolescents (10- to 19-year-olds) are at greatest risk for STDs because of a greater biologic susceptibility to infection and a greater likelihood of having multiple sexual partners and unprotected sexual encounters. Minority groups such as African-Americans and Hispanic-Americans have the highest STD rates.

STDs and HIV infections share common risk factors for transmission. Genital ulcer disease increases the risk of HIV acquisition and transmission by two- to five-fold; urethritis and cervicitis increase the risk by five-fold. Treatment and control of STDs at the population level may result in decreases in HIV incidence among populations with high rates of STDs. STD control should be considered an important component of HIV prevention in public health, as well as clinical practice.

Effective clinical management of STDs should include screening sexually active individuals with appropriate laboratory tests and providing definitive diagnosis and treatment, client-centered risk reduction and education, and evaluation and treatment of partners. Screening asymptomatic patients is of utmost importance in preventing sequelae. Screening for STDs among sexually active women, especially pregnant women, is essential because roughly 70% of chlamydial infections and 50% of gonococcal infections are asymptomatic in this population.

Unfortunately, the barriers to effective STD prevention are multiple, including the biologic characteristics of STDs, lack of public awareness regarding STDs, inadequate training of health professionals, and sociocultural norms related to sexuality that can lead to misperception of recognized risk and consequences. Primary care clinicians, from whom most patients with STDs seek care, have a vital role in the struggle to overcome these barriers. However, <50% of primary care physicians take histories of sexual practices of new patients. The primary care clinician can assist by increasing both self- and patients' awareness of sexual health issues and STDs, implementing guidelines of the Centers for Disease Control and Prevention (CDC) for management of STDs, and providing comprehensive STD-related services, education, and counseling, especially for those at high risk.

SUGGESTED READING

Centers for Disease Control and Prevention. 1998 guidelines for treatment of sexually transmitted diseases. MMWR 1998; 47 (RR-1): 1-111.

Holmes KK, Mårdh PA, Sparling PF, et al, eds. Sexually Transmitted Diseases. 3rd ed., New York: McGraw-Hill; 1999.

Peeling RW, Sparling PF. Sexually Transmitted Diseases: Methods and Protocols. Totowa, NJ: Humana Press; 1999.

TABLE 16-1
Clinical Features of Sexually Transmitted Pathogens That Cause Genital Diseases

Disease	Genital herpes simplex	Primary syphilis	Chancroid
Organism	Herpes simplex virus	*Treponema pallidum*	*Haemophilus ducreyi*
Number of lesions	Multiple	Usually one	Usually one to three
Genital lesion	Shallow, grouped vesicles, pustules, or ulcers, typically on an erythematous base; ulcers with smooth base	Deep, well-defined ulcer with a smooth, erythematous base	Well-defined or irregular ulcer with a rough base; presence of purulence; undermined edge of ulcer
Induration*	None	Present ("hard chancre" with cartilaginous feel)	None
Tenderness	Common with primary episode	None	Common
Inguinal lymphadenopathy	Bilateral and tender with primary episode	Unilateral or bilateral; nontender	Unilateral or bilateral; tender or nontender; may suppurate
Constitutional symptoms	Present with the primary episode; may have problems with bladder or bowel control because of sacral root involvement	Absent	Absent

Ross MW, Channon-Little LD, Rosser BR. Sexual Health Concerns: Interviewing and History Taking for Health Practitioners. 2nd ed., Philadelphia: F.A. Davis; 2000.

Stanberry LR, Bernstein DI, eds. Sexually Transmitted Diseases: Vaccines, Prevention and Control. San Diego: Academic Press; 2000.

St. Louis ME, Workowski KA, eds. 1998 guidelines for the treatment of sexually transmitted diseases. Clin Infect Dis 1999; 28 (Suppl 1): S1-S90.

Genital Ulcer Diseases: Overview

A genital ulcer is defined as a breach in the skin or mucosa of the genitalia. Genital ulcers may be single or multiple and may be associated with inguinal or femoral lymphadenopathy. Genital ulcer diseases (GUD) account for 2% to 5% of all STD clinic visits in Europe and North America; in Africa and Asia they account for 20% to 70% of all STD clinic visits. Sexually transmitted pathogens that cause GUD are herpes simplex virus (HSV), *Treponema pallidum, Haemophilus ducreyi,* L serovars of *Chlamydia trachomatis,* and *Calymmatobacterium granulomatis.*

Genital ulcer diseases facilitate enhanced HIV transmission among sexual partners. In the presence of genital ulcers the susceptibility to HIV is increased five-fold. In addition, HIV-infected individuals with GUD may transmit HIV to their sexual partners more efficiently.

Presentation and Progression
Cause

HSV is the most common cause of GUD among young, sexually active persons in the United States. *T. pallidum* is the next most common cause of GUD and should be considered in most situations despite the decline in cases of syphilis nationwide. Chancroid, which is caused by *H. ducreyi,* has been infrequently associated with cases of GUD in the United States but has been isolated in up to 10% of genital ulcers diagnosed from STD clinics in Memphis and Chicago. Chancroid is the most common genital ulcer disease in many developing countries. Lymphogranuloma venereum (LGV) caused by L serovars of *C. trachomatis* and granuloma inguinale (donovanosis) caused by *C. granulomatis* are endemic in tropical countries and should be considered in the differential diagnosis of genital ulcers from a native of the tropics or those with history of tropical travel.

The prevalence of pathogens that cause GUD varies according to the geographic area and the patient population. A single patient can have genital ulcers caused by more than one pathogen. Despite laboratory testing, approximately 25% of genital ulcers have no identifiable cause.

Presentation

Considerable overlap can be seen in the clinical presentation of herpes, primary syphilis, and chancroid, the three most common causes of genital ulcers in the United States (Table 16-1). Inguinal lymphadenopathy is present in about 50% of the patients with genital ulcer diseases. Genital herpes is characterized by multiple, shallow ulcers and bilateral lymphadenopathy. Primary syphilis can usually be differentiated from genital herpes by the presence of a single deep, defined ulcer with induration. A distinction may be made between syphilis and chancroid; unlike syphilis, chancroid commonly causes a painful, undermined ulcer with a purulent base and tender lymphadenopathy.

BOX 16-1
Recommended Tests in the Evaluation of Genital Ulcer Disease

- Dark-field examination or direct immunofluorescence and serology for *Treponema pallidum* (all patients need serologic tests)
- Culture or serologic for herpes simplex virus (see discussion)
- Culture for *Haemophilus ducreyi* (not widely available)
- Test for human immunodeficiency virus, especially for patients with documented *T. pallidum* or *H. ducreyi* infection (it should also be considered for those who have genital herpes)

Diagnosis

The cause of genital ulcers cannot be based on clinical findings alone. Diagnosis based on the classic presentation is only 30% to 34% sensitive but 94% to 98% specific. Therefore, diagnostic testing should be performed when possible (Box 16-1). Serologic testing for syphilis should be considered even when lesions appear atypical. If available, dark-field examination or direct immunofluorescence on the lesion material should be performed as the definitive tests for *T. pallidum*. Genital herpes can be diagnosed in the presence of typical lesions or positive serologic tests, but herpes culture should be performed when the diagnosis is uncertain.

The differential diagnosis that should be considered in GUD includes malignancy, trauma, fixed drug eruption, Behçet's disease, and Reiter's syndrome. Rare infectious causes of genital ulcers include tuberculosis, histoplasmosis, tularemia, and amebiasis. Primary HIV infection should also be considered in the differential diagnosis of mucocutaneous ulcers and a mononucleosis-like syndrome.

Treatment
Methods

An algorithmic approach to treatment is based on the history, physical examination, and selected laboratory tests (Figure 16-1). Directed treatment for specific causes of GUD is discussed later in the chapter. The World Health Organization has provided algorithms for the syndromic management of GUD in settings where diagnostic laboratory testing is not available. However, serologic testing for syphilis should be performed in all cases. Patients should be referred to an expert if no improvement is noted at follow-up.

Expected Response

Treatment based on a correct diagnosis is usually successful, although genital herpes is notoriously prone to recurrence.

 ## KEY POINTS

GENITAL ULCER DISEASES: OVERVIEW

- Genital herpes, syphilis, and chancroid cause genital ulcers in the United States.
- LGV and granuloma inguinale should be considered in the differential diagnosis of GUD among travelers to and immigrants from developing countries.

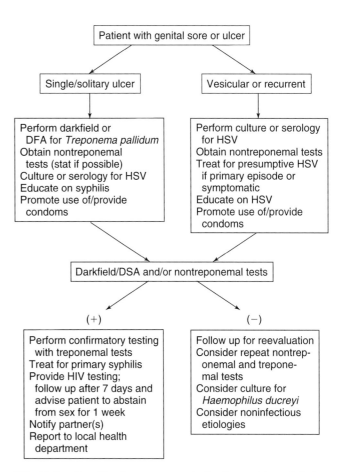

FIG. 16-1   Algorithm for management of patients with genital ulcer disease.

- Laboratory testing for diagnosis should be performed when possible, especially to rule out syphilis.
- Coinfection with more than one pathogen is not uncommon.

SUGGESTED READING

Ballard RC. Genital ulcer adenopathy syndrome. In: Holmes KK, Mardh PA, Sparling PF, et al, eds. Sexually Transmitted Diseases. 3rd ed., New York: McGraw-Hill; 1999: 887-892.

Cohen MS. Sexually transmitted diseases enhance HIV transmission: no longer a hypothesis. Lancet 1998; 351 (Suppl 3): 5-7.

DiCarlo RP, Martin DH. The clinical diagnosis of genital ulcer disease in men. Clin Infect Dis 1997; 25: 292-298.

Seña AC, Behets FM-T, Fox KK, Cohen MS. Sexually Transmitted Diseases. In: Guerrant RL, Walker DH, Weller PF, eds. Tropical Infectious Diseases: Principles, Pathogens, and Practice. Philadelphia: Churchill Livingstone: 1999: 1569-1585.

Genital Herpes Simplex

Genital HSV infection affects up to 60 million people in the United States and can be caused by both herpes simplex virus type 1 (HSV-1) and type 2 (HSV-2). The seroprevalence of HSV-2 has increased over the past three decades to 22% among individuals 15 to 74 years of age. Behavioral factors correlated with seroprevalence include cocaine use, multiple sexual partners, and early sexual activity. Approximately 40% of patients infected with genital HSV-2 and 60% of patients infected with HSV-1 are asymptomatic. Thus genital herpes is often acquired from individuals whose herpes has never been clinically diagnosed. Transmission of HSV between sexual partners has been estimated at 12% of previously uninfected partners per year but can be as high as 30% among women who are partners of infected men. Women have a 5% to 10% higher seroprevalence of HSV-2 than men, suggesting the increased risk of acquisition.

Presentation and Progression

Cause

Genital lesions acquired through sexual contact are typically caused by HSV-2, while oropharyngeal lesions acquired through nongenital personal contact are most commonly due to HSV-1. However, both viruses can cause genital and oral infections. HSV-2 causes the vast majority of genital herpes in the United States, but HSV-1 accounts for 5% to 30% of first episode cases.

After mucosal or cutaneous contact, HSV replicates in the dermis and epidermis and ascends through the sensory nerve fibers to the dorsal root ganglia. Once established in the sensory ganglia, the virus remains latent for life with periodic reactivation and spreads through the peripheral sensory nerves to the mucocutaneous sites.

Presentation

Most patients seropositive for HSV-2 have subclinical, undiagnosed genital herpes. About one fourth of the patients with a first episode of genital herpes have positive HSV-2 serology, suggesting prior asymptomatic infection. Thus the first clinical episode of genital herpes could be due either to a primary infection or to a first recognized episode of past infection.

Primary infection with HSV-2 is characterized by a prodrome of systemic symptoms, including fever, chills, headache, and malaise. Pain and paresthesia around the outbreak site precede the appearance of lesions by 12 to 48 hours. The hallmark of genital herpes consists of grouped vesicles or pustules that lead to shallow ulcers (Figure 16-2). Atypical lesions of genital herpes include linear fissures of the vulva, cervical ulcerations, vaginal discharge, papules, and crusts. Patients may have accompanying tender inguinal lymphadenopathy. Urethritis, rectal, or perianal symptoms may be present if there is urethral or rectal involvement. Immunocompromised patients may have extensive perianal and rectal manifestations. Extragenital manifestations of HSV include ulcerative lesions of the buttock, groin, and thighs; pharyngitis; aseptic meningitis; transverse myelitis; and sacral radiculopathy.

Primary infection with HSV-1 is manifested as genital ulcers in about one third of patients. Another one third may have orolabial lesions or pharyngitis, and the remaining patients are asymptomatic. The genital lesions caused by HSV-1 are indistinguishable from those of HSV-2.

Recurrent genital herpes is usually a milder syndrome than primary infection. The recurrence of genital herpes caused by HSV-2 is much more frequent than with HSV-1. The recurrence rate of orolabial infection caused by HSV-1 is much more greater than the recurrence rate with HSV-2.

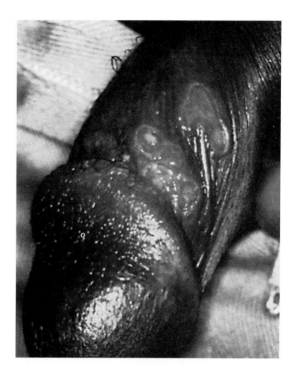

FIG. 16-2 Primary genital herpes simplex virus infection, with two clusters of shallow ulcers on the penile shaft. Groups of vesicles rupture to form multiple small ulcers, which often coalesce, forming larger ulcers as shown here. (Courtesy of Dr. Michael F. Rein.)

Diagnosis

Genital herpes is diagnosed on the basis of a positive HSV culture from the mucocutaneous lesions. Culture is more sensitive during the vesicle stage (100%) than the ulcer stage (33%). Vesicles should be unroofed, and the base should be swabbed for culture. The overall sensitivity of culture is about 50% and can be increased by use of the same swab for multiple lesions. If culture is not available, a Tzanck smear can be performed by scraping the base of the ulcer and staining the material with Wright's stain. The presence of multinucleated giant cells is pathognomonic of HSV.

Other diagnostic tests such as antigen detection or type-specific serologic tests are available. Several antigen detection kits are available, but they do not distinguish between HSV-1 and HSV-2. Newly approved type-specific serologic tests (Diagnology's POCkit HSV-2 Rapid Test, Meridian Diagnostics' Premier HSV-1 or HSV-2 IgG ELISA Test, Microbiology Reference Laboratory's [MRL] HSV-1 or HSV-2 IgG ELISA, and MRL's HSV-1 and HSV-2 Differentiation Immunoblot) differentiate between HSV-1 and HSV-2 infection. The sensitivity of type-specific serologic tests for HSV-2 ranges from 70% to 90%, and the specificity ranges from 95% to 99%. The POCkit HSV-2 Rapid Test is a rapid office-based test and can detect antibodies, on average, 2 weeks after symptoms first appear. Its sensitivity and specificity range from 96% to 100% and 97% to 99%, respectively. The Premier test's sensitivity and specificity range from 80% to 98% and 94% to 99%, respectively. This test has low sensitivity in the first 6 months after infection. The positive predictive value of the type-specific tests is high in populations with high likelihood of disease such as patients with recurrent infection with a false-negative viral culture, sexually active gay men, and sex partners of people with genital herpes. These tests can identify people with asymptomatic infection but do not distinguish oral from genital herpes. They are not recommended for mass screening of the general population, children, or babies. MRL's test may soon be approved for use in pregnant women, but the other type-specific tests mentioned here are not recommended for pregnant women. Other causes of GUD should also be considered when evaluating patients with genital lesions.

Natural History
Expected Outcome

Genital herpes is an incurable disease because of the latency in the sensory ganglia. After the resolution of the primary infection in 7 to 10 days, reactivation with new vesicles is common in the first month after healing of the primary lesions. Most patients have recurrence of the disease, although the incidence of recurrence decreases with time after the initial episode. Recurrent genital lesions are less severe and usually not preceded by prodromal symptoms. The majority of patients with genital herpes have intermittent asymptomatic viral shedding even without the presence of lesions. Recent polymerase chain reaction (PCR) evidence suggests that persons with asymptomatic viral shedding can shed virus on up to 10% to 12% of the days sampled. Sexual transmission can occur both during the genital ulcer stage and during the time of asymptomatic viral shedding.

Treatment
Methods

Treatment consists of antiviral therapy (Box 16-2), education, and counseling. Patients should be counseled about recurrent disease, asymptomatic viral shedding, sexual transmission, condom use, and risk of neonatal infection. Sex partners of patients with genital herpes who are symptomatic should be evaluated and treated. Asymptomatic sex partners should be evaluated, counseled, and encouraged to examine themselves for genital lesions.

All patients with first episode genital herpes should be considered for antiviral therapy, which can reduce the duration and severity of symptoms. Patient-initiated treatment should begin at the first sign of the prodrome or within 1 day after the onset of genital lesions for recurrent disease. Recurrent episodes of genital herpes may be treated episodically or with continuous suppressive therapy. Condoms are effective for decreasing the transmission between discordant couples.

Expected Response

The first clinical episode of genital herpes responds well to antiviral therapy with the resolution of constitutional symptoms within 48 hours. Herpetic lesions may take up to 21 days for complete resolution. Treatment of the first episode does not change the long-term natural history of the disease.

Treatment of recurrent disease with daily suppressive therapy reduces the frequency of recurrences (especially among patients with 4 to 12 episodes per year), decreases the duration of viral shedding, and improves the quality of life. After 1 year, the need for continued therapy should be

---

BOX 16-2
Treatment of Genital Herpes Simplex Infection

FIRST EPISODE OF GENITAL HERPES
- Acyclovir 400 mg PO t.i.d. for 7 to 10 days *or*
- Acyclovir 200 mg PO five times per day for 7 to 10 days *or*
- Famciclovir 250 mg PO t.i.d. for 7 to 10 days *or*
- Valacyclovir 1 g PO b.i.d. for 7 to 10 days

RECURRENT EPISODES
Episodic Treatment
- Acyclovir 400 mg PO t.i.d. for 5 days *or* acyclovir 200 mg PO 5 times per day for 5 days *or* acyclovir 800 mg PO b.i.d. for 5 days *or*
- Famciclovir 125 mg PO b.i.d. for 5 days *or*
- Valacyclovir 500 mg PO b.i.d. for 5 days *or* valacyclovir 1000 mg PO qd for 5 days

Daily Suppressive Therapy
- Acyclovir 400 mg PO b.i.d. *or*
- Famciclovir* 250 mg PO b.i.d. *or*
- Valacyclovir* 500 mg PO qd *or* valacyclovir* 1000 mg PO qd

*Insufficient experience precludes the use of these drugs for more than 1 year.

---

reassessed because the frequency of recurrences decreases with time.

Complications

Therapy with acyclovir, famciclovir, or valacyclovir is well tolerated. Famciclovir and valacyclovir have greater bioavailability than acyclovir. Acyclovir should be dose adjusted in patients with impaired creatinine clearance. The most common adverse effects are headache, nausea, and diarrhea. The safety of acyclovir in pregnant women has not been determined.

When to Refer

Patients with severe first-episode genital herpes or with symptoms of fever, headache, vomiting, photophobia, and nuchal rigidity should be hospitalized. Intravenous acyclovir is recommended for encephalitis caused by HSV (see Chapter 6).

Immunocompromised and pregnant patients should be referred because they are at high risk of dissemination, leading to diffuse cutaneous disease, pneumonitis, hepatitis, or central nervous system (CNS) infection.

 KEY POINTS

GENITAL HERPES SIMPLEX
- ⊃ Genital herpes is the most common STD in the United States.
- ⊃ Most people with genital herpes have asymptomatic disease and serve as the reservoir for sexual transmission.
- ⊃ Determining whether genital herpes infection is caused by HSV-1 or HSV-2 has prognostic implications.
- ⊃ Treatment consists of antiviral therapy and education regarding the natural history of disease.
- ⊃ Genital herpes is a lifelong disease. Treatment with antiviral agents does not eradicate infection.

⊃ Control strategies include abstinence or condom use in all sexual encounters.

SUGGESTED READING

Ashley RL, Wald A. Genital herpes: review of the epidemic and potential use of type-specific serology. Clin Microbiol Rev 1999; 12: 1-8.

Corey L, Wald A. Genital herpes. In: Holmes KK, Mardh PA, Sparling PF, et al, eds. Sexually Transmitted Diseases. 3rd ed., New York: McGraw-Hill; 1999: 285-306.

Fleming DT, McQuillan GM, Johnson RE, et al. Herpes simplex type II in the United States, 1976 to 1994. N Engl J Med 1997; 337: 1105-1111.

Handsfield HH. Public health strategies to prevent genital herpes: where do we stand? Curr Infect Dis Rep 2000; 2: 25-30.

Lafferty WE, Coombs RW, Benedetti J, et al. Recurrences after oral and genital herpes simplex virus infection: influence of site of infection and viral type. N Engl J Med 1987; 316: 1444-1449.

Langenberg AG, Corey L, Ashley RL, et al. A prospective study of new infections with herpes simplex virus type 1 and type 2. N Engl J Med 1999; 341:1432-1438.

Syphilis

T. pallidum, a spirochete that is the main cause of syphilis, is a major public health concern because of the complications of untreated disease. In the United States the rates of primary and secondary syphilis have declined significantly in the past 30 years. Some racial and ethnic groups such as African-Americans, Native Americans, and Alaskan natives continue to have disproportionately high rates of syphilis. The incidence of primary and secondary syphilis in non-Hispanic blacks remains high at 17 cases per 100,000 persons, which is 34 times greater than the rate for non-Hispanic whites. In the United States the Southeast has the highest rates of syphilis, perhaps because of unemployment, poor access to health care, and the stigma associated with discussion of STDs. Untreated syphilis infection in pregnancy can lead to congenital syphilis in 70% of the cases (see Chapter 5).

The prevalence of syphilis in HIV-infected individuals ranges from 14% to 22%. Syphilis, along with other genital ulcer diseases, facilitates transmission of HIV. A syphilitic chancre not only increases transmission of HIV by causing a breakdown of the skin, but also increases the number of inflammatory cells receptive to HIV. The transmission rate of syphilis from an infected sexual partner has been estimated at 30%.

Presentation and Progression

Cause

T. pallidum is an exclusive human pathogen that can be visualized by dark-field microscopy. It appears as a spiral bacterium with corkscrew motility. After inoculation through abraded skin or mucous membranes it attaches to the host cells and is disseminated within a few hours to the regional lymph nodes and eventually to the internal organs and the CNS.

Presentation

The clinical presentation of syphilis is divided into primary, secondary, early latent, late latent, and tertiary stages based on

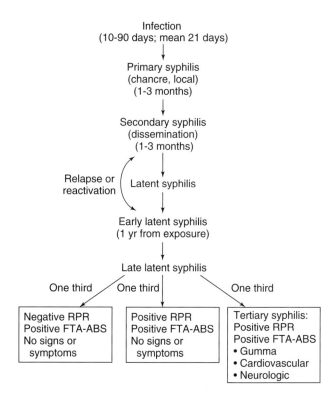

FIG. 16-3   Natural history of untreated syphilis.

infectiousness. The staging is used for therapeutic decisions and disease intervention strategies (Figure 16-3).

Primary Syphilis. After an incubation period of 2 to 6 weeks after exposure, a papule develops at the site of inoculation and then ulcerates into the characteristic syphilitic chancre. The classic chancre is a painless, indurated ulcer with well-defined borders and a clean base (Table 16-1 and Figure 16-4). A chancre can develop on the oral or anorectal mucosa, as well as on the genital mucosa. Prior application of topical antibiotics or the use of systemic antimicrobial agents may change the typical appearance of the lesion. Nontender lymphadenopathy may be present.

Secondary Syphilis (see also Chapter 7). Manifestations of secondary syphilis develop in 60% to 90% of patients with untreated primary syphilis. Secondary syphilis is a systemic disease that results from dissemination of the treponemes. Systemic symptoms include generalized lymphadenopathy, fever, headache, sore throat, and arthralgias. Numerous clinical manifestations occur 4 to 10 weeks after the chancre disappears (or 2 to 6 months after sexual contact). These involve dermatologic, central nervous (aseptic meningitis, cranial neuropathy), ocular (iritis, uveitis, or conjunctivitis), hepatic (hepatitis), and renal (immune complex glomerulonephritis) systems.

The most common manifestation of secondary syphilis is a skin rash characterized by macules and papules distributed on the head, neck, trunk, and extremities, including the palms and soles. The rash may be confused with pityriasis rosea, psoriasis, or drug eruption. Condylomata lata are large, raised whitish lesions that are seen in warm, moist areas, occur before or soon after the rash, and are highly infectious (Figure 16-5). These need to be distinguished from condylomata acuminata or human papillomavirus infections. Mucous

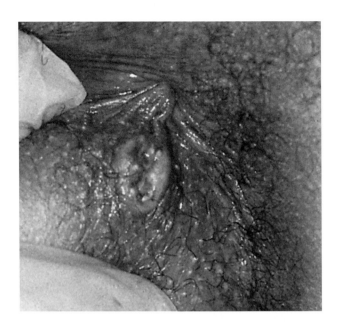

FIG. 16-4   Chancre of primary syphilis near the anus in a woman who had practiced receptive anal intercourse. (From Mandell GL, Rein MF. Atlas of Infectious Diseases. Volume 5. Sexually Transmitted Diseases. Philadelphia: Churchill Livingstone; 1996.)

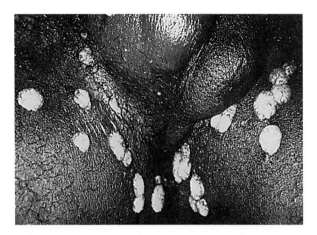

FIG. 16-5   Condylomata lata of secondary syphilis in the scrotal region. These lesions are highly contagious because of the presence of numerous spirochetes. (From Mandell GL, Rein MF. Atlas of Infectious Diseases. Volume 5. Sexually Transmitted Diseases. Philadelphia: Churchill Livingstone; 1996.)

patches are shallow, painless ulcerations that can be found on the oral or anorectal mucosa.

Latent Syphilis. Latent syphilis is defined by reactive serologic tests in the absence of clinical signs or symptoms. After resolution of early (primary or secondary) syphilis, mucocutaneous lesions can recur for up to 1 to 2 years in 25% of patients. Early latent syphilis is defined as a 1-year period after the suspected exposure when the patient is still at risk for relapse of the manifestations of secondary syphilis. Late latent syphilis is defined as a time period of a year or more after the primary infection and before the onset of tertiary syphilis. Late latent syphilis may follow the "rule of thirds," in which one third of patients may revert to a negative rapid plasma reagin (RPR) card test and a positive fluorescent treponemal antibody absorption (FTA-ABS) test with no clinical manifestations, one third may retain a positive RPR and a positive FTA-ABS test with no clinical manifestations, and one third may progress to tertiary syphilis with positive serologic tests (Figure 16-3). Syphilis of unknown duration is used to define patients with serologic evidence of syphilis but no history of prior exposure, disease, or treatment to determine the stage of disease.

Tertiary Syphilis. Tertiary syphilis or late syphilis can occur after primary, secondary, or latent syphilis. In the preantibiotic era, tertiary syphilis developed in 25% to 40% of patients with syphilis. The presentation of tertiary syphilis may include cardiovascular manifestations, gummatous lesions, and CNS disease. Cardiovascular manifestations include aortic aneurysms, aortic insufficiency, and coronary stenosis. Gummatous lesions are focal inflammatory areas that can involve any organ but usually involve the skin and bones. Neurologic disease during the tertiary stage includes general paresis and tabes dorsalis (discussed later in the chapter).

Neurosyphilis. The CNS can be infected by the treponemes at any time during the course of syphilitic infection. In 15% to 40% of patients with untreated primary and secondary syphilis, *T. pallidum* was found in the cerebrospinal fluid (CSF) by animal inoculation studies. Treponemal invasion of the CNS during untreated early syphilis may have the following outcomes: spontaneous resolution, asymptomatic neurosyphilis (at any time during syphilitic infection), acute syphilitic meningitis (in the first year), meningovascular syphilis (5 to 12 years after primary infection), and parenchymatous neurosyphilis (18 to 25 years after primary infection).

Acute syphilitic meningitis may occur with headache, nausea, vomiting, stiff neck, cranial nerve palsies, sensorineural hearing loss, and tinnitus. Meningovascular syphilis can lead to hemiparesis, hemiplegia, aphasia, and seizures caused by cerebral infarctions from syphilitic endarteritis. The manifestations of parenchymatous syphilis include general paresis, tabes dorsalis, and CNS gumma. General paresis results from meningoencephalitis, which can lead to seizures, memory loss, personality changes, emotional lability, paranoia, defective judgment, and lack of insight. Tabes dorsalis is characterized by lightning pains in the lower extremities, ataxia, bowel and bladder incontinence, impaired vibratory and position sense, impaired touch and pain sensation, Charcot's joints, and absence of ankle and knee jerks. Pupillary changes such as the Argyll Robertson pupil (fixed, small pupils that are unable to react to light but are able to react to accommodation) can occur in both general paresis and tabes dorsalis.

Diagnosis
Primary Syphilis
The definitive diagnosis of primary syphilis is based on visualization of treponemes by dark-field microscopy (Figure 16-6) or

by direct immunofluorescence. The yield of these tests is high provided that the patient has had no prior topical or systemic antibiotic treatment and that the examination is done by an experienced person. To obtain a specimen, the practitioner can gently abrade the lesion with gauze. The serous exudate is then applied to a glass slide. Direct or indirect immunofluorescence is recommended for oral lesions because nonpathogenic treponemes may be confused with *T. pallidum* on dark-field microscopy.

Serologic tests are the most widely used tests for syphilis and are categorized into treponemal and nontreponemal tests. The nontreponemal tests detect anticardiolipin antibodies and include the RPR card test, toluidine red unheated serum test (TRUST), reagin screen test (RST), Venereal Disease Research Laboratory (VDRL) test, and unheated serum reagin (USR) test. The sensitivity of the nontreponemal tests varies from 70% in primary syphilis to 100% in secondary syphilis (Table 16-2). These tests have the advantages that they are inexpensive and applicable for screening purposes and their titers tend to correlate with disease activity. However, confirmation of the nontreponemal tests is necessary with the specific treponemal tests. The FTA-ABS, microhemagglutination–*Treponema pallidum* assay (MHA-TP), and *Treponema pallidum*–particle agglutination assay (TP-PA) are 80% to 100% sensitive, depending on the stage of disease. However, a positive MHA-TP alone does not establish the diagnosis of primary syphilis in a patient with a genital ulcer because the MHA-TP can remain positive for life. Patients with suspected primary syphilis but with a negative dark-field examination, RPR, and MHA-TP should have follow-up serologic tests in 2 weeks because detection by direct microscopy depends on specimen collection and the expertise of the microscopist and serologic tests can be negative in the first 2 weeks after a chancre appears. False-positive nontreponemal and treponemal tests can occur in a variety of conditions, including acute viral infections, autoimmune diseases, vaccination, drug addiction, and malignancy.

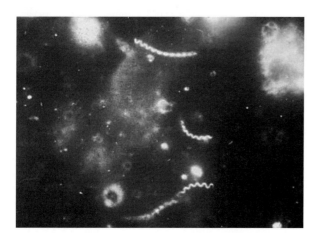

FIG. 16-6 *Treponema pallidum* spirochetes on dark-field examination. (From Centers for Disease Control and Prevention.)

TABLE 16-2
Sensitivity and Specificity of Serologic Tests for Untreated Syphilis, by Stage of the Disease

	SENSITIVITY BY STAGE OF SYPHILIS (%)				
	Primary	Secondary*	Latent	Late	Specificity: all stages (%)
NONTREPONEMAL TESTS†					
VDRL	74-87	100	88-100	37-94	96-99
RPR	77-100	100	95-100	73	99
USR	72-88	100	88-100	N/A	99
TRUST	77-100	100	95-100	N/A	98-99
TREPONEMAL TESTS‡					
FTA-ABS	70-100	100	100	96	94-100
MHA-TP	69-90	100	97-100	94	98-100
TP-PA	N/A†				

FTA-ABS, Fluorescent treponemal antibody absorption test; *MHA-TP*, microhemagglutination assay for *Treponema pallidum*; *N/A*, not applicable; *RPR*, rapid plasma reagin; *TP-PA*, *Treponema pallidum*–particle agglutination assay; *TRUST*, toluidine red unheated serum test; *USR*, unheated serum reagin; *VDRL*, Venereal Disease Research Laboratory.
*Rare cases of nonreactive serologic tests have been reported in persons with human immunodeficiency virus disease and secondary syphilis.
†The sensitivity of the TP-PA is slightly lower than that of the FTA-ABS in untreated primary syphilis but compares favorably in all other stages.

Secondary Syphilis

Treponemes can be differentiated from secondary syphilis skin lesions by dark-field examination. However, the RPR is 99% sensitive and MHA-TP is 100% sensitive. Thus a negative RPR or MHA-TP in a patient with rash essentially rules out secondary syphilis.

Latent and Tertiary Syphilis

Latent syphilis is diagnosed when a patient has a reactive RPR and confirmatory test in the absence of signs or symptoms. The duration of the disease from exposure can be estimated if the patient can recall specific signs or symptoms consistent with primary syphilis and has a history of exposure or previous positive serologic tests. However, the usual scenario is that of a patient with positive serologic findings and no clinical history suggestive of syphilis. Syphilis of unknown duration is the designation used for patients with serologic evidence of syphilis and no clinical history to determine the stage of syphilis. Tertiary syphilis is diagnosed when syphilitic gumma, cardiovascular disease, or neurologic disease is noted.

Neurosyphilis

The diagnosis of neurosyphilis is based on history, physical examination, serologic testing, and CSF examination. Although the sensitivity of the CSF VDRL varies widely (from 30% to 70%), a reactive CSF VDRL is highly specific for neurosyphilis unless the specimen is contaminated with blood. Although analysis of CSF with the FTA-ABS or the MHA-TP is not widely accepted, a negative FTA-ABS test of the CSF may help to eliminate the diagnosis of neurosyphilis. Other CSF findings include pleocytosis (10 to 100 white blood cells [WBCs]/mm^3 with predominance of lymphocytes) and an elevated protein level of 50 to 100 mg/dL.

The diagnosis of asymptomatic neurosyphilis, which can occur during both early and late syphilis, can be challenging. In a patient with positive serum treponemal and nontreponemal tests and CSF pleocytosis and a negative CSF VDRL, it is difficult to distinguish between a false-negative CSF VDRL and other causes of CSF pleocytosis. Patients with HIV infection pose a special problem in diagnosis because they have many other causes of CSF pleocytosis. Some clinicians opt for treatment of all patients with CSF pleocytosis and serologic evidence of syphilis, and others base treatment on high serologic titers and any signs and symptoms suggestive of neurosyphilis. Whether elderly patients with low-titer RPR (<1:2) should routinely undergo lumbar puncture for evaluation of neurosyphilis has not been determined.

Natural History
Expected Outcome

The syphilitic chancre heals within 3 to 6 weeks without treatment. Secondary syphilis leads to latent syphilis in approximately one third of untreated patients. In the early latent period (i.e., the first year), 25% of the patients may have reactivation of the skin lesions of secondary syphilis. Approximately 70% of untreated patients continue with lifelong latency, and 30% will have manifestations of tertiary syphilis as discussed previously.

Treatment
Methods

Treatment of syphilis depends on the stage (Table 16-3). Parenteral penicillin G is the mainstay of therapy for all stages. Doxycycline is the recommended alternative for penicillin-allergic patients. Recent evidence suggests that azithromycin may be an alternative to penicillin for early syphilis; it is undergoing clinical trials. Pregnant women or patients with neurosyphilis who are allergic to penicillin should be desensitized. All patients with syphilis should be tested for HIV. Patients with syphilis and their sex partners must be managed in conjunction with the health department. Recent (within the past 90 days) sex partners of patients with early syphilis should receive 2.4 million units of benzathine penicillin regardless of their serologic results.

Patients with latent syphilis should undergo CSF evaluation if there are neurologic, auditory, ophthalmic (iritis, uveitis), or cardiovascular signs (aortitis); treatment failure; HIV infection; or a nontreponemal titer >1:32. Patients with tertiary syphilis should undergo therapy with benzathine penicillin 2.4 million units IM each week for 3 weeks, as for late latent syphilis.

Patients with neurosyphilis who are allergic to penicillin should be desensitized. If aqueous penicillin G is not available, procaine penicillin IM should be considered. If the patient is unable to tolerate the intramuscular shots, alternative therapy with ceftriaxone 2 g IV for 10 to 14 days may be considered.

Expected Response

The nontreponemal titers should decrease four-fold (for example, from 1:32 to 1:8) within 6 months of therapy for primary and secondary syphilis. If this does not occur, treatment failure or reinfection may be assumed. In cases of treatment failure the following should be done: recheck HIV status, consider evaluation of CSF and treat accordingly, and treat again with weekly intramuscular doses of benzathine penicillin for 3 weeks. The decrease in titer after treatment for late syphilis may be slower than for primary syphilis. In cases of reinfection a repeat course of intramuscular benzathine penicillin should be administered. HIV-infected patients with primary and secondary syphilis may have a higher risk of serologic failure at 6 months and a slower decline in RPR titer than non–HIV-infected patients. They may need closer clinical and serologic follow-up at 3, 6, 9, 12, and 24 months.

Complications

Immediate hypersensitivity reaction (hives, respiratory distress, and anaphylactic shock) can occur to penicillin. This should be distinguished from the Jarisch-Herxheimer reaction, an acute febrile reaction characterized by headache, myalgias, tender lymphadenopathy, and pharyngitis. The Jarisch-Herxheimer reaction occurs within 2 to 8 hours after antimicrobial therapy for syphilis, especially during the primary and secondary stages. It may be treated with acetaminophen, but preventive measures are not known.

When to Refer

Patients with suspected neurosyphilis or tertiary syphilis and those who do not respond to treatment should be referred to an expert. Pregnant patients and HIV-infected patients may require consultation with an expert. All cases of syphilis must be reported to the local health department.

TABLE 16-3
Treatment Regimens for Syphilis

Stage of syphilis	Treatment	Follow-up	Expected response
Primary or secondary syphilis	Benzathine penicillin G 2.4 million units IM as one dose Penicillin-allergic patients: doxycycline 100 mg PO b.i.d. for 14 days *or* tetracycline 500 mg PO q.i.d. for 14 days	Repeat nontreponemal tests (e.g., RPR or VDRL) at 6 and 12 months	Four-fold decline in nontreponemal titer within 6 months (e.g., 1:32 to 1:8)
Early latent syphilis	Benzathine penicillin G 2.4 million units IM as one dose Penicillin-allergic patients: same as for primary syphilis	Repeat nontreponemal tests at 6 and 12 months	Four-fold decline in titer at 12 months
Late latent syphilis	Benzathine penicillin G 2.4 million units IM each week for 3 weeks Penicillin-allergic patients: doxycycline 100 mg PO b.i.d. for 4 weeks or tetracycline 500 mg PO q.i.d. for 28 days	Repeat nontreponemal tests at 6, 12, 24 months	Expect more gradual decline; 50% remain RPR positive at 2 years; reevaluate if a four-fold increase in titer occurs, if a titer >1:32 fails to decline at least four-fold within 1 to 2 years, or if signs or symptoms of syphilis occur
Neurosyphilis	Aqueous penicillin G, 3 to 4 million units IV q4h* *or* procaine penicillin 2 to 4 million units IM daily *plus* probenecid 500 mg PO q.i.d. for 10 to 14 days; both regimens followed by 2.4 million units of benzathine penicillin IM as one dose Penicillin-allergic patients: desensitize†	Repeat clinical examination and serum nontreponemal tests at 3, 6, and 12 months; repeat CSF examination every 6 months until cell count is normal	Cerebrospinal fluid serologic tests may remain positive for more than one year; pleocytosis resolves before the fall in CSF protein concentration

*Aqueous penicillin G can also be given by continuous IV infusion (18 to 24 million units per day). The dose should be adjusted in patients with renal failure to avoid neurotoxicity (see Chapter 19).
†"Desensitization" to penicillin G involves increasing the dose by small increments under close observation and should nearly always be carried out in the hospital setting.

 KEY POINTS

SYPHILIS

⊃ Syphilis is a systemic illness caused by *T. pallidum*. It has primary, secondary, latent, and tertiary stages.
⊃ Primary syphilis should be suspected in patients seeking treatment for genital ulcers.
⊃ The classic presentation of primary syphilis is a painless, indurated ulcer with a clean base (hard chancre). Direct visualization of spirochetes can be performed by dark-field examination or direct immunofluorescence.
⊃ Secondary syphilis is the only stage of the disease in which nontreponemal serologic tests such as the RPR and VDRL are nearly 100% sensitive.
⊃ Secondary syphilis should be suspected in patients with unexplained skin rash, aseptic meningitis, glomerulonephritis, or systemic illness with combinations of lymphadenopathy, fever, headache, sore throat, and arthralgias.

⊃ Patients with latent syphilis (reactive serologic tests without symptoms) follow one of three courses in roughly equal numbers: reversion to a nonreactive RPR (VDRL); persistence of a reactive RPR but without clinical manifestations; and tertiary syphilis manifested as neurosyphilis, cardiovascular syphilis, or gummas.
⊃ Penicillin G is the mainstay of treatment for all forms of syphilis.
⊃ Patients with syphilis should be reported to the health department for management of sexual partners, and treated patients should have follow-up serologic testing to ensure adequate response to treatment.

SUGGESTED READING

Blocker ME, Levine WC, St. Louis ME. HIV prevalence in patients with syphilis, United States. Sex Transm Dis 2000; 27: 53-59.
Hook EW, Marra CM. Acquired syphilis in adults. N Engl J Med 1992; 326: 1060-1069.

Larsen SA, Steiner BM, Rudolph AH. Laboratory diagnosis and interpretation of tests for syphilis. Clin Microbiol Rev 1995; 8: 1-21.

Rolfs RT, Joesoef MR, Hendershot EF, et al. A randomized trial of enhanced therapy for early syphilis in patients with and without human immunodeficiency virus infection. N Engl J Med 1997; 337: 307-314.

Singh AE, Romanowski B. Syphilis: review with emphasis on clinical, epidemiologic, and some biologic features. Clin Microbiol Rev 1999; 12: 187-209.

Chancroid

The incidence of chancroid has been steadily decreasing in the United States. The disease is endemic in some areas (New York City and Texas) and tends to occur as outbreaks in other parts of the United States. Chancroid is a major cause of genital ulcer diseases in the tropics.

Presentation and Progression
Cause

H. ducreyi is a gram-negative rod that requires abraded skin to penetrate the epidermis and cause infection. It is spread by sexual contact, but autoinoculation of other sites can occur.

Presentation

After an incubation period of 3 to 10 days, a papule surrounded by erythema develops at the site of inoculation. The papule evolves to a pustule over 24 to 48 hours and then ulcerates (Table 16-1). Men tend to have significant pain with the ulcer, whereas women may not notice the ulcer. About 50% of patients note tender unilateral inguinal adenopathy (buboes). Buboes can become fluctuant, undergo spontaneous drainage, and result in large ulcers. Systemic symptoms are usually not a feature of chancroid.

Diagnosis

Chancroid is a clinical diagnosis based on a tender, painful ulcer with ragged borders; tender lymphadenopathy; a negative dark-field examination of the ulcer for *T. pallidum* (or a negative serologic test for syphilis performed at least 7 days after onset of the ulcer); and a negative test for HSV. The presence of a painful ulcer along with tender lymphadenopathy and suppuration is highly indicative of chancroid. A definitive diagnosis is based on culture of *H. ducreyi,* but appropriate culture media are not widely available. Cotton or calcium alginate swabs can be used to swab the base of the ulcer; these require transport in a special medium. Culture of the bubo pus is usually sterile. Patients should be tested for HIV at the time of diagnosis of chancroid; HIV testing should be repeated 3 months later if initially negative.

Natural History
Expected Outcome

Untreated ulcers from *H. ducreyi* can persist for a long time. Complete resolution of ulcers after therapy does not afford protection from future outbreaks.

Treatment
Methods

Antimicrobial therapy is the mainstay of treatment. Options consist of azithromycin 1 g PO as a single dose; ceftriaxone 250 mg IM as a single dose; ciprofloxacin 500 mg PO b.i.d.

for 3 days (contraindicated in persons <18 years of age and in pregnant or lactating women); and erythromycin base 500 mg PO q.i.d for 7 days. Patients with fluctuant lymph nodes >5 cm require aspiration for resolution of symptoms. Sex partners of patients with chancroid should be treated regardless of the symptoms if the contact occurred 10 days before the onset of symptoms in the index case.

Expected Response

Cure rates for chancroid treated with appropriate regimens range from 87% to 100%. Patients should be reexamined in 3 to 7 days for resolution of symptoms. Most ulcers resolve in 7 days, although larger ones may take up to 2 weeks. If treatment seems to have failed, coinfection with *T. pallidum* or HSV should be considered. HIV-infected persons and uncircumcised men may not respond well to therapy and need close follow-up.

Complications

Antimicrobials used for the treatment of chancroid are well tolerated. Patients receiving azithromycin or erythromycin may have nausea.

When to Refer

Patients with large inguinal nodes may be referred for incision and drainage.

 KEY POINTS

CHANCROID

- Chancroid is a genital ulcer disease that must be differentiated from syphilis and genital herpes simplex.
- Diagnosis is based on clinical examination, which reveals a tender ulcer with ragged, undermined edges and a base covered with a gray, necrotic exudate that frequently bleeds on scraping.
- Definitive diagnosis can be based on isolation of *H. ducreyi,* but the media are not widely available.
- Syphilis and HSV infection should be excluded in every case, and HIV serologic tests should be performed.
- Treatment with appropriate regimens is usually curative.

SUGGESTED READING

Ronald AR, Albritton W. Chancroid and *Haemophilus ducreyi.* In: Holmes KK, Mardh PA, Sparling PF, et al, eds. Sexually Transmitted Diseases. 3rd ed., New York: McGraw-Hill; 1999: 515-523.

Schmid GP. Treatment of chancroid, 1997. Clin Infect Dis 1999; 28 (Suppl 1): S14-S20.

Seña AC, Behets F M-T, Fox KK, Cohen MS. Sexually Transmitted Diseases. In: Guerrant RL, Walker DH, Weller PF, eds. Tropical Infectious Diseases: Principles, Pathogens, and Practice. Philadelphia: Churchill Livingstone; 1999: 1569-1585.

Urethritis in Women: Overview

The symptoms of urethritis in women consist of dysuria, urinary frequency, and lower abdominal pain. Dysuria may be classified as internal or external dysuria (caused by contact of urine with inflamed perineum). Women with urethritis may also have concomitant cervicitis and vaginitis. Urethritis should be differentiated from acute cystitis, which is associated with abrupt onset of dysuria accompanied by frequency and urgency of urination, suprapubic tenderness, or low back pain. Acute cystitis may also be complicated by pyelonephritis, which is associated with fever and costovertebral angle tenderness (see Chapter 14).

Urethritis is most commonly caused by *N. gonorrhoeae, C. trachomatis,* and HSV. Cystitis is most commonly caused by *Escherichia coli.* Among women who seek treatment for dysuria and urinary frequency, urethritis caused by STDs should be considered along with bacterial urinary tract infections (Figure 16-7). A history of sexual activity can predispose to either disease, but a detailed history regarding risk factors for STDs may assist in the differential diagnosis. In patients with STD, urinalysis may reveal pyuria and a positive leukocyte esterase level caused by urethral inflammation from an STD. Urinalysis for a patient with cystitis should have accompanying nitrite or blood tests and a positive urine culture with ≥100 colony-forming units/mL of urogenital pathogens. Additional information can be obtained by appropriate STD screening and urine microscopy.

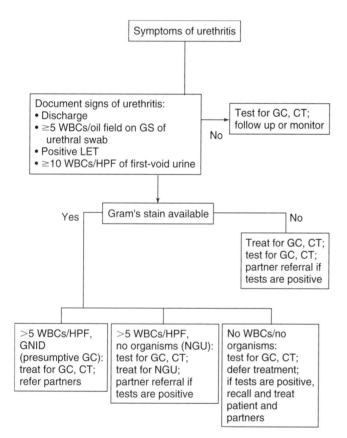

FIG. 16-7 Algorithm for the diagnosis and management of urethritis. *CT, Chlamydia trachomatis; GC,* gonococci; *GNID,* gram-negative intracellular diplococci; *GS,* Gram stain; *HPF,* per high-power field; *LET,* leukocyte esterase test; *NGU,* nongonococcal urethritis. (Modified from Burstein GR, Zenilman JM. Nongonococcal urethritis: a new paradigm. Clin Infect Dis 1999; 28 [Suppl 1]: S66-S73.)

Vaginal Discharge (Vaginitis): Overview

Vaginal discharge is a frequent gynecologic complaint, accounting for more than 10 million office visits annually (see also Chapter 5). Physiologic vaginal discharge is white and odorless and increases during midcycle because of estrogen. Abnormal vaginal discharge may result from vaginitis or vaginosis, cervicitis, and occasionally endometritis. Vaginitis manifests itself as an increase in the amount, odor, or color of discharge and may be accompanied by itching, dysuria, dyspareunia, edema, or irritation of the vulva. The three most common causes of vaginal discharge are bacterial vaginosis (BV) (40% to 50% of cases), vulvovaginal candidiasis (20% to 25% of cases), and trichomoniasis (15% to 20% of cases). Although trichomoniasis is an STD, bacterial vaginosis occurs both in women with high rates of STDs and in women who have never been sexually active. Vaginitis may also result from infection with group A streptococci, *Staphylococcus aureus* toxic shock syndrome, and severe HSV infection. Noninfectious causes of vaginal discharge include chemical or irritant vaginitis, trauma, pemphigus, collagen-vascular diseases, and Behçet's disease. Vaginal discharge may result from cervicitis caused by *N. gonorrhoeae* and *C. trachomatis* (see sections on gonorrhea and chlamydia). Severe genital herpes infection can cause both cervicitis and vaginitis.

A patient's history and physical examination findings alone are not sufficient for accurate diagnosis of the etiology of vaginitis. The simple office-based tests (wet mount preparation, pH measure, and potassium hydroxide [KOH] preparation) are valuable tools, but they are underused for the diagnosis of vaginitis (Figure 16-8). An algorithmic approach to the patient

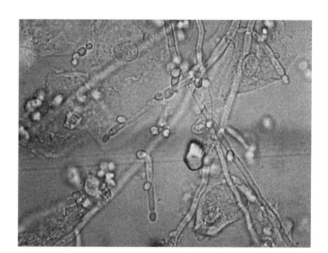

FIG. 16-8 Saline microscopy of vaginal secretions (wet prep), low-power magnification. The most common method is to obtain a swab specimen of secretions from the middle third of the vagina. The specimen is immediately placed in a test tube containing 0.5 mL of saline, from which a single drop is then placed on a clean glass slide and a coverslip applied. Hyphae (shown here), polymorphonuclear neutrophils, and motile trichomonads can be identified under low-power magnification. High-power magnification is then used to identify clue cells (see Figure 16-10). (From Mandell GL, Bleck TP, Brook I, et al., eds. Essential Atlas of Infectious Diseases for Primary Care. Philadelphia: Churchill Livingstone; 1997.)

with vaginal discharge can be based largely on observations made during a thorough pelvic examination (Figure 16-9).

Candida Vulvovaginitis

Vulvovaginal candidiasis (VVC) is not considered an STD in the traditional sense, but it is discussed in this chapter because it is frequently diagnosed in women with abnormal vaginal discharge. By age 25 half of all college women have had at least one episode of *Candida* vaginitis. In some studies up to 75% of premenopausal women have had at least one episode of VVC. Increased risk of vaginal candidiasis is associated with use of vaginal sponges, intrauterine devices, oral contraceptives with high levels of estrogens, and antibiotics, as well as with uncontrolled diabetes mellitus.

Presentation and Progression
Cause

Candida albicans causes 80% to 92% of cases of acute VVC. Uncomplicated episodes are primarily due to *C. albicans* and respond quickly to short-term antifungal therapy. Increased frequency of other *Candida* species (especially *C. glabrata*) is being reported, especially in complicated episodes. This may be due to inappropriate use of over-the-counter antifungal agents or short-term courses of topical and oral agents.

Presentation

The symptoms of VVC include acute vulvar pruritus and vaginal discharge that may appear white and curdlike or as a thin, watery liquid. Other symptoms include vaginal soreness, external dysuria, and dyspareunia. However, none of these symptoms are specific for the diagnosis.

Vulvovaginal candidiasis can be classified as uncomplicated (acute, sporadic, or nonrecurrent) and complicated (severe local or recurrent disease in an abnormal host or disease caused by *C. glabrata*). Uncomplicated episodes represent those caused by *C. albicans* and those that quickly respond to short-term antifungal therapy. Recurrent VVC is defined as four or more episodes per year unrelated to antibiotic use. Recurrent disease is more common in women with uncontrolled diabetes and immunosuppression, including HIV infection, but a majority of women with recurrent disease have no specific risk factors. Candidiasis recurs in 5% of healthy women.

Diagnosis

A clinical diagnosis of candidal vulvovaginitis is based on the presence of erythema and a white curdlike discharge. Self-diagnosis of VVC is only about 50% accurate. Supporting laboratory findings include the finding of yeasts or pseudo-hyphae in a wet mount or Gram stain of vaginal discharge, or a positive culture for yeast. The pH of the vaginal discharge is normal ($\leq$4.5) in vulvovaginal candidiasis. The addition of 10% KOH to the wet mount preparation increases the visualization of yeast and hyphae by destroying other cellular material. About 10% to 20% of healthy women harbor *Candida* species and other yeasts in the vagina, and therefore a positive culture for *Candida* should not prompt treatment in asymptomatic women. Patients with recurrent VVC should

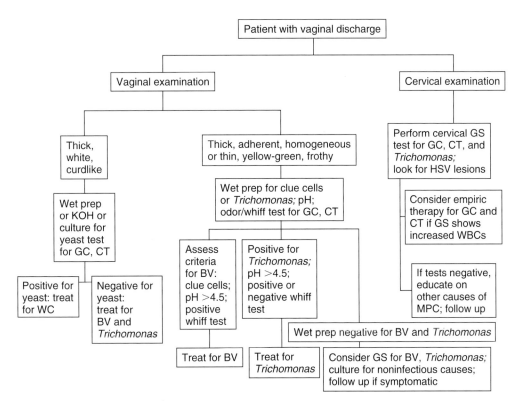

FIG. 16-9 Algorithm for management of vaginal discharge. *BV*, Bacterial vaginosis; *CT*, *Chlamydia trachomatis*; *GC*, gonococci; *GS*, Gram stain; *HSV*, herpes simplex virus; *KOH*, potassium hydroxide preparation; *MPC*, mucopurulent cervicitis; *VVC*, vulvovaginal candidiasis.

BOX 16-3
Treatment of Candida Vulvovaginitis

UNCOMPLICATED CANDIDA VULVOVAGINITIS
- Fluconazole is given as 150 mg PO in a single dose. Women with severe infection may need more than one dose of oral fluconazole.
- Intravaginal agents (creams, ointments or suppositories) such as butoconazole,* clotrimazole,* miconazole,* tioconazole,* or terconazole are administered for 3 to 7 days based on the product recommendations.

COMPLICATED VULVOVAGINAL CANDIDIASIS
Severe Candida Vulvovaginitis
- A 7-day course of topical azole therapy is superior to single-dose fluconazole therapy.
- A second dose of 150 mg of fluconazole 72 hours after the initial dose may be more clinically effective than a single dose.

Recurrent Vulvovaginal Candidiasis
- Initial intensive regimen is topical or oral agents for 10 to 14 days.
- Maintenance therapy with fluconazole 100 to 150 mg per week, ketoconazole 100 mg per day, itraconazole 400 mg monthly, or clotrimazole 500-mg vaginal suppositories once a week for 6 months. Some women have recurrences after stopping maintenance therapy.
- Non-*albicans* VVC may be treated with longer duration of azoles (7 to 14 days) or 600 mg of boric acid as intravaginal capsules for 14 days.

---

*Butoconazole, clotrimazole, and miconazole creams and tioconazole ointment are available over the counter.

---

have a vaginal culture for yeast to confirm the diagnosis and identify unusual species. Women with VVC may also harbor other STDs and must therefore be screened in high-risk cases.

Treatment
Methods

Nystatin (one 100,000-unit tablet inserted into the vagina for 14 days) has been largely replaced by the newer azole compounds, which are more convenient (Box 16-3). Cure rates with nystatin and the azole compounds are roughly comparable. Pregnant women should be treated with a 7-day course of the topical azoles, such as miconazole (see Chapter 5). The treatment of VVC in HIV-infected individuals is the same as for noninfected persons.

Expected Response

The overall efficacy of the azole agents ranges from 80% to 90%. Self-medication with topical azoles should be recommended only for women who have been previously diagnosed with vulvovaginal candidiasis and have recurrence of the same symptoms. About 3% to 10% of male sexual partners have *Candida* balanitis, and these men should also be treated. Recurrence is unfortunately common. Most studies indicate that recurrence is not to be attributed to resistance to antifungal drugs. There is no evidence to support that the ingestion of yogurt containing live *Lactobacillus acidophilus* reduces recurrence rates of *Candida* vaginitis.

Complications

The topical azoles are usually well tolerated except for occasional cases of burning and irritation of the vagina. Oral ketoconazole and itraconazole may be associated with systemic complications. The oral azoles have significant potential for drug interactions (see Chapter 21).

When to Refer

Recurrent candidal vulvovaginitis can be frustrating, and selected patients may benefit from referral to an infectious disease specialist.

 KEY POINTS

CANDIDA VULVOVAGINITIS

- *Candida* vulvovaginitis is a common disease, occurring in up to 75% of premenopausal women.
- *C. albicans* causes 80% or more of cases. The frequency of other species, such as *C. glabrata*, seems to be increasing, possibly because of inappropriate use of over-the-counter antifungal drugs.
- The diagnosis is made clinically by the presence of erythema and a white curdlike discharge and is supported by the demonstration of yeasts by wet mount, Gram stain, and culture.
- Between 10% and 20% of women harbor *Candida* as part of the normal vaginal flora. Treatment is unnecessary for healthy, asymptomatic persons.
- Underlying diabetes mellitus and immunosuppression should be considered in patients with recurrent vulvovaginal candidiasis and no obvious precipitating factors.
- About 3% to 10% of male sex partners have *Candida* balanitis and should be treated.

SUGGESTED READING
Nyirjesy P. Chronic vulvovaginal candidiasis. Am Fam Physician 2001; 63: 697-702.
Reef SE, Levine WC, McNeil MM, et al. Treatment options for vulvovaginal candidiasis, 1993. Clin Infect Dis 1995; 20 (Suppl 1): S80-S90.
Sobel JD. Vaginitis. N Engl J Med 1997; 337: 1896-1903.
Sobel JD, Faro S, Force RW, et al. Vulvovaginal candidiasis: epidemiologic, diagnostic, and therapeutic considerations. Am J Obstet Gynecol 1998; 178: 203-211.

Bacterial Vaginosis

BV is the most common cause of vaginitis in women of reproductive age. The prevalence varies among clinical settings: 17% to 19% in family planning or student health clinics, 24% to 37% in STD clinics, and 10% to 29% among pregnant women. The risk factors associated with BV include multiple sexual partners, intrauterine device use, nonwhite race, douching, and prior pregnancy. The specific causative agent of BV is unclear, and whether BV is a sexually transmitted infection remains incompletely understood. The prevalence of BV in women who have never been sexually active is very low.

BOX 16-4
Clinical Criteria for Diagnosis of Bacterial Vaginosis

Three of the following four criteria must be met to diagnose bacterial vaginosis:
- Homogeneous discharge that smoothly coats the vaginal walls
- Clue cells on wet mount examination
- pH greater than 4.5
- Fishy odor with or without the addition of potassium hydroxide (the whiff test)

Presentation and Progression
Cause

BV results from replacement of the normal *Lactobacillus* species of the vagina with anaerobes (*Prevotella* and *Mobiluncus* species), *Gardnerella vaginalis,* and *Mycoplasma hominis.* Which organism is the specific etiologic agent of BV is unclear, and the pathogenesis is incompletely understood. In the "normal vagina," hydrogen peroxide–producing lactobacilli predominate and are thought to suppress the BV-associated organisms. One viewpoint is that BV is a synergistic infection involving mainly *G. vaginalis* and anaerobes, hence the synonym "anaerobic vaginosis."

Presentation

Women with BV may have a malodorous ("fishy-smelling") vaginal discharge, but many women are asymptomatic. The vaginal discharge is grayish or white, homogeneous, and uniformly adherent to the vaginal walls. It may contain small bubbles. Inflammation and pruritus are not present. BV does not result in an inflammatory discharge. Thus the disease is usually milder than vaginal candidiasis and trichomoniasis.

Diagnosis

BV is diagnosed on the basis of clinical and Gram stain criteria (Box 16-4). The presence of clue cells (epithelial cells with obscured borders because of adherent bacteria) is the best predictor of BV (Figure 16-10). The Gram stain criterion has a sensitivity of 86% to 89% and a specificity of 94% to 96%. A scoring system of 0 to 10 points is based on the most important bacterial morphotypes—lactobacilli, *G. vaginalis,* and *Mobiluncus* species—for which high interobserver variability has been shown. Vaginal culture is not recommended for the diagnosis of BV. The vaginal pH is >4.5 in about 90% of patients. Addition of 10% of 20% KOH to the vaginal discharge (either on the speculum blade or on a glass slide) generates a typical pungent or fishy odor. This procedure, known as the whiff test, is about 70% sensitive for BV but is not entirely specific because positive test results sometimes occur in trichomoniasis.

Natural History
Expected Outcome

The diagnosis of bacterial vaginosis in pregnancy has adverse outcomes. Bacterial vaginosis is associated with premature rupture of membranes, preterm labor and birth, low birth weight, chorioamnionitis, and postcesarean and postpartum

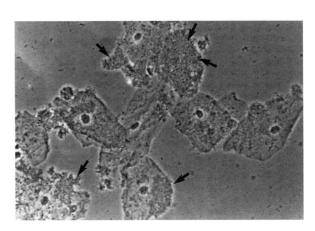

FIG. 16-10   Clue cells in bacterial vaginosis (*arrows*), demonstrated by examination of a wet mount preparation of vaginal fluid under high-power microscopy (×400). A clue cell is a squamous epithelial cell with indistinct borders and a granular appearance caused by the attachment of various aerobic and anaerobic bacteria. A clue cell–positive specimen is defined by the presence of at least one clue cell per five squamous epithelial cells. (From Mandell GL, Bleck TP, Brook I, et al., eds. Essential Atlas of Infectious Diseases for Primary Care. Philadelphia: Churchill Livingstone; 1997.)

BOX 16-5
Recommended Treatment Regimens for Bacterial Vaginosis

STANDARD REGIMENS
- Metronidazole 500 mg PO b.i.d. for 7 days *or*
- Clindamycin cream 2%, 5 g (one full applicator) intravaginally at bedtime for 7 days (clindamycin cream is oil based and may weaken condoms) *or*
- Metronidazole gel 0.75%, 5 g (one full applicator) at bedtime for 7 days

ALTERNATIVE REGIMENS
- Metronidazole 2 g PO in a single dose *or* clindamycin 300 mg PO b.i.d. for 7 days. The single-dose regimen of metronidazole is less efficacious than the 7-day regimen (the Food and Drug Administration has approved Flagyl ER 750 mg PO daily for 7 days).

endometritis. Bacterial pathogens associated with bacterial vaginosis have been known to cause upper genital tract disease, including PID (see later discussion).

Treatment
Methods

In nonpregnant women topical metronidazole or clindamycin regimens are as efficacious as the oral regimens (Box 16-5). Asymptomatic women who may undergo abortion benefit from screening and treatment of BV to reduce the risk of endometritis. The treatment of women undergoing invasive gynecologic procedures with antimicrobial agents that cover anaerobes leads to decreased postsurgical infections.

Universal screening of asymptomatic pregnant women at low risk (i.e., women with no history of premature delivery) is not recommended. Women at high risk of preterm delivery should be screened during the earliest part of the second trimester and, if BV is found, treated with metronidazole. Topical agents are not recommended during pregnancy, but evidence is increasing that topical clindamycin may be safe and effective when used during the first trimester of pregnancy (see Chapter 5).

Expected Response

A scheduled follow-up appointment is not necessary. The cure rate of bacterial vaginosis at 4 weeks after completion of therapy ranges from 75% to 84%. Symptoms recur within 3 months in 30% percent of patients. Recurrent episodes can be treated with a 10- to 14-day course of antimicrobial agents. Alternative treatments for BV with yogurt containing lactobacilli or purified *Lactobacillus* species in suppositories have varied widely in efficacy, and their value has yet to be proved in well-controlled clinical trials.

Complications

Adverse effects of metronidazole include metallic taste, headache, dizziness, nausea, vomiting, seizures, and transient neutropenia (7.5%). Drugs that interact with metronidazole include oral anticoagulants, hydantoins, phenobarbital, and alcohol (which results in a disulfiram-like reaction). Rare cases of anaphylaxis have been reported.

 KEY POINTS

BACTERIAL VAGINOSIS

- ⟳ BV is the most common cause of vaginitis in women of reproductive age.
- ⟳ The precise pathogenesis is unclear, but it involves displacement of the normal *Lactobacillus* species in the vagina by *G. vaginalis,* anaerobic bacteria, and possibly other organisms.
- ⟳ The disease is usually milder than *Candida* vulvovaginitis and trichomoniasis.
- ⟳ A foul or "fishy" odor is a common presenting symptom.
- ⟳ Diagnosis is based on finding three of the following four criteria: characteristic discharge, clue cells on wet mount examination, pH >4.5, and fishy odor with or without the addition of KOH (whiff test).
- ⟳ Occurrence during pregnancy can have adverse consequences (see Chapter 5).

SUGGESTED READING

Hill GB. The microbiology of bacterial vaginosis. Am J Obstet Gynecol 1993; 169: 450-454.

Joesoef MR, Schmid GP, Hillier SL. Bacterial vaginosis: review of treatment options and potential clinical indications for therapy. Clin Infect Dis 1999; 28 (Suppl 1): S57-S65.

Nugent RP, Krohn MA, Hillier SL. Reliability of diagnosing bacterial vaginosis is improved by a standardized method of Gram stain interpretation. J Clin Microbiol 1991; 29: 297-301.

Seña AC, Behets F M-T, Fox KK, Cohen MS. Sexually Transmitted Diseases. In: Guerrant RL, Walker DH, Weller PF, eds. Tropical Infectious Diseases: Principles, Pathogens, and Practice. Philadelphia: Churchill Livingstone; 1999: 1569-1585.

Sobel, JD. Vaginitis. N Engl J Med 1997; 337: 1896-1903.

Trichomoniasis

Trichomoniasis is the most common nonviral STD worldwide. In the United States more than 8 million new cases are diagnosed each year. Many women and men infected with *Trichomonas* remain asymptomatic and serve as reservoirs for transmission. Transmission of *Trichomonas* is primarily by sexual contact. *Trichomonas vaginalis* has been isolated in 67% to 100% of female partners of infected men and in 14% to 60% of male partners of infected women.

Presentation and Progression
Cause

T. vaginalis is a flagellated protozoan that infects the cervical and vaginal epithelial cells and leads to vaginitis and cervicitis. It has also been isolated from the urethra, Bartholin's gland, and Skene's gland in women. In men *T. vaginalis* infection may lead to urethritis, prostatitis, balanoposthitis, and epididymitis.

Presentation

Trichomoniasis may be an acute, chronic, or asymptomatic infection. The incubation period may range from 4 to 28 days. Women with acute vaginitis may have a frothy, yellow or green, mucopurulent discharge with symptoms of pruritus, dysuria, and dyspareunia. The chronic form is characterized by scanty vaginal discharge with mild pruritus and dyspareunia. Up to 25% to 50% of infected women remain asymptomatic, but symptoms may develop within 6 months in 50% of these women.

The majority of men with *Trichomonas* infection remain asymptomatic. Men may be classified into three clinical groups: asymptomatic carriers, those with acute purulent urethritis, and those with nongonococcal urethritis.

Diagnosis

The diagnosis of *Trichomonas* vaginitis is based on clinical examination, wet mount preparation, and culture. Pelvic examination may reveal diffuse vulvitis with copious, yellow or green, frothy, purulent discharge and vaginal and vulvar erythema. Punctate hemorrhages may be noted on the vaginal wall and cervix (colpitis macularis, or "strawberry cervix"). However, the signs and symptoms associated with *Trichomonas* have very low sensitivity. Colpitis macularis is a highly specific sign, but it is noted in only 2% of women with trichomoniasis.

Trichomoniasis is diagnosed on the basis of the presence of motile trichomonads on the wet mount preparation of the vaginal discharge (Figure 16-11). A vaginal pH >4.5 and a positive whiff test following the addition of KOH may be noted in trichomoniasis and BV and thus is not specific for trichomoniasis. Wet mount preparation of vaginal discharge reveals motile trichomonads. The sensitivity of a wet mount preparation for the diagnosis of trichomoniasis ranges from 38% to 82%, and the yield is much higher with purulent vaginal fluid. Broth culture method is the "gold standard" for the diagnosis of trichomoniasis, but it is not readily available in most clinical settings. Culture has greater sensitivity (90% to 97%) than the wet mount preparation. Molecular diagnostic techniques are being developed for the diagnosis of trichomoniasis.

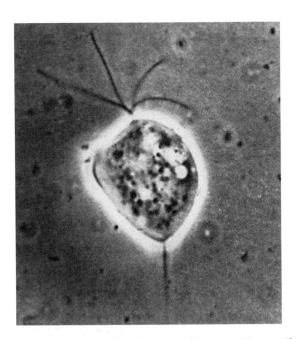

FIG. 16-11 *Trichomonas vaginalis* appears in wet mount preparations as a pear-shaped organism with four anterior flagella and a fifth (posterior) flagellum embedded in an undulating membrane. (From Mandell GL, Rein MF. Atlas of Infectious Diseases. Volume 5. Sexually Transmitted Diseases. Philadelphia: Churchill Livingstone; 1996.)

Natural History
Expected Outcome

In women trichomoniasis is associated with PID and infertility. In pregnant women trichomoniasis is associated with premature rupture of membranes, premature labor, and low birth weight infants (see Chapter 5).

Treatment (Box 16-6)
Methods

Pregnant women with trichomoniasis may be treated with the single 2-g dose of metronidazole. Sex partners of patients with trichomoniasis should be treated regardless of symptoms.

Expected Response

The cure rate of trichomoniasis with the metronidazole regimen is approximately 90% to 95%. If therapy with the single dose or the 7-day regimen fails, patients should be treated with another 7-day course. Treatment of sex partners is recommended to increase the probability of cure.

Complications

The complications of metronidazole therapy are discussed under "Bacterial Vaginosis" earlier in the chapter.

When to Refer

Some patients have refractory trichomoniasis and may not respond to repeated courses of therapy. Metronidazole-resistant trichomoniasis should be considered in such cases, and a consultation with the CDC should be obtained for determination of metronidazole susceptibility (telephone number 404-639-8371).

BOX 16-6
Treatment of Trichomoniasis

STANDARD REGIMEN
• Metronidazole 2 g PO in a single dose

ALTERNATIVE REGIMENS
• Metronidazole 500 mg PO b.i.d. for 7 days
• Flagyl 375 mg PO b.i.d. for 7 days (this drug has been approved by the Food and Drug Administration, but there are no published clinical trials)

 KEY POINTS

TRICHOMONIASIS
- Trichomoniasis is the most common STD worldwide. It may be acute, chronic, or asymptomatic.
- In women trichomoniasis has been associated with PID and infertility.
- Diagnosis can be made by finding motile trichomonads in a wet mount preparation of vaginal discharge, but the sensitivity of the wet mount is only 38% to 82%. Culture remains the "gold standard" for diagnosis.
- Trichomoniasis is associated with an elevated pH and a positive whiff test, which can also be observed in BV.
- Many women and men infected with *Trichomonas* remain asymptomatic and serve as reservoirs for transmission; thus treatment of partners is essential.
- The cure rate with metronidazole is 90% to 95%.

SUGGESTED READING
Petrin D, Delgaty K, Bhatt R, et al. Clinical and microbiological aspects of *Trichomonas vaginalis*. Clin Microbiol Rev 1998; 11: 300-317.
Wolner-Hanssen P, Krieger JN, Stevens CE, et al. Clinical manifestations of vaginal *Trichomonas*. JAMA 1989; 261: 571-576.

Cervicitis: Overview

Cervicitis (inflammation of the cervix) is a common but poorly understood condition that has been found in 32% to 45% of women attending STD clinics. Cervicitis can generally be classified as endocervicitis or ectocervicitis. Endocervicitis refers to the presence of inflammation in the columnar epithelium of the endocervical canal beyond the squamocolumnar junction. Inflammation of the cervix should be distinguished from the normal condition of the zone of ectopy (or ectropion) that results from the symmetric extension of the columnar cervical epithelium over the os and is frequently found among adolescents and women taking oral contraceptives. Cervicitis may be secondary to STDs, as well as systemic illnesses such as autoimmune diseases, Stevens-Johnson syndrome, measles, neoplasia, and mechanical or chemical trauma. In many cases the exact cause is not found.

The presence of mucopurulent cervicitis (MPC) has been used as a basis for presumptive diagnosis of chlamydial or gonococcal infection in settings where the prevalence of these infections is high and the patients are unlikely to return for follow-up. MPC is defined as the presence of a mucopurulent discharge noted from the endocervix and friability or easily induced bleeding with the first endocervical swab. Some experts further define MPC by the presence of WBCs on an endocervical Gram stain. MPC is a diagnosis of exclusion and should be made after the infectious etiologies discussed under "Cause" are ruled out.

Presentation and Progression
Cause

Endocervicitis may be caused by *N. gonorrhoeae* or *C. trachomatis.* The most common cause of ectocervicitis is *T. vaginalis.* Infection with HSV may result in both endocervicitis and ectocervicitis. MPC has been most strongly associated with *C. trachomatis* and *N. gonorrhoeae,* but 38% of cases of MPC have no identifiable pathogens.

Presentation

Cervicitis can be asymptomatic or can result in vaginal discharge, postcoital bleeding, or deep dyspareunia. Pelvic examination may reveal an increased amount of mucus, pus, or mucopus at the cervical os and easily inducible cervical bleeding (Figure 16-12). Frank ulcerations may be present on the cervix in the case of HSV infection.

Diagnosis

Microscopic examination and culture of the cervical discharge are helpful in reaching a diagnosis of the exact etiologic agent (Figure 16-9). When an endocervical specimen for Gram stain is collected, care should be taken to avoid contamination of the endocervical swab with vaginal secretions. A cervical Gram stain with >10 WBCs per high-power field has been reported to have a sensitivity of approximately 64% and specificity of 69% for chlamydial infection, depending on the prevalence of *C. trachomatis* in the population. Cervical Gram stain has limited (30% to 60%) sensitivity for

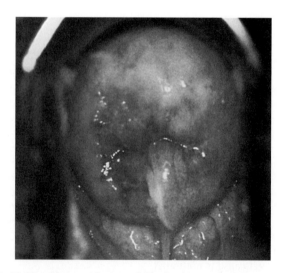

FIG. 16-12 Mucopurulent cervicitis is characterized by a yellow-green discharge from the endocervical os. This finding is highly characteristic of infection with *Chlamydia trachomatis* but also occurs in gonorrhea. (Courtesy of Dr. David E. Soper.)

N. gonorrhoeae (intracellular gram-negative diplococci), and the presence of extracellular gram-negative diplococci may represent normal genital flora. Testing for *N. gonorrhoeae, C. trachomatis,* and *T. vaginalis* should be performed and a culture for HSV collected when suspect lesions are present.

Natural History
Expected Outcome

Cervicitis may persist in women despite treatment of exact infectious causes, especially when associated with undetected systemic diseases, trauma, or other causes. The implications and management of persistent cervicitis with respect to sexually transmitted pathogens are unclear.

Treatment

Patients with cervicitis should be considered for presumptive treatment of *C. trachomatis* or *N. gonorrhoeae,* especially when the patient is at high risk or in high-prevalence settings. Otherwise, treatment should be based on laboratory testing for the etiologic agents. Management of sexual partners should be based on the suspected or detected infection in the index patient if contact occurred within the preceding 60 days.

 KEY POINTS

CERVICITIS: OVERVIEW
- Cervicitis is present in 32% to 45% of women attending STD clinics but is often poorly understood.
- Mucopurulent cervicitis can be caused by *N. gonorrhoeae, C. trachomatis, T. vaginalis,* or HSV.
- In settings where the prevalence of *N. gonorrhoeae* and *C. trachomatis* is high, empiric therapy for these pathogens is warranted.
- Management of sexual partners should be based on the suspected or detected infection in the index patient if contact occurred within the preceding 60 days.

SUGGESTED READING

Holmes KK, Stamm WE. Lower genital tract infection syndromes in women. In: Holmes KK, Mardh PA, Sparling PF, et al, eds. Sexually Transmitted Diseases. 3rd ed., New York: McGraw-Hill; 1999: 761-782.

Ryan CA, Courtois BN, Hawes SE, et al. Risk assessment, symptoms and signs as predictors of vulvovaginal and cervical infections in an urban U.S. STD clinic: implications for use of STD algorithms. Sex Transm Infect 1998; 74 (Suppl 1): S59-S76.

Gonorrhea

In the United States 355,642 cases of gonorrhea were diagnosed in 1998, the first increase since 1985. This increase is thought to result from expansion of screening programs, improved surveillance, increased sensitivity of new diagnostic tests, and an increase in morbidity. The risk factors for gonorrhea include young age (15- to 19-year-old age group in women and 20- to 24-year-old age group in men), low socioeconomic status, early onset of sexual activity, unmarried status, history of gonorrhea, and male homosexuality. Recently an increased incidence of rectal gonorrhea has been reported among men who have sex with men. The rates of gonorrhea are highest among minority races such as African-Americans, Hispanics, Asians, and Pacific Islanders. The southeastern region of the United States has the highest rates of gonorrhea in the nation.

Transmission efficiency of *N. gonorrhoeae* depends on the anatomic site of infection and the number of sexual exposures. Transmission by penile-vaginal intercourse has been reported to be 50% to 90% among women who are sexual contacts of infected men and 20% among men who are sexual contacts of infected women. The latter rate can increase to 60% to 80% after four exposures. Transmission of rectal and pharyngeal gonococcal infection is less well defined but appears to be relatively efficient.

Presentation and Progression
Cause

N. gonorrhoeae, the etiologic agent of gonorrhea, is almost always transmitted sexually except in cases of neonatal transmission. It causes a spectrum of mucosal diseases, including pharyngitis, conjunctivitis, urethritis, cervicitis, and proctitis. It also causes disseminated gonococcal infection (DGI), septic arthritis, endocarditis, meningitis, and PID. Up to 30% people infected with gonorrhea have concomitant infection with *C. trachomatis.*

Presentation

After an incubation period of 1 to 14 days, the classic presentation of gonorrhea in men is the presence of pus at the urethral meatus accompanied by symptoms of dysuria, edema, or erythema of the urethral meatus. However, one fourth of the patients have only scant, mucoid exudate or no exudate at all. Complications of gonococcal urethritis in men include epididymitis and acute or chronic prostatitis. Men who have sex with men may also have rectal gonorrhea, which is usually asymptomatic but may be associated with tenesmus, discharge, and rectal bleeding. Oropharyngeal gonorrhea is often asymptomatic but may be manifested as acute pharyngitis or tonsillitis.

In women the primary site of infection is the endocervical canal. Presenting symptoms include purulent or mucopurulent discharge, erythema, edema, and friability of the cervix. Concurrent urethritis and infection of the periurethral gland (Skene's gland) or Bartholin's gland may be present (Figure 16-13). Symptoms of gonococcal infection in women may include vaginal discharge, dysuria, menorrhagia, or intermenstrual bleeding. However, the majority of women with gonorrhea have few symptoms. Approximately one third of women with gonococcal cervicitis also have positive rectal cultures, usually because of perineal contamination with gonococci or because of rectal intercourse. Acute salpingitis or PID develops in 10% to 20% of women with acute gonorrhea (see later section on pelvic inflammatory disease).

Systemic complications of gonorrhea include perihepatitis (Fitz-Hugh–Curtis syndrome), DGI, endocarditis, and in rare instances meningitis. The incidence of DGI is 0.5% to 3% among patients with untreated gonorrhea. Bacteremia begins 7 to 30 days after infection. In the majority of patients mucosal infection is asymptomatic, which may lead to underdiagnosis of DGI. The most common areas of involvement are the skin and joints, which leads to arthralgias or arthritis, tenosynovitis, and tender necrotic nodules with an erythematous base in the distal extremities. Patients with DGI should also be examined for endocarditis or meningitis.

Diagnosis

Presumptive diagnosis of gonorrhea can be made by the identification of gram-negative intracellular diplococci from an endocervical or urethral swab specimen. The sensitivity of the Gram stain for men with symptomatic infection is 90% to 95%. The sensitivity decreases with asymptomatic infections, endocervical, and anorectal infections. Definitive diagnosis is based on a positive culture on modified Thayer-Martin medium and confirmation by specific biochemical tests. Culture is required for determination of antimicrobial susceptibility. Culture of blood, synovial fluid, skin lesions, the anogenital area, or the pharynx can be performed in cases of DGI.

Nonculture tests for the diagnosis of gonorrhea are being widely used in the United States. The nonamplified DNA probe test (Gen-Probe PACE 2) is comparable to culture. Amplified nucleic acid tests recently approved by the Food and Drug Administration include the PCR and the ligase chain reaction (LCR). The LCR test (LC$_x$) is as sensitive as culture for detection of *N. gonorrhoeae* on urethral and endocervical swabs and first void urine (the first 15 to 20 mL) from symptomatic and asymptomatic males and females. The PCR test (Amplicor) is approved for endocervical and urethral swabs from symptomatic patients and male urine specimens.

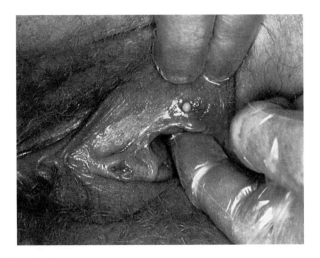

FIG. 16-13 Bartholinitis, showing expression of purulent discharge from the duct of Bartholin's gland by application of pressure. Bartholinitis, which can be caused by gonococcal infection, produces an acute, painful swelling of the labia. Physical examination often reveals a discrete mass. (From Mandell GL, Bleck TP, Brook I, et al., eds. Essential Atlas of Infectious Diseases for Primary Care. Philadelphia: Churchill Livingstone; 1997.)

Natural History
Expected Outcome

Untreated gonorrhea results in spontaneous resolution in several weeks, and 95% of the patients become asymptomatic in 6 months. Immunity does not develop from an episode of gonorrhea, and reinfection can occur from an infected partner.

Treatment
Methods

All patients receiving treatment for gonorrhea should also be treated for *Chlamydia* (unless *Chlamydia* has been rigorously excluded). The combination antimicrobial regimens noted in Box 16-7 include coverage for *Chlamydia*. Many other antimicrobials are effective against gonococci. Nearly 30% of gonococcal isolates in the United States are now resistant to penicillin, tetracycline, or both, and approximately 1% are resistance to ciprofloxacin. Quinolone-resistant *N. gonorrhoeae* is more common in Asia and the Pacific, including Hawaii. Therefore, quinolones are not recommended for travelers who acquired gonorrhea in these regions. All sex partners of the patient within 60 days prior to the onset of symptoms should be evaluated and treated. Pregnant women or children less than 18 years of age should not be treated with fluoroquinolones. Doxycycline is contraindicated in pregnancy.

Expected Response

The regimens of antimicrobial agents in Box 16-7 are 97% to 99% curative for uncomplicated cases of urogenital and anorectal infections. Gonococcal infections of the pharynx are less responsive to therapy, with a cure rate of no more than 90%.

Complications

Patients treated with the recommended regimens need not return for a test of cure. However, if patients have persistent symptoms (and no reexposure has taken place), a culture for *N. gonorrhoeae* should be obtained and tested for antibiotic susceptibility. Fluoroquinolones are not recommended for patients under 18 years of age or pregnant women.

When to Refer

Patients with disseminated gonococcal infection, meningitis, endocarditis, and PID (see later discussion) should be hospitalized for intravenous therapy.

 KEY POINTS

GONORRHEA

⊃ The incidence of gonorrhea has been increasing in recent years.

⊃ The majority of women with gonorrhea have few or no symptoms, and up to 5% of men with gonorrhea are asymptomatic.

⊃ Untreated gonorrhea can lead to significant morbidity from acute salpingitis or PID.

⊃ Up to 30% of patients with gonorrhea have concomitant infection with *C. trachomatis*; thus treatment regimens should include empiric coverage against *Chlamydia* unless the latter can be rigorously excluded.

⊃ Gram stain of urethral discharge is 90% to 95% sensitive in symptomatic men but is less helpful in women.

⊃ Widely used nonculture tests include the DNA probe test, PCR, and LCR.

⊃ Several antimicrobial regimens are useful; ceftriaxone is appropriate therapy for both complicated and uncomplicated forms of gonorrhea.

BOX 16-7
Treatment of Gonorrhea

UNCOMPLICATED GONOCOCCAL INFECTION OF THE CERVIX, URETHRA, AND RECTUM
- Cefixime 400 mg PO as one dose *or*
- Ceftriaxone 125 mg IM as one dose *or*
- Ciprofloxacin 500 mg PO as one dose *or*
- Ofloxacin 400 mg PO as one dose *plus either* azithromycin 1 g PO as one dose or doxycycline 100 mg PO b.i.d. for 7 days

GONOCOCCAL INFECTION OF THE PHARYNX
- Ceftriaxone *or* ciprofloxacin *plus either* azithromycin *or* doxycycline (same dosages as above)

GONOCOCCAL CONJUNCTIVITIS
- Ceftriaxone 1 g IM as one dose along with irrigation

DISSEMINATED GONOCOCCAL INFECTION
- Recommended initial regimen: ceftriaxone 1g IM (or IV) daily for 24 to 48 hours until improvement followed by either cefixime 400 mg PO b.i.d. *or* ciprofloxacin 500 mg PO b.i.d. *or* ofloxacin 400 mg PO b.i.d. to complete a full week of therapy
- Alternative initial regimen: cefotaxime 1 g IV q8h or ceftizoxime 1 g IV q8h followed by a full week of a PO regimen as recommended
- Treatment of all patients for concurrent chlamydial infection unless excluded by testing

GONOCOCCAL MENINGITIS AND ENDOCARDITIS
- Ceftriaxone 1 to 2 g IV q12h: 10 to 14 days for meningitis and at least 4 weeks for endocarditis

---

SUGGESTED READING

Centers for Disease Control and Prevention. 1998 Guidelines for treatment of sexually transmitted diseases. MMWR 1998; 47 (RR-1): 1-111.

Ehret JM, Judson FN. Quinolone-resistant *Neisseria gonorrhoeae*: the beginning of the end? Report of quinolone-resistant isolates and surveillance in the southwestern United States, 1989 to 1997. Sex Transm Dis 1998; 25: 522-526.

Fox KK, Whittington WL, Levine WC, et al. Gonorrhea in the United States, 1981-1996: demographic and geographic trends. Sex Transm Dis 1998; 25: 386-393.

Hook EW III, Handsfield HH. Gonococcal infections in the adult. In: Holmes KK, Mardh PA, Sparling PF, et al, eds. Sexually Transmitted Diseases. 3rd ed., New York: McGraw-Hill; 1999: 451-466.

Chlamydia Trachomatis Infection

Infections caused by *C. trachomatis* are among the most prevalent STDs. The rates of *Chlamydia* infection among males and females are highest between 15 and 24 years of age. The majority of *Chlamydia* urethritis in men and cervicitis in women is asymptomatic. Women endure the greatest morbidity and the most costly outcomes of *Chlamydia* infection because of PID, ectopic pregnancy, tubal infertility, and chronic pelvic pain. In men *Chlamydia* was formerly considered to be the cause of most cases of nongonococcal urethritis (NGU), but recent data suggest that only 10% to 20% of cases of NGU are caused by *Chlamydia* (see the section on urethritis in men).

Transmissibility of *C. trachomatis* has not been well studied. However, a recent study has shown that 68% of male partners of infected women and 70% of female partners of infected men are positive by PCR for *C. trachomatis,* which suggests that transmission from men and women is equally efficient.

Presentation and Progression
Cause

C. trachomatis infects the columnar or squamocolumnar epithelium of the urethra, cervix, rectum, conjunctiva, and respiratory tract (in the neonate). All chlamydiae contain DNA, RNA, and cell walls that resemble those of gram-negative bacteria, and all require multiplication in eukaryotic cells. *C. trachomatis* causes a spectrum of lower and upper genital tract diseases in women: urethritis, bartholinitis, cervicitis, endometritis, salpingitis, tuboovarian abscess, ectopic pregnancy, pelvic peritonitis, and perihepatitis (Fitz-Hugh–Curtis syndrome). About 75% to 90% of cases of chlamydial cervicitis are asymptomatic and may persist for years. Among women with gonorrhea, 30% to 50% have concomitant *Chlamydia* infection. Approximately 40% to 50% of men with chlamydial urethritis may be symptomatic with dysuria or minimal urethral discharge. In 1% of men urethritis leads to epididymitis.

C. trachomatis serovars L1-3 cause lymphogranuloma venereum (LGV), which is characterized by a genital papule followed by unilateral tender inguinal lymphadenopathy. Other genital ulcer diseases such as syphilis, chancroid, and herpes should be considered in the differential diagnosis of LGV. Although LGV is common in tropical countries, it is uncommon in the United States.

Presentation

The majority of women with chlamydial cervicitis are asymptomatic. Some women have symptoms of acute urethritis with dysuria and urinary frequency, postcoital or intermenstrual bleeding, or, less commonly, vaginal discharge. Symptoms of urethritis and the presence of pyuria and a negative bacterial culture in a urine specimen should prompt the diagnosis of *Chlamydia* infection. About 60% to 80% of women with chlamydial urethritis also have cervical infection. On examination the presence of pus, mucus, or mucopus at the cervical os and edema or friability of the cervix may be noted. Many cases of chlamydial upper genital tract disease cause mild or no symptoms despite ongoing tubal scarring and inflammation, which is thus termed "silent salpingitis." Perihepatitis should be considered in the differential diagnosis of young, sexually active women with right upper quadrant pain, fever, nausea, and vomiting.

Men with chlamydial infection often have asymptomatic urethritis. Proctitis, epididymitis (see section on epididymi-

tis), and Reiter's syndrome can also result from *Chlamydia* infection (see Chapter 15).

Diagnosis

Numerous molecular diagnostic tests have been recently developed for the diagnosis of chlamydial infection. Traditional culture techniques are expensive and require tissue culture and stringent specimen transport guidelines. The widely available antigen detection tests such as direct immunofluorescence assay (DFA) or enzyme immunoassay (EIA) are less sensitive (60% to 85%) and specific than culture.

More recently, molecular diagnostic tests that entail nuclei acid amplification—PCR, LCR, and transcription-mediated amplification (TMA, developed by Gen-Probe)—have been developed and are highly sensitive (90% to 95%) and specific (99%). Furthermore, the nucleic acid amplification tests can be performed on urethral or cervical swabs or first void urine (the first 20 mL of voided urine) or self-collected vaginal swab specimens. The sensitivity and specificity of PCR and LCR vary depending on the type of specimen and are most sensitive with first void urine specimens.

Natural History
Expected Outcome

Women and men may have asymptomatic infections for many years and can have recurrent infection with the same strain or a new strain. About 20% to 40% of untreated chlamydial genital infections lead to upper tract disease. Asymptomatic upper genital tract disease is three times as common as symptomatic PID. Long-term consequences of untreated chlamydial infection include tubal infertility, ectopic pregnancy, and chronic pelvic pain (see later section on pelvic inflammatory disease). Some evidence suggests that chlamydial infection, especially multiple exposures to different serotypes, may be a risk factor for carcinoma of the cervix.

Treatment (Box 16-8)
Methods

Treatment with antimicrobial agents is recommended for infected patients, pregnant women, and sexual partners. Sexual partners should be treated if the exposure occurred 60 days before the onset of symptoms in the index case. Furthermore, patients in whom gonorrhea is diagnosed should be treated for concomitant *Chlamydia* infection.

Given that the majority of chlamydial infections in men and women are asymptomatic, screening of high-risk

---

BOX 16-8
Treatment of Chlamydia Trachomatis Infection

RECOMMENDED REGIMENS
- Azithromycin 1g PO in a single dose on an empty stomach *or*
- Doxycycline 100 mg PO b.i.d. for 7 days

ALTERNATIVE REGIMENS
- Erythromycin base 500 mg PO q.i.d for 7 days *or*
- Erythromycin ethylsuccinate 800 mg PO q.i.d. for 7days *or*
- Ofloxacin 300 mg PO b.i.d. for 7 days

individuals should be undertaken for effective control. Individuals at high risk for chlamydial infection are sexually active persons who are between 15 and 25 years of age, have a new sexual partner or multiple sexual partners, or do not use condoms. In fact, cervical screening and treatment of *Chlamydia* infection in selected women at a health maintenance organization led to a substantial decrease in symptomatic PID.

Expected Response

Patients do not need a test of cure after completion of therapy except when erythromycin is used for therapy, since it is less efficacious than azithromycin, doxycycline, or ofloxacin.

Complications

Compliance with erythromycin may be less than with the other regimens because of gastrointestinal toxicity.

When to Refer

The major basis for referral of patients with chlamydial infection is PID (see later discussion).

 KEY POINTS

CHLAMYDIA TRACHOMATIS INFECTION

⊃ *C. trachomatis* infection is one of the most prevalent STDs and frequently coexists with gonococcal infection and other STDs.

⊃ Up to 90% of women with chlamydial cervicitis and up to 50% of men with chlamydial urethritis are asymptomatic; thus screening of sexually active individuals is essential.

⊃ In women symptoms of urethritis with pyuria and a sterile urine culture suggest chlamydial infection.

⊃ In about 20% to 40% of women with untreated chlamydial infection, upper tract disease develops, which can lead to tubal infertility, ectopic pregnancy, chronic pelvic pain, or PID. Some evidence suggests that chlamydial infection may be a risk factor for carcinoma of the cervix.

⊃ About 80% of cases of Reiter's syndrome (urethritis, conjunctivitis, arthritis, and skin lesions) are associated with chlamydial infection.

⊃ Diagnosis is increasingly made with molecular techniques such as PCR, LCR, or TMA. EIA has limited sensitivity.

⊃ All patients with gonorrhea should be treated for possible concomitant chlamydial infection.

SUGGESTED READING

Anttila T, Saikku P, Koskela P, et al. Serotypes of *Chlamydia trachomatis* and risk of development of cervical squamous cell carcinoma. JAMA 2001; 285: 47-51.

Black CM, Morse SA. The use of molecular techniques for the diagnosis and epidemiologic study of sexually transmitted infections. Curr Infect Dis Rep 2000; 2 (1): 31-43.

Marrazzo JM, Stamm WE. New approaches to the diagnosis, treatment, and prevention of chlamydial infection. Curr Clin Top Infect Dis 1998; 18: 37-59.

Scholes D, Stergachis A, Heidrich FE, et al. Prevention of pelvic inflammatory disease by screening for cervical chlamydial infection. N Engl J Med 1996; 334: 1362-1366.

Stamm WE. *Chlamydia trachomatis* infections: progress and problems. J Infect Dis 1999; 179 (Suppl 2): S380-S383.

Pelvic Inflammatory Disease

PID signifies inflammation of the upper female genital tract and its related structures. PID can manifest as endometritis, salpingitis, adnexitis, tuboovarian abscess, pelvic peritonitis, or perihepatitis. The most common manifestation of PID is salpingitis, and the terms are used synonymously in the literature. PID is one of the most common causes of hospitalization among women of reproductive age. Risk factors for PID include young age, multiple sexual partners, use of intrauterine devices, vaginal douching, tobacco smoking, BV, HIV infection, and STDs with gonorrhea or *Chlamydia* infection. Use of oral contraceptives has been associated with a decreased rate of PID, especially that associated with *C. trachomatis* infection.

Presentation and Progression
Cause

Most cases of PID are related to *C. trachomatis* or *N. gonorrhoeae* infection. *C. trachomatis* is the most common cause of PID in the United States. *C. trachomatis* is implicated in "silent salpingitis" or subclinical PID. Acute PID develops in approximately 10% of women with chlamydial cervicitis and between 10% and 19% of women with gonococcal cervicitis. The pathogenesis of PID is not well understood. The chronic sequelae of *Chlamydia*-induced PID, such as ectopic pregnancy and tubal infertility, are thought to be due to an inflammatory reaction to the chlamydial heat shock protein (HSP-60). Certain characteristics of gonococcal strains such as the serovar, the formation of transparent colonies on agar, and penicillin resistance have been correlated with a propensity for causing tubal infection. Women with PID and gonococcal infection tend to have pain during the first part of the menstrual cycle, suggesting that the gonococci ascend into the upper genital tract through a cervix with scant mucus during the menstrual cycle.

Microorganisms that are part of the vaginal flora such as group B streptococci, *Haemophilus influenzae, G. vaginalis,* anaerobes, and genital mycoplasmas (e.g., *Mycoplasma hominis* and *Ureaplasma urealyticum*) have also been isolated from the lower genital tract of women with PID. The organisms that result in bacterial vaginosis have been associated with endometritis and PID primarily after invasive gynecologic procedures. PID is frequently a result of mixed infection with facultative, anaerobic, and sexually transmitted pathogens. Multiple pathogens including several species of anaerobic bacteria are nearly always present in severe complications such as tuboovarian abscess.

Upper genital tract infections can also be caused by hematogenous dissemination of *Mycobacterium tuberculosis,* contiguous spread from intraabdominal sepsis, ascending infection from intrauterine devices, and postsurgical instrumentation.

Presentation

The presentation of PID varies from asymptomatic infection to mild endometritis or salpingitis to generalized peritonitis. Two thirds of women with infertility caused by postinfection tubal scarring report no history of PID. Asymptomatic PID from *C. trachomatis* is estimated to be three times more common than symptomatic disease.

Symptomatic PID may cause lower abdominal pain, deep dyspareunia, vaginal discharge, menstrual irregularities, or systemic symptoms of fever, chills, and malaise. Women with gonococcal PID may have abdominal pain of less than 3 days' duration when seen for treatment, whereas women with chlamydial PID tend to have had abdominal pain for more than 1 week at presentation. The clinical findings may consist of lower abdominal tenderness, cervical motion tenderness, adnexal tenderness, and mucopurulent cervical discharge. Furthermore, extragenital spread of *N. gonorrhoeae* and *C. trachomatis* can lead to infection of serosal surfaces, resulting in symptoms and signs of periappendicitis and perihepatitis.

Diagnosis

The diagnosis of PID is usually made clinically, which is imprecise because it is based on signs and symptoms alone. In fact, only 67% of the women in whom PID was diagnosed clinically had laparoscopic evidence of PID. The sensitivity and specificity of any one clinical finding or laboratory test is low for the diagnosis of PID. The 1998 STD guidelines issued by the CDC have therefore established criteria to assist in the diagnosis (Box 16-9).

Differential diagnosis of PID includes ectopic pregnancy and other gynecologic conditions (ovarian cyst rupture, bleeding, or torsion), acute appendicitis, urinary tract infection, renal or ureteral stones, mesenteric lymphadenitis, and inflammatory bowel disease.

Natural History
Expected Outcome

The major sequelae of acute PID are infertility, ectopic pregnancy, and chronic pelvic pain. The risk for tubal factor infertility after one episode of PID is 7%. The risk increases to 16% after two episodes and to 28% after three or more episodes. Furthermore, women with PID have a 7- to 10-fold increased risk of ectopic pregnancy, which accounts for 9% of all pregnancy-related deaths. Chronic pelvic pain occurs in 24% to 75% of women with PID, and women with PID have higher rates of hysterectomy.

Treatment
Methods

The approach to treatment of PID includes the decision to hospitalize, patient education, follow-up, and treatment of sex partners. Treatment should be initiated based on the minimal criteria, since a delay in therapy may lead to untoward long-term sequelae. The decision of whether to hospitalize is discussed under "When to Refer." Antimicrobial therapy should include coverage against *N. gonorrhoeae, C. trachomatis,* anaerobes, streptococci, and gram-negative bacteria (Box 16-10). Because of the concern about the role of anaerobes in PID, all regimens should include adequate anaerobic coverage.

Other antimicrobial agents effective in the treatment of PID are meropenem and azithromycin plus metronidazole. Patients treated with an outpatient regimen for PID should have a follow-up visit within 72 hours. Improvement in physical signs such as fever, abdominal tenderness, cervical motion tenderness, and adnexal tenderness should be noted at this time.

BOX 16-9
Criteria for Diagnosis of Pelvic Inflammatory Disease from the Centers for Disease Control and Prevention

MINIMAL CRITERIA*
- Lower abdominal tenderness
- Adnexal tenderness
- Cervical motion tenderness

ADDITIONAL CRITERIA THAT SUPPORT THE DIAGNOSIS OF PELVIC INFLAMMATORY DISEASE
- Oral temperature ≥101° F (38.3° C)
- Abnormal cervical or vaginal discharge
- Elevated erythrocyte sedimentation rate or C-reactive protein level
- Documentation of cervicitis with *Neisseria gonorrhoeae* or *Chlamydia trachomatis*

DEFINITIVE CRITERIA
- Histopathologic evidence of endometritis on endometrial biopsy
- Transvaginal ultrasonography or magnetic resonance imaging with evidence of fluid-filled tubes with or without free pelvic fluid or tuboovarian complex
- Laparoscopic abnormalities (hyperemia of tubal surface, edema of the tubal wall, and sticky exudate on the tubal surface or fimbriae)

*Empiric treatment should be initiated if all of these are present.

BOX 16-10
Treatment of Pelvic Inflammatory Disease

OUTPATIENT REGIMENS
Regimen A
- Ofloxacin 400 mg PO b.i.d. for 14 days *plus* metronidazole 500 mg PO b.i.d. for 14 days

Regimen B
- Ceftriaxone 250 mg IM (or cefoxitin 2 g IM and probenecid 1 g PO in a single dose concurrently) *plus* metronidazole 500 mg PO b.i.d. for 14 days *plus* doxycycline 100 mg PO b.i.d. for 14 days

Regimen C
- Levofloxacin 500 mg PO daily for 14 days

INPATIENT REGIMENS*
Regimen A
- Cefotetan 2 g IV q12h (or cefoxitin 2 g IV q6h) *plus* doxycycline 100 mg IV or PO b.i.d.

Regimen B
- Clindamycin 900 mg IV q8h *plus* gentamicin 1.5 mg/kg IV q8h

Alternative Regimens
- Ofloxacin 400 mg IV q12h *plus* metronidazole 500 mg IV q8h *or*
- Ampicillin-sulbactam 3 g IV q6h *plus* doxycycline 100 mg IV or PO q12h *or*
- Ciprofloxacin 200 mg IV q12h *plus* doxycycline 100 mg IV or PO q12h *plus* metronidazole 500 mg IV q8h

*Note: Both of these parenteral regimens (i.e., regimens A and B) should be continued for 24 hours after improvement followed by an oral regimen consisting of doxycycline 100 mg PO b.i.d. or clindamycin 450 mg PO q.i.d. for a total of 14 days of therapy. Some clinicians use metronidazole *plus* doxycycline in cases of tuboovarian abscess.

Patients with PID should abstain from intercourse until all symptoms have resolved. Sex partners of patients with PID who had contact with the patient 60 days before the onset of symptoms should be evaluated and treated empirically with regimens effective against *N. gonorrhoeae* and *C. trachomatis.*

Expected Response

The efficacy of the antimicrobial regimens ranges from 81% to 94%. A delay in treatment greater than 3 days results in a three-fold higher risk of infertility.

Complications

Intravenous doxycycline is associated with pain during infusion. Thus doxycycline should be prescribed for oral administration when possible, given the similarities in bioavailability for the oral and intravenous formulations.

When to Refer

The decision to hospitalize should be based on the presence of any of the following: severe illness with nausea, vomiting, or high fever; pregnancy; immunosuppressed state; suspected tuboovarian abscess; inability to exclude surgical emergency; inability to tolerate or follow an outpatient regimen; and lack of clinical improvement on the outpatient regimen. Patients with PID may also require referral for complications such as infertility and chronic pelvic pain.

 KEY POINTS

PELVIC INFLAMMATORY DISEASE

⟳ The most common manifestation is salpingitis; others are endometritis, adnexitis, tuboovarian abscess, pelvic peritonitis, and perihepatitis.

⟳ Most cases are related to *C. trachomatis* (the most common cause in the United States) or *N. gonorrhoeae* infection. However, the role of anaerobes is an increasing concern.

⟳ Many cases are asymptomatic. About two thirds of women with infertility caused by postinfection tubal scarring report no history of PID.

⟳ The diagnosis is usually made clinically, based on imprecise symptoms and signs.

⟳ Empiric treatment for PID should be initiated in patients with the triad of lower abdominal tenderness, adnexal tenderness, and cervical motion tenderness. Additional criteria that support the diagnosis include fever, abnormal discharge, elevated sedimentation rate, and documentation of chlamydial or gonococcal cervicitis.

⟳ Treatment includes the decision of whether to hospitalize, patient education, close follow-up, and treatment of sex partners.

SUGGESTED READING

Munday PE. Clinical aspects of pelvic inflammatory disease. Hum Reprod 1997; 12 (Suppl 11): 121-126.
Munday PE. Pelvic inflammatory disease—an evidence-based approach to diagnosis. J Infect 2000; 40: 31-41.
Paavonen J. Pelvic inflammatory disease: from diagnosis to prevention. Dermatol Clin 1998; 16: 747-756.
Simms I, Stephenson JM. Pelvic inflammatory disease epidemiology: what do we know and what do we need to know? Sex Transm Infect 2000; 76: 80-87.

Urethritis in Males

Urethritis (inflammation of the urethra) is characterized by a burning sensation during urination or itching or discharge at the urethral meatus. The exudate may be mucoid, mucopurulent, or purulent. Traditionally, urethritis has been divided into gonococcal and nongonococcal urethritis. When *N. gonorrhoeae* cannot be detected, the syndrome is called nongonococcal urethritis (NGU). In the United States the rates of NGU have surpassed those of gonococcal urethritis in the past 20 to 30 years. The 20- to 24-year-old age group has the highest incidence of gonococcal and nongonococcal urethritis.

Presentation and Progression
Cause

Up to 25% to 30% of men with gonococcal urethritis also have concurrent *Chlamydia* infection. In the past, the prevalence of *C. trachomatis* as the cause of NGU has ranged from 23% to 55%. Recent studies showed that up to two thirds of cases of NGU remain undiagnosed. *U. urealyticum, Mycoplasma genitalium,* and occasionally *T. vaginalis* and HSV have also been shown to cause NGU. Both gonococcal and chlamydial infections can cause asymptomatic urethritis, which is especially important from a public health perspective because these infections can increase HIV transmission by increasing HIV shedding in the genital secretions. Rare causes of urethral discharge include endourethral syphilitic chancre and warts from human papillomavirus. Urethritis caused by coliform bacteria may occur in association with bacterial prostatitis, urethral stricture, and instrumentation of the urethra. Other pathogens that cause urethritis are *S. aureus, Streptococcus pyogenes, H. influenzae,* and *Moraxella catarrhalis.*

Presentation

Gonococcal urethritis is characterized by a purulent discharge and dysuria, whereas NGU usually causes a scant, mucoid discharge. In some patients the inflammatory exudate may not be apparent on examination. Patients with NGU may have a discharge that is noted only in the morning, as crusting at the meatus, or as a stain on the underwear. It is difficult to distinguish gonococcal from nongonococcal urethritis based on physical examination alone. Patients with gonococcal urethritis seek treatment for acute urethritis within 4 days of onset of symptoms. Patients with nongonococcal urethritis may seek treatment 1 to 5 weeks after infection. Both groups may have asymptomatic infection. Some patients have recurrent urethritis characterized by persistent symptoms or frequent recurrences. The symptoms of classic urinary tract infection, such as fever, chills, urinary frequency and urgency, and hematuria, are not features of urethritis. Differential diagnosis of cystitis, prostatitis, epididymitis, Reiter's syndrome, and bacterial cystitis should be considered when evaluating a patient with urethritis.

Diagnosis

If no urethral discharge is apparent on physical examination, the urethra should be milked from the base to the meatus. The presence of urethritis should be confirmed by one or more of the following findings: mucopurulent or purulent discharge, ≥5 WBCs per oil immersion field from the Gram stain of a urethral swab, and either a positive leukocyte esterase test on first voided urine or the presence of ≥10 WBCs per high-power field in the spun sediment of the first voided urine. If no obvious discharge is found on examination, a specimen for Gram stain and culture should be obtained by inserting a urethral swab 2 to 3 cm into the urethra. All patients with urethritis should be tested for gonorrhea and chlamydia (see sections on gonorrhea and chlamydia). Gonococcal urethritis is diagnosed by the finding of gram-negative intracellular diplococci in the urethral exudate. NGU is diagnosed on the basis of absence of gram-negative intracellular diplococci in an inflammatory exudate. An approach to suspected urethritis is shown in Figure 16-7.

Asymptomatic urethritis is difficult if not impossible to diagnose. Selective screening by urine LCR or PCR for *N. gonorrhoeae* and *C. trachomatis* may be indicated in certain cases. Asymptomatic men who are sexual partners of women with gonorrhea and chlamydia should be treated.

Among patients with recurrent urethritis, the presence of urethritis should be documented by objective criteria as stated previously. Retreatment is indicated if the patient was noncompliant with the original regimen or had reexposure to an infected partner. If there is no such history, testing for *T. vaginalis* should be performed. In addition, a prostatic focus or anatomic abnormality of the genitourinary tract should be considered.

Natural History
Expected Outcome

In approximately two thirds of men with untreated asymptomatic urethritis, symptomatic disease will develop within the next 4 to 5 months. Complications of urethritis include epididymitis, orchitis, and urethral strictures.

Treatment
Methods

Treatment of urethritis involves antimicrobial therapy (Box 16-11), education, and management of sexual partners within the preceding 60 days. Patients should also be screened for syphilis and offered tests for HIV.

Expected Response

Treatment of urethritis with appropriate antibiotics results in alleviation of symptoms and microbiologic cure by the end of treatment period in 95% of the patients (provided the patients are not reexposed). Follow-up is not needed unless symptoms persist or recur. In cases of treatment failure, the physician should consider therapy with erythromycin for tetracycline-resistant *Ureaplasma* or evaluate for *Trichomonas*.

 KEY POINTS

URETHRITIS IN MALES
- NGU is now more common than gonococcal urethritis in the United States
- *C. trachomatis* is a major cause of NGU, but others include *U. urealyticum, M. genitalium,* and, occasionally, *T. vaginalis* and HSV.

- Up to 30% of men with gonococcal urethritis have concurrent chlamydial infection.
- Gonococcal urethritis usually causes purulent discharge and dysuria, whereas NGU usually causes a scant, mucoid discharge. Up to two thirds of cases of NGU go undiagnosed.
- Diagnosis of urethritis is based on one or more of the following: mucopurulent or purulent discharge, five or more WBCs per oil immersion field on Gram stain from a urethral swab, and pyuria in a first voided urine sample.
- In about two thirds of men with untreated asymptomatic urethritis, symptomatic disease will develop. Complications include epididymitis, orchitis, and urethral strictures.
- Treatment includes antimicrobial therapy, education, and management of sex partners.

SUGGESTED READING
Burstein GR, Zenilman JM. Nongonococcal urethritis—a new paradigm. Clin Infect Dis 1999; 28 (Suppl 1): S66-S73.
Erbelding EJ, Quinn TC. Urethritis treatment. Dermatol Clin 1998; 16: 735-738.
Handsfield HH, Lipman TO, Harnisch JP, et al. Asymptomatic gonorrhea in men: diagnosis, natural course, prevalence and significance. N Engl J Med 1974; 290: 117-123.

Epididymitis

Inflammation of the upper male genital tract may lead to epididymitis, orchitis, epididymoorchitis, and prostatitis.

Presentation and Progression
Cause

Epididymitis is usually a complication of urethritis from *N. gonorrhoeae* or *C. trachomatis* in men <35 years of age. The urethritis is often asymptomatic. About 70% of cases of epididymitis among young, sexually active men are caused by *C. trachomatis* infection. In men >35 years of age, the

---

BOX 16-11
Treatment of Urethritis in Males

GONOCOCCAL URETHRITIS
- See section on gonorrhea.

NONGONOCOCCAL URETHRITIS
- A single-dose regimen is preferable because of improved compliance.
- Azithromycin 1 g PO as one dose *or* doxycycline 100 mg PO b.i.d. for 7 days
- Alternative regimen: erythromycin base 500 mg PO q.i.d. for 7 days *or* erythromycin ethylsuccinate 800 mg PO q.i.d. for 7 days *or* ofloxacin 300 mg PO b.i.d. for 7 days

RECURRENT OR PERSISTENT URETHRITIS
- Metronidazole 2 g PO (one dose) *plus either* erythromycin base 500 mg PO q.i.d. for 7 days *or* erythromycin ethylsuccinate 800 mg PO q.i.d. for 7 days

usual causes of epididymitis are enteric gram-negative bacteria such as *E. coli* and *Proteus mirabilis*. Enteric gram-negative rods also cause epididymitis in insertive partners of homosexual men, men who have undergone recent urinary tract instrumentation or surgery, and men with anatomic abnormalities of the genitourinary tract.

Presentation

The usual presenting symptom of epididymitis is acute, unilateral scrotal and inguinal pain. Unilateral epididymitis may soon progress to bilateral epididymoorchitis. Physical examination may reveal an erythematous scrotum with a tender, swollen epididymis. Concurrent urethritis may be present. Testicular torsion, a surgical emergency, must be considered in evaluating a patient with testicular pain. Testicular torsion is more common among adolescents and may be associated with sudden, severe pain.

Diagnosis

In the evaluation of a patient with testicular pain and swelling, documentation of urethritis supports the diagnosis of epididymitis. Urethritis may be evidenced by the presence of urethral discharge, ≥5 WBCs per high-power field of an endourethral swab Gram stain, or a positive leukocyte esterase on a first voided urine specimen (see earlier discussion). Urinalysis with culture and tests for *N. gonorrhoeae* and *C. trachomatis* should be obtained. Serologic tests for syphilis and HIV counseling and testing are also needed. If the diagnosis of epididymitis is uncertain, consultation with an expert is recommended and emergency testing may be indicated.

Natural History
Expected Outcome

Untreated epididymitis may lead to orchitis, epididymoorchitis, and prostatitis.

Treatment
Methods

Empiric therapy is recommended while culture results are awaited. Ceftriaxone 250 mg IM in a single dose *plus* doxycycline 100 mg PO b.i.d. is the treatment regimen for epididymitis thought to be caused by *N. gonorrhoeae* or *C. trachomatis*. Ofloxacin 300 mg PO b.i.d. for 10 days is recommended for patients who are allergic to β-lactam drugs or for cases most likely caused by enteric organisms. In addition, scrotal elevation, analgesics, and ice packs will help lead to resolution. Sex partners of patients with epididymitis caused by *N. gonorrhoeae* or *C. trachomatis* should be evaluated and treated.

Expected Response and Complications

The symptoms should improve within 3 days. If the symptoms do not resolve with the completion of antibiotic therapy, evaluation for tumor, abscess, and infarction or mycobacterial or fungal disease should be pursued.

When to Refer

Patients in whom testicular torsion cannot be excluded should be referred to a surgeon, as should patients with suspected tumor or abscess.

KEY POINTS

EPIDIDYMITIS

- ⊃ Epididymitis is usually caused by *N. gonorrhoeae* or *C. trachomatis* in men <35 years of age and by enteric gram-negative rods in older men.
- ⊃ The disease typically is manifested as acute, unilateral scrotal and inguinal pain.
- ⊃ Documentation of urethritis supports the diagnosis of epididymitis.
- ⊃ Testicular torsion, which is more common among adolescents, should be considered. Testicular torsion often begins with sudden, severe pain and is a surgical emergency.
- ⊃ Untreated epididymitis can lead to orchitis, epididymoorchitis, and prostatitis.

SUGGESTED READING

Centers for Disease Control and Prevention. Gonorrhea—United States, 1998. MMWR 2000; 49: 538-542.

Seña AC, Behets F M-T, Fox KK, Cohen MS. Sexually Transmitted Diseases. In: Guerrant RL, Walker DH and Weller PF, eds. Tropical Infectious Diseases: Principles, Pathogens, and Practice. Philadelphia; Churchill Livingstone; 1999: 1569-1585.

Proctitis

Proctitis (inflammation of the rectum) is usually seen among patients who practice unprotected anal intercourse. Proctocolitis (inflammation of the rectum and colon) is usually acquired from indirect or direct fecal-oral contact. Symptoms of proctitis include tenesmus, anorectal pain, mucopurulent or bloody anal discharge, and constipation. Proctocolitis is associated with diarrhea and cramps in addition to the symptoms of proctitis. Sexually transmitted pathogens that cause proctitis include *N. gonorrhoeae, C. trachomatis*, HSV, and *T. pallidum*. Warts from human papillomavirus can also be noted in the anorectal area. Enteric pathogens such as *Salmonella, Shigella, Campylobacter, Giardia*, and *Entamoeba histolytica* are associated with proctocolitis. Anoscopy may reveal rectal exudates or rectal bleeding.

Evaluation of patients with symptoms of acute proctitis includes diagnostic procedures such as anoscopy or sigmoidoscopy and stool culture. In a person with acute proctitis with pus and a history of recent unprotected anal intercourse, presumptive therapy for gonorrhea and chlamydia is indicated.

Human Papillomavirus Infection

Human papillomavirus (HPV) infection is the most common viral STD worldwide. The prevalence ranges from 20% to 46% in young women worldwide. In the United States an estimated 1% of sexually active persons between the ages of 15 to 49 years have genital warts from HPV. The incidence of HPV infection is high among college students (35% to 43%), especially among minority races, individuals with multiple sexual partners, and those who consume alcohol. Immunocompromised persons, including those with HIV infection, have increased prevalence of HPV infection.

Most genital HPV infections are subclinical and are transmitted through sexual contact. Several transmission studies noted that 75% to 95% of male partners of women with HPV genital lesions also had genital HPV infection. Vertical transmission can cause laryngeal papillomatosis in infants and children. Digital transmission of genital warts can also occur.

Presentation and Progression

Cause

HPV is a double-stranded DNA virus that infects the squamous epithelium. It causes a spectrum of clinical disease ranging from asymptomatic infection, benign plantar and genital warts, and squamous intraepithelial neoplasia (bowenoid papulosis, erythroplasia of Queyrat, or Bowen's disease of the genitalia) to frank malignancy (Buschke-Lowenstein tumor, a form of verrucous squamous cell carcinoma) in the anogenital region. External genital warts have various morphologic manifestations such as condylomata acuminata (cauliflower-like, smooth, dome-shaped papular warts), keratotic warts, and flat warts (squamous intraepithelial neoplasia). Condylomata acuminata tend to occur on moist surfaces, whereas the keratotic and smooth warts occur on fully keratinized skin. Flat warts can occur on either surface.

Approximately 100 types of HPV have been identified. The 30 types that infect the anogenital area can be divided into low-risk (e.g., 6, 11, 42, 43, 44) and high-risk types (e.g., 16, 18, 31, 33, 35, 39, 45, 52, 55, 56, 58) based on their association with anogenital cancer. Types 6 and 11 are commonly associated with external genital, cervical, vaginal, urethral, and anal warts, as well as conjunctival, nasal, oral, and laryngeal warts. Although HPV types 6 and 11 are found in 90% of condylomata acuminata, they are rarely associated with squamous cell carcinoma of the external genitalia. On the other hand, HPV types 16, 18, 31, 33, and 35 have been associated with malignant transformation, squamous intraepithelial neoplasia, and squamous cell carcinoma of the vulva, vagina, cervix, penis, and anus. About 95% of squamous cell carcinomas of the cervix contain HPV DNA. Most HPV infections do not cause clinical manifestations, and mixed HPV types can be found in each lesion.

Presentation

Most genital warts are asymptomatic, but they may cause itching, burning, pain, and bleeding. Condylomata acuminata can appear as multiple nodules or large, exophytic, pedunculated, cauliflower-like lesions in the anogenital area. They are usually noted on the penis, vulva, vagina, cervix, perineum, and anal region. Flat condylomas are usually subclinical and not visible to the naked eye. They are most commonly noted on the cervix, but may also be present on the vulva and penis. They may also occur as white, plaquelike lesions in the anogenital region.

Diagnosis

Diagnosis of HPV infection is based on clinical examination, pathologic findings (Papanicolaou [Pap] smear), or HPV DNA detection, which can be used to determine whether high-risk serotypes are present (see Chapter 2). The clinical diagnosis is based on the dermatologic appearance of lesions on visual examination, which may be enhanced by a bright light and magnifying glass. Routine use of the acetowhite test (brief soaking of skin with 3% to 10% acetic acid), which causes HPV lesions to appear white, is not recommended because this test is not specific for HPV. When the diagnosis is uncertain, the patient should be referred to an expert. Biopsy of the lesions is recommended when the lesions are ulcerated, fixed to the underlying tissue, indurated, or >1 cm in diameter. Biopsy is also recommended if the warts do not respond to therapy or become worse. Cervical flat warts are not visible to the naked eye and require cytologic or colposcopic examination. All women with external genital warts or a history of contact with external genital warts should have cervical cytologic screening.

Differential diagnosis of papular genital warts includes condylomata lata of secondary syphilis, molluscum contagiosum, normal pearly papules of the glans penis, seborrheic keratosis, Crohn's disease, lichen planus, and melanocytic nevi. Differential diagnosis of flat warts includes erythema from psoriasis, seborrheic dermatitis, circinate balanitis of Reiter's syndrome, Bowen's disease, squamous intraepithelial neoplasia, or carcinoma.

Natural History

Expected Outcome

Many studies have shown that HPV infection can be detected only transiently. In a study that prospectively followed 608 females, the duration of new infection as detected by HPV DNA was 7 to 10 months. Persistent infection has been associated with HPV type 16 and older age. Hormones, pregnancy, and cigarette smoking may also have an impact on the course of HPV infection.

Treatment

Methods

The goal of treatment of external genital warts is to eliminate the physical symptoms and relieve the emotional distress associated with the presence of lesions. Treatment of external genital warts does not cure the infection, may not decrease infectivity, and may not alter the course of infection. Treatment may result in wart-free periods in most patients. Untreated genital warts may persist or resolve on their own. Sexual partners of patients with genital warts should be counseled and evaluated for other STDs. Female sex partners of patients with genital warts should be encouraged to receive Pap smears for cervical cancer screening.

The treatment modality of genital warts should be based on patient preference, provider experience, and available resources. All modalities are equally efficacious. Treatment of nonexophytic genital warts or subclinical warts is not recommended in the absence of squamous intraepithelial neoplasia. In general, the treatment of external genital warts is divided into patient applied and provider applied (Box 16-12).

Expected Response

If the lesions fail to respond to a treatment regimen, an alternative modality should be pursued. Immunosuppressed patients may not respond as well as immunocompetent patients and may have more recurrences. Examination of sex partners is unnecessary because they are most likely subclinically infected with HPV. The benefit of condom use to prevent sexual transmission to new partners is unknown.

BOX 16-12
Treatment of Human Papillomavirus Infection

PATIENT-APPLIED TREATMENTS
- Podofilox (Condylox) 0.5% solution or gel is applied twice a day for 3 days followed by 4 days of no therapy. This cycle can be repeated up to four times. The total wart area should not exceed 10 cm², and the total volume of podofilox used should not exceed 0.5 mL per treatment. Most patients (45% to 82%) achieve resolution of the warts within 4 to 6 weeks.
- Imiquimod (Aldara) 5% cream is applied at bedtime 3 days a week up to 16 weeks. The treated area should be washed with soap and water 6 to 10 hours after the application. A majority of patients (37% to 85%) are wart free at 8 to 10 weeks after therapy.

PROVIDER-APPLIED TREATMENTS
- Cryotherapy with liquid nitrogen or cryoprobe can be applied and repeated every 1 to 2 weeks. Cryotherapy is safe to use in pregnancy.
- Podophyllin resin (10% to 25% in compound tincture of benzoin) is applied to each wart, allowed to air-dry, and thoroughly washed off 1 to 4 hours after the application. This can be repeated weekly. As with podofilox, the area of treatment should be less than 10 cm² and the total volume of podophyllin used should not exceed 0.5 mL per treatment.
- Trichloroacetic acid or bichloroacetic acid 80% to 90% is applied to each wart and allowed to air-dry (a white frosting may be noted at this time). This may be repeated weekly. If there is intense pain or excess acid, it can be neutralized with liquid soap or sodium bicarbonate.
- Surgical removal has the advantage of removing all warts in one visit but requires significant training.
- Intralesional interferon has had variable results. Parenteral interferon has not been shown to be beneficial.
- Laser surgery may be used.

Complications

Complications of treatment vary with the therapeutic modality undertaken. Adverse effects associated with podophyllin and podofilox treatment include skin irritation, ulceration, erythema, phimosis, and preputial tightening, burning, and soreness. Imiquimod is associated with localized burning, pain, erythema, tenderness, and ulcerations. Cryotherapy can lead to tissue sloughing and destruction. Pain, necrosis, and blistering may occur after application. Treatment of a large area of warts or large warts may create wound care problems. Imiquimod, podophyllin, and podofilox should not be used during pregnancy.

When to Refer

The treatment of warts on mucosal surfaces such as cervical, intravaginal, and rectal areas should be managed in consultation with an expert.

 KEY POINTS

HUMAN PAPILLOMAVIRUS INFECTION
- ⊃ HPV infection is the most common viral STD worldwide; 1% of sexually active persons between the ages of 15 and 49 years in the United States are estimated to have genital warts from HPV.

- ⊃ Most cases of HPV are subclinical.
- ⊃ About 95% of squamous cell carcinomas of the cervix contain HPV DNA, which is usually of a high-risk serotype.
- ⊃ Diagnosis is based on clinical examination, pathologic findings (Pap smear), or HPV DNA detection, which can be used to determine whether high-risk serotypes are present. Routine use of the acetowhite test is not recommended.
- ⊃ The differential diagnosis of warts in the genital area is broad.
- ⊃ Treatment of warts on mucosal surfaces such as the cervical, intravaginal, and rectal areas should be carried out in consultation with an expert.
- ⊃ HPV infection is incurable.

SUGGESTED READING

Beutner KR, Reitano MV, Richwald GA, et al. External genital warts: report of the American Medical Association Consensus Conference. Clin Infect Dis 1998; 27: 796-806.

Beutner KR, Wiley DJ, Douglas JM, et al. Genital warts and their treatment. Clin Infect Dis 1999; 28(Suppl 1): S37-S56.

Hagensee ME. Infection with human papillomavirus: update on epidemiology, diagnosis and treatment. Curr Infect Dis Rep 2000; 2: 18-24.

Ho GY, Bierman R, Beardsley L, et al. Natural history of cervicovaginal papillomavirus infection in young women. N Engl J Med 1998; 338: 423-428.

Sedlacek TV. Advances in the diagnosis and treatment of human papillomavirus infections. Clin Obstet Gynecol 1999; 42: 206-220.

Ectoparasites: Scabies and Human Lice

Infestations with scabies mites and pubic lice are common in the United States (see Chapter 23 for further discussion and methods of treatment). Pubic lice are transmitted between humans primarily through sexual contact, while head and body lice may be transmitted by other intimate contact, such as sharing personal items. Pubic lice may also be transmitted by toilet seats and bedding. The highest rates of pubic lice occur in persons aged 15 to 25 years. Scabies is transmitted both by sexual contact and by close contact among family members (through skin-to-skin contact or fomites).

Infection with pubic lice causes itching that can lead to scratching, erythema, and inflammation. Some patients report seeing the lice or nits (eggs) around their pubic area. Scabies usually causes intense pruritus, which is generally worse at night or after a hot shower. Diagnosis of scabies and pubic lice is based on the history and physical examination, and these possibilities should be considered in all patients with pruritic skin lesions. The lice and nits are visible to the naked eye, but use of a magnifying glass is helpful (Figure 16-14). Pubic lice can appear as crusts (scabs) over papules. The presence of tiny, white nits, which should be differentiated from white flakes caused by seborrheic dermatitis, confirms the diagnosis. Presumptive diagnosis of scabies is based on finding burrows. A scraping is collected from the burrows or from under the fingernails for microscopic examination.

Treatment is outlined in Box 16-13.

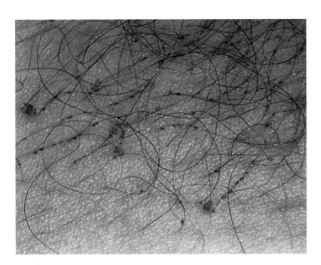

FIG. 16-14   Crab lice (*Phthirus pubis*). Several lice are attached to the skin between the hairs, which contain numerous nits. The nits secure themselves to the base of the hair shaft and grow out with the hair. (From Mandell GL, Bleck TP, Brook I, et al., eds. Essential Atlas of Infectious Diseases for Primary Care. Philadelphia: Churchill Livingstone; 1997.)

SUGGESTED READING

Billstein SA, Mattaliano VJ. The "nuisance" sexually transmitted diseases: molluscum contagiosum, scabies, and crab lice. Med Clin North Am 1990; 74: 1487-1505.

Platts-Mills TAE, Rein MF. Scabies. In: Holmes KK, Mardh PA, Sparling PF, et al, eds. Sexually Transmitted Diseases. 3rd ed., New York: McGraw-Hill; 1999: 645-650.

Molluscum Contagiosum

Infections caused by the molluscum contagiosum virus, a member of the *Poxviridae*, have been increasing in the United States since the 1960s. The virus is transmitted through close skin-to-skin contact and results in small, firm, umbilicated papules. Genital molluscum is usually sexually transmitted and peaks in the 20- to 29-year-old age group. The lesions are pearly or flesh colored, vary in size from few millimeters up to a centimeter, and occasionally itch. The

---

BOX 16-13
Treatment of Pubic Lice and Scabies

PUBIC LICE*
- Permethrin 1% cream rinse (Nix) applied to affected areas and washed off after 10 minutes *or*
- Lindane 1% shampoo applied for 4 minutes to the affected area and then washed off (this regimen is contraindicated in pregnant or lactating women or children <2 years of age) *or*
- Pyrethrins with piperonyl butoxide applied for 10 minutes to the affected area and washed off (a second application of these products is recommended in 7 to 10 days if there is no response to the first application)

SCABIES*
- Permethrin 5% cream (Elimite) applied to all areas of the body from the neck down and washed off after 8 to 14 hours *or*
- Lindane 1% (gamma benzene hexachloride) 1 oz. of lotion or 30 g of cream applied thinly to all areas of the body from the neck down and thoroughly washed off after 8 hours *or*
- Ivermectin 200 μg/kg PO as a single dose or as two doses separated by 1 to 2 weeks

*Sexual partners and close household contacts should also be treated. Patients should be advised about environmental disinfection (e.g., wash all clothing and bed linens in hot water).

---

lesions contain a milky white material that consists of virus particles and epidermal cells. Hematoxylin and eosin stains of molluscum lesions reveal intracytoplasmic inclusion bodies. The lesions of molluscum may be confused with keratoacanthomas, warts, syringomas, or pyoderma.

The lesions last for a few months and spontaneously resolve. Treatment approaches include removal by curettage, liquid nitrogen ablation, and expression of the lesion core by direct pressure followed by electrodesiccation or chemical agents such as phenol, silver nitrate, and trichloroacetic acid. Therapy hastens resolution, but recurrences are common.

SUGGESTED READING

Billstein SA, Mattaliano VJ. The "nuisance" sexually transmitted diseases: molluscum contagiosum, scabies, and crab lice. Sex Transm Dis 1990; 74: 1487-1505.

17 Human Immunodeficiency Virus Disease and Acquired Immunodeficiency Virus Syndrome

BOSKO POSTIC, CHARLES S. BRYAN

It is generally accepted that about 1 million people in the United States are infected with the human immunodeficiency virus (HIV-1). New advances, especially the introduction of highly active antiretroviral therapy (HAART), bring new hope for HIV-infected persons but have also introduced new complexities into the optimum management of the disease. Primary care clinicians are pivotal to the early recognition of HIV infection and should play a major role in the comprehensive care of these patients, especially with regard to ensuring compliance with complicated drug regimens and helping patients cope with anxiety, depression, and difficult life adjustments. Primary care clinicians who wish to assume responsibility for all aspects of the disease should strive to stay current with the rapid developments in this area of med-

icine. An optimum approach consists of having patients with HIV disease establish a relationship with an infectious disease specialist or other physician who makes this disease a substantial part of his or her practice. The patient can then see the specialist in acquired immunodeficiency syndrome (AIDS) periodically (in our practice, one to four times a year, depending on the primary care clinician's preference) or on an as-needed basis for major decisions concerning antiretroviral therapy and for complications. Enormous advances in the recognition, diagnosis, treatment, and prevention of complications of AIDS have occurred during the past 20 years and are summarized in this chapter.

When to Refer

In a study published in 1996 (based on data before the introduction of today's highly active antiretroviral therapy), it was shown that survival of patients with AIDS correlated with the extent of the treating physician's experience with the disease.

SUGGESTED READING

Bartlett JG, Gallant JE. 2001-2002 Medical Management of HIV Infection. Baltimore: Johns Hopkins University; 2001. (For updates, see The Johns Hopkins University AIDS Service website: http://www.hopkins-aids.edu.)

Cohen PT, Sande MA, Volberding PA. The AIDS Knowledge Base: A Textbook on HIV Disease from the University of California, San Francisco, and San Francisco General Hospital. 3rd ed., Philadelphia: Lippincott Williams & Wilkins; 1999.

Dolin R, Masur H, Saag MS, eds. AIDS Therapy. New York: Churchill Livingstone; 1999.

Kitahata MM, Koepsell TD, Deyo RA, et al. Physicians' experience with the acquired immunodeficiency syndrome as a factor in patients' survival. N Engl J Med 1996; 334: 701-706.

Merigan TC Jr, Bartlett JG, Bolognesi D, eds. Textbook of AIDS Medicine. Baltimore: Williams & Wilkins; 1999.

Sande MA, Volberding PA, eds. The Medical Management of AIDS. 6th ed., Philadelphia: W.B. Saunders Company; 1999.

Sepkowitz KA. AIDS—the first 20 years. N Engl J Med 2001; 344: 1764-1772.

Ungvarski PJ, Flaskerud JH, eds. HIV/AIDS: A Guide to Primary Care Management. 4th ed., Philadelphia: W.B. Saunders Company; 1999.

Wormser GP, eds. AIDS and Other Manifestations of HIV Infection. 3rd ed., Philadelphia: Lippincott-Raven; 1998.

Cause

HIV-1 is now classified as a lentivirus, which belongs to the retroviruses (Figure 17-1). The RNA genome of retroviruses encodes for a reverse transcriptase enzyme, which results in a complementary DNA copy of the viral RNA. The main

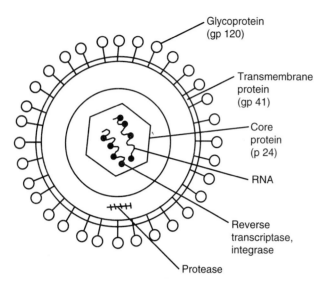

Glycoprotein
(gp 120)

Transmembrane
protein
(gp 41)

Core
protein
(p 24)

RNA

Reverse
transcriptase,
integrase

Protease

FIG. 17-1 Key components of the human immunodeficiency virus, showing the location of major proteins including enzymes.

cellular target for HIV is the CD4$^+$ helper T lymphocyte, a pivotal cell to the immune response. HIV also infects other cell types: megakaryocytes, peripheral white blood cells, follicular dendritic cells in the lymph nodes, epidermal Langerhans cells, astrocytes and other glial cells, cytotoxic lymphocytes known as CD8 cells, the cellular lining of the cervical uterus, the rectal mucosa, and the retinal lining.

Diagnostic Tests for HIV Infection

Antibodies to HIV (anti-HIV) can be recognized within weeks to several months after infection. The standard test for screening is the enzyme immunoassay (EIA) or enzyme-linked immunosorbent assay (ELISA). Anti-HIV is nearly always demonstrable within 3 to 6 months of infection. The Western blot assay, which identifies antibodies to the proteins in the core and in the envelope of HIV, is used to confirm a positive EIA screening test. Tests are usually performed on peripheral blood. Other body fluids, such as oral secretions or urine, may also be tested for antibodies to HIV.

The sensitivity of the ELISA for HIV is up to 99%. Most false-negative results are the result of early (primary) HIV infection, immunosuppression, and errors in specimen processing. Repeatedly positive ELISA tests are about 99% specific. The combined use of the ELISA and Western blot assays is >99% sensitive and specific for HIV infection. Autoimmune disorders including connective tissue diseases sometimes cause false-positive results from either or both of these assays.

Nucleic acid tests for HIV DNA or RNA use the polymerase chain reaction. Quantitative PCR-based assays (viral load tests) measure the number of copies of viral RNA genome circulating in blood and are used for staging the illness and following the response to treatment. The most frequently used quantitative test for viral load is currently the reverse transcriptase polymerase chain reaction (RT-PCR), followed by the branched DNA (bDNA) test. An ultrasensitive assay can detect 50 copies of the RNA genome of HIV and is used for treated and re-

sponding patients. The dynamic range of this test is between 50 and 75,000 copies. The viral load may be greater in some patients; for an unknown viral load the "standard assay" is preferred, since it detects 400 to 750,000 copies of HIV RNA. These PCR-based tests have replaced testing for the viral core p24 antigen, which is relatively insensitive.

A qualitative test for HIV, known as HIV DNA PCR, is used occasionally when the ELISA and Western blot methods yield equivocal results. The results are reported as positive or negative. The HIV DNA PCR is useful when recent (within 6 months) HIV infection is suspected and the screening tests for antibodies are negative. However, the HIV DNA PCR test is not approved by the Food and Drug Administration (FDA) as a screening test for HIV disease.

When interpreting test results for HIV antibodies, the physician must always remember that the likelihood of a false-positive test result varies inversely with the pretest probability (Bayes' theorem; see Chapter 1). The HIV DNA PCR test can occasionally be false positive at low levels owing to contamination of the specimen. Moreover, some patients who are HIV infected (perhaps as many as 12%) have undetectable viral loads even without treatment.

► KEY POINTS

DIAGNOSTIC TESTS FOR HIV INFECTION

⊃ The usual screening test for HIV infection is an enzyme immunoassay (EIA or ELISA) for anti-HIV antibodies. The usual confirmatory test is the Western blot method. Combined use of the ELISA and Western blot tests is >99% sensitive and specific for HIV infection. A qualitative test for HIV virus, known as HIV DNA PCR, can be useful when the ELISA and Western blot methods yield equivocal results.

⊃ A viral load test (usually a RT-PCR assay) measures the number of copies of the HIV genome in blood and is useful for staging the disease and following the response to treatment.

SUGGESTED READING

Centers for Disease and Prevention. Revised guidelines for HIV counseling, testing, and referral and revised recommendations for HIV screening of pregnant women. MMWR 2001; 50 (RR-19): 1-85.

Centers for Disease Control and Prevention. Guidelines for laboratory test result reporting of human immunodeficiency virus type 1 ribonucleic acid determination: recommendations from a CDC working group. MMWR 2001; 50 (RR-20): 1-12.

Mylonakis E, Paliou M, Lally M, et al. Laboratory testing for infection with the human immunodeficiency virus: established and novel approaches. Am J Med 2000; 109: 568-576.

Pathogenesis of HIV Infection

Infection with HIV occurs through sexual contact; through parenteral introduction of blood by transfusion, clotting factors, or injecting drug use; or from the infected mother to the child. Infection entails the entry of the virus into the body, replication of the virus after adhesion to susceptible cells, and the immune response to the virus. Antibodies to HIV occur in

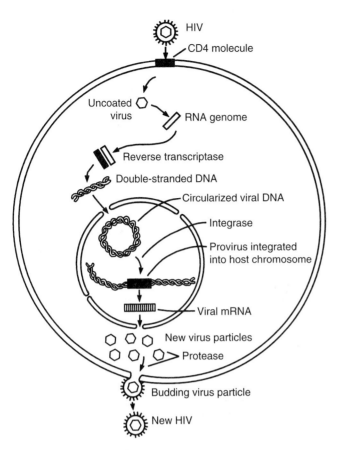

FIG. 17-2 Life cycle of the human immunodeficiency virus in the infected cell.

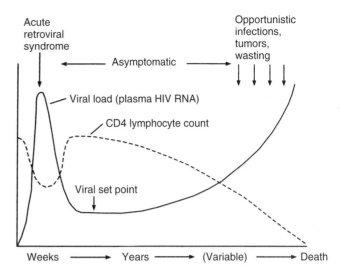

FIG. 17-3 Course of the human immunodeficiency virus (HIV) infection as determined by the CD4 lymphocyte count and the viral load as measured by quantitative assay for HIV RNA.

most individuals by 2 months after infection and in nearly all infected persons by 6 months. The HIV life cycle consists of the following steps (Figure 17-2):

- Adhesion of HIV to the cell (CD4) receptor, followed by viral penetration into the cell and then uncoating of the virus with presentation of its RNA genome.
- Synthesis of complementary DNA from the viral RNA by the infected cell's machinery, which is made possible by the viral enzyme reverse transcriptase.
- Integration of newly made double-stranded HIV DNA (provirus) into the host cell genome, which is made possible by another viral enzyme known as integrase.
- Synthesis of new viral RNA and peptide viral subunits by processes known as transcription and translation.
- Assembly of new virus particles followed by their release from the infected cell. The protease enzyme, which is also part of the HIV virion, is involved in the assembly and release of the infected virion.

Current drug therapies for HIV disease are directed at the steps involving the reverse transcriptase and protease enzymes, but other steps in the viral life cycle might also be amenable to intervention.

In the weeks after initial infection with HIV, replication results in a high level of viremia. The peak viral load (measured as circulating HIV-1 RNA copies) occurs within months and is followed by a gradual decline. However, production of the virus remains continuous for years at a plateau level known as the viral set point (Figure 17-3). The viral set point (which is also measured as viral load) varies from case to case. Between 1 billion and 10 billion new viral particles are made each day in most infected patients. CD4 lymphocytes, the main target cells of HIV infection, are destroyed through several mechanisms. These include the direct effects of virus replication, autoimmunity, and programmed cell death (known as apoptosis). Initially, increased production of CD4 lymphocytes serves to offset the losses. Eventually, the number of circulating CD4 lymphocytes declines, leading to immunodeficiency and opportunistic infections.

The variable viral load (or viral set point) from case to case has clinical implications. When the CD4 count and the viral load are both measured, as is done in current practice, a better estimate of prognosis can be made (Table 17-1). The viral load and the CD4 count are also both important for determining the effectiveness of treatment. These concepts can be explained to patients by asking them to envision a train heading down a track with a destroyed trestle waiting down the line. The CD4 count expresses the distance to the disaster, and the viral load expresses how fast the train is going. Few major diseases can be staged with blood tests alone to the extent that HIV disease can now be staged by use of the CD4 count and viral load in combination.

On the clinical level the chain of events leads from the acute retroviral syndrome, often present during the first few months of infection, to a clinically silent period that may last several years. Once the decline in CD4 count approaches 200/mm³, the resulting immunodeficiency state becomes expressed as opportunistic infections and tumors. During the long clinical latency period the virus localizes in lymph nodes, particularly follicular dendritic cells. Later in the course of disease, lymph nodes become depleted (i.e., cytopenic) and the virus escapes into the bloodstream, enhancing the viremia in the final phases of disease.

HIV infection causes immunodeficiency that affects most cell types involved in the response to infection. The resulting

TABLE 17-1
Likelihood of Development of AIDS Within 3 Years Based on the Viral Load and CD4 Lymphocyte Count*

CD4 count/mm³	VIRAL LOAD BY RT-PCR† (COPIES/MM³)				
	<1500 (%)	1500-7000 (%)	7000-20,000 (%)	20,000-55,000 (%)	>55,000 (%)
<200				40	86
201-350			8	40	64
351-500		2	8	16	48
501-750	2	2	8	16	33
>750		2	3	10	33

Modified from Mellors JW, Muñoz A, Giorgi JV, et al. Plasma viral load and CD4+ lymphocytes as prognostic markers of HIV-1 infection. Ann Intern Med 1997; 126: 946-954.
*For example, a patient with CD4 count <200/mm³ and viral load between 20,000 and 55,000 copies/mm³, if untreated, has a 40% chance that an AIDS-defining condition (opportunistic infection, malignancy, or wasting syndrome) will develop within 3 years.
†Viral loads as determined by branched-chain viral DNA are approximately one half of the levels determined by RT-PCR, as shown here.

immune incompetence opens the door to opportunistic pathogens and the formation and spread of tumors.

 KEY POINTS

PATHOGENESIS OF HIV INFECTION

⊃ After infection there is an initial burst of viral replication with a high level of viremia. This is followed by a plateau phase or set point. Between 1 billion and 10 billion new viral particles are made each day in most HIV-infected patients.

⊃ The CD4 lymphocyte count is a useful marker for defining the severity of HIV disease as it will be expressed clinically. The viral load (usually measured as quantitative HIV by RT-PCR) indicates the rate of viral replication and provides a discriminating prognostic tool.

⊃ Patients should learn to follow their CD4 lymphocyte counts and viral loads. A useful metaphor for teaching these concepts is that of a train heading toward a destroyed trestle. The CD4 count expresses the distance (or time) to the disaster, while the viral load expresses the rate at which the disease is progressing.

SUGGESTED READING

Ho DD, Neumann AU, Perelson AS, et al. Rapid turnover of plasma virions and CD4 lymphocytes in HIV-1 infection. Nature 1995; 373: 123-126.

Mellors JW, Rinaldo CR Jr, Gupta P, et al. Prognosis in HIV-1 infection predicted by the quantity of virus in plasma. Science 1996; 272: 1167-1170.

Acute Retroviral Syndrome

The acute retroviral syndrome (see also Chapters 7 and 8) occurs within weeks of infection and may have one of these presentations:

■ Heterophil-negative mononucleosis; occasionally the Monospot test can be false positive (see Chapter 8)

■ An influenza-like illness without the respiratory component, but occasionally with a maculopapular rash that is faint and centripetal (see Chapter 11)

■ Aseptic meningitis ("viral meningitis")

In a majority of HIV-infected persons the acute retroviral syndrome develops, which may be recognized when the exposure event is known, such as a freak accident in a health care setting. The acute retroviral syndrome is recognized less frequently when the exposure event (such as a sexual encounter) is not recognized to be a high risk. Overall, about 50% of recently infected persons remain asymptomatic. Highly active antiretroviral therapy (HAART) should be considered for patients with the acute retroviral syndrome. Although definitive data are lacking, aggressive treatment at this stage offers, theoretically, an opportunity to conserve the immune reserve and thus modify the natural history of the disease. When a diagnosis of acute retroviral syndrome is made, referral to a center with a research protocol should be considered; a list of available sites is available at http://aiedrp.fhcrc.org.

SUGGESTED READING

Capiluppi B, Ciuffreda D, Quinzan GP, et al. Four drug-HAART in primary HIV-1 infection: clinical benefits and virologic parameters. Journal of Biological Regulators & Homeostatic Agents 2000; 14: 58-62.

Carpenter CCJ, Cooper DA, Fischl MA, et al. Antiretroviral therapy in adults: updated recommendations of the International AIDS Society—USA Panel. JAMA 2000; 283: 381-390.

Geise R, Maenza J, Celum CL. Clinical challenges and diagnostic approaches to recognizing acute human immunodeficiency virus infection. Am J Med 2001; 111: 237-238.

Poggi C, Profizi N, Djediouane A, et al. Long-term evaluation of triple nucleoside therapy administered from primary HIV-1 infection. AIDS 1999; 13: 1213-1220.

Manifestations of HIV Disease

Previously, distinctions were made between AIDS-related complex (ARC) and acquired immunodeficiency syndrome (AIDS). However, it is more useful to think of the manifestations of HIV disease as a continuum. Here we review some of the disease manifestations that can occur relatively early in the disease (i.e., before the CD4 count falls below 200/mm³). Recognition of these manifestations should frequently prompt the primary care clinician to obtain a test for HIV antibodies.

Constitutional symptoms such as fatigue, malaise, episodic fever, night sweats, anorexia, and weight loss may occur at a variable time after infection with HIV and are usually progressive. When the CD4 count drops below 500/mm³, oral hairy leukoplakia may appear as white spikelike lesions at the lateral edges of the tongue. These represent crystals of Epstein-Barr virus relapsing from a latent stage. Although hairy leukoplakia may be unattractive, it is seldom symptomatic and does not require treatment. Oropharyngeal candidiasis is the most frequent of the mucous membrane manifestations. Most commonly, oral candidiasis appears as a flaky, cottage cheese–like thrush. However, erythema with small erosions may be the sole manifestation. When oral thrush is associated with dysphagia, a presumptive diagnosis of esophageal candidiasis is usually justified. Definitive diagnosis is reached by endoscopy (Figure 17-4). Candidiasis involving the genitalia is also common in HIV disease, especially in women. Aphthous stomatitis is bothersome in HIV-infected patients. Aphthae last longer in HIV-infected persons than in other persons, usually for weeks or months, are quite painful, and may lead to malnutrition. Treatment with short courses of corticosteroids is usually effective.

Herpes zoster in a person under age 50 should raise the possibility of HIV infection and necessitates screening for HIV antibodies.

In patients with advanced AIDS, herpes simplex virus (HSV) causes painful perianal or genital ulcers that can evolve into a major, disabling opportunistic infection. Often an even more painful herpes proctitis is associated with HSV. It is diagnosed by proctoscopy or sigmoidoscopy and virus culture, usually yielding HSV type 2. With an imprint slide (Tzanck preparation), characteristic giant cells with inclusions may be demonstrated. In most instances the diagnosis is based on a favorable response to an empiric trial with an antiviral agent, such as acyclovir (see Chapters 16 and 20). Some HSV-2 isolates are resistant to acyclovir. Foscarnet and ganciclovir represent alternative therapies.

Genital warts (condyloma acuminatum) caused by the human papillomavirus (HPV) are common, may be the first manifestations of HIV disease, and can be extensive. HPV is associated with uterine cervical and intraepithelial neoplasia in women and with penile carcinoma in men.

Other sexually transmitted diseases are common in patients with HIV infection and should be aggressively sought. Syphilis is the most important because of its implications. Early neurosyphilis (neurosyphilis within 2 years of infection by *T. pal-*

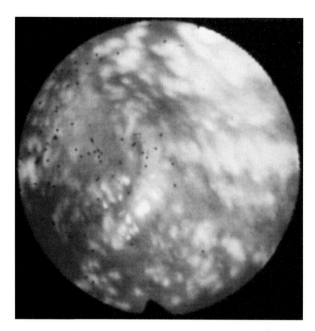

FIG. 17-4 Endoscopic view of the esophagus with the entire mucosa covered with white thrush. Yeast cells and pseudohyphae were seen on the smear, and *Candida albicans* grew luxuriously on fungal culture medium.

lidum) is often characterized by meningitis, cranial nerve abnormalities, or stroke. A seizure disorder in an HIV-infected individual may be due to neurosyphilis. Neurosyphilis in HIV-infected persons often occurs within 4 years of primary syphilis, whereas neurosyphilis in patients not infected with HIV generally occurs 15 years or more after the primary infection. A positive Venereal Disease Research Laboratory (VDRL) test on the cerebrospinal fluid (CSF) of a patient with serum antibodies to *Treponema pallidum* most conclusively makes the diagnosis of neurosyphilis. Unfortunately, the CSF VDRL test, although specific, is not sensitive. The most common CSF abnormality, lymphocytic pleocytosis, is only 70% sensitive. The diagnosis may be achieved by the demonstration of spirochetes in the CSF or the nervous tissue. A PCR method for demonstrating treponemal DNA has superior sensitivity, but standardization is lacking.

Tuberculosis is relatively common in HIV disease. The presentations of tuberculosis are frequently subtle and atypical in patients with advanced HIV disease. Infiltrates can occur in any lung segment and tend to be noncavitary, especially in patients with low CD4 counts. The tuberculin skin test is often suppressed in persons with CD4 counts <500/mm³. Therefore it is important to date the tuberculin test and interpret the result in the context of the patient's CD4 count. Induration of ≥5 mm with the standard Mantoux skin test is considered a positive reaction in HIV-infected patients. Performing simultaneous anergy skin testing is not especially useful (see Chapter 22). When pneumonia in a patient with HIV disease fails to respond to conventional antibiotics, tuberculosis should be considered. Disseminated (miliary) tuberculosis occurs in more than 25% of HIV-infected persons with tuberculosis. In some patients the chest x-ray film is clear despite the presence of endobronchial tuberculosis.

Regional mycoses, most notably histoplasmosis and coccidioidomycosis (see Chapter 21), assume great importance in patients with HIV disease because these infections have a penchant for dissemination. Disseminated histoplasmosis usually occurs with CD4 count <200/mm^3 and often is manifested as fever. Oral and genital ulcers, lymphadenopathy and hepatosplenomegaly, and a maculopapular, erythematous rash on the face, trunk, and extremities are possible associated findings. Occasionally a diagnosis of histoplasmosis can be made by finding yeast cells within polymorphonuclear leukocytes on a peripheral blood smear. Bone marrow aspiration and biopsy are often useful because they demonstrate granulomas and yeast cells and provide material for fungal culture. Histoplasmosis can occur in the brain, and brain biopsy may be necessary for diagnosis. An assay for heat-stable antigen in urine and serum is useful because it is about 90% sensitive for diagnosis of disseminated histoplasmosis.

Generalized, asymptomatic lymphadenopathy is common at all stages of HIV infection but especially during the earlier stages, before lymphocyte depletion causes the nodes to atrophy. Lymphadenopathy involves especially the cervical, axillary, and inguinal nodes. It is usually symmetric. Asymmetric lymphadenopathy, especially when one or more of the involved nodes is unusually large, hard, or fixed to underlying tissue, raises the suspicion of malignant disease, including lymphoma.

Of the dermatologic manifestations of HIV disease (Table 17-2), seborrheic dermatitis is especially common. Superinfection by dermatophytes sometimes occurs, complicating treatment. Xerosis (dry skin), ichthyosis (dry skin with fissuring to form a fish scale–like pattern), and atopic dermatitis occur more frequently in HIV-infected patients. Psoriasis affects about 5% of patients with HIV disease and can be severe. Another cause of pruritus is a condition known as eosinophilic folliculitis. Clinically, this resembles folliculitis caused by *Staphylococcus aureus;* punch skin biopsy can be helpful. Eosinophilic folliculitis is greatly annoying to the patient but is rarely progressive. Other dermatologic manifestations include mucocutaneous fungal infections (e.g., histoplasmosis, blastomycosis, and coccidioidomycosis; see Chapter 7), molluscum contagiosum, herpes zoster, HSV infection, and genital warts. An opportunistic tumor, Kaposi's sarcoma, is best diagnosed by biopsy of the deeply pigmented raised or nodular skin lesions (see later discussion). It must be distinguished from a systemic illness known as bacillary angiomatosis or, when it involves the liver, peliosis hepatis. Bacillary angiomatosis and peliosis hepatitis are usually caused by *Bartonella henselae* (the agent of cat scratch disease; see Chapter 8) when acquired from cats or fleas and by *Bartonella quintana* when acquired from lice. In AIDS patients these pathogens cause a generalized febrile illness with abdominal pain, lymphadenopathy and hepatosplenomegaly, and painful erythematous skin plaques and nodules. These lesions can be distinguished from Kaposi's sarcoma by demonstration of the organisms in biopsy specimens stained with Warthin-Starry stain (Table 17-2).

Aseptic meningitis can be caused by HIV, but its recognition should prompt consideration of other diseases, including secondary syphilis and, rarely, meningitis caused by *Listeria monocytogenes.* Peripheral neuropathy is relatively common and usually develops gradually as a distal sensory polyneuropathy with pain, impaired sensation, and dysesthesias beginning in the feet. Headaches in patients with HIV disease should raise suspicion of cryptococcal meningitis, toxoplasmic encephalitis, and tumor, including primary CNS lymphoma.

Psychiatric disorders are common in persons with HIV disease. About 60% of patients experience a depressive episode, and many develop major depression. Other frequent psychiatric diagnoses include adjustment disorder (generally manifested as demoralization), behavioral disorder (including substance abuse), and personality disorders. Clinicians must inquire about psychiatric symptoms, exclude organic disease (including AIDS dementia, discussed later in the chapter), and in many instances refer patients for psychological or psychiatric care and support.

KEY POINTS

MANIFESTATIONS OF HIV DISEASE

⊃ The diverse manifestations of HIV infection should prompt a high index of suspicion for the disease. Constitutional symptoms include fatigue, malaise, episodic fever, night sweats, anorexia, and weight loss.

⊃ Sexually transmitted diseases are, in general, more common in HIV-infected patients. Syphilis is important to recognize because it is curable with specific therapy.

⊃ Neurosyphilis in HIV-infected persons often occurs within 2 to 4 years after the primary infection (in contrast to the usual 15 or more years in persons without HIV disease) and can cause meningitis, cranial nerve abnormalities, stroke, or seizure.

⊃ Tuberculosis is relatively common in patients with HIV disease and is often atypical and likely to be extrapulmonary (>25% of cases).

⊃ Regional mycoses (e.g., histoplasmosis, coccidioidomycosis, and blastomycosis) should always be considered in HIV-infected patients who have unusual symptoms and live in an endemic zone.

⊃ Psychiatirc disorders are commom in HIV-affected persons, and clinicians should be alert to such problems as major depression.

SUGGESTED READING

Chiao EY, Ries KM, Sande MA. AIDS and the elderly. Clin Infect Dis 1999; 28: 740-745.

Gendelman HE, Lipton SA, Epstein L, Swindells S, eds. The Neurology of AIDS. New York: Chapman & Hall; 1998.

Masur H. Respiratory Infections in Patients with HIV. Philadelphia: Lippincott Williams & Wilkins; 1999.

Ramos-Gomez FJ. Oral aspects of HIV infection in children. Oral Dis 1997; 3 (Suppl 1): S31-S35.

Samet JH, Muz P, Cabral P, et al. Dermatologic manifestations in HIV-infected patients: a primary care perspective. Mayo Clin Proc 1999; 74: 658-660.

Semple SJG, Miller RF. AIDS and the Lung. Oxford: Blackwell Science, Ltd.; 1997.

Treisman GJ, Angelino AF, Hutton HE. Psychiatric issues in the management of patients with HIV infection. JAMA 2001; 286: 2857-2864.

Vassilopoulos D, Calabrese LH. Rheumatologic manifestations of HIV-1 and HTLV-1 infections. Cleve Clin J Med 1998; 65: 436-441.

Laboratory Findings

Baseline laboratory tests in persons with newly recognized HIV disease ideally include the following:

■ CD4 lymphocyte count and viral load (quantitative HIV-1 by RT-PCR) to stage the disease (see earlier discussion).

TABLE 17-2
Some Dermatologic Manifestations of HIV Disease

Manifestation	Clinical features	Diagnosis
Seborrheic dermatitis	Although common in the general population, is especially prominent in many patients with HIV disease. Superinfection with dermatophytes may occur.	Clinical appearance (erythema and scaling of midline areas of forehead, face, groin, and elsewhere).
Psoriasis	Affects about 5% of patients with HIV disease, with scaly, hyperkeratotic, lichenified, sharply demarcated plaques occurring most typically on the elbows, knees, scalp, and lower back. Onycholysis and nail separation may also be present.	Skin biopsy is confirmatory in doubtful cases.
Molluscum contagiosum	Occurs more often in patients with AIDS than in the general population, often with multiple lesions in patients with low CD4 counts. Is manifested as small, firm, pearly white or flesh-colored papules with central umbilication on face, trunk, and genital areas, sparing the palms and soles.	Distinctive clinical appearance. Skin lesions of cryptococcosis (and in parts of Asia, *Penicillium marneffei),* basal cell carcinoma, and pyogenic granuloma. Biopsy is therefore sometimes desirable. Treatment is usually with liquid nitrogen.
Herpes simplex virus infection	Infections recur more commonly and are more severe in patients with HIV disease. Painful erythematous papules become vesicles that ulcerate, sometimes leading to chronic ulcers with jagged edges.	Tzanck preparation; culture or fluorescent assay for HIV; however, standard practice is often to use a therapeutic trial of acyclovir or a similar drug (see Chapters 16 and 20).
Herpes zoster	Shingles, defined by vesicles on an erythematous base in a unilateral dermatomal distribution, can be the presenting manifestation of HIV and occurs in about 5% to 10% of patients annually.	Diagnosis is usually made on clinical grounds, followed by treatment with acyclovir or a similar drug (see Chapters 7 and 20). Viral culture or fluorescent assay is confirmatory in doubtful cases.
Syphilis	Secondary syphilis typically presents as erythematous macules and papules involving the trunk and extremities, including the palms and soles, but can mimic a variety of skin diseases, including psoriasis and pityriasis rosea.	Secondary syphilis should be suspected in any patient with HIV disease and generalized rash. The RPR (VDRL) is nearly always positive (rare false-negative results have been reported in patients with HIV disease).
Bacterial folliculitis	May be localized or disseminated in patients with HIV disease and is prone to relapse. *Staphylococcus aureus* is the usual pathogen.	Gram stain shows gram-positive cocci in clusters; culture reveals *S. aureus.*
Eosinophilic folliculitis	Sometimes called "itchy folliculitis," this lesion occurs as raised, pruritic papules with pustular heads on an erythematous base. Usually occurs in patients with advanced disease.	Skin biopsy enables the distinction of this lesion from bacterial folliculitis (clinically, the two lesions can be identical).
Drug reaction (dermatitis medicamentosa)	Classically, an erythematous papular or maculopapular rash especially over the trunk, but severe reactions including Stevens-Johnson syndrome (see Chapter 7) occur.	Drug reactions most commonly occur between 7 and 10 days after initiation of a new drug but can occur at any time, especially if there has been previous exposure. Resolution after the drug is stopped suggests the diagnosis.
Kaposi's sarcoma	Firm, subcutaneous, violaceous or brown-black plaques, papules, or nodules, 0.5 to 2 cm in diameter	Clinical appearance is distinctive, but biopsy is desirable, especially to distinguish this lesion from bacillary angiomatosis.
Bacillary angiomatosis	Usually occurs as one or several purple-red papules, nodules, or plaques that bear a strong resemblance to Kaposi's sarcoma. Hepatic involvement (peliosis hepatis) and involvement of other organs also occur.	Skin biopsy with Warthin-Starry stain shows organisms consistent with *Bartonella henselae* or *Bartonella quintana.*

- Complete blood count (CBC), which not infrequently shows one or more cytopenias. Leukopenia may be the most common, even in untreated patients. Anemia is occasionally profound even in the absence of bone marrow suppression from antiretroviral therapy. Severe anemia is occasionally caused by parvovirus B19 infection (diagnosis is by parvovirus B19 DNA PCR or IgM serology; see Chapter 7), in which case the anemia responds to intravenous immune globulin (400 mg/kg/day for 5 to 7 days). Platelet abnormalities are usually due to autoimmunity but vary in their appearance and occasionally show spontaneous improvement.

- Complete metabolic panel, including renal and liver function tests, electrolytes, lipase analysis, and urinalysis. Polyclonal hypergammaglobulinemia is due to the lack of helper lymphocyte regulatory function on immunoglobulin production by plasma cells. Elevated blood urea nitrogen or serum creatinine levels, proteinuria, and hypoalbuminemia suggest renal involvement that can lead to renal failure. The underlying pathologic condition is usually a focal sclerosing glomerulonephritis, which is seen particularly in persons of African ancestry who are infected with HIV. Serologic tests for syphilis (RPR or VDRL) should ideally be repeated annually.

- Tuberculin skin test, which, if nonreactive, should ideally be repeated annually. Persons with reactivity ($\geq$5 mm of induration) should be given isoniazid (INH) prophylaxis (see Chapter 22).

- Pelvic examination and Pap smear for HIV-infected women.

- Toxoplasmosis IgG (not IgM) serologic test. Patients with reactive serologic tests are at risk for CNS toxoplasmosis. Patients with nonreactive serologic tests should be advised about risk factors for toxoplasmosis and ways to prevent it. These include using disposable gloves when handling cat litter, sand, or soil (as in gardening); cleaning cat litter pans daily by soaking in near-boiling water; avoiding ingestion of raw eggs, unpasteurized milk, and meat that is not cooked "well done"; and carefully washing the hands after handling raw meat or vegetables.

- Cytomegalovirus IgG (not IgM) serologic test. Patients with reactive serologic tests are at risk of cytomegalovirus (CMV) retinitis and other complications. Since CMV IgG antibodies are highly prevalent ($\geq$95%) among men who have sex with men and injecting drug users, a case can be made that these patients need not be tested. Careful retinal examination should be a routine part of the clinic visit for every HIV-infected patient with a positive CMV serologic test, and periodic examination by an ophthalmologist is recommended.

- Chest x-ray examination. All patients should have a baseline chest x-ray film.

- Screening test for glucose-6 phosphate dehydrogenase (G6PD) deficiency. G6PD deficiency is found in about 10% of African-American men, up to 2% of African-American women, and men of Mediterranean ancestry, from the Indian subcontinent, and from Southeast Asia. Oxidant drugs, especially dapsone and primaquine, may cause a hemolytic anemia of varying intensity in patients with this deficiency. Sulfonamides (albeit with some oxidant capacity) rarely cause hemolysis in such patients.

- Serologic tests for hepatitis B and hepatitis C.

Results of baseline laboratory tests should be recorded prominently in the patient's database. A flowchart showing the patient's CD4 count and viral load, antiretroviral therapy, and other key parameters such as body weight is useful.

 KEY POINTS

LABORATORY FINDINGS
- ⊃ Minimum baseline laboratory tests include CD4 count and viral load, serologic test for syphilis (RPR), tuberculin skin test, chest x-ray examination, and (in women) a Pap smear.
- ⊃ Other desirable tests are CBC, metabolic panel, IgG serologic tests for toxoplasmosis and CMV, and serologic tests for hepatitis B and hepatitis C.
- ⊃ A qualitative screening test for G6PD deficiency is useful for patients of African, Mediterranean, Indian subcontinent, or Southeast Asian ancestry.

SUGGESTED READING
Koduri PR, Kumapley R, Valladares J, et al. Chronic pure red cell aplasia caused by parvovirus B19 in AIDS: use of intravenous immunoglobulin—a report of eight patients. Am J Hematol 1999; 61: 16-20.

Mildvan D, Landay A, De Gruttola V, et al. An approach to the validation of markers for use in AIDS clinical trials. Clin Infect Dis 1997; 24: 764-774.

Mitsuyasu R. Hematologic disease. In: Dolin R, Masur H, Saag MS. AIDS Therapy. Philadelphia: Churchill-Livingstone; 1999: 666-679.

Major Opportunistic Infections

The clinician caring for patients with HIV disease should be familiar with several opportunistic infections that occur on a regular basis.

Pneumocystis Carinii Pneumonia

Pneumocystis carinii pneumonia (PCP) is the classical opportunistic infection affecting patients with CD4 counts <200/mm^3. The presentation is often subtle. Clinicians caring for patients with HIV should be thoroughly familiar with this disease.

Presentation and Progression

Cause. *Pneumocystis carinii* is now considered a fungus rather than a protozoan as was once thought. Some researchers believe that *P. carinii* colonizes healthy persons for long, perhaps indefinite periods and that clinical disease is caused by reactivation of such latent infection when host defenses fail. Others believe that *P. carinii* colonization is transient but that nearly everyone is reexposed to the organism on a frequent basis. Unfortunately, the organism cannot be isolated in the laboratory, at least by conventional culture methods.

Presentation. PCP usually begins slowly with low-grade fever and cough over several weeks or even months before progressing to sustained fever and hypoxemia. Physical examination often reveals fever, tachypnea, and tachycardia, but the lungs are surprisingly clear to auscultation, even when diffuse infiltrates are present on the chest x-ray film. The chest x-ray film can be normal when the patient is first seen (up to 30% of patients), at which point mild hypoxemia and elevation of serum lactic dehydrogenase (LDH) levels provide valuable clues. The chest film frequently shows reticular nodular infiltrates, but unilateral or bilateral pneumonia (Figure 17-5) and a tumorlike appearance may also be present. The latter is seen in persons undergoing prophylaxis with pentamidine by

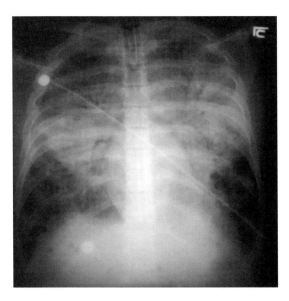

FIG. 17-5 Massive bilateral *Pneumocystis carinii* pneumonia with air bronchograms.

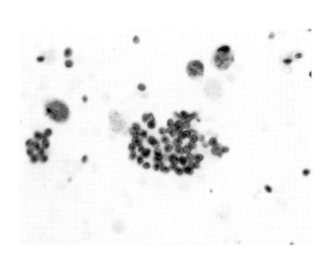

FIG. 17-6 Clusters of *Pneumocystis carinii* shown by Giemsa stain on a specimen obtained by bronchoalveolar lavage.

inhalation, which may be unevenly distributed and thus miss poorly ventilated lung segments. Since efficient prophylaxis against PCP is now available, it is important to ascertain that the patient has been taking TMP/SMX or other appropriate medications. If not, PCP becomes the primary consideration in any patient with HIV disease and CD4 count <200/mm³, especially if hypoxemia is present (PaO_2 ≤ 70 mm Hg).

Diagnosis

Sputum should be induced by nebulization with hypertonic (10%) saline and submitted to the laboratory for Gram stain, routine bacterial culture, acid-fast bacillus (AFB) stain and culture, fungal stain and culture, and cytologic examination for *P. carinii,* which is usually performed with a silver stain. For a patient with a CD4 count <200/mm³ and symptoms and signs consistent with PCP who has not been taking effective prophylactic measures against this disease, a common strategy is to begin empiric therapy.

Invasive diagnostic procedures are indicated if the patient has been taking effective prophylactic medication against PCP, such as TMP/SMX or dapsone; if epidemiologic or clinical features suggest an alternative diagnosis such as tuberculosis; and if little or no response to empiric therapy occurs within 72 to 96 hours of initiation. These procedures include bronchoscopy, bronchoalveolar lavage, transbronchial biopsy, or a pleural tap or biopsy, if applicable. Since *P. carinii* infiltration is an alveolar process, a bronchoalveolar lavage undertaken by a trained pulmonologist may be the most sensitive method (Figure 17-6). Fluorescent antibodies for the PCP antigen enhance the diagnostic sensitivity. Transbronchial biopsy is also an effective diagnostic method, since it may be used to diagnose a granulomatous disease, such as tuberculosis or histoplasmosis, or a tumor (Kaposi's sarcoma). A PCR test for *P. carinii* has been developed and appears highly promising.

Natural History

Expected Outcome. Untreated PCP is uniformly fatal in patients with AIDS and was the major cause of death be-

fore the development of new approaches to diagnosis and therapy.

Treatment

Methods. Treatment for PCP is usually begun empirically in a patient with suggestive symptoms and signs, including some degree of hypoxemia and elevation of the serum LDH level. Trimethoprim-sulfamethoxazole (TMP/SMX), at a dose of 15 to 20 mg/kg/day (based on the trimethoprim component) and given orally or intravenously, is the drug of choice for patients who do not have a history of hypersensitivity to sulfa drugs. In hypoxemic patients (PaO_2 ≤70 mm Hg), high-dose corticosteroid therapy should precede high-dose intravenous TMP/SMX. Corticosteroids are usually given as prednisone, 40 mg b.i.d. for 5 days, then 40 mg daily for 5 days, then 20 mg daily for the duration of treatment. In patients with milder disease (PaO_2 >70 mm Hg), corticosteroids are unnecessary and TMP/SMX can be given by mouth. Several alternative regimens are available for patients who cannot tolerate TMP/SMX. For mild to moderately severe cases of PCP treated in the outpatient setting, these include atovaquone 750 mg as an oral suspension b.i.d. with food and trimethoprim 15 to 20 mg/kg/day plus dapsone 100 mg/day. For more severe cases of PCP, alternative regimens include intravenously administered pentamidine, intravenously administered trimetrexate, and clindamycin plus primaquine. The usual duration of treatment for an acute episode of PCP is 21 days. The induction regimen is followed by a maintenance regimen, usually TMP/SMX in the same doses used for prophylaxis (see "Prophylaxis and Therapy of Opportunistic Infections" later in the chapter).

Expected Response. Patients with mild to moderately severe disease (PaO_2 >70 mm Hg) usually show improvement within 5 to 7 days of initiation of therapy. Overall, 80% to 90% of patients survive the disease. Patients are at risk of relapse, and patients who recover from PCP are at risk of pneumothorax.

A frequent problem with therapy for PCP is the development of allergic reactions to TMP/SMX, which require a change of therapy in up to 50% of patients. Stevens-Johnson syndrome and toxic epidermal necrolysis (see Chapter 7) may occur. Other problems include cytopenias, pancreatitis, metabolic acidosis, and hepatitis. It is sometimes possible to counter the milder side effects with judicious use of corticosteroids.

When to Refer

Patients with mild to moderately severe PCP (Pao$_2$ >70 mm Hg) can often be treated as outpatients provided compliance is ensured. Patients with more severe disease should be hospitalized.

 KEY POINTS

PNEUMOCYSTIS CARINII PNEUMONIA

⊃ PCP in HIV-infected persons usually occurs when the CD4 count falls below 200/mm^3.

⊃ Onset is often insidious over weeks to even months with cough, shortness of breath, and low-grade fever. Chest x-ray examination classically shows diffuse bilateral infiltrates but may be normal initially in up to 30% of patients.

⊃ Patients with Pao$_2$ >70 mm Hg can often be treated empirically as outpatients after initial diagnostic studies. Patients with Pao$_2$ ≤70 mm Hg should be hospitalized.

SUGGESTED READING

Arozullah AM, Yarnold PR, Weinstein RA, et al. A new preadmission staging system for predicting inpatient mortality from HIV-associated *Pneumocystis carinii* pneumonia in the early highly active antiretroviral therapy (HAART) era. Am J Respir Crit Care Med 2000; 161: 1081-1086.

Fishman JA. Prevention of infection due to *Pneumocystis carinii*. Antimicrob Agents Chemother 1998; 42: 995-1004.

Fishman JA. Treatment of infection due to *Pneumocystis carinii*. Antimicrob Agents Chemother 1998; 42: 1309-1314.

Kovacs JA, Gill VJ, Meshnick S, et al. New insights into transmission, diagnosis, and drug treatment of Pneumocystis carinii pneumonia. JAMA 2001; 286: 2450-2460.

Safrin S, Finkelstein DM, Feinberg J, et al. ACTG 108 Study Group. Comparison of three regimens for treatment of mild to moderate *Pneumocystis carinii* pneumonia in patients with AIDS: a double-blind, randomized trial of oral trimethoprim-sulfamethoxazole, dapsone-trimethoprim, and clindamycin-primaquine. Ann Intern Med 1996; 124: 792-802.

Thomas CF Jr, Limper AH. *Pneumocystis* pneumonia: clinical presentation and diagnosis in patients with and without acquired immune deficiency syndrome. Semin Respir Infect 1998; 13: 289-295.

Toxoplasmosis

Toxoplasmosis (see Chapters 8 and 23) is a common infection of humans that, in AIDS patients, is most frequently expressed as encephalitis with multiple CNS mass lesions if CD4 counts are <100/mm^3. The presentation usually includes some combination of headache, focal neurologic defect, seizure, and fever. In about 15% to 25% of cases the onset is acute and may include intracranial hemorrhage or seizures. In most instances the onset is subacute. Occasionally the first disease manifestations are neuropsychiatric, such as impaired memory or reasoning ability, anxiety, agitation, or paranoid psychosis. Up to 89% of patients have focal neurologic deficits such as hemiparesis, speech impairment, cranial nerve deficits, sensory abnormalities, and cerebellar signs. Numerous unusual manifestations have been described. Toxoplasmic chorioretinitis develops in occasional patients with HIV disease. Pulmonary toxoplasmosis sometimes occurs in patients with HIV disease and can be indistinguishable from PCP in its presentation.

Diagnosis of CNS toxoplasmosis is often presumptive, based on the clinical picture, a positive computed tomography (CT) or magnetic resonance imaging (MRI) scan of the brain, and the presence of IgG antibodies to *T. gondii*. Multiple ring enhancing lesions are often found on CT scan. MRI imaging is more sensitive than CT scanning, especially if contrast media is used, and sometimes shows multiple lesions that are not apparent on CT scan. However, use of contrast media is risky for patients with serum creatinine levels ≥2 mg/dL. The definitive diagnosis of cerebral toxoplasmosis can be established by brain biopsy through a burr hole. This is now seldom done in practice. Most patients with advanced HIV disease and multiple ring enhancing lesions are treated empirically, especially if *Toxoplasma* IgG antibodies are present in serum (which occurs in about 90% of patients with CNS toxoplasmosis).

Problems in diagnosis arise when only a single brain lesion is identified (about 20% of patients) and when no response to empiric therapy occurs. Primary CNS lymphoma is frequently a single lesion (about 50% of cases). Lumbar puncture, if safe to perform, can provide useful information. A PCR assay is now available for *T. gondii* DNA and is reported to be 11% to 77% sensitive (but 100% specific) for CNS toxoplasmosis in AIDS. Other useful studies of the CSF include PCR for the JC virus (the cause of progressive multifocal leukoencephalopathy), Epstein-Barr virus (a cause of primary CNS lymphoma), and CMV (which causes ventriculitis), and cryptococcal antigen for cryptococcosis (which can sometimes cause brain lesions, as well as meningitis). However, brain biopsy may be needed to resolve the diagnosis.

Natural History

Expected Outcome. Untreated toxoplasmic encephalitis in AIDS patients is uniformly fatal.

Treatment

Methods. Patients with suspected CNS toxoplasmosis should nearly always be hospitalized. Treatment usually consists of pyrimethamine PO 200 mg loading dose, then 50 to 75 mg daily; folinic acid (leucovorin) PO, IV, or IM, usually 10 to 20 mg daily but up to 50 mg daily if necessary; and sulfadiazine 1 to 1.5 g PO q6h. Clindamycin, usually 600 mg q6h if PO, up to 1200 mg q6h if IV, can be substituted for sulfadiazine. Several alternative regimens are also available. Empiric therapy is usually continued for 10 days to 3 weeks provided that no clinical deterioration occurs. CT or (preferably) MRI scanning is then repeated. Treatment is continued for 4 to 6 weeks after all signs and symptoms of the disease have resolved, which may require several months (sometimes >6 months). Because relapse occurs in about 80% of patients after treatment is discontinued, maintenance therapy (e.g., pyrimethamine 25 to 50 mg/day plus sulfadiazine 500 mg q.i.d.) is continued indefinitely or until marked immunologic improvement has occurred as a result of antiretroviral therapy (see "Prophylaxis and Therapy of Opportunistic Infections" later in the chapter). Appropriate therapy, if begun sufficiently early in the course of the disease, is usually but not always successful. About 90% of patients who respond to therapy recover at least half of their lost function within 2 weeks.

KEY POINTS

TOXOPLASMOSIS

⊃ Encephalitis with multiple CNS mass lesions is the most common presentation of toxoplasmosis in patients with AIDS. Clinical manifestations include altered mental state, focal neurologic signs, and seizures.

⊃ Empiric therapy is warranted for a patient with multiple ring enhancing lesions on CT or MRI scans and positive serologic tests for IgG *Toxoplasma* antibodies.

⊃ Primary CNS lymphoma, progressive multifocal leukoencephalopathy, and other specific infections should be considered in the differential diagnosis, especially if no response to empiric therapy occurs within 1 to 3 weeks.

SUGGESTED READING

Antinori A, Ammassari A, DeLuca A, et al. Diagnosis of AIDS-related focal brain lesions: a decision making analysis based on clinical and neuroradiologic characteristics combined with polymerase chain reaction assays in CSF. Neurology 1997; 48: 687-694.

Ashburn D, Davidson MM, Joss AW, et al. Improved diagnosis of reactivated toxoplasmosis. Mol Pathol 1998; 51: 105-109.

Chang KH, Han MH. MRI of CNS parasitic diseases. J Magn Reson Imaging 1998; 8: 297-307.

Torre D, Casari S, Speranza F, et al. Italian Collaborative Study Group. Randomized trial of trimethoprim-sulfamethoxazole versus pyrimethamine-sulfadiazine for therapy of toxoplasmic encephalitis in patients with AIDS. Antimicrob Agents Chemother 1998; 42: 1346-1349.

Cryptococcosis

Cryptococcosis (see Chapter 21) in patients with AIDS can manifest itself as pulmonary disease or disseminated disease affecting many organs, including the skin, but more commonly causes meningitis. Cryptococcal meningitis is the AIDS-defining illness in up to 5% of patients in the United States and occurs in up to 10% of AIDS patients at some point, usually when the CD4 count falls below $100/mm^3$ and typically when it is $<50/mm^3$. Onset can be acute but is more commonly subacute or chronic. The onset is often progressive headache and low-grade fever. Stiff neck is uncommon. Many patients have symptoms of brain dysfunction, such as impaired mental ability or confusion, irritability, somnolence, dizziness, or nausea. Impaired vision is relatively common, and impaired hearing from eighth nerve involvement also occurs. Seizures can occur but are seldom the presenting manifestation. Physical examination is usually unremarkable but may show cranial nerve abnormalities, hyperreflexia, ankle clonus, or Babinski's sign.

Diagnosis is by lumbar puncture, which should be performed in any patient with HIV disease, CD4 count $<200/mm^3$, headache, or evidence of brain dysfunction. The finding of multiple, small, nonenhancing mass lesions on CT or MRI scan should not negate lumbar puncture, since these lesions can reflect cryptococcomas. The CSF should be submitted to the laboratory for cell count, protein and glucose levels, fungal and AFB cultures, India ink preparation, and cryptococcal antigen test. The India ink test, if performed properly, has a 25% to 50% sensitivity for cryptococcal meningitis and can provide a rapid diagnosis. The cryptococcal antigen test on CSF is believed to be at least 90% sensitive for this disease and becomes increasingly specific for the disease with higher titers ($\geq$1:8). The cryptococcal antigen test can also be performed on serum, and cryptococcal disease is reasonably excluded if the antigen is absent from both CSF and serum. The diagnosis is confirmed by isolation of *Cryptococcus neoformans* from CSF by culture.

Occasionally, cryptococcosis in patients with AIDS can cause overwhelming, diffuse pneumonia with respiratory failure. An assay for serum cryptococcal antigen provides a means of rapid diagnosis.

Fluconazole has been shown to be effective initial therapy for patients with AIDS and cryptococcal meningitis who do not have adverse prognostic factors. Adverse prognostic factors include impaired mental function, a positive India ink preparation on CSF, CSF cryptococcal antigen titer $>$1:128, and positive blood cultures for *C. neoformans*. At present most patients with newly diagnosed cryptococcal meningitis and AIDS are treated for at least 2 weeks with amphotericin B 0.7 mg/kg/day. Flucytosine 25 mg/kg q.i.d. is often added. When flucytosine is used, the potential for severe cytopenias must be considered. The dose should be reduced when the serum creatinine level is elevated or becomes elevated during therapy. After 2 weeks of amphotericin B, most patients are changed over to fluconazole 400 mg daily for 8 weeks and then 200 mg indefinitely. In the event of intractable headaches, confusion, or altered consciousness, lumbar punctures should be repeated, with 20 to 30 mL of CSF removed at each lumbar puncture with the aim of reducing the CSF opening pressure to $<$200 mm of CSF. This procedure can be lifesaving.

Initial treatment of cryptococcal meningitis in patients with AIDS is now usually successful in the absence of adverse risk factors at the time of presentation. The overall fatality rate, however, is as high as 30%, and up to 25% have a relapse unless continuous prophylaxis is maintained (see "Prophylaxis and Therapy of Opportunistic Infections" later in the chapter).

Most patients with cryptococcal meningitis should be hospitalized.

KEY POINTS

CRYPTOCOCCOSIS

⊃ Cryptococcal meningitis is relatively common in patients with advanced HIV disease. Symptoms and signs include headache, low-grade fever, and evidence of brain dysfunction such as declining mental function, somnolence, irritability, and nausea. Lumbar puncture should be performed in patients with CD4 counts $<200/mm^3$, headache, and symptoms or signs of brain dysfunction.

⊃ Cryptococcosis should also be considered in patients with AIDS who have unexplained diffuse pneumonia; demonstration of cryptococcal antigen in serum can provide rapid diagnosis.

SUGGESTED READING

Saag MS, Graybill RJ, Larsen RA, et al. Infectious Diseases Society of America. Practice guidelines for the management of cryptococcal disease. Clin Infect Dis 2000; 30: 710-718.

Saag MS, Powderly WG, Cloud GA, et al. The NIAID Mycosis Study Group and the AIDS Clinical Trials Group. Comparison of amphotericin B with fluconazole in the treatment of acute AIDS-associated cryptococcal meningitis. N Engl J Med 1992; 326: 83-89.

van der Horst CM, Saag MS, Cloud GA, et al. Treatment of crypto-coccal meningitis associated with the acquired immunodeficiency syndrome. N Engl J Med 1997; 337: 15-21.

Visnegarwala F, Graviss EA, Lacke CE, et al. Acute respiratory failure associated with cryptococcosis in patients with AIDS: analysis of predictive factors. Clin Infect Dis 1998; 27: 1231-1237.

Cytomegalovirus Infection

CMV infection (see Chapters 8 and 20) in HIV-infected patients is most often manifested clinically as retinitis. The other relatively common syndromes caused by CMV are polyradiculitis and colitis.

CMV retinitis usually appears late in the course of HIV disease and correlates with a CD4 count <50/mm³. The disease advances rapidly, leading to progressive vision loss if untreated. The diagnosis of CMV retinitis is usually based on the distinctive, "brushfire" appearance of perivascular hemorrhages and exudates on ophthalmoscopic examination.

Other CNS manifestations of CMV include polyradiculopathy; peripheral neuropathy, including mononeuritis multiplex; myelopathy; and encephalopathy. Polyradiculopathy often begins as low back pain followed by ascending weakness of the lower extremities and loss of deep tendon reflexes. Loss of bowel and bladder control occurs later in the illness. Peripheral neuropathy is often painful. Patients with CMV encephalopathy show evidence of brain dysfunction and frequently have periventricular linear accentuation on MRI scan. When CMV polyradiculopathy, myelopathy, peripheral neuropathy, or encephalopathy is suspected, lumbar puncture should be performed and the CSF should be tested by PCR for CMV DNA by using a quantitative assay. A parallel quantitative PCR for CMV DNA in plasma is also useful. The CSF formula in patients with polyradiculopathy characteristically shows a moderate mononuclear pleocytosis with slightly elevated protein and slightly lowered glucose content. CMV colitis and CMV esophagitis are discussed later in the chapter ("Gastrointestinal Diseases Associated with AIDS"). CMV can also cause pneumonia in AIDS patients. CMV commonly infects the adrenal glands, and rare cases of adrenal insufficiency have been reported.

Drugs useful for treatment of CMV disease include ganciclovir, foscarnet, and cidofovir (see Chapter 20). Ganciclovir and foscarnet are sometimes given in tandem. Patients with CMV retinitis should be referred to an ophthalmologist for consideration of injecting antiviral drugs directly into the vitreous. New drugs (such as fomivirsen) have been developed for this purpose. Intraocular ganciclovir implants do not protect the contralateral eye and should therefore be supplemented with systemic therapy during the initial treatment. The course of CMV retinitis can often be arrested by aggressive treatment directed against both CMV and HIV. The prevalence of severe CMV retinitis has decreased markedly since the introduction of HAART. When the CD4 count rises and is maintained above 100/mm³ in patients receiving HAART, CMV retinitis often becomes and remains inactive even without maintenance therapy directed against HIV. However, new complications may arise, such as immune recovery–associated retinitis, vitreal abnormalities, and, in the retina, a cystoid change in the macula and edema of the optic disc. Manifestations of CMV other than retinitis, when severe, tend to occur late in the course of HIV disease, and referral is often indicated.

 KEY POINTS

CYTOMEGALOVIRUS INFECTION

⊃ The most common opportunistic viral pathogen in AIDS, CMV caused retinitis leading to blindness in up to 40% of patients before the introduction of highly active antiretroviral therapy (HAART).

⊃ CMV retinitis causes vision loss. Diagnosis is made by the characteristic "brushfire" appearance on ophthalmoscopic examination of the retina.

⊃ CMV polyradiculopathy often begins with low back pain and features a progressive weakness. Other manifestations of CMV are myelopathy, peripheral neuropathy, colitis, and esophagitis.

SUGGESTED READING

Macdonald JC, Karavellas MP, Torriani FJ, et al. Highly active antiretroviral therapy–related immune recovery in AIDS patients with cytomegalovirus retinitis. Ophthalmology 2000; 107: 877-881.

McCutchan JA. Clinical impact of cytomegalovirus infections of the nervous system in patients with AIDS. Clin Infect Dis 1995; 21 (Suppl 2): S196-S201.

Torriani FJ, Freeman WR, Macdonald JC, et al. CMV retinitis recurs after stopping treatment in virological and immunological failures of potent antiretroviral therapy. AIDS 2000; 14: 173-180.

Mycobacterium Avium Complex Disease

Mycobacterium avium complex (MAC) infection (see Chapter 22) was the leading bacterial infection in patients with AIDS and carried an extremely poor prognosis before the introduction of newer therapies. Its onset is usually as an undifferentiated febrile illness.

MAC infection includes both *M. avium* and *Mycobacterium intracellulare; M. avium* is the usual pathogen in AIDS. The organism is ubiquitous in the environment. In contrast to most of the opportunistic infections in AIDS, *M. avium* disease nearly always reflects recent acquisition of the organism rather than reactivation of latent infection. Person-to-person transmission does not seem to occur. In striking contrast to MAC infection in immunocompetent persons, in whom the disease is nearly always confined to the lungs, MAC infection in patients with AIDS is widespread. Numerous organs contain foamy histiocytes stuffed with acid-fast bacilli. The liver and spleen are typically massively infected, and the intestinal mucosa is also heavily involved.

Early symptoms and signs point to systemic illness. The clinical hallmarks are fever, drenching night sweats, and weight loss. Anorexia, malaise, and diarrhea are also common. Physical examination confirms wasting and may show lymphadenopathy, hepatomegaly, and splenomegaly. Laboratory findings include anemia; abnormal liver function tests, including elevation of the alkaline phosphatase level; and frequently elevation of the LDH level. Since the introduction of HAART, a more subtle presentation of MAC infection has been reported in which focal lymphadenitis dominates the clinical picture.

AFB blood culture is the single most useful test. A single AFB blood culture is 90% to 95% sensitive for MAC. Therefore one blood culture (rather than three, as are usually recommended for sepsis and for endocarditis, respectively) is a cost-effective approach in this setting. Bone marrow aspiration for AFB smear and culture can be useful, and lymph node biopsy is sometimes helpful as well. When the clinical presentation strongly suggests MAC as a possibility (unexplained febrile illness in a person with CD4 count <50/mm³), a prudent approach is to initiate presumptive therapy for MAC while awaiting the results of AFB cultures, which can take up to 3 months. In patients with diarrhea a positive AFB smear on stool suggests the diagnosis.

Recommended therapy for disseminated MAC in AIDS patients currently consists of clarithromycin 500 mg b.i.d. and ethambutol 15 mg/kg/day, sometimes with rifabutin 300 mg/day. Azithromycin 500 mg/day is sometimes used in place of clarithromycin. Fluoroquinolones may also have a role in therapy. Some clinicians also include intravenous administration of amikacin (10 mg/kg/day with adjustment of the dose for renal insufficiency) for 10 to 20 days to enhance the response. A concomitant attempt should be made to reduce the viral load and raise the CD4 count by aggressive therapy for the underlying HIV disease.

Response to therapy is often excellent provided the underlying HIV disease can be controlled with HAART. Resistance to the macrolide antibiotics (clarithromycin and azithromycin) is now described and is a problem.

Patients with disseminated MAC are usually extremely ill, both from the opportunistic infection and from the underlying HIV disease. They may benefit from infectious disease consultation.

 KEY POINTS

MYCOBACTERIUM AVIUM COMPLEX DISEASE

⊃ Before the advent of HAART, *M. avium* was the most common opportunistic bacterial pathogen in AIDS and carried a high mortality. Disseminated infection usually occurs when the CD4 count is <50/mm³.

⊃ Systemic signs and symptoms usually predominate and include drenching sweats, fever, weight loss, diarrhea, and hepatosplenomegaly. MAC is an extremely important cause of unexplained fever in patients with advanced HIV disease.

⊃ A single AFB blood culture has a sensitivity of 90% to 95% for disseminated MAC disease in AIDS patients. In patients with diarrhea a positive AFB culture on stool suggests the diagnosis.

⊃ Empiric therapy for MAC is often advisable while awaiting the results of AFB blood cultures and other studies. Patients with disseminated MAC disease are usually extremely ill and may benefit from an infectious disease consultation.

SUGGESTED READING

Cinti SK, Kaul DR, Sax PE, et al. Recurrence of *Mycobacterium avium* infection in patients receiving highly active antiretroviral therapy and antimycobacterial agents. Clin Infect Dis 2000; 30: 511-514.

Dube MP, Torriani FJ, See D, et al. California Collaborative Treatment Group. Successful short-term suppression of clarithromycin-resistant *Mycobacterium avium* complex bacteremia in AIDS. Clin Infect Dis 1999; 28: 136-138.

Kirk O, Gatell JM, Mocroft A, et al. EuroSIDA Study Group JD. Infections with *Mycobacterium tuberculosis* and *Mycobacterium avium* among HIV-infected patients after the introduction of highly active antiretroviral therapy. Am J Respir Crit Care Med 2000; 162: 865-872.

Race EM, Adelson-Mitty J, Kriegel GR, et al. Focal mycobacterial lymphadenitis following initiation of protease-inhibitor therapy in patients with advanced HIV-1 disease. Lancet 1998; 351: 252-255.

AIDS-Related Tumors

Patients with HIV disease, like other immunosuppressed patients, are especially vulnerable to malignancy. Tumors that are especially associated with AIDS include Kaposi's sarcoma, non-Hodgkin's lymphoma, and primary lymphoma of the central nervous system (CNS). Other tumors are also relatively more common than in the general population, including carcinoma of the cervix.

Kaposi's Sarcoma

Kaposi's sarcoma affected nearly 50% of gay and bisexual men with AIDS during the early years of the epidemic. The incidence is now declining, but it continues to be the most common malignancy associated with AIDS. A strong association between Kaposi's sarcoma and human herpesvirus type 8 (HHV-8) was identified in 1994, and HHV-8 is now generally accepted as the likely cause. Kaposi's sarcoma usually becomes manifest on the skin or mucous membranes as a firm, lightly raised or nodular, 0.5- to 2-cm violaceous or dark red lesion that does not blanch on pressure. In contrast to Kaposi's sarcoma in patients without AIDS, which is usually an indolent tumor involving the lower extremities of elderly men of Eastern European or Mediterranean ancestry, Kaposi's sarcoma in AIDS patients tends to be multicentric and aggressive. Lesions occur especially on the face, lower extremities, and oral mucosa. Lesions in the oral cavity are often predictive of lesions in the gastrointestinal tract. In about 15% of cases visceral involvement occurs without the telltale skin and oral cavity lesions. The most serious visceral lesions are those that affect the lung. Symptoms of lung involvement include cough, bronchospasm, and dyspnea. The chest x-ray film often shows diffuse interstitial infiltrates indistinguishable from those caused by *P. carinii*. Other chest radiographic patterns include hilar lymphadenopathy (about one half of patients), reticulonodular infiltrates (about one third of patients), and pleural effusions. Extensive pulmonary involvement, which usually occurs in patients with numerous skin lesions, carries a poor prognosis.

Diagnosis of Kaposi's sarcoma is usually based on skin biopsy, which is necessary because the lesion must be distinguished from bacillary angiomatosis (see preceding discussion and Table 17-2). When pulmonary Kaposi's sarcoma is suspected, bronchoscopy can be confirmatory but biopsy of the lesions should be avoided because of the risk of life-threatening pulmonary hemorrhage. Treatment of Kaposi's sarcoma, which is usually intended to be palliative rather than curative, should be individualized. Patients with advanced disease should be referred to an oncologist. The lesions of Kaposi's sarcoma often improve dramatically with highly active antiretroviral therapy (HAART) alone.

Non-Hodgkin's Lymphoma

Non-Hodgkin's lymphoma may occur in up to 8% of persons with HIV disease and is sometimes the initial AIDS diagnosis. Most of these tumors are of B-cell origin. About 60% of cases are large cell lymphomas, and about three fourths of cases are high grade. About 40% of systemic non-Hodgkin's lymphomas are associated with the Epstein-Barr virus (EBV) (i.e., EBV DNA sequences can be demonstrated in the lesions). Non-Hodgkin's lymphoma in patients with AIDS is usually characterized by widespread extranodal disease. The gastrointestinal tract, liver, bone marrow, and CNS are frequently involved. Diagnosis is made by biopsy. Patients with non-Hodgkin's lymphoma should be referred to an oncologist for aggressive chemotherapy. Patients with systemic non-Hodgkin's lymphoma (as opposed to primary CNS lymphoma; see subsequent section) often have CD4 counts $\geq 100/mm^3$ and therefore can be expected to benefit from HAART after treatment of the lymphoma.

Primary Lymphoma of the Central Nervous System

Primary lymphoma of the CNS is associated with AIDS. This lymphoma, which is usually confined to the CNS, is strongly associated with EBV; indeed, EBV DNA can be found in virtually 100% of lesions. Patients with primary CNS lymphoma typically have CD4 counts $\leq 50/mm^3$. Presenting symptoms are similar to those of toxoplasmic encephalitis and include impaired mental function, personality change, headache, and focal neurologic symptoms and signs. CT or MRI scan shows single or multiple lesions that enhance with contrast media. Multiple lesions are present in about one half of cases. The usual quandary is whether the lesions represent lymphoma or toxoplasmosis. Cytologic tests of CSF are positive for lymphoma in about 20% of affected patients. An emerging approach to the diagnosis of primary CNS lymphoma is to obtain a thallium scan (i.e., thallium-201 single photon emission CT scanning) and a PCR on CSF for EBV DNA. Data from small series suggest that the combination of a positive thallium CT scan and a positive assay for EBV DNA in CSF have a strong positive predictive value for primary CNS lymphoma and a strong negative predictive value for CNS toxoplasmosis. However, brain biopsy remains the "gold standard" for diagnosis. Patients with primary CNS lymphoma should be referred to an oncologist for aggressive treatment, which usually includes both chemotherapy and irradiation therapy. The previously dismal prognosis for AIDS patients with primary CNS lymphoma has improved since the advent of HAART.

Other Tumors

Carcinoma of the cervix is highly correlated with infection by oncogenic types of the human papillomavirus (HPV) and is now an AIDS-defining condition. Hence, Pap smears are indicated for all HIV-infected women, and those with abnormalities should have close follow-up. A relationship also exists between HIV infection, HPV infection, and carcinoma of the anus. Whether Pap smears will prove useful as a screening tool for anal neoplasia is being studied. Some evidence suggests that the incidence of Hodgkin's disease is increased in patients with AIDS.

When to Refer

Patients with neoplastic disease should generally be referred to an oncologist. The exception is some patients with Kaposi's sarcoma, who may improve with HAART alone.

 KEY POINTS

AIDS-RELATED TUMORS

⊃ Kaposi's sarcoma, which is now attributed to human herpesvirus type 8, causes firm, usually painless, 0.5- to 2-cm, violaceous or dark red lesions of the skin and mucous membranes. Visceral involvement is extremely common and can be serious when it involves the lungs. Diagnosis is usually made by skin biopsy. Effective treatment of HIV disease with HAART sometimes leads to dramatic regression of Kaposi's sarcoma.

⊃ Non-Hodgkin's lymphoma in patients with AIDS is most typically a high-grade large cell lymphoma, although many types of lymphoma occur. Extranodal involvement is usually present and is widespread. Most patients should be referred to an oncologist for aggressive chemotherapy.

⊃ Primary lymphoma of the CNS is strongly associated with AIDS (the relative risk is 1000-fold higher than in the general population), EBV, and advanced HIV disease (CD4 count $\leq 50/mm^3$). Although a positive thallium CT scan and PCR assay for EBV DNA in CSF are strongly predictive of primary CNS lymphoma, brain biopsy is recommended for diagnosis.

⊃ Carcinoma of the cervix occurs more frequently in patients with HIV disease and is now an AIDS-defining condition.

SUGGESTED READING

Aboulafia DM. The epidemiologic, pathologic, and clinical features of AIDS-associated pulmonary Kaposi's sarcoma. Chest 2000; 117: 1128-1145.

Goedert JJ. The epidemiology of acquired immunodeficiency syndrome malignancies. Semin Oncol 2000; 27: 390-401.

Levine AM. Acquired immunodeficiency syndrome–related lymphoma: clinical aspects. Semin Oncol 2000; 27: 442-453.

Gastrointestinal Diseases Associated with HIV Disease

Most patients with HIV disease have gastrointestinal symptoms at some point during their course.

Esophageal Manifestations

Candida esophagitis, causing dysphagia and odynophagia, often with retrosternal pain and constitutional symptoms, can be the presenting manifestation of HIV disease. It is usually associated with oral candidiasis (thrush) and treated empirically with fluconazole 100 to 200 mg daily. Failure of the symptoms to resolve within 7 to 10 days is an indication for endoscopy. In about three fourths of these patients endoscopy reveals ulcers of one etiology or another. Specific etiologies that should be sought at endoscopy are CMV, HSV, and fluconazole-resistant *Candida* species. HSV tends to cause superficial, confluent ulcers in the distal esophagus, whereas CMV tends to cause numerous, large, shallow ulcers. Idiopathic ulcers, which are also called aphthous ulcers, are large, shallow ulcers that resemble those caused by CMV and are therefore a diagnosis of exclusion. Idiopathic ulcers usually respond to corticosteroid therapy (prednisone

60 mg daily, with slow tapering of the dose). Thalidomide is also effective on an investigational basis. Other causes of esophageal symptoms in patients with HIV disease include medication (notably zidovudine, zalcitabine, and doxycycline), tumors (including Kaposi's sarcoma), and gastroesophageal reflux disease (the same type found in the general population).

Diarrhea

Diarrhea is a common manifestation of HIV disease and AIDS, and the pathogens involved sometimes correlate with the stage of the disease. The typical clinical manifestations of small bowel disease (infrequent, painless, high-volume, watery diarrhea or "runs") and colonic diarrhea (frequent, painful, small bowel diarrhea or "trots") can point toward one or another etiologic group, but some patients have overlapping features (panenteritis).

Salmonellosis can occur at any stage of the disease as enterocolitis or sometimes as enteric fever, in which case blood cultures are positive. About one half of patients with *Salmonella* infection and HIV disease have positive blood cultures. Quinolones (e.g., ciprofloxacin) are currently the drugs of choice; others are TMP/SMX and (for enteric fever) ceftriaxone. *Campylobacter* species can also cause diarrhea, sometimes bloody, at any stage of the disease.

When diarrhea occurs in patients with CD4 counts <200/mm^3, the liquid stool specimen should be submitted to the laboratory for the following tests:

- Fecal leukocytes (examination with methylene blue stain)
- Ova and parasites
- Intestinal bacterial pathogens (by culture)
- *C. difficile* toxin assay (since this infection can occur in the absence of antimicrobial therapy in HIV-infected patients)
- AFB smear and culture (looking mainly for MAC)
- Smear for *Cryptosporidia, Cyclospora,* and *Isospora* (modified acid-fast stain)
- Smear for *Microsporidia*

When all of these studies fail to reveal the cause of diarrhea, endoscopic biopsies are necessary. Sigmoidoscopy or colonoscopic virus may reveal CMV; jejunal biopsy may reveal microsporidiosis and giardiasis.

Parasitic diarrheas tend to occur in patients with advanced HIV disease (CD4 count <100/mm^3) and are often extremely troubling. *Cryptosporidium,* identified on modified AFB smear of stool as a large, round or ovoid parasite, causes massive colonization of the small bowel mucosa in persons with advanced AIDS and leads to disabling, watery diarrhea. Paromomycin has proved to be no better than a placebo, but its combined use with azithromycin shows promise. Patients with CD4 counts <100/mm^3 and cryptosporidiosis were treated for 4 weeks with paromomycin 1 g b.i.d. plus azithromycin 600 mg daily, followed by azithromycin alone for 8 weeks. Patients thus treated had reduced frequency of stools and reduced parasite burden (fewer oocytes in stool) by 12 weeks of therapy. However, optimum treatment is HAART, since spontaneous recovery may occur when the CD4 count rises above 200/mm^3. Diarrhea caused by *Microsporidia* is often difficult to diagnose and treat. Occasionally metronidazole provides temporary relief. Albendazole (400 to 800 mg b.i.d. for 4 weeks) is effective treatment against one microsporidial species, *Septata intestinalis. Isospora belli* can be treated effectively with TMP/SMX (see Table 23-4). *Cyclospora cayetanensis,* a coccidian parasite associated with various foods, including raspberries (but not strawberries) and potato salad, is another cause of diarrhea that responds to TMP/SMX (one double-strength tablet b.i.d. for 7 days).

CMV colitis likewise occurs in patients with advanced disease (CD4 count <100/mm^3) and can be extremely troubling. Presenting features include fever, crampy abdominal pain, and bloody diarrhea. Intestinal obstruction can occur, and rarely, intestinal perforation or toxic megacolon supervenes. Colonoscopy rather than sigmoidoscopy is recommended, since the disease can be confined to the right side of the colon. The usual finding is severe inflammation with shallow ulcerations, and biopsy confirms typical CMV inclusions. Treatment is with ganciclovir or foscarnet.

MAC is an important cause of diarrhea in patients with CD4 counts <50/mm^3, most of whom have disseminated MAC disease with positive blood cultures. Organisms are usually abundant on AFB smear of the stool.

Diseases of the Liver, Gallbladder, and Pancreas

Hepatitis B (HBV) and hepatitis C (HCV) viruses often coexist with HIV, especially in injecting drug users. About 10% of HIV-infected persons are coinfected with hepatitis B. Immunodeficiency impairs the clearance of hepatitis B viremia (antigenemia), resulting in a high frequency of HBV chronic carriers among HIV-infected persons. However, symptomatic hepatitis B is uncommon in HIV-infected persons, since progression to liver disease requires a host immune response (immunocompetence). HIV-infected persons may show impaired response to hepatitis B vaccine, especially when their CD4 count is <350/mm^3. However, the vaccine should be offered to persons with negative serologic markers for past HBV infection.

Hepatitis C virus (HCV) infection is becoming increasingly important in HIV-infected persons, up to 40% of whom may be coinfected with this virus. In contrast to HBV, HCV disease is accelerated in patients who are immunodeficient. Thus about 80% to 90% of HIV-infected persons who are coinfected with HCV have evidence of liver disease. Progression to cirrhosis may occur within 5 to 10 years, or about one-third to one-half the time in immunocompetent persons. Cirrhosis can be complicated by hepatocellular carcinoma. Recognition of HCV begins with a test for HCV antibodies by EIA. If EIA is positive, the viral load can be determined by the quantitative HCV RNA PCR. Patients with HCV infection and high viral loads can be treated with interferon and ribavirin (see Chapter 13). Recent experience suggests that treatment with ribavirin may increase the risk of mitochondrial toxicity from antiretroviral drugs (see later discussion).

Biliary tract disease (cholangiopathy) in patients with HIV disease includes acalculous cholecystitis and sclerosing cholangitis. The onset of sclerosing cholangitis in patients with AIDS is characterized by fever, abdominal pain, and a pattern of obstructive jaundice. It is diagnosed by endoscopic cholangiography. Causes of sclerosing cholangitis in HIV-infected patients include CMV, cryptosporidiosis, microsporidiosis, and MAC infection. HIV cholangiopathy can also involve the juxtaampullary portion of the pancreatic duct. Pancreatitis in patients with HIV disease is sometimes caused by drugs (especially didanosine, zalcitabine, and pentamidine).

When to Refer

Referral to a gastroenterologist is often indicated for endoscopy and management of HIV disease involving the gastrointestinal tract.

 KEY POINTS

GASTROINTESTINAL DISEASES ASSOCIATED WITH HIV DISEASE

⊃ *Candida* esophagitis, producing dysphagia, odynophagia, or retrosternal pain, can be the first manifestation of AIDS and is accompanied by oral candidiasis (thrush). Endoscopy should be performed if a therapeutic trial of fluconazole for 7 to 10 days fails to bring about improvement.

⊃ Esophagitis caused by HSV is characterized by superficial, confluent ulcers of the distal esophagus, whereas esophagitis caused by cytomegalovirus tends to cause large, shallow ulcerations.

⊃ Idiopathic (aphthous) ulcers of the esophagus, a diagnosis of exclusion, resemble CMV esophagitis but respond to prednisone therapy.

⊃ When diarrhea occurs in patients with advanced HIV disease (CD4 count $<200/mm^3$), stool should be examined for fecal leukocytes, bacteria, *C. difficile* toxin, mycobacteria, and ova and parasites, including special stains for *Cryptosporidium* and *Microsporidia*.

⊃ Although patients coinfected with HIV and hepatitis B virus commonly become hepatitis B carriers, progression to cirrhosis is infrequent.

⊃ Patients coinfected with HIV and hepatitis C virus are at high risk for cirrhosis, which may develop within 5 to 10 years. Aggressive diagnosis and treatment are therefore warranted. Ribavirin therapy for hepatitis C may increase the risk of mitochondrial toxicity from antiretroviral drugs.

SUGGESTED READING

Anastasi JK, Capili B. HIV and diarrhea in the era of HAART: 1998 New York State hospitalizations. Am J Infect Control 2000; 28: 262-266.

Dancygier H. AIDS and the gastrointestinal tract. Endoscopy 1998; 30: 222-229.

Filippini P, Coppola N, Scolastico C, et al. Can HCV affect the efficacy of anti-HIV treatment? Arch Virol 2000; 145: 937-944.

Lafeuillade A, Hittinger G, Chadapaud S. Increased mitochondrial toxicity with ribavirin in HIV/HCV coinfection. Lancet 2001; 357: 280-281.

Smith NH, Cron S, Valdez LM, et al. Combination drug therapy for cryptosporidiosis in AIDS. J Infect Dis 1998; 178: 900-903.

Wasting Syndrome

Involuntary weight loss of >10% has been a diagnostic requirement for this syndrome as a manifestation of AIDS. Laboratory abnormalities include hypercholesterolemia and hypertriglyceridemia. The abnormalities may reflect the effect of a cytokine, the tumor necrosis factor (TNF). Since the introduction of the wasting syndrome as an AIDS-defining condition by the Centers for Disease Control and Prevention (CDC) in 1993, the abnormality has been further defined. Even a 5% weight loss portends a poor prognosis in HIV-infected individuals. The body cell mass includes nonadipose and adipose (fat) cells and is estimated by bioelectric impedance, a sensitive and reliable method for the degree of wasting.

Wasting relates to inadequate caloric intake, anorexia, malabsorption, and altered metabolism. The latter seems to be the major contributor for the malnutrition in the HIV infected. Testosterone levels may be reduced but can be corrected with administration of this hormone. Many HIV patients with hypogonadism or malnutrition have a functional resistance to human growth hormone. Even if the level of growth hormone may be normal in HIV-infected individuals, exogenous synthetic growth hormone may overcome the acquired resistance to this hormone. This therapy is very expensive and should be a last resort when other factors are considered and treatment is initiated as described previously.

Therapy for malnutrition associated with AIDS requires first HAART and treatment of the associated opportunistic infections. Gastrointestinal problems, such as ulcer disease, concurrent small bowel disease, or colitis, should be diagnosed and treated.

SUGGESTED READING

Nemechek PM, Polsky B, Gottlieb MS. Treatment guidelines for HIV-associated wasting. Mayo Clin Proc 2000; 75: 386-394.

AIDS Dementia (Encephalopathy)

In up to 30% of patients with AIDS a progressive loss of cognitive ability develops late in the course of the disease. The onset of this abnormality is variable. Patients become unable to carry out tasks for their daily existence. Loss of memory can be prominent, but the patients preserve alertness and social graces until deep into the course of deterioration. Although opportunistic infections, including CMV encephalitis, may be associated with dementia, cognitive loss is the leading symptom and sign of AIDS dementia. It may be coupled with slow movements, impaired balance, ataxia, and spasticity resulting from the associated myelopathy. The diagnosis is made by excluding opportunistic infections and tumors of the CNS through a combination of CT or MRI scanning and special studies on CSF.

Progressive multifocal leukoencephalopathy, which can begin as subtle mental status changes with weakness, can be distinguished from AIDS dementia by MRI scan (which shows multiple nonenhancing subcortical white matter lesions) and demonstrating the JC virus in CSF by a PCR assay. Recent studies suggest that dementia may correlate with CSF HIV viral load. Cocaine use seems to increase the likelihood of dementia by making the blood-brain barrier more penetrable to the virus. Patients with AIDS dementia ultimately become bedridden and incontinent of urine and feces. The case-fatality rate exceeds 50% within 6 to 12 months of onset. AIDS encephalopathy may be associated with intense, steady pain of various body parts. The patients may require continuous intravenous morphine and a referral to a pain management specialist. Peripheral neuropathy and myelopathy coexist with AIDS dementia and encephalopathy. No specific therapy is available for this entity. HAART offers the hope of improvement in some patients.

SUGGESTED READING

Childs EA, Lyles RH, Selnes OA, et al. Plasma viral load and CD4 lymphocytes predict HIV-associated dementia and sensory neuropathy. Neurology 1999; 52: 607-613.

Krivine A, Force G, Servan J, et al. Measuring HIV-1 RNA and interferon-alpha in the cerebrospinal fluid of AIDS patients: insights into the pathogenesis of AIDS dementia complex. J Neurovirol 1999; 5: 500-506.

Roullet E. Opportunistic infections of the central nervous system during HIV-1 infection: emphasis on cytomegalovirus disease. J Neurol 1999; 246: 237-243.

Zhang L, Looney D, Taub D, et al. Cocaine opens the blood-brain barrier to HIV-1 invasion. J Neurovirol 1998; 4: 619-626.

Classification of HIV Infection, HIV Disease, and AIDS

HIV infection, HIV disease, and AIDS are parts of a chain of events in the infected individual. The CDC classification is offered in an abbreviated form in Table 17-3. Clinical categories A, B, and C are determined by severity, with 1, 2, and 3 referring to the CD4 counts. Diseases in the "C" category, irrespective of the CD4 count, qualify as cases of AIDS. Even if these diseases are not present, a CD4 count $<200/mm^3$ is diagnostic of AIDS for purposes of reporting the disease.

Prophylaxis and Therapy of Opportunistic Infections

Primary prophylaxis aims at preventing a first episode of opportunistic infection in HIV-infected patients with CD4 counts $<200/mm^3$ (Table 17-4). Secondary prophylaxis is designed to prevent recurrence of the same opportunistic infection (Table 17-5). Before the advent of HAART, secondary prophylaxis was usually continued for the remainder of the patient's life. HAART often sufficiently improves the immune response, as reflected by the rise in CD4 count, to allow prophylaxis to be discontinued in some instances (Table 17-5).

SUGGESTED READING

Freedberg KA, Scharfstein JA, Seage GR III, et al. The cost-effectiveness of preventing AIDS-related opportunistic infections. JAMA 1998; 279: 130-136.

Ledergerber B, Mocroft A, Reiss P, et al. Discontinuation of secondary prophylaxis against *Pneumocystis carinii* pneumonia in patients with HIV infection who have a response to antiretroviral therapy. N Engl J Med 2001; 344: 168-174.

Soriano V, Dona C, Rodriguez-Rosado R, et al. Discontinuation of secondary prophylaxis for opportunistic infections in HIV-infected patients receiving highly active antiretroviral therapy. AIDS 2000; 14: 383-386.

TABLE 17-3

Classification for HIV Infection and Disease, and AIDS Case Definition for Adults

CD4 cell count	CLINICAL CATEGORIES*		
	(A)	(B)	(C)
(1) ≥500/mm³	A1	B1	C1
(2) 200-499/mm³	A2	B2	C2
(3) <200/mm³	A3	B3	C3
	Asymptomatic HIV infection	*Symptomatic, not (A) or (C) conditions (formerly AIDS-related complex)*	*AIDS-indicator (opportunistic) conditions*
	Acute (primary) HIV infection Persistent generalized lymphadenopathy Acute retroviral syndrome	Candidiasis, oral or recurrent vaginal Cervical dysplasia Constitutional symptoms (such as fever or diarrhea) for more than 1 month Hairy leukoplakia, oral Herpes zoster infection Idiopathic thrombocytopenia purpura Listeriosis Pelvic inflammatory disease	Candidiasis, pulmonary or esophageal Cervical cancer Cryptococcosis, extrapulmonary Cryptosporidiosis Cytomegalovirus, retinitis or esophageal Histoplasmosis Isosporiasis Kaposi's sarcoma Lymphoma *Mycobacterium avium* infection, disseminated Tuberculosis *Pneumocystis carinii* pneumonia, recurrent Progressive multifocal leukoencephalopathy Salmonellosis, recurrent

Modified from Centers for Disease Control and Prevention. 1993 Revised classification system for HIV infection and extended surveillance case definitions for AIDS among adolescents and adults. MMWR 1992; 41: 1-19.

*This is an abbreviated list. All conditions under C, B3, and A3 have been classified as AIDS since January 1, 1993.

TABLE 17-4
Primary Prophylaxis of Opportunistic Infection in Adults Infected with HIV

Pathogen	INDICATION CD count/mm³	Other	First-choice drug and dose (mg/day or as noted)	Alternative drugs and doses (mg/day or as noted)	Criteria for stopping in patients receiving HAART
Pneumocystis carinii	<200	Oropharyngeal candidiasis	TMP/SMX 160/800*	TMP/SMX 80/400† *or* Dapsone 100 *or* Atovaquone 1500 *or* Pentamidine aerosol 300/month	CD4 >200/mm³ for 3 months
Toxoplasma gondii	<100	—	TMP/SMX 160/800*	TMP/SMX 80/400† Dapsone 50 *plus* pyrimethamine 75 *plus* leucovorin 25 weekly Atovaquone 1500	CD4 >200/mm³ for 3 months
Mycobacterium tuberculosis (INH sensitive)	Any	PPD >5 mm induration	INH 300 *plus* B6 50 for 9 months	Rifabutin 300 *plus* pyrazinamide 1500 for 6 months	N/A
M. tuberculosis (INH resistant)	Any	Same	Rifampin 600 *plus* pyrazinamide 1500 for 2 months	Rifabutin 300 *plus* pyrazinamide 1500 for 4 months	N/A
Mycobacterium avium complex	<50	—	Azithromycin 1200 weekly *or* clarithromycin 1000 in two divided doses	Azithromycin 1200 weekly *or* clarithromycin 1000 in two divided doses *plus* rifabutin 300	CD4 >100/mm³ for 3-6 months

Data from 1999 USPHS/IDSA Guidelines; Kovacs JA, Masur H. Prophylaxis against opportunistic infections in patients with human immunodeficiency virus. N Engl J Med 2000; 342: 1416-1429; and Bartlett JG, Gallant JE. 2001-2002 Medical Management of HIV Infection. Baltimore: Johns Hopkins University; 2001. *HAART,* Highly active antiretroviral therapy; *INH,* isoniazid; *N/A,* not applicable; *PPD,* purified protein derivative; *TMP/SMX,* trimethoprim-sulfamethoxazole.
*TMP/SMX 160/800 = one double-strength (DS) tablet.
†TMP/SMX 80/400 = one regular-strength tablet.

Antiretroviral Drug Therapy

Treatment of HIV disease is increasingly facilitated by the introduction of new antiviral drugs and the refinement of old ones. Generic names, commercial names, and abbreviations for the available antiretroviral drugs are summarized in Table 17-6. Currently available drugs fall into four categories: nucleoside reverse transcriptase inhibitors (NRTI), a single nucleotide reverse transcriptase inhibitor (tenofovir, released in October 2001), nonnucleoside reverse transcriptase inhibitors (NNRTI), and protease inhibitors (PI). The NRTI drugs act by terminating the elongation of DNA chains in the HIV provirus. The NNRTI drugs bind directly to the hydrophobic pocket of the viral reverse transcriptase enzyme and block its function. The PI drugs interfere with the assembly of new virions, resulting in deficient viral particles that are unfit for infecting a susceptible cell.

Initiation of Antiretroviral Drug Therapy

The decision to start antiretroviral drug therapy must be carefully thought out for each patient because adherence to therapy requires a lifelong commitment. Patients must realize

that compliance is all important. They should understand the goals of treatment and should become conversant with the concepts of CD4 count and viral load. They should also thoroughly understand the possible side effects of the different regimens and the importance of taking their medications on a regular schedule without "catching up." Nurses specializing in HIV care and other health professionals can help ensure compliance by taking the time in multiple encounters to explain again and again the goals of therapy and the need for strict adherence. Recruitment of family and friends to support and uphold the treatment plan is often worthwhile.

The International AIDS Society–USA Panel continues to issue updated recommendations for antiretroviral therapy. Therapy is initiated according to the CD4 count and viral load expressed as plasma HIV RNA copies per cubic millimeter.

Current guidelines for starting treatment are as follows:
- When the CD4 count is <350/mm³ at any viral load
- When the viral load is >55,000/mm³ by RT PCR or >30,000/mm³ by bDNA at any CD4 count

TABLE 17-5
Secondary Prophylaxis Against Opportunistic Infections

Pathogen	First-choice drug and dose (mg/day or as noted)	Alternative drugs and doses (mg/day or as noted)	Criteria for stopping in patients receiving HAART*
Pneumocystis carinii	TMP/SMX 160/800	Dapsone 100 Atovaquone 1500 aerosol Pentamidine 300/month	Possibly when CD4 >200/mm³ for 3 months
Toxoplasma gondii	Pyrimethamine 25-75 *plus* sulfadiazine 2-4 g *plus* folinic acid (leucovorin)10†	Clindamycin 1200 *plus* pyrimethamine 25-75 *plus* leucovorin 10	Possibly when CD4 >200/mm³ for 3 months and HIV-RNA <5000/mm³
Mycobacterium avium complex (MAC) (disseminated disease)	Clarithromycin 1000 *plus* ethambutol 15 mg/kg *with or without* rifabutin 300	Azithromycin 500 *plus* ethambutol 15 mg/kg *with or without* rifabutin 300	When MAC has been treated for 1 year and CD4 >100/mm³ for 6 months in an asymptomatic patient
Cytomegalovirus retinitis	Ganciclovir 5-6 mg/kg IV (5-7 days/week) *plus* foscarnet 90-120 IV *plus* ganciclovir intraocular implant (every 6-9 months) *plus* oral ganciclovir 3000 to 4500 in three divided doses	Cidofovir 5 mg/kg IV every other week	CD4 >100-150/mm³ for more than 30 weeks and no evidence of active disease in a patient undergoing regular opthalmologic examination
Cryptococcus neoformans	Fluconazole 200	Itraconazole 200	Not applicable; therapy is lifelong
Histoplasma capsulatum	Itraconazole 400	Itraconazole 200	Insufficient data for recommendation; probably lifelong

Data from 1999 USPHS/IDSA Guidelines; Kovacs JA, Masur H. Prophylaxis against opportunistic infections in patients with human immunodeficiency virus. N Engl J Med 2000; 342: 1416-1429; and Bartlett JG, Gallant JE. 2001-2002 Medical Management of HIV Infection. Baltimore: Johns Hopkins University; 2001.
HAART, Highly active antiretroviral therapy; *TMP/SMX,* trimethoprim-sulfamethoxazole.
*Criteria for discontinuing secondary prophylaxis in patients whose CD4 counts and viral loads have improved markedly while receiving HAART therapy, based on published evidence.
†The combination of pyrimethamine, sulfadiazine, and folinic acid (leucovorin) is effective for prophylaxis of *P. carinii* pneumonia. Therefore TMP/SMX is not required in this context.

- When symptoms are present, irrespective of the CD4 count and viral load

Treatment may be safely deferred in asymptomatic patients with CD4 counts of >350/mm³ and viral load <5000/mm³. However, if the decision is made to defer treatment, the CD4 count and viral load should be monitored more frequently (e.g., every 2 months). Treatment should also be considered in patients with the acute retroviral syndrome (see "Acute Retroviral Syndrome" earlier in the chapter).

The current standard of care is to begin treatment with three antiretroviral drugs. Monotherapy with any antiretroviral drug is inappropriate. From the classes of drugs and the individual agents shown in Table 17-6, drug combinations or "partners" can be selected as follows:

- Three RTI drugs: AZT and 3TC (as Combivir) plus abacivir (ABC) (AZT, 3TC, and ABC are now available as Trizivir). If the viral load is >100,000/mm³, failures may occur. Another such "set" would be d4T, ddI, and ABC or 3TC.
- Two NRTIs and one NNRTI (EFV is recommended; NVP and DLV are alternative choices).

- Two NRTIs and one PI (for example, Combivir plus nelfinavir).

In selecting one or another regimen, the clinician can take into account such factors as the results of ongoing trials, the ease of administration, and the presence of comorbid conditions and concomitant medications that might cause drug interactions. Other useful combinations include 3TC plus AZT (Combivir) combined with a protease inhibitor and dual protease inhibitor combinations.

Certain drug combinations should *not* be offered:

- d4T and AZT, because these thymidine analogs compete for intracellular activation via phosphorylation
- SQV and IDV (virologically antagonistic)
- ddc and 3TC (weak combination)
- ddI and ddC (lead to enhanced peripheral nerve toxicity)

Because of the rapid pace of new information about the efficacy, toxicity, and interactions of the antiretroviral drugs, clinicians making decisions about treatment for patients should stay current.

An effective drug regimen should result in a substantial (three-fold or greater) fall in the viral load within 2 weeks of

TABLE 17-6
Antiretroviral Drugs*

Category	Generic name	Trade name	Abbreviation	Usual adult dose
Nucleoside reverse transcriptase inhibitors (NRTIs)	Zidovudine	Retrovir	AZT (ZDV)	300 mg q12h
	Stavudine	Zerit	d4T	40 mg q12h
	Didanosine	Videx	ddI	200 mg q12h
	Lamivudine	Epivir	3TC	150 mg q12h
	Zalcitabine	Hivid	ddC	0.75 mg q8h
	Abacavir	Ziagen	ABC	300 mg q12h
	Zidovudine plus lamivudine	Combivir	AZT + 3TC	1 tablet q12
	Zidovudine plus lamivudine plus abacavir	Trizivir	AZT + 3TC + ABC	1 tablet q12h
Nonnucleoside reverse transcriptase inhibitor	Tenofovir disoprosil fumarate†	Viread	TDF	300 mg daily
Nonnucleoside reverse transcriptase inhibitors (NNRTIs)	Nevirapine	Viramune	NVP	200 mg q12h
	Elavirdine	Rescriptor	DLV	400 mg q8h or 600 mg q12h
	Efavirenz	Sustiva	EFV	600 mg q24h
Protease inhibitors (PIs)	Saquinavir (hard gel)	Invirase	SQV (HG)	600 mg q8h
	Saquinavir (soft gel)	Fortovase	SQV (SG)	1200 mg q8h
	Ritonavir	Norvir	RTV	600 mg q12h
	Indinavir	Crixivan	IDV	800 mg q8h
	Nelfinavir	Viracept	NFV	1250 mg q8h
	Amprenavir	Agenerase	APV	1200 mg q12h
	Lopinavir†	Kaletra	LPV/RTV	400 mg LPV/100 mg RTV q12h

Modified from Postic B, Horvath JA, Green PA, Bryan CS. Antiretroviral therapy, 1998. J SC Med Assoc 1998; 94: 207-217.
*ddI is taken 1 hour before or 2 hours after a meal. Indinavir is taken 1 hour before or 2 hours after a meal, but not concurrently with ddI. Patients taking indinavir should drink 1.5 liters of water daily. The other drugs listed in the table are to be taken with or within 1 hour after a meal.
†The combination of zidovudine, lamivudine, and abacavir, consisting of three nucleoside reverse transcriptase inhibitors, was released in 2001. Tenofovir was also released in 2001. Lopinavir is a dual protease inhibitor released in September 2000. One capsule contains 133 mg LPV and 33 mg RTV.

initiation of therapy. The maximal effect of therapy, assuming excellent compliance, is achieved within 4 to 5 months. A good practice is to start a flowchart with columns for the date, CD4 count, viral load, and drug regimens. In practice the CD4 count and viral load are measured between 4 and 8 weeks after the start of a new regimen. These parameters are assayed every 3 to 4 months, along with a review of medication side effects. The importance of compliance should be emphasized at each office visit.

Problem of Resistance to Antiretroviral Drugs and Attempts to Overcome It (Salvage)

Combination antiretroviral therapy has a dual rationale: to enhance efficacy and avoid or postpone the emergence of resistant viral strains. The aim of therapy is to reduce the plasma viral load to levels that are undetectable with the use of an ultrasensitive PCR-based assay. Resistant viral strains emerge through mutations because of the high replication rate of HIV and faulty proofreading for errors in viral biosynthesis. Since mutations conferring resistance to one drug may be independent of those that confer resistance to others, standard practice is to use three or more drugs to avoid or delay the selection of mutants.

HIV isolates can now be characterized by their phenotype and genotype with molecular and computer-assisted methods. These assays are expensive and may require an expert's insight for optimum interpretation. Evidence suggests that when drug therapy fails as indicated by a rising viral load despite compliance, genotyping or phenotyping is useful in designing a salvage therapy regimen. Before either genotyping or phenotyping is ordered, the patient must be taking antiretroviral drug therapy and the plasma viral load must be at least 1000 copies/mm³. If the patient is on a "drug holiday," wild-type virus (the original strain) tends to take over and obscure the minority population of resistant mutants (quasi-species).

The genotype reflects whether the patient's virus exhibits mutations that encode for resistance to a particular drug. HIV DNA is obtained from the patient's mononuclear blood cells and analyzed in a sequenator. The DNA sequence is determined by use of fluorescent labels attached to the four bases of DNA. Nucleotide sequences that are recognized in this assay include the genotypes for the viral enzymes, reverse transcriptase, and protease. Common mutations that confer resistance are classified as major (primary) and secondary. Major mutations affect specific HIV codons and correlate with high-level resistance and therapeutic ineffectiveness. Secondary mutations contribute to resistance, and a series of such mutations can have a cumulative effect. Assays for genotyping are commercially available (e.g., as HIV-1 GenotypR PLUS, # 7480, Specialty Laboratories, Santa Monica, California, 1-800-421-4449).

The phenotype reflects whether the patient's virus is sensitive or resistant to a particular drug. The virus is grown in cell culture in the presence of varying concentrations of the drug. The inhibitory concentration is thus determined. This concentration should exceed the minimal drug level at the end of the dosage interval. Phenotyping is akin to determining the minimum inhibitory concentration of bacteria to antibiotics (see Chapter 19). Phenotyping is more precise than genotyping, but more expensive.

What drugs should be employed in salvage regimens? The following are some general recommendations:

- Optimally, salvage regimens are selected on the basis of genotyping (or phenotyping), include at least two drugs the patient has not previously taken, and take into account compliance issues and convenience in administration.
- Some treated patients show an unexpected rise in the viral load from an undetectable level to a low but detectable level (<1000 HIV RNA copies/mm³). It is prudent to continue the patient's regimen, reinforcing compliance, and to monitor the viral loads every 2 to 3 months. Such unexpected "blips" often resolve spontaneously. If not, the patient may benefit from intensification of the regimen, for example, by adding a single drug (such as abacavir or an NNRTI) or by introducing a dual protease inhibitor regimen (discussed later). Should the viral load rise to >1000 HIV RNA copies/mm³, it is best to change the patient's entire regimen after reviewing the genotype.
- Dual–protease inhibitor regimens that incorporate low doses of ritonavir are useful. Ritonavir is a potent inhibitor of the liver cytochrome P450 enzyme system. Low doses of ritonavir (100 to 200 mg b.i.d.) are usually well tolerated.

Although the plasma levels achieved by ritonavir at these levels are subinhibitory, the plasma levels of the second protease inhibitor are substantially increased. Such dual regimens also permit b.i.d. doses, promoting compliance. Regimens given twice daily and postprandially include (1) ritonavir 100 to 200 mg plus saquinavir 1 g to 800 mg, (2) ritonavir 100 to 200 mg plus indinavir 800 mg, and (3) ritonavir 100 mg plus amprenavir 600 mg (to reiterate, all of these doses are b.i.d. and postprandially). A new protease inhibitor, lopinavir, was released in September 2000 coformulated with ritonavir at the dose of 400 mg of lopinavir/100 mg of ritonavir (Kaletra). Lopinavir requires five or more serial mutations in the protease gene to become ineffective therapeutically and is therefore useful for salvage regimens.

- Combinations of an NNRTI and a PI can be pharmacokinetically advantageous. For example, efavirenz enhances nelfinavir at full doses of either drug, thus introducing two potentially effective drugs for salvage regimens. Similarly, delavirdine (at 600 mg b.i.d.) enhances saquinavir (at doses of 1200 to 1400 mg b.i.d.), offering another effective combination. On the other hand, efavirenz reduces the plasma levels of other protease inhibitors, except for nelfinavir. Adding small doses of ritonavir (see the previous bulleted item) overcomes this obstacle.
- The clinician may find the best solution to resistance of substantial magnitude to be referral to a center where researchers have numerous protocols for investigational drugs.

Antiretroviral Therapy for Patients Undergoing Hemodialysis

Some of the current national and international guidelines for antiretroviral therapy do not cover the issue of hemodialysis. Consultation with a clinical pharmacist is recommended, particularly when patients on hemodialysis have concurrent liver disease. Monitoring of predialysis drug levels can be useful. Short of an accepted guideline, the following is suggested: (1) use of protease inhibitors and nonnucleotide RTIs at full daily doses and (2) use of one half of the usual dose for RTIs. Hepatitis C and HIV often coexist in patients with end-stage renal failure. Unfortunately, ribavirin is contraindicated and interferon alone would be ineffective.

Adverse Effects of Antiretroviral Drugs

The clinician caring for HIV-infected patients should have a general familiarity with antiretroviral drugs and keep in mind the possibility of drug toxicity as the cause of new symptoms. The following are major side effects.

Zidovudine (AZT) causes significant bone marrow toxicity manifested as anemia and neutropenia. Headaches can occur early and may respond to acetaminophen. Another side effect of AZT is myopathy, suspected on the basis of muscle weakness and associated with an increase in the plasma creatinine phosphokinase level. An esthetically unpleasant effect is pigmentation of the nails.

Didanosine (ddI) is associated with increases in serum lipase and amylase levels and may cause clinical, sometimes life-threatening, pancreatitis. Another side effect is peripheral neuropathy. Gastrointestinal intolerance is manifested as nausea and vomiting.

Zalcitabine (ddC) causes significant peripheral neuropathy and also mouth ulcers, which necessitate discontinuation of the drug.

Stavudine (d4T) has relatively few side effects except for peripheral neuropathy, which may persist after the discontinuation of this medication. Deep tendon reflexes should be evaluated at each office visit.

Lamivudine (3TC) is usually extremely well tolerated. Like other NRTIs, however, it may be involved in the pathogenesis of lactic acidosis (discussed later in the chapter).

Abacavir causes a specific and potentially severe hypersensitivity reaction in about 3% to 5% of patients, usually during the first 6 weeks of therapy. The full syndrome includes fever, rash, lymphadenopathy, nausea, vomiting, malaise, diarrhea, headache, fatigue, myalgia, and arthralgia. The drug should be stopped and the patient not rechallenged.

Tenofovir disoprosil fumarate (TDF) caused mild to moderately severe nausea, diarrhea, vomiting, and flatulence in about 11% of patients in clinical trials. These symptoms were severe enough to cause about 1% of patients to discontinue the drug.

Efavirenz causes a rash that, although usually not menacing, can progress to Stevens-Johnson syndrome. Like other NNRTs, this drug can cause elevations of aminotransferase levels and other biochemical abnormalities. Patients should know about the potential CNS effects of efavirenz, the most important of which are insomnia and bizarre dreams. These occur in about one fourth of patients, usually during the first months of use. Later they tend to decrease.

Nevirapine may cause hepatotoxicity, which is occasionally serious.

The protease inhibitors are frequently associated with gastrointestinal side effects. Nelfinavir, for example, often causes diarrhea. Loperamide, up to 8 mg per day, may help regulate it. Amprenavir causes nausea and occasionally vomiting and diarrhea. Indinavir is associated with nephrolithiasis and hyperbilirubinemia, which can be tolerated unless the bilirubin level is higher than 6 mg/dL. Hydration with at least 2 liters of fluid per day is recommended. Ritonavir causes more side effects than the other protease inhibitors, especially when used at doses $\geq$300 mg b.i.d. Intestinal intolerance, nausea, and vomiting are common. Ritonavir is the most potent inhibitor of P450 enzymes in the liver, thereby elevating levels of many drugs and rendering them potentially toxic.

Untoward reactions to antiretrovirals tend to be class specific. All NRTIs can cause mitochondrial toxicity, leading to lactic acidosis. This should be suspected when the serum electrolytes show an anion gap (sodium $-$ [bicarbonate $+$ chloride] $>$ 18). The order of frequency seems to be ddC $>$ d4T $>$ ddI $>$ AZT. Mitochondrial toxicity should be suspected in cases of myopathy, neuropathy, pancreatitis, cardiomyopathy, and occasionally hepatomegaly with steatosis and lipoatrophy. The syndrome is confirmed by an increased plasma lactic acid level. The offending drugs should be discontinued.

Protease inhibitors are associated with lipodystrophy at varying rates, but 40% or more of patients are affected in some series and lipodystrophy usually develops in patients who have been treated for long durations. Lipodystrophy can be manifested as fat depletion or accumulation. Hyperlipidemia, insulin resistance, elevated lactic acid levels, and osteoporosis have been noted. Patients may lose subcutaneous fat in the face, buttocks, and extremities, with veins becoming more visible. Concurrently, adipose augmentation may occur in the viscera and breasts and over the upper thoracic spine ("buffalo hump"). Lipodystrophy affects both genders. Since the pathophysiology

of the abnormality remains incompletely understood, finding a protease inhibitor–sparing alternative to treatment is considered first. Hypolipidemic agents, such as atorvastatin, and drugs enhancing endogenous insulin may be helpful.

 KEY POINTS

ANTIRETROVIRAL DRUG THERAPY

- ⊃ Initiating antiretroviral drug therapy is a major decision, since it entails a lifelong commitment by the patient.
- ⊃ Compliance is all important. Patients must understand the goals of therapy, the concepts of CD4 count and viral load, and the need to take their drugs on a regular schedule to delay or prevent the emergence of resistant viral strains.
- ⊃ Treatment is initiated when the CD4 count is $<$350/mm^3 at any viral load, when the viral load is $>$55,000 copies/mm^3 by RT-PCR at any CD4 count, or when patients are symptomatic.
- ⊃ Current treatment recommendations call for at least three drugs. Examples include use of three reverse transcriptase inhibitors or two nucleoside reverse transcriptase inhibitors plus a protease inhibitor.
- ⊃ Examples of drug combinations that should *not* be used are d4T and AZT, ddC and 3TC, ddI and d4T or ddC, and saquinavir plus indinavir.
- ⊃ The goal of antiretroviral therapy is to reduce the viral load to an undetectable level.
- ⊃ HIV-1 genotyping or phenotyping can be useful in the design of optimum salvage regimens for patients whose treatment has failed.
- ⊃ Occasionally, unexpected rises (or "blips") in the viral load ($<$1000/mm^3) resolve spontaneously or can be suppressed by intensifying the patient's regimen.
- ⊃ A general knowledge of the side effects of antiretroviral drugs is essential.

SUGGESTED READING

Baxter JD, Mayers DL, Wentworth DN, et al. A randomized study of antiretroviral management based on plasma genotype antiretroviral resistance testing in patients failing therapy. AIDS 2000; 14: F83-F93.

Carr A, Cooper DA. Adverse effects of antiretroviral therapy. Lancet 2000; 356: 1423-1430.

Department of Health and Human Services/Henry J. Kaiser Family Foundation. Panel on Clinical Practices for the Treatment of HIV Infection, February 2001 (available at www.hivatis.org or 1-800-448-0440).

Freedberg KA, Losina E, Weinstein MC, et al. The cost effectiveness of combination antiretroviral therapy for HIV disease. N Engl J Med 2001; 344: 824-831.

Grabar S, Le Moing V, Goujard C, et al. Clinical outcome of patients with HIV-1 infection according to immunologic and virologic response after 6 months of highly active antiretroviral therapy. Ann Intern Med 2000; 133: 401-410.

Hanna GJ, D'Aquila RT. Clinical use of genotypic and phenotypic drug resistance to monitor antiretroviral therapy. Clin Infect Dis 2001; 32: 774-782.

Max B, Sherer R. Management of the adverse effects of antiretroviral therapy and medication adherence. Clin Infect Dis 2000; 30 (Suppl 2): S96-S116.

O'Brien WA. Resistance against reverse transcriptase inhibitors. Clin Infect Dis 2000; 30 (Suppl 2): S185-S192.

Piscitelli SC, Gallicano KD. Interactions among drugs for HIV and opportunistic infections. N Engl J Med 2001; 984-996.

Rabkin JG, Ferrando SJ, Lin SH, et al. Psychological effects of HAART: a 2-year study. Psychosom Med 2000; 62: 413-422.

Staszewski S, Keiser P, Montaner J, et al. Abacavir-lamivudine-zidovudine vs indinavir-lamivudine-zidovudine in antiretroviral-naive HIV-infected adults: a randomized equivalence trial. JAMA 2001; 285: 1155-1163.

Prevention of HIV Transmission from Mother to Child (see also Chapter 4)

Transmission of HIV can occur either during pregnancy (transplacentally) or during labor and delivery. The latter accounts for about 70% of such transmissions. Infection of the infant can also occur postnatally through breast-feeding. Following the demonstration that zidovudine (AZT) can prevent the mother-to-infant transmission, antiretroviral prophylaxis became a standard of care. For women who are already receiving antiretroviral combination therapy, the effective regimen should be continued after a discussion of the uncertainty of the teratogenicity of particular drugs. Current FDA categories for use in pregnancy are as follows:

- Category B: didanosine, saquinavir, ritonavir, nelfinavir, and tenofivir
- Category C: most of the remaining antiretroviral drugs, including efavirenz (which is best avoided because it has caused birth defects in primates)
- Category D: hydroxyurea (cytotoxic and therefore contraindicated)

Viral load determinations are of value in pregnant women, since high viral loads increase the probability of transmission to the fetus and newborn. In small series of cases, no transmission occurred from mothers with undetectable virus. However, perinatal transmission of HIV to the infant has been reported in women with undetectable viral loads. Thus all HIV-infected pregnant women, irrespective of their viral loads and CD4 counts, should receive combination chemotherapy (HAART), either by continuing an ongoing, effective regimen or by initiating therapy with a potent and relatively safe regimen such as AZT plus 3TC (Combivir) plus nevirapine (Viramune). Previously treated women may, of course, develop drug-resistant HIV strains. In such cases an effective regimen should be designed on the basis of the HIV genotype (see earlier discussion).

Cesarean section has been shown to decrease the risk of HIV transmission to the infant. It should therefore be considered by the mother and her obstetrician, especially when the viral load is at a detectable level. Breast-feeding should be avoided to prevent the transmission of HIV via milk.

Clinicians treating HIV-infected pregnant women are strongly encouraged to report their data to a confidential national registry kept for this purpose: Antiretroviral Pregnancy Registry, 1410 Commonwealth Drive, Wilmington, NC (telephone 1-800-258-4263; fax 1-800-800-1052).

SUGGESTED READING

Anderson JR. A guide to the clinical care of women with HIV, 2001. HIV/AIDS Bureau.www.hab.hrsa.gov.

Andiman WA. Medical management of the pregnant woman infected with human immunodeficiency virus type 1 and her child. Semin Perinatol 1998; 22: 72-86.

Department of Health and Human Services/Henry J. Kaiser Family Foundation. Guidelines for the Use of Antiretroviral Agents in HIV-Infected Adults and Adolescents, January 2000. Available at http://www.hivatis.org or by telephone at 1-800-448-0440.

U.S. Public Health Service Perinatal HIV Guidelines Update, February 25, 2000, HIV/AIDS Treatment Information Service (ATIS). Available at: http://www.hivatis.org.

HIV Postexposure Issues

These issues are discussed in Chapter 26.

Other Human Retroviruses: HTLV-I and HTLV-II

Two retroviruses known as human T-cell lymphotropic viruses types I and II (HTLV-I and HTLV-II) were isolated between 1979 and 1981. Serologic screening of blood donors for antibodies to these viruses sometimes yields positive results, creating a dilemma for primary care clinicians.

Presentation and Progression

Cause

HTLV-I and HTLV-II belong to a group of viruses known as primate T-cell leukemia-lymphoma viruses. Both viruses are transmitted mainly by sexual intercourse, injecting drug use or administration of blood products, and mother-to-child transfer, which occurs mainly through breast-feeding. Sexual transmission of HTLV-I occurs in about 60% of women exposed over 10 years to an infected male partner but in only 0.4% of men exposed to an infected female partner for a similar duration. HTLV-II is transmitted mainly among injecting drug users and their sexual partners.

HTLV-I infects up to 20 million people worldwide, mainly in the southeastern United States (notably Florida), the Caribbean, and parts of Latin America, West Africa, the Middle East, India, and Melanesia. HTLV-II is endemic among injecting drug users in the United States and elsewhere and is also found in certain Native American populations.

Presentation

HTLV-I and HTLV-II most commonly come to the attention of primary care clinicians as a result of serologic testing of blood donors. HTLV-I is associated with two distinctive diseases: adult T-cell leukemia and myelopathy (also known as chronic progressive myelopathy or tropical spastic paraparesis). Adult T-cell leukemia-lymphoma has a variable presentation, including lymphadenopathy, hepatosplenomegaly, skin lesions (papules, nodules, plaques, and erythroderma), lytic bone lesions, hypercalcemia, and abnormal lymphocytes in the peripheral blood. HTLV-I–associated myelopathy causes gait abnormalities, weakness, and stiffness of the lower extremities. HTLV-II has not been definitively associated with any disease, although suggestive evidence links this virus with certain rare hematologic malignancies.

Diagnosis

Diagnosis of HTLV-I and HTLV-II infection depends on serologic testing similar to testing for HIV. ELISA assays are used to screen for antibodies, and the Western blot method is used for confirmation. PCR can be used to distinguish between HTLV-I and HTLV-II.

Natural History

Expected Outcome

An estimated 1% to 4% of carriers of HTLV-I will eventually develop adult T-cell leukemia and that <5% will eventually develop myelopathy.

Treatment and Prevention

Adult T-cell leukemia is treated primarily with chemotherapy, but there appears to be a role for antiretroviral therapy as well. There is no standardized treatment for HTLV-I–associated myelopathy.

CDC guidelines for persons testing positive for HTLV-I and HTLV-II include use of latex condoms to prevent sexual transmission, avoidance of needle sharing and blood donation, and avoidance of breast-feeding.

When to Refer

Patients with adult T-cell leukemia or myelopathy should be referred to appropriate specialists.

 KEY POINTS

OTHER HUMAN RETROVIRUSES: HTLV-I AND HTLV-II

⊃ HTLV-I and HTLV-II usually come to the attention of primary care clinicians as a result of serologic screening of blood donors.

⊃ PCR can be used to confirm infection and to distinguish between HTLV-I and HTLV-II.

⊃ HTLV-I carries a 1% to 4% lifetime risk of adult T-cell leukemia and a <5% lifetime risk of chronic myelopathy.

⊃ HTLV-II has not been clearly associated with any disease.

⊃ Persons testing positive for HTLV-I or HTLV-II should be advised to use latex condoms, to avoid needle sharing and blood donation, and to refrain from breast-feeding of infants.

SUGGESTED READING

Centers for Disease Control and Prevention and the U.S.P.H.S. Working Group. Guidelines for counseling persons infected with human T-lymphotropic virus type I (HTLV-I) and type II (HTLV-II). Ann Intern Med 1993; 118: 448-454.

Gotuzzo E, Arango C, de Queiroz-Campos A, et al. Human T-cell lymphotropic virus-I in Latin America. Infect Dis Clin North Am 2000; 14: 211-239.

18 Chronic Fatigue Syndrome

NILI GUJADHUR, JOSEPH F. JOHN, JR.

Case Definition and Epidemiology
Cause
Presentation
Diagnosis
Treatment
Outcomes and Disability
Summary

Chronic fatigue syndrome (CFS) is an illness currently defined by unexplained persisting or relapsing fatigue and other debilitating symptoms of at least 6 months' duration. There are no pathognomonic physical findings or definitive laboratory tests. Whether most cases of CFS will ultimately prove to have a single cause is unclear, but authorities agree that a quantum leap forward in our understanding of this enigmatic syndrome will be necessary to provide specific therapy. In the meantime, CFS challenges the ability of primary care clinicians to provide appropriate supportive management in the face of uncertainty about the nature of the underlying process.

Case Definition and Epidemiology

Fatigue is a common complaint, accounting for up to 25% of all primary care office visits. Numerous medical conditions can have fatigue as a chief complaint (Table 18-1). In most instances a diagnosis will be established or the fatigue will resolve within 6 months. The current U.S. case definition of CFS, established by the Centers for Disease Control and Prevention (CDC) in 1994 on the basis of extensive conferences and consultations, requires that the fatigue be of at least 6 months' duration and that at least four of eight minor symptoms be present (Box 18-1). Several aspects of this case definition deserve emphasis:

- The case definition was established in part because of the need for a standardized definition in conducting epidemiologic and clinical studies.
- Insistence that fatigue be of at least 6 months' duration before assigning a diagnosis of CFS is an important rule, especially in view of the publicity and controversy surrounding this disorder.
- The fatigue can fluctuate from year to year, month to month, day to day, and even hour to hour.
- Specific diseases should be excluded by thorough history and physical examination with selected laboratory tests.

The 1994 case definition was proposed to replace a previous case definition, published in 1988, that incorporated overrestrictive criteria and relied on nonspecific physical signs. The newer definition resolves the confounding issue of neuropsychiatric syndromes, which may have similar symptoms.

CFS is by no means a new condition. In the mid-19th century George Miller Beard, a New York City neurologist, coined the term "neurasthenia," by which he meant exhaustion of nervous energy. Other diagnostic labels proposed through the years include postviral fatigue, chronic mononucleosis, and myalgic encephalomyelitis. It is likely that the term CFS will be abandoned in the future for a more appropriate name. Various subtle perturbations of the immune system have been described, prompting activists in the United States to lobby for "chronic fatigue and immune deficiency syndrome" as the best appellation. CFS has been associated with numerous infectious etiologies, including Epstein-Barr virus (EBV), human

TABLE 18-1
Some Medical Conditions That Can Cause Fatigue

Category of illness	Examples
Endocrinopathies	Hypothyroidism; diabetes mellitus; Cushing's syndrome; adrenal insufficiency
Chronic inflammatory disease	Wegener's granulomatosis; sarcoidosis
Psychiatric disorders	Depression; bipolar disorder; anxiety disorder
Infections	Toxoplasmosis (see Chapter 8); infectious mononucleosis caused by Epstein-Barr virus (see Chapter 8); infectious mononucleosis caused by cytomegalovirus (see Chapter 8)
Malignancies	Leukemias; lymphomas
Cardiopulmonary	Sleep apnea syndrome; chronic lung disease; heart failure
Liver disease	Chronic hepatitis or cirrhosis
Medication side effects	Antidepressants; antihistamines; antineoplastic agents

BOX 18-1
Case Definition of Chronic Fatigue Syndrome by the Centers for Disease Control and Prevention

- Clinically evaluated, unexplained chronic fatigue of >6 months' duration that is not the result of ongoing exertion and is not substantially alleviated by rest. The fatigue is associated with a significant reduction in occupational, educational, social, or personal activities.
- Four or more of the following symptoms:
  - Impaired memory or concentration
  - Sore throat
  - Tender cervical or axillary lymph nodes
  - Muscle pain
  - Pain in multiple joints (polyarthralgia)
  - New headaches
  - Unrefreshing sleep
  - Postexertional malaise

herpesvirus type 6 (HHV-6), *Brucella* species, influenza, and malaria. Extensive research has yet to provide convincing data in favor of one or another infectious agent, and even the most ardent advocate of a specific cause must acknowledge that Koch's postulates (in either the classic or molecular version) remain unfilled. Thus, despite years of research, rhetoric, and reproach, CFS is fraught with controversy and uncertainty.

Based on the 1994 CDC definition, the prevalence of CFS has been determined to be as high as 230 cases per 100,000 persons. CFS disproportionately affects females by ratios of 7 to 1 (using the older criteria) to 3 to 1 (using the newer criteria), and cases tend to cluster during the fourth and fifth decades of life. However, the premise that CFS is mainly a disease of white upper-middle-class women in their thirties and forties has been challenged by recent studies, in which CFS has also been found to be common in African-Americans, Hispanics, and persons of lower socioeconomic status. Strong evidence suggests that CFS has a worldwide distribution.

 KEY POINTS

CHRONIC FATIGUE SYNDROME: CASE DEFINITION AND EPIDEMIOLOGY

⊃ Fatigue accounts for up to 25% of primary care office visits, but most cases have an apparent cause or prove to be self-limited.

⊃ Clinicians must insist that fatigue be of at least 6 months' duration before rendering a diagnosis of chronic fatigue syndrome, and the CDC criteria (Box 18-1) should be consulted.

⊃ CFS is not a new disease. Synonyms over the years include neurasthenia, postviral fatigue, chronic mononucleosis, and myalgic encephalomyelitis.

⊃ The prevalence of CFS, using the newer definition, is up to 230 cases per 100,000, or about 1 in 40 persons.

SUGGESTED READING

Fukuda K, Straus SE, Hickie I, et al. International Chronic Fatigue Syndrome Study Group. The chronic fatigue syndrome: a comprehensive approach to its definition and study. Ann Intern Med 1994; 121: 953-959.

Goshorn RK. Chronic fatigue syndrome: a review for clinicians. Semin Neurol 1998; 18: 237-242.

Jason LA, Richman JA, Rademaker AW, et al. A community-based study of chronic fatigue syndrome. Arch Intern Med 1999; 159: 2129-2137.

Wessely S. Chronic fatigue: symptom and syndrome. Ann Intern Med 2001; 134: 838-843.

Cause (Figure 18-1)

The cause is unknown. The heterogeneous nature of the syndrome suggests that CFS may not be a discrete disease caused by a single agent. Many researchers believe that CFS represents a common set of symptoms triggered by a variety of infectious or noninfectious factors. The search for one or more etiologies has been focused especially on infectious agents, the immune system, the central nervous system, and the cardiovascular system. The possibility that both psychological factors and chemical sensitivities might predispose to CFS continues to be studied, most recently in veterans of the Gulf War.

Infections

A majority of patients with CFS date their symptoms to an apparent viral infection. Much effort has been given to finding a viral etiology. Reports during the mid-1980s incriminated EBV. Subsequent controlled studies, based on seroepidemiology, have failed to validate this hypothesis. There is no clear correlation between CFS and serologic markers of EBV infection. However, a majority of patients with CFS have a high antibody titer to the viral capsid antigen (anti-VCA) or EBV and also have antibodies to the early antigen (EA) and nuclear antigen (NA) (see Chapter 8). Other implicated viruses are human T-cell leukemia virus types 1 and 2 (HTLV-1 and HTLV-2), enteroviruses, and HHV-6 and other herpesviruses (herpes simplex virus [HSV] and cytomegalovirus [CMV]), but, again, antibody titers against these viruses do not differ between patients with CFS and persons without CFS.

Immunologic Factors

Extensive studies suggest that patients with CFS may have one or more defects in their immune systems. These include low immunoglobulin levels, increased levels of circulating immune complexes, increased levels of interleukins 1 and 6 and transforming growth factor-β, and quantitative alterations among lymphocyte subpopulations. In Japan CFS is often called "cytokine disease" (*New York Times*, February 3, 2000). Recent studies suggest that patients with CFS have up-regulation of a set of enzymes that are involved in the degradation of single-stranded RNA by the enzyme ribonuclease L (RNase L). Patients with CFS may also have increased levels of a novel 37-kilodalton binding protein. Whether these and other observations will prove useful for diagnosis and management of CFS remains to be established.

Central Nervous System Abnormalities and Exercise Capacity

Various abnormalities in hypothalamic function have been described in patients with CFS. Blunting of diurnal variation occurs, and these patients typically have lower morning cortisol levels, higher evening cortisol levels, and decreased urinary free cortisol compared with control subjects. A response profile similar to that seen in patients with neurally medi-

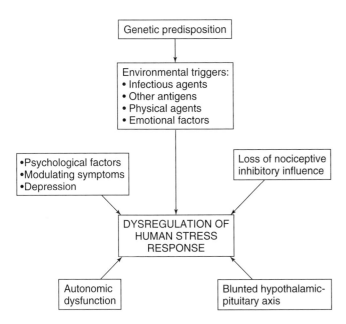

FIG. 18-1 Chronic fatigue syndrome, according to prevailing opinion, may represent dysregulation of the human stress response brought about by one or more of several factors.

ated hypotension, with abnormalities of the sympathetic and parasympathetic systems on tilt table testing, has been demonstrated. Some researchers have found white matter abnormalities on magnetic resonance imaging (MRI) of the brain to be more common in patients with CFS than in healthy subjects. Similarly, single photon emission computed tomography (SPECT) shows hypoperfusion abnormalities more often in these patients.

Some patients with CFS have marked impairment in their functional capacity. In a recent study the exercise capacity of patients with CFS was markedly lower than that of healthy sedentary women without CFS symptoms. Compared with the healthy control subjects, patients with CFS had higher resting heart rates but lower maximal heart rates at the end of exercise. Maximal oxygen uptake was also reduced in patients with CFS, suggesting a physiologic basis for their complaints of reduced energy and ability to work. However, whether these physiologic observations reflect the cause of CFS or are merely the result of deconditioning has not been determined.

 KEY POINTS

CAUSE

⊃ The cause of CFS is unknown. The heterogeneous nature of the syndrome argues against the notion that CFS is a discrete disease caused by a single agent.

⊃ Various immunologic abnormalities have been described. Symptoms of CFS can be reproduced in volunteers by administration of interleukin-1 (IL-1).

⊃ Some patients with CFS have abnormalities that suggest neurally mediated hypotension on tilt table testing. Some patients with CFS have impaired functional capacity on exercise testing, but whether this observation reflects the cause of the illness or is merely the result of deconditioning is unclear.

SUGGESTED READING

De Becker P, Roeykens J, Reynders M, et al. Exercise capacity in chronic fatigue syndrome. Arch Intern Med 2000; 160: 3270-3277.

De Meirleir K, Bisbal C, Campine I, et al. A 37 kDa 2-5A binding protein as a potential biochemical marker for chronic fatigue syndrome. Am J Med 2000; 108: 99-105.

Fiedler N, Lange G, Tiersky L, et al. Stressors, personality traits, and coping of Gulf War veterans with chronic fatigue. J Psychosom Res 2000; 48: 525-535.

Ottenweller JE, Sisto SA, McCarty RC. Hormonal responses to exercise in chronic fatigue syndrome. Neuropsychobiology 2001; 43: 34-41.

Streeten DH, Thomas D, Bell DS. The roles of orthostatic hypotension, orthostatic tachycardia, and subnormal erythrocyte volume in the pathogenesis of chronic fatigue syndrome. Am J Med Sci 2000; 320: 1-8.

Wallace HL II, Natelson B, Gause W, et al. Human herpesviruses in chronic fatigue syndrome. Clin Diagn Lab Immunol 1999; 6: 216-223.

Presentation

Onset of CFS can be abrupt or gradual, but most patients describe a "trigger" event. About one third of patients date the onset of CFS to an acute, flulike illness. Other trigger events include emotional trauma, physical trauma, childbirth, or surgery. Less than 20% of patients describe no specific events before the onset.

Fatigue

Persistent disabling fatigue is the hallmark of CFS. Fatigue can last hours to days and occur with minimal exertion. Patients report lack of energy and inability to carry out their daily activities. Some patients report inability to assume an upright posture. At certain periods in their disease some patients remain bedfast much of the day. They characteristically report a sense of profound muscle fatigue with or without pain in muscle, joint, or bone that sends a signal to cease their current activity. For some patients even slight motions like flipping the page of a book produce fatigue. Escalation of fatigue after intense physical or social interaction is characteristic, leading patients to describe a typical "payback" for expenditure of energy.

Sleep Disorders

Sleep disorders are common and may consist mainly of insomnia or of excessive sleeping. Patients report that on awakening, they feel exactly as they did when they went to sleep. Sleep is often interrupted or described as very light. Some patients sleep for 12 to 18 hours at a stretch. Few patients with CFS dream normally. Absence of stage 4 non–rapid eye movement (REM) sleep is often found when a sleep study is undertaken. Some studies indicate that patients with CFS have a defect in their sleep-wake pattern caused by serotonin deficiency. The sleep apnea syndrome should be considered as a possible cause of CFS, especially in heavyset patients who snore.

Cognition

Neurocognitive difficulties are common and, although often subtle, may cause disability. Patients describe difficulty with concentration and short-term memory. They may have problems with information processing, word finding, or serial number recall. Many patients forgo reading complex novels or nonfiction, an activity that once was routine, because of inability to retain theoretical material. Few patients attempt crossword puzzles. Patients also report paresthesias, disequilibrium, blurred vision, and photophobia, although neurologic signs are extremely uncommon. Sophisticated neuropsychological testing indicates that impaired cognition cannot be attributed solely to psychiatric conditions.

Febrile Episodes

Flulike symptoms, frequently present at the onset of CFS, may recur frequently. Patients complain intermittently of sore throat, low-grade fever, tender lymphadenopathy, generalized myalgia, arthralgia, and headache. Many patients describe facial pain, especially over the paranasal sinuses, with or without fever.

Dizziness and Headaches

Orthostatic postural hypotension in CFS is usually neurally mediated. Dizziness is a common symptom, and patients may report this as intermittent or severe. Patients learn to change position slowly from lying to sitting and from sitting to standing. Some patients feel a sense of vertigo or whirling. Others report a buzzing or vibration of the inner body. Headache is also common. Patients sometimes describe classic migraine but more often report a dull and persistent occipital pain. Headache often worsens with fatigue and can be associated with other symptoms, such as arthralgias and myalgias.

Allergy

Some researchers have found that allergy is more common in patients with CFS than in the general population. Some patients have allergies for years before the onset of CFS, whereas others report worsening of their allergic symptoms soon after the onset of CFS. Up to 50% of persons with CFS may have atopy.

Other Symptoms

Other symptoms that may accompany fatigue or be debilitating themselves include diarrhea, sensitivity to light, daytime somnolence, shortness of breath, and urinary urgency.

 KEY POINTS

PRESENTATION

⊃ Onset can be abrupt or gradual. About 80% of patients report a "trigger" event, most commonly a flulike illness. Flulike symptoms tend to recur during the course of CFS.
⊃ Persistent disabling fatigue is the hallmark of CFS. Some patients report inability to assume an upright posture. Orthostatic postural hypotension is common and is usually neurally mediated. Dizziness, headache, sleep disorders, and neurocognitive difficulties are also common. Patients have difficulty concentrating and impairment of short-term memory.

SUGGESTED READING

DeLuca J, Johnson SK, Ellis SP, et al. Cognitive functioning is impaired in patients with chronic fatigue syndrome devoid of psychiatric disease. J Neurol Neurosurg Psychiatry1997; 62: 151-155.
Fischler B, Dendale P, Michiels V, et al. Physical fatigability and exercise capacity in chronic fatigue syndrome: association with disability, somatization, and psychopathology. J Psychosom Res 1997; 42: 369-378.
Morriss RK, Wearden AJ, Battersby L. The relation of sleep difficulties to fatigue, mood, and disability in chronic fatigue syndrome. J Psychosom Res 1997; 42: 597-605.
Straus SE, Dale JK, Wright R, et al. Allergy and the chronic fatigue syndrome. J Allergy Clin Immunol 1988; 81: 791-795.

Diagnosis

Diagnosis of CFS is based on specific criteria (Box 18-1) when the patient's symptoms cannot be explained by coexisting illnesses. The clinician should insist on the criterion of severe fatigue of at least 6 months' duration without alternative explanation. In a recent study only 2.5% of patients seeking medical treatment for fatigue or psychiatric symptoms or both met this criterion, since most patients became well or an alternative diagnosis became apparent during 6 months of observation.

No laboratory tests are diagnostic. The clinical features of CFS overlap considerably with those of fibromyalgia, mild systemic lupus erythematosus (SLE), early multiple sclerosis, and depression. Symptoms of CFS and fibromyalgia often coexist in the same patient. Moreover, the relationship of CFS to depression is problematic. The clinician should keep open the possibility that an alternative diagnosis may eventually become apparent.

The initial history and physical examination should be supplemented with selected baseline laboratory tests. These include a complete blood count with differential, chemistry profile (including creatinine, glucose, serum potassium, calcium, and liver enzymes), erythrocyte sedimentation rate (ESR), sensitive thyroid-stimulating hormone assay, morning cortisol level (as an initial screen for adrenal insufficiency), human immunodeficiency virus (HIV) antibody test, urinalysis, and chest x-ray examination. Usually test results are normal. Additional tests to exclude alternative diagnoses should be guided by the patient's history and physical examination. Some potential areas of investigation include the following:

- Endocrine abnormalities. Endocrine disease should always be considered as a cause of fatigue, since it is nearly always treatable. The major possibilities are hypothyroidism, hypoadrenalism, and abnormalities in the hypothalamic-pituitary-ovarian axis.
- Immune dysregulation. Results of immunologic tests are of dubious, if any, value in the diagnosis and management of CFS. Various abnormalities such as low CD4 lymphocyte counts or abnormal CD4/CD8 ratios may be useful for substantiating disability claims (see later discussion).
- Viral studies. HIV causes persistent fatigue, and thus HIV infection should be excluded, especially if risk factors are present. EBV titers are frequently misused in clinical practice, and neither EBV titers nor HHV-6 titers should be used as the basis for the diagnosis of CFS. A diagnosis of CFS can be supported to some extent by high antibody titers to the various EBV antigens and also by high IgG titers to HHV-6 or by the presence of IgM antibodies to HHV-6 (found in a recent study to be present in 57% of patients with CFS compared with 16% of healthy blood donors).
- Sleep study. Sleep studies are expensive but may be useful to document lack of REM sleep and sleep fragmentation and to make an occasional diagnosis of sleep apnea syndrome.

- Tilt table testing. Many patients are found to have neurally mediated hypotension. Some of these patients respond to treatment with fludrocortisone (Florinef) or β-blockers, although the benefit of this approach has not been established by controlled trials.
- Neuroimaging. Abnormalities on MRI and SPECT imaging have been described, but the findings are inconsistent and nonspecific.
- Psychological and psychiatric evaluations. Major depression and CFS have many symptoms in common, and depression is much more amenable to drug therapy than is CFS. Although some persons believe that depression underlies most cases of CFS, various studies suggest significant differences between these entities. Formal psychological testing instruments such as the Minnesota Multiphasic Personality Inventory (MMPI) often provide information that is useful for counseling. Many patients with CFS react to stress in ways that are less than optimal. Patients can often be helped by cognitive behavior therapy.

 KEY POINTS

DIAGNOSIS

- Diagnosis of CFS is based on specific criteria (Box 18-1) after other explanations for the patient's symptoms have been excluded.
- Features of CFS overlap with those of fibromyalgia, mild systemic lupus erythematosus, early multiple sclerosis, and depression, but no disease fully mimics the classic constellation of CFS symptoms. The clinician should keep open the possibility that an alternative diagnosis might ultimately become apparent.
- Patients with CFS should have a complete history and physical examination, supplemented with selective laboratory tests.

SUGGESTED READING

Bates DW, Buchwald D, Lee J, et al. Clinical laboratory test findings in patients with chronic fatigue syndrome. Arch Intern Med 1995; 155: 97-103.

Deale A, Wessely S. Diagnosis of psychiatric disorder in clinical evaluation of chronic fatigue syndrome. J R Soc Med 2000; 93: 310-312.

Jacobson SK, Daly JS, Thorne GM, et al. Chronic parvovirus B19 infection resulting in chronic fatigue syndrome: case history and review. Clin Infect Dis 1997; 24: 1048-1051.

Lawrie SM, MacHale SM, Cavanagh JT, et al. The difference in patterns of motor and cognitive function in chronic fatigue syndrome and severe depressive illness. Psychol Med 2000; 30: 433-442.

Scott LV, Dinan TG. Urinary free cortisol excretion in chronic fatigue syndrome, major depression and in healthy volunteers. J Affect Disord 1998; 47: 49-54.

Van der Linden G, Chalder T, Hickie I, et al. Fatigue and psychiatric disorder: different or the same? Psychol Med 1999; 29: 863-868.

Treatment

No cure has been found for CFS, and the long-term effects of available treatments are largely unknown. Most patients gradually improve or at least compensate for their disability (see below). Studies suggest that a multidisciplinary approach that incorporates cognitive behavioral therapy may be worthwhile. At present, management must be individualized (Box 18-2).

Supportive Physician-Patient Relationship

A trustful, supportive clinician-patient relationship is paramount. The significance of the patient's symptoms should not be dismissed. The patient must understand that the diagnosis of CFS is made in part by excluding other disorders and that the possibility of an alternative diagnosis will be kept open. Office visits should be scheduled on a regular basis, initially every 2 to 4 months and then less frequently when the illness stabilizes. The clinician must keep an open mind about the nature of the disorder and should review information the patient might obtain from various sources, including the Internet, but should generally discourage the patient from spending his or her resources on unproved therapies, including CFS clinics that claim unique expertise.

The clinician should be familiar with the patient's social context. The patient should be encouraged strongly to set specific long-term goals, *in writing,* in the major areas of life (e.g., health, education, family, finances, friends, outside interests, and spiritual growth). The physician should outline a definite management plan, and a concerted effort should be made to rehabilitate the patient toward a near normal lifestyle. The primary care clinician may wish to utilize various consultants, but should not abdicate responsibility for ongoing care and interest.

Activity, Exercise, and Sleep

Inactivity resulting from fatigue leads to deconditioning, causing loss of social interaction and thus perpetuating a vicious cycle. However, muscle performance seems to be normal in these patients. A graded exercise program therefore should be slowly introduced after the patient is told that this may lead initially to an exacerbation of symptoms but they often will improve with time. Graded exercise was shown to improve functional work capacity and fatigue in a recent controlled trial. The benefit of rehabilitation programs for patients with CFS is unclear, despite the apparent benefit for patients with clear-cut postviral syndromes. In our practice we find the benefit of prolonged physical therapy to be minimal at best. We encourage daily aerobic activity and advise patients that such activity is not harmful and can be graded to produce a minimum of postexercise fatigue. We also encourage patients to keep an hourly journal of how they feel for at least several weeks. Such a journal forms the basis for planning high-priority

---

BOX 18-2
Management of Chronic Fatigue Syndrome

- Establish trustful rapport.
- Provide a definite treatment plan.
- Use a team approach.
- Encourage a graded exercise program.
- Suggest physical rehabilitation.
- Refer for cognitive therapy as indicated.
- Provide symptomatic relief.*
- Consider Ampligen or other investigational drugs.
- Give emotional support.

*Antiinflammatory drugs, antidepressants, and stimulants in selected patients.

activities during the time of day that they usually feel the best. The clinician should demonstrate interest in the patient's accomplishments, which are necessary for self-esteem.

Sleep is often impaired in patients with CFS, just as it is in patients with fibromyalgia. Patients with CFS typically spend a great deal of time in bed, which often exacerbates daytime fatigue. The therapeutic goal should be a regular sleeping pattern, which limits the amount of time spent in bed. If simple measures fail, tricyclic antidepressants or hypnotics may be helpful.

Cognitive Behavior Therapy

Cognitive therapy helps patients to understand CFS and gradually increase their activity. Studies of the value of cognitive behavior therapy have yielded conflicting results. In one study patients receiving cognitive behavior therapy and patients receiving only standard care had similar outcomes. In other studies, however, cognitive behavior therapy seemed beneficial. Therapists with special interest and expertise in CFS can be extremely helpful to some patients, and some therapists have formed support groups.

Nonsteroidal Antiinflammatory Drugs and Benzodiazepines

Nonsteroidal antiinflammatory drugs (NSAIDs) can alleviate such symptoms as myalgias, arthralgias, and headaches. Benzodiazepines can be useful for management of insomnia, anxiety, and panic attacks.

Antidepressants

Few large randomized trials address the use of antidepressants in patients with CFS. In uncontrolled studies and in our clinical experience, up to 70% or 80% of patients with CFS benefit from antidepressants. Explanations for the efficacy of antidepressants in many patients include the high prevalence of depression in patients with CFS and also the efficacy of antidepressants for patients with fibromyalgia, which often coexists with CFS. Patients with CFS often tolerate tricyclic antidepressants poorly because of the sedative and anticholinergic effects of these drugs. Serotonin reuptake inhibitors (SSRIs) are often used. In a double-blinded study, fluoxetine (Prozac) was not beneficial. Low doses of phenelzine, a monoamine oxidase inhibitor, were shown to be superior to placebo in a small study.

Antiviral Agents

The possibility that antiviral drugs might benefit patients with CFS was suggested after the reported association with EBV (now generally disregarded; see earlier discussion). The effect of acyclovir was identical to that of placebo, although, interestingly, 40% of patients in each group improved with therapy. Some patients with reactivation of HHV-6 might benefit from intermittent therapy with acyclovir or similar drugs, but this intervention has not been proved successful.

Ampligen, a polymer of inosine and cytosine (poly I-poly C), is an experimental double-stranded RNA preparation that has both antiviral and immunomodulatory effects. Patients receiving this compound had a significant improvement in exercise performance and quality of life compared with patients receiving placebo over a 26-week period, but the durability of the improvement was not evaluated after the end of therapy. Currently a double-blinded, placebo-controlled trial is near completion to determine the safety and efficacy of Ampligen 200 mg twice weekly. Amantadine (Chapter 20) has also been studied, but thus far its benefit seems to be limited.

Treatment of Patients with Postural Hypotension

After the report that many patients with CFS have neurally mediated hypotension as determined by a positive tilt table test, pharmacologic treatment has received much interest. Some patients with positive tilt table tests report marked improvement with fludrocortisone (Florinef). However, no controlled studies have documented the efficacy of fludrocortisone for this purpose, and a recent study suggested no demonstrable effect. Fludrocortisone often causes mild edema but otherwise is generally well tolerated. As an alternative to fludrocortisone, increased dietary salt and water intake can be prescribed. Some patients with CFS use this tactic on a daily basis. Another approach to these patients is to prescribe β-blockers such as atenolol in low doses. Midodrine HCl (Pro-Amatine) has been used to help sustain blood pressure in some patients, but this drug should be used with great care because of its potential to cause supine hypertension.

Other Forms of Treatment

The following are some of the many forms of treatment that have been tried or are currently being studied:

- Intravenous immune globulin (IVIG), given with the rationale that it provides passive immunity and modulates antigen-antibody responses, was beneficial in one placebo-controlled study and has been used in children and adolescents with CFS. However, its role in CFS, if any, remains uncertain. Isoprinosine, an older immune modulator, is widely used in Europe and is scheduled to enter U.S. trials in the near future.

- Corticosteroids in low doses have been used with the rationale that mild hypocortisolism is sometimes present in patients with CFS. No benefit has been clearly established by randomized trials. Dehydroepiandrosterone (DHEA) was reported to be helpful in preliminary studies, but the benefit was not confirmed. Hence, its use should be considered experimental.

- Nicotinamide adenine dinucleotide (NADH) has been used with the rationale that it facilitates generation of adenosine triphosphate (ATP), which may be depleted in patients with CFS. In a small randomized trial, patients receiving NADH 10 mg per day showed improvement compared with those receiving placebo.

- Other treatments such as dietary manipulation, vitamins, herbal preparations, and avoidance of environmental toxins have not been supported by solid data. Essential fatty acids (evening primrose oil and fish oil) were reported to be of benefit, as was parenteral infusion of magnesium. However, these and similar claims have not been substantiated by larger trials. Claims are frequently made that herbal preparations are useful for patients with CFS, but only primrose oil has been evaluated in a controlled study, and with largely negative results.

▶ KEY POINTS

TREATMENT

⊃ The clinician-patient relationship is paramount. The patient should have regular, scheduled follow-up appointments and a definite management plan. Patients should be given reassurance and exhorted to set goals for themselves in writing. Daily aerobic exercise and good sleep hygiene should be encouraged.

- ➲ Cognitive behavior therapy is sometimes useful, especially if a therapist with interest and expertise in CFS is available.
- ➲ Symptomatic drug therapy is often useful and includes NSAIDs, antidepressants (especially the SSRIs), and benzodiazepines.
- ➲ Patients with positive tilt table test results sometimes report benefit from fludrocortisone or low-dose β-blockers, although the value of these therapies has not been established by well-controlled trials.
- ➲ The clinician should keep an open mind about the potential value of new therapies but should discourage patients from trying remedies that are not only unproved by well-controlled studies but also expensive or potentially harmful.

SUGGESTED READING

Ang DC, Calabrese LH. A common-sense approach to chronic fatigue in primary care. Cleve Clin J Med 1999; 66: 343-350, 352.

Marlin RG, Anchel H, Gibson JC, et al. An evaluation of multidisciplinary intervention for chronic fatigue syndrome with long-term follow-up, and a comparison with untreated controls. Am J Med 1998; 105 (3A): 110S-114S.

Morriss RK, Ahmed M, Wearden AJ, et al. The role of depression in pain, psychophysiological syndromes and medically unexplained symptoms associated with chronic fatigue syndrome. J Affect Disord 1999; 55: 143-148.

Prins JB, Bleijenberg G, Bazelmans E, et al. Cognitive behaviour therapy for chronic fatigue syndrome: a multicentre randomised controlled trial. Lancet 2001; 357: 841-847.

Rowe PC, Calkins H, DeBusk K, et al. Fludrocortisone acetate to treat neurally mediated hypotension in chronic fatigue syndrome: a randomized controlled trial. JAMA 2001; 285: 52-59.

Sharpe M. Cognitive behavior therapy for chronic fatigue syndrome: efficacy and implications. Am J Med 1998; 105 (3A): 104S-109S.

Vollmer-Conna U, Hickie I, Hadzi-Pavlovic D, et al. Intravenous immunoglobulin is ineffective in the treatment of patients with chronic fatigue syndrome. Am J Med 1997; 103: 38-43.

Wearden AJ, Morriss RK, Mullis R, et al. Randomised, double-blind, placebo-controlled treatment trial of fluoxetine and graded exercise for chronic fatigue syndrome. Br J Psychiatry 1998; 172: 485-490.

Werbach MR. Nutritional strategies for treating chronic fatigue syndrome. Altern Med Rev 2000; 5: 93-108.

Outcomes and Disability

Patients should be told at the onset that the prognosis for full recovery is uncertain. Observations concerning the natural history of CFS include the following:

- Older age at onset of symptoms correlates with a less favorable prognosis. The prognosis for CFS in children and adolescents is good; in a recent study based on 3 years of follow-up, the illness resolved in 43% of patients, improved in 52%, and remained unchanged in only 5%.
- Gradual onset of symptoms as opposed to abrupt onset of symptoms correlates with a higher rate of concurrent psychiatric disease and a less favorable prognosis.
- More severe symptoms at the time of the initial clinic visit correlate with a less favorable prognosis.
- The presence of a comorbid psychiatric condition correlates with a less favorable prognosis.
- Having a supportive, solicitous "significant other" correlates with a less favorable prognosis, although the cause-and-effect relationship is unclear.

- Some (but not other) studies suggest that clinging to the belief that the disease has a purely physical cause is an unfavorable sign.

Among adults who meet stringent criteria for CFS and who have had at least several years of follow-up, full recovery has occurred in about 5% to 12% according to various studies. Many patients improve, but others are unable to work and must resort to filing for disability payments.

Disability

Primary care clinicians should be familiar with some of the issues involved in filing for disability payments. Under U.S. Social Security law, an individual is considered disabled in the following circumstances:

- The person is unable to do any substantial gainful work activity because of a medical condition (or conditions) that has lasted, or can be expected to last, for at least 12 months, or that is expected to result in death *or*
- In the case of an individual under the age of 18, he or she suffers from any medically determinable physical or mental impairment of comparable severity.

The medical condition(s) must be shown to exist by means of medically acceptable clinical and laboratory findings. Under the law, symptoms alone cannot be the basis for a finding of disability, although the effects of symptoms may be an important factor in deciding whether a person is disabled. The Social Security law requires that a disabling impairment be documented by medically acceptable clinical and laboratory findings. There is an emerging role in documentation for biologic markers, tilt table tests, and, if validated by further studies, the 37-kilodalton protein mentioned previously.

In addition to a thorough medical history and pertinent clinical and laboratory findings, the Social Security Administration requires longitudinal records and detailed historical notes discussing the course of the disorder, including treatment and response. Patients should apply for disability when they believe their condition will preclude them from working for at least 1 year. In our experience, the counsel of an experienced disability lawyer is invaluable in facing the Social Security system. Physicians who enter disability claims with their patients should anticipate the sizable amount of time required to complete this task.

 KEY POINTS

EXPECTED OUTCOME AND DISABILITY

- ➲ Adverse prognostic signs in CFS include older age at onset, more severe disease at onset, gradual rather than abrupt onset, and comorbid psychiatric conditions. Only about 4% to 12% of adults who meet rigorous criteria for CFS recover completely within several years. Many patients, however, are improved and can continue to function at home and at work.
- ➲ Some patients with CFS are unable to work and must file for disability insurance payments. Under Social Security law, symptoms alone cannot be the basis for a finding of disability. There is an emerging role for biologic markers of CFS, such as altered CD4/CD8 ratios, and potentially for the results of tilt table tests and other studies.

⊃ Detailed medical records that include documentation of symptoms and therapeutic interventions may be useful for the patient applying for disability payments.

SUGGESTED READING

Anderson JS, Ferrans CE. The quality of life of persons with chronic fatigue syndrome. J Nerv Ment Dis 1997; 185: 359-367.

Bell DS, Jordan K, Robinson M. Thirteen-year follow-up of children and adolescents with chronic fatigue syndrome. Pediatrics 2001; 107: 994-998.

Deale A, Chalder T, Wessely S. Illness beliefs and treatment outcome in chronic fatigue syndrome. J Psychosom Res 1998; 45 (1 Spec No): 77-83.

DeLuca J, Johnson SK, Ellis SP, et al. Sudden vs. gradual onset of chronic fatigue syndrome differentiates individuals on cognitive and psychiatric measures. J Psychiatr Res 1997; 31: 83-90.

Hill NF, Tiersky LA, Scavalla VR, et al. Natural history of severe chronic fatigue syndrome. Arch Phys Med Rehabil 1999; 80: 1090-1094.

Joyce J, Hotopf M, Wessely S. The prognosis of chronic fatigue and chronic fatigue syndrome: a systematic review. QJM 1997; 90: 223-233.

Schmaling KB, Smith WR, Buchwald DS. Significant other responses are associated with fatigue and functional status among patients with chronic fatigue syndrome. Psychosom Med 2000; 62: 444-450.

Summary

CFS remains enshrouded in uncertainty, causing many persons, including physicians, to question the existence of this entity. Such skepticism, although appropriate, does the patient little good. Clinicians should not hesitate to make a diagnosis of CFS when, after careful study and prolonged observation, no alternative physical or psychiatric disorder explains the patient's symptoms. Clinicians should also be sympathetic to patients who, seeking medical legitimacy for their condition, bring to the office information gleaned from the Internet, support groups, and other sources beyond the realm of randomized, controlled trials published in the peer-reviewed medical literature. CFS brings out the ambiguous interface between mind and body. Validation of the patient's symptoms is important. The clinician should acknowledge that "we just don't know yet" the precise etiology and specific treatment while seeking ways to help the patient cope with this frustrating and often debilitating disorder.

SUGGESTED READING

Aronowitz RA. From myalgic encephalitis to yuppie flu: a history of chronic fatigue syndromes. In: Rosenberg CE, Golden J, eds. Framing Disease: Studies in Cultural History. New Brunswick, NJ: Rutgers University Press; 1992: 155-181.

Clarke JN. The search for legitimacy and the "expertization" of the lay person: the case of chronic fatigue syndrome. Soc Work Health Care 2000; 30: 73-93.

Demitrack MA. Chronic fatigue syndrome and fibromyalgia: dilemmas in diagnosis and clinical management. Psychiatr Clin North Am 1998; 21: 671-692.

Fuller NS, Morrison RE. Chronic fatigue syndrome: helping patients cope with this enigmatic illness. Postgrad Med 1998; 103: 175-176, 179-184.

Lloyd AR, Hickie I, Peterson PK. Chronic fatigue syndrome: current concepts of pathogenesis and treatment. Curr Clin Top Infect Dis 1999; 19: 135-159.

Richman JA, Jason LA, Taylor RR, et al. Feminist perspectives on the social construction of chronic fatigue syndrome. Health Care Women Int 2000; 21: 173-185.

Whiting P, Bagnall A-M, Sowden AJ, et al. Interventions for the treatment and management of chronic fatigue syndrome: a systematic review. JAMA 2001; 286: 1360-1368.

19 Principles of Antimicrobial Therapy, and Antibacterial Drugs

CHARLES S. BRYAN, JOSEPH E. KOHN

The purpose of this chapter is to provide a framework for antimicrobial prescribing and to discuss the major antibacterial drugs. Antiviral, antifungal, antimycobacterial, and antiparasitic drugs, and use of antimicrobials for preexposure and postexposure prophylaxis, are discussed elsewhere (see Chapters 20 to 23 and 26).

Overview of Antibacterial Drugs

A general knowledge of antimicrobial pharmacology facilitates appreciation of how bacteria develop resistance, why some drugs are predominantly bactericidal whereas others are predominantly bacteriostatic, why combination therapy can be helpful or harmful, and what the basis is for manufacturers' competing claims.

Available antimicrobials target one or another component of the bacterial cell, as follows:

- Inhibition of peptidoglycan synthesis in the cell wall by agents such as the β-lactams (penicillins, cephalosporins, carbapenems, monobactams, and others), the glycopeptides (vancomycin and teicoplanin), cycloserine, and bacitracin
- Inhibition of protein synthesis inside the bacterial cell by agents such as the macrolides, azalides, and ketolides (erythromycin, clarithromycin, azithromycin, and telithromycin) clindamycin, chloramphenicol, streptogramin A and B (present in Synercid), oxazolidinones (linezolid), aminoglycosides (e.g., gentamicin, tobramycin, and amikacin), aminocyclitols (spectinomycin), tetracycline, fusidic acid, and mupirocin (Bactroban)
- Increase in the permeability of the cell membrane by colistin and polymyxin B
- Inhibition of enzymes involved in nucleic acid (DNA and RNA) synthesis by metronidazole (Flagyl), the quinolones (nalidixic acid, oxolinic acid, and the potent fluoroquinolones such as ciprofloxacin and levofloxacin), rifampin, and rifabutin
- Inhibition of folic acid synthesis by the sulfonamides and trimethoprim

With this framework in mind, some properties of antimicrobial drugs (Table 19-1) can be reviewed:

- The minimum inhibitory concentration (MIC) refers to the lowest concentration needed to inhibit growth in the laboratory of a standardized inoculum of a microorganism. The minimum lethal concentration (MLC; also called minimum bactericidal concentration, or MBC) refers to the lowest concentration needed to kill (rather than merely inhibit) the microorganism (Figure 19-1). The terms "cidal" (short for bactericidal) and "static" (short for bacteriostatic) allude to the relationship between the MIC and the MLC. A drug is cidal if the MIC and the MLC are the same or virtually the same—that is, the lowest concentration that inhibits growth also destroys the microorganism. A drug is static if the MLC is considerably higher (at least four-fold higher) than the MIC—that is, the organism remains viable even though growth is inhibited. Cidal and static are relative terms, and the same drug can fall into either category depending on the organism and other factors.

- Tolerance refers to the situation in which a drug that is usually cidal proves to be only static (the MLC exceeds the MIC by 32-fold or greater). This phenomenon may be clinically relevant, especially in chronic staphylococcal infections such as osteomyelitis, because long-term therapy with β-lactam antibiotics encourages the survival of "tolerant" mutants.

- The inoculum effect refers to instances in which the MIC and MLC values are less impressive when susceptibility testing is carried out with a large inoculum of bacteria (10^7 colony-forming units [CFUs]/mL) rather than the conventional inoculum (10^5 CFUs/mL). Production of extended-spectrum β-lactamases by gram-negative bacteria may become apparent only when a high level of inoculum is used in testing.

TABLE 19-1
Some Terms and Abbreviations Pertaining to Antimicrobial Therapy

Term	Definition
Bioavailability	The percentage of a drug, following a dose, that reaches the systemic circulation
V_d	*Volume of distribution:* a mathematically derived expression of the extent to which a drug, following a dose, is distributed throughout the body's tissues and fluids
MIC	*Minimum inhibitory concentration:* the lowest concentration of a drug needed to inhibit growth of a standardized inoculum of a microorganism; usually used in reference to antibacterial and antifungal drug therapy
MIC_{90}	The concentration of a drug required to inhibit 90% of strains (or clinical isolates) of a given microbial species
MLC	*Minimum lethal concentration:* the lowest concentration of a drug needed to destroy entirely a standardized inoculum of a microorganism; also called MBC (minimum bactericidal concentration) or MFC (minimum fungicidal concentration)
IC_{50}	*Inhibitory concentration* for 50% of all isolates of a strain of virus; also called EC_{50} (effective concentration for 50% of all isolates of a strain of virus)
C_{max}	*Maximum serum concentration* (or peak concentration) of an antimicrobial agent after a dose
$T_{1/2}$	*Serum half-life:* the time required for the C_{max} to be reduced by one half
AUC	*Area under the curve:* the magnitude and duration of serum levels of a drug plotted against time after a single dose, usually measured over a 24-hour period
C_{max}/MIC	The ratio of maximum (peak) serum concentration to the MIC, or "inhibitory ratio" (sometimes called "kill ratio")
SBT	*Serum bactericidal titer:* the maximum dilution of a patient's serum capable of sterilizing a standardized inoculum of an infecting microorganism (for a drug with a bactericidal mechanism of action, this value should in theory be the inverse of the C_{max}/MIC)
AUC/MIC	The ratio of the area under the curve (usually for 24 hours) to the MIC; that is, the magnitude and the duration of serum levels in relation to the MIC
Time > MIC	The amount of time the serum level of a drug exceeds the MIC after a dose
PAE	*Postantibiotic effect:* a persistent inhibitory effect of an antimicrobial agent against a microorganism after concentrations have fallen below the MIC

KEY POINTS

OVERVIEW OF ANTIBACTERIAL DRUGS

⊃ The major mechanisms of action of antimicrobials include inhibition of cell wall synthesis (e.g., β-lactams and glycopeptides), inhibition of protein synthesis (e.g., tetracyclines, macrolides, and aminoglycosides), inhibition of DNA or RNA synthesis (fluoroquinolones, metronidazole, rifampin), and inhibition of folic acid synthesis (sulfonamides, trimethoprim).

⊃ MIC and MLC refer, respectively, to the lowest concentration of drug needed to inhibit or destroy a given organism. Related terms include cidal, static, tolerance, and the inoculum effect.

SUGGESTED READING

Gregg CR. Drug interactions and anti-infective therapies. Am J Med 1999; 106: 227-237.

Kucers A, Crowe SM, Grayson ML, Hoy JF, eds. The use of antibiotics: a clinical review of antibacterial, antifungal and antiviral drugs. 5th ed., Oxford: Butterworth-Heinemann; 1997.

O'Grady F, Lambert HP, Finch RG, Greenwood D, eds. Antibiotic and chemotherapy: anti-infective agents and their use in therapy. New York: Churchill Livingstone; 1997.

Piscitelli SC, Roodvold KA, eds. Drug interactions in infectious diseases. Totowa, NJ: Humana Press; 2001.

Schossberg D, ed. Current therapy of infectious disease. 2nd ed., St. Louis: Mosby; 2001.

Pharmacokinetics and Pharmacodynamics

Pharmacokinetics denotes the absorption, distribution, and elimination of a drug and is usually expressed as the relationship of serum levels to time. Pharmacodynamics denotes the relationship between the serum level and the observed clinical effects of the drug, both desired and undesired (Figure 19-2). From the MIC against a specified microorganism, the peak serum level after a dose (C_{max}), and the magnitude and duration of serum levels over time after a dose, three relationships can be derived (Figure 19-3):

■ The ratio of the peak serum level to the MIC (C_{max}/MIC), sometimes called the kill ratio

■ The relationship of the magnitude and duration of serum levels (area under the curve, or AUC) to the MIC (AUC/MIC)

■ The amount of time during which the serum level exceeds the MIC after a dose (time > MIC)

Two patterns of antimicrobial activity are based on these relationships:

■ Time-dependent killing, meaning that the amount of time during which the serum level exceeds the MIC (time > MIC) matters more than the magnitude of the serum level. This pattern characterizes the β-lactam antibiotics, vancomycin, the macrolides, and clindamycin. With these agents sustained therapeutic serum levels are more important than high peak serum levels.

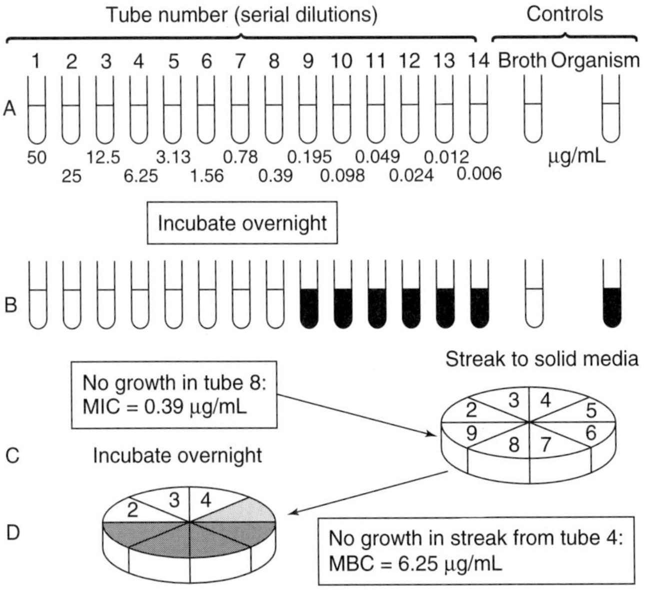

FIG. 19-1 Classic two-fold dilution method for determining the minimum inhibitory concentration (MIC) and minimum bactericidal concentration (MBC) of an antibiotic against a standardized inoculum of a given microorganism. Note that the end point for the MIC determination is the absence of visible growth after overnight inoculation (step B), whereas the end point for the MBC determination is the absence of growth on solid media after subculturing from the tubes that showed no visible growth (step D).

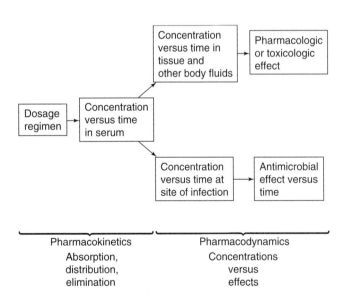

FIG. 19-2 Pharmacokinetics denotes the absorption, distribution, and elimination of a drug; pharmacodynamics denotes the relationship between the serum level and the observed clinical effects, both desired and undesired. (From Craig WA. Pharmacokinetic/pharmacodynamic parameters: rationale for antibacterial dosing of mice and men. Clin Infect Dis 1998; 26: 1-12.)

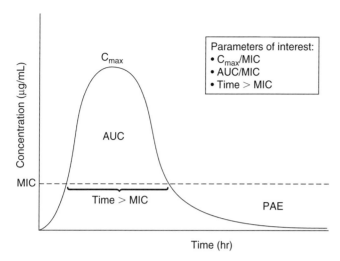

FIG. 19-3 Relationship of the serum concentration of a drug to the minimum inhibitory concentration (MIC) of a microorganism. The relationship of both the peak serum concentration (C_{max}) and the area under the curve (AUC) to the MIC expresses the potential therapeutic usefulness of the drug, as does the amount of time that the serum concentration exceeds the MIC (time > MIC). The postantibiotic effect (PAE) denotes the potential usefulness of the drug even at subinhibitory concentrations.

■ Concentration-dependent killing, meaning that the height of the serum level (C_{max}/MIC and AUC/MIC) matters more than the time during which the serum level exceeds the MIC. This pattern characterizes the fluoroquinolones, metronidazole, and the aminoglycosides.

A persistent inhibitory effect at levels below the MIC is called the postantibiotic effect (PAE) (Figure 19-3). All antimicrobials exert a PAE, at least in vitro, against susceptible gram-positive bacteria. A prolonged PAE against gram-negative bacteria is characteristic mainly of drugs that inhibit protein, DNA, or RNA synthesis such as tetracyclines, macrolides, chloramphenicol, and rifampin. For the quinolones the 24-hour AUC/MIC ratio is now thought to be the best predictor of therapeutic efficacy. For the tetracyclines, azithromycin, vancomycin, and quinupristin-dalfopristin, the AUC/MIC ratio is thought to be the key predictor of efficacy even though little concentration-dependent killing occurs, possibly because these drugs produce long PAEs compared, for example, with the β-lactams.

In the treatment of systemic infections, a common general goal is to provide peak serum concentrations at least four-fold greater than the MIC of the infecting microorganism (i.e., C_{max}/MIC ≥4). A higher C_{max}/MIC is desired in the treatment of endocarditis and infections of tissues or body fluids in which penetration of the drug is expected to be poor. A lower C_{max}/MIC ratio is permissible when treating urinary tract infections (UTIs) (for antibiotics that are concentrated in the urine) and for drugs with unusual pharmacologic properties such as azithromycin, which is highly concentrated within phagocytic cells. The concepts of time-dependent killing, concentration-dependent killing, and postantibiotic effect are often taken into account in formulating specific dosage regimens.

 KEY POINTS

PHARMACOKINETICS AND PHARMACODYNAMICS

⊃ Pharmacokinetics denotes serum levels over time, while pharmacodynamics denotes the relationship of serum levels to observed effects, both desired and undesired.

⊃ The β-lactams, vancomycin, macrolides, and clindamycin exhibit time-dependent killing, meaning that the amount of time during which the serum level exceeds the inhibitory concentration (time > MIC) matters more than the magnitude of the serum level.

⊃ The fluoroquinolones, metronidazole, and the aminoglycosides exhibit concentration-dependent killing, meaning that the height of the serum level (C_{max}/MIC or AUC/MIC) matters more than the duration of the serum level.

⊃ A common general goal of antimicrobial therapy is to provide a C_{max}/MIC of 4 or greater. However, the concepts of time-dependent killing, concentration-dependent killing, and postantibiotic effect are taken into account in formulating specific regimens.

SUGGESTED READING

Craig WA. Pharmacokinetic/pharmacodynamic parameters: rationale for antibacterial dosing of mice and men. Clin Infect Dis 1998; 26: 1-12.

Levison ME. Pharmacodynamics of antibacterial drugs. Infect Dis Clin North Am 2000; 14: 281-291.

Li RC. New pharmacodynamic parameters for antimicrobial agents. Int J Antimicrob Agents 2000; 13: 229-235.

Schentag JJ. Antimicrobial action and pharmacokinetics/pharmacodynamics: the use of AUIC to improve efficacy and avoid resistance. J Chemother 1999; 11: 426-439.

Oral Therapy Versus Parenteral Therapy

Bioavailability represents the extent to which serum levels of a drug (measured as AUC) after nonparenteral administration approximate the levels achieved after an intravenous dose. For example, oral bioavailability is 87% if the AUC after a 1-g oral dose is 87% of the AUC after a 1-g intravenous dose. Certain drugs such as the aminoglycosides and vancomycin are poorly absorbed from the gastrointestinal tract. Drugs with excellent oral bioavailability include the short-acting sulfonamides, trimethoprim, the quinolones, chloramphenicol, metronidazole, and linezolid (Table 19-2). Most gastrointestinal absorption takes place in the proximal jejunum and in the ileum. A few antimicrobials—metronidazole is perhaps the best example—provide excellent bioavailability even when given as rectal suppositories. It is now possible to provide oral therapy for many, and perhaps most, serious infections at a fraction of the cost of parenteral therapy and with greater convenience to the patient.

Several caveats apply to oral therapy:

■ Food inhibits the absorption of some drugs, such as the antistaphylococcal penicillins.

■ Antacids and H₂-receptor antagonists inhibit the absorption of some drugs, such as the antifungal agents ketoconazole and itraconazole.

■ Polyvalent cations (e.g., those present in magnesium-, aluminum-, or calcium-containing antacids or in zinc and iron

TABLE 19-2
Oral Bioavailability of Selected Antimicrobials

Drug (representative brand name)	Oral bioavailability (%)	Comments
Amoxicillin (Polymox)	89	Peak serum concentrations are 2 to 2.5 times higher than those attained with an equivalent dose of amoxicillin.
Amoxicillin-clavulanate (Augmentin)	89	Minimal concentrations are achieved in CSF in patients with uninflamed meninges.
Ampicillin (Principen and others)	50	Presence of food in the GI tract greatly decreases the rate and extent of absorption.
Azithromycin (Zithromax)	37	Tissue concentrations exceed plasma concentrations 10- to 100-fold after single-dose administration.
Cefaclor (Ceclor)	93	Peak concentrations are lower and attained later when administered with food, although the total amount of the drug remains unchanged.
Cefdinir (Omnicef)	16-25	Distribution into the CSF is unknown.
Cefixime (Suprax)	40-50	Presence of food in the GI tract greatly decreases the rate but not the extent of absorption.
Cefpodoxime (Vantin)	41-64	Presence of food in the GI tract increases the bioavailability of tablets but does not affect the suspension.
Cefprozil (Cefzil)	89-95	Distribution into the CSF is unknown.
Ceftibutin (Cedax)	80	Food decreases the rate and extent of absorption; however, food has a greater effect on absorption when given as a suspension instead of tablets.
Cefuroxime axetil (Ceftin)	39-52	Tablets and suspension are not bioequivalent and therefore cannot be substituted on a milligram per kilogram basis.
Cephalexin (Keflex)	90-99	Peak serum concentrations are lower and attained later when the drug is administered with food, although the total amount of drug absorbed remains unchanged.
Ciprofloxacin (Cipro)	60-80	Quinolones bind to divalent cations (Ca^{2+}, Mg^{2+}, Al^{2+}, and Fe^{2+}) in the GI tract and form an insoluble complex; concurrent administration with antacids, dairy products, and other drugs containing these products should be avoided.
Clarithromycin (Biaxin)	50	The extent of absorption is either increased or unaffected by food.
Clindamycin (Cleocin)	90	Only small amounts diffuse into the CSF, even with inflamed meninges.
Dicloxacillin (Dynapen)	60-80	The presence of food in the GI tract markedly decreases the rate and extent of absorption.
Dirithromycin (Dynabac)	6-14	Absorption is slightly enhanced with concomitant antacids.
Doxycycline (Vibramycin)	90-100	Doxycycline chelates divalent cations (Ca^{2+}, Mg^{2+}, Al^{2+}, and Fe^{2+}). Concurrent administration of antacids, dairy products, or other drugs containing these cations may decrease oral absorption. Doxycycline has a low affinity for Ca^{2+}.
Erythromycin (Ery-Tab)	18-45	Bioavailability depends on the particular erythromycin derivative, dosage formulation, acid stability, presence of food in the GI tract, and gastric emptying time.
Gatifloxacin (Tequin)	96	Quinolones bind to divalent cations (Ca^{2+}, Mg^{2+}, Al^{2+}, and Fe^{2+}) in the GI tract and form an insoluble complex; avoid concurrent administration with antacids, dairy products, and other drugs containing these products.

Continued

TABLE 19-2—cont'd
Oral Bioavailability of Selected Antimicrobials

Drug (representative brand name)	Oral bioavailability (%)	Comments
Levofloxacin (Levaquin)	99	Quinolones bind to divalent cations (Ca^{2+}, Mg^{2+}, Al^{2+}, and Fe^{2+}) in the GI tract and form an insoluble complex; avoid concurrent administration with antacids, dairy products, and other drugs containing these products.
Linezolid (Zyvox)	90	Maximum plasma concentrations are reached 1 to 2 hours after dose.
Loracarbef (Lorabid)	90	Peak serum concentrations occur within 1 hour.
Metronidazole (Flagyl)	100	Peak serum concentrations are lower and attained later when administered with food, although the total amount of the drug absorbed remains unchanged.
Minocycline (Minocin)	90	Minocycline chelates divalent cations (Ca^{2+}, Mg^{2+}, Al^{2+}, and Fe^{2+}). Concurrent administration of antacids, dairy products, and other drugs containing these products should be avoided.
Moxifloxacin (Avelox)	90	Quinolones bind to divalent cations (Ca^{2+}, Mg^{2+}, Al^{2+}, and Fe^{2+}) in the GI tract and form an insoluble complex; avoid concurrent administration with antacids, dairy products, and other drugs containing these products.
Nitrofurantoin (Macrodantin)	87-94	Food or delayed gastric emptying increases the extent of absorption by increasing the dissolution rate of macrocrystals.
Penicillin V (Pen Vee K)	25-50	Penicillin V is more resistant to acid-catalyzed inactivation than is penicillin G.
Rifampin (Rifadin)	90-95	Rifampin is widely distributed into most body tissues and fluids, including liver, lungs, bile, prostate, seminal fluid, CSF, saliva, tears, ascitic fluid, and bone.
Telithromycin (Ketek)	57%	Telithromycin is well absorbed without regard to meals, is concentrated in phagocytic cells, and penetrates rapidly into respiratory tissues and fluids.
Tetracycline (Sumycin)	60-80	Tetracycline chelates divalent cations (Ca^{2+}, Mg^{2+}, Al^{2+}, and Fe^{2+}). Concurrent administration of antacids, dairy products, or other drugs containing these cations may decrease oral absorption.
Trimethoprim-sulfamethoxazole (Bactrim, Septra)	90-100	In patients with inflamed meninges, trimethoprim and sulfamethoxazole concentrations are 50% and 40%, respectively, of concurrent serum concentrations.

CSF, Cerebrospinal fluid; *GI,* gastrointestinal.

preparations) inhibit the absorption of some drugs, notably the tetracyclines, by forming unabsorbable complexes.

■ Coadministration of other drugs inhibits the absorption of some drugs. For example, the quinolones are inactivated when coadministered with compounds such as sucralfate (Carafate) or ddI (didanosine; Videx).

■ Anatomic or physiologic disease of the upper gastrointestinal tract, including active vomiting, can profoundly affect oral bioavailability.

 KEY POINTS

ORAL VERSUS PARENTERAL THERAPY

⊃ Oral bioavailability is the extent to which the serum levels (measured as AUC) after an oral dose approximate those achieved after an intravenous dose.

⊃ Certain antimicrobials provide oral bioavailability that approaches 100%. Examples include the short-acting sulfonamides and trimethoprim (including trimethoprim-sulfamethoxazole [TMP/SMX]), some of the newer quinolones, chloramphenicol, metronidazole, and linezolid.

⊃ Oral bioavailability can be reduced by food, antacids, H_2-antagonists, polyvalent cations, various drugs, and anatomic or physiologic disease of the upper gastrointestinal tract.

SUGGESTED READING

Joshi N. Oral antibiotics: are the old still gold? Hosp Pract Off Ed 1999; 34: 117-122.

MacGregor RR, Graziani AL. Oral administration of antibiotics: a rational alternative to the parenteral route. Clin Infect Dis 1997; 24: 457-467.

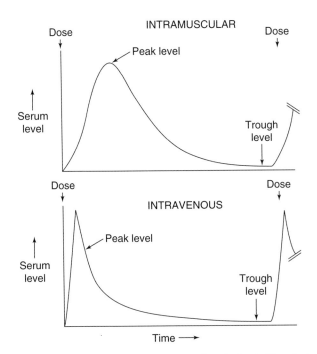

FIG. 19-4 Peak serum levels are usually obtained 60 minutes after an intramuscular dose of an antibiotic or 30 minutes after an intravenous dose. Especially after an intravenous dose, the value of the peak level is critically dependent on accurate timing of the dose and the blood sample, since the time-serum concentration curve is falling rapidly. Trough levels, obtained just before the next anticipated dose, allow more leeway. Peak levels, if they are to be determined at all, must be obtained with great care. We consider trough levels to be more reliable and useful in daily clinical practice.

Singh BN. Effects of food on clinical pharmacokinetics. Clin Pharmacokinet 1999; 37: 213-235.

Monitoring of Antibiotic Serum Levels

Monitoring of antibiotic serum levels in primary care is indicated mainly when aminoglycoside antibiotics (e.g., gentamicin or tobramycin) are administered on an outpatient basis because of the potential ototoxicity. Vancomycin also causes eighth nerve neurotoxicity, but the risk appears to be lower than with the aminoglycosides, and the case for monitoring levels is less clear.

The measurement of "peak and trough" serum levels has become customary. This practice became popular during the late 1960s on the basis of extensive studies with gentamicin, mainly after intramuscular administration. Peak levels were obtained 1 hour after an intramuscular injection of gentamicin. Today, parenteral antimicrobials are usually given intravenously rather than intramuscularly, at least in most practices, and peak levels are customarily obtained 30 minutes after an intraveous infusion (Figure 19-4). Our preference for most patients is to obtain only trough levels for several reasons. First, the validity of peak serum levels has never been rigorously established outside of research settings. Second, an accurate peak level after intravenous administration requires extremely close attention to the tim-

ing and rate of infusion of the dose and the sample. Third, trough levels (i.e., levels obtained just before the next scheduled dose) are obtained at a time when the serum level is falling much more gradually (Figure 19-4). We recommend the following protocol:

- Prescribe the drug on a weight (mg/kg) basis, recognizing that there is a tendency to undermedicate, especially with the aminoglycosides.
- Specify that the first dose each day be given at 8 AM.
- Obtain a trough blood level before administering the morning dose. Simultaneous measurement of the serum creatinine level is customary.
- Reduce the dose if the trough level exceeds 2 μg/mL for gentamicin or tobramycin or 10 to 20 μg/mL for vancomycin. (With vancomycin, trough levels <10 μg/mL were recommended in the past, but a case is now being made for pushing the trough level up to 15 μg/mL or even 20 μg/mL in critical situations such as pneumonia.)

The frequency of monitoring trough levels is a matter of individual preference. With the aminoglycosides, this might vary from weekly to every other day, depending on renal function and the severity of illness. With vancomycin, less frequent monitoring of trough levels (e.g., weekly or even every other week in patients with stable renal function) is suggested provided the dosage has been planned correctly.

Trough levels are measured mainly to reduce the risk of toxicity, whereas peak levels are measured mainly to ensure therapeutic efficacy. Situations in which peak levels are sometimes indicated include difficult-to-treat infections such as pneumonia caused by *Pseudomonas aeruginosa* or endocarditis caused by drug-resistant microorganisms and the desire to document adequate absorption of a drug during oral therapy. Neither of these circumstances is common in primary care. The issue of peak-versus-trough levels is controversial, and some authorities strongly believe that both peak and trough levels should be obtained.

▶ KEY POINTS

MONITORING OF ANTIBIOTIC SERUM LEVELS
- ↻ Monitoring serum levels is indicated mainly during aminoglycoside (gentamicin or tobramycin) therapy because of the risk of permanent auditory or vestibular neurotoxicity.
- ↻ Trough levels (measured just before the next dose is due) are more reliable than peak levels (30 minutes after an intravenous dose) in ambulatory practice because the validity of peak levels is crucially dependent on accurate timing of the dose, rate of infusion, and timing of the sample.

SUGGESTED READING
Begg EJ, Barclay ML, Kirkpatrick CJ. The therapeutic monitoring of antimicrobial agents. Br J Clin Pharmacol 1999; 47: 23-30.

James CW, Gurk-Turner C. Recommendations for monitoring serum vancomycin concentrations. Baylor Univ Med Center Proc 2001; 14: 189-190.

Moellering RC Jr. Monitoring serum vancomycin levels: climbing the mountain because it is there? Clin Infect Dis 1994; 18: 544-546.

Special Considerations in Selected Patients

Patients Requiring Bactericidal Therapy or Synergistic Combinations

Is it necessary to kill all of the infecting microorganisms to cure infection? The answer is no for most primary care settings. Antimicrobials help tilt the battle in favor of the patient, and host defense mechanisms do the rest of the work. Therefore bacteriostatic (as opposed to bactericidal) therapy usually suffices.

Bactericidal therapy is necessary in four situations: endocarditis, meningitis, infections in patients who are granulocytopenic, and infections in patients with disorders of polymorphonuclear function (granulocytopathies). The common denominator of these four conditions is poor functioning of the patient's phagocytes: white cell access to bacteria is limited in endocarditis; help from opsonizing antibodies is lacking in meningitis; white cell numbers are deficient in granulocytopenia; and white cells malfunction in the primary leukocyte disorders.

When two or more antimicrobials are given simultaneously, the effect can be synergistic, antagonistic, or indifferent. The terms "synergism" and "antagonism" have operational definitions based on in vitro studies. Synergism is the phenomenon in which greater killing (at leat four-fold) occurs when the drugs are used in combination than when either drug is used separately. With antagonism, joint use of the antimicrobials has a lesser effect than the sum of the drugs' individual effects. The combination of two bactericidal drugs with different mechanisms of action often results in synergism. A classic example is the combination of penicillin and an aminoglycoside for treatment of endocarditis; penicillin damages the cell wall of the bacterium, allowing more of the aminoglycoside to penetrate the cell's interior. The combination of a bactericidal drug with a bacteriostatic drug often results in antagonism. Synergistic combinations of antibiotics are seldom required in the treatment of bacterial infections in the primary care setting. Overuse of aminoglycosides such as gentamicin to achieve synergism is a major cause of drug toxicity.

Patients with Impaired Renal Function

The only known advantage of renal failure is the slower elimination rate of many drugs, which enables lower and less frequent doses. This dosage reduction is more convenient to the patient and lowers the cost of antimicrobial therapy. A more important reason to consider renal function is the need to minimize unwanted effects resulting from excessive blood and tissue concentrations. Elderly patients may also need lower doses, largely for the same reason. The glomerular filtration rate declines naturally with age, so that age must be considered when estimating the creatinine clearance on the basis of the serum creatinine level (Table 19-3). The standard equation for creatinine clearance based on age (known as the Cockcroft and Gault equation) is as follows:

For men:
$$\text{Creatinine clearance (mL/min)} = \frac{(140 - \text{Age})\,(\text{Weight in kg})}{72 \times \text{Serum creatinine}}$$

For women:
$$\text{Creatinine clearance (mL/min)} = \frac{0.85 \times [(140 - \text{Age})\,(\text{Weight in kg})]}{72 \times \text{Serum creatinine}]}$$

Corrections for lean body weight in obese patients are discussed in the section "Obese Patients."

Numerous articles and nomograms address the issue of how best to reduce drug doses in renal failure. One approach is to use a single nomogram for all antimicrobials that follow first-order elimination kinetics (Table 19-3 and Figure 19-5). This nomogram enables calculation of the daily dose for any antimicrobial if the practitioner knows the serum half-life in normal subjects and in anephric subjects receiving hemodialysis. Detailed information about dose reduction in renal failure is widely available in standard sources such as the *Physician's Desk Reference.*

Patients with Impaired Liver Function

Patients with advanced liver disease also need dose reduction of some antimicrobial agents. No currently available liver function test permits estimation of antibiotic elimination in liver disease to the extent that this information is available for patients with renal disease. Therefore these estimates must be made on clinical grounds. Fortunately, the margin of error (i.e., the risk of toxicity from doses exceeding the therapeutic dose) is usually large for drugs that are eliminated mainly by the liver, compared with some of the drugs (e.g., the aminoglycosides and vancomycin) that are eliminated mainly by the kidneys.

The following drugs are frequently given by the oral route in primary care and require dose reduction in *severe* liver disease (but not necessarily in moderately severe liver disease):

- Erythromycin. The dose interval should be increased from q6h or q8h to q12h or even q24h.
- Clindamycin. The dose interval (for dosages of 150 to 300 mg) should be increased from q6h to q8h or q12h.
- Metronidazole. The dose interval should be increased from q8h to q12h or q24h.
- Rifampin. The dose and dose interval should be changed from 600 mg q24h to 6 to 8 mg/kg twice weekly in patients with elevated serum bilirubin levels (>2.9 mg/dL).
- Tetracycline. The dose interval should be increased from q6h to q12h. Use of tetracycline should be avoided if possible in patients with severe liver disease.
- Chloramphenicol (which should not be used if safer alternatives are available). The dose and dose interval should be changed from 1 to 2 g q6h to 25 mg/kg q24h.

Drugs that are given parenterally and require dose reduction in *moderately severe* liver disease include cefoperazone and mezlocillin. Drugs that given parenterally and require dose reduction in *severe* liver disease include clindamycin, erythromycin, and quinupristin-dalfopristin (Synercid).

Obese Patients

Physiologic changes in obesity that may affect antimicrobial pharmacokinetics include increased cardiac output and blood volume, increased renal function, changes in serum protein levels, and changes in liver metabolism. One proposed method for adjusting drug doses is based on the actual body weight (ABW) and ideal body weight (IBW), as follows:

1. Determine IBW from the Devine formula, as follows:

For men:
IBW (in kg) = 50 + (2.3 × Height in inches over 60 inches)

For women:
IBW (in kg) = 45 + (2.3 × Height in inches over 60 inches)

2. Add a dose weight correction factor (DWCF), as follows:

DWCF = 0.3 (ABW − IBW) + IBW

TABLE 19-3
Dose Reduction of Antimicrobials in Renal Disease (Dose Lines to Be Used with Figure 19-6)*

Drug	Dose line	Drug	Dose line	Drug	Dose line
Acyclovir	B	Ceftibuten	B	Ketoconazole	F
Amikacin	A	Ceftriaxone	F	Levofloxacin	B
Amoxicillin	B	Cefuroxime	A	Linezolid	H
Amoxicillin-clavulanate	B	Cephalexin	A	Loracarbef	A
Amphotericin B	See note†	Chloramphenicol	F	Meropenem	C
Ampicillin	B	Ciprofloxacin	F	Metronidazole	E
Ampicillin-sulbactam	B	Clarithromycin	See note§	Minocycline	G
Azithromycin	H‡	Clindamycin	A	Moxifloxacin	H
Aztreonam	C	Dalfopristin-quinupristin	B	Nafcillin	E
Cefaclor	D	Dicloxacillin	F	Nitrofurantoin	F
Cefadroxil	A	Dirithromycin	See note‡	Ofloxacin	C
Cefamandole	B	Doxycycline	F	Penicillin G	A
Cefazolin	A	Erythromycin	C	Piperacillin-tazobactam	C
Cefepime	B	Ethambutol	D	Rifampin	E
Cefixime	C	Famciclovir	B	Sulfamethoxazole	C
Cefonicid	A	Fluconazole	E	Tetracycline	B
Cefoperazone	G	Foscarnet	A	Ticarcillin	B
Cefotaxime	A	Ganciclovir	D	Ticarcillin-clavulanate	B
Cefotetan	B	Gatifloxacin	D	Tobramycin	A
Cefoxitin	A	Gentamicin	A	Trimethoprim	D
Cefpodoxime	B	Imipenem	D	Valacyclovir	C
Cefprozil	D	Isoniazid	F	Vancomycin	A
Ceftazidime	A	Itraconazole	H		

*Dose line as shown in Figure 19-5. Dose lines are determined on the basis of the fraction of the normal dose (i.e., the dose for persons with normal renal function) appropriate for patients with end-stage renal failure. The dose fraction for functionally anephric persons is the quotient, serum $T_{1/2}$ in persons with normal renal function/serum $T_{1/2}$ in anephric patients. For principles behind this approach, see Bryan CS, Stone WJ. Antimicrobial therapy in renal failure: a unifying nomogram. Clin Nephrol 1997; 7: 81-84. This and other nomograms should be considered as approximations. Consulting the manufacturer's recommendations is always helpful.

†Amphotericin B does not follow the first-order elimination kinetics on which the nomogram shown in Figure 19-6 is based. Amphotericin B is nephrotoxic but, paradoxically, does not give higher plasma levels in patients with renal failure. For a detailed discussion of amphotericin B pharmacology, see Chapter 21.

‡Biliary elimination is the major route of elimination.

§Extent of renal excretion depends on the dose and formulation.

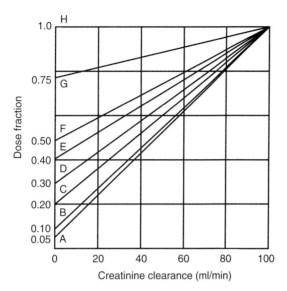

FIG. 19-5 *Nomogram for calculating the dose of an antimicrobial agent for patients with any degree of impaired renal function. The method is as follows: (1) Determine or estimate the creatinine clearance (see text). (2) Determine the dose line from Table 19-3 (if the dose line is not given or if different serum half-life values are used, the dose line can be determined from the following formula: Dose fraction for anephric patients = $T\frac{1}{2}$ (normal renal function)/$T\frac{1}{2}$ (anephric patients). Based on the patient's creatinine clearance and the appropriate dose line, determine the patient's dose fraction from the figure. (4) Calculate the patient's total daily dose, as follows: Dose = Usual dose (for a patient with normal renal function) × Patient's dose fraction. (5) Divide the total daily dose into portions (e.g., q8h, q12h) based on dose intervals considered to be both convenient and effective. (From Bryan CS, Stone WJ. Antimicrobial dosage in renal failure: a unifying nomogram. Clin Nephrol 1977; 7: 81-84.)*

This equation is based on the observation that about 30% of adipose tissue is water. Empiric evidence suggests that the DWCF should be about 40% (or 0.4 in the equation) for aminoglycosides and about 45% (or 0.45 in the equation) for quinolones.

3. Determine the dose (mg/kg) on the basis of the "corrected body weight," which is the sum of the IBW and the DWCF. Few data are available to confirm this approach for β-lactam antibiotics. However, these antibiotics usually have a wide margin of safety. When markedly obese patients require therapy with drugs that have a relatively narrow therapeutic index, such as the aminoglycosides or vancomycin, monitoring of serum levels is often desirable.

Pregnant Patients

Considerations for antimicrobial therapy in pregnancy are summarized in Chapter 5.

 KEY POINTS

SPECIAL CONSIDERATIONS IN SELECTED PATIENTS

⊃ Bacteriostatic (rather than bactericidal) therapy suffices in most ambulatory patients.

⊃ For patients with impaired renal function (including elderly persons, even when their serum creatinine values are normal), dosage of antibiotics should often be reduced depending on the toxicity of the drug and the extent to which the drug is eliminated by the kidneys.

⊃ For patients with impaired liver function, dosage of some drugs should be reduced, although the guidelines are less precise than they are for renal disease.

⊃ For markedly obese patients, it may be appropriate to calculate the weight on which dosage should be based using a dose weight correction factor.

SUGGESTED READING

Bearden DT, Rodvold KA. Dosage adjustments for antibacterials in obese patients: applying clinical pharmacokinetics. Clin Pharmacokinet 2000; 38: 415-426.

Bryan CS, Stone WJ. Antimicrobial dosage in renal failure: a unifying nomogram. Clin Nephrol 1977; 7: 81-84.

Livornese LL Jr, Slavin D, Benz RL, et al. Use of antibacterial agents in renal failure. Infect Dis Clin North Am 2000; 14: 371-390.

Rodighiero V. Effects of liver disease on pharmacokinetics: an update. Clin Pharmacokinet 1999; 37: 399-431.

Wurtz R, Itokazu G, Rodvold K. Antimicrobial dosing in obese patients. Clin Infect Dis 1997; 25: 112-118.

β-Lactam Antibiotics: An Overview

Broad spectrums of activity, relative safety, and favorable pharmacokinetics make the β-lactam antibiotics perennial favorites for many of the common syndromes in primary care. These diverse drugs have in common a β-lactam ring (Figure 19-6). The β-lactam antibiotics also share a common mechanism of action and common mechanisms of resistance.

Mechanisms of Action and Resistance

The β-lactam antibiotics are usually bactericidal against susceptible organisms. Bacteria become resistant by three mechanisms:

■ Production of β-lactamases that destroy the β-lactam ring, including extended-spectrum β-lactamases.

■ Alterations in penicillin-binding proteins (PBPs), causing antibiotics to bind less avidly to the target enzymes. Altered PBPs account for methicillin-resistant staphylococci and penicillin-resistant pneumococci. Enterococci, gonococci, and *Haemophilus influenzae* also acquire resistance by this mechanism.

■ Decreased penetrability of the cell wall, inhibiting the entry of antibiotics into gram-negative bacteria because of changes in holes in the outer bacterial membranes known as porin channels. Such "permeability mutants" explain, for example, the resistance of *P. aeruginosa* to many β-lactam drugs.

Contraindications

The main contraindication to β-lactam antibiotic therapy is a history of type I hypersensitivity reaction in recent years, as defined in the following section.

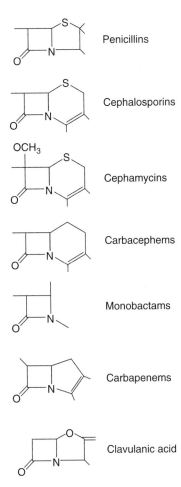

FIG. 19-6   Structural overview of seven therapeutically useful classes of β-lactam compounds. In each instance, the rectangle represents the β-lactam ring.

Toxicity and Adverse Reactions

Allergic Reactions to β-Lactam Antibiotics. It is important to ask patients whether they have ever previously received β-lactam antibiotics and, if so, whether an adverse reaction occurred, what type of adverse reaction occurred, and when. Immunologically mediated reactions include the following:

- Type I allergic reactions (IgE mediated). Anaphylaxis, angioedema, bronchospasm, and urticaria occur typically within 60 minutes of administration, but they can occur at any time. The risk of anaphylaxis after penicillin G is reported to be somewhere between 1 in 7000 cases and 1 in 25,000 cases, with death occurring in about 1 in 32,000 to 1 in 100,000 courses of therapy.
- Type II reactions (IgG mediated). Autoimmune hemolytic anemia sometimes occurs during high-dose parenteral β-lactam therapy.
- Type III reactions (immune complex mediated). Symptoms similar to serum sickness (fever, rash that is usually urticarial, lymphadenopathy, and arthritis) often begin 7 to 10 days after initiation of therapy.
- Type IV reactions (T lymphocyte mediated). Contact dermatitis may occur.

The basis for the familiar morbilliform (measleslike) rash, sometimes called dermatitis medicamentosa, is less well char-

acterized. A morbilliform rash occurs regularly when patients with infectious mononucleosis receive ampicillin. Other reactions include erythema multiforme, exfoliative dermatitis, hypersensitivity angiitis, and photosensitivity; diarrhea; hypersensitivity hepatitis (especially with antistaphylococcal penicillins); unusual pulmonary reactions; and neurotoxicity with high doses.

Whether patients with history of penicillin allergy can be given other β-lactam antibiotics, such as the cephalosporins, is discussed frequently. Between 3% and 20% of people give a history of penicillin allergy, but only about 5% to 10% of these reactions represent type I allergy manifested by IgE. The risk of an allergic reaction to cephalosporins is increased up to eight-fold in patients with history of penicillin allergy, but only a small fraction of these reactions are IgE mediated. Cross-reactivity between the penicillins and cephalosporins occurs in about 3% to 5% of cases. Again, only a small fraction of these reactions are IgE mediated. It has been shown that skin testing with reliable agents enables the clinician to predict which patients are likely to have type I reactions from penicillin G. Unfortunately, wide application of skin testing in the United States is limited because of the unavailability of a standardized commercially available preparation of the most relevant antigens (known as the minor determinant mixture). Moreover, skin test reagents to the other β-lactam antibiotics are not available. With the exception of the monobactam compounds (of which aztreonam is the only available representative), IgE-mediated cross-allergenicity should be anticipated. The following rules are derived largely from the literature:

- When a history is obtained of recent (within two decades) type I allergy to β-lactam antibiotics (anaphylaxis, angioedema, urticaria, or bronchospasm), it is usually best to avoid all of these drugs with the sole exception of the monobactams (aztreonam).
- The newer cephalosporins should not be considered exceptions to this rule even though the likelihood of fatal anaphylaxis is probably low.
- When it is determined that the risk/benefit ratio is favorable for giving β-lactam antibiotics despite a history of allergy, the following precautions should be taken:
  - Documenting that the risks and benefits have been reviewed with the patient
  - Having someone observe the patient during the first dose
  - In some situations, keeping epinephrine (conveniently available as EpiPen) available

Occasionally "desensitization" of the patient to penicillin G is appropriate because of a clinical situation such as syphilis during pregnancy or endocarditis, despite a history of type I, IgE-mediated allergy. Such desensitization should be undertaken in the hospital setting with resuscitation equipment readily available.

 KEY POINTS

β-LACTAM ANTIBIOTICS: AN OVERVIEW

⊃ β-Lactam antibiotics are usually bactericidal by inhibiting cell wall synthesis.

⊃ Alteration of the target enzymes known as PBPs has emerged as an important mechanism of resistance, including methicillin-resistant *Staphylococcus aureus* and penicillin-resistant *Streptococcus pneumoniae*.

⊃ Allergy to β-lactam antibiotics occurs by several mechanisms, of which the most important is type I, IgE-mediated allergy (anaphylaxis, urticaria, angioneurotic edema, or bronchospasm).

⊃ Use of β-lactam antibiotics for patients with a history of penicillin allergy is generally safe when the latter was not clearly manifested by a type I, IgE-mediated reaction.

⊃ With the sole exception of aztreonam, β-lactam antibiotics should not be given to patients with history of type I, IgE-mediated reactions to penicillin or to other drugs of this class.

SUGGESTED READING

Bryan CS. Antibiotic therapy in penicillin-allergic patients. In Cunha BA, ed. Infectious Diseases in Critical Care Medicine. New York: Marcel Dekker, Inc.; 1998: 803-810.

MacGowan AP, Bowker KE. Continuous infusion of β-lactam antibiotics. Clin Pharmacokinet 1998; 35: 391-402.

Salkind AR, Cuddy PG, Foxworth JW. Is this patient allergic to penicillin? An evidence-based analysis of the likelihood of penicillin allergy. JAMA 2001; 285: 2498-2505.

Penicillin G and Penicillin V

Phenoxymethyl penicillin V for oral therapy and penicillin G for parenteral therapy continue to be important drugs in primary care.

Spectrum of Activity, Clinical Indications, Pharmacokinetics, and Pharmacodynamics

Penicillin remains the drug of choice or an acceptable alternative drug for many microorganisms, including most of the streptococci, many gram-positive anaerobic bacteria, *Neisseria meningitidis*, *Listeria monocytogenes*, *Treponema pallidum*, and unusual pathogens such as *Capnocytophaga canimorsus*, *Erysipelothrix rhusiopathiae*, and *Pasteurella multocida*. It is important to match the clinical indication with the appropriate preparation and dose.

Phenoxymethyl penicillin V potassium (Pen-Vee K and many other preparations) is used for oral therapy because, unlike penicillin G, it is acid stable. Penicillin V is less active than penicillin G against many pathogens and especially against gram-negative bacteria.

Penicillin G procaine and penicillin G benzathine are repository salts used for IM injection that were developed to provide more sustained blood levels. These preparations should never be given intravenously, nor should they be used to irrigate wounds. Penicillin G procaine (Crysticillin A.S.; Wycillin) is slowly absorbed, resulting in a peak serum concentration within 1 to 4 hours that can persist within the therapeutic range for highly susceptible bacteria for up to 24 hours. Penicillin G benzathine (Bicillin; Permapen) is even more slowly absorbed, resulting in a peak serum concentration within 12 hours to 24 hours that (depending on the dose) can persist within the therapeutic range for up to 4 weeks. Crystalline penicillin G in aqueous penicillin G (Pfizerpen-AS, also called aqueous or crystalline penicillin) is now seldom used in primary care settings but continues to be useful for treatment of endocarditis, meningitis, and other serious infections that require hospitalization. The short serum half-life of aqueous penicillin G in persons with normal renal function makes it inconvenient for

ambulatory patients unless a special infusion pump is employed for continuous administration.

Unwanted Effects

The major unwanted effect is allergy, especially type I hypersensitivity reactions (see earlier discussion). Dose-related complications occur mainly in patients receiving high-dose intravenous penicillin G therapy. These complications include neurotoxicity (confusion, encephalopathy, multifocal myoclonus, and seizures), hemolytic anemia, bleeding diathesis caused by an effect on platelets, and potassium or sodium overload (depending on the salt administered). Penicillin has relatively few drug interactions. Tetracyclines can reduce the therapeutic efficacy of penicillin, and penicillins can possibly reduce the efficacy of oral contraceptives.

Administration

Oral penicillin is best given on an empty stomach because food decreases the rate and extent of absorption. Probenecid (Benemid) is sometimes given with penicillin G procaine or penicillin G benzathine to slow the renal elimination of the drug and thereby enhance blood levels. Probenecid should never be given during intravenous therapy with crystalline penicillin G because this combination can result in dangerously high blood levels that can lead to neurotoxicity. Intravenous penicillin G must be given at frequent intervals to patients with normal renal function (q3-4h). We prefer to give intravenous penicillin by continuous infusion, which is made practical by various systems now available for this purpose.

Penicillin V potassium is available as 250- and 500-mg tablets and also as a liquid suspension (125 mg/5 mL and 250 mg/5 mL). The usual adult dose is 125 to 500 mg q6-8h. The usual pediatric dose is 25 to 50 mg/kg/day in divided doses every 6 to 8 hours (to a maximum of 3 g per day).

 KEY POINTS

PENICILLIN G AND PENICILLIN V

⊃ Penicillin continues to be a drug of choice or acceptable alternative drug for many bacterial infections.

⊃ Penicillin G procaine and penicillin G benzathine should never be given intravenously and should never be used to irrigate wounds.

⊃ Probenecid can be used to increase the blood levels (and thus the therapeutic efficacy) of orally or intramuscularly administered penicillin but should never be given with intravenous penicillin because of the risk of neurotoxicity.

SUGGESTED READING

Bryan CS, Stone WJ. "Comparably massive" penicillin G therapy in renal failure. Ann Intern Med 1975; 82: 189-195.

Kelkar PS, Li J T-C. Cephalosporin allergy. N Engl J Med 2001; 345: 804-808.

Wright AJ. The penicillins. Mayo Clin Proc 1999; 74: 290-307.

Aminopenicillins (Ampicillin, Amoxicillin, and Others)

Ampicillin and amoxicillin are among the most commonly used drugs in primary care. Overuse of these drugs is thought to have contributed to the emergence of penicillin-resistant strains of *S. pneumoniae* and other pathogens.

Spectrum of Activity, Clinical Indications, Pharmacokinetics, and Pharmacodynamics

This group of compounds extends the usefulness of penicillins G and V to include various gram-negative bacteria, including many strains of *H. influenzae* and *Escherichia coli.* Many bacteria, including strains of *H. influenzae, E. coli,* and *Salmonella* species, have developed resistance based on β-lactamase production. Compared with penicillin G, these compounds are slightly less active against *Streptococcus pyogenes* (group A streptococci), *Streptococcus agalactiae* (group B streptococci), and *S. pneumoniae;* similar in activity against *N. meningitidis,* clostridia, and *Actinomyces* species; slightly more active against enterococci; and more active against *L. monocytogenes.*

Amoxicillin differs from ampicillin by a single hydroxyl group. It is significantly better absorbed, and food does not interfere with its absorption, unlike the situation with ampicillin. Thus amoxicillin's peak blood levels are about twice as high as those achieved with ampicillin. Amoxicillin is therefore superior to ampicillin for most indications other than UTI (in which the high serum levels are unnecessary if renal function is relatively normal).

Cyclacillin (Cylapen) is a slight modification of ampicillin with similar activity. Bacampicillin (Spectrobid) is an ester of ampicillin with no inherent antibacterial activity. However, like amoxicillin, it is better absorbed than ampicillin. Food actually enhances the absorption of bacampicillin, which is completely hydrolyzed to free ampicillin after absorption. The advantage of bacampicillin is that it can be given every 12 hours rather than every 6 to 8 hours. Clinical trials suggest that the in vivo efficacy of bacampicillin is similar to that of ampicillin.

Unwanted Effects

Compared with other penicillins, the aminopenicillins are more commonly associated with maculopapular rashes. Patients with infectious mononucleosis from Epstein-Barr virus and also patients with cytomegalovirus mononucleosis nearly always develop a rash during therapy. Patients with other viral infections are also more likely to have an ampicillin rash, as are patients with lymphocytic leukemia, hyperuricemic patients, and patients who are receiving allopurinol. "Ampicillin rash" is not an absolute contraindication or even a strong relative contraindication to future β-lactam therapy.

Diarrhea is relatively common after ampicillin administration (up to 12% of cases), and ampicillin has been associated fairly commonly with pseudomembranous colitis caused by *Clostridium difficile.* Diarrhea is less commonly associated with amoxicillin, bacampicillin, and other aminopenicillins.

Administration

Coadministration with food reduces the absorption of ampicillin, has no effect on amoxicillin, and may actually increase the absorption of bacampicillin. Parenteral ampicillin is widely used in hospitalized patients for treatment of enterococcal infections, meningitis, endocarditis, and other infections that are caused by susceptible bacteria.

Ampicillin is available as 125-, 250-, and 500-mg capsules, as 125- and 250-mg chewable tablets, and as a liquid suspension (100 mg/mL, 125 mg/5 mL, 250 mg/5 mL, and 500 mg/

5 mL). The usual adult dose is 250 to 500 mg q6h. The usual pediatric dose is 50 to 100 mg/kg/day in divided doses q6h (maximum 2 to 3 g per day). Amoxicillin is available as 125-, 250-, and 500-mg capsules and also as a liquid suspension (50 mg/mL, 125 mg/5 mL, and 250 mg/5 mL). The usual adult dose is 250 to 500 mg q8h or 500 to 875 mg q12h. The usual pediatric dose is 20 to 50 mg/kg/day in divided doses q8h.

 KEY POINTS

AMINOPENICILLINS (AMPICILLIN, AMOXICILLIN, AND OTHERS)

⊃ Wide use of ampicillin and amoxicillin has led to the emergence of resistance owing to β-lactamase production by many bacteria such as *H. influenzae* and *E. coli.*

⊃ Better oral absorption and higher blood levels make amoxicillin preferable to ampicillin for most systemic infections.

⊃ A generalized maculopapular rash is common during aminopenicillin therapy and probably has a nonimmunologic basis. "Ampicillin rash" is extremely common in patients with mononucleosis and also occurs in patients with viral infections, lymphocytic leukemia, or hyperuricemia and in patients who are receiving allopurinol.

Amoxicillin-Clavulanate and Other β-Lactam–β-Lactamase Inhibitor Combinations

Amoxicillin-clavulanate (Augmentin) and ampicillin-sulbactam (Unasyn) use β-lactamase inhibitors to expand the spectrum of amoxicillin and ampicillin, respectively. Amoxicillin-clavulanate, an oral preparation, is a valuable drug in primary care.

Spectrum of Activity and Clinical Indications

β-Lactamase inhibitors are compounds that have little antibacterial activity of their own but, when used with a β-lactam antibiotic, expand the spectrum of activity by negating the effect of β-lactamase enzymes produced by bacteria. The three β-lactamase inhibitors available in the United States are clavulanate, sulbactam, and tazobactam. These agents are combined in one oral preparation (amoxicillin-clavulanate [Augmentin]) and in three preparations for parenteral therapy: ampicillin-sulbactam (Unasyn), ticarcillin-clavulanate (Timentin), and piperacillin-tazobactam (Zosyn).

Amoxicillin-clavulanate is active against most strains of methicillin-sensitive *S. aureus,* most strains of *H. influenzae,* some Enterobacteriaceae (e.g., *E. coli*), and many anaerobic bacteria. This combination is useful in primary care for treatment of upper respiratory infections (including sinusitis and otitis media), lower respiratory infections, UTIs, and bite wounds. Ampicillin-sulbactam is the parenteral equivalent of amoxicillin-clavulanate and has been used for prophylaxis and treatment of intraabdominal and pelvic infections and for treatment of diabetic foot ulcers. Many physicians use ampicillin-sulbactam to treat lower respiratory tract infections, especially when aspiration pneumonia is suspected. Ticarcillin-clavulanate and piperacillin-tazobactam are generally used in the treatment of hospitalized patients in complicated clinical settings.

Unwanted Effects

The β-lactamase inhibitor compounds are remarkably free of side effects. Orally administered clavulanate sometimes causes nausea or diarrhea.

Administration

Like amoxicillin, amoxicillin-clavulanate can be given with or without food and is well absorbed. Amoxicillin-clavulanate is available as 125-, 200-, 250-, 400-, 500-, and 875-mg tablets, based on the amoxicillin component, and also as a liquid suspension (125, 200, 250, and 400 mg/5 mL). The usual adult dose is 250 to 500 mg q8h or 875 mg q12h. The usual dose for children ≤40 kg is 20 to 40 mg/kg/day in divided doses q8h or 45 mg/kg/day in divided doses q12h. Children >40 kg can received the same dosage as adults.

KEY POINTS

AMOXICILLIN-CLAVULANATE AND OTHER β-LACTAM–β-LACTAMASE INHIBITOR COMBINATIONS

⊃ β-Lactamase inhibitors (clavulanate, sulbactam, and tazobactam) have little antibiotic activity of their own but negate the effect of β-lactamases produced by bacteria.
⊃ Amoxicillin-clavulanate (Augmentin) expands the activity of ampicillin to include methicillin-sensitive strains of *S. aureus*, most *H. influenzae* strains, some *E. coli* strains, and many anaerobic bacteria.
⊃ Ampicillin-sulbactam (Unasyn), the parenteral equivalent of amoxicillin-clavulanate, is useful for treating intraabdominal and pelvic infections, diabetic foot ulcers, and respiratory infections.

SUGGESTED READING

Lee NLS, Yuen KY, Kumana CR. β-Lactam antibiotic and β-lactamase inhibitor combinations. JAMA 2001; 285: 386-388.

Antistaphylococcal Penicillins (Dicloxacillin, Cloxacillin, Oxacillin, and Nafcillin)

Methicillin is no longer used because of its tendency to cause interstitial nephritis. However, because staphylococci resistant to one of the antistaphylococcal penicillins are almost invariably resistant to the others, it is customary to speak of staphylococci as being methicillin sensitive or methicillin resistant. In the United States, dicloxacillin and cloxacillin are the preferred antistaphylococcal penicillins for oral therapy, whereas oxacillin and nafcillin are used for parenteral therapy, usually in the hospital setting.

Spectrum of Activity, Clinical Indications, Pharmacokinetics, and Pharmacodynamics

Nafcillin, dicloxacillin, cloxacillin, and oxacillin are indicated mainly for treatment of *S. aureus* infections caused by methicillin-sensitive strains. These antibiotics are usually active against streptococci and pneumococci, but they have less intrinsic activity than penicillin G against most bacteria other than *S. aureus*. Some bacteria that are susceptible to penicillin G, such as the enterococci, *L. monocytogenes*, *Neisseria* species, and anaerobic species, are nearly always resistant to the antistaphylococcal penicillins.

Variable absorption after oral administration makes the use of oral antistaphylococcal penicillins a challenging proposition. Food markedly impairs absorption of these drugs. Even on an empty stomach, absorption of dicloxacillin is usually less than 75%, and absorption of cloxacillin and oxacillin is often less than 50%. Many prescribers prefer dicloxacillin because it results in serum levels about twice those of cloxacillin, which are in turn greater than those of oxacillin. Another limitation of these drugs is that all of them are highly protein bound.

Nafcillin and oxacillin are generally reserved for therapy for life-threatening *S. aureus* infections in patients who require hospitalization. Abundant experience indicates that the antistaphylococcal penicillins are superior to cefazolin and vancomycin for therapy of serious *S. aureus* infections caused by mutually susceptible strains.

Unwanted Effects

The effects are similar to those of the other penicillins.

Administration

The oral antistaphylococcal penicillins should be taken on an empty stomach 1 hour before or 2 hours after meals. Probenecid (500 mg t.i.d. or 1 g b.i.d.) is a useful adjunct for raising blood levels. Dicloxacillin is available as 125-, 250-, and 500-mg capsules and as a liquid suspension (62.5 mg/5 mL). The usual adult dose is 125 to 250 mg q6h. The usual dose for children ≤40 kg is 12.5 to 25 mg/kg/day in divided doses q6h. Children >40 kg can receive the same dosage as adults.

KEY POINTS

ANTISTAPHYLOCOCCAL PENICILLINS (DICLOXACILLIN, CLOXACILLIN, OXACILLIN, AND NAFCILLIN)

⊃ The antistaphylococcal penicillins are the drugs of choice for infections caused by methicillin-sensitive, penicillin-resistant staphylococci.
⊃ These agents have less activity than penicillin G against many bacteria, including enterococci, *Neisseria* species, and *L. monocytogenes*.
⊃ Absorption after oral administration is variable. Dicloxacillin should be given on an empty stomach 1 hour before meals and at bedtime, with no food intake in the previous 3 hours. Probenecid is a useful adjunct for raising dicloxacillin serum levels.

Antipseudomonal Penicillins (Carbenicillin, Ticarcillin, and Others)

The antipseudomonal penicillins have a limited role in primary care. Carbenicillin indanyl sodium can be used to treat UTIs caused by *P. aeruginosa* and other pathogens, but its use has diminished markedly since introduction of the fluoroquinolones.

Spectrum of Activity, Clinical Indications, Pharmacokinetics, and Pharmacodynamics

The antipseudomonal penicillins are active against many strains of *P. aeruginosa,* other difficult-to-treat gram-negative rods, and many anaerobic bacteria, including *Bacteroides* species. However, many strains of *P. aeruginosa* have developed resistance.

Carbenicillin indanyl sodium (Geocillin) is the only member of this group available for oral use. Only about 30% to 40% of an orally administered dose is absorbed, and therapeutic serum and tissue concentrations are not achieved. However, the drug is highly concentrated in the urine (unless renal insufficiency is present) and is therefore useful for treatment of urinary infections and prostatitis. Fluoroquinolones offering similar coverage with more convenient dosage and fewer side effects have largely replaced carbenicillin indanyl sodium.

Ticarcillin, being more active than carbenicillin against *P. aeruginosa* on a weight basis, has replaced carbenicillin for parenteral therapy. Azlocillin, mezlocillin, and piperacillin, sometimes called second-generation antipseudomonal penicillins, are in general more active than ticarcillin against *P. aeruginosa* and provide a slightly expanded spectrum of coverage. All of these drugs are susceptible to β-lactamases. Ticarcillin-clavulanate (Timentin) and piperacillin-tazobactam (Zosyn) are combinations that include β-lactamase inhibitors, making them useful for treatment of hospitalized patients with complicated infections.

Unwanted Effects

Carbenicillin indanyl sodium causes diarrhea in more than 10% of recipients, and other gastrointestinal side effects, including nausea, vomiting, and flatulence, are relatively common. Complications of parenteral antipseudomonal penicillins include bleeding caused by platelet dysfunction, sodium overload, hypokalemia, neutropenia, and neurotoxicity.

Administration

Carbenicillin indanyl sodium is available as 382-mg tablets; the usual adult dose is 1 to 2 tablets q6h for UTIs or 2 tablets q6h for prostatitis. The tablets have a bitter taste and should be given with a full glass of water.

 KEY POINTS

ANTIPSEUDOMONAL PENICILLINS (CARBENICILLIN, TICARCILLIN, AND OTHERS)

⊃ Carbenicillin indanyl sodium can be used for treatment of UTI and prostatitis caused by *P. aeruginosa* in patients with relatively normal renal function, although it has largely been replaced by fluoroquinolones for this purpose.

⊃ Carbenicillin indanyl sodium does not provide adequate serum and tissue levels for treatment of systemic infection.

First-Generation Cephalosporins (Cephalexin, Cephradine, Cefadroxil, and Cefazolin)

Cephalosporins and certain closely related compounds such as the cephamycins and carbacephems are commonly grouped into four "generations" according to their spectrums of activity against gram-positive and gram-negative bacteria. Compared with the newer agents, the older, first-generation cephalosporins such as cephalothin (Keflin) and cephalexin (Keflex) have equal or superior activity against gram-positive cocci but less activity against aerobic gram-negative rods.

Spectrum of Activity, Clinical Indications, and Pharmacokinetics

The first-generation cephalosporins available for oral use are cefadroxil, cephalexin, and cephradine. They are less active than some of the newer cephalosporins against *S. pneumoniae* and *H. influenzae* and should therefore probably not be used for upper respiratory tract infections such as sinusitis and acute otitis media. Cefadroxil has a slightly longer serum half-life than the others, permitting twice-daily or even once-daily dosing for less severe infections.

The first-generation cephalosporins available for parenteral use are cefazolin and cephradine (cephalothin and cephapirin are no longer available in the United States). Cefazolin (Ancef, Kefzol, Zolicef) has a relatively long serum half-life, making it a perennial favorite for prophylactic antibiotic therapy before surgical procedures. Cefazolin is useful for definitive treatment of *S. aureus* infections but is less effective than the antistaphylococcal penicillins. Cefazolin is somewhat susceptible to staphylococcal β-lactamases and, like all of the older cephalosporins, penetrates poorly into cerebrospinal fluid (CSF).

Unwanted Effects

Diarrhea occurs in up to 10% of patients. Hypersensitivity reactions include anaphylaxis, angioedema, rashes (including not only the typical maculopapular rash of dermatitis medicamentosa but also urticaria, erythema multiforme, and Stevens-Johnson syndrome), and fever. Uncommon adverse reactions to the cephalosporins include pseudomembranous colitis, abdominal pain, abnormal liver function tests (elevated aminotransferase levels), cholestasis, vaginitis, neutropenia or agranulocytosis, and thrombocytopenia. Rare reactions attributed to the cephalosporins include toxic epidermal necrolysis, renal dysfunction including toxic nephropathy, hemolytic anemia, aplastic anemia, pancytopenia, prolonged partial thromboplastin time and sometimes hemorrhage, and seizures.

Administration

Cephalexin is best given on an empty stomach to improve absorption. The absorption of cefuroxime axetil is actually enhanced by food.

Cephalexin, cephradine, and cefadroxil are available as 250-, 500-, and 1000-mg capsules and also as liquid suspensions (125 and 250 mg/5 mL for all three agents; also, 500 mg/5 mL for cefadroxil and cephalexin). The usual adult doses are 250 to 1000 mg q6h for cephalexin; 250 to 1000 mg q6-12h for cephradine; and 500 to 1000 mg q12-24h for cefadroxil. The usual pediatric doses are 20 to 100 mg/kg/day in divided doses q6h (to a maximum 3 g per day) for cephalexin; 25 to 50 mg/kg/day in divided doses q6h for cephradine; and 30 to 50 mg/kg/day in divided doses q12-24h for cefadroxil (to a maximum of 2 g per day).

KEY POINTS

FIRST-GENERATION CEPHALOSPORINS (CEPHALEXIN, CEPHRADINE, CEFADROXIL, AND CEFAZOLIN)

⊃ The oral first-generation cephalosporins are less active than some of the newer cephalosporins against *S. pneumoniae* and *H. influenzae* and should therefore not be used for upper respiratory infection such as sinusitis and otitis media.

⊃ Although the first-generation cephalosporins are usually active against methicillin-sensitive *S. aureus* strains, they are less effective than the antistaphylococcal penicillins for definitive treatment of life-threatening *S. aureus* disease.

SUGGESTED READING

Anne S, Reisman RE. Risk of administering cephalosporin antibiotics to patients with histories of penicillin allergy. Ann Allergy Asthma Immunol 1995; 74: 167-170.

Marshall WF, Blair JE. The cephalosporins. Mayo Clin Proc 1999; 74: 187-195.

Second-Generation Cephalosporins (Cefaclor, Ceprozil, Cefuroxime, Loracarbef, Cefoxitin, and Others)

The so-called second-generation cephalosporins are a diverse group of compounds: true cephalosporins, cephamycins (cefoxitin, cefotetan, and cefmetazole), and a carbacephem (loracarbef).

Spectrum of Activity, Clinical Indications, and Pharmacokinetics

Cefaclor, cefprozil, cefuroxime, and loracarbef, the four compounds available for oral use, have generally superior activity against *H. influenzae* and *S. pneumoniae* compared with the first-generation cephalosporins. However, none is superior against *S. pneumoniae* strains with reduced susceptibility to penicillin.

Cefuroxime has significantly enhanced activity against *H. influenzae* and penicillin-susceptible *S. pneumoniae* strains. Although the bioavailability of cefuroxime axetil after an oral dose is only 37% to 52%, it is probably the second-generation cephalosporin of choice for empiric treatment of upper respiratory tract infections based on its pharmacokinetics and its in vitro activity profile. Cefaclor, although widely used in clinical practice, has only moderately increased activity against *H. influenzae* and *S. pneumoniae* compared with the first-generation cephalosporins. Moreover, cefaclor is destroyed by two of the β-lactamases produced by *H. influenzae* and *Moraxella catarrhalis*. The activity of cefprozil against *H. influenzae* is similar to that of cefaclor and less than that of cefuroxime and loracarbef.

The second-generation cephalosporins available for parenteral use are divided into two groups: the true cephalosporins (cefamandole, cefuroxime, and cefonicid) and the cephamycins (cefoxitin, cefotetan, and cefmetazole). In the hospital cefuroxime is useful for treatment of serious upper and lower respiratory tract infections. Ceftriaxone would generally be preferred, however, because of its better activity against penicillin-resistant *S. pneumoniae* strains. The cephamycins have reasonably good activity against anaerobic bacteria, including *Bacteroides fragilis,* and are therefore useful in the treatment and prevention of intraabdominal and pelvic infections.

Unwanted Effects

The unwanted effects are similar to those of the first-generation cephalosporins. Cefamandole and cefotetan have the methylthiotetrazole (MTT) moiety that has been associated with bleeding diathesis.

Administration

The absorption of cefuroxime axetil is increased when the drug is given during or shortly after a meal. The extended-release preparation of cefaclor (Ceclor CD) must be taken with food.

Cefaclor is available as 250- and 500-mg capsules and as a liquid suspension (125 and 250 mg/5 mL). The usual adult dose is 250 to 500 mg q8h; the usual pediatric dose is 20 to 40 mg/kg/day in divided doses q8-12h (to a maximum of 2 g per day). Cefprozil is available as 250-mg tablets and as a liquid suspension (125 and 250 mg/5 mL). The usual adult dose is 250 mg q12h or 500 mg q12-24h; the usual pediatric dose is 7.5 to 20 mg/kg/day. Cefuroxime is available as 125-, 250-, and 500-mg tablets and as a suspension (125 and 250 mg/5 mL). The usual adult dose is 125 to 500 mg q12h, and the usual pediatric dose is 20 to 30 mg/kg/day in divided doses q12h (to a maximum of 1 g per day). Loracarbef is available as 200- and 400-mg capsules and as a suspension (100 and 200 mg/5 mL). The usual adult dose is 200 to 400 mg q12-24h; the usual pediatric dose is 7.5 to 15 mg/kg q12h.

KEY POINTS

SECOND-GENERATION CEPHALOSPORINS (CEFACLOR, CEPROZIL, CEFUROXIME, LORACARBEF, CEFOXITIN, AND OTHERS)

⊃ The second-generation cephalosporins available for oral use (cefaclor, cefprozil, cefuroxime, and loracarbef) are in general more active than the first-generation cephalosporins against *H. influenzae* and *S. pneumoniae*.

⊃ For empiric oral therapy of respiratory infections, cefuroxime axetil is probably the drug of choice among this group of agents based on its pharmacokinetics and in vitro susceptibility activity.

⊃ None of these agents provides adequate coverage against penicillin-resistant *S. pneumoniae* strains.

⊃ The cephamycin group of compounds (cefoxitin, cefotetan, and cefmetazole) is active against most anaerobic bacteria, including *B. fragilis,* and is therefore used in the treatment and prevention of intraabdominal and pelvic infections.

Third-Generation Cephalosporins (Cefixime, Cefpodoxime, Cefdinir, Ceftibuten, Ceftriaxone, and Others) and Fourth-Generation Cephalosporins (Cefepime)

The third-generation cephalosporins are a diverse group of compounds available for oral and parenteral therapy. Compared with older cephalosporins, they offer superior activity (for some of the agents) against *S. pneumoniae, H. influenzae,* and many gram-negative bacilli. In general, these agents are more valuable for treatment of inpatients than of outpatients. Ceftriaxone (Rocephin), although available only for parenteral use, is a valuable drug in primary care because of its long serum half-life and activity against pathogens associated with life-threatening community-acquired infection. Cefepime is a fourth-generation cephalosporin that is discussed here only briefly because its main use is in the hospital setting.

Spectrum of Activity, Clinical Indications, Pharmacokinetics, and Pharmacodynamics

Third-generation cephalosporins now available for oral use include cefixime, cefpodoxime, cefdinir, and ceftibuten. These agents have excellent activity against penicillin-susceptible *S. pneumoniae, H. influenzae,* and *M. catarrhalis* with one exception (ceftibuten has only weak activity against *S. pneumoniae*). Cefixime (Suprax), which can be given as a single daily dose, is highly active against the more common gram-negative bacteria encountered in primary care; its limitation is poor activity against *S. aureus.*

The third-generation cephalosporins available for parenteral therapy can be divided into those with little or no activity against *P. aeruginosa* (cefotaxime, ceftizoxime, and ceftriaxone) and those that provide some coverage against this problem pathogen (cefoperazone and ceftazidime). In the former group, cefotaxime and ceftriaxone differ mainly in that ceftriaxone has a longer serum half-life, permitting once-a-day dosage. Cefoperazone is now seldom used because of its MTT side chain, but ceftazidime is a useful drug for serious infections caused by *P. aeruginosa.*

Cefepime, the first fourth-generation cephalosporin, is like ceftazidime in that it is highly active against gram-negative rods, including *P. aeruginosa.* Cefepime is also effective against methicillin-susceptible *S. aureus* and against *S. pneumoniae,* including strains with relative resistance to penicillin G.

Unwanted Effects

In addition to the other adverse effects of cephalosporins (as previously identified), the third-generation cephalosporins predispose patients to enterococcal superinfection.

Administration

Ceftibuten must be given at least 2 hours before or 1 hour after a meal. Cefpodoxime should be given with food. Cefixime can be given with or without food.

Cefixime is available as 200- and 400-mg tablets and as a liquid suspension (100 mg/5 mL). The usual adult dose is 200 mg q12h or 400 mg q24h. The usual pediatric dose is 8 mg/kg/day in divided doses q12h or q24h. Cefpodoxime is available as 100- and 200-mg tablets and as a liquid suspension (50 and 100 mg/5 mL). The usual adult dose is 100 to 400 mg q12h; the usual pediatric dose is 10 mg/kg/day in

divided doses q12h or q24h. Cefdinir is available as 300-mg capsules and as a liquid suspension (125 mg/5 mL). The usual adult dose is 300 mg q12h or 600 mg q24h; the usual pediatric dose is 7 mg/kg q12h or 14 mg/kg q24h. Ceftibutin is available as a 400-mg capsule and a liquid suspension (90 and 180 mg/5 mL). The usual adult dose is 400 mg daily; the usual pediatric dose is 9 mg/kg/day as a single dose.

 KEY POINTS

THIRD-GENERATION CEPHALOSPORINS (CEFIXIME, CEFPODOXIME, CEFDINIR, CEFTIBUTEN, CEFTRIAXONE, AND OTHERS) AND FOURTH-GENERATION CEPHALOSPORINS (CEFEPIME)

➲ Compared with other cephalosporins, the third-generation cephalosporins have, as a group, better activity against *S. pneumoniae* (with exceptions), *H. influenzae,* and aerobic gram-negative rods.

➲ The relative role of the oral third-generation cephalosporins in primary care is uncertain. For most common infections the spectrum of activity is unnecessarily broad and may predispose patients to complications such as *C. difficile* colitis.

➲ Ceftriaxone is a third-generation cephalosporin with an unusually long serum half-life, making it useful in primary care for initial treatment of potentially life-threatening infection.

➲ Ceftriaxone is also useful for once-daily therapy on an outpatient basis.

➲ Ceftazidime and cefepime (which is a fourth-generation cephalosporin) are active against *P. aeruginosa.* These drugs are used mainly in the hospital setting.

➲ Overuse of third-generation cephalosporins promotes enterococcal superinfection and the emergence of resistant organisms.

SUGGESTED READING

Esposito S. Parenteral cephalosporin therapy in ambulatory care: advantages and disadvantages. Drugs 2000; 59 (Suppl 3): 19-28.

Francioli P, Etienne J, Hoigne R, et al. Treatment of streptococcal endocarditis with a single daily dose of ceftriaxone sodium for 4 weeks: efficacy and outpatient treatment feasibility. JAMA 1992; 267: 264-267.

Nathwani D. Place of parenteral cephalosporins in the ambulatory setting: clinical evidence. Drugs 2000; 59 (Suppl 3): 37-46.

Tice AD. Pharmacoeconomic considerations in the ambulatory use of parenteral cephalosporins. Drugs 2000; 59 (Suppl 3): 29-35.

Monobactams and Carbapenems (Aztreonam, Imipenem, and Meropenem)

Brief mention is made here of two classes of β-lactam antibiotics useful mainly in the treatment of hospitalized patients: the monobactams (of which aztreonam is the only clinically available drug) and the carbapenems (represented by imipenem-cilastatin and by meropenem).

Aztreonam (Azactam) is a monobactam compound, which means that its β-lactam ring is not fused to an adjacent ring (Figure 19-6). Aztreonam is available only for parenteral use. It is highly active against most aerobic gram-negative bacteria but has essentially no activity against gram-positive bacteria or against anaerobic bacteria. Thus aztreonam can be used to treat infections caused by many gram-negative rods while leaving most of the body's normal bacterial flora intact. Another novel aspect of aztreonam is its lack of type I cross-allergenicity with the other β-lactam antibiotics. With the possible exception of patients with cystic fibrosis, aztreonam can be given safely even when the patient has a history of anaphylaxis, angioedema, bronchospasm, or urticaria to other β-lactam antibiotics.

Imipenem and meropenem are active against nearly all aerobic gram-positive and gram-negative bacteria and against most anaerobic pathogens, including *B. fragilis*. The major bacteria resistant to these agents are methicillin-resistant *S. aureus*, the enterococcus *Streptococcus faecium*, *Stenotrophomonas maltophilia*, *Burkholderia cepacia*, and *C. difficile*. Problems include development of resistance (especially by *P. aeruginosa*) and central nervous system (CNS) toxicity (especially with imipenem). Imipenem is inactivated by a brush border enzyme in the kidneys and is therefore combined with another compound, cilastatin, which counters this effect. Meropenem, the newer of the two agents, is not inactivated in the kidneys and has less neurotoxicity.

KEY POINTS

MONOBACTAMS AND CARBAPENEMS (AZTREONAM, IMIPENEM, AND MEROPENEM)

⊃ Aztreonam, imipenem, and meropenem are used almost exclusively for parenteral therapy in hospitalized patients.

⊃ Aztreonam, a monobactam antibiotic, is active only against aerobic gram-negative rods and can be given safely to patients with a history of type I allergy to other β-lactam antibiotics.

SUGGESTED READING

Hellinger WC, Brewer NS. Carbapenems and monobactams: imipenem, meropenem, and aztreonam. Mayo Clin Proc 1999; 74: 420-434.

Quinolones

The first quinolone, nalidixic acid, was used mainly for UTIs. Since the 1970s, structural modifications have resulted in many new compounds, some of which are extremely useful in

TABLE 19-4
Relative In Vitro Activity of Oral Quinolones Against Bacteria Commonly Encountered in Primary Care*

Microorganism	Ciprofloxacin	Ofloxacin	Levofloxacin	Sparfloxacin	Trovafloxacin	Gatifloxacin	Moxifloxacin
Streptococcus pneumoniae, PCN-sensitive†	+	+	+ +	+ + +	+ + +	+ +	+ + +
S. pneumoniae, PCN-intermediate†	+	+	+ +	+ + +	+ + +	+ +	+ + +
S. pneumoniae, PCN-resistant†	+	+	+ +	+ + +	+ + +	+ +	+ + +
S. pyogenes (group A streptococcus)	+ +	+	+ +	+ +	+ + +	+ +	+ + +
Streptococcus agalactiae (group B streptococcus)	+ +	+	+ +	+ +	+ + +	+ +	+ + +
Staphylococcus aureus, methicillin-sensitive	+ +	+ +	+ +	+ + +	+ + +	+ + +	+ + +
S. aureus, methicillin-resistant	0	0	0	0	+†	0	+‡
Haemophilus influenzae	+ + + +	+ + +	+ + + +	+ + + +	+ + + +	+ + + +	+ + +
Moraxella catarrhalis	+ + +	+ + +	+ + +	+ + + +	+ + + +	+ + + +	+ + +
Escherichia coli	+ + + +	+ + +	+ + +	+ + +	+ + +	+ + +	+ + + +

primary care (Table 19-4). The newer fluoroquinolones are bactericidal and active against a wide variety of bacteria and other pathogens such as *Mycoplasma pneumoniae* and *Chlamydia pneumoniae*. Resistance is becoming a problem. Moreover, clinical experience with temafloxacin (withdrawn from the market because of hemolytic anemia), grepafloxacin (withdrawn from the market because of cardiac arrhythmias), and trovafloxacin (usage markedly curtailed because of deaths from liver failure) illustrates the need to temper initial enthusiasm for all newly introduced drugs.

Spectrum of Activity and Clinical Indications

The spectrum of clinically useful activity continues to increase as newer quinolones are developed. This includes activity against the following:

- Aerobic gram-negative bacteria. Ciprofloxacin (Cipro), the first of the newer quinolones to be introduced in the United States, continues to be the most active of these drugs against gram-negative bacteria and especially against *P. aeruginosa*. All of the newer fluoroquinolones provide good coverage against *E. coli* and most other Enterobacteriaceae, and all are effective against *H. influenzae* and *M. catarrhalis*.

- Aerobic gram-positive bacteria. The activity of ciprofloxacin against *S. pneumoniae* is often marginal, and failures of therapy occur. Some of the newer quinolones such as sparfloxacin, gatifloxacin, and moxifloxacin are more active against *S. pneumoniae*, including penicillin-resistant strains. Most methicillin-sensitive staphylococci are also susceptible to the fluoroquinolones, but these agents are not the drugs of choice for *S. aureus* infections.

- Pathogens causing atypical pneumonia. Most of the quinolones and especially levofloxacin, sparfloxacin, gatifloxacin, and moxifloxacin are highly active against *Legionella pneumophila*, *M. pneumoniae*, and *C. pneumoniae*.

- Sexually transmitted pathogens. The newer quinolones are active against the major sexually transmitted pathogens, including *Neisseria gonorrhoeae*, *Chlamydia trachomatis*, *Ureaplasma urealyticum*, and *Mycoplasma hominis*. However, *T. pallidum* is resistant.

- Mycobacteria. Some of the newer quinolones—notably ciprofloxacin, ofloxacin, levofloxacin, and sparfloxacin—are active against *Mycobacterium tuberculosis* and also against some of the nontuberculous mycobacteria such as *Mycobacterium kansasii*, *Mycobacterium fortuitum*, and

TABLE 19-4—cont'd
Relative In Vitro Activity of Oral Quinolones Against Bacteria Commonly Encountered in Primary Care*

Microorganism	Ciprofloxacin	Ofloxacin	Levofloxacin	Sparfloxacin	Trovafloxacin	Gatifloxacin	Moxifloxacin
Proteus species	+++	++	+++	++	++	+++	+++
Klebsiella species	+++	++	+++	+++	+++	+++	+++
Pseudomonas aeruginosa	+§	0	+	+	+	0	0
Salmonella species	++++	+++	+++	+++	+++	+++	+++
Shigella species	++++	+++	++++	++++	++++	++++	++++
Legionella pneumophila	++++	+++	++++	++++	++++	++++	+++
Neisseria gonorrhoeae	++++	+++	+++		++++	++++	
Mycoplasma pneumoniae	+	+	++	+++	+++	+++	+++
Chlamydia pneumoniae	+	++	++	++	++	+++	+++

PCN, Penicillin.

*Scale is determined from published values for minimum inhibitory concentration for 90% of isolates (MIC$_{90}$), as follows: 0, MIC$_{90}$ > 4 μg/mL; +, MIC$_{90}$ 2 to 4 μg/mL; ++, MIC$_{90}$ 0.5 to 1 μg/mL; +++, MIC$_{90}$ 0.06 to 0.25 μg/mL; and ++++, MIC$_{90}$ ≤ 0.03 μg/mL. For representative MIC$_{90}$ values, see Pickerill KE, Paladino JA, Schentag JJ. Comparison of the fluoroquinolones based on pharmacokinetic and pharmacodynamic parameters. Pharmacotherapy 2000; 20: 417-428.

†Penicillin sensitive is defined as MIC to penicillin G ≤0.06 μg/mL, penicillin intermediate as MIC 0.12 to 1 μg/mL, and penicillin resistant as MIC ≥ 2 μg/mL.

‡Fluoroquinolones should not be used for treatment of methicillin-resistant *S. aureus*.

§Ciprofloxacin is the drug of choice among the quinolones for infections caused by *P. aeruginosa* (MIC$_{90}$ 2 μg/mL versus 4 μg/mL for levofloxacin, sparfloxacin, and trovafloxacin).

some strains of *Mycobacterium chelonei*. Activity against *Mycobacterium avium-intracellulare* is limited.

■ Anaerobic bacteria. Trovafloxacin, moxifloxacin, and some of the fluoroquinolones currently under development have increased activity against anaerobic bacteria.

Wide use of quinolones seems to promote the emergence of resistance, especially among strains of *P. aeruginosa* and methicillin-resistant *S. aureus*. Reports of increasing resistance among *N. gonorrhoeae* in areas of the United States and among *S. pneumoniae* strains in Canada are also grounds for concern.

The clinical indications for fluoroquinolones are similarly broad and are expanding, even though the quinolones are considered the drugs of choice for relatively few situations. These include UTIs (see Chapter 14), community-acquired pneumonia (see Chapter 11), gastroenteritis (see Chapter 16), skin and soft tissue infections (see Chapter 15), and sexually transmitted diseases (see Chapter 16). Quinolones have been used with variable success in the treatment of intraabdominal infections, osteomyelitis, mycobacterial diseases, endocarditis, meningitis, and other systemic infections.

Mechanisms of Action and Resistance

The newer fluoroquinolones are bactericidal by inhibiting two enzymes required for the assembly of DNA: DNA gyrase and topoisomerase IV. Resistance to the quinolones develops by mutations that affect the two target enzymes and also by mutations that reduce the ability of the drug to enter the cell. *S. aureus* and *P. aeruginosa* develop resistance at a frequency of 1 in 10^7 to 1 in 10^9 cells.

Pharmacokinetics and Pharmacodynamics

The quinolones are well absorbed from the upper gastrointestinal tract. The oral bioavailability is about 70% for ciprofloxacin, 90% for moxifloxacin, and >95% for gatifloxacin, levofloxacin, and ofloxacin. With several of the quinolones, the time-serum concentration curves after oral and intravenous administration are virtually identical. Peak serum concentrations after standard oral doses vary, from as low as 1.1 μg/mL with sparfloxacin to as high as 6.4 μg/mL with levofloxacin. Tissue concentrations often exceed serum concentrations in lung, prostate, bile, and stool. Tissue concentrations are lower than serum concentrations, however, in CSF, bone, saliva, and prostatic fluid (as opposed to prostate tissue). Fluoroquinolones are concentrated in phagocytic cells. Against gram-negative bacteria, fluoroquinolones have a significant postantibiotic effect. Half-lives and routes of administration vary among the quinolones, and these pharmacokinetic parameters provide one basis for comparison. The agents that are eliminated mainly by the kidneys (e.g., ofloxacin, levofloxacin, and moxifloxacin) may possibly have less toxicity than those that are converted by the liver to metabolites (e.g., ciprofloxacin, norfloxacin, and enoxacin), but this point is not well established.

Unwanted Effects
Contraindications

The quinolones are not recommended for routine use in children under age 18 years because of damage to cartilage observed in animal models. Although quinolones have now been used in children and adolescents with cystic fibrosis and other conditions without evidence of permanent damage to joints or cartilage, use in children should be justified on the basis of the risk/benefit ratio. Safety in pregnancy has not been established.

Toxicity and Adverse Reactions

Adverse effects of the quinolones include the following, in approximate order of frequency:

■ Gastrointestinal side effects. These side effects are common. Nausea, vomiting, anorexia, and abdominal discomfort occur in up to 17% of patients but are generally mild. Diarrhea occurs, but antibiotic-associated colitis is uncommon or rare.
■ CNS side effects. Mild headaches, dizziness, insomnia, or mood alterations occur in up to 11% of patients. Seizures have occurred in patients who were receiving quinolones, theophylline, and nonsteroidal antiinflammatory agents (NSAIDs).
■ Phototoxicity. This side effect occurs with all of the quinolones but is less common with some of the newer agents than with older drugs such as sparfloxacin and lomefloxacin. Extensive exposure to ultraviolet light should be avoided with all of the quinolones.
■ Nonspecific symptoms. Up to 2.2% of patients have a rash. Sparfloxacin has been associated with photosensitivity. Anaphylactoid reactions, drug fever, angioedema, urticaria, vasculitis, serum sickness, and interstitial nephritis are all uncommon.
■ QT interval prolongation and arrhythmias. Torsades de pointes and other ventricular arrhythmias have been reported with sparfloxacin and also with moxifloxacin. With the latter drug, the prolongation is only slight, and its significance is unclear.
■ Liver toxicity. This side effect has proved to be a major problem with trovafloxacin, with 14 cases of acute liver failure and six deaths during postmarketing surveillance.
■ Tendinitis and tendon rupture. Usually affecting the Achilles tendon, this problem can occur during therapy with the quinolones or even months after treatment has been completed. It is thought to reflect a toxic effect on connective tissue.

Other occasional side effects include leukopenia, eosinophilia, and mild elevations of liver enzyme levels (aminotransferases).

Drug Interactions

Quinolones reduce the elimination of theophylline and caffeine to a variable extent, apparently by inhibiting hepatic cytochrome P450 isoenzyme 1A2. Serum theophylline levels should be monitored mainly in patients receiving enoxacin or ciprofloxacin, which have the greatest effects in this regard. NSAIDs enhance the CNS stimulant effects of quinolones, which can lead to seizures.

Preparations and Dosage

Food does not substantially reduce quinolone absorption. However, the bioavailability of quinolones is markedly reduced when they are given concomitantly with antacids. This effect is most prominent when quinolones are given with aluminum- or magnesium-containing antacids, but it also occurs with calcium-containing antacids. Sucralfate (Carafate) also reduces the absorption of quinolones. There have been reports that iron sulfate preparations, including zinc-containing mineral preparations, and the buffered formulation of dideoxyinosine (ddI) reduced quinolone absorption.

Nalidixic acid (NegGram) is available as 250- and 500-mg tablets and as a liquid suspension (250 mg/mL); the usual adult dose is 1 g q.i.d., and the usual pediatric dose is 55 mg/kg/day in divided doses q6h. Ciprofloxacin (Cipro) is available as 100-, 250-, 500-, and 750-mg tablets and as a liquid suspension (250 and 500 mg/5 mL); the usual adult dose is 250 to 750 mg q12h. The other fluoroquinolones are available as follows: cinoxacin (Cinobac, 250- and 500-mg capsules, with the usual adult dose 1 g per day in two or four divided doses; enoxacin (Penetrex), as 200- and 400-mg tablets, with the usual adult dose 200 to 400 mg b.i.d.; gatifloxacin (Tequin), 200- and 400-mg tablets, with the usual adult dose 400 mg daily; levofloxacin (Levaquin), 250- and 500-mg tablets, with the usual adult dose 250 to 500 mg daily; lomefloxacin (Maxaquin), 400-mg tablets, with the usual adult dose 400 mg daily; moxifloxacin (Avelox), 400-mg tablets, with the usual adult dose 400 mg daily; norfloxacin (Noroxin), 400-mg tablets, with the usual adult dose 400 mg q12h; ofloxacin (Floxin), 200-, 300-, and 400-mg tablets, with the usual adult dose 200 to 400 mg q12h; sparfloxacin (Zagam), 200-mg tablets, with the usual adult dose 400 mg on the first day and then 200 mg/day; and trovafloxacin (Trovan), 100- and 200-mg tablets, with the usual adult dose 200 mg/day.

Ciprofloxacin, ofloxacin, trovafloxacin, moxifloxacin, levofloxacin, and gatifloxacin are also available for parenteral administration.

 KEY POINTS

QUINOLONES

⊃ The quinolones have a wide spectrum of activity but are the drugs of choice against relatively few pathogens.

⊃ Of the currently available quinolones, ciprofloxacin (Cipro) is the most potent against gram-negative rods, including *P. aeruginosa*. It should not be used for respiratory infections.

⊃ The "respiratory quinolones" such as levofloxacin, gatifloxacin, and moxifloxacin have excellent activity against respiratory pathogens, including *S. pneumoniae, H. influenzae, M. catarrhalis, L. pneumophila, M. pneumoniae,* and *C. pneumoniae.*

⊃ Frequent side effects include nausea, anorexia, headache, and dizziness. Phototoxicity has occurred with all the quinolones, and patients should be advised to avoid extensive ultraviolet light exposure. Several of the drugs prolong the QT interval. Seizures can occur when quinolones are given with theophylline or NSAIDs. Prolonged use of fluoroquinolones can cause rupture of the Achilles tendon.

⊃ Withdrawal of two quinolones from the market and marked curtailment of a third because of adverse reactions (hemolytic anemia, cardiac arrhythmias, death from liver failure) should temper the initial enthusiasm for still-newer drugs.

⊃ *S. aureus* and *P. aeruginosa* develop resistance to quinolones by one-gene mutations. The fluoroquinolones should seldom if ever be used as monotherapy for serious *S. aureus* infections.

SUGGESTED READING

Casparian JM, Luchi M, Moffat RE, et al. Quinolones and tendon ruptures. South Med J 2000; 93: 488-491.

Hooper DC. New uses for new and old quinolones and the challenge of resistance. Clin Infect Dis 2000; 30: 243-254.

O'Donnell JA, Gelone SP. Fluoroquinolones. Infect Dis Clin North Am 2000; 14: 489-513.

Pickerill KE, Paladino JA, Schentag JJ. Comparison of the fluoroquinolones based on pharmacokinetic and pharmacodynamic parameters. Pharmacotherapy 2000; 20: 417-428.

Walker RC. The fluoroquinolones. Mayo Clin Proc 1999; 74: 1030-1037.

Tetracyclines

The tetracyclines, especially doxycycline (Vibramycin and other trade names), are extremely versatile drugs for primary care with two caveats: they should not be used in children <8 years of age or during pregnancy except in rare circumstances, and many bacteria are now resistant, including some pneumococcal strains and many gonococcal strains. The available tetracyclines in the United States are tetracycline, oxytetracycline, demeclocycline, doxycycline, and minocycline.

Spectrums of Activity and Clinical Indications

The wide activity of tetracyclines includes the following:

■ Many gram-positive bacteria (although *S. pneumoniae* strains with reduced susceptibility to penicillin are also more resistant to tetracyclines)

■ Many gram-negative bacteria (although penicillin-resistant *N. gonorrhoeae* strains are usually resistant to the tetracyclines)

■ Some of the agents of atypical pneumonia, including *M. pneumoniae, C. pneumoniae,* and *Chlamydia psittaci* (the agent of psittacosis)

■ Some of the agents of sexually transmitted disease, including *C. trachomatis* (including the serovars that cause lymphogranuloma venereum), *T. pallidum, Calymmatobacterium granulomatis* (granuloma inguinale), and various agents of nongonococcal urethritis

■ *Rickettsia* species, including *Rickettsia rickettsii* (the cause of Rocky Mountain spotted fever), and *Coxiella burnetii* (the cause of Q fever)

■ A host of miscellaneous pathogens, including *Borrelia burgdorferi* (Lyme disease), *Borrelia recurrentis* (relapsing fever), *Ehrlichia* species (ehrlichiosis), *Brucella* species (brucellosis), *Vibrio* species (*V. cholerae, V. parahaemolyticus,* and *V. vulnificus*), and, to some extent, malaria parasites and *Entamoeba histolytica* (amebiasis)

Their broad spectrum of activity makes the tetracyclines drugs of choice for numerous conditions that are occasionally encountered in primary care practices (Table 19-5 and Appendix 1). Minocycline has an important role in the management of acne.

Mechanisms of Action and Resistance

Tetracyclines are bacteriostatic antibiotics that inhibit protein synthesis by binding irreversibly to the 30S ribosomal subunit. All tetracyclines have essentially the same spectrum of activity, although minocycline is generally more active than the other compounds because of its slightly greater lipid solubility. Resistance develops mainly by mutations that prevent tetracyclines

Text continued on p. 463

TABLE 19-5
Precise (Specific) Antimicrobial Therapy for Bacterial, Mycoplasmal, Chlamydial, Rickettsial, and Spirochetal Pathogens

Microorganism	Drugs of choice in primary care	Effective alternative drugs and drugs for seriously ill patients	Comments
BACTERIA: AEROBIC GRAM-POSITIVE COCCI			
Streptococcus pyogenes (group A streptococci)	Penicillin V or G; amoxicillin	First- or second-generation cephalosporin; erythromycin; azithromycin; clarithromycin; clindamycin. IV penicillin G is drug of choice for hospitalized patients.	For necrotizing fasciitis or toxic shock syndrome, IV penicillin G plus clindamycin used.
β-Hemolytic streptococci, groups B, C, and G	Penicillin V or G; amoxicillin	First- or second-generation cephalosporin; erythromycin; azithromycin; clarithromycin; clindamycin. IV penicillin G is drug of choice for hospitalized patients.	Gentamicin is often added for serious group B streptococcal infections (generally treated in the hospital).
Streptococci, viridans group	(Hospitalization usually indicated)	IV penicillin G ± gentamicin (first choice); first- or second-generation cephalosporin; vancomycin	Viridans streptococci are associated mainly with serious infections (notably endocarditis) that require hospitalization.
Streptococcus bovis	(Hospitalization usually indicated)	IV penicillin G; first- or second-generation cephalosporin; vancomycin	*S. bovis* is associated mainly with bacteremia and endocarditis (generally treated in the hospital); carcinoma of the colon should be excluded.
Staphylococcus aureus, methicillin-sensitive	Dicloxacillin (or other penicillinase-producing penicillin)	First- or second-generation cephalosporin; clindamycin; macrolide or quinolone. For hospitalized patients, first-choice therapy is IV nafcillin or oxacillin ± gentamicin.	Probenecid can be used to increase the serum level of dicloxacillin. Macrolides and quinolones, although effective in vitro, should probably not be used for serious infection. *S. aureus* infection with symptoms and signs consistent with bloodstream infection calls for hospitalization.
S. aureus, methicillin-resistant	Vancomycin (IV) or linezolid (PO)	Quinupristin-dalfopristin (Synercid). For hospitalized patients, IV vancomycin is drug of choice.	*S. aureus* strains resistant to methicillin and other β-lactam agents are becoming more common in the community. Vancomycin must be given IV, and linezolid is expensive. Cephalosporins are usually ineffective even when the organism is "sensitive" in vitro.
Staphylococcus epidermidis, methicillin-sensitive	Dicloxacillin; first- or second-generation cephalosporin	In seriously ill patients or patients with prosthetic devices, treatment usually requires vancomycin (often with gentamicin or rifampin) and frequently requires removal of the infected device.	In primary care, *S. epidermidis* is encountered most often as UTI in chronically ill patients. Relapse or recurrence is common. Susceptibility test results can be misleading (see below).
S. epidermidis, methicillin-resistant	(Hospitalization often indicated)	Vancomycin is the drug of choice and is often combined with gentamicin or rifampin. Removal of infected devices is frequently required.	Many authorities hold that all serious infections caused by *S. epidermidis* should be considered methicillin resistant, since susceptibility testing can be misleading owing to the "heteroresistance" phenomenon.
Staphylococcus saprophyticus	TMP/SMX; ampicillin or amoxicillin; fluoroquinolones	First- or second-generation cephalosporin; tetracycline	UTI caused by *S. saprophyticus* usually responds to the same antibiotics used to treat *Escherichia coli* UTI

TABLE 19-5—cont'd
Precise (Specific) Antimicrobial Therapy for Bacterial, Mycoplasmal, Chlamydial, Rickettsial, and Spirochetal Pathogens

Microorganism	Drugs of choice in primary care	Effective alternative drugs and drugs for seriously ill patients	Comments
Enterococci	Ampicillin or amoxicillin	For hospitalized patients, IV ampicillin or high-dose penicillin G; alternatives include vancomycin, linezolid, and quinupristin-dalfopristin (see "Comments")	Treatment of serious enterococcal infection (e.g., endocarditis or wound infection) should be based on susceptibility testing and usually requires combination IV therapy with penicillin G, ampicillin, or vancomycin plus an aminoglycoside. Ampicillin and amoxicillin are often effective for enterococcal UTI. Linezolid and quinupristin-dalfopristin are expensive alternatives generally reserved for vancomycin-resistant strains.
Streptococcus pneumoniae, penicillin-susceptible (MIC ≤0.1 μg/mL)	Penicillin V, amoxicillin, or penicillin G	For hospitalized patients, high-dose IV penicillin G is still effective; alternatives include first- or second-generation cephalosporin; "respiratory fluoroquinolones" (e.g., levofloxacin, gatifloxacin, gemifloxacin, or moxifloxacin), erythromycin, azithromycin, clarithromycin, and doxycycline.	Pneumococcal strains are becoming increasingly resistant to penicillin G, with important regional differences within the United States (see Chapter 11).
S. pneumoniae, intermediate resistance to penicillin G (MIC 1 to 2 μg/mL)	"Respiratory fluoroquinolone" (e.g., levofloxacin, gatifloxacin, gemifloxacin, or moxifloxacin)	Clindamycin	High-dose aqueous penicillin G (12 to 24 million units/day for adults), ceftriaxone, cefotaxime, and vancomycin are effective drugs when parenteral therapy is indicated.
S. pneumoniae, high-level resistance to penicillin G (MIC ≥2 μg/mL)	"Respiratory fluoroquinolone" ceftriaxone (see comments)	For hospitalized patients, vancomycin + ceftriaxone is appropriate initial therapy; "respiratory fluoroquinolones" can be used for pneumonia; alternatives include imipenem, meropenem, clindamycin, quinupristin-dalfopristin, and linezolid.	Vancomycin plus ceftriaxone and in some cases rifampin is used for meningitis. Hospitalization is often indicated for patients with risk factors for pneumococcal strains exhibiting high-level resistance to penicillin G.
BACTERIA: AEROBIC GRAM-POSITIVE RODS			
Bacillus anthracis	(Hospitalization usually indicated)	Penicillin G (historically the drug of choice); erythromycin; tetracycline; ciprofloxacin	Anthrax is a notifiable disease. When bioterrorism is suspected, health officials should be consulted for current susceptibility patterns.
Bacillus cereus	(Hospitalization usually indicated)	Vancomycin (drug of choice); imipenem or meropenem; clindamycin	*B. cereus* is usually resistant to penicillin; treatment should ideally be based on in vitro susceptibility testing.
Corynebacterium diphtheriae	(Hospitalization usually indicated)	Erythromycin or penicillin G	Antitoxin is the mainstay of therapy. Erythromycin and penicillin G are essentially equivalent (some authorities prefer erythromycin because it is slightly better than penicillin for eradication of the carrier state). Parenteral penicillin G is acceptable initial therapy.

Continued

TABLE 19-5—cont'd
Precise (Specific) Antimicrobial Therapy for Bacterial, Mycoplasmal, Chlamydial, Rickettsial, and Spirochetal Pathogens

Microorganism	Drugs of choice in primary care	Effective alternative drugs and drugs for seriously ill patients	Comments
Corynebacterium jeikeium	(Hospitalization usually indicated)	Vancomycin; penicillin G + gentamicin; erythromycin	An emerging cause of nosocomial sepsis, especially in oncology patients; successful treatment often requires removal of a prosthetic device.
Erysipelothrix rhusiopathiae	(Hospitalization usually indicated)	High-dose penicillin G is drug of choice; alternatives include erythromycin, cephalosporins, and fluoroquinolones.	Most strains are resistant to vancomycin. Consider endocarditis especially in older males. Susceptibility tests should be performed.
Listeria monocytogenes	(Hospitalization usually indicated)	Ampicillin ± vancomycin (regimen of choice); TMP/SMX; trimethoprim	Many authorities consider ampicillin to be slightly superior to penicillin G. Combination therapy is often used for serious infections, since both ampicillin and vancomycin may be bacteriostatic.

BACTERIA: AEROBIC GRAM-NEGATIVE COCCI

Microorganism	Drugs of choice in primary care	Effective alternative drugs and drugs for seriously ill patients	Comments
Moraxella catarrhalis (Branhamella catarrhalis)	TMP/SMX	Amoxicillin–clavulanic acid; erythromycin; tetracyclines; second- and third-generation cephalosporins; "respiratory" fluoroquinolones; azithromycin; clarithromycin	Nearly all strains now produce β-lactamase and are therefore resistant to penicillin, ampicillin, and amoxicillin.
Neisseria gonorrhoeae	Third-generation cephalosporin (ceftriaxone or cefixime); ciprofloxacin; ofloxacin; gatifloxacin	Spectinomycin; penicillin G	Penicillin is appropriate for non–β-lactamase–producing strains; spectinomycin is usually reserved for pregnant patients with β-lactam allergy.
Neisseria meningitidis	(Hospitalization usually indicated)	IV penicillin G (drug of choice); alternatives include third-generation cephalosporins (e.g., ceftriaxone or cefotaxime) and fluoroquinolone	Hospitalization is nearly always indicated (see Chapter 6).

BACTERIA: AEROBIC GRAM-NEGATIVE RODS

Microorganism	Drugs of choice in primary care	Effective alternative drugs and drugs for seriously ill patients	Comments
Acinetobacter species	(Hospitalization usually indicated)	Imipenem or meropenem (drugs of choice); aminoglycosides (gentamicin, tobramycin, amikacin); ciprofloxacin; TMP/SMX; ceftazidime; antipseudomonal penicillins	Usually encountered as an opportunistic pathogen in hospitalized patients or in patients who have received multiple antibiotics. Susceptibility testing should be performed.
Aeromonas hydrophila	TMP/SMX	Gentamicin or tobramycin; fluoroquinolone; imipenem	Susceptibility testing should be performed. Antibiotics may be useful for patients with diarrhea caused by Aeromonas species. Hospitalization is often indicated for patients with Aeromonas wound infections.
Agent of bacillary angiomatosis and peliosis hepatis (Bartonella henselae or Bartonella quintana)	Erythromycin	Doxycycline; azithromycin	Encountered mainly in HIV-infected patients (see Chapter 17). Lesions need to be distinguished from Kaposi's sarcoma.

TABLE 19-5—cont'd
Precise (Specific) Antimicrobial Therapy for Bacterial, Mycoplasmal, Chlamydial, Rickettsial, and Spirochetal Pathogens

Microorganism	Drugs of choice in primary care	Effective alternative drugs and drugs for seriously ill patients	Comments
B. henselae (cat scratch disease)	Ciprofloxacin	Azithromycin; TMP/SMX; gentamicin; rifampin	The efficacy of antibiotics in cat scratch disease has not been firmly established.
Bordetella pertussis (whooping cough)	Erythromycin	TMP/SMX	Hospitalization should be considered especially in infants <1 year of age. Many authorities recommend erythromycin estolate. Azithromycin and clarithromycin are promising.
Brucella species	Doxycycline + rifampin	TMP/SMX ± gentamicin; chloramphenicol	Brucellosis is a reportable disease. Doxycycline plus streptomycin is the most effective regimen; gentamicin can be substituted for streptomycin, but the optimum regimen has not been determined.
Burkholderia cepacia (*Pseudomonas cepacia*)	TMP/SMX	Ceftazidime; fluoroquinolone; imipenem or meropenem	In primary care, encountered especially in patients with cystic fibrosis. Susceptibility testing is advised.
Calymmatobacterium granulomatis (granuloma inguinale)	TMP/SMX	Doxycycline; ciprofloxacin; erythromycin (during pregnancy)	Treat until lesions have healed; failures with doxycycline and TMP/SMX have been reported.
Campylobacter fetus	(Hospitalization usually indicated)	Imipenem or meropenem (drugs of choice); gentamicin	In contrast to *Campylobacter jejuni*, *C. fetus* typically causes a bacteremic illness requiring hospitalization.
Campylobacter jejuni	Erythromycin; azithromycin; fluoroquinolone (e.g., ciprofloxacin)	Tetracyclines; gentamicin	Susceptibility testing is advised, since resistance is often a problem.
Capnocytophaga canimorsus (CDC group DF-2)	Penicillin G; clindamycin	Third-generation cephalosporins (e.g., ceftriaxone); imipenem or meropenem; fluoroquinolones; vancomycin	Usually encountered in dog and cat bites. Asplenic patients should be hospitalized.
Citrobacter species (*Citrobacter diversus, Citrobacter freundii*)	Fluoroquinolone (e.g., ciprofloxacin); TMP/SMX; cefepime	Tetracycline; for seriously ill patients, parenteral drugs include imipenem or meropenem, aminoglycosides, and third- and fourth-generation cephalosporins (e.g., ceftriaxone, cefepime).	In primary care, *Citrobacter* species are encountered most often in UTIs of chronically ill patients. In vitro susceptibility tests are advised.
Enterobacter species	Fluoroquinolones (e.g., ciprofloxacin); TMP/SMX	For seriously ill or septic patients, parenteral drugs include imipenem, meropenem, aminoglycosides (gentamicin, tobramycin), antipseudomonal penicillins, and cephalosporins (e.g., cefepime).	Patients with *Enterobacter* infections are often seriously ill or have had previous exposure to antibiotics, especially cephalosporins. Cefepime is now the cephalosporin of choice for parenteral therapy.
Escherichia coli	TMP/SMX; first- or second-generation cephalosporins; fluoroquinolones (e.g., ciprofloxacin); amoxicillin-clavulanate	Nitrofurantoin; trimethoprim. Parenteral drugs for septic patients include aminoglycosides, aztreonam, imipenem, meropenem, antipseudomonal penicillins (e.g., ticarcillin), and third-generation cephalosporins.	In primary care, *E. coli* is encountered most commonly in UTI (see Chapter 14) and gastroenteritis (see Chapter 12). A high percentage (30% or more) of community-acquired isolates are now resistant to ampicillin.

Continued

TABLE 19-5—cont'd
Precise (Specific) Antimicrobial Therapy for Bacterial, Mycoplasmal, Chlamydial, Rickettsial, and Spirochetal Pathogens

Microorganism	Drugs of choice in primary care	Effective alternative drugs and drugs for seriously ill patients	Comments
Francisella tularensis (tularemia)	(Hospitalization usually indicated)	Streptomycin (or gentamicin) is drug of choice; alternatives include tetracycline and ciprofloxacin.	Patients with tularemia should usually be hospitalized.
Gardnerella vaginalis (bacterial vaginosis)	Metronidazole	Clindamycin. Topical metronidazole or clindamycin is often effective.	Bacteremia from *G. vaginalis* occurs occasionally but often has a benign course, sometimes resolving without therapy.
Haemophilus influenzae	TMP/SMX (for upper respiratory infections and bronchitis treated on an outpatient basis)	Ampicillin or amoxicillin; amoxicillin-clavulanate; azithromycin; clarithromycin; fluoroquinolones; third-generation cephalosporins (e.g., ceftriaxone) especially for septic patients	Amoxicillin is still recommended by many authorities for otitis media and sinusitis despite rising resistance (see Chapter 10).
Helicobacter pylori	Tetracycline + metronidazole + bismuth subsalicylate	Amoxicillin + clarithromycin; tetracycline + clarithromycin + bismuth subsalicylate; amoxicillin + metronidazole + bismuth subsalicylate	Eradication of *H. pylori* is useful in the treatment of peptic ulcer but is of questionable value in many circumstances. Recommendations in this area change rapidly.
Klebsiella pneumoniae	A fluoroquinolone (e.g., ciprofloxacin) or TMP/SMX	For seriously ill or septic patients, parenteral drugs include third- and fourth-generation cephalosporins (e.g., ceftriaxone; cefepime), aminoglycosides (gentamicin; tobramycin); imipenem or meropenem, aztreonam, and piperacillin-tazobactam.	Most patients with *K. pneumoniae* infection are seriously ill and require hospitalization.
Legionella species	Azithromycin or a fluoroquinolone or erythromycin, ± rifampin	Doxycycline ± rifampin; TMP/SMX	Patients with legionnaire's disease are usually seriously ill; hospitalization should be considered.
Pasteurella multocida	Penicillin G	Amoxicillin-clavulanate; tetracycline; second- or third-generation cephalosporin	Usually encountered in animal bites (see Chapter 26); presence of anaerobic pathogens should be considered.
Proteus mirabilis	Ampicillin	First- or second-generation cephalosporins; fluoroquinolones; TMP/SMX. Parenteral drugs for septic patients are the same as for *E. coli.*	In primary care, *P. mirabilis* is encountered most often in UTI; struvite stone should be considered.
Proteus, indole-positive species (e.g., *Proteus vulgaris*), and closely related bacteria (*Morganella morganii, Providencia rettgeri,* and *Providencia stuartii*)	Fluoroquinolone (e.g., ciprofloxacin); TMP/SMX	For seriously ill or septic patients, options for parenteral therapy include third- and fourth-generation cephalosporins (e.g., ceftriaxone, cefepime), imipenem or meropenem, aminoglycosides, aztreonam, and antipseudomonal penicillins.	In primary care, these organisms are most often encountered as UTI in chronically ill patients, often with indwelling catheters, who have received previous courses of antibiotics. Susceptibility testing is advised, as resistance is a common problem.
Pseudomonas aeruginosa	Ciprofloxacin	For seriously ill or septic patients, ceftazidime or cefepime; aminoglycosides (gentamicin or tobramycin), aztreonam, antipseudomonal penicillins, imipenem or meropenem. Combination therapy (e.g., a β-lactam agent + an aminoglycoside) is often advisable.	In primary care, *P. aeruginosa* is encountered most often as UTI in a patient with a history of urologic intervention; dermatitis associated with whirlpools; or osteomyelitis following nail puncture wounds (see Chapter 15). Susceptibility testing is advised.

TABLE 19-5—cont'd
Precise (Specific) Antimicrobial Therapy for Bacterial, Mycoplasmal, Chlamydial, Rickettsial, and Spirochetal Pathogens

Microorganism	Drugs of choice in primary care	Effective alternative drugs and drugs for seriously ill patients	Comments
Salmonella enteritidis	Fluoroquinolone (e.g., ciprofloxacin)	TMP/SMX; ampicillin or amoxicillin; for septic patients, a third-generation cephalosporin (ceftriaxone or cefotaxime) is commonly used.	Most cases of gastroenteritis due to *Salmonella enteritidis* resolve without antimicrobial therapy. In vitro susceptibility testing is advised.
Salmonella typhi (typhoid fever)	(Hospitalization usually indicated)	Ciprofloxacin or ceftriaxone (drugs of choice); alternatives include TMP/SMX, ampicillin, and chloramphenicol.	For carriers, a fluoroquinolone or amoxicillin. Susceptibility testing should be performed.
Serratia marcescens	Fluoroquinolone (e.g., ciprofloxacin); TMP/SMX	For seriously ill or septic patients, options include third- and fourth-generation cephalosporins (e.g., ceftriaxone, cefepime), aminoglycosides, aztreonam, and antipseudomonal penicillins.	In primary care, these organisms are most often encountered as UTI in chronically ill patients, often with indwelling catheters, who have received previous courses of antibiotics. Susceptibility testing is advised.
Shigella species	TMP/SMX or a fluoroquinolone (e.g., ciprofloxacin)	Azithromycin; amoxicillin; for seriously ill patients, a third-generation cephalosporin (ceftriaxone or cefotaxime)	Authorities differ on whether TMP/SMX or a quinolone is the drug of first choice. Shigellosis is highly contagious and should be treated aggressively. Susceptibility testing is advised. Azithromycin has been successful against multiresistant strains.
Spirillum minus (rat-bite fever) (see also *Streptobacillus moniliformis*)	(Hospitalization usually indicated)	IV penicillin G (drug of choice); tetracyclines or streptomycin	Untreated, usually resolves within 2 to 3 months, but endocarditis can occur. Rat-bite fever caused by *S. minus* is rare in the United States.
Stenotrophomonas maltophilia (*Pseudomonas maltophilia; Xanthomonas maltophilia*)	TMP/SMX	Fluoroquinolone (e.g., ciprofloxacin); minocycline; for seriously ill patients, ceftazidime or ticarcillin-clavulanate	Usually encountered as an opportunistic pathogen in patients who have received broad-spectrum antimicrobial therapy. Susceptibility testing is advised.
Streptobacillus moniliformis (rat-bite fever)	(Hospitalization usually indicated)	IV penicillin G (drug of choice); tetracyclines or streptomycin	*S. moniliformis* is the usual cause of rat-bite fever in the United States. Mortality without treatment is up to 13%, and endocarditis can occur.
Vibrio cholerae	Doxycycline (for children, TMP/SMX or erythromycin; for pregnant women, erythromycin)	A fluoroquinolone (e.g., ciprofloxacin); TMP/SMX	Fluid and electrolyte replacement is the mainstay of treatment; antibiotics have a secondary role. Tetracycline-resistant strains are relatively common common in some areas. Quinolones are effective against these strains, but ciprofloxacin-resistant strains have been reported.
Vibrio vulnificus	Doxycycline (+ ceftazidime for severe infection)	Cefotaxime; fluoroquinolone	Patients with wound infection or sepsis should usually be hospitalized.
Yersinia enterocolitica	TMP/SMX; fluoroquinolone (e.g., ciprofloxacin)	Third-generation cephalosporin; aminoglycoside	Neither enterocolitis nor mesenteric lymphadenitis caused by *Y. enterocolitica* usually requires treatment.

Continued

TABLE 19-5—cont'd
Precise (Specific) Antimicrobial Therapy for Bacterial, Mycoplasmal, Chlamydial, Rickettsial, and Spirochetal Pathogens

Microorganism	Drugs of choice in primary care	Effective alternative drugs and drugs for seriously ill patients	Comments
Yersinia pestis (plague)	(Hospitalization is usually required)	Streptomycin is drug of choice. Alternatives include gentamicin, tetracycline, TMP/SMX, and chloramphenicol.	Aminoglycosides other than streptomycin (e.g., gentamicin and tobramycin) have not been rigorously tested but should be effective. Dual therapy (e.g., an aminoglycoside + tetracycline) is often recommended, but rationale is debatable.

ANAEROBIC AND MICROAEROPHILIC BACTERIA

Microorganism	Drugs of choice in primary care	Effective alternative drugs and drugs for seriously ill patients	Comments
Anaerobic streptococci (peptostreptococci)	Penicillin G	IV penicillin G is drug of choice for serious infections; clindamycin; first- or second-generation cephalosporin; vancomycin	Syndromes involving anaerobic streptococci (such as brain abscess or cervical soft tissue infection) generally require hospitalization.
Bacteroides and *Prevotella* species (oral strains)	Amoxicillin–clavulanic acid	Metronidazole; clindamycin; cefoxitin, cefotetan, and cefmetazole; doxycycline; chloramphenicol	Resistance to penicillin is increasing because of β-lactamase production. In patients with clenched-fist injuries, suspect coinfection with *Eikenella corrodens* and other bacteria (see Chapter 26).
Bacteroides fragilis	Metronidazole or clindamycin	Imipenem or meropenem; ampicillin-sulbactam, amoxicillin–clavulanic acid, ticarcillin–clavulanic acid, or piperacillin-tazobactam; cefoxitin, cefotetan, or cefmetazole; high-dose penicillin G; chloramphenicol	Metronidazole and clindamycin are probably equally effective. Metronidazole carries less risk of antibiotic-related colitis caused by *Clostridium difficile*; however, *C. difficile* colitis can occur during metronidazole therapy.
Clostridium perfringens	Penicillin G	Clindamycin; metronidazole; imipenem or meropenem; chloramphenicol	Many strains of *C. perfringens* are resistant to cephalosporins, which should therefore not be used. *C. perfringens* can cause life-threatening infections but also colonizes healthy tissues and is frequently a contaminant of cultures.
Clostridium tetani	Penicillin G	Tetracycline	Primary therapy consists of tetanus immune globulin.
Clostridium difficile	Metronidazole	Vancomycin	Most authorities recommend metronidazole, especially for hospitalized patients, to minimize the emergence of vancomycin-resistant enterococci. Vancomycin can then be used if the patient fails to respond to metronidazole. Some authorities also use vancomycin as initial therapy for seriously ill patients.
Eikenella corrodens	Ampicillin	Amoxicillin-clavulanate; ampicillin-sulbactam; ceftriaxone; erythromycin; doxycycline	Occasional strains produce β-lactamase; susceptibility testing is advised. Often associated with clenched-fist injuries (see Chapter 26).
Fusobacterium species	(Hospitalization usually required)	Penicillin G (drug of choice); metronidazole; clindamycin; cefoxitin; chloramphenicol	Typically associated with necrotizing soft tissue infections or septic thrombophlebitis of the internal jugular vein (Lemierre syndrome).

TABLE 19-5—cont'd
Precise (Specific) Antimicrobial Therapy for Bacterial, Mycoplasmal, Chlamydial, Rickettsial, and Spirochetal Pathogens

Microorganism	Drugs of choice in primary care	Effective alternative drugs and drugs for seriously ill patients	Comments
MYCOPLASMA			
Mycoplasma pneumoniae ("primary atypical pneumonia")	Doxycycline; erythromycin; clarithromycin; azithromycin	"Respiratory fluoroquinolones" (levofloxacin, moxifloxacin, gemifloxacin, gatifloxacin)	Tetracyclines (e.g., doxycycline) and erythromycin have been shown to shorten the duration of illness. Erythromycin is often poorly tolerated. Clarithromycin and azithromycin are better tolerated but more expensive. The fluoroquinolones are less active than the macrolides against *M. pneumoniae*. There is also concern that wide use of fluoroquinolones might limit their usefulness against *Streptococcus pneumoniae*.
Ureaplasma urealyticum, Mycoplasma hominis, and *Mycoplasma genitalium* ("genital mycoplasmas")	Erythromycin (see comments; some authorities use doxycycline as first-line therapy)	Doxycycline; clarithromycin	These are the most common of eight mycoplasmas that have been isolated from the genital tract. Doxycycline (100 mg b.i.d. for 7 days) is recommended by many authorities with the caveat that about 10% of strains are resistant. Patients who do not respond to doxycycline could then be treated with a macrolide.
CHLAMYDIA			
Chlamydia pneumoniae (TWAR agent of atypical pneumonia)	Doxycycline	Erythromycin; clarithromycin; azithromycin; "respiratory fluoroquinolones"	Persistence or relapse is common, and second courses of therapy are often necessary. Doxycycline, clarithromycin, and azithromycin are usually better tolerated than erythromycin. "Respiratory quinolones" may be effective (levofloxacin was 98% effective in one trial), but are not currently considered the drugs of choice.
Chlamydia psittaci (psittacosis)	Doxycycline	Erythromycin; chloramphenicol	Treatment lowers the mortality rate from about 20% to about 1%. Erythromycin may be less effective than doxycycline for severe cases. Endocarditis can occur.
Chlamydia trachomatis (trachoma)	Azithromycin	A tetracycline (e.g., doxycycline) topically plus PO; a sulfonamide topically plus PO	
Chlamydia trachomatis (neonatal inclusion conjunctivitis)	Erythromycin (oral or IV)	A sulfonamide	Erythromycin therapy is about 80% effective for neonatal inclusion conjunctivitis. Retreatment may be necessary.
Chlamydia trachomatis (pneumonia)	Erythromycin	A sulfonamide	Treatment of infant pneumonia caused by *C. trachomatis* is similar to that of neonatal inclusion encephalitis.

Continued

TABLE 19-5—cont'd
Precise (Specific) Antimicrobial Therapy for Bacterial, Mycoplasmal, Chlamydial, Rickettsial, and Spirochetal Pathogens

Microorganism	Drugs of choice in primary care	Effective alternative drugs and drugs for seriously ill patients	Comments
Chlamydia trachomatis (urethritis, cervicitis)	Azithromycin or doxycycline	Erythromycin; ofloxacin; amoxicillin	Azithromycin as a single 1-g dose has been found to be as effective as a 7-day course of doxycycline 100 mg b.i.d.; however, recurrences after erythromycin therapy have been reported. Ofloxacin (300 mg PO b.i.d. for 7 days) is now approved by the Food and Drug Administration for this indication.
Chlamydia trachomatis (lymphogranuloma venereum; LGV biovars [L_1, L_2, L_3])	Doxycycline	Erythromycin; sulfisoxazole	Doxycycline 100 mg PO b.i.d. is the standard therapy for lymphogranuloma venereum.
RICKETTSIA AND RELATED ORGANISMS			
Rickettsia rickettsii (Rocky Mountain spotted fever)	Doxycycline	Chloramphenicol; fluoroquinolone	Hospitalization is usually indicated for patients with severe manifestations. The mortality with doxycycline treatment is about 5%.
Rickettsia akari (rickettsialpox)	Doxycycline		Usually a mild illness. Clinical findings include an eschar at the site of the bite, regional lymphadenopathy, and a papulovesicular rash.
Coxiella burnetii (Q fever)	Doxycycline	Chloramphenicol; erythromycin; a fluoroquinolone. For endocarditis, doxycycline + hydroxychloroquine.	Spectrum of illness ranges from a self-limited fever to serious disease such as hepatitis or endocarditis. Consultation or hospitalization is usually advised.
Rickettsia prowazekii (epidemic or louseborne typhus)	Doxycycline	Chloramphenicol; fluoroquinolone	Mortality rates up to 40% have been reported.
Rickettsia typhi (murine typhus)	Doxycycline	Chloramphenicol; fluoroquinolone	Presentation often suggests another diagnosis.
Orientia tsutsugamushi (scrub typhus)	Doxycycline	Chloramphenicol; fluoroquinolone	Relapse may occur.
Ehrlichia chaffeensis (human monocytotropic ehrlichiosis)	Doxycycline	Chloramphenicol	Hospitalization is frequently indicated. Severe complications can occur, and mortality with treatment is up to 3%.
Agent of human granulocytic ehrlichiosis (*Ehrlichia phagocytophila* group)	Doxycycline	Rifampin has been successful in pregnancy.	Hospitalization is frequently indicated.
SPIROCHETES			
Treponema pallidum (syphilis)	Penicillin G	Doxycycline; ceftriaxone	See Chapter 16.

TABLE 19-5—cont'd
Precise (Specific) Antimicrobial Therapy for Bacterial, Mycoplasmal, Chlamydial, Rickettsial, and Spirochetal Pathogens

Microorganism	Drugs of choice in primary care	Effective alternative drugs and drugs for seriously ill patients	Comments
Treponema pertenue (yaws)	Penicillin G	A tetracycline	Yaws is rare in the United States.
Borrelia burgdorferi (Lyme disease)	Doxycycline; amoxicillin; cefuroxime axetil	Ceftriaxone or cefotaxime; IV penicillin G; azithromycin; clarithromycin	See Chapter 7.
Borrelia recurrentis (louseborne relapsing fever) and *Borrelia* species (tickborne relapsing fever)	Tetracycline	Penicillin G; erythromycin; chloramphenicol	Tetracycline as a single 0.5-g dose has been used for louseborne relapsing fever; erythromycin is effective alternative therapy for children and pregnant women. Tickborne relapsing fever is treated with longer courses of tetracycline or erythromycin because of a higher rate of relapse.
Leptospira species	Doxycycline (mild cases)	IV penicillin G (more severe cases)	Impact of treatment of the natural history of the disease is arguable, but data indicate that IV penicillin G or ampicillin is efficacious for severe cases and doxycycline for mild cases.
ACTINOMYCETES			
Actinomyces israelii (actinomycosis)	(Hospitalization usually indicated)	IV penicillin G; tetracyclines; erythromycin; clindamycin	For all but the mildest cases, high-dose IV penicillin G is given for 2 to 6 weeks followed by an oral regimen.
Nocardia species	(Hospitalization usually indicated)	TMP/SMX (drug of choice); amikacin; tetracycline; imipenem or meropenem; cycloserine	Treatment is based in part on location and extent of disease; consultation is frequently advisable.
Rhodococcus equi	(Hospitalization usually indicated)	Vancomycin (drug of choice); erythromycin + rifampin	*R. equi* is an emerging pathogen in HIV-infected patients, most commonly causing pneumonia. It develops resistance to β-lactam antibiotics, which therefore should not be used.
Tropheryma whippelii (Whipple's disease)	TMP/SMX (usually after an initial course of ceftriaxone)	IV ceftriaxone 2 g day for 2 weeks, given initially to patients with severe disease; penicillin G; a tetracycline	Recommendations for treatment continue to evolve. For most patients treatment with TMP/SMX is continued for at least 1 year.

Data from various sources, especially Bartlett JG. Pocket Book of Infectious Disease Therapy. 10th ed., Philadelphia: Lippincott Williams & Wilkins; 2000: 20-41; Moellering RC. Principles of anti-infective therapy. In: Mandell GL, Bennett JE, Dolin R, eds. Mandell, Douglas, and Bennett's Principles and Practice of Infectious Diseases. 5th ed., Philadelphia: Churchill Livingstone; 2000: 223-235; Spach DH, Lyles WC. Antimicrobial therapy for bacterial diseases. In: Root RK, Waldvogel F, Corey L, Stamm WE, eds. Clinical Infectious Diseases: A Practical Approach. New York: Oxford University Press; 1999: 337-348; and The choice of antibacterial drugs. Med Lett 2001; 43: 69-78; and Gilbert DN, Moellering RC Jr, Sande MA. The Sanford Guide to Antimicrobial Therapy. 31st ed., 2001; Antimicrobial Therapy, Inc.
HIV, Human immunodeficiency virus; *MIC,* minimum inhibitory concentration; *TMP/SMX,* trimethoprim-sulfamethoxazole; *UTI,* urinary tract infection.

from entering the target cell. Resistance to one tetracycline usually implies resistance to all other drugs included in this class.

Pharmacokinetics and Pharmacodynamics

The tetracyclines are, in general, "concentration-dependent" antibiotics in that the 24-hour AUC/MIC ratio correlates best

with activity. Absorption occurs mainly in the stomach and proximal small intestine. On the basis of their serum half-lives, tetracyclines are sometimes grouped as short acting (tetracycline HCl, oxytetracycline), intermediate acting (demeclocycline), and long acting (doxycycline and minocycline). Tissue distribution is generally good with all tetracyclines, with especially good penetration into the maxillary sinuses. The tetracyclines have varying routes of elimination. Tetracycline HCl is eliminated mainly by renal excretion. Doxycycline, which is eliminated mainly in the intestinal tract, is the drug of choice for patients with renal failure. Minocycline is metabolized extensively in the liver, but no accumulation is seen in patients with liver failure.

Unwanted Effects
Contraindications

With rare exception, tetracyclines should not be given to children <8 years of age or to women during pregnancy because of their accumulation in bone and teeth, which can lead to darkening of the teeth, hypoplasia of enamel, and depression of skeletal growth. Rare exceptions include diseases such as Rocky Mountain spotted fever, in which tetracyclines might be safer than the alternative drug (chloramphenicol). Tetracyclines other than doxycycline should not be given to patients with renal failure. Minocycline, like doxycycline, is eliminated mainly through the hepatobiliary system; however, data are insufficient to support use of minocycline in patients with renal failure.

Toxicity and adverse reactions

The tetracyclines have irritative properties, an effect that has been used therapeutically in the management of neoplastic pleural effusions. Both tetracycline and doxycycline have caused esophageal ulcers that can lead to stricture. Taking the drug with a large glass of water reduces this risk. Other gastrointestinal side effects such as nausea, vomiting, abdominal pain and discomfort, and diarrhea are common. Photosensitivity can occur with all tetracyclines, especially with demeclocycline. Allergy to tetracyclines is uncommon. Tetracyclines other than doxycycline can cause worsening of azotemia and even irreversible renal damage in patients with impaired renal function. Demeclocycline can cause nephrogenic diabetes insipidus. Minocycline causes vertigo, especially in women, which usually resolves after the drug is stopped. Hematologic side effects are uncommon.

Drug Interactions

Absorption of tetracycline is decreased by calcium-, aluminum-, and magnesium-containing antacids, milk, iron preparations, multivitamin preparations, sucralfate, and didanosine (ddI). The half-life of doxycycline is shortened significantly by phenytoin, barbiturates, and carbamazepine (Tegretol). Chronic alcoholism shortens the half-life of doxycycline but not of tetracycline. The tetracyclines may potentiate the effect of warfarin (Coumadin).

Preparations and Dosage

Doxycycline (Vibramycin and others) is preferred by many prescribers for most indications because it lacks the antianabolic activity of the other compounds. Doxycycline is available as 50- and 100-mg capsules and as a liquid suspension (25 and 50 mg/5 mL). The usual adult dose is 100 to 200 mg/day, as one or two doses. The usual dose for children <45 kg is 2 to 5 mg/kg/day in one or two doses; doses for larger children are the same as for adults. Use of tetracycline (Achromycin V, Sumycin, and others) and oxytetracycline (Terramycin, Urobiotic) should be avoided in pregnant women. Tetracycline is available as 250- and 500-mg capsules and as a suspension (125 mg/5 mL); the usual adult dose is 250 to 500 mg q6h, and the usual pediatric dose is 25 to 50 mg/kg/day in divided doses q6h.

Oxytetracycline is available as 250-mg capsules; the usual adult dose is 200 to 500 mg q6h to q12h, and the usual pediatric dose is 40 to 50 mg/kg/day in divided doses q6h (to a maximum of 2 g per day). Minocycline (Minocin) is available as 50- and 100-mg capsules and also as a liquid suspension; the usual adult dose is 200 mg initially, then 100 mg q12h, not to exceed 400 mg/day, and the usual pediatric dose is 4 mg/kg initially, then 2 mg/kg q12h. Demeclocycline (Declomycin) is available as 75-, 150-, and 300-mg capsules; the usual adult dose is 150 mg q.i.d. or 300 mg b.i.d., and the usual pediatric dose is 8 to 12 mg/kg/day in divided doses q6h or q12h.

KEY POINTS

TETRACYCLINES

⊃ Tetracyclines have broad activity against many pathogens, including gram-positive and gram-negative bacteria, rickettsiae, spirochetes, vibrios, and the agents of atypical pneumonia.

⊃ Except under exceptional circumstances (e.g., Rocky Mountain spotted fever), tetracyclines should not be given to children under 8 years of age or during pregnancy because these drugs accumulate in bones and teeth.

⊃ Tetracyclines other than doxycycline should not be given to patients with impaired renal function.

⊃ Doxycycline, the tetracycline of choice for most indications, can cause esophageal ulcerations. This risk can be minimized by taking the drug with a large glass of water and by not taking the drug at bedtime.

⊃ Tetracyclines are bacteriostatic rather than bactericidal and should not be combined with bactericidal antibiotics if possible (antagonism has been documented in the treatment of pneumococcal meningitis; whether it occurs in other situations is unknown).

SUGGESTED READING

Smilack JD. The tetracyclines. Mayo Clin Proc 1999; 74: 727-729.
Sum PE, Sum FW, Projan SJ. Recent developments in tetracycline antibiotics. Curr Pharm Des 1998; 4: 119-132.

Macrolides (Erythromycin, Clarithromycin, Telithromycin, Azithromycin, and Others)

Erythromycin is widely used in primary care because of its spectrum of activity, favorable pharmacokinetics, and safety. Clarithromycin (a macrolide, like erythromycin) and azithromycin (an azalide) have, compared with erythromycin, expanded spectrums of activity and fewer gastrointestinal side effects, but they are more expensive. Telithromycin, a ketolide compound developed to address the problem of resistance to erythromycin, is scheduled for marketing at the time of this writing.

Spectrums of Activity and Clinical Indications

The spectrum of activity of the macrolides, azalides, and ketolides includes many gram-positive bacteria, selected gram-negative bacteria, and various "atypical" pathogens:

■ A majority of group A streptococci and pneumococci are susceptible to the macrolides. However, heavy use of erythromycin promotes the emergence of resistance, and up to 65% of *S. pneumoniae* strains with high-level resistance to penicillin (MIC ≥2 μg/mL are resistant to the macrolides. Telithromycin is active against nearly all strains of erythromycin-resistant pneumococci tested to date. Compared with the activity of erythromycin against streptococci, clarithromycin is about two to four times more active; azithromycin is about two to four times less active.

- Methicillin-sensitive *S. aureus* strains are often susceptible, but resistance can emerge during therapy.
- Most strains of *H. influenzae* and *M. catarrhalis* are susceptible. Azithromycin is the most active of the three agents.
- Against the causes of atypical pneumonia, erythromycin is about 50 times more potent than tetracycline against *M. pneumoniae*. Azithromycin and clarithromycin are slightly more active than erythromycin against some *L. pneumophila* strains.
- All four of these drugs are active against *C. trachomatis;* azithromycin is especially active.
- Clarithromycin, azithromycin, and telithromycin (but not erythromycin) have substantial activity against the *M. avium-intracellulare* complex.

Erythromycin is active against many anaerobic bacteria, making it useful for bowel preparation before surgery. Aerobic gram-negative rods such as *E. coli* are usually resistant to erythromycin but can sometimes be rendered susceptible by an alkaline pH.

Mechanisms of Action and Resistance

The macrolides are usually bacteriostatic by inhibiting protein synthesis. They are sometimes bactericidal against *S. pyogenes*, *S. pneumoniae*, and *H. influenzae*. However, resistance to the macrolides by these same bacteria is now being reported. Microorganisms can become resistant to the macrolides in at least four ways, including decreased permeability into the cell, active extrusion of the drug, enzymatic alterations of the drug, and decreased affinity of the ribosome.

Pharmacokinetics and Pharmacodynamics

All four of these compounds are well absorbed from the gastrointestinal tract. Food decreases the absorption of erythromycin, except for the estolate preparation. Clarithromycin and telithromycin are the best absorbed of these agents (50% and 57% bioavailability, respectively). Peak serum concentrations are lower with azithromycin than with the other three drugs, but azithromycin has the unusual property of being extremely concentrated within phagocytic cells. As a result, the tissue half-life (as opposed to the serum half-life) of azithromycin is 2 to 4 days. This feature allows one-dose treatment of some sexually transmitted diseases, 3- to 5-day regimens for upper respiratory infections, and weekly prophylaxis against *M. avium-intracellulare* infection in patients with HIV disease. Telithromycin is also concentrated within phagocytic cells and, compared with the macrolides, provides a higher AUC/MIC ratio against many common pathogens.

Unwanted Effects
Contraindications

Relative contraindications to erythromycin include severe liver disease, known hypersensitivity, and concomitant use of certain antihistamines, pimozide, midazolam, or cisapride (see the section on drug interactions).

Toxicity and Adverse Reactions

Erythromycin causes dose-related abdominal cramping, nausea and vomiting, and diarrhea. These side effects are attributed in part to increased gastrointestinal motility (a motilin-simulating effect) and occur more often in children and young adults than in older patients. The gastrointestinal side effects of clarithromycin, azithromycin, and telithromycin are typically milder. Cholestatic hepatitis has been associated with erythromycin estolate. Intravenous erythromycin has been associated with transient hearing loss and, rarely, with polymorphic ventricular tachycardia (torsades de pointes). True allergy to these compounds is rare.

Drug Interactions

Erythromycin has a number of potentially clinically significant drug interactions as a result of its interference with their hepatic metabolism through the cytochrome P450 enzyme system, including the following:

- Elevations of levels of certain antihistamines (e.g., terfenadine and astemizole, both of which have been taken off the market), causing serious ventricular arrhythmias
- Elevated levels of triazolam and midazolam, causing unconsciousness
- Elevated levels of theophylline, causing theophylline toxicity
- Elevated levels of felodipine (and certain other calcium antagonists), leading to cardiac toxicity
- Elevated levels of cisapride, carbamazepine, cyclosporine, and other drugs, including some of the protease inhibitors used in the management of AIDS
- Potentiation of the effect of warfarin

Clarithromycin similarly increases the serum levels of certain drugs that are metabolized in the liver by the CYP3A enzyme system. These include carbamazepine, cisapride, cyclosporine, pimozide, rifampin, rifabutin, ritonavir, terfenadine, and zidovudine. Azithromycin does not appear to inactivate these key enzyme systems.

Preparations and Dosage

The vulnerability of erythromycin base to gastric acid led to the development of various preparations designed to improve absorption, such as enteric-coated granules, tablets, and preparations (notably the estolate), the absorption of which is unaffected by food. Erythromycin (which is irritating to veins) and azithromycin are both available for intravenous administration.

Availability and usual doses are as follows:

- Azithromycin (Zithromax), 250- and 600-mg tablets and liquid suspension (100 mg and 200 mg/5 mL and 1 g packet). The usual adult dose is 500 mg on day 1, then 250 mg daily on days 2 through 5, with higher doses used for *M. avium-intracellulare* treatment and prophylaxis. The usual dose for children 6 months to 2 years of age is 10 mg/kg/day on day 1 followed by 5 mg/kg/day on days 2 through 5 (to a maximum 250 mg/day). For children ≥2 years, the usual dose is 12 mg/kg/day for 5 days (to a maximum of 500 mg/day).
- Clarithromycin (Biaxin), 250- and 500-mg tablets and liquid suspension (125 mg and 250 mg/5 mL). The usual adult dose is 250 to 500 mg q12h.
- Dirithromycin (Dynabac), 250-mg tablets. The usual adult dose is 500 mg/day for 5 to 14 days.
- Erythromycin base (ERYC, E-Mycin, and others): 250-, 333-, and 500-mg tablets and capsules as a suspension (200 mg and 400 mg per 5 mL). The usual adult dose is 250 to 500 mg q6-12h. The usual pediatric dose is 30 to 50 mg/kg/day in divided doses q6-8h.

- Erythromycin stearate (Erythrocin, others): 250- and 500-mg tablets. The usual adult dose is 250 mg q6h or 500 mg q12h. The usual pediatric dose is 30 to 50 mg/kg/day in divided doses.
- Erythromycin ethylsuccinate (E.E.S., Ery Ped), 200- and 400-mg tablets and also as a suspension (200 and 400 mg/5 mL). The usual adult dose is 400 to 800 mg q6-12h. The usual pediatric dose is 30 to 50 mg/kg/day in divided doses.
- Erythromycin estolate (Ilosone), 250- and 500-mg capsules and also as a liquid suspension (125 and 250 mg/5 mL). The usual adult dose is 250 to 500 mg q6-12h. The usual pediatric dose is 30 to 50 mg/kg/day in divided doses.
- Telithromycin (Ketek) is, at the time of this writing, in the process of being marketed. The usual adult dose in clinical trials was 800 mg daily.

 KEY POINTS

MACROLIDES, AZALIDES, AND KETOLIDES (ERYTHROMYCIN, CLARITHROMYCIN, AZITHROMYCIN, TELITHROMYCIN, AND OTHERS)

- ⟳ The macrolides, azalides, and ketolides are broadly active against many streptococci, respiratory pathogens, *C. trachomatis,* and other pathogens encountered in primary care.
- ⟳ Because the macrolides and azalides have little activity against penicillin-resistant *S. pneumoniae* strains, which are becoming more prevalent in the United States, they should no longer be considered first-line therapy for suspected pneumococcal pneumonia.
- ⟳ Telithromycin, a new ketolide compound, is active against most pneumococcal strains that are resistant to the macrolides and azalides.
- ⟳ Macrolides are effective therapy against the usual causes of "atypical" pneumonia: *M. pneumoniae, C. pneumoniae,* and *L. pneumophila.*
- ⟳ Erythromycin increases the levels of many drugs that undergo metabolism in the liver by the cytochrome P450 system, with results that are sometimes fatal. Clarithromycin increases the levels of a smaller list of drugs.
- ⟳ Azithromycin and clarithromycin cause less gastrointestinal distress than erythromycin.

SUGGESTED READING

Alvarez-Elcoro S, Enzler MJ. The macrolides: erythromycin, clarithromycin, and azithromycin. Mayo Clin Proc 1999; 74: 613-634.

Balfour JA, Figgitt DP. Telithromycin. Drugs 2001; 61: 815-829.

Garey KW, Amsden GW. Intravenous azithromycin. Ann Pharmacother 1999; 33: 218-228.

Kelley MA, Weber DJ, Gilligan P, et al. Breakthrough pneumococcal bacteremia in patients being treated with azithromycin and clarithromycin. Clin Infect Dis 2000; 31: 1008-1111.

Pai MP, Graci DM, Amsden GW. Macrolide drug interactions: an update. Ann Pharmacother 2000; 34: 495-513.

Principi N, Esposito S. Comparative tolerability of erythromycin and newer macrolide antibacterials in paediatric patients. Drug Saf 1999; 20: 25-41.

Stratton CW. Get a handle on resistance before it gets a handle on you: the PROTEKT US Surveillance Study. Prospective Resistant Organism Tracking and Epidemiology for Ketolide Telithromycin. South Med J 2001; 94: 891-892.

Zuckerman JM. The newer macrolides: azithromycin and clarithromycin. Infect Dis Clin North Am 2000; 14: 449-462.

Clindamycin

Clindamycin is a potent antibiotic against gram-positive bacteria, anaerobic bacteria including *B. fragilis,* and certain other pathogens, but it is not used widely in primary care because of the small but definite risk of pseudomembranous colitis caused by *C. difficile* (see Chapter 12).

Spectrum of Activity and Clinical Indications

Clindamycin is active against most pneumococci and streptococci and is usually active against *S. aureus.* However, resistant isolates of *S. pneumoniae* and *S. pyogenes* have been reported, and up to one third of methicillin-resistant *S. aureus* strains are clindamycin resistant. The major role of clindamycin has been in the therapy of life-threatening infections outside the CNS that are likely to involve *B. fragilis,* such as serious intraabdominal and pelvic infections and lung abscess from aspiration of oral flora. Short courses of clindamycin are commonly used for odontogenic infections such as dental abscess. Evidence that clindamycin inhibits production of certain potent toxins produced by *S. aureus* and *S. pyogenes* has led to use of clindamycin for both staphylococcal and streptococcal toxic shock syndromes.

Mechanisms of Action and Resistance

Clindamycin is primarily bacteriostatic by inhibiting protein synthesis through binding to the 50S ribosomal subunit. However, clindamycin is often bactericidal against gram-positive bacteria and anaerobic pathogens. Resistance develops by several mechanisms, including alteration of the target ribosome.

Pharmacokinetics and Pharmacodynamics

Orally administered clindamycin is about 90% bioavailable. Distribution into tissues other than the CSF is reasonably good. Clindamycin penetrates well into bone, making it useful in the treatment of osteomyelitis. It also penetrates well into inflammatory cells and, at least experimentally, into abscesses.

Unwanted Effects

Oral clindamycin causes diarrhea in up to 20% of patients, in some of whom pseudomembranous colitis caused by *C. difficile* toxin develops. The reported incidence of *C. difficile* colitis ranges widely (0.01% to 10% of treated patients). Clindamycin causes rash, fever, and reversible abnormalities of liver function tests (mainly aminotransferase levels).

Preparations and Dosage

Clindamycin is available as 75-, 150-, and 300-mg capsules. The usual adult dose is 150 to 300 mg q6h. The usual pediatric dose is 8 to 16 mg/kg/day in divided doses. Capsules should be taken with a full glass of water to avoid esophageal irritation.

 KEY POINTS

CLINDAMYCIN

- ⟳ Use of clindamycin in primary care is limited by the occasional but potentially fatal occurrence of *C. difficile* colitis.
- ⟳ Short courses of clindamycin are sometimes used for odontogenic infections such as dental abscess, and clindamycin is an effective alternative drug for infections caused by gram-positive bacteria.

➲ In the hospital setting, clindamycin is used in combination with other agents to treat life-threatening infections, including intraabdominal sepsis and the toxic shock syndromes.

SUGGESTED READING

Kasten MJ. Clindamycin, metronidazole, and chloramphenicol. Mayo Clin Proc 1999; 74: 825-833.

Metronidazole

Although metronidazole (Flagyl) was introduced as an antiparasitic drug, it is now considered the most potent drug against anaerobic bacteria, including *B. fragilis*. Since it is relatively safe, it can be used to advantage by the primary care clinician.

Spectrum of Activity and Clinical Indications

Metronidazole is bactericidal against nearly all anaerobic and microaerophilic bacteria. Exceptions are *Propionibacterium* and *Actinomyces* species, *Actinobacillus actinomycetemcomitans,* and *Eikenella corrodens.* Activity against aerobic bacteria is limited. Metronidazole is often combined with a second antibiotic (e.g., a β-lactam) to excellent advantage in the treatment of mixed aerobic-anaerobic bacterial infections, including diabetic foot ulcers (see Chapter 15). It is a first-line drug for *C. difficile* colitis (see Chapter 12), *Trichomonas vaginalis,* giardiasis, and amebiasis. Topical metronidazole is also useful for treatment of acne rosacea.

Mechanisms of Action and Resistance

Metronidazole generates toxic compounds within the cell that damage DNA and possibly other large molecules. Acquired resistance to metronidazole is rare, apparently requiring several mutations. There is some evidence that anaerobic bacteria are becoming less susceptible.

Pharmacokinetics and Pharmacodynamics

Metronidazole is almost completely absorbed from the gastrointestinal tract, has a large volume of distribution, and penetrates well into most tissues and body fluids, including CSF. The drug is metabolized by the liver to at least five major products, and the dose should probably be reduced by about 50% in patients with severe liver disease.

Unwanted Effects

Metronidazole can cause a disulfiram (Antabuse) reaction in patients who use alcohol while taking the drug (this effect is generally accepted in the literature, although its existence has recently been questioned). It occasionally causes peripheral neuropathy during prolonged therapy. Rare but serious adverse effects include seizures, encephalopathy, cerebellar dysfunction, pseudomembranous colitis, and pancreatitis. More common adverse reactions include nausea and epigastric distress, headache, confusion, depression, vertigo, rash, and a variety of oral effects: metallic taste, furring of the tongue, glossitis, stomatitis, and dry mouth. Metronidazole potentiates the action of warfarin (Coumadin).

Preparations and Dosage

Metronidazole is available as 250- and 500-mg tablets, as a 375-mg capsule, and as a 750-mg extended release tablet.

The usual adult doses are 250 to 750 mg q8h (for doses in bacterial vaginosis, see Chapter 16). The usual pediatric dose is 15 to 50 mg/kg/day in divided doses.

 KEY POINTS

METRONIDAZOLE

➲ Metronidazole is the most potent drug available against anaerobic bacteria, including *B. fragilis.*
➲ Orally administered metronidazole has nearly 100% bioavailability and diffuses well into most tissues and body fluids, including CSF.
➲ Metronidazole can be combined with other agents (e.g., β-lactam antibiotics) to great advantage in the treatment of mixed aerobic and anaerobic infections.
➲ Adverse effects include a disulfiram (Antabuse)-like reaction in patients who use alcohol while taking the drug, potentiation of warfarin, and—rarely—peripheral neuropathy, encephalopathy, pseudomembranous colitis (even though metronidazole is a drug of choice for treatment of this condition), and pancreatitis.

SUGGESTED READING

Kasten MJ. Clindamycin, metronidazole, and chloramphenicol. Mayo Clin Proc 1999; 74: 825-833.
Lamp KC, Freedman CD, Klutman NE, et al. Pharmacokinetics and pharmacodynamics of the nitroimidazole antimicrobials. Clin Pharmacokinet 1999; 36: 353-373.
Samuelson J. Why metronidazole is active against both bacteria and parasites. Antimicrob Agents Chemother 1999; 43: 1533-1541.
Williams CS, Woodcock KR. Do ethanol and metronidazole interact to produce a disulfiram-like reaction? Ann Pharmacother 2000; 34: 255-257.

Chloramphenicol

Were it not for the occurrence of irreversible and usually fatal aplastic anemia in 1 in 24,000 to 1 in 41,000 treated patients, chloramphenicol would continue to be a popular antibiotic for primary care because of its broad spectrum of activity and excellent pharmacokinetic profile. It is well absorbed from the gastrointestinal tract; gives excellent tissue and fluid levels, including CSF penetration; and inhibits growth of the majority of pathogenic aerobic and anaerobic bacteria and rickettsiae. Some authorities still prefer chloramphenicol for treatment of life-threatening Rocky Mountain spotted fever. In general, however, patients taking chloramphenicol should be considered for hospitalization or referral.

SUGGESTED READING

Kasten MJ. Clindamycin, metronidazole, and chloramphenicol. Mayo Clin Proc 1999; 74: 825-833.

Rifampin

Rifampin, which revolutionized the treatment of tuberculosis (see Chapter 22), is sometimes useful in the management of bacterial infections. Its nearly 100% oral bioavailability, its wide distribution into tissues and fluids, including bone and phagocytic cells, and its potent bactericidal activity against most of the gram-positive cocci would suggest that rifampin might indeed be extremely valuable in primary care. Unfortunately, bacteria rapidly develop resistance to rifampin when the drug is used as a sole agent. Infectious disease specialists often use rifampin as a second or third drug for management of serious staphylococcal infections such as endocarditis and osteomyelitis, but consultation is probably advisable before such use. Rifampin can sometimes antagonize the action of other antibiotics. It has also been combined with other antibiotics for eradication of the nasal carriage of *S. aureus* and pharyngeal carriage of *S. pyogenes*. Rifampin is usually well tolerated, but it has many important drug interactions and sometimes causes major side effects, including hepatitis and renal failure (see Chapter 22).

Aminoglycosides (Gentamicin, Tobramycin, Amikacin, and Others)

The aminoglycosides are potent, bactericidal antibiotics active against most aerobic gram-negative rods and also, to a lesser extent, against staphylococci and some mycobacteria. For many years they have been the durable drugs of choice for certain difficult-to-treat pathogens such as *Klebsiella*, *Enterobacter*, and *Serratia* species and *P. aeruginosa* in the hospital setting. They are poorly absorbed and therefore, with rare exception (notably for bowel cleansing or for treatment of hepatic encephalopathy with neomycin), must be given parenterally. Administration requires careful attention to dose amount and frequency, taking into account the severity of the infection and the patient's renal function, because of the relatively narrow therapeutic index (i.e., the ratio of the therapeutic dose to the toxic dose). Ototoxicity is the major complication and can be vestibular or cochlear. Older patients, who often have subclinical high-frequency hearing deficits, are especially vulnerable to clinically apparent ototoxicity. Complete deafness has resulted from even the use of aminoglycosides as irrigating solutions or from administration of neomycin orally to patients with impaired renal function. Nephrotoxicity also occurs, especially in critically ill patients. Age, shock, and liver disease are risk factors. Other toxicities of the aminoglycosides include neuromuscular paralysis (especially in patients given certain anesthetics or in patients with myasthenia gravis), allergic reactions, and acute brain syndromes. The latter include confusion, delirium, and psychosis—findings easily misattributed to other causes in the seriously ill.

The major aminoglycosides in clinical use in the United States are gentamicin, tobramycin, and amikacin. Others are neomycin and paromomycin (for oral use), sisomicin, netilmicin, and streptomycin. Indications for aminoglycosides include empiric treatment of suspected severe sepsis (see Chapter 6); specific therapy for certain problem pathogens, including not only hospital-acquired gram-negative rods but also *Yersinia pestis* (plague) and *Francisella tularensis* (tularemia); combination therapy with other antibiotics in the treatment of enterococcal infections, endocarditis, mycobacterial disease (including notably the use of amikacin for *M. avium-intracellulare* complex disease); and preventive (prophylactic) therapy in patients undergoing genitourinary or gastrointestinal surgical procedures who are at high risk of enterococcal bacteremia. Because of the risk of complications, aminoglycosides are seldom used in most primary care settings. However, the growing trend to treat sicker patients as outpatients, the increasing popularity of once-daily administration of aminoglycosides, and the possibility that gram-negative rods will become increasingly resistant to the β-lactams and fluoroquinolones make it possible that aminoglycosides will someday surface as important drugs in primary care. Clinicians using these potent but toxic agents in the ambulatory care setting should become thoroughly familiar with their pharmacology and adverse effects.

SUGGESTED READING

Edson RS, Terrell CL. The aminoglycosides. Mayo Clin Proc 1999; 74: 519-528.

Fisman DN, Kaye KM. Once-daily dosing of aminoglycoside antibiotics. Infect Dis Clin North Am 2000; 14: 475-487.

Gonzalez LS 3rd, Spencer JP. Aminoglycosides: a practical review. Am Fam Physician 1998; 58: 1811-1820.

Santucci RA, Krieger JN. Gentamicin for the practicing urologist: review of efficacy, single daily dosing and "switch" therapy. J Urol 2000; 163: 1076-1084.

Swan SK. Aminoglycoside nephrotoxicity. Semin Nephrol 1997; 17: 27-33.

Vancomycin

The emergence of methicillin-resistant staphylococci moved vancomycin to the forefront of antimicrobial therapy in the hospital setting. Now, vancomycin-resistant enterococci and staphylococci with reduced susceptibility to vancomycin threaten to undermine its value. Although vancomycin is rarely used in the primary care setting, some familiarity is desirable because many patients are discharged from the hospital to receive home therapy with vancomycin (see Chapter 27) and because further spread of methicillin-resistant *S. aureus* strains in the community may enhance the need to use vancomycin as part of an initial regimen for severe sepsis of unknown origin.

Vancomycin is a glycopeptide antibiotic active against nearly all gram-positive bacteria but with little or no activity against gram-negative bacteria or against anaerobic bacteria. It is less active than the antistaphylococcal penicillins (e.g., nafcillin and oxacillin) against mutually susceptible strains. The major unwanted effect of vancomycin is ototoxicity. Like the aminoglycosides, vancomycin can cause permanent hearing loss through destruction of hair cells in the organ of Corti. Whether vancomycin is intrinsically nephrotoxic remains unsettled, but vancomycin seems to enhance the nephrotoxicity of other drugs such as the aminoglycosides. An unusual side effect is the "red man syndrome," characterized by flushing of the upper body, hypotension, itching, and occasionally chest pain and muscle spasm. Slowing the rate of vancomycin infusion (it should always be given over 60 minutes) reduces the risk of red man syndrome. Vancomycin is eliminated almost entirely by glomerular filtration, and the maintenance dose should be based on the calculated or estimated creatinine clearance. Serum levels should be monitored, at least in certain patients (see Chapter 27).

Justifications for vancomycin include serious infection from β-lactam–resistant gram-positive bacteria such as methicillin-resistant *S. aureus;* gram-positive bacterial infections in patients with a history of type I allergy to β-lactam agents; prophylaxis of endocarditis in certain situations, especially when prosthetic heart valves are in place; and empiric therapy for sepsis in patients with indwelling vascular catheters or in patients with suspected life-threatening infections likely to involve methicillin-resistant staphylococci or penicillin-resistant pneumococci. Oral vancomycin is effective therapy for colitis caused by the *C. difficile* toxin. Some authorities maintain that vancomycin is preferable to metronidazole for unusually severe cases of pseudomembranous colitis.

SUGGESTED READING

Wilhelm MP, Estes L. Vancomycin. Mayo Clin Proc 1999; 74: 928-935.

Streptogramins (Quinupristin-Dalfopristin)

Quinupristin-dalfopristin (Synercid) is a combination of two semisynthetic derivatives of pristinamycin, a streptogramin compound. The streptogramins inhibit protein synthesis by binding to the 50S ribosome unit. Quinupristin and dalfopristin are bacteriostatic when given separately, but the combination is often bactericidal. This preparation has some activity against anaerobic bacteria and a few grain-negative bacteria, but its main activity is against gram-positive cocci.

Administration of the drug is complicated by dose-dependent toxicity to veins. Arthralgias and myalgias are common side effects, and elevations of the serum bilirubin level, anemia, or thrombocytopenia develops in some patients.

Quinupristin-dalfopristin received early approval from the Food and Drug Administration for treatment of infections caused by the vancomycin-resistant enterococcus *S. faecium.* Although about 70% successful against *S. faecium,* it has little activity against *Streptococcus faecalis,* which is more common. *S. faecium* can develop resistance during therapy. Arthralgias and myalgias are relatively common side effects, occurring in up to 25% of patients. For the present, quinupristin-dalfopristin has an exceedingly limited role in primary care. Like linezolid, however, its use may expand if vancomycin-resistant enterococci continue to become more prevalent.

SUGGESTED READING

Lundstrom TS, Sobel JD. Antibiotics for gram-positive bacterial infections: vancomycin, teicoplanin, quinupristin/dalfopristin, and linezolid. Infect Dis Clin North Am 2000; 14: 463-474.

Oxazolidinones (Linezolid)

The oxazolidinones are a new class of antibiotics active against gram-positive bacteria, including methicillin-resistant staphylococci and the vancomycin-resistant enterococcus *S. faecium.* Linezolid (Zyvox), the first approved agent in this class, is bacteriostatic against staphylococci and enterococci but bactericidal against most streptococcal strains. Certain anaerobic bacteria (*Clostridium, Prevotella,* and *Peptostreptococcus* species) and also *M. tuberculosis* are often susceptible as well. These drugs apparently inhibit protein synthesis at an early stage by a unique mechanism. Linezolid is now available for both oral and intravenous use, and another drug in this class (eperezolid) is being developed. Although the oxazolidinones are effective therapy for community-acquired pneumonia caused by *S. pneumoniae* and for complicated

skin and skin structure infections, these drugs should probably be reserved for the treatment of difficult-to-treat infections involving methicillin-resistant staphylococci or vancomycin-resistant enterococci. For the foreseeable future the oxazolidinones will have a limited role in primary care.

Sulfonamides

Use of sulfonamides as sole agents in primary care is largely confined to UTI and topical therapy. However, the combination of sulfamethoxazole with trimethoprim (TMP/SMX, discussed later in the chapter) has numerous indications. Life-threatening adverse reactions include bone marrow depression and hypersensitivity.

Activity and Clinical Indications

Sulfonamides are bacteriostatic against a wide range of gram-negative and gram-positive bacteria and also against *Nocardia asteroides, C. trachomatis, Plasmodium* species, and *Actinomyces* species. Current use takes advantage mainly of the activity against gram-negative bacteria such as *E. coli* and *Proteus mirabilis.* Sulfonamides are useful and inexpensive drugs for treatment of uncomplicated UTIs. However, increasing resistance of uropathogens to sulfonamides makes other agents, including TMP/SMX, the preference of many physicians. Special situations calling for sulfonamides include nocardiosis (see Chapter 7), *M. kansasii* infection caused by rifampin-resistant strains (see Chapter 22), toxoplasmosis (see Chapter 23), and nongonococcal urethritis caused by *C. trachomatis* (see Chapter 16). Dapsone is a sulfone derivative (closely related to the sulfonamides) used most frequently in primary care for prophylaxis against *P. carinii* and toxoplasmosis (see Chapter 17); it is also useful in the management of leprosy, dermatitis herpetiformis, malaria prophylaxis, leishmaniasis, various rheumatic and connective tissue disorders, inflammatory bowel disease, and brown recluse spider bites. Sulfasalazine is used in the treatment of inflammatory bowel disease.

Mechanisms of Action and Resistance

Sulfonamides interfere with microbial folic acid synthesis by competing with paraaminobenzoic acid (PABA) for a key enzyme, dihydropteroate synthetase. Reduced folic acid synthesis reduces the synthesis of bacterial nucleotides and thus inhibits growth. Microorganisms develop resistance to sulfonamides by overproducing PABA or by reducing the affinity of dihydropteroate. Bacterial mutants with decreased permeability to sulfonamides have also been described. Unfortunately, resistance to sulfonamides is now widespread. In recent years plasmid-mediated resistance has been observed in many countries.

Pharmacokinetics and Pharmacodynamics

Sulfonamides are usually given by mouth and, with certain exceptions (e.g., sulfasalazine and sulfonamides developed especially for activity within the gastrointestinal tract), are well absorbed. In serum they are variably bound to proteins (45% for sulfadiazine to up to 98% with sulfadoxine) but widely distributed into tissues and body fluids. Sulfonamides undergo acetylation and glucuronidation in the liver. Metabolites of sulfonamides appear in the urine. Renal excretion seems to involve both glomerular filtration and tubular secretion.

Unwanted Effects
Contraindications

Sulfonamides should not be given during the third trimester of pregnancy because of the risk of kernicterus in the newborn. Sulfonamides should not be given to newborn infants (<2 months of age) except for treatment of congenital toxoplasmosis. Sulfonamides must be used carefully in patients with renal insufficiency, and dosage should be reduced according to the level of renal function. Other relative contraindications include porphyria, glucose-6 phosphate dehydrogenase (G6PD) deficiency, and previous hypersensitivity to sulfonamides. Patients should avoid sunscreens and local anesthetics that contain PABA because absorbed PABA can decrease the activity of sulfonamides.

Toxicity and adverse reactions

Relatively common side effects include fever, dizziness, headache, itching, rash, photosensitivity, anorexia, nausea, vomiting, and diarrhea. Adequate fluid intake should be encouraged to reduce the risk of crystalluria with tubular deposits that can cause renal insufficiency, even though this effect is much less frequent than with the early sulfa drugs. Uncommon but serious adverse effects include serum sickness, drug-induced lupus, liver necrosis, acute pancreatitis, acute nephropathy, hemolytic anemia (especially in patients with G6PD deficiency), bone marrow depression (aplastic anemia, leukopenia or agranulocytosis, and thrombocytopenia), hypersensitivity reactions, and kernicterus in the newborn. Erythema multiforme, including the life-threatening Stevens-Johnson syndrome, is probably the most common severe hypersensitivity reaction to sulfonamides. Other serious hypersensitivity reactions include anaphylaxis and a vasculitis syndrome that can mimic polyarteritis nodosa and toxic epidermal necrolysis.

Drug Interactions

Competition for serum albumin–binding sites explains many of the drug interactions that occur with sulfonamides. Sulfonamides increase the effect or toxicity of oral anticoagulants, oral hypoglycemic agents, uricosuric drugs (e.g., probenecid), phenytoin, some of the thiazide diuretics, and methotrexate. Conversely, the effect of sulfonamides can be increased by salicylates, indomethacin, phenylbutazone, probenecid, and sulfinpyrazone. Compounds that include PABA such as certain sunscreens and local anesthetics (procaine, proparacaine, tetracaine) can reduce the activity of sulfonamides.

Preparations and Dosage

Sulfonamides are often grouped according to serum half-life as short acting, medium acting, and long acting. Short-acting and medium-acting sulfonamides in current usage include the following:

- Sulfisoxazole (Gantrisin, others), available as 500-mg tablets and as a liquid suspension (500 mg/5 mL), with usual adult dose 1 to 2 g q.i.d.
- Sulfamethoxazole (Gantanol, Urobak), available as 500- and 1000-mg tablets and as a liquid suspension (500 mg/5 mL), with usual adult dose 500 mg to 1 g b.i.d. or t.i.d.
- Sulfadiazine USP (Microsulfon, available from Eon Labs, 1-800-366-1595) as 500-mg tablets, with usual adult dose 500 mg to 1 g q.i.d.

- Sulfamethizole USP (Thiosulfil), available as 500-mg tablets, with usual dose 500 mg to 1 g q.i.d.

Phenazopyridine (Pyridium), a urinary analgesic, is combined with short-acting sulfonamides in preparations such as Azo Gantrisin (with sulfisoxazole) and Azo Gantanol (with sulfamethoxazole). Especially with sulfisoxazole and sulfamethoxazole, alkalinization of the urine promotes solubility of the drug.

Long-acting sulfonamides have been withdrawn from the market in the United States because of a high association with Stevens-Johnson syndrome, with the exception of sulfadoxine (Fansidar), which is used in the treatment and prophylaxis of malaria caused by chloroquine-resistant strains of *Plasmodium falciparum* (see Chapters 23 and 24).

Salicylazosulfapyridine, also known as sulfasalazine (Azulfidine), is a compound used in the treatment of ulcerative colitis.

KEY POINTS

SULFONAMIDES

⊃ Sulfonamides are now used mainly for treatment of UTIs and for topical applications.
⊃ Oral administration results in excellent absorption and distribution.
⊃ The physician should watch for hypersensitivity reactions, including Stevens-Johnson syndrome.
⊃ Patients should be advised to drink plenty of fluids to reduce the risk of crystalluria.
⊃ Sulfonamides should not be administered during the last trimester of pregnancy or to neonates.

Trimethoprim

Trimethoprim (Proloprim, Trimpex), although usually given with sulfamethoxazole as TMP/SMX (as discussed later in this chapter), can be used alone for treatment of UTIs and certain other infections.

Spectrum of Activity and Clinical Indications

Trimethoprim has broad activity against most gram-negative rods and many gram-positive cocci. Organisms that are typically resistant include *P. aeruginosa,* most anaerobic bacteria including *Bacteroides* species, *Mycoplasma* species, and *T. pallidum.* In primary care trimethoprim is used primarily for treatment of uncomplicated and recurrent UTI. It can also be incorporated into strategies to prevent recurrent UTIs (see Chapter 14). Some authorities prefer trimethoprim alone to TMP/SMX for these indications because use of trimethoprim alone avoids the risk of unwanted effects caused by sulfonamides. Others point out, however, that resistance to trimethoprim emerges fairly rapidly. Trimethoprim is sometimes combined with dapsone for treatment of *P. carinii* pneumonia.

Mechanisms of Action and Resistance

Trimethoprim inhibits the enzyme dihydrofolate reductase, thereby blocking the synthesis of tetrahydrofolate, a key precursor to purine and DNA synthesis. Bacteria acquire resistance through alterations in dihydrofolate reductase, cell wall permeability, or drug-binding capacity.

Pharmacokinetics and Pharmacodynamics

Trimethoprim is absorbed almost completely from the gastrointestinal tract and is widely distributed in body tissues and fluids. About 60% to 80% is excreted in the urine by tubular secretion.

Unwanted Effects
Contraindications

Trimethoprim should be used with care in patients with impaired hepatic or renal function, possible folate deficiency, or previous severe hypersensitivity.

Toxicity and Adverse Reactions

Long-term, high-dose therapy can cause megaloblastic anemia. Rash is relatively common (3% to 7% of patients). Other side effects include pruritus, fever, nausea, vomiting, and epigastric discomfort. Uncommon complications include cytopenias, cholestatic jaundice, abnormal liver function tests, azotemia, and hyperkalemia. Hyperkalemia is attributed to an effect on potassium excretion in the distal tubule. Slight elevations of the serum creatinine level are sometimes seen, caused by inhibition of tubular secretion of creatinine; these are usually unimportant.

Drug Interactions

Trimethoprim increases serum levels of phenytoin, leading to increased drug effects and toxicity. Trimethoprim can increase the levels of digoxin, and it increases the extent of myelosuppression in patients receiving methotrexate.

Preparations and Dosage

Trimethoprim as a single agent is available only for oral use. The usual dose for adults is 100 mg q12h or 200 mg q24h.

KEY POINTS

TRIMETHOPRIM
➲ Trimethoprim is used mainly for treatment of UTI.
➲ Use of trimethoprim alone (rather than TMP/SMX) avoids the risk of sulfonamide toxicity; however, resistance can emerge fairly rapidly.

Trimethoprim-Sulfamethoxazole (TMP/SMX; Co-Trimoxazole)

Synergistic activity against a wide spectrum of microorganisms makes the combination of trimethoprim and sulfamethoxazole a versatile addition to the primary care practitioner's armamentarium. TMP/SMX has been widely used in the United States (an estimated 25 million courses each year). However, severe reactions, including fatal Stevens-Johnson syndrome, sometimes occur, and resistance among common bacteria is increasing. In the United Kingdom, the Committee on Safety of Medicines Control Agency limited the indications for TMP/SMX to UTIs and acute exacerbations of chronic bronchitis in selected patients.

Spectrum of Activity and Clinical Indications

TMP/SMX is active against most aerobic gram-negative rods likely to be encountered in primary care, with the notable exception of *P. aeruginosa*. It is also active against most (but not all) strains of *H. influenzae*, many strains of *N. gonorrhoeae* and *N. meningitidis*, and most aerobic gram-positive cocci. Resistance is emerging among *S. pneumoniae* strains in some localities, and the effects against enterococci are variable. TMP/SMX is active against *P. carinii*, *N. asteroides*, *Toxoplasma gondii*, and some of the nontuberculous mycobacteria.

TMP/SMX is a first-line agent for treatment and prevention of UTIs (see Chapter 14) and of *P. carinii* pneumonia (see Chapter 17). It is also useful for management of upper respiratory tract infections (see Chapter 10), acute exacerbations of chronic bronchitis (see Chapter 11), gastrointestinal infections (see Chapter 12), sexually transmitted diseases (see Chapter 16), and infections caused by nontuberculous mycobacteria (see Chapter 22). Indications for TMP/SMX that are less likely to be encountered in primary care include brucellosis, malaria, melioidosis, Whipple's disease, and Wegener's granulomatosis. TMP/SMX has little or no activity against *B. fragilis* and other anaerobic bacteria, *Campylobacter* species, *P. aeruginosa*, and rickettsiae. It is not effective against *S. pneumoniae* strains with reduced susceptibility to penicillin G. Increasing resistance is being shown by *H. influenzae* and *Salmonella typhi* strains. Although sometimes active in vitro against methicillin-resistant *S. aureus*, TMP/SMX is not considered to be a drug of choice for staphylococcal infections.

Mechanisms of Action and Resistance

Sulfamethoxazole and trimethoprim block sequential steps in the synthetic pathway that produces folic acid, a key precursor to purine and DNA synthesis. Microorganisms develop resistance modification of the target enzymes (tetrahydropteroic acid synthetase for sulfonamides; dihydrofolate reductase for trimethoprim), altering cell wall permeability, altering drug-binding sites, or overproducing PABA. Emerging resistance of *S. pneumoniae* to TMP/SMX sharply limits the usefulness of this drug in pneumonia. Resistance of *E. coli* to TMP/SMX is becoming a problem in the treatment of UTIs (see Chapter 14).

Pharmacokinetics and Pharmacodynamics

As previously noted, both agents are well absorbed from the upper gastrointestinal tract; moreover, neither drug interferes with the absorption of the other. Both are widely distributed in body fluids and tissues. Sulfamethoxazole is partially metabolized in the liver; trimethoprim is not metabolized. About 85% of sulfamethoxazole is recovered in the urine (30% of free drug), and most of the trimethoprim component is excreted in the urine.

Unwanted Effects

The main unwanted effects are those of the sulfonamides and of trimethoprim alone, as previously reviewed.

Contraindications

Contraindications are the same as for the sulfonamides and as for trimethoprim alone. TMP/SMX should be used with extreme caution if at all in patients receiving methotrexate because of the risk of severe pancytopenia.

Toxicity and Adverse Reactions

The reactions are the same as for the sulfonamides and for trimethoprim alone. Hypersensitivity reactions occur in 3% to 5% of patients and should be taken seriously because of the risk of Stevens-Johnson syndrome. Patients with HIV disease are more likely to experience adverse reactions, including rashes. Some data suggest that patients with HIV disease who have adverse reactions from TMP/SMX are at risk of accelerated progression to AIDS and its complications. Elderly patients are more likely to develop cytopenias. Elevation of the serum creatinine sometimes occurs (see the Trimethoprim section), and TMP/SMX can cause hyperkalemia in patients with renal insufficiency. Uncommon but potentially life-threatening complications include pseudomembranous colitis, fulminant hepatic failure, pancreatitis, and drug-induced hypoglycemia. Unusual complications include aseptic meningitis, meningoencephalitis, renal tubular acidosis, anterior uveitis, retinal hemorrhage, and angle-closure glaucoma.

Drug Interactions

Interactions are the same as for the sulfonamides and for trimethoprim alone. TMP/SMX can cause marked elevations of the serum phenytoin level and can also cause elevations of the serum rifampin level. TMP/SMX inhibits the metabolism of some of the antiretroviral drugs, but the effect may be minimal.

Preparations and Dosage

TMP/SMX is available as single-strength tablets (Bactrim, Septra, Sulfatrim, and others) containing 80 mg of TMP and 400 mg of SMX, as double-strength tablets (Bactrim DS, Septra DS, Sulfatrim DS, and others) containing 160 mg of TMP and 800 mg of SMX, and as an oral suspension containing 40 mg of TMP and 200 mg of SMX per 5 mL. The usual adult dose for most indications is 1 double-strength tablet q12h, with higher doses for sepsis and for *P. carinii* pneumonia. The usual pediatric dose is 8 mg (based on the trimethoprim component) per kilogram per day in divided doses q12h. TMP/SMX is also available in parenteral formulations.

Because of excellent absorption of TMP/SMX from the gastrointestinal tract, the parenteral preparation is seldom necessary in primary care. The dose should be reduced in patients with moderate or severe renal failure. One recommendation is to give half the standard dose q12h or the full dose q24h to patients with creatinine clearance between 10 and 50 mL/min.

 KEY POINTS

TRIMETHOPRIM-SULFAMETHOXAZOLE (TMP/SMX)
- ⊃ The combination has a wide range of indications in primary care.
- ⊃ Uropathogens such as *E. coli* are showing increased resistance to TMP/SMX.
- ⊃ About 3% to 5% of patients develop severe hypersensitivity reactions, which can progress to life-threatening Stevens-Johnson syndrome.

- ⊃ Patients with HIV disease are more likely than others to have hypersensitivity reactions.
- ⊃ Dosage should be reduced in patients with moderately severe to severe renal insufficiency.

SUGGESTED READING

Huovinen P. Resistance to trimethoprim-sulfamethoxazole. Clin Infect Dis 2001; 32: 1608-1614.

Smilack JD. Trimethoprim-sulfamethoxazole. Mayo Clin Proc 1999; 74: 730-734.

Veenstra J, Veugelers PJ, Keet IP, et al. Rapid disease progression in human immunodeficiency virus type 1–infected individuals with adverse reactions to trimethoprim-sulfamethoxazole prophylaxis. Clin Infect Dis 1997; 24: 936-941.

Nitrofurantoin

Nitrofurantoin (Furadantin; Macrodantin; Macrobid) is a synthetic compound used exclusively for treatment and prevention of UTI. Serum levels after an oral dose are low or undetectable, but sufficient concentrations are achieved in the urine to inhibit most strains of *E. coli* and *Staphylococcus saprophyticus,* the usual causes of acute uncomplicated UTI in otherwise healthy younger women. Activity is unreliable against most of the bacteria that cause complicated UTI, such as the enterococcus *S. faecium* and *Klebsiella, Enterobacter, Serratia,* and *Pseudomonas* species. Comparative studies of 3-day regimens for acute uncomplicated cystitis in young women suggest that nitrofurantoin compares favorably with amoxicillin and cefadroxil but is less effective than TMP/SMX. Nitrofurantoin is not recommended for treatment of acute uncomplicated pyelonephritis because of a relatively high failure rate. For long-term suppressive therapy against recurrent UTI, nitrofurantoin (100 mg/day) compares favorably with low-dose TMP/SMX.

Nitrofurantoin frequently causes nausea and vomiting, which often limit its use. Patients receiving long-term suppressive therapy should be warned about the possibility of pulmonary and hepatic toxicity. Both of these toxicities are rare but can lead to disability or death. Nitrofurantoin toxicity can be acute, subacute, or chronic. The acute form is characterized by fever, cough, shortness of breath, myalgia, and lower lobe infiltrates, with pleural effusions present in about 20% of cases. The subacute and chronic forms are manifested as cough, dyspnea, and interstitial pulmonary infiltrates that can progress to irreversible pulmonary fibrosis. Similarly, hepatic toxicity can cause acute hepatitis, sometimes with cholestasis, or a smoldering chronic active hepatitis that progresses to cirrhosis. Other side effects attributable to nitrofurantoin include hemolytic anemia (usually in patients with G6PD deficiency) and peripheral neuropathy. Nitrofurantoin is available as 25-, 50-, and 100-mg capsules.

Methenamine

Methenamine is a compound used exclusively for suppression or prophylaxis of recurrent UTI. It is a synthetic compound available in three forms: as a salt of mandelic acid (Mandelamine, Uroquid-Acid), as a salt of hippuric acid (Urex), or as a compound with neither of these acids (Urised; Prosed). If the urine is acid (pH < 6), methenamine is converted in urine into ammonia and formaldehyde. Free formaldehyde has broad-spectrum activity against most urinary pathogens. When methenamine is used, it is necessary to ascertain that the urine pH is <6. Ascorbic acid is often given with methenamine to ensure urine acidification, but high doses of ascorbic acid may be necessary.

Methenamine provides inadequate therapy for acute uncomplicated pyelonephritis, and its usefulness for treatment of acute cystitis is not well documented. The main role of methenamine is prophylaxis or long-term suppressive therapy. In comparative trials, however, methenamine has been less effective than TMP/SMX, trimethoprim, or nitrofurantoin. Attempts to determine whether methenamine can be used to suppress UTI in patients who require intermittent bladder catheterization have been mixed. Methenamine should not be used in patients with advanced liver disease because of its ammonia-generating capacity, and it is not recommended for patients with renal failure because of the risk of acidosis.

Methenamine mandelate is available as 500-mg and 1-g tablets. Methenamine hippurate is available in 1-g tablets.

Topical Antibacterial Preparations

Topical antibacterial agents (Table 19-6) offer several advantages over oral and parenteral agents: ease of administration, ability to deliver high concentrations of drug to infected sites, patient acceptability, less potential for adverse reactions, and, in some but not all instances, reduced cost. Topical therapy is useful mainly when the infection is localized in superficial layers of tissue such as the epidermis or papillary dermis of the skin, the conjunctiva, the external ear canal, or the vagina. Topical therapy for eye and ear infections is discussed elsewhere (see Chapters 9 and 10).

Antibacterials Used Largely as Skin Disinfectants

Several preparations with antibacterial activity are used almost exclusively as skin disinfectants. These include alcohols, chlorhexidine, and iodophors. Alcohols are bactericidal but irritating, especially with repeated use or when applied to

TABLE 19-6
Some Topical Antimicrobials Useful in Primary Care

Primary indication	Antimicrobial	Concentration	Application frequency
Acne vulgaris	Azeleic acid (Azelex)	20% cream	2 times daily
	Benzoyl peroxide	2.5% to 10%	1 to 2 times daily
	Clindamycin (Cleocin)	1% to 2%	2 times daily
	Erythromycin (ATS; Emgel; Erycette)	2%	2 times daily
	Erythromycin–benzoyl peroxide (Benzamycin)	3%	2 times daily
Burns; skin grafting	Mafenide (Sulfamylon)	—	2 times daily
	Nitrofurazone (Furacin)	0.2%	1 time daily
	Silver sulfadiazine (SSD; Silvadene)	1%	1 to 2 times daily
Skin infections; elimination of nasopharyngeal carriage of *S. aureus*	Fusidic acid (Fucidin)	2%	3 times daily
	Mupirocin (Bactroban)*	2%	2 times daily
Inflammatory pustules, papules, and rosacea; bacterial vaginosis	Metronidazole (MetroGel; Metrocream)	0.75%	2 times daily
Corticosteroid-responsive dermatoses with secondary infection	Neomycin-dexamethasone (NeoDecadron) Polymyxin B–neomycin–hydrocortisone (Cortisporin)	3.5 mg/g (0.1%) 10,000 units/g of polymyxin B; 3.5 mg/g of neomycin base; 0.5% (cream) or 1% (ointment) of hydrocortisone	3 to 4 times daily 2 to 4 times daily
Skin infections; treatment of minor cuts and scrapes	Bacitracin Gentamicin (Garamycin) Polymyxin B–bacitracin–neomycin (Neosporin)	500 units/g 0.1% 5000 units/g – 400 units/g – 3.5 mg/g	3 to 4 times daily 1 to 3 times daily

*Mupirocin (Bactroban) is available as a 2% ointment and as a 2% ointment for intranasal use only (Bactroban nasal).

damaged skin. Chlorhexidine (Hibiclens and others) works by disrupting microbial cell membranes and cell contents. With a broad antibacterial spectrum, rapid cidal activity, minimal systemic absorption, and persistent activity when used repeatedly, chlorhexidine is the near-ideal agent for skin cleaning and surgical scrubs. Chlorhexidine has largely replaced hexachlorophene (pHisoHex) for this purpose. Iodophors such as povidone-iodine (Betadine and others) are complexes consisting of iodine and a carrier (i.e., polyvinylpyrrolidone) that slowly liberate iodine on reduction. These agents exert their antibacterial effect by penetrating the cell wall and substituting the microbial contents with free iodine. Iodophors have a broad spectrum of activity, although antibacterial activity does not persist on the skin and the preparation may be inactivated by body fluids. The iodophors are widely used for preoperative skin preparation, hand scrubbing, and prevention of skin infections.

Other Antibacterial Preparations Used Topically

The therapeutic use of topical antibacterial drugs requires an understanding of their spectrum of activity. Those used in the treatment of pyodermas must be effective against *S. aureus* and *S. pyogenes* (group A streptococci), the most important pathogens.

Bacitracin has broad activity against gram-positive bacteria, has been used for many years, and is inexpensive. Small studies support its use for self-treatment after minor cuts and abrasions, and it is sold over the counter for this purpose. However, the efficacy of bacitracin has never been established in rigorous clinical trials.

Neomycin is active against staphylococci but less active against streptococci. It is broadly active against most gram-negative bacilli with the exceptions of *P. aeruginosa* and obligate anaerobes. Neomycin is often combined with bacitracin to provide broad-spectrum coverage against both gram-positive and gram-negative bacteria. Systemic absorption of neomycin can result in toxicity in persons with impaired renal function (see "Toxicity of Topical Antibacterial Agents").

Polymyxin B, which is often combined with bacitracin and neomycin, is active against aerobic gram-negative bacilli, including *P. aeruginosa*, but has little or no activity against gram-positive bacteria. The triple combination of bacitracin, neomycin, and polymyxin B is available for broad-spectrum topical therapy.

Gentamicin, an aminoglycoside similar to neomycin, inhibits staphylococci, *S. pyogenes*, and aerobic gram-negative bacilli, including *P. aeruginosa*. Gentamicin is often avoided for topical treatment because sensitization to this agent would deprive the patient of its later usefulness for systemic infection.

Mupirocin (pseudomonic acid) is an important, relatively new agent intended only for topical use. An antibacterial substance produced by *Pseudomonas fluorescens*, mupirocin is highly active against all species of staphylococci, including methicillin-resistant *S. aureus*, and most species of streptococci, including *S. pyogenes*. Mupirocin inhibits bacterial RNA and protein synthesis and is bactericidal at high concentrations. It is ineffective against most gram-positive bacilli, anaerobes, and aerobic gram-negative bacilli. This aspect, however, is therapeutically useful because it results in relative sparing of much of the normal protective skin flora (e.g., *Propionibacterium*, *Corynebacterium*, and *Micrococcus* species).

Mupirocin is used mainly for treatment of skin infections caused by *S. aureus* and *S. pyogenes*, such as impetigo and folliculitis. Mupirocin is also useful for the staphylococcal nasal carrier state (see "Staphylococcal Nasal Carriage").

Clindamycin, tetracycline, and erythromycin are effective agents in the topical treatment of acne, specifically against *Propionibacterium acnes*. Topical erythromycin and clindamycin are equally effective but not superior to tretinoin and benzoyl peroxide, two other topical agents for acne. Also, the topical agents are equal but not superior to oral tetracycline. The response of acne to topical antibiotics is more impressive for inflammatory lesions than for comedones, nodules, and cysts. Because the frequency of adverse effects among the different options for acne is approximately equivalent, the choice usually depends on other factors such as cost, convenience, and personal preference.

Fluoroquinolones have been developed for topical therapy of eye and ear infections. They should probably not be used for skin infections, especially because resistance develops rapidly in *S. aureus*.

Metronidazole is available as a 1% cream and as a 0.75% gel for topical administration. The broad activity of metronidazole against anaerobic pathogens makes it useful for topical therapy of rosacea, and its antiparasitic activity makes it useful against vaginal trichomoniasis (see Chapters 5 and 16).

Rosacea

Topical metronidazole is effective for rosacea. It reduces papules, pustules, and erythema, but not telangiectasias. Topical metronidazole is equivalent to oral tetracycline 500 mg daily when given for 2 months. The rapidity of improvement may be higher with tetracycline, but the frequency and speed of relapse after the agents are discontinued may be lower with topical metronidazole. The mechanism of action of metronidazole in rosacea is unclear. However, inhibition of anaerobic bacteria and against *Demodex folliculorum* (a hair follicle mite) may be important because metronidazole has little effect against aerobic pathogens.

Impetigo

Treatment of impetigo with topical neomycin, bacitracin, gentamicin, or mupirocin is better than use of a skin disinfectant or soap alone but is less effective than systemic therapy with erythromycin or penicillin. Bacitracin is sometimes effective in mild cases of impetigo but is less effective than mupirocin. Reliance on topical agents is inappropriate for extensive disease, for bullous impetigo, or for children with poststreptococcal glomerulonephritis. Other drawbacks of topical therapy for impetigo include inability to eradicate streptococci from the respiratory tract and difficulty applying topical agents to extensive lesions.

Minor Skin Trauma

Despite studies advocating the use of topical agents in the treatment of simple abrasions or lacerations, the efficacy of topical antibiotics in the prevention of infection in clean wounds remains controversial. It is likely, however, that topical antibiotics will continue to be used in this situation. For superficial wounds topical antibiotics are used for several days until the integrity of the epidermis has been reestablished.

Staphylococcal Nasal Carriage

S. aureus is present in the anterior nares in up to 20% to 40% of normal adults. It is usually asymptomatic but can be a reservoir for furunculosis and other infections, including postoperative wound infection. Several topical antibiotics are effective at eliminating nasal carriage of *S. aureus*. Mupirocin (Bactroban nasal, b.i.d. for 5 days) is the most effective among these agents, eliminating nasal carriage in most patients. However, recolonization commonly occurs after discontinuation of treatment (up to 60% of patients at 12 weeks) and is sometimes rapid. Resistance to mupirocin is common in patients who have been treated for long periods and in clinical settings where mupirocin is used heavily as a strategy to reduce nosocomial *S. aureus* infections. Limited data suggest that mupirocin therapy for staphylococcal nasal carriage may be useful for treatment of patients with furunculosis.

Toxicity of Topical Antibacterial Agents

Topically applied antibacterial agents seldom cause significant toxicity. Bacitracin has rarely caused anaphylaxis when applied to extensive open lesions. Systemic absorption of neomycin, polymyxin B, or bacitracin can cause neurotoxicity, including ototoxicity and nephrotoxicity, when applied to large areas of denuded skin in patients with impaired renal function. Topical neomycin has occasionally caused complete deafness (which is more common when neomycin is used as an irrigating solution for wounds). Neomycin is also the topical agent most commonly associated with allergic contact sensitization, which occurs in about 1% of patients. The cream is reported to be less sensitizing than the ointment. Contact sensitivity reactions to topical bacitracin, clindamycin, erythromycin, gentamicin, mupirocin, and polymyxin B are rare.

 KEY POINTS

TOPICAL ANTIBACTERIAL THERAPY

⊃ Topical therapy is useful for some superficial infections because of ease of administration, low risk for adverse reactions, and clinical efficacy.

⊃ Agents used for disinfection of skin include alcohols, chlorhexidine, and iodophors.

⊃ Bacitracin is broadly active against gram-positive bacteria and inexpensive. However, its efficacy has never been established by rigorous trials.

⊃ Neomycin is broadly active against most gram-negative bacteria, but it is not generally recommended for superficial skin infections because of its relatively high incidence of skin sensitization and the potential for systemic toxicity. The use of topical gentamicin is similarly discouraged.

⊃ Mupirocin (Bactroban) is a unique antimicrobial agent active especially against staphylococci and streptococci. It is relatively inactive against many organisms present in the normal skin flora.

⊃ Some of the indications for topical antibacterial therapy include acne vulgaris, rosacea, mild cases of impetigo, and the staphylococcal nasal carriage state.

SUGGESTED READING

Bass JW, Chan DS, Creamer KM, et al. Comparison of oral cephalexin, topical mupirocin, and topical bacitracin for treatment of impetigo. Pediatr Infect Dis J 1997; 16: 708-710.

Kaye ET, Kaye KM. Topical antibacterial agents. Infect Dis Clin North Am 1995; 9: 547-559.

Langford JH, Artemi P, Benrimoj SI. Topical antimicrobial prophylaxis in minor wounds. Ann Pharmacother 1997; 31: 559-563.

Morden NE, Berke EM. Topical fluoroquinolones for eye and ear. Am Fam Physician 2000; 62: 1870-1876.

Raz R, Miron D, Colodner R, et al. A 1-year trial of nasal mupirocin in the prevention of recurrent staphylococcal nasal colonization and skin infection. Arch Intern Med 1996; 156: 1109-1112.

Wain AM. Metronidazole vaginal gel 0.75% (MetroGel-Vaginal): a brief review. Infect Dis Obstet Gynecol 1998; 6: 3-7.

Summary of Therapy Against Bacterial and Other Pathogens

A summary of drugs of choice against bacterial, mycoplasmal, chlamydial, rickettsial, and spirochetal pathogens is shown in Table 19-5.

20 Viral Diseases and Antiviral Drugs for Non–Human Immunodeficiency Virus Viral Infections

STEPHEN B. GREENBERG

Herpesviruses
Herpes Simplex Viruses 1 and 2
Varicella-Zoster Virus
Epstein-Barr Virus
Cytomegalovirus
Human Herpesviruses 6, 7, and 8
Respiratory Viruses
Influenza Viruses
Respiratory Syncytial Virus and Other
Respiratory Viruses
Hepatitis Viruses
Viruses That Cause Meningitis or Encephalitis
Causes of Aseptic Meningitis
Arbovirus Encephalitis
Colorado Tick Fever Dengue and Yellow Fever
Other Viral Diseases
Viruses Causing Gastroenteritis
Viruses Causing Exanthems
Mumps Virus
Parvovirus B19
Human Papillomavirus
Exotic Viral Diseases
Antiviral Drugs: Overview
Drugs Active Mainly Against Herpesviruses
Acyclovir (Zovirax)
Valacyclovir (Valtrex)
Penciclovir (Denavir)
Famciclovir (Famvir)
Ganciclovir (Cytovene) and
Valganciclovir (Valcyte)
Foscarnet (Foscavir)
Cidofovir (Vistide)
Trifluridine (Viroptic) and Vidarabine (Vira-A)
Drugs Active Mainly Against Respiratory Viruses
Amantadine (Symmetrel)
Rimantadine (Flumadine)
Zanamivir (Relenza)
Oseltamivir (Tamiflu)
Ribavirin (Virazole, Rebetol)
Interferons

parenteral therapy of acute and chronic viral infections. More than 12 drugs have been approved for treatment of non–human immunodeficiency virus (HIV) viral infections (Table 20-1). Effective therapy is available for specific viral infections affecting the central nervous system (CNS), eye, respiratory tract, liver, and skin. Because antiviral agents are usually effective at only one specific stage of virus replication, they often have a restricted spectrum of activity. The availability of antiviral drugs and also the increased prevalence of patients at risk for serious viral infections (e.g., patients who have received organ transplants and patients with HIV disease) enhance the desirability of early, specific diagnosis of viral infections.

Molecular techniques such as the polymerase chain reaction (PCR) are being introduced into clinical medicine at a rapid rate. Clinical virology will almost surely become a more important component of primary care medicine during the 21st century. A presumptive diagnosis of viral infection is usually based on the history and physical examination. Laboratory confirmation is unnecessary when disease is self-limited (e.g., the common cold) and when the physical findings are pathognomonic (e.g., herpes zoster in a dermatomal distribution). The clinician should, however, have a general appreciation of diagnostic procedures that are now available. These include cell culture, antigen detection systems (fluorescent antibody [FA] staining, immunoperoxidase antibody staining, and enzyme immunoassay [EIA]), nucleic acid detection (PCR and other methods), cytology, histology, serology, and electron microscopy (see Chapter 2). Against this background, in this chapter are reviewed the major groups of viruses relevant to primary care, beginning with the viral diseases for which therapy is now available and specific diagnosis therefore desirable.

SUGGESTED READING

Balfour HH Jr. Antiviral drugs. N Engl J Med 1999; 340: 1255-1268.
Drugs for non-HIV viral infections. Med Lett 1999; 41: 113-120.
Fields BN, Knipe DM, Howley PM. Virology. 3rd ed., Philadelphia: Lippincott Williams & Wilkins; 1996.
Keating MR. Antiviral agents for non-human immunodeficiency virus infections. Mayo Clin Proc 1999; 74: 1266-1283.
Margo KL, Shaughnessy AF. Antiviral drugs in healthy children. Am Fam Physician 1998; 57: 1073-1077.
Richman DD, Whitley RJ, Hayden FG, eds. Clinical Virology. New York: Churchill Livingstone; 1997.
Storch GA. Diagnostic virology. Clin Infect Dis 2000; 31: 739-751.
Wagner EK, Hewlett MJ. Basic Virology. Oxford, England: Blackwell Science; 1999.

Primary care clinicians now have at their disposal an expanded list of approved antiviral drugs for topical, oral, or

TABLE 20-1
Approved Antiviral Drugs for Viral Infections Other Than Human Immunodeficiency Virus*

ANTIVIRAL DRUG			
Generic name	Trade name	Viruses inhibited	Chapter
Amantadine	Symmetrel	Influenza A	11
Rimantadine	Flumadine	Influenza A	11
Oseltamivir	Tamiflu	Influenza A and B	11
Zanamivir	Relenza	Influenza A and B	11
Ribavirin	Virazole; Rebetol	Hepatitis C, Lassa virus, Hantavirus, respiratory syncytial virus	4, 13
Interferon-alfa	Alferon-N, Roferon-A, Intron-A	Hepatitis B and C, papillomavirus	13, 16
Lamivudine (3TC)	Epivir	Hepatitis B	13
Acyclovir	Zovirax	Herpes simplex, varicella-zoster, cytomegalovirus	6, 7, 13
Valacyclovir	Valtrex	Herpes simplex, varicella-zoster, cytomegalovirus	7, 16
Pencilovir	Denovir	Herpes simplex	16
Famciclovir	Famvir	Herpes simplex, varicella-zoster	7, 16
Ganciclovir	Cytovene	Cytomegalovirus	17
Valgancilovir	Valcyte	Cytomegalovirus	
Foscarnet	Foscavir	Cytomegalovirus, herpes simplex, varicella-zoster	17
Cidofovir	Vistide	Cytomegalovirus, herpes simplex, and varicella-zoster	17

*Not shown on this table are three drugs approved only for therapy of herpes simplex keratoconjunctivitis: trifluridine, vidarabine, and idoxuridine (Chapter 9).

Herpesviruses

The herpesviruses are large DNA viruses that establish life-long latent infection by poorly understood processes. Transmission usually involves direct person-to-person contact with transfer of an infected body fluid onto a susceptible tissue such as the eye, mouth, respiratory tract, or urogenital mucosa. Herpesviruses are fragile and do not survive long on objects. Disease results from various combinations of direct destruction of tissues (as in the familiar "fever blister" of herpes simplex), immunologic responses (as in Epstein-Barr virus mononucleosis), and promotion of neoplasia (as in primary CNS lymphoma and Kaposi's sarcoma in persons with HIV disease). Nearly 100 herpesviruses have been isolated from various animal species. The eight currently recognized human herpesviruses are the two herpes simplex viruses, varicella-zoster virus, Epstein-Barr virus, cytomegalovirus, and human herpesviruses 6, 7, and 8 (Table 20-2).

Herpes Simplex Viruses 1 and 2

Herpes simplex viruses 1 and 2 (HSV-1 and HSV-2) cause genital tract lesions (see Chapter 16), oral ulcers (herpes labi-alis and herpes stomatitis; see Chapter 10), keratitis (see Chapter 9), skin lesions (e.g., herpetic whitlow, involving the fingers, or herpes gladiatorum, involving any part of the body), meningitis, encephalitis (see Chapter 6), congenital disease of the newborn (see Chapter 5), and rarely pneumonia. The characteristic skin or mucosal lesion is a vesicle on an erythematous base. Serologic diagnosis is generally unhelpful, and the extent to which other diagnostic measures (notably culture and PCR) are desirable depends on the circumstances. An attempt should be made to confirm the diagnosis of genital herpes simplex virus infection because of the therapeutic and social implications. Culture and FA staining have traditionally been used for this purpose. PCR is now available and is extremely sensitive, but it is expensive; the issue of cost-effectiveness in primary care has yet to be resolved (see Table 20-2). PCR of cerebrospinal fluid (CSF) has revolutionized the diagnosis of herpes simplex encephalitis. Antiviral drugs now available for treatment of HSV infection include acyclovir, valacyclovir, and famciclovir for parenteral use and penciclovir for topical use (Table 20-3). Acyclovir, valacyclovir, and famciclovir have equal efficacy. Acyclovir has a long safety record, but famciclovir and valacyclovir require fewer doses.

TABLE 20-2
Herpesvirus Infections: Current Methods Of Diagnosis

Virus (synonyms)	Setting	Method	Comments
Herpes simplex virus (HSV-1 and HSV-2; human herpesviruses 1 and 2)	Skin and mucous membranes	Culture	80% sensitivity for genital lesions; higher for vesicular and pustular lesions than for crusted lesions. Sensitivity is about 10^5 virions/mL. Cytopathic effect usually becomes apparent within 2 to 4 days.
		FA staining	Staining enables early diagnosis.
		PCR	Recently shown to be more sensitive than culture; may find wider application. Can detect as few as 5 virions.
		Cytology	Tzanck preparation (Wright or Giemsa stain) or Papanicolaou stain shows giant cells or inclusions consistent with the diagnosis but not specific.
	Viral encephalitis or meningitis	PCR of CSF	Sensitivity reported to be 96% with 99% specificity.
	Any setting	Acute and convalescent serology	Allows demonstration of HSV-1 or HSV-2 seroconversion. Primary usefulness is for identifying asymptomatic carriers.
Varicella-zoster virus (VZV; human herpesvirus 3)	Skin and mucous membranes	Culture	VZV is more labile than HSV; culture is less sensitive for diagnosis and slower, usually requiring 4 to 10 days.
		FA staining	More sensitive than culture for diagnosis of VZV infection.
	Viral encephalitis or meningitis	PCR of CSF	VZV has recently been reported to cause meningitis in the absence of skin lesions.
Epstein-Barr virus (EBV; human herpesvirus 4)	Infectious mononucleosis	Serology	IgM VCA is ~100% sensitive for infectious mononucleosis. IgG VCA persists lifelong and is therefore more useful for surveillance than for diagnosis of acute infectious mononucleosis. Other serologic tests are sometimes useful (see Chapter 8).
		Culture	Culture of throat washings or circulating lymphocytes is 80% to 90% sensitive for acute infectious mononucleosis but is not specific (since asymptomatic shedding from past infection is common) and is of little practical use.
	Primary CNS lymphoma (HIV disease)	PCR of CSF	PCR is 97% sensitive and 97% specific for EBV-associated primary CNS lymphoma in persons with AIDS.
Cytomegalovirus (CMV; human herpesvirus 5)	Documentation of immune status	IgG serology	Useful for documenting previous infection with CMV. In patients with HIV disease and also in patients undergoing organ transplantation, identifies those at risk of complications.
	Mononucleosis, immunocompetent person	IgM serology	IgM serology for EBV should be obtained simultaneously, since some patients with acute EBV mononucleosis have false-positive IgM serologic tests for CMV.
		PCR and other molecular methods	Potentially useful for diagnosis of CMV mononucleosis (see below), but expensive and probably unnecessary for this purpose.
	Systemic infection, immunocompromised person	pp65 antigen assay on blood	The assay for pp65 antigenemia probably offers better sensitivity and specificity than the other approaches to diagnosis.
		Quantitative PCR for CMV DNA	The qualitative PCR for CMV DNA is not useful in this setting (highly sensitive but not specific); however, a high titer of CMV DNA copies (viral load) correlates with severe disease.
		Other methods of nucleic acid detection	These include the hybrid capture assay and nucleic acid sequence–based amplification (NASBA).

Continued

TABLE 20-2—cont'd
Herpesvirus Infections: Current Methods Of Diagnosis

Virus (synonyms)	Setting	Method	Comments
	CNS infection (encephalitis or radiculopathy)	PCR of CSF	PCR is reported to be 82% sensitive and 98% specific for CMV disease of the central nervous system.
	Congenital CMV infection, in utero	Culture or PCR of amniotic fluid	Useful for prenatal diagnosis (see Chapter 5).
	Congenital CMV infection, newborn	Urine culture for CMV	Maternally derived antibodies would cause false-positive serologic tests.
	CMV disease of gastrointestinal tract, lungs, or other organs	Biopsy	Diagnosis is made by finding the characteristic intranuclear inclusions and can be confirmed by immunochemistry.
Human herpesvirus 6 (HHV-6)	Exanthem subitum (roseola infantum); associated encephalitis	Serology	IgM serologic testing is useful for diagnosis of acute HHV-6 in young children. An alternative is demonstration of seroconversion (acute and convalescent IgG serologic tests).
		Culture or PCR of blood	Culture or PCR of peripheral blood mononuclear cells can be used for diagnosis (when IgG antibody is absent), but value in practice is unclear.
Human herpesvirus 7 (HHV-7)	Role in disease unclear	Serology, culture, PCR	Diagnostic methods are available, but value is unclear because the role of HHV-7 in human disease, if any, is largely undetermined.
Human herpesvirus 8 (HHV-8; Kaposi's sarcoma–associated virus)	Kaposi's sarcoma; multicentric Castleman's disease; B-cell lymphoma of body cavities	Culture, PCR	Reliable tests are generally not available, and utility of diagnosis is unclear.

AIDS, Acquired immunodeficiency syndrome; *CSF*, cerebrospinal fluid; *FA*, fluorescent antibody; *PCR*, polymerase chain reaction; *VCA*, viral capsid antigen.

Varicella-Zoster Virus

Varicella (chickenpox) usually affects young children but occasionally affects adults. Varicella in adults is a more severe illness and warrants treatment. Varicella during pregnancy carries a high risk of maternal complications and also of transmission to the fetus. Herpes zoster (shingles) is the reactivation form of latent varicella-zoster virus (VZV) infection. The incidence of herpes zoster increases with age. The most frequent complication is persistent pain (postherpetic neuralgia).

Diagnosis of varicella (chickenpox) and herpes zoster (shingles) is usually based on the characteristic skin lesions. The evolution of the rash of chickenpox distinguishes this disease from smallpox, which has not been reported since 1977 but remains a potential agent of bioterrorism (see Chapter 4). In smallpox the rash progresses uniformly (maculopapules, then vesicles, then pustules, then scabs) over 1 to 2 weeks, whereas in chickenpox lesions occur simultaneously in all stages of development. The rash of herpes zoster is distinguished on the basis of its unique dermatomal distribution. Disseminated herpes zoster (see Chapter 7), which nearly always occurs in immunocompromised persons, must be distinguished from other lesions, and diagnostic tests are therefore useful in this setting (Table 20-2).

Acyclovir reduces the duration of symptoms in varicella when initiated within 24 hours of onset of the skin lesions (Table 20-4). Adults with varicella, and especially pregnant women, should be treated. Although acyclovir, valacyclovir, and famciclovir shorten the duration of rash in herpes zoster, only a few researchers were able to demonstrate a reduced incidence of postherpetic neuralgia. Nevertheless, patients >50 years of age should be offered acyclovir, valacyclovir, or famciclovir if seen within 72 hours of onset of the rash. Ophthalmic zoster should be treated in all age groups. In recent controlled trials the use of corticosteroids in combination with acyclovir did not reduce the incidence of postherpetic neuralgia compared with acyclovir alone. Immunocompromised patients should be given acyclovir intravenously if seen within 5 days after onset of the rash because treatment reduces the incidence of cutaneous and visceral dissemination. Measures used to treat postherpetic

TABLE 20-3
Regimens for Treatment of Herpes Simplex Virus (HSV-1 and HSV-2) Infection

Syndrome	Regimen*	Duration (days)	Cost of total therapy† ($)
Primary genital herpes	Acyclovir 400 mg PO t.i.d. Valacyclovir 1 gram PO b.i.d. Famciclovir 250 mg PO t.i.d.	10 10 5 to 10	65 135 105
Recurrent genital herpes	Acyclovir 400 mg PO t.i.d. Valacyclovir 500 mg PO b.i.d. Famciclovir 125 mg PO b.i.d.	5 5 5	33 34 31
Chronic recurrent genital herpes (suppression)	Acyclovir 200 to 400 mg PO b.i.d. to t.i.d. Valacyclovir 500 mg to 1 g PO daily Famciclovir 125 mg to 250 mg PO b.i.d. (see note‡)	Up to 365 Up to 365 Up to 365	800 to 2000 1200 to 2400 2200 to 2500
Orolabial herpes (herpes labialis)	Penciclovir cream, 1%, applied q2h during the day Acyclovir cream, 5%, applied q3h, 6 times a day Docosanol cream, 10%, applied 5 times a day	4	23 56
Keratoconjunctivitis (HSV keratitis)	Trifluridine, 1%, 1 drop q2h	10	80
Encephalitis or meningitis	Acyclovir 10 to 15 mg/kg IV q8h	14 to 21	1300 to 3000
Neonatal herpes simplex	Acyclovir 10 to 15 mg/kg IV q8h	14	
Mucocutaneous herpes simplex infection in an immunocompromised patient	Acyclovir 5 mg/kg q8h Acyclovir 400 mg PO t.i.d.§ Valacyclovir 1 g PO t.i.d.§ Famciclovir 500 mg PO b.i.d.§ Foscarnet 400 mg IV b.i.d. to t.i.d.§¶	7 7 7 7 7 to 21	900 45 140 98 2400 to 3600

*In patients with renal insufficiency, drug dosages of systemic agents shown here should be reduced in accordance with the manufacturer's recommendations. In some instances the doses shown here are according to common usage rather than the manufacturer's recommendations.
†Based on average wholesale price, 2000.
‡Because famciclovir has been shown to be carcinogenic in animals, some authorities advise against its use for long-term suppressive therapy (in contrast to short-term therapy for primary or recurrent disease).
§Not approved by the Food and Drug Administration for this indication.
¶Recommended only for patients with acyclovir-resistant strains of HSV.

neuralgia include tricyclic antidepressants, topical lidocaine, gabapentin, and opiates.

Epstein-Barr Virus

The Epstein-Barr virus (EBV) causes infectious mononucleosis (see Chapter 8) and has also been associated with Burkitt's lymphoma, other lymphomas (including primary CNS lymphoma in persons with HIV disease), nasopharyngeal carcinoma, and a lymphoproliferative syndrome in recipients of solid organ and bone marrow transplants. In general, serologic tests are used for diagnosis of EBV infection in immunocompetent persons and molecular techniques are used for diagnosis of EBV infection in immunocompromised persons (Table 20-2). Serologic testing of patients with chronic fatigue syndrome for EBV infection is discouraged because a causal relationship remains hypothetical at best (see Chapter 18). In vitro, EBV replication is inhibited by several antiviral drugs, including acyclovir, and also by interferon-α. However, no clear benefit from antiviral therapy has been observed. Corticosteroids are sometimes used for severe complications of EBV mononucleosis such as impending airway obstruction, thrombocytopenia, hemolytic anemia, CNS involvement, or myocarditis. Corticosteroids are not recommended for the vast majority of patients with infectious mononucleosis caused by EBV, which is a self-limited disease.

Cytomegalovirus

Cytomegalovirus (CMV) is the usual cause of heterophilnegative mononucleosis (see Chapter 8) and causes substantial morbidity and mortality in immunocompromised patients.

TABLE 20-4
Recommendations for Treatment of Varicella-Zoster Virus (VZV) Infection

Syndrome	Regimen*	Duration (days)	Cost of total therapy† ($)
Varicella (chickenpox) in normal host	Acyclovir 20 mg/kg (maximum, 800 mg) PO q.i.d.	5	84 (maximum)
Varicella in immunocompromised host	Acyclovir 10 mg/kg IV q8h‡	7 to 10	216 to 309
Herpes zoster in normal host (especially age >50 years or with involvement of ophthalmic branch of fifth nerve)§	Acyclovir 800 mg PO 5 times daily Valacyclovir 1 g PO t.i.d. Famciclovir 500 mg PO t.i.d.	7 to 10 7 7	140 to 210 92 to 160 160
Herpes zoster in immunocompromised host	Acyclovir 10 mg/kg IV q8h	7	216

*In patients with renal insufficiency, drug dosages of systemic agents shown here should be reduced in accordance with the manufacturer's recommendations.
†Based on average wholesale price.
‡Not approved by the Food and Drug Administration for this indication.
§In other settings, treatment is optional (see text).

Serologic testing is used for the diagnosis of CMV infection in immunocompetent persons and also for determining whether immunocompromised patients are at risk for CMV-related complications. Patients with advanced HIV disease who are CMV antibody–positive are at risk for retinitis, colitis, polyradiculopathy, and other complications. Patients undergoing organ transplantation who are CMV antibody positive from previous infection or who receive an organ from a CMV antibody–positive donor are at high risk for complications, including CMV pneumonitis (see Chapter 3). Molecular techniques are now used for the diagnosis of CMV complications. Quantitation of CMV virus in blood by PCR or other methods is being used increasingly as a guide to therapy of CMV infection in immunocompromised persons (Table 20-2).

Preventive therapy has been shown to be effective in recipients of renal, liver, heart, and bone marrow allografts (Table 20-5). Prophylaxis is usually given for at least 3 months. Intravenous administration of ganciclovir or foscarnet is recommended for symptomatic organ involvement by CMV in immunocompromised patients. Cidofovir is a new nucleoside analog approved for treatment of CMV retinitis in immunocompromised persons. Evaluation by an infectious disease specialist is recommended for most patients requiring antiviral therapy for CMV infection. Evaluation by an ophthalmologist with special interest in CMV retinitis is recommended for most patients with this complication.

Human Herpesviruses 6, 7, and 8

Human herpesviruses 6 and 7 (HHV-6 and HHV-7) are ubiquitous viruses affecting primarily children. HHV-6 infects nearly all children by 2 years of age and HHV-7 nearly all children by 5 years of age. Most children are asymptomatic. HHV-6 causes most cases of exanthem subitum, or sixth disease (see Chapter 4), and more commonly causes fever without rash. HHV-6 is a major cause of febrile seizures in adults and sometimes causes encephalitis. Investigations of the possible role of HHV-6 as a cause of infections in immunocompromised per-

sons or a cause of the chronic fatigue syndrome have been largely inconclusive. There is no clear indication that HHV-7 causes disease. Human herpesvirus 8 (HHV-8) is strongly associated with Kaposi's sarcoma and also with a form of lymph node hyperplasia known as Castleman's disease (see Chapter 8). Recent data indicate significant oral shedding of HHV-8, suggesting that oral exposure to saliva is a risk factor for acquisition of HHV-8 among men who have sex with men.

SUGGESTED READING

Alper BS, Lewis PR. Does treatment of acute herpes zoster prevent or shorten postherpetic neuralgia? J Fam Pract 2000; 49: 255-264.

Chiu SS, Cheung CY, Tse CY, et al. Early diagnosis of primary human herpesvirus 6 infection in childhood: serology, polymerase chain reaction, and virus load. J Infect Dis 1998; 178: 1250-1256.

Cohen JI, Brunell PA, Straus SE, et al. Recent advances in varicella-zoster virus infection. Ann Intern Med 1999; 130: 922-932.

Drew WL, Lalezari JP. Cytomegalovirus: disease syndromes and treatment. Curr Clin Top Infect Dis 1999; 19: 16-29.

Eddleston M, Peacock S, Juniper M, et al. Severe cytomegalovirus infection in immunocompetent patients. Clin Infect Dis 1997; 24: 52-56.

Moore PS. The emergence of Kaposi's sarcoma–associated herpesvirus (human herpesvirus 8). N Engl J Med 2000; 343: 1411-1413.

Pauk J, Huang M-L, Brodie SJ, et al. Mucosal shedding of human herpesvirus 8 in men. N Engl J Med 2000; 343: 1369-1377.

Schmader K. Herpes zoster in older adults. Clin Infect Dis 2001; 32: 1481-1486.

Spruance SL, Rea TL, Thoming C, et al. Penciclovir cream for the treatment of herpes simplex labialis: a randomized, multicenter, double-blind, placebo-controlled trial. JAMA 1997; 277: 1374-1379.

Tebas P, Nease RF, Storch GA. Use of the polymerase chain reaction in the diagnosis of herpes simplex encephalitis: a decision analysis model. Am J Med 1998; 105: 287-295.

Whitley RJ, Roizman B. Herpes simplex virus infections. Lancet 2001; 357: 1513-1518.

TABLE 20-5
Recommendations for Treatment of Cytomegalovirus (CMV) Infection

Syndrome	Regimen*	Duration (days unless specified)	Cost (total therapy unless specified)† ($)
Prevention of CMV infection in patients undergoing organ or bone marrow transplantation	Acyclovir 800 mg PO q.i.d. (renal transplant)‡	90	1440
	Valacyclovir 2 g PO q.i.d. (renal transplant)‡	90	3150
	Ganciclovir 1 g PO t.i.d. §	Up to 98	4700
Colitis, esophagitis, pneumonitis, hepatitis, or other organ diseases	Ganciclovir 5 mg/kg IV q12h‡	14 to 21	680 to 1000
	Foscarnet 60 mg/kg IV q8h or 90 mg/kg IV q12h‡	14 to 21	24,000 to 37,000
Retinitis	Ganciclovir 5 mg/kg IV q12h§		50 per day
	Foscarnet 60 mg/kg IV q8h or 90 mg/kg IV q12h		1760 per day
	Cidofovir 5 mg/kg IV once weekly	2 doses	1420
Suppression of retinitis	Ganciclovir 1 g PO t.i.d.§	Indefinite	
	Ganciclovir 5 mg/kg IV daily or 6 mg/kg IV 5 times/week§	Indefinite	
	Foscarnet 90 to 120 mg/kg IV daily	Indefinite	
	Cidofovir 5 mg/kg IV every 2 weeks	Indefinite	

*In patients with renal insufficiency, drug dosages of systemic agents shown here should be reduced in accordance with the manufacturer's recommendations.
†Based on average wholesale price.
‡Not approved by the Food and Drug Administration for this indication.
§Valganciclovir may replace ganciclovir for these indications; the literature should be watched.

Respiratory Viruses

Influenza Viruses

Influenza virus infection is discussed in Chapter 11. Although yearly vaccination is recommended for high-risk individuals, including all persons >50 years of age, antiviral drugs have an important complementary role in preventing and treating this serious infection. Amantadine and rimantadine are approved for treatment of influenza A but not influenza B. Their use is limited by development of resistant viruses and potential CNS side effects. In 1999 two neuraminidase inhibitors, zanamivir and oseltamivir, were approved for treatment of both influenza A and B. They are also approved for prophylaxis, including protection of household contacts. Side effects and cost of these new agents must be considered before they are used during influenza outbreaks.

Respiratory Syncytial Virus and Other Respiratory Viruses

Respiratory syncytial virus (RSV) is the leading cause of pneumonia, bronchiolitis, and tracheobronchitis in young children, affecting nearly everyone during the first several years of life (see Chapter 4). Immunity acquired as a result of infection is incomplete, and therefore the risk for RSV infection is lifelong. Healthy adults have mild RSV infections, but serious infections can occur among the elderly and the immunocompromised. Antigen detection tests are now widely used for rapid diagnosis in pediatric practice. The most commonly used methods are FA staining and EIA. Viral culture is also available. Ribavirin is the only currently available drug approved for treatment. However, aerosolized ribavirin has not been shown to decrease mortality or hospital stay in

hospitalized children with RSV bronchiolitis or pneumonia. Ideally an infectious disease specialist should consult with the pediatrician for children admitted to the hospital for treatment of bronchiolitis.

Many viruses are associated with the common cold and other respiratory tract infections. Antigen detection systems are available for rapid diagnosis of parainfluenza viruses and adenoviruses but not for rhinoviruses or coronaviruses. No specific antiviral drug therapy is available for treatment of rhinovirus or coronavirus infection, the two most commonly identified causes of the common cold.

SUGGESTED READING

Domachowske JB, Rosenberg HF. Respiratory syncytial virus infection: immune response, immunopathogenesis, and treatment. Clin Microbiol Rev 1999; 12: 298-309.

Falsey AR, Walsh EE. Respiratory syncytial virus infection in adults. Clin Microbiol Rev 2000; 13: 371-384.

Hall CB. Respiratory syncytial virus and parainfluenza virus. N Engl J Med 2001; 344: 1917-1928.

Malhotra A, Krilov LR. Influenza and respiratory syncytial virus: update on infection, management, and prevention. Pediatr Clin North Am 2000; 47: 353-372.

Hepatitis Viruses

Hepatitis viruses, major causes of chronic liver disease, are increasingly amenable to therapy, although progress has been slow (see Chapter 13). Up to 10% of patients infected with hepatitis B become chronic carriers, and significant liver disease develops in at least 20% of these patients over 20 years.

Hepatitis C leads to chronic infection in about 85% of infected patients, and according to current data, cirrhosis will eventually develop in about 20% of infected persons. Interferon-α and lamivudine (3TC) have been used for hepatitis B infection. Combined use of interferon-α and ribavirin for hepatitis C results in sustained virologic response in about 40% of patients. Referral of patients with hepatitis B or hepatitis C to a physician with special interest in this area is usually desirable (see Chapter 13).

Viruses That Cause Meningitis or Encephalitis

Aseptic meningitis is relatively common in primary care; encephalitis is uncommon and generally calls for hospitalization (see Chapter 6). Newer diagnostic tests often facilitate specific diagnosis. With the notable exception of acyclovir therapy for herpes simplex encephalitis, specific therapies are largely unavailable or are disappointing (Table 20-6).

Causes of Aseptic Meningitis

Enteroviruses and HSV-2 are the most commonly identified causes of aseptic meningitis. PCR technology for early, specific diagnosis of enteroviral meningitis potentially represents a major advance because it will reduce the need for empiric antibiotic therapy for possible bacterial meningitis. Unfortunately, this technology is not widely available. Other important causes of the aseptic meningitis syndrome include the lymphocytic choriomeningitis (LCM) virus and the mumps virus. A low CSF glucose (hypoglycorrhachia) is present in up to 33% of cases of aseptic meningitis caused by LCM and

TABLE 20-6
Viruses That Cause Meningitis or Encephalitis: Current Diagnosis and Treatment

Virus	Usual syndromes	Diagnosis	Treatment
Enteroviruses	Aseptic meningitis	RT-PCR of CSF	Supportive
Lymphocytic choriomeningitis virus	Aseptic meningitis	Serology (serum); culture (CSF and blood)	Supportive
Herpes simplex virus type 2	Aseptic meningitis	PCR of CSF	Supportive
Herpes simplex virus type 1	Encephalitis	PCR of CSF	Acyclovir (see Table 20-3)
Varicella-zoster virus	Aseptic meningitis in immunocompetent persons; encephalitis or myelitis in immunocompromised persons	PCR of CSF	Acyclovir for immunocompromised persons (see Table 20-4)
Mumps virus	Aseptic meningitis; encephalitis	Serology (mumps-specific IgM); culture (CSF, saliva, urine)	Supportive
Measles virus	Subacute sclerosing panencephalitis	Serology	Supportive
Arboviruses	Encephalitis	Serology of both CSF and serum (specifying IgM serology for specific viruses)	Supportive
Colorado tick fever	Encephalitis	Serology for virus-specific IgM; PCR of whole blood; FA staining; culture	Supportive
Cytomegalovirus	Encephalitis or radiculomyelitis in immunocompromised persons	PCR of CSF (see Table 20-2)	Ganciclovir alone or with foscarnet
JC virus	Progressive multifocal leukoencephalopathy in immunocompromised persons	PCR of CSF	Largely supportive (various drugs have been tried; none approved)
Rabies	Encephalitis	Culture (saliva), serology (CSF, serum); RT-PCR (saliva, skin), FA staining (skin)	Supportive

CSF, Cerebrospinal fluid; *FA,* fluorescent antibody; *PCR,* polymerase chain reaction; *RT-PCR,* reverse transcriptase polymerase chain reaction.

30% of cases caused by mumps. CSF pleocytosis occurs in about one half of patients with mumps, but encephalitis is rare. Antiviral drug treatment is not available for most causes of aseptic meningitis.

Arbovirus Encephalitis

HSV-1 is currently the most important cause of sporadic viral encephalitis in the United States, especially because of its therapeutic implications (see Chapter 6). Numerous viruses for which specific therapy is not currently available also cause encephalitis. Most of these viruses are known as arboviruses (for "arthropod-borne") or, more specifically, as alphaviruses, flaviviruses (*flavus* is Latin for "yellow"; yellow fever is, historically, the most important flavivirus), or bunyaviruses. Fewer than 200 cases of arboviral encephalitis are reported each year to the Centers for Disease Control and Prevention (CDC), but many milder cases no doubt go undetected. The more important arboviruses causing encephalitis in the United States and some prominent clinical features are as follows:

- St. Louis encephalitis virus. The most important cause of arboviral encephalitis in the United States, the St. Louis encephalitis virus disproportionately affects elderly persons and homeless persons. Outbreaks have been reported from nearly every state, typically involving older neighborhoods with breeding habitats for the northern or southern house mosquitoes, *Culex pipiens* and *Culex quinquefasciatus*. An outbreak should be suspected when cases of "summer stroke" with fever occur. The illness begins with fever, headache, myalgias, nausea, vomiting, or a combination of these symptoms. Subsequent clinical findings include lethargy, confusion, tremor, ataxia, and focal neurologic signs. Leukocytosis is often present. Seizures portend a poor prognosis, and nonconvulsive status epilepticus can occur. Mortality is 8% overall, but it is up to 20% in persons >60 years of age.
- California (La Crosse) encephalitis virus. Belonging to the genus *Bunyavirus*, California encephalitis virus is second only to St. Louis encephalitis as a cause of arboviral encephalitis in the United States. The La Crosse virus is the most common antigenic variant of this serogroup of viruses. California encephalitis affects mainly children <15 years of age, and in the United States it is the most commonly reported CNS viral infection of childhood. The principal vector is *Aedes triseriatus*, a forest-dwelling, tree hole–breeding mosquito virus. Initial symptoms include fever, headache, nausea, and vomiting. Severity of CNS disease ranges from aseptic meningitis to severe encephalitis resembling HSV encephalitis. Leukocytosis is common. Mortality is about 1%, but behavioral residua occur. The Jamestown Canyon virus, another virus in this serogroup, is widely distributed in the United States and may be more common than was previously thought.
- Eastern, western, and Venezuelan equine encephalitis viruses. These viruses are alphaviruses that cause encephalitis in both children and adults. Transmitted by mosquitoes, they cause outbreaks of disease in horses. The number of human cases in the United States has been declining. Encephalitis from the western equine encephalitis virus or the Venezuelan equine encephalitis is typically mild. Eastern equine encephalitis causes

a much more severe disease (mortality up to 20% in cases with clinical encephalitis, and up to 70% in outbreaks). Eastern equine encephalitis is surpassed only by rabies in the rapidity of the disease progression. Brawny edema of the face and extremities is found in about 10% of patients. Magnetic resonance imaging (MRI) and computed tomography (CT) often reveal focal lesions in the basal ganglia, thalami, and brainstem. Neurologic sequelae are more common in children than in adults.

- West Nile encephalitis virus. Recognized in the United States in 1999, the West Nile encephalitis is a flavivirus carried by various migrating birds and transmitted to humans principally by *Culex* mosquitoes. The disease disproportionately affects children, the elderly, and immunocompromised persons. As with the other arboviral encephalitides, symptoms typically begin with low-grade fever, myalgias, and weakness, sometimes accompanied by sore throat, eye pain, nausea, vomiting, diarrhea, abdominal pain, or a combination of these symptoms. In up to 50% of patients, and especially children, a rash develops that is usually concentrated over the trunk but may involve the face and upper extremities. Physical findings may include conjunctival suffusion, pharyngitis without exudates, cervical (especially submental) or generalized lymphadenopathy, hepatomegaly, splenomegaly, muscle weakness, diminished deep tendon reflexes, and, in about 10% of cases, a diffuse flaccid paralysis. Laboratory findings include leukopenia, lymphocytopenia, elevated sedimentation rate, and elevated aspartate aminotransferase and alanine aminotransferase levels.

Diagnosis of arboviral encephalitis is usually made by serologic testing. Virus-specific IgM antibodies can be detected in CSF and serum in nearly all cases by the 10th day of illness. No specific treatment is available.

Colorado Tick Fever

Colorado tick fever is an important cause of self-limited illness at high altitudes in the western United States. Classified as a coltivirus, the Colorado tick fever virus and related viruses usually cause a self-limited febrile illness in children <15 years of age. The virus infects circulating erythrocytes. The disease is transmitted by *Dermacentor andersoni*, the wood tick, in mountainous areas of the western United States. A history of tick bite is obtained in about 90% of cases. Aseptic meningitis or encephalitis develops in about 5% to 10% of patients, and the clinical course is typically biphasic. Initial symptoms are fever, chills, severe headache, and myalgias. A maculopapular rash that can suggest Rocky Mountain spotted fever develops in about 15% of patients. Other findings may include conjunctival suffusion, lymphadenopathy, splenomegaly, and leukopenia. The acute symptoms resolve within 7 days but may be followed several days later by the reappearance of fever with symptoms and signs of aseptic meningitis or encephalitis. Most patients make a full recovery, but persons >30 years of age may have prolonged fatigue. Diagnosis is made by PCR analysis on a whole blood clot (whole blood rather than serum because of the virus's predilection for erythrocytes), FA staining, or serologic demonstration of virus-specific IgM. No specific treatment is available, but mortality is rare.

Dengue and Yellow Fever

Dengue virus and yellow fever virus are both flaviviruses transmitted mainly by *Aedes aegypti* (the common household mosquito) but also by other mosquito vectors. In the United States both diseases should be suspected in returning travelers with undiagnosed fever. Anecdotal reports suggest that about 25 imported cases of dengue occur in the United States each year. Two cases of yellow fever have been reported in the United States in recent years. The hallmark of dengue is severe musculoskeletal pain (hence its nickname, "breakbone fever"), but occasionally a life-threatening illness with hemorrhage and hypovolemic shock (dengue hemorrhagic fever–dengue shock syndrome) develops. Like dengue, yellow fever is often asymptomatic but can be a severe illness with features of hemorrhagic fever, liver failure, encephalitis, or a combination of these illnesses. Diagnosis of both dengue and yellow fever is usually made by serologic tests, especially demonstration of IgM antibodies. A PCR assay for dengue virus is available in specialized laboratories.

 KEY POINTS

HEPATITIS VIRUSES

⊃ Enteroviruses and HHV-2 are the most common proven causes of aseptic meningitis. PCR of CSF enables early, specific diagnosis of enteroviral meningitis; introduction of this test into clinical practice should simplify patient management.

⊃ Aseptic meningitis caused by LCM or mumps virus is sometimes associated with low CSF glucose (hypoglycorrhachia).

⊃ The most important arboviruses causing encephalitis in the United States are the California encephalitis viruses, St. Louis encephalitis virus, equine encephalitis viruses (eastern, western, and Venezuelan), and West Nile virus. Diagnosis is by serologic testing (IgM-specific antibodies in serum and CSF).

⊃ Colorado tick fever is an important cause of acute illness with aseptic meningitis or encephalitis at high altitudes in the western United States.

⊃ Dengue and yellow fever should be suspected in cases of undiagnosed illness in returning travelers.

SUGGESTED READING

Balkhy HH, Schreiber JR. Severe La Crosse encephalitis with significant neurologic sequelae. Pediatr Infect Dis J 2000; 19: 77-80.

Centers for Disease Control and Prevention. Arboviral infections of the central nervous system—United States, 1996-1997. MMWR 1998; 47: 517-522.

Deresiewicz RL, Thaler SJ, Hsu L, et al. Clinical and neuroradiographic manifestations of eastern equine encephalitis. N Engl J Med 1997; 336: 1867-1874.

McJunkin JE, Khan RR, Tsai TF. California–La Crosse encephalitis. Infect Dis Clin North Am 1998; 12: 83-93.

Nash D, Mostashari F, Fine A, et al. The outbreak of West Nile virus infection in the New York City area in 1999. N Engl J Med 2001; 344: 1807-1814.

Rappole JH, Derrickson SR, Hubalek Z. Migratory birds and spread of West Nile virus in the Western Hemisphere. Emerg Infect Dis 2000; 6: 319-328.

Wasay M, Diaz-Arrastia R, Suss RA, et al. St. Louis encephalitis: a review of 11 cases in a 1995 Dallas, Tex, epidemic. Arch Neurol 2000; 57: 114-118.

Other Viral Diseases

Several other groups of viruses discussed elsewhere in this book are briefly mentioned here.

Viruses Causing Gastroenteritis

The four viruses now identified as major causes of gastroenteritis are classified as rotaviruses, caliciviruses, enteric adenoviruses, and astroviruses (see Chapter 12). No specific treatment is available for any of these causes of viral diarrhea.

Viruses Causing Exanthems

Common exanthems are discussed in Chapters 4 and 7. Diagnosis of acute infection from measles and rubella can be made by detection of IgM antibody.

Mumps Virus

Mumps is a vaccine-preventable illness affecting mainly children and adolescents and causing more severe disease in adults. Mumps virus is a paramyxovirus, related to the human parainfluenza viruses and respiratory syncytial virus. Epidemics occurred every 2 to 5 years in the United States before the introduction of live attenuated mumps vaccine in 1967. Symptoms typically begin with fever, anorexia, malaise, and headache, followed by earache and tenderness over one or both parotid glands. High fever and pain on chewing are common. About 10% of patients have involvement not only of the parotid glands but also of the submandibular glands, sublingual glands, or both, which can be mistaken for anterior cervical lymphadenopathy. In about one half of patients, CSF pleocytosis is found when sought; aseptic meningitis is relatively common, but encephalitis is rare (see previous discussion). Epididymoorchitis, which can cause sterility, develops in about 25% of adult men with mumps, and oophoritis develops in about 5% of adult women. Diagnosis is usually confirmed serologically by demonstration of IgM antibodies. The virus can also be isolated from saliva until 4 to 5 days after the onset of parotitis. No specific treatment is available.

Parvovirus B19

Parvovirus B19 (see Chapter 7) is an important cause of rash in children (fifth disease) and of arthritis with rash in adults. This virus is also of great concern during pregnancy because it affects developing erythrocytes (see Chapter 4). Demonstration of parvovirus B19 IgM antibodies is used to diagnose acute infection and also congenital, postpartum infection. Demonstration of parvovirus B19 DNA by PCR is the preferred method for diagnosis of chronic infection, aplastic crisis, and in utero infection. No specific treatment is available, but intravenously administered immune globulin is useful for patients who are immunosuppressed and those with aplastic crisis.

Human Papillomavirus

More than 70 types of human papillomaviruses (HPVs) have been described. These viruses cause laryngeal papillomas and genital warts (see Chapter 16). Most external genital warts are caused by HPV types 6 and 11 and are sexually transmissible.

Juvenile laryngeal papillomatosis occurs in children whose mothers had a history of genital warts. Recurrences of genital warts are common but improve with specific treatment. There is little evidence that any available treatment modality (see Chapter 16) decreases infectivity.

Exotic Viral Diseases

Diagnosis and management of exotic viral diseases such as Lassa fever, Ebola, and other hemorrhagic fevers should be undertaken in consultation with the state health department. Cases seen in the United States are nearly always associated with a history of recent travel to a developing nation. Newer diagnostic methods include IgM serology and PCR. Treatment is supportive. Special patient isolation and infection control measures are needed in all suspected cases.

SUGGESTED READING

Bausch DG, Rollin PE, Demby AH, et al. Diagnosis and clinical virology of Lassa fever as evaluated by enzyme-linked immunosorbent assay, indirect fluorescent-antibody test, and virus isolation. J Clin Microbiol 2000; 38: 2670-2677.

Colebunders R, Borchert M. Ebola haemorrhagic fever—a review. J Infect 2000; 40: 16-20.

Fisher-Hoch SP, Hutwagner L, Brown B, et al. Effective vaccine for Lassa fever. J Virol 2000; 74: 6777-6783.

Peters CJ, LeDuc JW. An introduction to Ebola: the virus and the disease. J Infect Dis 1999; 179 (Suppl 1): ix-xvi.

Porterfield JS, ed. Exotic viral infections. London: Chapman & Hall Medical; 1995.

Schwartz DA. Emerging and reemerging infections: progress and challenges in the subspecialty of infectious disease pathology. Arch Pathol Lab Med 1997; 121: 776-784.

Spear PG. A welcome mat for leprosy and Lassa fever. Science 1998; 282: 1999-2000.

Suresh V. The enigmatic haemorrhagic fevers. J R Soc Med 1997; 90: 622-624.

Antiviral Drugs: Overview

Useful agents for treatment of viral infections are of three types: virucidal agents, including agents such as podophyllin that destroy viruses and host tissues simultaneously; antiviral drugs that inhibit viral replication at the cellular level; and immunomodulating agents such as interferons that alter the host response to infection. Antiviral drugs usually target nucleic acid synthesis. None of the approved antiviral drugs can eliminate nonreplicating or latent viruses from the body. Pharmacokinetic and pharmacodynamic considerations are similar to those that apply to antibacterial drugs. Many antiviral drugs are excreted mainly by the kidneys, and therefore the dose must be adjusted for patients with renal insufficiency (Table 20-7; see also Chapter 19). Viral strains that are resistant to available antiviral drugs are becoming a problem, especially among immunocompromised patients. These include acyclovir-resistant strains of HSV and VZV, ganciclovir-resistant strains of CMV, and amantadine- and rimantadine-resistant strains of influenza virus.

TABLE 20-7
Usual Adult Doses of Antiviral Drugs in Patients with Normal and Impaired Renal Function*

Drug	Indication and dose	Normal renal function	Moderately impaired renal function (creatinine clearance 30 to 50 mL/min)	Markedly impaired renal function (creatinine clearance 11 to 29 mL/min)	End-stage impairment of renal function function (creatinine clearance <10 mL/min)
Acyclovir	Low-dose, PO (primary or recurrent genital herpes)	200 mg 5 times daily	No adjustment	No adjustment	200 mg q12h
	High-dose, PO (herpes zoster)	800 mg 5 times daily	No adjustment	800 mg q8h	800 mg q12h
	Suppressive therapy, PO	400 mg b.i.d.	No adjustment	No adjustment	200 mg q12h
	IV (herpes encephalitis)	10 to 15 mg/kg q8h	10 to 15 mg/kg q12h	10 to 15 mg/kg q24h	5 to 7.5 mg/kg q24h
Valacyclovir	High-dose, PO (primary genital herpes)	1 g q12h	No adjustment	1 g q24h	500 mg q24h
	Higher-dose, PO (herpes zoster)	1 g q8h	1 gram q12h	1 g q24h	500 mg q24h
	Low-dose, PO (recurrent genital herpes)	500 mg q12h	No adjustment	500 mg q24h	500 mg q24h
	Suppressive therapy, PO	500 mg to 1 g q24h	No adjustment	500 mg q24h to q48h	500 mg q24h to q48h

Continued

TABLE 20-7—cont'd
Usual Adult Doses of Antiviral Drugs in Patients with Normal and Impaired Renal Function*

Drug	Indication and dose	Normal renal function	Moderately impaired renal function (creatinine clearance 30 to 50 mL/min)	Markedly impaired renal function (creatinine clearance 11 to 29 mL/min)	End-stage impairment of renal function function (creatinine clearance <10 mL/min)
Famciclovir	High-dose, PO (herpes zoster)	500 mg q8h	500 mg q12h to q24h	250 mg to 500 mg q24h	250 mg q24h or after each dialysis treatment
	Low-dose, PO (primary genital herpes)†	250 mg q8h	250 mg q12h	250 mg q24h	125 mg q24h or after each dialysis treatment
	Lower-dose, PO (recurrent genital herpes)	125 mg q12h	125 mg q24h	125 mg q24h	125 mg q24h or after each dialysis treatment
	Suppressive therapy, PO	250 mg q12h	125 mg to 250 mg q12h	125 mg q12h to q24h	125 mg q24h or after each dialysis treatment
	Recurrent infection in AIDS patients, PO	500 mg q12h	500 mg q12h to q24h	250 mg q24h	250 mg q24h or after each dialysis treatment
Ganciclovir	IV for CMV retinitis	5 mg/kg q12h	2.5 mg/kg q24h	1.25 mg/kg q24h	1.25 mg/kg 3 times/week
Valganciclovir	PO for CMV retinitis	900 mg daily	450 mg daily		
Foscarnet	High-dose, IV (CMV retinitis)	60 mg/kg q8h or 90 mg/kg q12h	40 mg/kg q12h or 60 to 80 mg/kg q24h	50 to 60 mg/kg q24h	Not recommended
Cidofovir	IV for CMV retinitis	5 mg/kg/weekly	Do not use	Do not use	Do not use
Amantadine	PO, prophylaxis‡	200 mg daily or 100 mg b.i.d.‡	100 mg daily to every other day	100 mg every 3 days	100 or 200 mg weekly, alternate weeks
Rimantadine	PO, prophylaxis	200 mg daily	No adjustment	No adjustment	100 mg daily
Zanamivir	Inhalation	10 mg b.i.d.	10 mg b.i.d.	10 mg b.i.d.	No data
Osteltamivir	PO, prophylaxis	75 mg b.i.d.	75 mg b.i.d.	75 mg daily	No data
Ribavirin	Aerosol	1.1 g/day	No adjustment	No adjustment	

AIDS, Acquired immunodeficiency syndrome; *CMV,* cytomegalovirus.
*Based on manufacturer's recommendations. In some instances doses shown here differ from those shown in Table 20-3. The differences are explained by common usage (as recommended by various authorities) versus doses approved by the Food and Drug Administration (FDA). For example, for primary genital herpes infection, 200 mg five times daily is FDA approved (as shown here), whereas 400 mg t.i.d. is recommended by various authorities on the basis of greater convenience with apparently equivalent efficacy. Doses are for immunocompetent persons unless otherwise indicated.
†Not approved by the FDA for this indication.
‡For persons >65 years of age, an amantadine dose of 100 mg/day is recommended.

Drugs Active Mainly Against Herpesviruses

Drugs active against the herpesviruses, of which acyclovir is the prototype, inhibit viral synthesis of DNA by inhibiting viral DNA polymerase.

Acyclovir (Zovirax)

Acyclovir is a guanosine analog that is activated by viral thymidine kinase (TK), which inhibits viral DNA polymerase

and thereby blocks DNA synthesis. Its greatest activity and clinical utility are against HSV-1, HSV-2, and EBV. Acyclovir is the drug of choice for HSV encephalitis, neonatal herpes, and VZV infection. It is also approved for HSV mucocutaneous disease, including genital herpes. It can be shown to inhibit EBV and, at high concentrations, CMV, but it has no clear clinical utility in EBV or CMV infections.

Viral strains that have low or absent TK activity are resistant to acyclovir. Acyclovir-resistant HSV isolates generally make up <1% of the total virus population in immunocompetent persons but are more common (up to 8% of the total virus population) in immunocompromised patients. Emergence of acyclovir-resistant HSV does not seem to be a problem during long-term suppressive therapy for genital HSV in immunocompetent persons. However, emergence of resistance has been a major problem in immunocompromised persons, and especially those with advanced HIV disease. Acyclovir-resistant HSV-2 sometimes causes painful, necrotizing perirectal ulcers in patients with advanced HIV disease.

The oral bioavailability of acyclovir is only about 15% to 20% and actually decreases as the dose of the drug is increased. The drug is widely distributed throughout the body, with CSF concentrations about one half of plasma levels. Plasma levels are about 15% to 20% higher in older patients, mainly because of reduced renal function. Unmetabolized acyclovir (60% to 90%) is excreted through the kidneys by glomerular filtration and tubular secretion. The serum half-life is about 3 hours in persons with normal renal function but increases to nearly 20 hours in persons who are functionally anephric. Therefore the dose must be reduced in patients with renal insufficiency. Acyclovir is removed by hemodialysis but not by peritoneal dialysis.

Drug interactions with acyclovir include increased nephrotoxicity from cyclosporine, increased lethargy with zidovudine (AZT), increased plasma levels when given with probenecid, and decreased renal clearance of methotrexate. Adverse effects of topically applied acyclovir (which is minimally absorbed) include burning, itching, and, rarely, contact dermatitis. Adverse effects of orally administered acyclovir include nausea, diarrhea, rash, and headache. Adverse effects of intravenously administered acyclovir include reversible renal dysfunction from crystalline nephropathy, phlebitis, and neurotoxicity.

Valacyclovir (Valtrex)

Valacyclovir, the L-valyl ester of acyclovir, is a prodrug that is rapidly and almost completely converted (>99%) to acyclovir after oral administration by an enzyme present in the intestines and liver. The oral bioavailability of valacyclovir is three to five times that of acyclovir, resulting in plasma levels similar to those achieved with intravenously administered acyclovir. No intravenous preparation of valacyclovir is available. Valacyclovir is used mainly for genital herpes infection and VZV infection. Valacyclovir compares favorably with acyclovir for treatment of herpes zoster in immunocompetent persons. Drug interactions and adverse effects are similar to those seen with acyclovir. A thrombotic thrombocytopenic purpura–hemolytic-uremic syndrome has been observed in severely immunocompromised patients.

Penciclovir (Denavir)

Penciclovir is an acyclic guanine analog similar to acyclovir. The mechanism of action differs slightly from that of acyclovir, but cross-resistance occurs. Like acyclovir, penciclovir is active against HSV-1, HSV-2, and VZV, is less active against EBV, and has limited activity against CMV. It has been shown to inhibit the hepatitis B virus and to be synergistic with lamivudine (3TC) against hepatitis B virus in

vitro. Penciclovir has poor oral bioavailability. It is available in the United States as a 1% cream for treatment of herpes labialis.

Famciclovir (Famvir)

Famciclovir, a diacetyl ester of penciclovir, is a prodrug that is converted to the active form (penciclovir) by an enzyme in the intestines and the liver. Famciclovir has 77% oral bioavailability. Unmetabolized famciclovir (70%) is excreted by the kidneys, and dose reduction is necessary in persons with renal insufficiency. No clinically important drug interactions have been identified. Adverse reactions to famciclovir include headache, nausea, diarrhea, rash (especially in the elderly), hallucinations or confusion, and neutropenia, which occurs in about 5% of patients. Famciclovir is approved for treatment of genital herpes, mucocutaneous herpes, and herpes zoster.

Ganciclovir (Cytovene) and Valganciclovir (Valcyte)

Ganciclovir is a guanine analog that differs from acyclovir only by the addition of a hydroxymethyl group to the acyclic side chain. This small chemical difference confers dramatic differences in spectrum of activity and extent of toxicity. Compared with acyclovir, ganciclovir is equally potent against HSV and VZV but is 10-fold more potent against CMV and EBV. It also has some activity against HHV-6. The major clinical indications for ganciclovir are treatment and chronic suppression of CMV retinitis in immunocompromised patients (especially those with advanced HIV disease) and prevention of CMV disease in transplant recipients. CMV strains that are highly resistant to ganciclovir have been recovered during prolonged therapy.

The oral bioavailability of ganciclovir is about 5% in the fasting state and is increased slightly by administration with food. Intravenous administration of ganciclovir (5 mg/kg) gives peak plasma levels of about 10 μg/mL. CSF levels are up to 70% of plasma levels. Unmetabolized ganciclovir (>90%) is excreted by the kidneys, and the dose must be reduced severely in patients with renal insufficiency.

Valganciclovir is an L-valyl ester (prodrug) of ganciclovir with superior bioavailability (about 60% after administration with food). Once-daily oral administration of valganciclovir (900 mg) results in plasma levels of ganciclovir comparable to those achieved with intravenously administered ganciclovir (10 mg/kg per day). For these reasons valganciclovir will probably replace ganciclovir for most indications.

Bone marrow suppression is the most important adverse reaction to ganciclovir and valganciclovir. Neutropenia occurs in about 40% of patients and thrombocytopenia in up to 20% of patients. Side effects include headache, confusion, psychosis, and coma. Ganciclovir is also mutagenic and carcinogenic. Data from animal studies suggest that ganciclovir might cause permanent sterility. Coadministration of zidovudine (AZT) increases the risk for myelosuppression; moreover, AZT antagonizes the action of ganciclovir against CMV. Renal clearance of ganciclovir is reduced by probenecid. The nephrotoxicity of ganciclovir and valganciclovir is increased when the drugs are given with other agents.

Foscarnet (Foscavir)

Chemically unrelated to the preceding compounds, foscarnet is an inorganic pyrophosphate analog. It is active against most of the herpesviruses (HSV-1, HSV-2, VZV, EBV, and CMV) and also against influenza A and B viruses, hepatitis B virus, and HIV. Foscarnet blocks the binding site of viral polymerase and inhibits cleavage of pyrophosphate from deoxynucleotide triphosphates. Because this mechanism of action differs radically from that of acyclovir and compounds related to acyclovir, foscarnet is useful for therapy of acyclovir-resistant HSV infections and ganciclovir-resistant CMV infections. Resistance to foscarnet arises by point mutations in DNA polymerase of HSV and CMV.

Foscarnet provides poor oral bioavailability (7% to 9%) and is given intravenously (60 mg/kg q8h to persons with normal renal function). CSF levels average about two thirds of plasma levels. Unmetabolized foscarnet (80%) is excreted by the kidneys.

Foscarnet has significant nephrotoxicity. During therapy about one third of patients have impaired renal function, such as elevated blood urea nitrogen (BUN) and serum creatinine levels, proteinuria, and occasionally acute tubular necrosis and nephrogenic diabetes insipidus. Nephrotoxicity is enhanced when the drug is given with aminoglycosides, pentamidine, acyclovir, cyclosporine, or amphotericin B. Coadministration of foscarnet with AZT increases the severity of anemia. Metabolic abnormalities are common during foscarnet therapy and include hypocalcemia (up to 35% of patients) or hypercalcemia, hypomagnesemia (up to 44% of patients), hypokalemia (up to 16% of patients), and hypophosphatemia or hyperphosphatemia. Other adverse reactions include fever, diarrhea, nausea, and genital ulcerations. Because of these significant toxicities, foscarnet is generally reserved for problematic cases that require consultation.

Cidofovir (Vistide)

Cidofovir is an acyclic nucleoside phosphonate derivative. It is active against all of the herpesviruses currently recognized to cause human disease and also against other DNA viruses, such as the adenoviruses, papillomaviruses, and poxviruses. Cidofovir is metabolized intracellularly to the active diphosphate form by cellular enzymes, and it acts by inhibiting viral DNA polymerase. Because activation of cidofovir does not depend on virus-specified enzymes, cidofovir is active against acyclovir- and ganciclovir-resistant strains. There is, however, some cross-resistance to ganciclovir. Oral bioavailability is low (about 5%). The drug is eliminated mainly by the kidneys and causes dose-related nephrotoxicity, which can be severe. Neutropenia occurs in about 20% of patients. Cidofovir is carcinogenic and teratogenic and therefore contraindicated during pregnancy. At present, cidofovir is reserved for treatment of CMV retinitis in patients with HIV disease. It may also have a role in the treatment of acyclovir-resistant HSV infections. Use of topical cidofovir for mucocutaneous HSV infection caused by acyclovir-resistant strains and intralesional cidofovir for genital warts is being studied.

Trifluridine (Viroptic) and Vidarabine (Vira-A)

Trifluridine (Viroptic) and vidarabine (Vira-A) are available in the United States for topical treatment of keratoconjunctivitis caused by HSV (see Chapter 9).

 KEY POINTS

DRUGS ACTIVE AGAINST HERPESVIRUSES: ACYCLOVIR, VALACLOVIR, PENCICLOVIR, FAMCICLOVIR, GANCICLOVIR, AND FOSCARNET

⊃ Acyclovir, the current drug of choice against life-threatening HSV and VZV infection, activates viral thymidine kinase (TK), resulting in the inhibition of viral DNA synthesis.

⊃ Resistance to acyclovir is more common in isolates from immunocompromised patients and is usually the result of virus variants with absent or deficient TK.

⊃ Valacyclovir, the L-valyl ester of acyclovir, is metabolized to acyclovir after oral administration, resulting in plasma levels resembling those achieved with intravenously administered acyclovir.

⊃ Penciclovir, which is chemically similar to acyclovir, is available in the United States as a topical preparation for treatment of cold sores (herpes labialis).

⊃ Famciclovir, a prodrug of penciclovir, provides 77% oral bioavailability and is approved for treatment of genital and mucocutaneous HSV infection and herpes zoster.

⊃ Ganciclovir, used for treatment or chronic suppression of CMV retinitis and for prevention of CMV in transplant patients, causes significant myelosuppression. Valganciclovir is a prodrug of ganciclovir with superior bioavailability after oral administration.

⊃ Foscarnet, an inorganic pyrophosphate analog, is used for treatment of acyclovir-resistant HSV infection and for difficult cases of CMV retinitis. Foscarnet causes significant nephrotoxicity and an array of metabolic abnormalities.

⊃ Cidofovir, which is nephrotoxic and potentially carcinogenic, is used mainly for treatment of CMV retinitis.

⊃ All of the preceding drugs are eliminated mainly by renal excretion. The dose should therefore be reduced in patients with renal insufficiency.

SUGGESTED READING

Acosta EP, Fletcher CV. Valacyclovir. Ann Pharmacother 1997; 31: 185-191.

Grose C, Wiedean J. Generic acyclovir vs. famciclovir and valacyclovir. Pediatr Infect Dis J 1997; 16: 838-841.

Martinez CM, Luks-Golger DB. Cidofovir use in acyclovir-resistant herpes infection. Ann Pharmacother 1997; 31: 1519-1521.

Noble S, Faulds D. Ganciclovir: an update of its use in the prevention of cytomegalovirus infection and disease in transplant recipients. Drugs 1998; 56: 115-146.

Ormrod D, Goa K. Valaciclovir: a review of its use in the management of herpes zoster. Drugs 2000; 59: 1317-1340.

Ormrod D, Scott LJ, Perry CM. Valaciclovir: a review of its long term utility in the management of genital herpes simplex virus and cytomegalovirus infections. Drugs 2000; 59: 839-863.

Plosker GL, Noble S. Cidofovir: a review of its use in cytomegalovirus retinitis in patients with AIDS. Drugs 1999; 58: 325-345.

Drugs Active Mainly Against Respiratory Viruses
Amantadine (Symmetrel)

Amantadine is a tricyclic amine compound active against influenza A viruses at low concentrations (<1 μg/mL). It has no activity against influenza B virus. At low concentrations amantadine inhibits the ion channel function of the M2 protein of influenza viruses, which inhibits viral uncoating. At high concentrations, amantadine also inhibits virus-induced membrane fusion. Resistant influenza A virus can be selected by virus passage in the presence of amantadine. About 30% of drug-treated patients shed resistant influenza virus after 5 days of treatment. Transmission of resistant influenza virus occurs.

Amantadine is well absorbed after oral administration. Levels in nasal secretions and saliva are similar to serum plasma levels, and CSF levels are about one half of plasma levels. Unmetabolized amantadine is excreted by the kidneys. The drug accumulates in patients with renal insufficiency, in whom the dose should be reduced. Amantadine is not cleared by hemodialysis.

CNS side effects are common (up to 33% of patients) during amantadine therapy and may reflect both adrenergic and anticholinergic activity. Relatively common dose-related side effects include nervousness, lightheadedness, difficulty concentrating, and insomnia. Seizures can occur, especially in persons with underlying seizure disorders. Life-threatening neurotoxicity, including seizures, coma, and cardiac arrhythmias, can develop with high plasma levels. This neurotoxicity usually occurs in patients with renal insufficiency who are given high doses. The CNS side effects are more common and more severe when antihistamines or anticholinergic drugs are given concomitantly. Increased CNS toxicity has been observed in patients given trimethoprim-sulfamethoxazole or triamterene-hydrochlorothiazide (Dyazide) concomitantly. Patients receiving minor tranquilizers or antidepressants may also be at risk for CNS side effects.

Rimantadine (Flumadine)

Rimantadine is structurally similar to amantadine. It is absorbed more slowly than amantadine after oral administration. Unlike amantadine, it is extensively metabolized before renal excretion. CNS side effects occur less frequently than with amantadine. Like amantadine, rimantadine has been shown to be useful in the prevention and treatment of influenza A.

Zanamivir (Relenza)

Zanamivir is a sialic acid analog, which explains its activity against influenza A and B viruses. For influenza viruses to be released from infected cells and spread within the respiratory tract, sialic acid residues must be cleaved from receptors on the host cell by the viral enzyme neuraminidase. As an analog of sialic acid, zanamivir competes successfully with neuraminidase for the active enzyme site. Resistant influenza virus strains have not yet been reported. Oral bioavailability is low. Zanamivir is given intranasally or by inhalation. No drug interactions are known, and the only significant adverse reaction thus far is occasional bronchospasm in persons with asthma.

Oseltamivir (Tamiflu)

Oseltamivir is similar to zanamivir but, unlike zanamivir, it is well absorbed when given orally. After absorption it is converted by an enzyme to an active compound (a sialic acid analog known as GS4071). Viruses with decreased neuraminidase susceptibility develop in 1% to 2% of treated patients. Oseltamivir is eliminated mainly by renal excretion.

The drug is usually well tolerated but causes mild nausea and vomiting in some patients.

Ribavirin (Virazole; Rebetol)

Ribavirin, a purine analog, has broad activity against both DNA and RNA viruses. Ribavirin acts by inhibiting viral messenger RNA formation. Ribavirin has been reported to be effective against influenza A and B; RSV; hepatitis A, B, and C; Lassa fever; and hemorrhagic fever. Viral resistance to ribavirin has not been demonstrated.

Ribavirin has an oral bioavailability of about 40%. The metabolism of ribavirin is complex. The drug is highly concentrated, as a triphosphate, in red blood cells; the erythrocyte/plasma ratio is about 40:1 or greater. About 40% of the drug is eliminated by renal excretion, but metabolism by the liver is also important.

Prolonged administration of ribavirin commonly causes a dose-related anemia. Other adverse reactions are headache, nausea, lethargy, and elevations of the serum bilirubin, iron, and uric acid levels. A major concern, especially with the use of aerosolized ribavirin, is its teratogenicity, mutagenicity, embryotoxicity, and gonadotoxicity. Ribavirin is contraindicated during pregnancy, and many physicians are reluctant to expose potentially pregnant health care workers to aerosolized ribavirin because of this concern.

Ribavirin is given by aerosol to hospitalized children with severe RSV bronchiolitis or pneumonia, but consultation is desirable (see earlier discussion). Oral ribavirin has been approved by the Food and Drug Administration (FDA) for treatment of chronic hepatitis C in combination with interferon-α-2b (see Chapter 13). Intravenous ribavirin can be obtained from the CDC for treatment of Lassa fever and the Hantavirus pulmonary syndrome, in which its efficacy is currently being investigated. Intravenous and aerosolized ribavirin have been used to treat severe influenza, but the drug is not FDA approved for this purpose.

 KEY POINTS

DRUGS ACTIVE MAINLY AGAINST RESPIRATORY VIRUSES: AMANTADINE, RIMANTADINE, ZANAMIVIR, OSTELTAMIVIR, AND RIBAVIRIN

⊃ Amantadine and rimantadine are active against influenza A viruses but not against influenza B. Resistant influenza A virus strains develop during treatment. Transmission of resistant virus has been reported.

⊃ Amantadine causes significant CNS side effects in up to one third of patients.

⊃ The dose of amantadine and rimantadine should be reduced in patients with renal insufficiency, including elderly patients.

⊃ Rimantadine, compared with amantadine, is more slowly absorbed, is metabolized before renal excretion, and is less likely to cause CNS side effects.

⊃ Zanamivir and oseltamivir are active against both influenza A and influenza B viruses and have been shown to be useful for prevention and treatment of influenza.

⊃ Ribavirin, used to treat selected cases of severe RSV bronchiolitis and pneumonia in children, causes anemia and is both teratogenic and mutagenic.

SUGGESTED READING

Bardsley-Elliot A, Noble S. Oseltamivir. Drugs 1999; 58: 851-860.

Dominguez KD, Mercier RC. Treatment of RSV pneumonia in adults: evidence of ribavirin effectiveness? Ann Pharmacother 1999; 33: 739-741.

Dunn CJ, Goa KL. Zanamivir: a review of its use in influenza. Drugs 1999; 58: 761-784.

Gubareva LV, Kaiser L, Hayden FG. Influenza virus neuraminidase inhibitors. Lancet 2000; 355: 827-835.

Hayden FG. Antivirals for pandemic influenza. J Infect Dis 1997; 176 (Suppl 1): S56-S61.

Treanor JJ, Hayden FG, Vrooman PS, et al. US Oral Neuraminidase Study Group. Efficacy and safety of the oral neuraminidase inhibitor oseltamivir in treating acute influenza: a randomized controlled trial. JAMA 2000; 283: 1016-1024.

Zimmerman RK, Ruben FL, Ahwesh ER. Influenza, influenza vaccine, and amantadine/rimantadine. J Fam Pract 1997; 45: 107-122.

Interferons

Interferons are glycoprotein cytokines made by cells in response to various stimuli. Three broad classes of human interferons, designated α, β, and γ, are currently recognized. Interferon-α and interferon-β are made by most cell types in response to viral infection and numerous other stimuli. Interferon-γ is made by T lymphocytes and natural killer cells in response to various stimuli. Interferons have no direct antiviral activity. However, they induce cellular proteins that inhibit viral protein synthesis, and by this mechanism they render cells resistant to viral infection. Interferon-γ, compared to interferon-α and interferon-β, exhibits less antiviral activity but more immunomodulating activity. Interferon-γ induces cytotoxic T lymphocytes, activates macrophages, promotes the expression of class II major histocompatibility antigens, and mediates local inflammation. Interferon-α, commonly known as interferon-alfa (or interferon-alpha), is now approved in various forms for several viral infections: chronic hepatitis B, chronic hepatitis C, Kaposi's sarcoma in HIV-infected persons, and condyloma acuminatum. Four preparations of interferon-α are available commercially.

Oral administration of interferons does not result in detectable serum levels. Interferons are therefore given intramuscularly, subcutaneously, intravenously, or by intralesional injection. Plasma levels are dose related, and CSF levels are about 1% of serum concentrations. Interferons, especially when given systemically rather than by intralesional injection, are associated with significant side effects. Most common is an influenza-like syndrome with fever, chills, headache, fatigue, myalgias, arthralgias, and dizziness. Major toxicities that limit the dose and duration of therapy are bone marrow suppression with neutropenia and thrombocytopenia; neurotoxicity with somnolence, confusion, behavioral disturbances, and depression; and cardiotoxicity with arrhythmias and cardiomyopathy. Interferons are also associated with thyroid dysfunction and autoimmune thyroiditis, abnormal liver function tests, hypertriglyceridemia, and impaired fertility in women.

 KEY POINTS

INTERFERONS

⊃ Interferons are glycoprotein cytokines made by cells in response to various stimuli.

⊃ Interferons have no direct activity against viruses. However, they induce cellular proteins that render cells resistant to viral infection.

⊃ Interferon-alfa (interferon-α) is approved for use in treatment of chronic hepatitis B, chronic hepatitis C, Kaposi's sarcoma in patients with AIDS, and condyloma acuminatum.

⊃ Major side effects, relatively low potency, and availability of alternative agents limit the wider applicability of interferons for treatment of viral infections.

SUGGESTED READING

Tilg H. New insights into the mechanisms of interferon-α: an immunoregulatory and anti-inflammatory cytokine. Gastroenterology 1997; 112: 1017-1021.

Woo MH, Burnakis TG. Interferon-α in the treatment of chronic viral hepatitis B and C. Ann Pharmacother 1997; 31: 330-337.

21 Fungal Infections and Antifungal Drug Therapy

AMAR SAFDAR, CHARLES S. BRYAN, JOHN R. GRAYBILL

Only about 150 of the nearly 250,000 identified species of fungi are known to cause disease in humans. Noninvasive, superficial fungal infections are relatively common in primary care. In recent years a near-exponential increase in the incidence of nosocomial fungal infections has occurred in the United States, attributed largely to the growing population of patients receiving immunosuppressive medications, broad-spectrum antibiotics, and indwelling intravascular devices. Opportunistic fungal infections may be seen initially in the primary care setting because of the trend toward outpatient, or ambulatory, management of high-risk patients. Primary care clinicians should also be familiar with the major regional mycoses (histoplasmosis, coccidioidomycosis, and blastomycosis) and with the major antifungal drugs.

SUGGESTED READING

Jacobs PH, Nall L, eds. Fungal diseases: biology, immunology, and diagnosis. New York: Marcel Dekker; 1997.
Jacobs PH, Nall L, eds. Antifungal drug therapy. New York: Marcel Dekker, 1990.
Richardson MD, Warnock DW. Fungal infections: diagnosis and management. New York: Blackwell Science; 1997.
Sarosi GA, Davies SF, eds. Fungal diseases of the lung. Philadelphia: Lippincott Williams & Wilkins; 2000.

Cutaneous and Mucocutaneous Fungal Infections: Overview

Fungal infections involving the skin and related structures are common and seen in all age groups. Tinea capitis is common in children, whereas tinea pedis is the most common fungal infection in adults. Cutaneous mycosis can lead to severe infection in immunocompromised persons. Dermatophytes and *Candida* species are the most common fungi affecting the skin and mucous membranes (Table 21-1). *Malassezia* species cause tinea versicolor and have also been implicated in the pathogenesis of seborrheic dermatitis. *Candida* species are common causes of nondermatophytic cutaneous infections in patients with certain risk factors, such as diabetes mellitus, prolonged corticosteroid therapy, severe burns, extended broad-spectrum antibiotic therapy, obesity, poor personal hygiene, and chronic skin maceration. Infrequently, systemic mycosis caused by *Fusarium, Aspergillus, Cryptococcus neoformans, Coccidioides immitis, Blastomyces dermatitidis,* and other fungi is manifested as skin lesions (see Chapter 7). Cutaneous manifestations from systemic mold infections are highly variable in appearance, and diagnostic skin biopsy is often required.

SUGGESTED READING

Goldstein AO, Smith KM, Ives TJ, et al. Mycotic infections: effective management of conditions involving the skin, hair, and nails. Geriatrics 2000; 55: 40-42, 45-47, 51-52.
Rudy SJ. Superficial fungal infections in children and adolescents. Nurse Pract Forum 1999; 10: 56-66.
Rupke SJ. Fungal skin disorders. Prim Care 2000; 27: 407-421.
Suhonen RE, Dawber RPR, Ellis D. Fungal infection of the skin, hair and nails. London: Martin Dunitz; 1999.

Fungal Infections of the Skin and Related Structures: Dermatophytosis

Dermatophytosis and cutaneous candidiasis are common in primary care and can be difficult to distinguish from each other.

Presentation and Progression
Cause

Dermatophytes are molds that cause disease by invading tissues containing keratin, namely the stratum corneum of the skin, hair, and nails. The three genera of medical importance are *Trichophyton, Microsporum,* and *Epidermophyton.*

TABLE 21-1
Dermatophytoses, Onychomycosis, and Other Superficial Mycoses

Diseases	Causative organisms	Clinical characteristics	Treatment
DERMATOPHYTOSES			
Tinea capitis (ringworm of scalp)	*Trichophyton tonsurans* (90% in U.S.); *Microsporum canis; Microsporum audouinii*	Noninflammatory scaling dermatosis of scalp with patchy alopecia, or inflammatory pustular lesions and regional lymphadenopathy.	Systemic agents: griseofulvin 500 mg b.i.d for 8 to 12 weeks; terbinafine 250 mg/day for 8 to 12 weeks; or itraconazole 5 mg/kg/day for 6 to 8 weeks. Topical sporicidal shampoo (in combination with systemic therapy): selenium sulfide 2.5%; ketoconazole; or zinc pyrithione
Tinea barbae	*Trichophyton verrucosum; Trichophyton mentagrophytes*	Inflammatory pustular folliculitis of beard and mustache area. Often heals with local scarring.	As above
Tinea faciei	*T. mentagrophytes; Trichophyton rubrum; M. canis*	Firm erythema, minimal scaling, involving face other than bearded area.	As above, for 2 to 4 weeks
Tinea corporis (ringworm)	*T. rubrum; T. mentagrophytes; M. canis; Epidermophyton floccosum*	Deep erythema with scaling, central clearing and well-demarcated margins. Minimal inflammatory response and often pruritic.	Topical agents: miconazole nitrate 2%, clotrimazole 1%, terbinafine %, or ketoconazole 2% for 2 to 4 weeks
Tinea cruris (jock itch)	*E. floccosum; T. rubrum; T. mentagrophytes*	Pruritic, well-demarcated scaly erythematous rash with central clearing. Involving inner thigh, perineum, and perianal areas; sparing scrotum, penis, and vagina.	As above, for 4 to 8 weeks
Tinea pedis (athlete's foot)	*E. floccosum; T. rubrum; T. mentagrophytes*	Interdigital web space maceration, fissures, erythema, and pruritus.	As above, for 8 to 12 weeks

Species that infect humans are classified as anthropophilic, geophilic, or zoophilic, depending on whether their major reservoir is humans, the soil, or animals.

The anthropophilic dermatophytes are acquired by close human contact, especially in the setting of disadvantaged socioeconomic situations such as overcrowding, poor personal hygiene, and malnutrition. Tinea capitis caused by *Trichophyton tonsurans* is an important example. *Trichophyton rubrum*, however, may be the most important organism of this group in most primary care practices. Anthropophilic dermatophytosis is usually of insidious onset, with minimal host inflammatory response.

The zoophilic dermatophytes are typically acquired by close household contact with animals, such as puppies and kittens. Children and young adults are often affected. Such exposure leads to infection involving the exposed body parts such as skin over the face and extremities. *Microsporum canis* and *Trichophyton mentagrophytes* are common examples.

The geophilic dermatophytes, such as *Microsporum gypseum, Microsporum fulvum,* and *Microsporum racemosum,*

tend to cause sporadic or incidental infections. These, along with zoophilic dermatophytic infections, are usually associated with an intense host inflammatory response.

Candida species also cause skin and nail infection that can be clinically indistinguishable from dermatophytosis. *Malassezia* species (previously known as *Pityrosporum* species) are lipophilic yeasts that commonly colonize the normal skin and occasionally cause infections (tinea versicolor and possibly seborrheic dermatitis) for reasons that are unclear.

Presentation

The most characteristic lesion of dermatophyte infection is an annular, scaling, erythematous patch. The margin is typically raised, and the central portion of the lesion shows less inflammation than the periphery. Dermatophyte lesions are usually called tinea (Latin for "gnawing worm") followed by reference to the anatomic region involved (Table 21-1). Tinea infections are sometimes difficult to recognize because of inappropriate use of medications, including steroid creams. Such lesions have been called tinea incognito.

TABLE 21-1—cont'd
Dermatophytoses, Onychomycosis, and Other Superficial Mycoses

Diseases	Causative organisms	Clinical characteristics	Treatment
ONYCHOMYCOSIS			
Tinea unguium	*T. rubrum; T. mentagrophytes;* (occasionally) *E. floccosum*	Multiple nails involved; hyperkeratosis, onycholysis, and nail thickening.	*Topical antifungals are not effective.* Itraconazole 200 mg daily or terbinafine 250 mg daily, for 6 weeks (fingernails) or 12 weeks (toenails)
Nondermatophytes: yeasts	*Candida* species	Single nail involvement; paronychia common.	Fluconazole 200 mg daily for 8 to 12 weeks (fingernails) or for 12 to 24 weeks (toenails)
Nondermatophytes: molds	*Acremonium, Aspergillus, Fusarium,* and *Scytahidium* species	Intense hyperkeratosis involving a single nail; onycholysis; nail thickening.	Itraconazole 200 mg daily for 8 to 12 weeks (fingernails) or for 12 to 24 weeks (toenails)
OTHERS			
Tinea versicolor	*Malassezia* species (*Pityrosporum* species*)*	Scaling dermatosis, hyperpigmentation or hypopigmentation involving trunk and upper extremities.	Topical agents: selenium sulfide shampoo (allowed to dry for 40 minutes before showering daily for 1 week); 1% clotrimazole cream b.i.d. for 3 to 4 weeks; 2% miconazole cream/solution b.i.d. for 3 to 4 weeks; 2% ketoconazole cream b.i.d. for 3 to 4 weeks Oral therapy (strongly resistant cases): ketoconazole 400 mg daily for 2 days
Seborrheic dermatitis	? *Malassezia* species (*Pityrosporum* species)	Red, greasy scaling rash involving central face, hairlines, ear, central chest, and back. Occasionally axillae and groin may be involved.	Topical agents: ketoconazole 2%; selenium sulfide; zinc pyrithione; mild steroid and keratolytic (such as salicylic acid or sulfur)

Tinea capitis (scalp ringworm) mainly affects children. Occasionally it affects elderly adults, in whom it may contribute to scarring alopecia (pseudopelade). The characteristic lesion is a noninflammatory scaling dermatosis with patchy alopecia. Two types of hair involvement are recognized: ectothrix and endothrix infections. In ectothrix infections, arthrospores are found on the outside of the hair shaft and the infected hairs tend to break off a few millimeters above the skin surface. In endothrix infections, spores are found within the hair itself and the infected hairs tend to break off at skin level, sometimes leaving stumps ("black-dot ringworm"). The involved area can become pustular, leading to a thick, exudative crust known as a kerion.

Tinea barbae (fungal infection of the neck and bearded area of the face) affects adults and usually consists of an inflammatory, pustular folliculitis that heals by local scarring. Tinea faciei (fungal infection of the nonbearded area of the face) usually causes pruritus and erythema with ill-defined margins.

Tinea corporis is found most often on the trunk and lower extremities. The classic lesion is a large, round or oval scaly plaque with a raised peripheral margin that contains papules or pustules, with less inflammation in the central portion. Lesions can be single or multiple. In some instances, and especially when *Trichophyton rubrum* is the causative mold, the lesions are poorly demarcated from the surrounding normal skin.

Tinea cruris (commonly known as jock itch) occurs mainly in young adult men and is characterized by a pruritic, well-demarcated, scaly erythematous rash with central clearing. When the disease occurs in women the lesions tend to be less well demarcated and sometimes involve the waist area. The inner thigh, perineum, and perianal areas are often involved, but the scrotum, penis, and vagina are usually spared.

Tinea pedis (athlete's foot) occurs mainly in adolescents and young adults who have used common shower facilities. Itching occurs between the toes or on the undersurface of the lateral aspects of the toes. Cracks and fissures develop in the skin, which can become macerated. The infection sometimes spreads to involve the dorsum of the feet. When *T. rubrum* is the causative mold, the infection may involve the lateral aspects of the feet and sometimes the entire sole.

Tinea manuum refers to dermatophytosis involving the hand, usually on the palmar surface and usually caused by *T. rubrum.* In some patients the soles are involved as well. Tinea manuum is usually unilateral.

Onychomycosis of the nails (tinea unguium) affects people of any age but is more common in older persons. In a recent study, culture-confirmed onychomycosis of the toenails was identified in 9% of patients and was more common in older men. Usually the skin adjacent to the nail is infected. The pattern of involvement of the nail plate varies according to the direction from which fungal invasion of the nail takes place. Most often, fungi invade the nail from the distal and lateral borders, leading to a subungual ("beneath the nail") onychomycosis. The nail plate becomes thickened and discolored (white, yellow, or brown). Less commonly, fungi invade the nail plate from its top surface, which becomes covered with white plaques. The least common pattern of invasion is from the proximal aspect of the nail plate. Non-*Candida* onychomycoses caused by *Acremonium, Aspergillus,* or *Fusarium* species are indistinguishable in appearance. Involvement of a single nail and accompanying paronychia are highly suggestive of nondermatophyte infection.

Tinea versicolor (pityriasis versicolor) is a scaling dermatosis with nonpruritic hyperpigmented or hypopigmented macules and plaques found most typically over the trunk and proximal aspects of the extremities.

Diagnosis

Microscopic examination of a potassium hydroxide (KOH) preparation of skin scrapings, nail scrapings, or hair strands often enables visualization of fungal hyphae and spores, leading to a rapid office diagnosis. Examination of the face and scalp with Wood's lamp is another method for rapid diagnosis in the outpatient setting. However, fungal cultures are necessary to identify species that may determine mode of transmission and help in the selection of appropriate therapy. Methods of diagnosis based on the polymerase chain reaction (PCR) are being developed.

Tinea capitis must be distinguished from seborrheic dermatitis. Seborrheic dermatitis usually affects older children, adolescents, or adults rather than young children. Moreover, it does not lead to hair loss. Tinea capitis must also be distinguished from alopecia areata, a skin disease with localized areas of hair loss. However, alopecia areata does not feature scaling lesions.

Tinea barbae must be distinguished from sycosis barbae, which also causes a pustular folliculitis of the bearded area of the face. Sycosis barbae is usually caused by *Staphylococcus aureus* and tends to be more localized than tinea barbae. Rarely, candidiasis causes a folliculitis-mimicking tinea barbae (folliculitis barbae candidomycetica). Tinea faciei can be difficult to recognize because of its indistinct borders and because commonly prescribed steroid creams mask the inflammatory response (tinea incognito).

Tinea corporis must be distinguished from nummular eczema, annular erythema, and psoriasis. Features that point to tinea corporis include the scaling margin of the lesion and the follicular prominence, but skin scrapings for KOH preparation and fungal culture are strongly advised. Tinea corporis is often confused with other skin diseases, especially when caused by *T. rubrum.*

Tinea cruris must be distinguished from candidiasis involving the groin. Candidiasis, but not tinea cruris, characteristi-

cally features small "satellite" pustules beyond the demarcation of the main body of the rash from the normal skin. Also, and in contrast to tinea cruris, candidiasis frequently involves the penis, scrotum, and vagina.

Tinea pedis must be distinguished from other pathogens that can cause the symptoms and signs of athlete's foot. These include *Corynebacterium minutissimum* (erythrasma), aerobic gram-negative rods (especially *Pseudomonas* and *Proteus* species), *S. aureus,* and fungi other than the dermatophytes. Bacterial cultures obtained from areas of fissuring and maceration can, however, be misleading because colonization of the lesions of tinea pedis is inevitable.

Tinea manuum must be distinguished from eczema. Eczema, however, is usually unilateral. Superinfection with dermatophytes often occurs in patients with tylosis (palmoplantar keratoderma).

Skin and nail *Candida* infections can be clinically indistinguishable from dermatophytosis. Yeast skin infections, however, tend to have ill-defined margins and satellite lesions and, unlike tinea cruris, commonly involve the scrotum, penis, and vulva.

Tinea versicolor (pityriasis versicolor) is often diagnosed on the basis of the typical appearance of the nonpruritic macules or plaques. Yellow-green fluorescence may occur under Wood's light, but the diagnosis is most easily confirmed by finding the typical "spaghetti and meatballs" fungal elements on microscopic examination of a KOH preparation of skin lesions.

Natural History

Tinea capitis, if untreated, usually remits after puberty. Hair loss is seldom permanent. Some of the other tinea infections tend to resolve spontaneously, but more commonly the lesions become chronic.

Treatment
Methods

Newer antifungal drugs have simplified the treatment and improved the prognosis for many of the common fungal infections of the skin and its related structures (Table 21-1). Topical therapy is often successful against dermatophytosis that does not involve the hair or nails. The allylamines (such as terbinafine) seem to be slightly more effective than the azole compounds (such as ketoconazole) but are also more expensive. Hair and nail dermatophytosis often requires systemic therapy because topical agents are ineffective. Duration of treatment was longer (6 to 12 months) with fungiostatic agents such as griseofulvin. However, since the introduction of itraconazole and terbinafine, which exhibit greater affinity for nail tissue, 6 weeks of therapy for fingernails to 12 weeks of therapy for toenails is often curative. Griseofulvin is still considered the systemic drug of choice for children, pending careful studies of the safety of the newer agents.

Expected Outcome

Treatment with the newer antifungal drugs is usually successful, although relapse occurs. Cure rates for onychomycosis of 70% to 80% have been reported with terbinafine, but relapse occurs in up to 40% of patients.

When to Refer

Difficult cases of dermatophytosis are often best managed by a dermatologist.

KEY POINTS

FUNGAL INFECTIONS OF THE SKIN AND RELATED STRUCTURES: DERMATOPHYTOSIS

⊃ Dermatophytes are molds that infect keratin in the stratum corneum of the epidermis, hair, and nails.

⊃ Dermatophyte infections are usually called "tinea," followed by reference to the region involved.

⊃ Tinea infections that are difficult to recognize, often because steroid creams have been used inappropriately, are sometimes called tinea incognito.

⊃ Tinea capitis (scalp ringworm) usually occurs in children and generally consists of a noninflammatory dermatosis with patchy alopecia.

⊃ Tinea barbae consists of an inflammatory pustular folliculitis of the neck, beard, and mustache area. It is usually more localized than sycosis barbae caused by *S. aureus.*

⊃ Tinea faciei consists of erythema with minimal scaling involving the nonbearded areas of the face. It can be difficult to recognize (tinea incognito).

⊃ Tinea corporis (body ringworm) usually presents as one or more round or oval scaly, erythematous plaques with raised margins over the trunk and extremities. When *T. rubrum* is the pathogen, the margins can be indistinct, leading to confusion with other skin diseases.

⊃ Tinea cruris (jock itch) must be distinguished from candidiasis. In candidiasis, but not in tinea cruris, satellite pustules sometimes form beyond the demarcation between inflamed and normal skin. The penis, scrotum, and vagina tend to be involved in candidiasis but not in tinea cruris.

⊃ Tinea pedis (athlete's foot) typically appears as itching with cracking and fissuring between the toes. Bacteria and other molds sometimes cause the same syndrome.

⊃ Tinea manuum (dermatophytosis involving the hand) is usually caused by *T. rubrum* and affects the palm. It must be distinguished from eczema and palmoplantar keratoderma (tylosis), in which superinfection with dermatophytes commonly occurs.

⊃ Skin and nail *Candida* infection can be clinically indistinguishable from dermatophytosis. Yeast skin infections, however, tend to have ill-defined margins and satellite lesions.

⊃ Onychomycosis due to dermatophytes typically involves multiple nails, with nail thickening and onycholysis.

⊃ Treatment of fungal infections of the skin and its supportive structures has been greatly improved in recent years on account of the introduction of new antifungal drugs such as the azole antifungal compounds and terbinafine.

SUGGESTED READING

Drake LA, Shear NH, Arlette JP, et al. Oral terbinafine in the treatment of toe nail onychomycosis: North American multicenter trial. J Am Acad Dermatol 1997; 37: 740-745.

Gupta AK, Einarson TR, Summerbell RC, et al. An overview of topical antifungal therapy in dermatomycoses: a North American perspective. Drugs 1998; 55: 645-674.

Liu V, Mackool BT. Current diagnosis and management of chronic fungal infection of the feet and nails. Curr Clin Top Infect Dis 1999; 19: 305-326.

Rodgers P, Bassler M. Treating onychomycosis. Am Fam Physician 2001; 63: 663-672, 677-678.

Summerbell RC. Epidemiology and ecology of onychomycosis. Dermatology 1997; 194 (Suppl 1): 32-36.

Mucocutaneous Candidiasis

Mucocutaneous candidiasis is a common problem in primary care.

Presentation and Progression
Cause

Candida species are ubiquitous in the environment as unicellular yeasts. They are present in soil, inanimate objects, and food. *Candida* species are part of cutaneous, oropharyngeal, gastrointestinal, and vaginal microflora. Most *Candida* infections are thought to arise from the patient's own flora. However, person-to-person transmission may occur.

Among the nearly 150 species of *Candida, Candida albicans* is most frequently associated with human infection. The frequency of oropharyngeal and vaginal yeast infections caused by *Candida* species other than *C. albicans* is increasing. The following *Candida* species may be encountered: *C. parapsilosis, C. tropicalis, C. glabrata, C. krusei, C. lusitaniae, C. guilliermondi,* and the recently identified *C. dubliniensis.* Factors that predispose individuals to superficial candidiasis include poor hygiene, chronic skin maceration, obesity, diabetes mellitus, burns, prolonged broad-spectrum antibiotic exposure, and cellular immune dysfunction.

Presentation

The following are the common clinical diseases associated with nonsystemic candidiasis.

Oral Candidiasis. Oral candidiasis can be manifested in a number of ways. The most characteristic is thrush, the presence of thick, white, cottage cheese–like or curdlike patches on the tongue and buccal mucosa. Removal of these patches by scraping reveals a raw, bleeding epithelial surface. Thrush is seen most commonly in patients who have received inhaled steroids or broad-spectrum antibiotics and in patients with advanced HIV disease or acquired immunodeficiency syndrome (AIDS). The other forms of oral candidiasis are chronic atrophic candidiasis ("denture sore mouth") in patients with dental plates, appearing as chronic inflammation; acute atrophic candidiasis, appearing as atrophy of the tongue; erosive candidiasis, occurring as shallow ulcerations and usually found in persons with HIV disease; angular cheilitis (inflammation at the corners of the mouth, from *Candida* and other causes); and *Candida* leukoplakia (white plaques on the cheek, lips, and tongue).

Candida Esophagitis. This disease usually occurs in patients with advanced HIV disease or malignancy. The major symptoms are central chest pain, odynophagia, and dysphagia.

Vulvovaginal Candidiasis. An extremely common problem (see Chapter 5), vulvovaginal candidiasis is most commonly associated with antibiotic therapy, pregnancy, and diabetes mellitus. However, an estimated 75% of women have this infection at some point during their lives. The most characteristic form is a thick, white, cottage cheese–like or curdlike discharge somewhat reminiscent of the lesions of thrush. However, the discharge can be scanty. Intense pruritus is nearly always present.

Intertrigo. This common skin infection caused by *Candida* typically involves skin folds, affecting areas under the breast, perineum, and abdominal wall. The warm, moist environment of these areas promotes invasion of the epidermis by the yeast cells. The process begins as vesicopustules that rupture, leading to maceration and fissuring of the skin. Satellite lesions are commonly seen beyond the advancing border of the rash.

Candida Folliculitis. Sometimes affecting the beard area, *Candida* folliculitis must be distinguished from tinea barbae and sycosis barbae (see preceding discussion). Widespread *Candida* folliculitis sometimes occurs in severely ill patients who have received multiple antibiotics. Secondary streptococcal and staphylococcal bacterial infections can occur.

Candida Balanitis. This form of candidiasis usually begins as vesicles on the penis that evolve into pruritic patches and often spread to the scrotum, perineum, and buttocks.

Chronic Mucocutaneous Candidiasis. This chronic, relapsing, or refractory infection involves the skin and mucous membranes, including the esophagus. It often leads to scarring and irreversible disfigurement. It most often presents in infancy as a congenital immunodeficiency syndrome involving a selective defect in T-lymphocyte response to *Candida* antigens. It is rarely encountered in persons over the age of 30 years.

Other Syndromes. Mucocutaneous candidiasis also occurs as diaper rash in infants, perianal candidiasis (as a cause of pruritus ani), and generalized cutaneous candidiasis, an uncommon infection occasionally seen in both children and adults.

Diagnosis

Candida species can be readily identified microscopically (KOH preparation, Gram stain, and other methods) and by culture. However, identification of *Candida* must be correlated with clinical findings because these yeasts can be a prominent part of the normal flora. Serologic tests and demonstration of *Candida* DNA by PCR are not helpful.

Thrush is usually diagnosed on the basis of the clinical appearance. The diagnosis can be confirmed by recognizing masses of hyphae, pseudohyphae, and yeast forms on a KOH preparation or Gram stain of material obtained by scraping. Culture is of no value in diagnosis. Thrush, if unexplained, is an indication for testing for HIV-1 antibodies.

Candida esophagitis, when suspected in a patient with HIV disease or cancer on the basis of such symptoms as substernal pain and odynophagia, is now usually diagnosed on the basis of response to a therapeutic trial of antifungal drugs such as fluconazole. Endoscopy is generally reserved for patients who fail to respond. Herpes simplex infection and nonspecific "aphthous" ulceration of the esophagus are other diagnostic considerations.

Vulvovaginal candidiasis must be distinguished from the other major causes of vaginitis (see Chapters 5 and 16).

Natural History
Expected Outcome

In immunocompetent hosts most of the syndromes of mucocutaneous candidiasis are self-limited, although relapse is common. Chronic mucocutaneous candidiasis is a persistent, disfiguring disease. Untreated *Candida* esophagitis in AIDS patients is uniformly fatal.

Treatment
Methods

Treatment of candidiasis has been simplified by the introduction of potent new antifungal drugs, notably triazole-based compounds such as fluconazole and itraconazole.

For thrush, topical therapy with clotrimazole troches 10 mg five times daily or nystatin 500,000 units q.i.d. for 7 to 14 days is usually effective. For persistent infections systemic therapy with azoles is recommended; examples are fluconazole 100 mg daily or itraconazole 200 mg daily for 7 to 14 days. In azole-refractory disease, parenteral amphotericin B 0.3 mg/kg/day may be necessary. For thrush related to dentures, careful disinfection of the dentures is critical to preventing relapse.

For esophageal candidiasis, topical antifungal therapy is not recommended. Treatment with fluconazole 100 mg daily or itraconazole 200 mg daily for 14 to 21 days is effective. In azole-refractory cases, parenteral amphotericin B 0.3 to 0.7 mg/kg/day is recommended.

For vulvovaginal candidiasis, topical treatment with several regimens of oral fluconazole is usually effective (see Chapter 5 for a full discussion).

For chronic mucocutaneous candidiasis, topical antifungal therapy has little benefit. Response to amphotericin B 0.4 to 0.7 mg/kg/day is slow and modest. Triazole-based agents have been used successfully, and treatment is often continued for years in an effort to prevent relapse.

Expected Results

Response to therapy in immunocompetent hosts is usually excellent.

When to Refer

Patients with refractory mucocutaneous candidiasis may benefit from referral.

 KEY POINTS

MUCOCUTANEOUS CANDIDIASIS

⊃ Of the nearly 150 species of *Candida, C. albicans* most commonly causes disease in humans. Other species are assuming importance, however, especially in the hospital setting.

⊃ Thrush is the most typical form of oral candidiasis and appears as white, curdlike patches on the buccal mucosa and tongue. Its recognition should prompt testing for HIV-1 antibodies. Other forms of oral candidiasis include chronic atrophic candidiasis ("denture sore mouth"), angular cheilitis, and *Candida* leukoplakia.

⊃ *Candida* esophagitis, manifested as chest pain and odynophagia, is seen most commonly in patients with advanced HIV disease or cancer.

⊃ Vulvovaginal candidiasis, which may affect up to 75% of women during their lifetimes, classically occurs with a white, curdlike discharge somewhat reminiscent of thrush. However, the discharge is often scanty.

⊃ Other syndromes of candidiasis are intertrigo, folliculitis, and balanitis.

⊃ Treatment of candidiasis has been simplified by the introduction of potent new agents such as the triazole-based antifungals. However, the possible emergence of drug resistance is a concern.

SUGGESTED READING

del Palacio A, Cuetara S, Garau M, et al. Topical treatment of dermatophytosis and cutaneous candidosis with flutrimazole 1% cream: double-blind, randomized comparative trial with ketoconazole 2% cream. Mycoses 1999; 42: 649-655.

Glick M, Siegel MA. Viral and fungal infections of the oral cavity in immunocompetent patients. Infect Dis Clin North Am 1999; 13: 817-831.

Rex JH, Walsh TJ, Sobel JD, et al. Infectious Diseases Society of America. Practice guidelines for the treatment of candidiasis. Clin Infect Dis 2000; 30: 662-678.

Histoplasmosis

Histoplasmosis is a fungal disease endemic to the Ohio and Mississippi river valleys. The infection is usually asymptomatic. Pulmonary infection and disseminated disease may occur. Dissemination is more common in the elderly, infants, and immunocompromised individuals. Multiorgan involvement may lead to significant morbidity and mortality.

Presentation and Progression
Cause

Histoplasma capsulatum is a dimorphic fungus endemic to soil of the Ohio and Mississippi river valleys but occasionally found throughout much of the world. Infection is acquired by inhalation of spores or rarely by direct inoculation. Bird droppings and bat guano in soil promote sporulation of *H. capsulatum,* and poorly ventilated spaces promote inhalation. Exploration of caves, archaeologic sites, or abandoned buildings therefore increases the risk of infection. Many outbreaks of acute histoplasmosis have been described; a typical scenario is acute disease in a community where soil underneath blackbird or starling roosts has been disturbed by bulldozing. Immunocompromised patients, especially those with advanced HIV disease, are at risk for disseminated histoplasmosis.

Presentation

In endemic areas most of the population acquires histoplasmosis without symptoms or with only a vague, flulike illness. Less than 10% of patients come to medical attention. The major syndromes of histoplasmosis are as follows.

Acute Pulmonary Histoplasmosis. This type of histoplasmosis typically occurs in persons exposed to large numbers of spores. Symptoms include cough, chest pain, fever, and arthralgias. Erythema nodosum or erythema multiforme is present in about 5% of patients, especially women. Physical examination usually shows few if any abnormalities. Chest x-ray examination may reveal one or a few patchy infiltrates. Hilar lymphadenopathy is often present. In patients who have inhaled massive numbers of spores, especially if they have some degree of immunity from previous exposure to *H. capsulatum,* widespread pneumonitis may develop in a miliary pattern that heals with a "buckshot" pattern of calcification throughout the lung fields.

Acute Pericarditis. Among patients with symptomatic acute histoplasmosis, acute pericarditis occurs in 5% to 10% and is commonly manifested as fever and precordial pain. About 75% of affected patients have a pericardial friction rub on physical examination.

Mediastinal Lymphadenopathy. Mediastinal lymphadenopathy frequently complicates acute histoplasmosis and occasionally becomes symptomatic. Compression of airways by enlarged lymph nodes predisposes patients to pneumonia and bronchiectasis. Mediastinal lymphadenopathy often evokes suspicion of malignancy, prompting unnecessary surgery. Mediastinal fibrosis (also known as fibrosing mediastinitis) may occur and cause progressive invasion and occlusion of the mediastinal great vessels and airways. Mediastinoscopy with biopsy in this setting can be dangerous because the fibrosis that is sometimes present may encase blood vessels and thus predispose patients to massive bleeding.

Histoplasmoma. Another complication of acute histoplasmosis, histoplasmoma begins as a coin lesion that gradually enlarges. Demonstration of a central core of calcification helps distinguish this lesion from malignancy.

Cavitary Pulmonary Histoplasmosis. This syndrome usually affects persons with underlying chronic obstructive pulmonary disease (COPD), especially men. The cavities are nearly always in the upper lobes, at least initially, and are associated with low-grade fever, dyspnea, productive cough, weight loss, and less frequently night sweats and hemoptysis.

Progressive Disseminated Histoplasmosis. This form of histoplasmosis is classified as acute, subacute, or chronic. Acute progressive disseminated histoplasmosis is seen mainly in immunocompromised patients, especially those with advanced HIV disease. Findings include fever, weight loss, lymphadenopathy, hepatosplenomegaly, skin and mucosal lesions (see Chapter 7), anemia, leukopenia, thrombocytopenia, and abnormal liver function tests. Chest x-ray films frequently show patchy pneumonitis with hilar lymphadenopathy. Multiorgan failure with shock occurs in severe cases.

Subacute progressive disseminated histoplasmosis is by definition a more subtle illness. Clinical features include oral ulcers that can easily be mistaken for malignancy (see Chapter 7), gastrointestinal ulcers, chronic meningitis and other central nervous system (CNS) syndromes, and adrenal insufficiency. Laboratory abnormalities are similar to those in the acute form of the disease but tend to be less striking.

Chronic progressive disseminated histoplasmosis presents with fever and malaise. A deep, painless mouth ulcer is found in about 50% of cases and is an important clue to diagnosis.

Histoplasmosis, like tuberculosis, can affect nearly every organ. Ocular histoplasmosis is relatively common in endemic zones.

Diagnosis

Definitive diagnosis depends on isolation and identification of *H. capsulatum* in cultures. Sputum cultures appear to be the least sensitive, except in patients with cavitary lesions. Cultures performed on bronchial specimens yield the organism in most severely immunocompromised patients (about 90%). Blood and bone marrow cultures are helpful in patients with disseminated infection but are positive in only about one half of instances. Detection of antibodies to *H. capsulatum* is useful in all forms of histoplasmosis, but nearly 50% of immunosuppressed patients are unable to form detectable antibody responses. Complement fixation (CF) serial dilution titers are commonly used. Titers >1:8 suggest acute infection, and titers ≥1:32 are consistent with systemic dissemination. Rarely, in overwhelming infections, as in patients with HIV disease, *H. capsulatum* can be visualized on peripheral blood smear (Figure 21-1).

Demonstration of *H. capsulatum* polysaccharide antigen in urine and serum is now widely used for diagnosis. The sensitivity is highest (90%) in the presence of a large yeast burden, as occurs in progressive disseminated histoplasmosis. In cases without clinically apparent dissemination, such as acute pulmonary histoplasmosis, the urine antigen test is often negative (80%). Even with cavitary pneumonia the diagnostic yield is <50%. Monitoring of the antigen level is used as a guide to therapeutic response and also for surveillance for relapse.

Natural History
Expected Outcome

Acute pulmonary histoplasmosis heals spontaneously in most cases without treatment. Cavitary pulmonary histoplasmosis is usually a slowly progressive disease. Many of the cavities (10% to 60%) resolve spontaneously; death usually results from the underlying lung disease or from pneumonia. Disseminated histoplasmosis has a high mortality rate (83% to 100%) if untreated.

Treatment
Methods

Asymptomatic infection does not need treatment. Acute pulmonary histoplasmosis with mild symptoms heals spontaneously. Treatment should be reserved for moderately symptomatic acute pulmonary histoplasmosis and for disseminated infections, in which the Infectious Diseases Society of America (IDSA) guidelines should be consulted. Diffuse pulmonary histoplasmosis in an immunocompromised host and severe progressive disseminated histoplasmosis are treated with amphotericin B. Itraconazole can be useful for chronic pulmonary histoplasmosis and for less severe cases of progressive disseminated histoplasmosis.

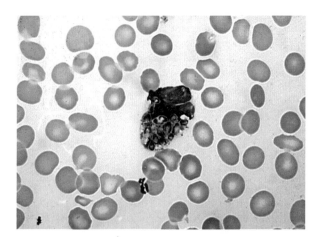

FIG. 21-1 Yeast cells consistent with *Histoplasma capsulatum* within the cytoplasm of a neutrophil on a peripheral blood leukocyte in a patient with advanced human immunodeficiency virus disease. (Courtesy of Dr. Bosko Postic.)

Treatment of patients with granulomatous mediastinitis is problematic. Itraconazole or amphotericin B is often used for those with severe obstructive symptoms. Surgery can be useful but is often technically difficult.

Expected Response

With treatment the mortality rate is decreased to 7% for disseminated histoplasmosis.

When to Refer

All patients with acute disseminated histoplasmosis should be hospitalized. Patients with suspected progressive disseminated histoplasmosis should usually be referred for diagnostic procedures.

 KEY POINTS

HISTOPLASMOSIS

⊃ Histoplasmosis is highly endemic in the soil of the Ohio and Mississippi river valleys, but occasionally it is found elsewhere.

⊃ Acute pulmonary histoplasmosis is usually a mild illness and comes to medical attention in <10% of cases, but it can cause high fever with headache, chest pain, and nonproductive cough. Chest x-ray films generally show patchy infiltrates.

⊃ Mediastinal lymphadenopathy often develops after acute histoplasmosis, and it can prompt unnecessary surgical exploration if the possibility of histoplasmosis is not considered.

⊃ Healed pulmonary histoplasmosis typically leaves pulmonary calcifications similar to healed tuberculosis. Inhalation of massive numbers of spores, especially if previous infection has conferred some degree of immunity, can cause miliary granulomatosis of the lungs that heals leaving a "buckshot" pattern of calcification.

⊃ Acute progressive disseminated histoplasmosis should be suspected in immunocompromised patients, especially those with HIV infection. If the disease is untreated, the mortality rate is 83% to 100%.

⊃ Subacute progressive disseminated histoplasmosis should be suspected in patients with combinations of fever, weight loss, localizing symptoms (e.g., symptoms pointing to the gastrointestinal tract or CNS), hepatosplenomegaly, mouth ulcers, and cytopenias.

⊃ Definitive diagnosis of histoplasmosis occurs by fungal culture.

⊃ Demonstration of the *H. capsulatum* polysaccharide antigen in urine and serum has become a valuable aid to diagnosis; the test is positive in up to 90% of patients with progressive disseminated histoplasmosis.

SUGGESTED READING

Bonifaz A, Cansela R, Novales J, et al. Cutaneous histoplasmosis associated with acquired immunodeficiency syndrome (AIDS). Int J Dermatol 2000; 39: 35-38.

Wheat LJ, Chetchotisakd P, Williams B, et al. Factors associated with severe manifestations of histoplasmosis in AIDS. Clin Infect Dis 2000; 30: 877-881.

Wheat J, Sarosi G, McKinsey D, et al. Infectious Diseases Society of America. Practice guidelines for the management of patients with histoplasmosis. Clin Infect Dis 2000; 30: 688-695.

Coccidioidomycosis

Coccidioidomycosis is a systemic fungal infection endemic to the southwestern United States and parts of Central and South America. It is especially prevalent in southern Arizona, central California, southern New Mexico, and western Texas. An estimated 100,000 new cases of coccidioidomycosis occur in the United States each year. Most of these (50% to 70%) are subclinical, and most of the clinically apparent infections are mild, but disseminated disease develops occasionally. As in histoplasmosis, disseminated coccidioidomycosis is more common in immunosuppressed patients, including those with advanced HIV disease.

Presentation and Progression
Cause

The etiologic agent of coccidioidomycosis is *C. immitis,* a dimorphic fungus confined to a few arid regions of the Western Hemisphere. Transmission to humans occurs through the inhalation of spores. Animals and the soil serve as sources of infection. Disseminated disease is more common in patients of African-American or Filipino decent. Other risk factors for dissemination are pregnancy, AIDS, hematologic malignancy, and organ or bone marrow transplantation.

Presentation

Mild symptoms of cough, malaise, chest pain, headache, and sore throat are common during the acute pulmonary infection, which is often self-limited. A nonpruritic papular rash sometimes occurs early in the illness, and some patients lose weight. Erythema nodosum and erythema multiforme occur occasionally, especially in women; the combination of fever, arthralgia, and erythema nodosum is known as desert fever. Laboratory evaluation often reveals an elevated erythrocyte sedimentation rate and eosinophilia. Chest x-ray examination frequently reveals patchy infiltrates, hilar lymphadenopathy, and pleural effusions. Some patients (about 8%) have thin-walled pulmonary cavities when first seen, and others (about 4%) have pulmonary nodules. Occasional patients, especially those with advanced HIV disease, have diffuse, life-threatening pneumonia with symptoms and signs suggesting septic shock. Chronic fibrocavitary pneumonia develops in a few patients, mainly those with underlying lung disease.

Disseminated infection may occur in the first few months of infection and is clinically apparent in about 0.5% of all infections. Disseminated infection may involve the skin, bone, joints, and CNS. Various skin lesions are encountered (see Chapter 7). Arthritis (especially of the knee) and osteomyelitis (especially of the vertebrae) are common sites of dissemination. The most feared complication is chronic meningitis, which develops within 6 weeks to 6 months of the acute infection and manifests itself by combinations of headache, vomiting, altered mental status, and cerebrospinal fluid (CSF) abnormalities.

Diagnosis

The diagnosis is usually suspected on the basis of the clinical presentation in a person who resides in or who has visited an endemic area. Recent reports highlight the need to consider coccidioidomycosis in travelers returning from the southwestern United States.

Definitive diagnosis is made by culture. Diagnosis can also be made by finding the pathognomonic spherules in bronchoalveolar lavage fluid or in biopsy specimens from lung, lymph node, or skin. Serologic diagnosis is based on an IgM-induced tube precipitin (TP) test, which is positive within 2 to 3 weeks after an acute infection. An IgG-based CF test is also commonly used. A high CF titer ($\geq$1:32) is consistent with disseminated infection. The CF titer is often used to monitor the response to treatment. The spherule-derived coccidioidin skin test remains positive for life and does not aid in diagnosis. Patients with systemic coccidioidomycosis may remain nonreactive to the skin test, and the presence of anergy is associated with a poor outcome.

Natural History
Expected Outcome

Acute pulmonary disease resolves spontaneously. About 50% of pulmonary cavities resolve spontaneously within 2 years. However, 50% of disseminated infections are fatal without treatment. Untreated coccidioidomycosis with meningeal involvement is uniformly fatal.

Treatment
Methods

Most acute pulmonary infections are self-limited and do not require treatment. However, periodic follow-up is important for patients with persistent pulmonary disease, including those with solitary lung nodules. Long-term antifungal drug therapy is indicated for patients with progressive, nonresolving pulmonary infection, meningeal involvement, systemic dissemination, and compromised cellular immune function. Options include amphotericin B 0.5 to 0.7 mg/kg/day, ketoconazole 400 to 800 mg daily, and fluconazole 400 to 800 mg daily. Itraconazole appears to be at least as effective as fluconazole for nonmeningeal coccidioidomycosis, but fluconazole is preferred for treatment for coccidioidal meningitis. The IDSA guidelines for management of coccidioidomycosis contain specific recommendations for methods and duration of therapy for the various syndromes of coccidioidomycosis.

Expected Response

The cure rate of coccidioidomycosis with amphotericin B is 50% to 70% with frequent relapses. The response rate to fluconazole and itraconazole is about 60%. For this reason treatment is aimed at remission instead of cure.

When to Refer

Patients with complications of coccidioidomycosis should be referred to a physician familiar with the subtleties of this difficult-to-treat disease.

 KEY POINTS

COCCIDIOIDOMYCOSIS
- Coccidioidomycosis is endemic in the southwestern United States and parts of Central and South America.
- It should be considered in the diagnosis of disease in tourists and other returning travelers.

⊃ The most common clinical presentation of primary infection is a mild, self-limited pulmonary illness. Laboratory findings may include an elevated erythrocyte sedimentation rate and eosinophilia. Chest x-ray examination often reveals patchy infiltrates with hilar lymphadenopathy, and pleural effusions, thin-walled cavities, or pulmonary nodules sometimes develop. Occasionally, especially in patients with advanced HIV disease, the primary infection appears as an acute diffuse pneumonia with respiratory failure.

⊃ Dissemination of coccidioidomycosis may involve the skin, bone, joints, and CNS.

⊃ Skin findings of disseminated coccidioidomycosis include papules, nodules, plaques, or ulcers.

⊃ Treatment of disseminated infection with amphotericin B should be instituted early to prevent significant morbidity and mortality.

SUGGESTED READING

Arsura EL, Kilgore WB. Miliary coccidioidomycosis in the immunocompetent. Chest 2000; 117: 404-409.

Cairns L, Blythe D, Kao A, et al. Outbreak of coccidioidomycosis in Washington State residents returning from Mexico. Clin Infect Dis 2000; 30: 61-64.

Chaturvedi V, Ramani R, Gromadzki S, et al. Coccidioidomycosis in New York State. Emerg Infect Dis 2000; 6: 25-29.

Galgiani JN, Ampel NM, Catanzaro A, et al. Infectious Diseases Society of America. Practice guideline for the treatment of coccidioidomycosis. Clin Infect Dis 2000; 30: 658-661.

Galgiani JN, Catanzaro A, Cloud GA, et al. Comparison of oral fluconazole and itraconazole for progressive, nonmeningeal coccidioidomycosis: a randomized, double blind trial. Ann Intern Med 2000; 133: 676-686.

Leake JA, Mosley DG, England B, et al. Risk factors for acute symptomatic coccidioidomycosis among elderly persons in Arizona. J Infect Dis 2000; 181: 1435-1440.

Rosenstein NE, Emery KW, Werner SB, et al. Risk factors for severe pulmonary and disseminated coccidioidomycosis: Kern County, California, 1995-1996. Clin Infect Dis 2001; 32: 708-715.

North American Blastomycosis

Blastomycosis is a fungal infection endemic to the Mississippi and Ohio river basins. The infection is asymptomatic in nearly one half of patients. If symptoms do occur, they are usually pulmonary. Skin disease, the most common extrapulmonary manifestation, may signal more extensive disease.

Presentation and Progression
Cause

The causative agent, *Blastomyces dermatitidis,* is a thermally dimorphic fungus. Its habitat is believed to be the soil. Transmission usually occurs by the inhalation of spores. The fungus may remain isolated in the lung or may disseminate through the bloodstream. The most common sites of dissemination are the skin, bone, genitourinary tract, and CNS. Direct inoculation rarely occurs.

Presentation

Nearly one half of all cases are asymptomatic. Initial symptoms may include fever, cough, chest discomfort, hemoptysis, and skin lesions. Acute pulmonary blastomycosis can be easily mistaken for influenza or community-acquired pneumonia. Pleural effusions and hilar lymphadenopathy are uncommon. When pulmonary blastomycosis is diagnosed, a slowly progressive chronic pneumonia is the usual presentation. The upper lobes are involved more often than the lower, and chest x-ray examination can suggest bronchogenic carcinoma. Extrapulmonary complications occur in 20% to 40% of cases. A variety of skin lesions may be present. The most characteristic fully developed lesion is a hyperkeratotic plaque that may show central ulceration or scarring and often occurs on the face or extremities (see Chapter 7). Patients with skin involvement commonly have involvement of multiple organs. Skeletal blastomycosis results in osteolytic lesions, paraspinous abscesses, osteomyelitis, and arthritis. Genitourinary involvement is manifested as urinary obstruction, pyuria, and prostatitis. Meningitis and brain lesions, including abscess, are relatively common (up to 40%) in patients with compromised immunity owing to cancer or AIDS.

Diagnosis

The most rapid method of diagnosis is visualization of budding yeast on KOH mounts of pus, skin scrapings, or sputum. The budding yeasts of *B. dermatitidis* have two distinctive characteristics: a refractile cell wall and a single, broad-based daughter yeast (in contrast to the narrow-based daughter cells of most budding yeasts, such as *H. capsulatum*). Serologic evaluation for acute and chronic blastomycosis is not recommended.

Natural History
Expected Outcome

Some patients with blastomycosis recover spontaneously, especially those with self-limited pulmonary disease. However, most patients in whom blastomycosis is diagnosed require therapy. Rarely, pulmonary blastomycosis leads to adult respiratory distress syndrome (ARDS) and death.

Treatment
Methods

Taking itraconazole 200 to 400 mg PO once daily for 6 months is generally adequate therapy for patients who are not seriously ill and who do not have CNS infection. Seriously ill patients, including immunocompromised patients with severe lung disease and all patients with CNS blastomycosis, should be treated with amphotericin B in accordance with the IDSA guidelines. Amphotericin B is the only drug approved by the Food and Drug Administration for treating blastomycosis during pregnancy.

Expected Response

Itraconazole therapy for patients who are not critically ill and who do not have CNS disease is successful in about 95% of cases. Amphotericin B therapy in seriously ill patients is curative in 70% to 90% of cases. Relapse is uncommon.

When to Refer

Patients with disseminated blastomycosis should be hospitalized.

KEY POINTS

NORTH AMERICAN BLASTOMYCOSIS

⊃ Blastomycosis is a fungal infection most commonly seen in the Mississippi and Ohio river basins.

⊃ The disease is acquired by inhalation of *B. dermatitidis* microconidia.

⊃ Pulmonary infections are self-limited in about one half of cases.

⊃ Acute pulmonary blastomycosis can be mistaken for influenza or community-acquired pneumonia.

⊃ Blastomycosis (and other fungal diseases) should be considered in cases of chronic pneumonia.

⊃ Extrapulmonary infections occur in 20% to 40% of cases and most commonly involve skin, bones, or the genitourinary system. Rarely, the CNS is involved.

⊃ Diagnosis is suggested by visualizing the characteristic budding yeasts with refractile cell walls and broad-based daughter yeasts. Diagnosis is confirmed by culture.

⊃ Itraconazole is the drug of choice for non–life-threatening blastomycosis in nonpregnant, immunocompetent persons.

⊃ Treatment of disseminated blastomycosis requires amphotericin B.

SUGGESTED READING

Chapman SW, Bradsher RW Jr, Campbell GD Jr, et al. Infectious Diseases Society of America. Practice guidelines for the management of patients with blastomycosis. Clin Infect Dis 2000; 30: 679-683.

Hanson JM, Spector G, El-Mofty SK. Laryngeal blastomycosis: a commonly missed diagnosis; report of two cases and review of the literature. Ann Otol Rhinol Laryngol 2000; 109: 281-286.

Lortholary O, Denning DW, Dupont B. Endemic mycoses: a treatment update. J Antimicrob Chemother 1999; 43: 321-331.

Tomecki KJ, Dijkstra JW, Hall GS, et al. Systemic mycosis. J Am Acad Dermatol 1989; 21: 1285-1293.

Weil M, Mercurio MG, Brodell RT, et al. Cutaneous lesions provide a clue to mysterious pulmonary process: pulmonary and cutaneous North American blastomycosis infection. Arch Dermatol 1996; 132: 822, 824-825.

Cryptococcosis

Like the other systemic fungal infections discussed thus far, cryptococcosis is usually a self-limited pulmonary infection. Meningitis, however, is the most common presentation. Before the AIDS epidemic about one half of cases of cryptococcal meningitis occurred in patients with apparently normal immunity. Today cryptococcosis is a frequent complication of AIDS (see Chapter 17). Infection may also involve the kidneys, prostate, bone, pericardium, peritoneum, skin, and other organs.

Presentation and Progression

Cause

C. neoformans is an encapsulated yeast found throughout the world. Virulent strains usually have large polysaccharide capsules. *C. neoformans* is found especially in areas where aged bird droppings accumulate, such as common roosting sites in attics and vacant old buildings. Transmission occurs through inhalation of aerosolized yeast. The infection is usually contained by intact host defenses. Factors predisposing individuals to disseminated disease include AIDS, systemic lupus erythematosus, sarcoidosis, lymphoreticular malignancies (lymphoma and leukemia), and hypercortisolism (Cushing's disease and Cushing's syndrome, including patients receiving corticosteroid therapy).

Presentation

The acute pulmonary infection is usually asymptomatic. Pulmonary cryptococcosis is sometimes discovered accidentally on a routine chest x-ray examination. Solitary or multiple pulmonary nodules can suggest malignancy, prompting unnecessary invasive procedures. Rarely, pulmonary cryptococcosis manifests itself as ARDS. Cryptococcal meningitis usually begins insidiously (Figure 21-2) but can be acute. The symptoms and signs include headache, fever, stiff neck, malaise, confusion, behavioral changes, and, in advanced cases, stupor or coma. Cranial nerve involvement is relatively common and is often manifested as impaired hearing or vision. Papilledema occurs in up to one third of patients. Skin lesions develop in up to 10% of patients (see Chapter 7). Papular lesions can resemble molluscum contagiosum, especially in AIDS patients.

Diagnosis

The diagnosis of cryptococcosis is made rapidly by an antigen detection assay in which latex agglutination is used on blood or CSF. In addition, direct microscopy with India ink or nigrosin mounts allows observation of the budding encapsulated yeast. Definitive diagnosis is made by culture of appropriate specimens such as CSF, blood, or tracheobronchial secretions.

Natural History
Expected Outcome

The mortality rate of untreated disseminated cryptococcosis is 70% to 80%.

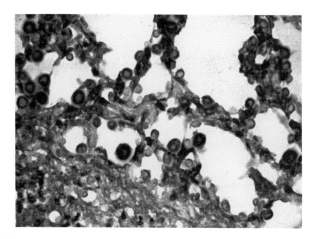

FIG. 21-2 Cryptococcal meningitis, with numerous yeast cells apparent on mucicarmine stain of the brain specimen at autopsy. Note the essential absence of an inflammatory response. A low white blood cell count in cerebrospinal fluid is one of the markers of poor prognosis in this disease.

Treatment
Methods

Cryptococcal disease confined to the lungs is often treated with 200 to 400 mg fluconazole for 3 to 12 months, depending on the severity of the disease. Patients who have undergone thoracic surgery (e.g., lobectomy or wedge resection of a coin lesion) for suspected neoplasm and who are found to have cryptococcosis should be treated with fluconazole because of the theoretical risk of dissemination to the meninges during the manipulation of pulmonary tissue at surgery. Patients with severe or progressive pulmonary infection are treated with amphotericin B 0.4 to 0.7 mg/kg per day for a total cumulative dose of 1 to 2 g.

Fluconazole, usually at a dose of 400 mg per day or higher, has been used successfully in patients with mild cases of cryptococcal meningitis, with or without AIDS as a risk factor. However, the supporting evidence for this approach is anecdotal. Most patients with cryptococcal meningitis are treated with amphotericin B plus flucytosine. However, the combination of amphotericin B plus flucytosine carries the risk of fatal bone marrow toxicity. Combination therapy with amphotericin B and flucytosine should be attempted on an outpatient basis with the greatest care, if at all. Most patients with cryptococcal meningitis should be hospitalized, and the IDSA guidelines for disease management should be consulted.

Expected Response

With treatment the mortality rate for cryptococcal meningitis is 10% to 15% in immunocompetent patients. In patients with AIDS the mortality rate can be up to 58% despite appropriate treatment, and relapse is common (50% to 65%) unless continuous prophylaxis is administered.

When to Refer

Most patients with cryptococcal meningitis should be hospitalized. Physicians assuming responsibility for these patients should be familiar with the IDSA guidelines.

 KEY POINTS

CRYPTOCOCCOSIS

⊃ Cryptococcosis is caused by an encapsulated yeast, *C. neoformans.*
⊃ It has wide geographic distribution.
⊃ The disease often occurs as an asymptomatic pulmonary infection, which is sometimes discovered accidentally on routine chest x-ray examination and which can resemble pneumonia.
⊃ Meningitis is the most common clinical manifestation. Onset is usually insidious. Features are headache, nausea, confusion, and cranial nerve involvement, including impaired hearing or vision.
⊃ Disseminated disease, including meningitis, frequently occurs in patients with compromised T-cell immunity. Between 80% and 90% of cases of cryptococcal meningitis occur in patients with AIDS. However, before the AIDS epidemic it was recognized that about one half of cases of cryptococcal meningitis occurred in persons with intact immunity.

⊃ Mortality of disseminated cryptococcosis is very high without treatment.
⊃ Treatment regimens include amphotericin B, with or without flucytosine, and fluconazole. Amphotericin B plus flucytosine is a standard regimen for initial treatment of cryptococcal meningitis. This regimen carries the potential for fatal bone marrow toxicity owing to the accumulation of flucytosine, especially if renal function is impaired before or as a result of therapy. Monitoring of flucytosine serum levels is important to prevent drug-related myelosuppression.
⊃ Most if not all patients with cryptococcal meningitis should be treated initially in the hospital.

SUGGESTED READING

Blanco P, Viallard JF, Beylot-Barry M, et al. Cutaneous cryptococcosis resembling molluscum contagiosum in a patient with non-Hodgkin's lymphoma. Clin Infect Dis 1999; 29: 683-684.

Durden FM, Elewski B. Cutaneous involvement with *C. neoformans* in AIDS. J Am Acad Dermatol 1994; 30: 844-848.

Núñez M, Peacock JE Jr, Chin R Jr. Pulmonary cryptococcosis in the immunocompetent host: therapy with fluconazole; a report of four cases and a review of the literature. Chest 2000; 118: 527-534.

Powderly WG. Current approach to the acute management of cryptococcal infections. J Infect 2000; 41:18-22.

Saag MS, Graybill JR, Larsen RA, et al. Infectious Diseases Society of America. Practice guidelines for the management of cryptococcal disease. Clin Infect Dis 2000; 30: 710-718.

Sporotrichosis

Sporotrichosis is encountered in primary care most commonly as the syndrome of nodular lymphangitis (see Chapter 8). Occasionally inhalation of microconidia causes pulmonary and systemic infection. This is especially likely to occur in patients with immunity compromised by cancer or AIDS. Pulmonary sporotrichosis sometimes occurs in middle-aged men with underlying COPD or alcoholism and manifests itself as chronic pneumonia or fibronodular cavitary disease. Sporotrichosis can also appear as chronic arthritis. Itraconazole has become the drug of choice for lymphocutaneous sporotrichosis and for milder forms of pulmonary disease, and it is effective in about 60% to 80% of patients with osteoarticular sporotrichosis. Amphotericin B continues to be the mainstay of therapy for patients with disseminated, life-threatening disease.

Aspergillosis

Aspergillus is a saprophytic mold found throughout the world. It frequently colonizes mucosal surfaces and is a relatively common laboratory contaminant. The term "aspergillosis" is currently used to denote invasive disease and allergic diseases attributed to this fungus. Invasive aspergillosis is uncommon in previously healthy persons but is a major cause of morbidity and mortality among severely immunocompromised individuals. More relevant to primary care are two syndromes attributed to allergy: allergic bronchopulmonary aspergillosis and allergic *Aspergillus* sinusitis.

Presentation and Progression
Cause

Aspergillus thrives especially in decaying vegetable matter. It is commonly found in air-conditioning duct systems, cellars, and potted plants and in certain foods such as peppers and other spices. *Aspergillus fumigatus* is the most frequent cause of human *Aspergillus* infection (approximately 90%) followed by *A. flavus* (approximately 10%), *A. niger* (approximately 2%), and *A. terreus* (approximately 2%). Infection is acquired by way of the respiratory tract in >90% of patients with aspergillosis. Colonization of the upper and occasionally the lower respiratory tract with *Aspergillus* is especially common in patients with congenital or acquired structural abnormalities because of such conditions as cystic fibrosis, severe bronchiectasis, silicosis, and pneumoconiosis. Intact polymorphonuclear leukocyte function is pivotal to host defense against invasive aspergillosis, and T-cell immunity has a lesser role. This observation may explain why invasive aspergillosis is an extremely important disease in severe granulocytopenia, especially in patients undergoing therapy for hematologic malignancy, but is a relatively uncommon pathogen in patients with AIDS. In severely immunocompromised hosts, *Aspergillus* commonly invades the walls of blood vessels, causing tissue infarction. Why allergic disease develops in some persons with *Aspergillus* colonization of the paranasal sinuses or lower respiratory tract and not in others remains a mystery.

Presentation

The various syndromes of aspergillosis are discussed in the approximate order of their importance in primary care practice.

Allergic Bronchopulmonary Aspergillosis. This hypersensitivity disease of the respiratory tract occurs especially in patients with asthma or cystic fibrosis. Patients often have worsening of preexisting asthma or mucoid impaction. Diagnostic criteria are discussed later in the chapter. An estimated 7% to 14% of patients with corticosteroid-dependent asthma in the United States have allergic bronchopulmonary aspergillosis. Patients may have recurrent episodes of eosinophilic pneumonia and tenacious, mucoid bronchial secretions. Allergic fungal sinusitis is discussed in Chapter 10.

Aspergilloma (Fungus Ball). Aspergilloma may develop within a preexisting lung cavity or in a paranasal sinus. In the past, pulmonary aspergillomas were encountered most commonly in patients with tuberculosis. Aspergillomas eventually develop in 15% to 25% of tuberculous cavities >2 cm in diameter. At present the most common predisposing conditions are sarcoidosis, healed cases of necrotizing pneumonia, and chronic *Pneumocystis carinii* infections in patients with AIDS. Pulmonary aspergillomas are often asymptomatic. Symptoms include chronic cough, wheezing, weight loss, and hemoptysis. Hemoptysis can be mild but is occasionally life threatening. Aspergilloma in a paranasal sinus cavity may lead to recurrent bacterial infection and carries the risk of locally invasive disease.

Superficial Aspergillosis. This form of aspergillosis most commonly occurs as chronic otitis externa. *A. niger* is the usual pathogen. Posttraumatic aspergillosis is encountered most commonly in ophthalmology practice as posttraumatic keratitis or endophthalmitis.

Invasive Aspergillosis. Invasive aspergillosis occurs most commonly in immunocompromised patients, usually appearing in the lungs (80% to 90% of cases). Acute invasive pulmonary aspergillosis is a fulminant, rapidly progressive infection. Most affected patients have severe granulocytopenia (absolute neutrophil count <150/mm³), have AIDS, or are bone marrow or organ transplant recipients. The presentation is often nonspecific, with fever and malaise as the only symptoms. The chest x-ray film may show consolidation, nodules, cavities, or diffuse infiltrates. High-resolution computed tomography (CT) of the chest showing a thick- or thin-walled cavitary lesion or a dense peripheral consolidation, often pleura based but without pleural effusion, is highly suggestive of invasive aspergillosis. Chronic invasive pulmonary aspergillosis, which is less common, pursues a more indolent course. Underlying conditions include diabetes mellitus, COPD treated with steroids, alcoholism, AIDS, or chronic granulomatous disease. Invasive *Aspergillus* sinusitis (see Chapter 10) usually begins with nonspecific symptoms, but extension to the orbit, brain, or palate can occur. Aspergillosis of the CNS is uncommon and is encountered most often in recipients of allogeneic (marrow or organ) transplantation.

Diagnosis

Seven diagnostic criteria are currently used for allergic bronchopulmonary aspergillosis: episodic bronchospasm or asthma, eosinophilia, early reactivity to *Aspergillus* antigen scratch test, elevated serum IgE levels, precipitating antibodies to *Aspergillus* antigens, history of pulmonary infiltrates, and central bronchiectasis. A minimum of six of these criteria is required to establish the diagnosis.

Pulmonary aspergilloma is suspected on the basis of its characteristic appearance on chest x-ray film or CT scan. Isolation of *Aspergillus* from sputum and demonstration of precipitating IgG antibodies in serum support the diagnosis.

For diagnosis of invasive aspergillosis, colonization must be distinguished from invasive disease. Demonstration of wide (2- to 4-μm) septate hyphae that branch at 45-degree angles in tissues, characteristically with invasion of blood vessels (Figure 21-3), is the most useful finding, especially when supported by isolation of *Aspergillus* in a culture specimen from lung. Unfortunately, a tissue diagnosis is often

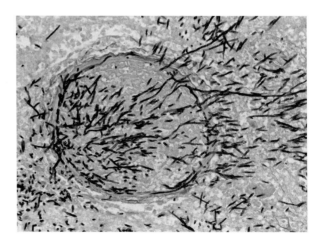

FIG. 21-3 Invasive aspergillosis, demonstrating massive infiltration of a blood vessel in brain tissue by branching, filamentous hyphae (Gomori methenamine-silver stain). Angioinvasive molds such as *Aspergillus* species and the agents of mucormycosis cause infarction of tissue by this mechanism.

difficult to secure. Open lung biopsy has a sensitivity of only about 50%, and thus resection of the involved lobe is often necessary to prove the diagnosis. A characteristic x-ray appearance in an appropriate clinical setting, however, is highly suggestive of the diagnosis, and positive tissue cultures for *Aspergillus* strengthen the presumptive diagnosis. Diagnosis of invasive fungal sinusitis is discussed in Chapter 10.

Natural History
Expected Outcome

Allergic bronchopulmonary aspergillosis is characterized by recurrent episodes of asthma that respond to brief courses of corticosteroids but evolve into steroid-dependent asthma. Central bronchiectasis and irreversible pulmonary fibrosis are late sequelae. About 10% of pulmonary aspergillomas resolve spontaneously. Acute invasive pulmonary aspergillosis is nearly uniformly fatal.

Treatment
Methods

Allergic Bronchopulmonary Aspergillosis. This form of aspergillosis is usually managed with oral corticosteroids during exacerbations (e.g., 0.5 mg/kg prednisone per day) and with high-dose inhaled corticosteroids for maintenance therapy to prevent exacerbations. Itraconazole, 10 mg/kg/day, can be used in refractory cases to reduce the *Aspergillus* colonization load. No convincing data have shown that steroids are useful in the management of allergic sinusitis caused by *Aspergillus* species.

Aspergilloma. Sometimes aspergilloma requires surgical resection. Indications include massive hemoptysis and patients perceived to be at risk for massive hemoptysis, such as immunocompromised patients, patients with sarcoidosis, and patients with increasing *Aspergillus*-specific IgG levels. However, surgical complications, including bronchopulmonary fistula, are relatively common. Some patients have been treated with intracavitary amphotericin B. Orally administered itraconazole may be helpful.

Invasive Sinusitis. Invasive sinusitis is usually treated with high-dose amphotericin B. Surgery has a role in acute management, and itraconazole may have a role in long-term maintenance therapy.

Expected Response

Appropriate management of allergic bronchopulmonary aspergillosis reduces the risk of progression to chronic lung disease. Morbidity and mortality rates from all forms of invasive aspergillosis can be reduced by aggressive approaches to diagnosis and treatment, but they remain high.

When to Refer

Patients with invasive aspergillosis should nearly always be hospitalized or referred for specialty care, and the IDSA guidelines for management should be consulted.

 KEY POINTS

ASPERGILLOSIS

⊃ *Aspergillus* species are widespread in nature, commonly colonize mucosal surfaces, and are frequent laboratory contaminants.

⊃ The term "aspergillosis" currently refers to invasive or allergic disease caused by *Aspergillus* species.

⊃ Allergic bronchopulmonary aspergillosis often appears as a hypersensitivity disease in patients with asthma or cystic fibrosis. It is estimated to affect 7% to 14% of patients with steroid-dependent asthma in the United States. Eosinophilia and the presence in serum of precipitating antibodies to *Aspergillus* antigens are important clues to the diagnosis.

⊃ Aspergilloma (fungus ball) can occur in old lung cavities and also in the paranasal sinuses. Pulmonary aspergilloma is often symptomatic, and complications include life-threatening massive hemoptysis. Surgical resection is definitive treatment, but complications of surgery are relatively common.

⊃ Invasive aspergillosis most commonly involves the lung (80% to 90% of cases), less commonly the paranasal sinuses, and rarely the brain.

⊃ Diagnosis of invasive aspergillosis should not be based solely on culture because *Aspergillus* is a common colonizer and laboratory contaminant. Optimally, diagnosis is based largely on demonstration of characteristic hyphae in tissue specimens in the appropriate clinical setting.

SUGGESTED READING

Latge JP. *Aspergillus fumigatus* and aspergillosis. Clin Microbiol Rev 1999; 12: 310-350.

Leon EE, Craig TJ. Antifungals in the treatment of allergic bronchopulmonary aspergillosis. Ann Allergy Asthma Immunol 1999; 82: 511-516.

Lin S-J, Schranz J, Teutsch SM. Aspergillosis case-fatality rate: systematic review of the literature. Clin Infect Dis 2001; 32: 358-366.

Patterson R, Greenberger PA, Harris KE. Allergic bronchopulmonary aspergillosis. Chest 2000; 118: 7-8.

Patterson TF, Kirkpatrick WR, White M, et al. I3 Aspergillus Study Group. Invasive aspergillosis: disease spectrum, treatment practices, and outcomes. Medicine (Baltimore) 2000; 79: 250-260.

Regnard JF, Icard P, Nicolosi M, et al. Aspergilloma: a series of 89 surgical cases. Ann Thorac Surg 2000; 69: 898-903.

Stevens DA, Kan VL, Judson MA, et al. Infectious Diseases Society of America. Practice guidelines for diseases caused by *Aspergillus*. Clin Infect Dis 2000; 30: 696-709.

Mucormycosis

The term "mucormycosis" denotes invasive tissue infection caused by one or another of a diverse group of fungi belonging to the order Mucorales. "Zygomycosis" and "phycomycosis" are less precise synonyms for these infections. Like *Aspergillus,* the Mucoraceae species are notorious for invading the walls of blood vessels and causing infarction and gangrene of tissues. Most patients with mucormycosis have a predisposing factor such as diabetes mellitus (poorly controlled or with a recent history of ketoacidosis), extensive trauma, burns, or an immunocompromised state. Occasionally, direct inoculation of abraded skin can lead to local or systemic infection.

Rhinocerebral mucormycosis as seen in primary care occurs mainly in patients with diabetes mellitus (see Chapter 3). Pulmonary mucormycosis, the other major form of the disease, occurs mainly in patients with prolonged granulocytopenia. All patients with rhinocerebral mucormycosis and most patients with other forms of the disease should be hospitalized for aggressive débridement and amphotericin B therapy.

SUGGESTED READING

Deshpande AH, Munshi MM. Rhinocerebral mucormycosis diagnosis by aspiration cytology. Diagn Cytopathol 2000; 23: 97-100.

Ferguson BJ. Mucormycosis of the nose and paranasal sinuses. Otolaryngol Clin North Am 2000; 33: 349-365.

Kontoyiannis DP, Wessel VC, Bodey GP, et al. Zygomycosis in the 1990s in a tertiary-care cancer center. Clin Infect Dis 2000; 30: 851-856.

Lee FY, Mossad SB, Adal KA. Pulmonary mucormycosis: the last 30 years. Arch Intern Med 1999; 159: 1301-1309.

Invasive Candidiasis

Primary care clinicians need to be familiar with invasive candidiasis because of two groups of patients: those released from the hospital after treatment of complicated problems, and those receiving outpatient intravenous therapy. *C. albicans* has traditionally been the major cause of invasive candidiasis, but other species are assuming increasing importance. These include *C. tropicalis, C. glabrata, C. parapsilosis, C. krusei* (which tends to be resistant to fluconazole), *C. lusitaniae* (which tends to be resistant to amphotericin B), and numerous other species. Nearly all patients with invasive candidiasis have one or more risk factors, such as large-bore intravascular devices, prolonged exposure to multiple broad-spectrum antibiotics, and granulocytopenia. The major expressions of the disease are as follows:

- Bloodstream infection, often associated with an infected intravascular access device and often leading to complications summarized in other items of this list. Hospitalized patients with positive blood cultures for *Candida* species have crude mortality rates ≥50%.
- *Candida* endophthalmitis occurs as a result of hematogenous dissemination in as many as 10% to even 35% of patients with fungemia. Ophthalmoscopic examination often shows the lesion before the onset of vision loss, which can be permanent.
- *Candida* peritonitis usually occurs as a result of infection of a peritoneal dialysis catheter. It also occurs in patients with intraabdominal infection or necrotizing pancreatitis who have had complicated hospital courses.
- *Candida* osteomyelitis and septic arthritis occur occasionally as complications of surgery (e.g., sternal osteomyelitis following median sternotomy) or as the result of candidemia caused by an infected vascular access device.
- Urinary tract candidiasis commonly follows instrumentation and is often associated with prior exposure to broad-spectrum antibiotics, especially in the geriatric population (see Chapter 14).
- *Candida* pulmonary infection is uncommon, except as part of widespread hematogenous dissemination.
- Hepatosplenic candidiasis is a syndrome of disseminated candidiasis that occurs in neutropenic patients. Remitting fever may be the only clinical sign. Multiple abscesses in the liver and spleen appear as well-circumscribed, hypodense lesions on CT scan.

Diagnosis is made by isolation of *Candida* from blood cultures or other clinical settings. However, the sensitivity of blood cultures for detecting candidemia may be as low as 50%. Numerous researchers have sought practical serologic markers for invasive candidiasis, but to date the results have been disappointing. Patients with invasive candidiasis should be hospitalized because most authorities agree that all patients with positive blood cultures for *Candida* species should be treated. Amphotericin B and fluconazole are the most useful drugs; for appropriate regimens the IDSA guidelines should be consulted.

SUGGESTED READING

Klepser ME, Lewis RE, Pfaller MA. Therapy of *Candida* infections: susceptibility testing, resistance, and therapeutic options. Ann Pharmacol Ther 1998; 32: 1353-1361.

Rex JH, Walsh TJ, Sobel JD, et al. Infectious Diseases Society of America. Practice guidelines for the treatment of candidiasis. Clin Infect Dis 2000; 30: 662-678.

Verduyn Lunel FM, Meis JF, Voss A. Nosocomial fungal infections: candidemia. Diagn Microbiol Infect Dis 1999; 34: 213-220.

Unusual Fungal Infections

Infections caused by several infrequently encountered fungal species are mentioned briefly here.

Fusarium Species (Fusariosis)

Fungi belonging to the genus *Fusarium* are commonly found in soil and organic debris. Disease in immunocompetent persons usually results from traumatic inoculation. The three major syndromes are fungal keratitis, onychomycosis, and chronic infections of skin, muscle, bone, or joints, including mycetoma. Mycetoma, which is also known as Madura foot, is a slowly progressive, often painful, destructive infection caused by various saprophytic soil fungi, including *Fusarium* species. It typically involves the hands and feet and is distinguished by small "grains" of fungal organisms that can be found in tissue biopsy specimens or in sinus tracts. Disseminated infection caused by *Fusarium* species (systemic fusariosis) occurs in immunocompromised patients, especially those who have undergone bone marrow transplantation or who have leukemia and chemotherapy-induced agranulocytosis. Clinical features of fusariosis include primary multicentric pneumonia, skin lesions (79% of patients), and positive blood cultures (40% of patients). On histologic examination, systemic fusariosis can be indistinguishable from aspergillosis and other invasive mold infections. Treatment consists of high-dose amphotericin B.

Pseudallescheria Boydii (Pseudallescheriasis) and Scedosporium Apiospermum

Pseudallescheria boydii (the sexual or perfect stage of the organism) and *S. apiospermum* (the asexual or imperfect stage of the same organism) occasionally cause disease in immunocompetent persons and can cause disseminated infection in immunocompromised hosts. In immunocompetent persons, penetrating trauma to the eye, bone, joints, brain, or other organisms can cause a localized, recalcitrant infection. *P. boydii* occasionally causes invasive fungal sinusitis (see Chapter 10), meningitis, or sinusitis. Disseminated infection most commonly involves the lungs, followed by the brain and eye. These fungi are histologically similar to other invasive molds. Correct identification by culture is crucial because the fungi are resistant to amphotericin B. Ketoconazole, miconazole, and itraconazole are the current drugs of choice, but the efficacy of drug therapy is not clearly established. Aggressive débridement is the key to a successful outcome.

Dematiaceous Fungi (Phaeohyphomycosis)

Alternaria, Bipolaris, Curvularia, Exserohilum, Fonsecaea, and various other fungal species are grouped together as dematiaceous fungi because of the presence of a melanin-like pigment in their cell walls that gives a dark-brown or black appearance to their hyphae or spores in tissue specimens and cultures. The term "phaeohyphomycosis" refers to infections caused by these molds, although some authorities recommend that this term be reserved for cases in which dark-walled fungi are found in biopsy specimens without confirmation of the organism by culture. These agents sometimes cause localized infection of the skin, nails, and subcutaneous tissues after minor trauma. More seriously, they occasionally cause invasive fungal sinusitis or brain abscess in immunocompetent persons. Dissemination can occur in immunocompromised patients. Treatment includes surgical excision and drug therapy with itraconazole (10 mg/kg/day). Use of amphotericin B alone has been associated with therapeutic failures.

SUGGESTED READING

De Hoog GS. Significance of fungal evolution for the understanding of their pathogenicity, illustrated with agents of phaeohyphomycosis. Mycoses 1997; 40 (Suppl 2): 5-8.

Fernandez M, Noyola DE, Rossmannn SN, Edwards MS. Cutaneous phaeohyphomycosis caused by *Curvularia lunata* and a review of *Curvularia* infections in pediatrics. Pediatr Infect Dis J 1999; 18: 727-731.

Hospenthal DR, Bennett JE. Miscellaneous fungi and Prototheca. In: Mandell GL, Bennett JE, Dolin R, eds. Mandell, Douglas, and Bennett's Principles and Practice of Infectious Diseases. 5th ed.; Philadelphia: Churchill Livingstone; 2000: 2772-2780.

Sugar AM. Miscellaneous fungi. In: Gorbach SL, Bartlett JG, Blackow NR, eds. Infectious Diseases. 2nd ed., Philadelphia: W.B. Saunders Company; 1998: 2387-2392.

Antifungal Drug Therapy: Overview

Systemic antifungal therapy has undergone great advances in the past 20 years. Amphotericin B remains the most generally effective drug with the broadest spectrum of activity and most rapid onset of activity; however, it is also the most toxic. There are three new lipid vehicle forms of amphotericin B. All reduce the nephrotoxicity of amphotericin B, and one reduces the infusion toxicity as well. The triazole compounds are the best-tolerated antifungal drugs now available, and they enable oral therapy for some mycoses that previously required amphotericin B and act against a variety of mycotic pathogens. Their major problems are a relatively slow mechanism of action and complex drug interactions. Terbinafine, flucytosine, and the echinocandins represent three additional classes that have more limited applications than amphotericin B or the triazoles.

SUGGESTED READING

Andriole VT. The 1998 Garrod lecture. Current and future antifungal therapy: new targets for antifungal agents. J Antimicrob Chemother 1999; 44: 151-62.

Bohme A, Karthaus M. Treatment of systemic fungal infections in patients with hematologic malignancies. Antibiot Chemother 2000; 50: 79-93.

Dismukes WE. Introduction to antifungal drugs. Clin Infect Dis 2000; 30: 653-657.

Polyenes (Amphotericin B and Related Compounds)

Amphotericin B remains the most useful drug for life-threatening fungal infection. Increasingly, it is given on an outpatient basis.

Mechanism of Action and Toxicity

All polyenes act by rapidly binding to ergosterol in fungal cell membranes. This disrupts the steric integrity of the membrane, permitting increased influx of sodium and efflux of potassium. Amphotericin B also binds to ergosterol in mammalian cell membranes, which explains much of the toxicity, such as impaired renal function, renal tubular acidosis, hemolysis, anemia, and cardiac arrhythmias. Binding to phagocytes and lymphocytes elicits the production of cytokines, which may cause the fever, chills, and thrombophlebitis associated with administration. Rarely, amphotericin B causes severe hypertension. These various properties make amphotericin B a valuable but difficult-to-use drug in clinical practice.

Administration

Absorption is insufficient to permit oral therapy for systemic infections. Amphotericin B solution has been used topically solely for local effect in bladder irrigation (50 mg/L) and for treatment of oral thrush. Amphotericin B has also been used for local injections into subcutaneous fungal lesions, for soaking packs for infected areas (e.g., invasive fungal sinusitis), for local injections subcutaneously applied in fungal lesions, and for intrathecal administration in coccidioidal meningitis. Local injections of amphotericin B are extremely painful, and intrathecal use is seldom indicated. The most common method of delivering amphotericin B is to dissolve (actually suspend, because it is a colloid) 50 mg of amphotericin B in 1 liter of 5% glucose and administer through a central venous line (to avoid causing thrombophlebitis). The daily dose varies, from 0.7 to 1 mg/kg/day for candidiasis, histoplasmosis, and cryptococcosis to 1 to 1.5 mg/kg/day for mucormycosis and aspergillosis.

Multiple problems attend the administration of amphotericin B. At doses of ≥1 mg/kg/day, renal failure supervenes within 1 to 2 weeks. The nephrotoxicity of amphotericin B is paradoxical, because the kidneys play only a small role (about 10%) in the excretion of the drug and renal failure does not influence pharmacokinetics. The dose for patients receiving dialysis is the same as for patients with normal renal function. How should amphotericin B be administered to patients with intermediate degrees of renal insufficiency? In the past, amphotericin B was customarily given at full doses until the serum creatinine level rose to >2 mg/dL, at which point therapy was interrupted for several days or the drug was given every other day. The underlying assumption was that "resting the kidneys" would allow renal function to improve. The consequences of amphotericin B nephrotoxicity are now known to be more profound and long lasting. Up to 30% of patients treated in such fashion may later require hemodialysis. A common strategy to delay onset of renal failure is to administer 1 liter of saline solution before each dose of amphotericin B (but not to mix the drug in the saline solution, since it precipitates). Experience is largely anecdotal, and exactly how much benefit this strategy yields is unclear.

A second area of difficulty concerns the rate of infusion for amphotericin B. Some favor giving the full dose in as short a time as 1 hour; others favor prolonged administration of up to 4 hours. There is agreement that rapid infusion of amphotericin B in patients with renal failure is dangerous, causing acute increases in potassium level, which may in turn cause lethal arrhythmias. Six hours or longer may be preferable for patients with renal insufficiency. Amphotericin B is not dialyzable and does not clear with peritoneal dialysis. Nevertheless, patients may require dialysis during administration of the drug to control dangerous hyperkalemia.

Recent Advances

Delivery of amphotericin B in high concentrations to sites of fungal infections and phagocytic cells is desirable, and delivery to the kidneys is undesirable. Formulation of amphotericin B in lipid vehicles accomplishes the goal of delivery to the desired sites; drug concentrations in reticuloendothelial organs such as the spleen are sharply increased, and kidney concentrations (and glomerular toxicity) are decreased. Three lipid vehicles for amphotericin B are available (Table 21-2).

TABLE 21-2
Characteristics of Licensed Amphotericin B Preparations for Systemic Use

	Amphotericin B deoxycholate	Amphotericin B lipid complex	Amphotericin B cholesteryl sulfate	Amphotericin B liposomal
Trade name	Fungizone	Abelcet	Amphotec	AmBisome
Manufacturer	Squibb; Apothecon	Lipsome Company	SEQUUS	Fujisawa; Gilead
Structure	Colloid	Ribbons	Polymorphous disks	"Bubbles"
Percentage of amphotericin B	>50	33 to 35	50	10
Maximum dose (mg/kg)	1.5	10+	5	10+
Nephrotoxicity				
Glomerular	+++++	++	++	+
Tubular	+++++	+++	+++	+++
Infusion reactions	+++++	+++	+++++	+
Arrhythmias	++	—	—	—
Serum concentration	+	+	+	++++
Kidney concentration	+++	+	+	+
Efficacy studies*				
Candidemia	+++	+++	+++	+++
Aspergillosis	+++	+++	+++	+++
Fusariosis	+	+++	—	+++
Mucormycosis	++	+++	++	+++
Cryptococcosis	+++	+++	+++	+++
Febrile neutropenia	+++	+++	—	+++

Toxicity is ranked here from "none recognized" (−) to "severe" (+++++). Efficacy is ranked from "marginal" (+) to "marked" (+++).
*Efficacy compared in limited studies of some drugs in candidemia, aspergillosis, febrile neutropenia, and cryptococcosis. Other conclusions are inferred from open studies.

All three somewhat or greatly reduce glomerular toxicity, but all have some tubular toxicity (manifested as hypokalemia and hypomagnesemia). All three preparations can be given in doses >5 mg/kg, which would be an acutely lethal dose for amphotericin B desoxycholate (Fungizone). These drugs are useful options for treatment of fungal disease in patients with underlying renal disease. When fungal disease involves the kidneys, however, these newer agents may be unreliable because of poor renal penetration.

Animal studies suggest that the lipid formulations are less active milligram for milligram than amphotericin B desoxycholate, and therefore higher doses have been recommended. AmBisome has been given safely in doses up to 15 mg/kg, but whether such heroic doses are more effective than lower doses is unclear. Indeed, no evidence has shown that the lipid formulations are more effective than amphotericin B desoxycholate in candidemia, and little evidence of increased efficacy in aspergillosis has been presented. The clearest indication for these preparations is for patients who have renal toxicity or are not responding to amphotericin B desoxycholate. The major problem is cost, which can exceed $800 per day for AmBisome and $300 per day for Abelcet. The third preparation, amphotericin B colloidal dispersion (Amphotec), is not used as often because of frequent infusion reactions.

Polyene Use in the Office

Polyene therapy is generally initiated while the patient is hospitalized, and care is continued in the office for infections, which require prolonged therapy. Commonly these include such diseases as the endemic mycoses and aspergillosis, or completion of treatment for mucormycosis. Unless renal failure occurs, for most indications the dose of amphotericin B desoxycholate is 0.6 mg/kg/day, or 50 mg every other day. Treatment is often continued until a total dose of ≥25 mg/kg is achieved. Our preference is to give the drug over 2 to 4 hours (or over a longer period if renal failure is present) and to monitor the serum creatinine and electrolyte levels three times per week. When the creatinine level rises above 1.5 mg/dL, the patient can be switched to amphotericin B lipid complex (Abelcet) at 3 mg/kg/day (or 5 to 10 mg/kg/day for aspergillosis). We prefer to infuse saline solution before amphotericin B desoxycholate but not before the lipid formulations. Abelcet causes infusion reactions more often than AmBisome; however, Abelcet is less expensive. Infusion reactions can be treated with acetaminophen and diphenhydramine and if necessary with meperidine (Demerol) 25 mg IV. Many clinicians give acetaminophen and diphenhydramine before the initial infusions of amphotericin preparations. Most infusion reactions subside in a day or two, and premedications can then be discontinued.

Duration of Therapy and Changeover to Azole Compounds

For mucormycosis and fusariosis, treatment is entirely with amphotericin B, to a total dose of 20 to 35 mg/kg for the course of treatment. This may take 2 months. For cryptococcosis the first 2 weeks involves treatment with amphotericin B, followed by a switch to fluconazole. For aspergillosis the switch is to itraconazole (or in the future posaconazole or voriconazole) but when to switch is less clear. Deterioration of renal function is a common basis for changing therapy from amphotericin B to a triazole compound.

 KEY POINTS

POLYENES (AMPHOTERICIN B AND RELATED COMPOUNDS)

⊃ Amphotericin B desoxycholate (Fungizone) remains the most useful drug for life-threatening fungal infection.

⊃ Toxicity of amphotericin B includes renal failure (which is paradoxical, because amphotericin B plays only a small role in the drug's elimination) and anemia, hypokalemia (and hyperkalemia with rapid infusion), and infusion reactions.

⊃ Newer lipid formulations of amphotericin B include amphotericin B lipid complex (Abelcet), amphotericin B cholesteryl sulfate (Amphotec), and amphotericin B liposomal (AmBisome).

⊃ The lipid formulations of amphotericin B are less active on a weight basis than amphotericin B desoxycholate (Fungizone), less nephrotoxic, and considerably more expensive.

⊃ Amphotericin B therapy is usually initiated in the hospital, but it can be continued in the outpatient setting with infusions every second day.

SUGGESTED READING

Bates DW, Su L, Yu DT, et al. Mortality and costs of acute renal failure associated with amphotericin B therapy. Clin Infect Dis 2001; 32: 686-693.

Patel R. Antifungal agents. Part I. Amphotericin B preparations and flucytosine. Mayo Clin Proc 1998; 73: 1205-1225.

Rowles DM, Fraser SL. Amphotericin B lipid complex (ABLC)-associated hypertension: case report and review. Clin Infect Dis 1999; 29: 1564-1565.

Wong-Beringer A, Jacobs RA, Guglielmo BJ. Lipid formulations of amphotericin B: clinical efficacy and toxicities. Clin Infect Dis 1998; 27: 603-618.

Flucytosine

Flucytosine is active against many *Candida* species, against *Cryptococcus neoformans,* and to a lesser extent against *Aspergillus* species and the agents of chromomycosis. Flucytosine was initially developed as an antimetabolite for oncology, and its toxicity is mainly that of an antimetabolite: gastrointestinal, hepatic, and hematopoietic. Myelotoxicity, including fatal bone marrow failure, is more likely to occur when flucytosine is used in combination with amphotericin B. Monitoring of the complete blood count (CBC) and liver function tests is essential, and the dose must be reduced in patients with renal failure. These toxicities limit the role of flucytosine in primary care.

SUGGESTED READING

Patel R. Antifungal agents. Part I. Amphotericin B preparations and flucytosine. Mayo Clin Proc 1998; 73: 1205-1225.

Vermes A, Guchelaar HJ, Dankert J. Flucytosine: a review of its pharmacology, clinical indications, pharmacokinetics, toxicity, and drug interactions. J Antimicrob Chemother 2000; 46: 171-179.

Allylamines (Terbinafine)

Terbinafine is the only currently available member of its class, the squalene oxidase inhibitors. Terbinafine is systemically administered at 250 or 500 mg per day. This drug was given initially only to treat dermatomycosis and onychomycosis, but more recently it has been used for sporotrichosis. It becomes concentrated in the skin and nail beds. Although multiple other species, such as *Aspergillus,* are susceptible in vitro, the value of terbinafine in more serious systemic infections is unclear. A common regimen for toe onychomycosis is to give 500 mg daily for 1 week each month for 6 or more months, until convincing evidence of a clear new toenail growing out is seen. Treatment does not have to continue until all involved toenails are clipped off.

SUGGESTED READING

Bryan CS, Smith CW, Berg DE, et al. *Curvularia lunata* endocarditis treated with terbinafine: case report. Clin Infect Dis 1993; 16: 30-32.

Hay RJ. Therapeutic potential of terbinafine in subcutaneous and systemic mycoses. Br J Dermatol 1999; 141(Suppl 56): 36-40.

Perez A. Terbinafine: broad new spectrum of indications in several subcutaneous and systemic mycoses and parasitic diseases. Mycoses 1999; 42 (Suppl 2): 111-114.

Azole Antifungals

Ketoconazole, the first azole antifungal, was useful especially in the treatment of candidiasis. Fluconazole and itraconazole are triazole-based compounds with expanded spectrums of activity. Azole compounds in clinical development include ravuconazole, voriconazole, and posaconazole. The agents have brought relative safety and convenience of administration to the treatment of several systemic mycoses, but drug interactions are a potential problem.

Mechanism of Action and Toxicity

All azoles act by binding to and inhibiting the activity of lanosterol demethylase. This is a cytochrome enzyme of the P450 group. Inhibition of the enzyme progressively blocks synthesis of ergosterol and leads to substitution of other intermediate sterols in fungal cell membranes. This causes breakdown of the steric integrity of the membrane, albeit much more slowly than with amphotericin B. The toxicity of these drugs derives largely from their similarity to mammalian P450 enzymes. Ketoconazole has considerable cross-reactivity, and it causes hepatic toxicity and impaired synthesis of several key hormones. Adverse effects include hypogonadism from low testosterone synthesis, impairment of menstrual cycles, hair loss, and adrenal insufficiency. Hypocholesterolemia has also been reported. In part because of these adverse effects, ketoconazole is now mainly used as a topical shampoo for dandruff and ointment for dermatophyte infections. Ketoconazole is cleared largely by hepatic degradation by the cytochrome (P450 isozyme) cyp3A4. Substrate competition by other drugs can increase ketoconazole levels sharply and cause toxicity, either from ketoconazole or from the other drugs. The newer triazole agents (fluconazole and itraconazole) have much more specificity for fungal enzymes and much less hepatotoxicity than ketoconazole.

Pharmacokinetics

Ketoconazole is available for topical and oral administration as 200-mg tablets, and it must be taken with food on an acid stomach to optimize absorption. Ingestion of acids, such as Coca-Cola, increases absorption, whereas buffers or proton pump inhibitors reduce absorption. Because ketoconazole is lipid soluble, ingestion of fat with a meal aids absorption. Doses of ≥600 mg/day saturate the enzymes of degradation, causing ketoconazole to accumulate, with a clearance half-life >24 hours.

Itraconazole is somewhat similar to ketoconazole in kinetics, except that one metabolite, hydroxy-itraconazole, is biologically active. Itraconazole metabolism also occurs via cyp3A4, an enzyme that is highly vulnerable to drug interactions (Table 21-3). All agents that induce enzyme activity induce more rapid clearance of itraconazole. These include rifampin derivatives (although less with rifabutin than rifampin). Usually 1 to 2 weeks is needed after discontinuing such drugs for the perturbations to decrease. This is a major problem in the treatment of HIV-infected patients for tuberculosis, if they are receiving either itraconazole for a fungal infection or protease inhibitors, which are similarly affected.

A more pernicious problem is the coadministration of drugs that are also metabolized by the cyp3A4 enzyme. These provide substrate competition, which may increase the serum and tissue concentrations of either or both drugs. Many classes of drugs are represented, and if the practitioner is unaware of these interactions, the consequences can be dangerous. For example, triazolam retention can cause profound somnolence. Lovastatin may accumulate as the acid form, causing rhabdomyolysis. Cyclosporine retention may cause renal failure. Terfenadine, astemizole, or cisapride retention may cause QT interval prolongation and lethal torsades de pointes. Digoxin toxicity may occur. Because of the risk, practitioners must be aware of concurrent medications and make dose adjustments or change drugs as necessary. Alcohol, when given with ketoconazole, can cause a disulfiram (Antabuse)-like reaction. Ketoconazole increases the effect of methylprednisolone but decreases the plasma level of theophylline.

Fluconazole

Two classes of triazoles have replaced ketoconazole (Table 21-4). Both have much less cross-reactivity with human cytochrome enzymes, and both are safer than ketoconazole. The first is represented only by fluconazole. Fluconazole is water soluble and well absorbed, can be given intravenously (at the same dose as the oral drug), has fewer drug interactions than ketoconazole, and has linear renal clearance. Doses up to 2 g/day can be given to patients with normal renal function, although the usual daily dose is 200 to 400 mg. The pharmacokinetic effects are predictable, with wide tissue distribution in the aqueous phase. Mild gastrointestinal intolerance is the major problem with fluconazole. Fluconazole may be useful for urinary tract infections. The downside of fluconazole is the relatively narrow spectrum (some *Candida* species and *C. neoformans,* as well as modest effect against endemic mycoses) and the emergence of resistant strains.

Resistance to fluconazole is innate to some yeasts, such as *C. krusei.* Resistance can induced in *C. albicans* and

TABLE 21-3
Common Drug Interactions of the Azole Antifungal Compounds (Partial List)

Drugs that accelerate hepatic metabolism of azoles (leading to decreased plasma levels of the azole and therefore decreased efficacy)	Inhibition of metabolism of other drugs by azoles (leading to increased plasma levels and therefore increased toxicity)
Rifampin and rifabutin* Rifabutin Rifapentine	Triazolam, alprazolam, midazolam (CNS toxicity)* Chlordiazepoxide (sedation)† Digoxin (digoxin toxicity)‡
Phenytoin§	Terfenadine (prolonged QT interval; torsades de pointes)*
Phenobarbital and other barbiturates§	Astemizole (prolonged QT interval; torsades de pointes)*
Carbamazepine‡	Warfarin (potentiation of anticoagulant effect)*
Didanosine‡	HMG-CoA reductase inhibitors (lovastatin, others) (rhabdomyolysis)*
Nevirapine	Cisapride (cardiotoxicity)*
Efavirenz	Cyclosporine (increased drug toxicity, including nephrotoxicity)*
Omeprazole, lansoprazole‡	Tacrolimus (increased drug toxicity, including nephrotoxicity)¶
Cimetidine*	Phenytoin (phenytoin toxicity) Nortriptyline (sedation, cardiac arrhythmias)¶ Loratadine (cardiac arrhythmias)§ Felodipine, nifedipine (edema)‡ Rifabutin (uveitis)¶ Zidovudine (AZT) (zidovudine toxicity)¶ Indinavir (indinavir toxicity)† Saquinavir (saquinavir toxicity)¶ Ritonavir (ritonavir toxicity)† Oral hypoglycemics (hypoglycemia)*

*Ketoconazole, itraconazole, and fluconazole.
†Ketoconazole only.
‡Itraconazole only.
§Ketoconazole and itraconazole.
¶Fluconazole only.

C. glabrata by chronic exposure to fluconazole and occurs by multiple mechanisms. Susceptible isolates have a minimum inhibitory concentration (MIC) of ≤8 μg/mL. Thrush responds to 100 mg/day. So-called dose-dependent isolates, named because a higher dose (400 to 800 mg/day) is needed, have an MIC of 16 to 32 μg/mL. Fully resistant isolates have an MIC of ≥64 μg/mL and may fail at 800 mg/day for thrush. *C. neoformans* may also develop resistance to fluconazole, but this is much less common than for *Candida* species.

Initially fluconazole was used most commonly for treatment and suppression of thrush, which is caused mainly by *C. albicans.* The more common use at present is for long-term suppression of cryptococcal meningitis and occasionally for treatment of coccidioidomycosis or histoplasmosis. Doses of 200 to 400 mg/day are usual and may be adjusted downward in severe renal failure. Because fluconazole is well tolerated up to 1600 mg/day in normal renal function, modest renal failure does not usually require a reduction in dose.

Itraconazole

Itraconazole is much more lipid soluble than is fluconazole. Optimal absorption after oral administration requires a vehicle. In the capsule form, itraconazole is absorbed optimally from an acid intragastric environment, shortly after a lipid-containing meal. The dose is 200 to 400 mg b.i.d. A new solution, with β-hydroxycyclodextrin to dissolve itraconazole, is absorbed optimally in a fasting state and does not require acid. However, the taste of the vehicle discourages some patients from prolonged therapy. The dose of this new solution is also 200 to 400 mg b.i.d. A new parenteral solution, also made with β-hydroxycyclodextrin as the vehicle, permits intravenous administration. The dose is approximately half that for the oral formulations, or about 200 mg/day for most patients. Itraconazole dosage does not require adjustment for renal failure. However, the cyclodextrin vehicle used for the intravenous drug may be partly cleared renally, and whether this must be dose adjusted is not yet clear. Severe hepatic failure may affect clearance of itraconazole.

TABLE 21-4
Spectrum of Activity of Triazole Compounds In Vitro

Fungus	Fluconazole	Itraconazole	Voriconazole*	Posaconazole*
Candida albicans, fluconazole-sensitive	+++++	+++++	+++++	+++++
C. albicans, fluconazole-resistant	+	+	+++	+++
Candida tropicalis	++++	+++++	+++++	+++++
Candida glabrata	++	++	++++	++++
Candida krusei	0	+	++++	++++
Cryptococcus neoformans	++++	++++	++++	++++
Aspergillus species	0	+++	+++	+++
Zygomycetes (agents of mucormycosis)	0	0	0	+++
Fusarium species	0	0	++	++
Alternaria and other Phaeohyphomycetes	0	+++	++++	++++

Activity is ranked from "none" (0) to "marked" (+++++).
*Investigational.

Because the hepatic enzymes degrading itraconazole can be saturated, not only by competing drugs but also by high doses of itraconazole, the clearance is not linear. At daily doses above 400 mg/day (capsules), the half-life may rise from between 24 and 30 hours to more than 45 hours. This may be useful for such conditions as aspergillosis brain abscess, but high doses are associated with an occasional syndrome of hypertension, edema, and hypokalemia. The cause of this syndrome is not known, but it can be managed with diuretics or a reduction in drug dose.

With all of the possible problems, why use itraconazole at all? The microbiologic spectrum of itraconazole and its potency are much greater than those of fluconazole (or for that matter ketoconazole). Itraconazole covers some fluconazole-resistant *Candida* species, most *Aspergillus* species, and all of the endemic dimorphic mycoses much more effectively than fluconazole does. Other mycoses, such as phaeohyphomycosis and chromomycosis, are also preferentially treated with itraconazole.

 KEY POINTS

AZOLE ANTIFUNGALS
⊃ Currently available agents include ketoconazole, fluconazole, and itraconazole.
⊃ Adverse effects are related in large part to the similarity of these drugs to mammalian P450 enzymes. Coadministra-

tion of drugs that are metabolized by the hepatic cyp3A4 enzyme can also result in serious interactions.
⊃ Fluconazole and itraconazole have largely replaced ketoconazole, the first drug in this class, for most indications.
⊃ Fluconazole is active mainly against *Candida* species and *C. neoformans*. *C. krusei* is inherently resistant to fluconazole, and resistant strains of other *Candida* species and *C. neoformans* occur.
⊃ Itraconazole is active against most *Aspergillus* species and against all of the endemic dimorphic mycoses (e.g., histoplasmosis, blastomycosis) with the exception of coccidioidal meningitis.

SUGGESTED READING
Graybill JR. Itraconazole: managing mycotic complications in immunocompromised patients. Semin Oncol 1998; 5(Suppl 7): 58-63.
Martin MV. The use of fluconazole and itraconazole in the treatment of *Candida albicans* infections: a review. J Antimicrob Chemother 1999; 44: 429-37.
Terrell CL. Antifungal agents. Part II. The azoles. Mayo Clin Proc 1999; 74: 78-100.

Echinocandins

Echinocandins are a new class of antifungal agents that target β (1,3)-D glucan synthase, a key enzyme in the synthesis of the fungal cell wall. The spectrum at present is all *Candida* species, *Aspergillus,* and some endemic mycoses and other mycelial pathogens (although not all). Caspofungin (Cancidas) is the first drug of this class to be approved for clinical use, with aspergillosis as the first approved indication. These drugs are extremely potent in mucosal candidiasis, and studies of candidemia and other mycoses are in progress. Other agents (versicor and FK 463) are being developed. These drugs will be useful against pathogens resistant to other antifungals. No nephrotoxicity and minimal liver toxicity are associated with the echinocandins. The main downside at present is limited clinical experience. Also, echinocandins must be given parenterally, penetrate CSF poorly, and are ineffective against *C. neoformans.* Adverse interaction with cyclosporine (but not

tacrolimus) is a potential problem. Echinocandins will probably emerge as a major alternative for systemic mycoses.

Summary: The Systemic Mycoses

The rising prevalence of susceptible and immunocompromised patients in the ambulatory population increases the potential that patients with systemic mycoses will appear initially in primary care practices. Therapy for these infections has been somewhat simplified by the introduction of new drugs. Awareness of the protean clinical manifestations of these infections improves the likelihood of early diagnosis, which in turn improves the prognosis.

22 Mycobacterial Diseases and Antimycobacterial Drugs

ERIC R. BRENNER, CHARLES S. BRYAN

Tuberculosis in the United States is now largely a disease of the disadvantaged: the frail elderly, immigrants from developing nations, the inner-city poor, migrant farm workers, injecting drug users, and persons infected with human immunodeficiency virus (HIV). However, primary care clinicians occasionally encounter tuberculosis (TB) even among the affluent, and mistakes in diagnosis and management of this disease are relatively common (see Chapter 1). Although tuberculosis is by far the most important mycobacterial disease, primary care clinicians in the United States are likely to encounter nontuberculous mycobacteria more frequently than

Mycobacterium tuberculosis. The purpose of this chapter is to provide a framework for diagnosis and management of these infections with special emphasis on treatment of latent tuberculosis infection (preventive therapy).

SUGGESTED READING

Centers for Disease Control and Prevention. Core curriculum on tuberculosis: what the clinician should know. 4th edition, Atlanta: Centers for Disease Control; 2000. This extremely useful document is available online at www.cdc.gov/nchstp/tb/pubs/corecurr/default.htm.
Espinal MA, Laszlo A, Simonsen L, et al. Global trends in resistance to antituberculous drugs. N Engl J Med 2001; 344: 1294-1303.
Iseman MD. A clinician's guide to tuberculosis. Philadelphia: Lippincott Williams & Wilkins; 2000.
Kato-Maeda M, Small PM. User's guide to tuberculosis resources on the Internet. Clin Infect Dis 2001; 32: 1580-1588.
Reichman LB, Hershfield ES. Tuberculosis: a comprehensive international approach. New York: Marcel Dekker; 2000.
Schlossberg D, ed. Tuberculosis and nontuberculous mycobacterial infections. Philadelphia: W.B. Saunders Company; 1999.

Tuberculosis: Overview, Cause, and Pathogenesis

Tuberculosis holds a special place in medical history, is responsible worldwide for a staggering toll of disease and death, remains relatively common in the United States, can humble master clinicians, and poses formidable challenges to public health authorities. Yet, paradoxically, it is both treatable and preventable. The World Health Organization, estimating that over 8 million cases and 2 million deaths from tuberculosis occur worldwide each year, has declared tuberculosis to be a "global public health emergency." Furthermore, persons with tuberculosis *disease* represent only the tip of the iceberg. The estimated 25% to 33% of the world's population (>1.5 billion persons) who have silent latent infection with *M. tuberculosis* constitute a formidable reservoir for future cases. In the United States every state health department has a division of tuberculosis control (DTC) that has ultimate legal responsibility for the control of tuberculosis. Services offered vary according to locality but generally include the following:

- Extensive records of previously treated patients with tuberculosis
- Assistance with diagnostic evaluation (e.g., outpatient chest x-ray examination; collection and laboratory examination of sputum specimens)
- Free antituberculous medications
- HIV testing
- Tuberculosis educational materials for patients and their families

515

- Direct or indirect access to expert consultation
- Case management (if desired), including directly observed therapy (DOT)
- Appropriate contact investigation
- Provision of preventive therapy (treatment of latent tuberculosis infection)

The DTC of each state health department operates as part of national network coordinated by the Division of Tuberculosis Elimination of the Centers for Disease Control and Prevention (CDC), which assists states with technical guidelines and consultation and serves as a conduit for federal funding for tuberculosis control activities. In most areas of the United States diagnosed cases can often be either completely turned over to the state or local tuberculosis program or managed in what must necessarily be a collaborative effort between the attending clinician and the tuberculosis control program.

In 1999 more than 17,000 cases of tuberculosis were reported in the United States. Cases were reported in every state, and drug-resistant cases, which present a major challenge, were identified in almost every state. Coinfection with *M. tuberculosis* and HIV has continued to emerge as a complex problem both for diagnosis and for therapy, and the estimated 10 million to 15 million persons who remain latently infected with *M. tuberculosis* constitute a reservoir from which, without intervention, up to 10% of persons will eventually develop active tuberculosis disease.

Cause

M. tuberculosis, commonly called *M. TB* or simply the tubercle bacillus, is a slightly curved or straight rod-shaped bacillus that requires special (acid-fast) stains to be visualized by routine microscopy. It is closely related to *Mycobacterium*

bovis, which, as the name implies, is primarily a pathogen of cattle and related animals. *M. tuberculosis* is also related to *Mycobacterium leprae,* the causative agent of leprosy, as well as to numerous other mycobacterial species, which are referred to collectively as nontuberculous mycobacteria (NTM; see later discussion). Infections caused by NTM are not spread from person to person and thus do not have the same community health importance as cases of tuberculosis.

Transmission and Pathogenesis

Tuberculosis is spread from person to person through the air by droplet nuclei 1 to 5 μL in diameter that have been expelled into the air by a person with pulmonary tuberculosis, usually unrecognized and untreated. Cough is the primary means by which tubercle bacilli are aerosolized, but singing, sneezing, or speaking may contribute to a lesser extent. Droplet nuclei, unlike larger respiratory droplets that rapidly fall to surfaces or to the ground, are small enough to remain suspended in the air for relatively long periods. Persons who share airspace with an individual with infectious tuberculosis are at risk for infection. The probability of transmission depends on numerous factors relating to the source case, the exposed contacts, and shared airspace.

Tuberculosis pathogenesis begins when a droplet containing viable tubercle bacilli is inhaled, transits the upper and middle airways without landing on ciliated respiratory epithelium, and reaches the alveolar surface, typically in a peripheral lower lobe location (Figure 22-1). The alveolar macrophage response often fails to halt bacillary multiplication, resulting in a local focus of infection. Bacilli then spread through the pulmonary lymphatics and reach hilar or mediastinal lymph nodes, which may become enlarged. Efferent lymphatics

FIG. 22-1   Usual pathogenesis of tuberculosis. Inhaled droplet nuclei containing *Mycobacterium tuberculosis* reach the alveoli (usually in the peripheral portion of a lower lobe) where they multiply, spread to regional lymph nodes (Ghon complex), and then reach the systemic arterial circulation by way of the thoracic duct. Hematogenous dissemination sometimes leads to miliary tuberculosis, but more commonly active immunity develops and contains the microorganisms. Thus 1 year after the infection most persons have latent tuberculosis manifested as a positive tuberculin skin test. Viable bacilli are present within macrophages at the apices of the lungs (Simon focus). Reactivation occurs when macrophages are no longer able to contain the organisms.

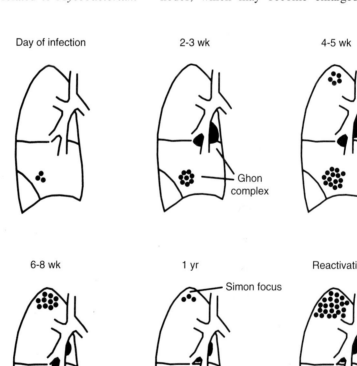

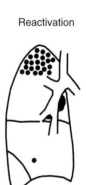

carry bacilli into the systemic circulation, permitting seeding of any organ in the body. Areas most commonly seeded include the apices of the lungs, the brain, the kidneys, and the bones. Tubercle bacilli replicate relatively slowly, having a dividing time on the order of 18 to 24 hours (compared with about 20 minutes for most common pathogens). Thus the aforementioned process of local, lymphatic, and eventual systemic spread typically requires several weeks. By that time the bacillary load has become sufficient to stimulate cell-mediated host defenses, which usually halts bacillary multiplication. Disease develops in only about 5% of apparently immunocompetent persons in the first year or two after infection. The remaining 95% remain infected and carry a lifelong risk of reactivation of latent infection, which occurs in another 5% of infected persons. Thus, on average in most populations, perhaps only 10% of persons infected with *M. tuberculosis* will have clinical disease in their lifetimes. However, the risk of progression from infection to disease is considerably higher in certain subpopulations. For example, persons with untreated HIV coinfection may progress from tuberculosis infection to tuberculosis disease at the rate of 10% per year. Infants and persons with immunologic, metabolic, or systemic copathologies are also more likely to develop disease once infected. This complex scenario explains why tuberculosis, although acquired by the airborne route, may affect any organ in the body and why certain vulnerable subpopulations are in need of targeted testing and treatment of latent tuberculosis infection.

 KEY POINTS

TUBERCULOSIS: OVERVIEW, CAUSE, AND PATHOGENESIS

⟳ In the United States about 17,000 cases of active tuberculosis occur each year. However, there are 10 million to 15 million cases of latent tuberculosis, and drug-resistant *M. tuberculosis* has been identified in nearly every state.

⟳ Although pulmonary tuberculosis represents >75% of all cases of active tuberculosis, tuberculosis is a systemic disease that can affect nearly every organ.

⟳ *M. tuberculosis* is transmitted by 1- to 5-µL droplet nuclei expelled by coughing, sneezing, speaking, or singing.

⟳ In about 5% of persons newly infected with *M. tuberculosis,* active disease will develop within 2 years. The remaining 95% of persons have latent tuberculosis, and of these about 5% will have active tuberculosis at some point during their lives. Thus the lifetime risk of active disease after infection with *M. tuberculosis* is about 10%. However, the risk is substantially higher in certain populations (up to 10% *per year* in patients with HIV disease).

SUGGESTED READING

American Thoracic Society. Diagnostic standards and classification of tuberculosis in adults and children. Am J Respir Crit Care Med 2000; 161: 1376-1395.

Efferen LS. Tuberculosis update: will good news become bad news? Curr Opin Pulm Med 1997; 3: 131-138.

Ellner JJ, Hirsch CS, Whalen CC. Correlates of protective immunity to *Mycobacterium tuberculosis* in humans. Clin Infect Dis 2000; 30 (Suppl 3): S279-S282.

Lauzardo M, Ashkin D. Phthisiology at the dawn of the new century. Chest 2000; 117: 1455-1473.

Schluger NW, Rom WN. The host immune response to tuberculosis. Am J Respir Crit Care Med 1998; 157: 679-691.

Latent Tuberculosis Infection: Diagnosis and Treatment (Preventive Therapy)

Recognition and treatment of selected subgroups from among the 10 million to 15 million persons in the United States with latent tuberculosis infection may be the primary care clinician's most important role in the national strategy for eventual elimination of tuberculosis as a public health problem. Unfortunately, and despite intensive efforts, no convenient serologic test is available for diagnosis of latent tuberculosis. Diagnosis therefore depends on tuberculin skin testing.

Formerly, widespread tuberculin skin testing was commonly performed in schools and other settings. Preventive therapy with isoniazid (INH) was offered to persons with a reactive test, defined as 10 mm of induration with the standard Mantoux skin test. In recent years three changes have occurred in the approach to latent tuberculosis infection. First, identification and treatment of all persons with a positive tuberculin skin test are now considered neither possible nor desirable. Targeted skin testing is now recommended for identifying persons at high risk for active tuberculosis (Box 22-1). Second, the need to vary interpretation of the test according to the patient population has now been recognized (Box 22-2). Third, the recommendations for treatment of latent tuberculosis infection have recently been modified (Table 22-1).

Tuberculin Skin Testing

The tuberculin skin test (TST) is the only tool currently available for diagnosis of latent tuberculosis infection. The Mantoux method, involving the intradermal administration of purified protein derivative (PPD), is preferred. Multiple puncture tests, although more convenient to administer, are less well standardized, less reliable, and not recommended. The Mantoux method calls for intradermal injection of 0.1 mL of 5TU PPD tuberculin, usually administered on the inner surface of the forearm. The injection should produce a discrete elevation of the skin (wheal) 6 to 10 mm in diameter. The reaction to the Mantoux test should be read 48 to 72 hours after injection. The reaction is recorded as millimeters of induration measured across the forearm (i.e., perpendicular to the long axis of the limb). Erythema (redness without induration) should not be measured. If no induration is present, the result should be recorded as "0 mm" rather than "negative." Depending on the clinical setting and local policies, tuberculin testing can sometimes be performed by a professional (e.g., employee health nurse, health department nurse) who has had special training and extensive experience in administering TSTs.

The TST is far from perfect. False-positive results can occur from previous infection (not necessarily accompanied by disease) with nontuberculous mycobacteria and also from prior vaccination with bacille Calmette-Guérin (BCG, as discussed in the section on BCG vaccine). Causes of false-negative results include the following:

■ Chronologic causes. The test may be performed too soon after infection (e.g., <2 to 10 weeks after the initial infection; see Figure 22-1) or, conversely, many years after the infection and after reactivity has waned. In some patients a second skin test performed immediately after interpretation of the first test result will give a positive result (booster phenomenon from the two-step method).

- Technical causes. Several possibilities exist: the tuberculin material may be outdated or the batch of tuberculin flawed; the test may be applied improperly; or the test may be interpreted improperly.
- Immunologic causes. Examples include recent immuno-suppressive illness or medication (e.g., prednisone at >15 mg per day for 2 to 4 weeks), HIV disease, recent viral illness or live virus vaccine, malnutrition, or severe wasting owing to any disease, including tuberculosis itself.

Anergy testing has been often used as a "control" to the tuberculin test, but it is not recommended for this purpose. Anergy testing has never been standardized, does not predict the risk of progression to active tuberculosis, and can be misleading. Anergy testing should be used only to answer specific questions (e.g., it may provide information about the person's nutritional status and is possibly useful in the diagnosis of sarcoidosis).

The previous criterion of 10 mm of induration for a positive tuberculin test was based mainly on the use of PPD for popula-tion surveys. The new criteria (Box 22-2) reject this "one size fits all" approach. Different "cut points" for different patient populations are now used as a guide to recommending treatment for latent tuberculosis infection. The mean reaction size of HIV-negative patients with active tuberculosis is about 15 mm, with about 85% of such patients having between 10 and 20 mm of induration. In nearly all published series of culture-proven tuberculosis, however, about 20% to 30% of patients failed to react at all to tuberculin. Thus, in a person being tested for latent tuberculosis infection, a large reaction (e.g., 15 mm of induration) is extremely likely to indicate past infection with *M. tuberculosis;* a somewhat smaller reaction (e.g., 10 to 14 mm or even 5 to

---

BOX 22-1
Persons for Whom Tuberculin Skin Testing Is Recommended (Targeted Tuberculin Testing)*

- Testing is recommended for close contacts of persons known or suspected to have tuberculosis (i.e., those sharing the same household or other enclosed environments).
- Foreign-born persons, including children, from areas that have a high tuberculosis incidence or prevalence (e.g., Asia, Africa, Latin America, Eastern Europe, Russia) should be tested.
- Residents and employees of high-risk congregate settings (e.g., correctional institutions, nursing homes, mental institutions, other long-term residential facilities, and shelters for the home-less) should be tested.
- Health care workers who serve high-risk clients should be tested.
- Some medically underserved, low-income populations as defined locally should be tested.
- Individuals from high-risk racial or ethnic minority populations, defined locally as having an increased prevalence of tuberculosis (e.g., Asians and Pacific Islanders, Hispanics, African-Americans, Native Americans, migrant farm workers, or homeless persons) should be tested.
- Infants, children, and adolescents exposed to adults in high-risk categories should be tested.
- Persons who inject illicit drugs should be tested, including any other locally identified high-risk substance users (e.g., crack cocaine users).
- Persons with human immunodeficiency virus (HIV) infection should be tested.
- Persons should be tested if they have medical conditions known to increase the risk for disease if infection occurs, such as diabetes, end-stage renal disease, silicosis, gastrectomy, jejunoileal bypass, or certain malignancies. Patients receiving prolonged therapy with corticosteroids and other immunosuppressive agents such as prednisone or its equivalent given >15 mg/day for 2 to 4 weeks should also be tested.

*Conceptually, this list consists of two subsets of persons: those at higher risk for tuberculosis exposure and infection (e.g., contacts to cases) and those at higher risk for tuberculosis once infected (e.g., persons with HIV infection).

BOX 22-2
Classification of the Tuberculin Reaction and Identification of Candidates for Treatment of Latent Tuberculosis Infection

1. A tuberculin reaction of ≥5 mm of induration is classified as positive in the following groups:
   - HIV-positive persons
   - Persons in recent contact with an individual with clinically active tuberculosis
   - Persons with fibrotic changes on chest radiograph consistent with old healed tuberculosis
   - Patients with organ transplants and other immunosuppressed patients (receiving the equivalent of prednisone ≥15 mg/day for ≥1 month)
2. A tuberculin reaction of ≥10 mm of induration is classified as positive in persons who do not meet the preceding criteria but who have other risk factors for tuberculosis. These include the following:
   - Individuals who are recent arrivals (<5 years) from high-prevalence countries
   - Injecting drug users
   - Residents and employees of high-risk congregate settings: prisons and jails, nursing homes and other long-term facilities for the elderly, hospitals and other health care facilities, residential facilities for patients with acquired immuno-deficiency syndrome, and homeless shelters
   - Persons with clinical conditions that place them at high risk
   - Children <4 years of age, or children and adolescents exposed to adults in high-risk categories
3. A tuberculin reaction of ≥15 mm of induration is classified as positive in persons with no known risk factors for tuberculosis. However, targeted skin testing programs should be conducted only among high-risk groups.
4. Persons found to be positive according to any of the preceding criteria should be considered for treatment of latent tuberculosis infection, as should the following:
   - High-risk tuberculin-negative contacts of an infected individual who have a high probability of having been infected but who may not have had sufficient time after infection for development of a "positive skin test" ("high-risk" in this setting refers, for example, to contacts <5 years of age or HIV-positive contacts); immunocompetent persons in these groups can be retested 2 months after last exposure to the infectious individual, and treatment of latent tuberculosis infection may be discontinued if the tuberculin skin test has remained negative
   - Persons who were recently infected with *Mycobacterium tuberculosis* (within the past 2 years), such as infants and very young children, health care workers (or others who have annual tuberculin skin tests), or individuals whose skin test converted to positive within the past 2 years

10 mm in certain subgroups) is consistent with past infection. An absent or small reaction (0 to 4 mm) is unhelpful.

BCG Vaccine

BCG (bacille Calmette-Guérin) is a live attenuated strain of *M. bovis* used in many countries as vaccine against tuberculosis. BCG has rarely been used in the United States because studies have shown it to be of variable effectiveness, because prior administration of BCG may interfere with the interpretation of subsequent TSTs, because much of the tuberculosis seen in the United States arises in persons previously infected with *M. tuberculosis* (for whom vaccination now would be too late), and because it is now appreciated that BCG cannot have a large-scale impact on the epidemiology and transmission of tuberculosis. BCG remains a valuable vaccine in developing countries, where the incidence of tuberculosis is much higher than in the United States and where its incorporation into infant immunization programs has been shown to decrease the incidence of severe disseminated tuberculosis (e.g., miliary, meningeal) in early childhood. Physicians who see large numbers of foreign-born children or adults in their practice need to be familiar with BCG and its interplay with tuberculin skin testing.

 KEY POINTS

BCG VACCINE

⊃ BCG vaccine is a live attenuated vaccine derived from *M. bovis* and commonly administered to children (and sometimes to other populations) in many countries.

⊃ Neither history of BCG vaccination (with or without documentation) nor a BCG scar (usually seen on the deltoid) is a contraindication to tuberculin skin testing if otherwise indicated.

⊃ Tuberculin reactions from BCG tend to be smaller than those from *M. tuberculosis* and to wane with time. Many persons who have had BCG in the past eventually become tuberculin negative.

⊃ In high-risk persons (e.g., persons in contact with an individual with clinically active tuberculosis, persons from countries where tuberculosis rates are high), history of prior BCG administration should not alter the interpretation of the TST.

TABLE 22-1
Recommended Regimens for Treatment of Latent Tuberculosis Infection

Option	Drug(s)	Regimen	STRENGTH OF CDC-ATS RECOMMENDATION* HIV−	HIV+	Comment
1	Isoniazid	Daily for 9 months	A	A	Regimen of choice especially for HIV infected patients, children, and those with fibrotic lesions seen on chest x-ray examination
2	Isoniazid	Twice weekly for 9 months	B	B	DOT strongly recommended with twice-weekly doses
3	Isoniazid	Daily for 6 months	B	C	Not indicated for HIV-infected patients, those with fibrotic lesions on chest x-ray examination, or children
4	Isoniazid	Twice weekly for 6 months	B	C	DOT strongly recommended with twice-weekly doses
5	Rifampin	Daily for 4 months	B	B	May be offered to persons who are contacts of patients with isoniazid-resistant, rifampin-susceptible tuberculosis or those who cannot take isoniazid
6	Rifampin *plus* pyrazinamide	Daily for 2 months	B	A	May be offered to persons who are contacts of patients with isoniazid-resistant rifampin-susceptible tuberculosis or those who cannot take isoniazid. However, this regimen should be used with great caution (see footnote†).
7	Rifampin *plus* pyrazinamide	Twice weekly for 2 to 3 months	C	B	DOT must be used with twice-weekly doses

Modified from Centers for Disease Control and Prevention. Targeted Tuberculin Testing and Treatment of Latent Tuberculosis Infection. MMWR 2000; 40 (RR-6). This document should be consulted for more detailed information.
ATS, American Thoracic Society; *CDC,* Centers for Disease Control and Prevention; *DOT,* directly observed therapy; *HIV,* human immunodeficiency virus.
*Strength of recommendation: *A,* preferred; *B,* acceptable alternative; *C,* offer when A and B cannot be given.
†Severe liver injury has been recently reported with this regimen. Physicians using the regimen should be thoroughly familiar with current recommendations. See Centers for Disease Control and Prevention. Update: fatal and severe liver injuries associated with rifampin and pyrazinamide for latent tuberculosis infection, and revisions in American Thoracic Society/CDC recommendations—United States 2001. MMWR 2001: 50: 733-735.

TABLE 22-2
Doses of First-Line Drugs Used in the Treatment of Tuberculosis

		DOSE (MG/KG) (MAXIMUM DOSE)					
		DAILY		**TWO TIMES PER WEEK***		**THREE TIMES PER WEEK***	
Drug	**Route**	**Children**	**Adults**	**Children**	**Adults**	**Children**	**Adults**
Isoniazid	PO, IM	10 to 20 (300 mg)	5 (300 mg)	20 to 40 (900 mg)	15 (900 mg)	20 to 40 (900 mg)	15 (900 mg)
Rifampin	PO, IV	10 to 20 (600 mg)	10 (600 mg)	10 to 20 (600 mg)	10 (600 mg)	10 to 20 (600 mg)	10 (600 mg)
Rifabutin†	PO, IV	10 to 20 (300 mg)	5 (300 mg)	10 to 20 (300 mg)	5 (300 mg)	Not known	Not known
Pyrazinamide	PO	15 to 20 (2 g)	15 to 30 (2 g)	50 to 70 (4 g)	50 to 70 (4 g)	50 to 70 (3 g)	50 to 70 (3 g)
Ethambutol‡	PO	15 to 25	15 to 25	50	50	25 to 30	25 to 30
Streptomycin	IM, IV	20 to 40 (1 g)	15 (1 g)	25 to 30 (1.5 g)	25 to 30 (1.5 g)	25 to 30 (1.5 g)	25 to 30 (1.5 g)

Modified from Centers for Disease Control and Prevention. Core Curriculum on Tuberculosis: What the Clinician Should Know. 4th ed., Atlanta: Centers for Disease Control and Prevention; 2000.
*Directly observed therapy (DOT; see text) should be used for all intermittent dosage regimens.
†If rifabutin is to be used for patients with human immunodeficiency virus disease, the clinician should be thoroughly familiar with the interactions between rifabutin and antiretroviral drugs. Rifabutin is contraindicated in patients who are taking hard-gel saquinavir or delavirdine.
‡The dose of ethambutol should always be calculated on a milligram per kilogram basis. In obese patients, ethambutol dosage should be based on lean body weight.

Treatment of Latent Tuberculosis Infection (Preventive Treatment)

Before treatment is prescribed for latent tuberculosis infection, active tuberculosis must be excluded. A chest x-ray examination suffices for this purpose if no symptoms or signs consistent with active tuberculosis are present. In children <5 years of age a lateral view should be obtained in addition to the standard posteroanterior (PA) view. Persons with positive tuberculin skin tests should be considered for treatment of latent tuberculosis infection if the history, physical examination, and chest x-ray examination produce no evidence of active tuberculosis. Formerly the only recommended treatment was INH given daily for 6 to 12 months. At present the CDC endorses seven different options according to the clinical setting (see Table 22-3). Recent investigators have addressed especially the issue of preventive treatment in persons with HIV disease. Data do not support preventive treatment of persons with HIV disease who are anergic and who have not been exposed to active tuberculosis. In tuberculin-positive persons with HIV disease a 2-month regimen of rifampin and pyrazinamide was shown to be similar in safety and efficacy to a 12-month regimen of INH alone.

The hepatotoxicity of INH, the mainstay of treatment for latent tuberculosis infection, has been controversial for many years. Current thinking holds that although INH causes elevations of alanine aminotransferase (ALT) and aspartate aminotransferase (AST) levels in 10% to 20% of patients, the elevations are usually transient and INH hepatitis develops in <1% of persons (although the incidence of INH hepatitis is age related; see later discussion). Baseline and periodic (e.g., after 1 month and 3 months of treatment) liver function tests are therefore recommended as a standard of care only in

patients at high risk for liver injury. These include patients with alcoholism and those with chronic hepatitis B or hepatitis C. Biochemical monitoring does not replace close questioning for signs and symptoms of hepatitis, which must be done at least once a month, and patients must be instructed to discontinue their medication and be evaluated if they have an onset of manifestations such as jaundice, unexplained anorexia, nausea, vomiting, or dark urine. Such clinical monitoring suffices for most adults whose baseline liver function tests were normal and who are not otherwise at risk of hepatic injury. Most children can be evaluated solely with clinical monitoring. Most health departments in the United States have well-established preventive therapy clinics to which physicians may refer patients for management of latent tuberculosis infection. In all cases patients must be seen at least monthly and should never be given more than a 1-month supply of medication.

 KEY POINTS

LATENT TUBERCULOSIS INFECTION: DIAGNOSIS AND TREATMENT (PREVENTIVE THERAPY)

⊃ Emphasis has shifted from widespread tuberculin skin testing to targeted testing for persons who are at high risk for either recent infection or active disease.
⊃ Criteria for interpreting the tuberculin skin test have been modified to take into account the patient category. Thus 5 mm of induration is considered a positive result in persons with HIV disease, but 15 mm of induration is required for a positive result in low-risk persons.

↺ Causes of false-positive tuberculin tests include nontuberculous mycobacterial infection and prior BCG vaccination.

↺ Causes of false-negative tuberculin tests include testing too soon after the initial infection or too late in the course of the illness, poor technical performance of the test, and immunosuppression from any cause.

↺ Routine "anergy" testing as a control to the tuberculin test is not recommended.

↺ The CDC currently endorses seven options for treatment of latent tuberculosis infection, depending on the circumstances.

↺ INH, the mainstay of preventive therapy, causes transient elevations of ALT and AST levels in about 10% to 20% of patients, but INH hepatitis is uncommon (<1% of treated patients). Routine biochemical monitoring is now recommended as a standard of care only for persons at high risk of liver toxicity from other diseases such as alcoholism, chronic hepatitis B, or chronic hepatitis C.

↺ Patients receiving treatment for latent tuberculosis infection should be seen monthly and never given more than a 1-month supply of medication. Most U.S. health departments have preventive therapy clinics to which patients can be referred for this purpose.

SUGGESTED READING

American Thoracic Society. Diagnostic standards and classification of tuberculosis in adults and children. Am J Respir Crit Care Med 2000; 161: 1376-1395.

Centers for Disease Control and Prevention. Prevention and treatment of tuberculosis among patients infected with human immunodeficiency virus: principles of therapy and revised recommendations. MMWR 1998; 47 (RR-20): 1-58.

Centers for Disease Control and Prevention. Targeted tuberculin testing and treatment of latent tuberculosis infection. MMWR 2000; 49 (RR-6): 1-51.

Centers for Disease Control and Prevention: The role of BCG vaccine in the prevention and control of tuberculosis in the United States. MMWR 1996; 45 (RR-4): 1-18.

Gammaitoni L, Gordin F, Chaisson RE, Matts JP, et al. Rifampin and pyrazinamide vs isoniazid for prevention of tuberculosis in HIV-infected persons: an international randomized trial. JAMA 2000; 283: 1445-1450.

Gordin FM, Matts JP, Miller C, et al. A controlled trial of isoniazid in persons with anergy and human immunodeficiency virus infection who are at high risk for tuberculosis. N Engl J Med 1997; 337: 315-320.

King AB. Accurately interpreting PPD skin test results. Nurse Pract 1999; 24: 144-147.

Nolan CM. Community-wide implementation of targeted testing for and treatment of latent tuberculosis infection. Clin Infect Dis 1999; 29: 880-887.

Slovis BS, Plitman JD, Haas DW. The case against anergy testing as a routine adjunct to tuberculin skin testing. JAMA 2000; 283: 2003-2007.

Pulmonary Tuberculosis

Worldwide, tuberculosis remains the most common cause of death from an infectious agent. Pulmonary tuberculosis is the most common manifestation and the form of the disease usually responsible for its transmission.

Presentation and Diagnosis

As tuberculosis has become less common in the United States, the diagnosis is easily overlooked or at least delayed, usually because tuberculosis is not considered initially in the differential diagnosis. The clinician must "think TB" (see Chapter 1). Once tuberculosis is considered, however, the approach to diagnosis is usually straightforward and includes a medical history, an epidemiologic history, an HIV status review, a physical examination, a Mantoux skin test, a radiographic examination of the chest, and bacteriologic examination of spontaneously coughed or induced sputum. In some instances ancillary radiologic examinations (e.g., thoracic computed tomography [CT] scans) or other procedures (e.g., bronchoscopy or lung biopsy) may be needed.

Medical History

At first visit to a primary care practice, the usual patient with pulmonary tuberculosis describes a history of several weeks of a progressive illness. The most important pulmonary symptom is cough, which initially may not be productive but which becomes productive of sputum as inflammation and tissue necrosis develop. Hemoptysis is variable and is more suggestive of advanced disease. Chest pain on deep inspiration or coughing suggests pleural involvement. Dyspnea is uncommon unless the patient has extensive disease or an underlying pulmonary pathologic condition. Constitutional complaints coexist and may predominate. These include fever, chills, night sweats, weight loss, appetite loss, and easy fatigability. Not all patients have all of these manifestations. Because neither the pulmonary symptoms nor the constitutional symptoms are specific for tuberculosis, the clinician often entertains more common diagnoses at first, such as bacterial pneumonia, carcinoma of the lung, or, especially if constitutional symptoms predominate, occult cancers or other systemic diseases. Often it is only when a patient has failed to improve after receiving one or more courses of oral antibiotics that tuberculosis is considered in the differential diagnosis.

Epidemiologic History

Helpful information to elicit in the history includes a prior episode of tuberculosis; contact (especially household contact) with a confirmed case of pulmonary tuberculosis; birth or sojourn in a country where tuberculosis is much more common than in the United States (e.g., many countries of sub-Saharan Africa, Southeast Asia, and Eastern Europe, including former republics of the Soviet Union); or incarceration in prison. Any of these factors, when combined with suggestive symptoms and signs of tuberculosis, increases the likelihood that positive findings from tuberculin skin testing, chest x-ray examination, or bacteriologic examination of sputum are true-positive rather than false-positive results.

Review of Human Immunodeficiency Virus Status

HIV has a profound effect on the natural history of tuberculosis infection, greatly increasing the risk that clinically silent latent infection will progress to overt tuberculosis disease. However, the diagnosis of tuberculosis in patients with HIV, especially profoundly immunosuppressed patients, can be difficult because coinfected patients are more likely to have small or even absent tuberculin skin test results and are less likely to show findings typical of tuberculosis on a chest radiograph. Thus documentation of a positive serologic test for HIV can help guide the diagnostic evaluation. Suspicion of tuberculosis is an indication for HIV antibody testing.

Physical Examination

Findings on physical examination can neither confirm nor exclude pulmonary tuberculosis but may provide information about the patient's overall condition.

Tuberculin Skin Testing

Tuberculin testing (see earlier discussion) must be carefully performed and interpreted. As mentioned previously, about 20% to 30% of persons with active tuberculosis have nonreactive skin tests.

Chest Radiograph

A PA radiograph of the chest is the standard view for detection of abnormalities that are due to pulmonary tuberculosis. Lateral, apical, lordotic, or other studies (e.g., CT scans) are occasionally helpful. Abnormalities are most commonly seen in the apical and posterior segments of the upper lobe or in the superior segments of the lower lobe—hence the rule learned by students that *TB is a disease of the apices of the lungs.* However, lesions of pulmonary tuberculosis can be present in any lung zone and may differ greatly in size, shape, density, and appearance (Figure 22-2). Patients who are coinfected with HIV often have atypical radiographic presentations, including isolated mediastinal or hilar lymphadenopathy (more commonly seen in HIV-negative children with early or primary tuberculosis infection) or disease that involves the middle or lower lung zones. Some patients with tuberculosis and advanced HIV disease have entirely normal-looking chest radiographs. Because of the overlapping radiologic presentations of numerous pulmonary conditions, it should be remembered that abnormalities on a chest radiograph can only suggest tuberculosis and are not diagnostic in and of themselves.

Bacteriologic Examination of Sputum

All patients with suspected pulmonary tuberculosis should have three or more sputum specimens examined for mycobacteria by smear and culture. Early morning sputum specimens are ideal because secretions have pooled overnight. However, specimens can also be collected whenever a patient is being seen. Because the vigorous cough needed to produce a good sputum specimen may aerosolize infectious droplet nuclei, specimens should be collected in an isolated, well-ventilated area, in a specially designed sputum collection booth, or even outdoors or at home. For patients who cannot spontaneously produce adequate sputum specimens, a series of progressively more invasive procedures may be required, including sputum induction, gastric aspiration (historically used more commonly for children), and bronchoscopy.

Detection of acid-fact bacilli (AFB) in stained smears often provides the first bacteriologic clue for tuberculosis. However, sputum smears for AFB have two shortcomings. First, they are less sensitive than sputum cultures; indeed, patients with tuberculosis sometimes have one or more positive sputum cultures despite having had negative AFB smears. Second, *M. tuberculosis* cannot be distinguished from nontuberculous mycobacteria on the basis of the smear alone. Thus positive AFB smears suggest but do not prove tuberculosis. The predictive value of a positive sputum smear depends on the relative prevalence of *M. tuberculosis* and nontuberculous mycobacteria in the patient population (see discussion of Bayes' theorem in Chapter 1). For example, a positive AFB smear in a young adult who has had household contact with a person in whom pulmonary tuberculosis has been diagnosed in a major U.S. metropolitan area almost certainly represents *M. tuberculosis.* However, a positive smear in a middle-aged smoker from a rural area of the Midwest who has not been exposed to tuberculosis is more likely to indicate a nontuberculous mycobacterium. From a practical point of view, both of these patients would be managed initially as though they had tuberculosis if other evidence pointed toward tuberculosis.

Most state and large metropolitan tuberculosis control programs can make sputum collection, smear services, and culture services available at no cost. Furthermore, these tuberculosis programs typically work with a major reference laboratory (e.g., their state laboratory) equipped to perform not only traditional smear and culture tests but also one or more modern mycobacteriology tests (e.g., nucleic acid amplification or DNA gene probes) for diagnosis of tuberculosis. Because *M. tuberculosis* grows slowly, culture and sensitivity results are often not available for up to 6 weeks after specimens have been submitted. Use of molecular methods, specifically the polymerase chain reaction (PCR), for early and specific diagnosis of tuberculosis is a current area of active investigation. In one recent study the sensitivity of PCR for culture-proven tuberculosis was 70% on specimens obtained by bronchial brushings, 76% on bronchial washings, and 90% when both samples were mixed together. Occasionally a single positive culture for *M. tuberculosis* is false positive because of contamination of the specimen.

Treatment
Methods

Treatment of pulmonary tuberculosis requires at least 6 months of therapy with several drugs. The importance of full compliance cannot be overemphasized. Current options endorsed by the American Thoracic Society (ATS) and the CDC for patients

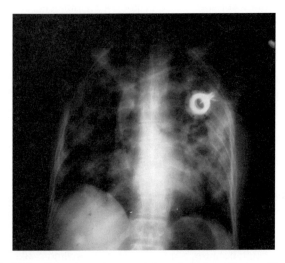

FIG. 22-2 Extensive pulmonary tuberculosis in a 74-year-old man who had recently undergone placement of a cardiac pacemaker. He had been treated recently for presumed right lower lobe pneumonia.

without HIV disease include the following (with dosages shown in Table 22-2):

- Option A. Eight weeks of daily isoniazid, rifampin, pyrazinamide, and ethambutol (or streptomycin), followed by 16 weeks of isoniazid and rifampin given daily, twice a week, or three times a week (if susceptibility to isoniazid and rifampin is demonstrated)
- Option B. Two weeks of isoniazid, rifampin, pyrazinamide, and ethambutol (or streptomycin), given daily at first, then twice a week for 6 weeks; followed by twice-weekly isoniazid and rifampin for 16 more weeks (if susceptibility to isoniazid and rifampin is demonstrated)
- Option C. Six months of isoniazid, rifampin, pyrazinamide, and ethambutol (or streptomycin) given three times a week throughout the course of treatment
- Option D. Two months of daily isoniazid, rifampin, and ethambutol (or streptomycin) followed by 7 months of daily or twice-weekly isoniazid and rifampin. (If susceptibility to isoniazid and rifampin is demonstrated, isoniazid and rifampin may be given twice weekly after an initial 4 to 8 weeks of daily treatment.)

Patients should be educated orally and in writing about tuberculosis, the dosage and possible adverse effects of medications (Table 22-3), and the importance to themselves, their

TABLE 22-3
Major Adverse Reactions to First-Line Drugs Used for Treatment of Tuberculosis and Recommendations for Monitoring

Drug	Major adverse reactions	Monitoring	Comments
Isoniazid	Rash, hepatic enzyme (AST, ALT) elevation, hepatitis, peripheral neuropathy, mild central nervous system effects, drug interactions resulting in increased phenytoin (Dilantin) or disulfiram (Antabuse) reactions	Baseline measurements of hepatic enzymes (AST, ALT) for adults. Repeat measurements if (1) baseline results are abnormal, (2) patient is at high risk for adverse reactions, or (3) patient has symptoms of adverse reactions.	Risk of hepatitis increases with age and alcohol consumption. Pyridoxine (vitamin B$_6$) may prevent peripheral neuropathy and central nervous system effects.
Rifampin	Gastrointestinal upset, multiple drug interactions, hepatitis, bleeding problems, flulike symptoms, rash, renal failure, fever	Baseline measurements of complete blood cell count, platelets, and hepatic enzymes (AST, ALT). Repeat measurements if baseline results are abnormal or if patient has symptoms of adverse reactions.	Significant drug interactions include methadone, oral contraceptives, and antiretroviral drugs. Rifampin colors body fluids orange and may permanently discolor soft contact lenses.
Rifabutin	Rash, hepatitis, fever, thrombocytopenia; increased rifabutin levels are associated with severe arthralgias, uveitis, and leukopenia	Same as with rifampin. Also, special care must be taken for patients receiving certain antiretroviral drugs.	Similar to rifampin. Rifampin is contraindicated in patients taking ritonavir or delavirdine, and great care must be taken with other antiretroviral drugs.
Pyrazinamide	Hepatitis, rash, gastrointestinal upset, joint pain, hyperuricemia (common), gout (rare)	Baseline measurements of uric acid and hepatic enzymes (AST, ALT). Repeat measurements if baseline results are abnormal and patient has symptoms of adverse reactions.	Treat hyperuricemia only if the patient has symptoms. Pyrazinamide can make glucose control more difficult in patients with diabetes mellitus.
Ethambutol	Optic neuritis; rash	Baseline and monthly tests of visual acuity and color vision. The patient should be advised to check vision in each eye daily.	Patients with impaired baseline vision should probably have follow-up by an ophthalmologist. Care must be taken with ethambutol dosage in patients with impaired renal function, including elderly patients.
Streptomycin	Ototoxicity (hearing loss or vestibular dysfunction); renal toxicity	Baseline hearing test (audiogram) and renal function tests; repeat as needed	Avoid use or reduce dose in persons ≥60 years of age. Ultrasound and warm compresses may reduce pain of IM injection.

Modified from Centers for Disease Control and Prevention. Core Curriculum on Tuberculosis: What the Clinician Should Know. 4th ed., Atlanta: Centers for Disease Control and Prevention; 2000.
ALT, Alanine aminotransferase; *AST,* aspartate aminotransferase.

families, and their coworkers of taking their medication. During therapy patients need to be monitored for adherence to the prescribed regimen, for adverse drug reactions, and for response to therapy. Response must be monitored through serial sputum specimens collected at least monthly until cultures convert to negative. Patients with positive sputum smears should initially be monitored even more closely.

With effective therapy the majority of patients should have sputum conversion after 8 weeks. Patients whose sputum has converted after 2 months of treatment should have at least one further sputum smear and culture performed at the completion of therapy. Complete blood count and measurement of liver enzymes and blood urea nitrogen or creatinine are useful as baselines against which to monitor patients for adverse drug reactions. During therapy patients must be monitored clinically at least monthly, although chemical and hematologic monitoring for adverse reactions may be individualized. Patients should be instructed to report adverse reactions such as onset of jaundice immediately, since they may be indicative of isoniazid-induced (or rifampin-induced) hepatotoxicity.

Most patients feel better after a few weeks of treatment and may thus be tempted to stop taking their medications. Failure to complete therapy as prescribed (noncompliance) is the major risk factor for subsequent relapse and emergence of drug-resistant organisms. Noncompliance is thus a major problem for clinicians, for tuberculosis control programs, and ultimately for the community. In recent years DOT has progressively emerged as the standard of care for patients with pulmonary tuberculosis. A health care worker (usually a public health nurse or other specially trained outreach worker) observes *every dose* of medication. Where resources are lacking to supervise every dose of medication for every patient with pulmonary tuberculosis in a community, *every patient must at least be considered for DOT* and resources allocated accordingly.

To facilitate adherence to therapy and to a DOT schedule, many health departments now have programs, supported by federal funds or the local Lung Association, that provide patients with incentives and "enablers" (e.g., persons who provide assistance with transportation). In most parts of the country physicians may refer patients with tuberculosis to the care of the local tuberculosis control program, which is staffed by a multidisciplinary team trained in management and community control of tuberculosis. Alternatively, physicians may prefer to maintain overall responsibility for the clinical management of their patients (e.g., monitoring for and managing adverse drug reactions, adjusting medications, managing coexisting medical problems), while leaving to the tuberculosis control program the management of the public health components that relate to every case of pulmonary tuberculosis, such as the technical and epidemiologic aspects of contact investigation and the provision of DOT. No matter which option is followed, optimal practice is for clinician and health department to agree on an explicit plan of care, follow-up, and division of responsibilities within a week of diagnosis.

Expected Results

Current regimens for pulmonary tuberculosis caused by drug-susceptible *M. tuberculosis* result in cure rates >95% if the drugs are taken exactly as prescribed. The duration of patients' contagiousness remains unclear. However, indirect evidence indicates that patients with active tuberculosis remain contagious for at least 2 weeks after initiation of therapy. Monitoring of therapy therefore includes regularly scheduled sputum AFB smears and cultures, usually coordinated by the health department.

Complications

Antituberculous drugs can cause significant adverse reactions (Table 22-3) that sometimes result in interruption of therapy.

When to Refer

Referral, consultation with an expert, or both are advisable for patients with laboratory-proven drug resistance, HIV coinfection, failure to show clinical or bacteriologic response to therapy, major drug toxicities, or nonadherence with the treatment program. Some patients with drug-resistant *M. tuberculosis* require surgical resection of diseased lung tissue for control of the infection.

 KEY POINTS

PULMONARY TUBERCULOSIS

⊃ The diagnosis is often overlooked when the patient is first seen and is typically considered only after the patient fails to respond to one or more courses of antibiotics.

⊃ About 20% to 30% of persons with active pulmonary tuberculosis have nonreactive tuberculin skin tests.

⊃ The classic x-ray appearance of pulmonary tuberculosis (apical cavitary disease) is not always present. Moreover, this appearance can be mimicked by other diseases such as carcinoma of the lung, lung abscess, and nontuberculous mycobacterial infection. In some patients the radiographic findings are subtle (e.g., middle or lower lung field infiltrates, retroclavicular infiltrates, and retrocardiac infiltrates). In patients with HIV disease the chest radiograph is occasionally normal.

⊃ The sputum AFB smear is customarily used to make a presumptive diagnosis of pulmonary tuberculosis.

⊃ Causes of a false-positive sputum AFB smear include nontuberculous mycobacterial infection and, rarely, infection with other AFB-positive bacteria (*Nocardia* species and certain "diphtheroid" organisms). In some populations positive AFB smears are now more commonly due to nontuberculous mycobacteria than to *M. tuberculosis*.

⊃ Patients with positive sputum AFB smears and clinical evidence of tuberculosis are usually treated with antituberculous drugs until definitive culture results are available. Newer molecular techniques (DNA probes, PCR) are being used to make an earlier specific diagnosis.

⊃ Current treatment regimens for pulmonary tuberculosis caused by drug-susceptible strains result in cure in >95% of patients.

⊃ Failure to complete the entire course of treatment (noncompliance) is the most common cause for relapse and also for the emergence of drug-resistant strains.

⊃ All patients with pulmonary tuberculosis should be managed in active collaboration with the health department.

⊃ DOT, in which a health care worker directly observes the administration of each dose of medication, is emerging as the standard of care for treatment of pulmonary tuberculosis.

SUGGESTED READING

Burman WJ, Reves RR. Review of false-positive cultures for *Mycobacterium tuberculosis* and recommendations for avoiding unnecessary treatment. Clin Infect Dis 2000; 31: 1390-1395.

Chaulk CP, Kazandjian VA. Directly observed therapy for treatment completion of pulmonary tuberculosis: consensus statement of the Public Health Tuberculosis Guidelines Panel. JAMA 1998; 279: 943-948.

Fennelly KP. Personal respiratory protection against *Mycobacterium tuberculosis*. Clin Chest Med 1997; 18: 1-17.

Hidaka E, Honda T, Ueno I, et al. Sensitive identification of mycobacterial species using PCR-RFLP on bronchial washings. Am J Respir Crit Care Med 2000; 161: 930-934.

Hirsch CS, Johnson JL, Ellner JJ. Pulmonary tuberculosis. Curr Opin Pulm Med 1999; 5: 143-150.

Horsburgh CR Jr, Feldman S, Ridzon R. Infectious Diseases Society of America. Practice guidelines for the treatment of tuberculosis. Clin Infect Dis 2000; 31: 633-639.

Jerant AF, Bannon M, Rittenhouse S. Identification and management of tuberculosis. Am Fam Physician 2000; 61: 2667-2678, 2681-2682.

Menzies D. Effect of treatment on contagiousness of patients with active pulmonary tuberculosis. Infect Control Hosp Epidemiol 1997; 18; 582-586.

Wisnivesky JP, Kaplan J, Henschke C, et al. Evaluation of clinical parameters to predict *Mycobacterium tuberculosis* in inpatients. Arch Intern Med 2000; 160: 2471-2476.

Woods GL. Molecular methods in the detection and identification of mycobacterial infections. Arch Pathol Lab Med 1999; 123: 1002-1006.

Extrapulmonary Tuberculosis

Extrapulmonary tuberculosis is less common than pulmonary tuberculosis but is usually more difficult to diagnose. Diagnosis usually requires invasive procedures or biopsies. Molecular methods of diagnosis such as PCR offer the promise of greater sensitivity than with traditional culture methods. On the other hand, extrapulmonary tuberculosis usually responds to treatment more readily than pulmonary tuberculosis because the density of *M. tuberculosis* organisms is usually much lower than that in the usual pulmonary cavitary lesion. The syndromes of extrapulmonary tuberculosis can be divided into three categories: miliary (disseminated) tuberculosis, serosal tuberculosis (i.e., affecting the linings of various spaces), and tuberculosis of solid organs.

SUGGESTED READING

Engin G, Acunas B, Acunas G, et al. Imaging of extrapulmonary tuberculosis. Radiographics 2000; 20: 471-488.

Maltezou HC, Spyridis P, Kafetzis DA. Extra-pulmonary tuberculosis in children. Arch Dis Child 2000; 83: 342-346.

Portillo-Gomez L, Morris SL, Panduro A. Rapid and efficient detection of extra-pulmonary *Mycobacterium tuberculosis* by PCR analysis. Int J Tuberc Lung Dis 2000; 4: 361-370.

Miliary (Disseminated) Tuberculosis

Miliary tuberculosis, so named because the individual lesions resemble millet seeds, represents lymphohematogenous dissemination of *M. tuberculosis* throughout the body. The clinical presentation can be dramatic or subtle, and autopsy studies indicate that about 20% of cases are never correctly diagnosed. Miliary tuberculosis is especially common in patients with HIV disease.

Presentation and Progression
Cause

Classically, miliary tuberculosis results from the passage of *M. tuberculosis* from the lungs to the thoracic duct and then into the systemic arterial circulation. This event occurs routinely shortly after primary *M. tuberculosis* infection and, although usually contained by host defenses (Figure 22-1), sometimes results in clinical disease. Miliary tuberculosis can also result from previous, untreated tuberculosis involving a solid organ. In immunocompetent persons the typical lesion is a small, well-formed, often caseating granuloma containing relatively few microorganisms. In severely immunocompromised patients, including those with advanced HIV disease, granulomas may fail to develop, and tissues as well as blood may contain numerous bacilli. Patients in whom miliary tuberculosis is more likely to occur include young children recently exposed to the disease, pregnant women, the elderly, persons suffering from alcoholism or liver disease, and persons who are immunosuppressed for any reason.

Presentation

Several clinical expressions of miliary tuberculosis are recognized.

Acute Miliary Tuberculosis. This form manifests itself with high fevers, night sweats, and other symptoms and signs of dramatic infectious illness. Occasionally patients have the acute respiratory distress syndrome, septic shock, and multiorgan failure. Localizing symptoms may point to organ involvement; examples include headache (meningitis), chest pain (pleurisy or pericarditis), and abdominal pain (peritonitis). Children tend have an acute illness. Young adults often have a subacute illness. Miliary lesions are often seen on chest radiograph (Figure 22-3), although they may not be present when the patient is first seen.

Chronic Miliary Tuberculosis. The chronic form is associated with various combinations of fever, anorexia, weight loss, or, especially in the elderly, simply failure to thrive. The term "cryptic miliary tuberculosis" applies to older patients with extremely subtle symptoms and signs that are usually attributed to another underlying disease process. Occasionally the disease occurs as a hematologic disorder such as a leukemoid reaction, thrombocytopenia, myelofibrosis, or polycythemia. Chronic miliary tuberculosis is an important cause of fever of unknown origin.

Tuberculosis in Persons Infected with Human Immunodeficiency Virus. Miliary tuberculosis occurs in about 10% of patients with pulmonary tuberculosis and up to 38% of patients with extrapulmonary tuberculosis. High fever is characteristic. Some HIV-infected patients exhibit a rare form of the disease known as nonreactive tuberculosis, in which sepsis may dominate the clinical picture and in which autopsy discloses abscesses teeming with *M. tuberculosis* but with little or no host response.

Diagnosis

Diagnosis of miliary tuberculosis is hampered by the nonspecificity of the clinical symptoms and signs in most cases and therefore hinges on a high index of suspicion. The TST is

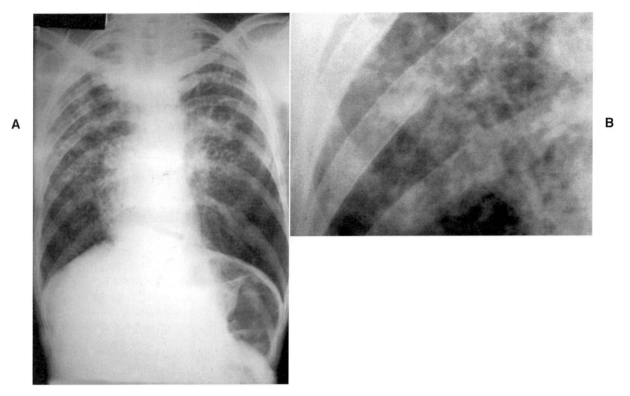

FIG. 22-3   A, Chest x-ray appearance of miliary tuberculosis. **B,** "Snowstorm" appearance of the fine reticulonodular infiltrate can sometimes be appreciated best by holding the film up to a strong light.

helpful if positive, but it is nonreactive in 47% to 72% of cases in various series. Physical examination of the chest is abnormal in about one half to three fourths of patients, but the findings are nonspecific (e.g., rales, rhonchi, rubs, and signs of pleural effusion). The following clinical findings should be aggressively sought:

- Choroidal tubercles, which appear as round white lesions on ophthalmoscopic examination
- Palpable lymph nodes (especially supraclavicular or scalene lymph nodes), biopsy of which sometimes reveals the diagnosis
- Hematologic abnormalities such as anemia (about one half of cases), leukopenia, and thrombocytopenia or thrombocytosis
- Hyponatremia (present in up to 78% of cases and a valuable clue)
- Elevation of the serum alkaline phosphatase level (up to 83% of cases) and other abnormal liver function test results
- Hypoxemia
- Sterile pyuria (present in about one third of cases)
- Miliary granulomas on chest radiograph or on high-resolution CT scanning of the chest (which is more sensitive than chest radiography for this purpose)

Sputum AFB smears are positive in about one third of cases, and cultures of gastric aspirates, urine, cerebrospinal fluid (CSF), and other body fluids are occasionally helpful. AFB blood cultures are typically positive in persons with HIV disease but are less frequently positive in immunocompetent patients. Bronchoscopy with transbronchial lung biopsy is probably the most useful diagnostic procedure. Liver and bone marrow biopsies can also be helpful. Recently PCR has been used for early diagnosis based on liver and bone marrow

biopsies, but more clinical experience is needed. When the diagnosis is strongly suspected in patients with life-threatening symptoms and signs of disease, a therapeutic trial of antituberculous drugs is often appropriate while the results of AFB cultures are awaited.

Natural History
Expected Outcome

Untreated miliary tuberculosis is almost uniformly fatal.

Treatment
Methods

Treatment consists of standard antituberculous drugs.

Expected Response

Response is usually dramatic, with about three fourths of patients becoming afebrile within 14 days of appropriate treatment.

When to Refer

When miliary tuberculosis is suspected, patients should usually be admitted to the hospital or referred for special studies.

 KEY POINTS

MILIARY TUBERCULOSIS

⊃ Miliary tuberculosis results from lymphohematogenous spread of *M. tuberculosis,* either from the lungs (as during primary tuberculous infection) or from a solid organ previously infected.

⊃ Symptoms include fever, night sweats, anorexia, weight loss, and localizing symptoms that reflect specific organ involvement such as headache (meningitis), chest pain (pleurisy or pericarditis), and abdominal pain (peritonitis).

⊃ Presentation varies from fulminant disease with the acute respiratory distress syndrome, septic shock, and multi-organ failure to a chronic or "cryptic" disease that can be extremely subtle and difficult to diagnose.

⊃ When miliary tuberculosis is suspected, hospitalization or referral is usually warranted.

SUGGESTED READING

Akcan Y, Tuncer S, Hayran M, et al. PCR on disseminated tuberculosis in bone marrow and liver biopsy specimens: correlation to histopathological and clinical diagnosis. Scand J Infect Dis 1997; 29: 271-274.

Del Giudice P, Bernard E, Perin C, et al. Unusual cutaneous manifestations of miliary tuberculosis. Clin Infect Dis 2000; 30: 201-204.

Gurkan F, Bosnak M, Dikici B, et al. Miliary tuberculosis in children: a clinical review. Scand J Infect Dis 1998; 30: 359-262.

Hong SH, Im JG, Lee JS, et al. High resolution CT findings of miliary tuberculosis. J Comput Assist Tomogr 1998; 22: 220-224.

Kim JH, Langston AA, Gallis HA. Miliary tuberculosis: epidemiology, clinical manifestations, diagnosis, and outcome. Rev Infect Dis 1990; 12: 583-590.

Maartens G, Willcox PA, Benatar SR. Miliary tuberculosis: rapid diagnosis, hematologic abnormalities, and outcome in 109 treated adults. Am J Med 1990; 89: 291-296.

Serosal Tuberculosis

"Serosal tuberculosis" is a convenient term to use in appreciating the pathogenesis, presentation, and diagnosis of five syndromes: tuberculous pleurisy, meningitis, pericarditis, peritonitis, and arthritis. The pleural, subarachnoid, pericardial, peritoneal, and synovial membranes define spaces that under normal circumstances contain small amounts of sterile fluid that lubricate the underlying tissues or allow freedom of movement. Tuberculosis results when *M. tuberculosis* organs gain access to the space. This can occur during hematogenous dissemination of *M. tuberculosis* or by extension into the membrane of a localized lesion such as a granuloma or tuberculous lymph node. Thus careful examination of the brain in fatal cases of tuberculous meningitis invariably reveals a subependymal tubercle (Rich focus) that has ruptured into the subarachnoid space. The clinical manifestations of serosal tuberculosis can reflect both or either of two processes: multiplication of *M. tuberculosis* within the space, and host inflammatory response to *M. tuberculosis* antigens (delayed hypersensitivity reaction). The latter of these processes often predominates. Experimentally, injection of *M. tuberculosis* into the pleural spaces of guinea pigs causes large pleural effusions only if the animals have been previously rendered tuberculin positive; otherwise, the animals die of miliary tuberculosis with minimal pleural effusion. Similarly, the symptoms and signs of tuberculous meningitis can be reproduced in tuberculin-positive human volunteers by instillation of tuberculin antigen into the CSF (intrathecal tuberculin reaction). These considerations help to explain the varied presentations of these syndromes and also the relatively low yield,

in some instances, of AFB smears and cultures for establishing the diagnosis. Molecular methods, notably PCR, are becoming increasingly useful for diagnosis of these syndromes, most cases of which warrant referral or hospitalization.

Tuberculous Pleurisy

Tuberculous pleurisy occurs in about 5% of all cases of tuberculosis and in 10% to 30% of cases of miliary tuberculosis. This diagnosis must be considered in all cases of unexplained pleural fluid exudates.

Presentation and Progression

Tuberculous pleurisy results from rupture of a subpleural focus of tuberculosis into the pleural space. In adolescents and younger adults the disease usually appears with fever, cough, pleuritic chest pain, and an obvious pleural effusion that is usually unilateral. This form of the disease often reflects primarily a hypersensitivity response to *M. tuberculosis* antigen. Therefore it is commonly self-limited. Before the advent of chemotherapy, studies showed that tuberculous pleural effusions resolved within several months in about 90% of patients; however, active tuberculosis developed at other sites within 5 years in about 65% of these patients. In older adults with underlying diseases such as heart failure or chronic liver disease, the presentation can be subtle and insidious. Tuberculous empyema (frank pus in the pleural space) can also occur but is rare.

Diagnosis

Tuberculous pleurisy is easily confused with pneumonia, pulmonary thromboembolism with infarction, tumor, and effusions resulting from connective tissue diseases. Initial tuberculin skin tests are reactive in 69% to 93% of cases. Repeating the skin test 2 months after a nonreactive result is worthwhile because conversion of the test to a positive result can be demonstrated in most immunocompetent persons with tuberculous pleurisy. Analysis of pleural fluid reveals an exudate with 500 to 2500 white blood cells (WBCs)/mm^3 (predominantly lymphocytes but sometimes predominantly polymorphonuclear neutrophils, elevated protein and lactate dehydrogenase levels, moderately low glucose level, and low pH (<7.3). Paucity of mesothelial cells on cytologic examination is a time-honored and valuable clue. The finding of <10% mesothelial cells in a pleural fluid cytology specimen is 95% sensitive for tuberculous pleurisy in HIV-negative patients, in whom a finding of >10% mesothelial cells virtually excludes tuberculosis. However, this statement does not apply to persons with HIV disease, whose tuberculous pleural effusions may contain substantial numbers of mesothelial cells.

AFB smears of pleural fluid are often positive (up to 50% of cases) for pleural effusions, complicating clinically apparent pulmonary tuberculosis, but are infrequently positive in patients with isolated tuberculous pleurisy resulting from post-primary *M. tuberculosis* infection. AFB cultures are positive in 28% to 58% (mean, 44%) of recent series of tuberculous pleurisy. Therefore the diagnosis frequently requires invasive procedures. Closed pleural needle biopsy should usually be carried out when tuberculous pleurisy is suspected because granulomatous histology consistent with tuberculosis can be demonstrated in about three fourths of patients by this method. Open pleural biopsy and pleuroscopy (thoracoscopy) are usually positive. To date, PCR has been disappointing for diagnosis of tuberculous pleurisy (only 42% to 81% sensitive), possibly because of the presence of inhibitors in pleural fluid. Numerous alternative diagnostic approaches have been suggested over the years. Recent interest centers on measurement of adenosine deaminase levels in pleural fluid; however, this method is not widely available in the United States.

Treatment

Patients with pleural exudates and a reactive tuberculin skin test should be treated for tuberculous pleurisy with standard antituberculous drugs unless tuberculosis is excluded by open pleural biopsy or pleuroscopy (thoracoscopy). Corticosteroids cannot be endorsed on the basis of available data. Some patients require chest tube drainage.

When to Refer

Referral is frequently needed for diagnostic procedures, and some patients need surgical drainage.

 KEY POINTS

TUBERCULOUS PLEURISY

⊃ Tuberculous pleurisy should be suspected in all patients with undiagnosed pleural exudates.

⊃ In some patients, especially adolescents and younger adults, tuberculous pleurisy appears as an acute illness with fever, pleuritic chest pain, and a large pleural effusion. In other patients, especially older adults with underlying disease such as heart failure or chronic liver disease, it can develop insidiously.

⊃ Misdiagnoses include pneumonia, pulmonary infarction, tumor, and effusion resulting from underlying disease (e.g., heart failure, chronic liver disease, connective tissue disease).

⊃ Open pleural biopsy or pleuroscopy (thoracoscopy) may be necessary to confirm the diagnosis.

SUGGESTED READING

Jones D, Lieb T, Narita M, et al. Mesothelial cells in tuberculous pleural effusions of HIV-infected patients. Chest 2000; 117: 289-291.

Merino JM, Carpintero I, Alvarez T, et al. Tuberculous pleural effusion in children. Chest 1999; 115: 26-30.

Morehead RS. Tuberculosis of the pleura. South Med J 1998; 91: 630-636.

Riantawan P, Chaowalit P, Wongsangiem M, et al. Diagnostic value of pleural fluid adenosine deaminase in tuberculous pleuritis with reference to HIV coinfection and a Bayesian analysis. Chest 1999; 116: 97-103.

Sahn SA, Iseman MD. Tuberculous empyema. Semin Respir Infect 1999; 14: 82-87.

Valdés L, Alvarez D, San José E, et al. Tuberculous pleurisy: a study of 254 patients. Arch Intern Med 1998; 158: 2017-2021.

Villena V, Rebollo MJ, Aguado JM, et al. Polymerase chain reaction for the diagnosis of pleural tuberculosis in immunocompromised and immunocompetent patients. Clin Infect Dis 1998; 26: 212-214.

Tuberculous Meningitis

Tuberculous meningitis is a life-threatening disease with serious sequelae.

Presentation and Progression

Tuberculous meningitis can occur as an isolated syndrome or as part of disseminated tuberculosis (miliary-meningeal tuberculosis). In children miliary tuberculosis usually develops during the initial lymphohematogenous dissemination of *M. tuberculosis* (Figure 22-1). About three fourths of children with tuberculous meningitis therefore have evidence of miliary tuberculosis, active pulmonary disease, or pleural effusion. In adults tuberculous meningitis can mimic acute bacterial meningitis but more commonly occurs as a subacute or chronic meningitis. Fever is usually but not always present. Other symptoms include headache, vomiting, confusion, meningismus, and focal neurologic signs. Numerous syndromes of central nervous system involvement occasionally complicate tuberculosis. Some symptoms and signs reflect localized mass lesions (tuberculomas); others reflect vasculitis with thrombosis and infarction of tissues; and others reflect the inflammatory response, which can result in cranial neuropathies, hydrocephalus, or both.

Diagnosis

Recent data suggest that CT scans are abnormal in more than 80% of patients; findings include hydrocephalus, parenchymal enhancement, contrast enhancement of the basal cisterns, brain infarction, and focal or diffuse brain edema. However, lumbar puncture remains the cornerstone of diagnosis. Tuberculous meningitis should be considered in all patients with unexplained lymphocytic CSF pleocytosis. In some patients the first CSF specimen may show a predominantly polymorphonuclear pleocytosis. Serial lumbar punctures are often helpful, especially because the CSF glucose level tends to fall with time. AFB smears on CSF are positive in about one third of cases, although the yield can be increased to 90% if four large-volume CSF specimens from sequential lumbar punctures are examined. PCR has proved to be extremely helpful for early, specific diagnosis of tuberculous meningitis, although false-negative tests occur.

Treatment

Treatment consists of standard antituberculous drugs, although some authorities recommend higher than usual doses of INH (10 mg/kg). Patients with confusion, stupor, coma, or focal neurologic deficits are now usually treated with prednisone 60 to 80 mg/day until improvement begins to occur. Despite the availability of effective chemotherapy, morbidity and mortality remain high. In one recent series mortality was 44% and only 31% of patients made a complete recovery.

When to Refer

Patients with suspected tuberculous meningitis should be admitted to the hospital.

 KEY POINTS

TUBERCULOUS MENINGITIS

⊃ Tuberculous meningitis may occur as an acute meningitis or, more commonly, as a subacute or chronic illness with headache, fever, vomiting, and meningismus.

⊃ In children it is often a postprimary infection (miliary-meningeal tuberculosis).

⊃ In older adults tuberculous meningitis often appears as a chronic meningitis.

⊃ The initial CSF specimen shows a polymorphonuclear pleocytosis in about one fourth of patients. Sequential CSF specimens usually show progressive lymphocytic pleocytosis and falling glucose levels (hypoglycorrhachia).

⊃ AFB smears of CSF are positive in only a minority of cases.

⊃ PCR is a promising method for early, specific diagnosis, but false-negative results occur.

SUGGESTED READING

Dube MP, Holtom PD, Larsen PA. Tuberculous meningitis in patients with and without human immunodeficiency virus infection. Am J Med 1992; 93: 520-524.

Haas DW. Current and future applications of polymerase chain reaction for *Mycobacterium tuberculosis*. Mayo Clin Proc 1996; 71: 311-313.

Hosoglu S, Ayaz C, Geyik MF, et al. Tuberculous meningitis in adults: an eleven-year review. Int J Tuberc Lung Dis 1998; 2: 553-557.

Ozates M, Kemaloglu S, Gurkan F, et al. CT of the brain in tuberculous meningitis: a review of 289 patients. Acta Radiol 2000; 41: 13-17.

Paganini H, Gonzalez F, Santander C, et al. Tuberculous meningitis in children: clinical features and outcome in 40 cases. Scand J Infect Dis 2000; 32: 41-45.

Shah GV. Central nervous system tuberculosis: imaging manifestations. Neuroimaging Clin North Am 2000; 10: 355-374.

Tuberculous Pericarditis

Tuberculous pericarditis results most commonly from extension of tuberculosis in a lymph node contiguous with the pericardial sac. Acute tuberculous pericarditis typically causes substernal chest pain, often made worse by inspiration and relieved by leaning forward. Chronic tuberculous pericarditis typically manifests itself as heart failure. Enlargement of the liver, ascites, and edema of the lower extremities may suggest cirrhosis. The tuberculin skin test is helpful when positive but may be nonreactive. In patients with suspected acute idiopathic ("viral") pericarditis the tuberculin test should be repeated in 2 months if initially nonreactive. Echocardiography in acute tuberculous pericarditis reveals an effusion that may show loculations. Pleural effusions are present in up to 39% of patients, and for these patients an aggressive approach to diagnosis should be pursued as previously outlined (see "Tuberculous Pleurisy").

Establishment of a specific diagnosis is often extremely difficult. AFB smears on pericardial fluid are seldom positive, and AFB cultures are positive in only about one half of cases. PCR of pericardial fluid can be helpful, but the sensitivity has not been clearly determined. In one study the overall sensitivity of PCR was 50% versus 70% for AFB culture; the sensitivity was higher for PCR on pericardial tissue specimens (80%) than on pericardial fluid (15%). For these reasons diagnostic pericardiocentesis is often deferred, especially because the procedure is potentially hazardous. Drug treatment usually consists of standard antituberculous therapy, often supplemented with corticosteroids. Small studies suggest that adjunctive steroids may improve survival, but the data are too scanty to permit definitive conclusions. Surgery is indicated for patients with hemodynamic compromise. Options include creation of a pericardial window and peri-

cardiectomy. Incomplete removal of the pericardium is associated with an increased risk of late complications.

Patients with suspected tuberculous pericarditis should nearly always be referred to a specialist or admitted to the hospital.

KEY POINTS

TUBERCULOUS PERICARDITIS

⊃ Tuberculous pericarditis can appear as acute idiopathic ("viral") pericarditis with effusion or as a chronic pericarditis with heart failure, sometimes resembling cirrhosis with ascites.

⊃ A tuberculin skin test should be performed on all patients with suspected acute idiopathic pericarditis, and if the test is nonreactive, it should be repeated in 2 months.

SUGGESTED READING

Cegielski JP, Devlin BH, Morris AJ, et al. Comparison of PCR, culture, and histopathology for diagnosis of tuberculous pericarditis. J Clin Microbiol 1997; 35: 3254-3257.

Hakim JG, Ternouth I, Mushangi E, et al. Double blind randomized placebo controlled trial of adjunctive prednisolone in the treatment of effusive tuberculous pericarditis in HIV seropositive patients. Heart 2000; 84: 183-188.

Hayashi H, Kawamata H, Machida M, et al. Tuberculous pericarditis: MRI features with contrast enhancement. Br J Radiol 1998; 71: 680-682.

Rana BS, Jones RA, Simpson IA. Recurrent pericardial effusion: the value of polymerase chain reaction in the diagnosis of tuberculosis. Heart 1999; 82: 246-247.

Strang JI. Tuberculous pericarditis. J Infect 1997; 35: 215-219.

Tuberculous Peritonitis

Tuberculous peritonitis is now uncommon in the United States, but it should be considered in cases of unexplained ascites or abdominal pain. It is often the result of tuberculosis involving an abdominal lymph node, but it can also be caused by miliary tuberculosis, tuberculosis of the gastrointestinal tract (which most commonly involves the ileocecal region), or tuberculous salpingitis (as spill-over from the fimbriated end of the fallopian tube). Classically the clinical presentation is one of two types: a serous type, manifested as ascites with or without signs of peritonitis such as tenderness with rebound accentuation, or a plastic type, with a "doughy abdomen" that gives the impression of tender masses. Peritoneal fluid usually reveals exudates with 500 to 2000 WBCs/mm³, most of which are lymphocytes. The AFB smear is only rarely positive, and AFB culture is positive in only about one fourth of cases. Gallium-67 scintigraphy may reveal diffuse or focal abdominal uptake with decreased hepatic accumulation of the isotope, and CT scan of the abdomen may show involvement of the gastrointestinal tract, lymph nodes, and various organs. Peritoneoscopy affords a diagnosis in up to 85% of cases, but fatal hemorrhages from the procedure have been reported. The diagnosis of tuberculous peritonitis is often overlooked in patients with cirrhosis and ascites. The clinical picture sometimes suggests ovarian cancer, and a high serum cancer antigen 125 (CA 125) concentration titer may be present. Recent data suggest that adjunctive corticosteroid therapy reduces the frequency and morbidity of complications such as intestinal obstruction and extensive adhesions, but more information is required for definitive recommendations in this regard.

 KEY POINTS

TUBERCULOUS PERITONITIS

⊃ Two classic clinical types are the serous type with ascites and the plastic type with a "doughy" abdomen.

⊃ Tuberculous peritonitis is often overlooked in patients with cirrhosis and ascites. It can also resemble ovarian cancer in its presentation, and many patients have high cancer antigen (CA 125) levels.

⊃ Analysis of peritoneal fluid typically shows exudates with predominance of lymphocytes, but positive AFB smears are uncommon.

SUGGESTED READING

Alrajhi AA, Halim MA, al-Hokail A, et al. Corticosteroid therapy of peritoneal tuberculosis. Clin Infect Dis 1998; 27: 52-56.

Brizi MG, Celi G, Scaldazza AV, e al. Diagnostic imaging of abdominal tuberculosis: gastrointestinal tract, peritoneum, lymph nodes. Rays 1998; 23: 115-125.

Haas DW. Is adjunctive corticosteroid therapy indicated during tuberculous peritonitis? Clin Infect Dis 1998; 27: 57-58.

Simsek H, Savas MC, Kadayifci A, et al. Elevated serum CA 125 concentration in patients with tuberculous peritonitis: a case-control study. Am J Gastroenterol 1997; 92: 1174-1176.

Suri S, Gupta S, Suri R. Computed tomography in abdominal tuberculosis. Br J Radiol 1999; 72: 92-98.

Panoskaltsis TA, Moore DA, Haidopoulos DA, et al. Tuberculous peritonitis: part of the differential diagnosis in ovarian cancer. Am J Obstet Gynecol 2000; 182: 740-742.

Wang HK, Hsueh PR, Hung CC, et al. Tuberculous peritonitis: analysis of 35 cases. J Microbiol Immunol Infect 1998; 31: 113-118.

Tuberculous Arthritis

Tuberculous arthritis is part of the spectrum of skeletal tuberculosis, discussed in more detail later in the chapter. Classically the disease is a slowly progressive arthritis involving a single joint, most commonly the knee or hip. A history of previous trauma to the joint is often obtained, as is a predisposing factor. More recently, multiple joint involvement has been emphasized. The joint space is typically preserved, which is explained by an absence of the proteolytic enzymes that characterize acute bacterial arthritis. Periarticular abscesses sometimes develop. Occasionally tuberculous arthritis appears as synovitis of the hand or wrist or as carpal tunnel syndrome. Diagnosis is usually based on biopsy with AFB culture, and chemotherapy with standard antituberculous drugs is usually successful.

SUGGESTED READING

Kim NH, Lee HM, Yoo JD, et al. Sacroiliac joint tuberculosis: classification and treatment. Clin Orthop 1999; 358: 215-222.

Muradali D, Gold WL, Vellend H, et al. Multifocal osteoarticular tuberculosis: report of four cases and review of the management. Clin Infect Dis 1993; 17: 204-209.

Skoll PJ, Hudson DA. Tuberculosis of the upper extremity. Ann Plast Surg 1999; 43: 374-378.

Tuberculosis of Solid Organs: Overview

Occasional reports document the occurrence of tuberculosis in nearly every organ. The disease can, for example, mimic breast cancer, metastatic cancer to the liver, or even acute myocardial infarction. Tuberculosis was formerly the usual cause of Addison's disease (adrenal insufficiency); this presentation is now rare. Several common or important organ involvements are reviewed here briefly.

Tuberculous Lymphadenitis (Scrofula)

Tuberculous lymphadenitis is the most common form of tuberculosis outside the chest cavity. Cervical lymphadenitis from mycobacteria in adults is caused by *M. tuberculosis* in about 90% of patients and nontuberculous mycobacteria in about 10% of patients (the reverse is true in children; see under "When to Suspect Nontuberculous Mycobacteria"). Patients with HIV disease often have generalized lymphadenopathy with fever, weight loss, and evidence of tuberculosis in the lungs or elsewhere. Fine-needle aspiration is now being used for diagnosis, but lymph node biopsy is often required. Rarely, tuberculous lymphadenitis causes fibrosing mediastinitis resembling that usually associated with histoplasmosis (see Chapter 21). Standard antituberculous drugs are used for all forms of tuberculous lymphadenitis (for further discussion and suggested reading, see Chapter 8).

Genitourinary Tuberculosis

The glomeruli are frequently infected in the course of the initial hematogenous dissemination of *M. tuberculosis,* often resulting in foci of tuberculosis in the renal cortex. These are frequently symptomatic, and indeed they have been an incidental finding at postmortem examination in about three fourths of patients with pulmonary tuberculosis. Genitourinary tuberculosis often becomes expressed clinically when the disease spills over into the renal medulla and then into other parts of the genitourinary tract. In males the organism can spread to the prostate, causing a form of prostatitis that may be chronic, subtle, and difficult to diagnose. Less commonly the seminal vesicles, epididymides, and testes become involved. In both male and female patients genitourinary infection can also result from direct hematogenous dissemination, such as to the prostate, testes, or fallopian tubes. Tuberculous salpingitis was formerly a major cause of infertility. Sterile pyuria is a classic finding in genitourinary tuberculosis. For diagnosis the customary approach is to obtain three morning urine specimens for AFB culture; the sensitivity for three urine cultures is about 80% to 90%. In a study from Egypt, AFB smears of urine, compared with urine cultures, had a 52% sensitivity and 97% specificity for *M. tuberculosis,* whereas PCR of urine had a 96% sensitivity and 98% specificity for *M. tuberculosis.* Treatment of genitourinary tuberculosis involves standard chemotherapy regimens, often supplemented with urologic intervention.

SUGGESTED READING

Carl P, Stark L. Indications for surgical management of genitourinary tuberculosis. World J Surg 1997; 21: 505-510.

Chung JJ, Kim MJ, Lee T, et al. Sonographic findings in tuberculous epididymitis and epididymo-orchitis. J Clin Ultrasound 1997; 25: 390-394.

Kostakopoulos A, Economou G, Picramenos D, et al. Tuberculosis of the prostate. Int Urol Nephrol 1998; 30: 153-157.

Moussa OM, Eraky I, El-Far MA, et al. Rapid diagnosis of genitourinary tuberculosis by polymerase chain reaction and nonradioactive DNA hybridization. J Urol 2000; 164: 584-588.

Valentini AL, Summaria V, Marano P. Diagnostic imaging of genitourinary tuberculosis. Rays 1998; 23: 126-143.

Weiss SG II, Kryger JV, Nakada SY, et al. Genitourinary tuberculosis. Urology 1998; 51: 1033-1034.

Tuberculous Osteomyelitis

Tuberculous osteomyelitis, like other forms of hematogenous osteomyelitis, classically involves the long bones in growing children and the spine in adults. Tuberculosis should be suspected in cases of osteomyelitis in which pyogenic bacteria are not isolated, or in which bacteria usually considered to be nonpathogenic (such as *Streptococcus epidermidis*) are isolated. Tuberculosis of the spine (Pott's disease) accounts for about 2% of all cases of tuberculosis and about one third of all cases of skeletal tuberculosis. The lower thoracic spine is involved most often, followed by the lumbar spine and then the cervical spine. Like other forms of hematogenous vertebral osteomyelitis the disease typically involves two adjacent vertebral bodies with anterior wedging (owing to disproportionate destruction of the anterior aspects of the vertebral bodies) and narrowing of the intervertebral disk space. Recent studies, however, suggest an atypical form of the disease in which disk involvement is not apparent. Physical examination often reveals localized tenderness and a prominence, known as a gibbus, over the involved vertebrae. A cold abscess develops alongside the spine in about 50% of patients, especially when the upper spine is involved, and it can gravitate downward as a psoas abscess. About one half of patients become paraplegic. The importance of attempting to secure the diagnosis with biopsy and AFB culture cannot be overemphasized, because vertebral osteomyelitis can have many causes (see Chapter 15) and specific therapy is mandatory. Use of PCR for rapid diagnosis is being investigated, but it has not been standardized for this purpose. In the past, neurosurgical intervention with laminectomy was usually advised. Studies from Africa establish that most patients improve without surgery if treated with appropriate chemotherapy and modified bed rest.

SUGGESTED READING

Harrington JT. The evolving role of direct amplification tests in diagnosing osteoarticular infections caused by mycobacteria and fungi. Curr Opin Rheumatol 1999; 11: 289-292.

Mousa HA. Tuberculosis of bones and joints: diagnostic approaches. Int Orthop 1998; 22: 245-246.

Pertuiset E, Beaudreuil J, Liote F, et al. Spinal tuberculosis in adults: a study of 103 cases in a developed country, 1980-1994. Medicine (Baltimore) 1999; 78: 309-320.

Watts HG, Lifesco RM. Tuberculosis of bone and joints. J Bone Joint Surg (Am) 1996: 78: 288-298.

Nontuberculous Mycobacteria: Overview

More than 50 species of the genus *Mycobacterium* are recognized as potential human pathogens. Species other than *M. tuberculosis* and *M. leprae* have been designated "atypical mycobacteria" or "mycobacteria other than *M. tuberculosis*" in the past and are now called simply "nontuberculous mycobacteria" (NTM). Many clinical laboratories in the United States now find that isolates of NTM outnumber isolates of *M. tuberculosis,* sometimes by a wide margin. This creates a dilemma for clinicians because the report of a positive AFB smear or preliminary culture result traditionally calls for prompt initiation of therapy for tuberculosis while definitive identification of the microorganism is awaited. Whereas isolation of *M. tuberculosis* always signifies disease (except for the rare instance of contamination in the laboratory), isolation of NTM, especially from pulmonary specimens, often has little or no clinical importance. The rising frequency of NTM isolates is explained only in part by the frequency of *M. avium-intracellulare* complex (MAC) in persons with advanced HIV disease (see Chapter 22). Possible explanations include improved microbiologic techniques, greater awareness among clinicians, environmental contamination, and an actual change in disease epidemiology. Primary care clinicians should have a general familiarity with the major syndromes caused by NTM microorganisms (Table 22-4), including when to order AFB cultures and when to specify lower than usual incubation temperatures. Here we briefly review the diverse clinical settings, microbiology, and diagnostic approaches to these microorganisms.

When to Suspect Nontuberculous Mycobacteria

Nontuberculous mycobacteria should be considered and AFB cultures requested in the following clinical settings:
- Chronic cavitary pulmonary disease of the upper lobes. The classic patient is a white man with chronic obstructive lung disease from heavy cigarette smoking; alcoholism is also common. MAC or *Mycobacterium kansasii* is the usual pathogen. The disease resembles tuberculosis but is typically milder and seldom spreads beyond the lungs.
- Reticulonodular pulmonary disease, or localized nodular bronchiectasis involving the middle lobes. The classic patient is a white woman, often ≥50 years of age and a nonsmoker. Nontuberculous mycobacterial disease is being seen in young women with increasing frequency; these patients tend to be thin and often have pectus excavatum, scoliosis, or mitral valve prolapse. The pathogen is usually MAC complex but can also be *M. kansasii* or *Mycobacterium abscessus.*
- Bronchiectasis. Nontuberculous mycobacteria are often isolated, especially in patients with underlying lung disease such as cystic fibrosis. The issue of infection versus colonization is frequently difficult to resolve. MAC and *M. abscessus* are common pathogens.
- Chronic lower lobe pneumonia or reticulonodular infiltrates in patients with esophageal disease, such as achalasia. Esophageal disease such as achalasia or chronic vomiting is a classic setting for subtle, slowly progressive aspiration pneumonia that often contains a component of mineral oil (lipoid pneumonia). Opportunistic mycobacteria are relatively

TABLE 22-4
Nontuberculous Mycobacteria Most Commonly Associated with Human Disease

Rate of growth	Runyon classification*	Microorganisms	Usual syndromes
Slow	Group 1 (photochromogens: form pigment when exposed to light)	M. kansasii	Pulmonary disease in immunocompetent persons; disseminated infection in patients with HIV disease
		M. marinum	Cutaneous infection, typically involving wounds exposed to water, including the lymphocutaneous syndrome
	Group 2 (scotochromogens: form pigment in the dark)	M. gordonae	Usually a contaminant of cultures or a clinically significant isolate; occasionally causes pulmonary disease and other syndromes
		M. scrofulaceum†	Cervical lymphadenitis in children
	Group 3 (nonchromogens: do not form pigment)	M. avium complex: M. avium, M. intracellulare, M. scrofulaceum†	Pulmonary disease in immunocompetent persons; disseminated infection in persons with HIV disease; cervical lymphadenitis in children
		M. terrae complex	Most commonly causes an indolent tenosynovitis of the upper extremity following trauma; also causes pulmonary disease
		M. ulcerans	Cutaneous disease in children
		M. xenopi	Pulmonary disease in persons who are immunocompromised or have underlying lung disease
Rapid	Group 4 (distinguished from the others by rapid growth)	M. fortuitum	Pulmonary disease in patients with esophageal infection; skin and soft tissue infections including surgical wound infections; rare cases of prosthetic valve endocarditis, cervical lymphadenitis, keratitis, and other infections
		M. chelonei	Similar to M. fortuitum
		M. abscessus	Chronic bronchopulmonary disease in immunocompetent adults

HIV, Human immunodeficiency virus.
*The Runyon classification is an older system for categorizing these microorganisms based on their growth patterns (rate of growth and presence or absence of pigment) on solid media. Improved methods of speciation have rendered this classification largely obsolete. However, knowledge of the basic growth patterns often facilitates communication with the microbiology laboratory with regard to preliminary culture results.
†Variable pigment formation.

common in this setting and include *Mycobacterium fortuitum, M. abscessus,* MAC, and *Mycobacterium smegmatis.*
- Cervical lymphadenitis in children. Children between the ages of 1 and 5 years may have painless, unilateral anterior cervical lymphadenopathy. The lymph nodes may enlarge rapidly, raising the suspicion of malignancy, and may be associated with fistulas. Although *M. tuberculosis* and *Mycobacterium scrofulaceum* are the traditional causes of this syndrome, MAC now causes about 80% of cases in the United States.
- Unusual localized skin lesions, often developing as multiple, small, violet papules in a patient who may give a history of a scratch, cut, or puncture wound that became contaminated with water. *Mycobacterium marinum* is the usual pathogen in this setting. The disease sometimes resembles lymphocutaneous sporotrichosis (see Chapter 8). The spectrum of cutaneous disease caused by nontuberculous mycobacteria is wide and continues to expand.

- Unusual rheumatologic infections, such as infections of tendon sheaths, bursae, and bones. Chronic tenosynovitis of the hand is sometimes caused by nontuberculous mycobacteria, especially MAC and *M. marinum.* Nontuberculous mycobacteria also cause granulomatous arthritis and bursitis and occasionally osteomyelitis, usually as a postoperative complication.
- Postoperative infections. Rapidly growing mycobacteria, now classified as the *M. fortuitum* group and the *M. chelonei/abscessus* group, occasionally cause postoperative infections, such as after cardiac or plastic surgery. A combination of aggressive débridement and chemotherapy may be necessary for cure.

When AFB cultures are obtained in one of the preceding settings, the laboratory should be advised to look for nontuberculous mycobacteria because some of these organisms require lower than usual incubation temperatures (82.4° or 86.8° F [28° or 30° C] rather than 95° F [35° C]).

Questions to Ask the Microbiology Laboratory About a Positive Acid-Fast Bacillus Culture Pending Definitive Identification

Diagnosis of NTM infection is crucially dependent on the microbiology laboratory. When the clinician receives a positive preliminary AFB culture report on a patient who might have NTM disease, four questions are appropriate:

- How rapidly did the culture "turn positive" and in what culture systems? With traditional culture systems using solid media, *M. tuberculosis* and most of the nontuberculous mycobacteria, including the MAC and *M. kansasii*, typically require 2 or more weeks' incubation to form mature colonies. *M. marinum* and *Mycobacterium gordonae* (a common isolate, usually of little clinical significance) generally form mature colonies within 7 to 10 days. Formation of mature colonies within 7 days suggests a "rapid grower" such as *M. fortuitum*, *M. chelonei*, or *M. abscessus*.

- Does the isolate "look like" *M. tuberculosis* or a nontuberculous mycobacterium? Experienced microbiologists can usually advise the clinician that an isolate has a high probability of being one of the "atypical" mycobacteria rather than *M. tuberculosis*, based on the appearance of colonies on agar and the presence or absence of "cording." *M. tuberculosis*, unlike most mycobacteria, is niacin positive (i.e., it produces niacin), is catalase positive (with the exception of INH-resistant strains, which do not produce catalase), and reduces nitrates.

- How soon will the results of nucleic acid probes or other identification systems become available? Older methods for determining the species of mycobacterial isolates usually required weeks to complete because they depended on subcultures and biochemical tests. Newer techniques that have been developed include specific nucleic acid probes that allow confirmation of the identity of some of the more common mycobacteria within hours. These include *M. tuberculosis*, MAC, *M. kansasii*, and *M. gordonae*.

- What should I do if susceptibility testing is desired? The susceptibility patterns of NTM vary widely, and in difficult cases in vitro susceptibility testing is often desirable. With MAC, in vitro susceptibility testing with clarithromycin is often desirable. Susceptibility testing can also help in the treatment of serious infections caused by one of the "rapid growers." Susceptibility testing is not always necessary, the results can be difficult to interpret, and in some instances in vitro susceptibility does not necessarily correlate with in vivo efficacy. However, the clinician should ascertain that the isolate will be saved for this purpose if necessary.

Because sophisticated laboratory methods for dealing with mycobacterial isolates are usually available only in larger hospitals or reference facilities, the primary care clinician frequently deals with laboratory personnel at a remote site. Communicating a knowledgeable and concerned interest in the preceding questions can be extremely helpful.

KEY POINTS

NONTUBERCULOUS MYCOBACTERIA: OVERVIEW
- More than 50 species of the genus *Mycobacterium* are potential pathogens in humans.

- Many laboratories in the United States now find that NTM are isolated from clinical specimens more frequently than is *M. tuberculosis*. This creates a dilemma for the clinician because a positive AFB smear or preliminary culture result is traditionally taken as grounds for starting treatment for presumed tuberculosis.
- Chronic pulmonary disease is the syndrome most frequently caused by NTM. Unlike in tuberculosis, a single positive AFB culture *does not* establish a diagnosis. Multiple positive cultures with clinical correlation are required.
- Other syndromes include cervical lymphadenopathy in children, skin and soft tissue infections after exposure to water, rheumatologic infections, and infections of postoperative wounds.
- When NTM are suspected, the laboratory should be requested to process the cultures at lower than usual incubation temperatures (82.4° or 86.8° F [28° or 30° C], as well as at the usual 95° F [35° C]).
- When a positive preliminary AFB culture report is received, four questions are appropriate to ask the microbiology laboratory: How soon did it grow out? Does it "look like" *M. tuberculosis*? When will the results of rapid identification tests be available? What do I do if I want susceptibility testing?

SUGGESTED READING
Brown BA, Wallace RJ Jr. Infections due to nontuberculous mycobacteria. In Mandell GL, Bennett JE, Dolin R. Mandell, Douglas, and Bennett's Principles and Practice of Infectious Diseases. 5th ed., Philadelphia: Churchill Livingstone; 2000: 2636.
Wallace RJ Jr, Cook JL, Glassroth J, et al. American Thoracic Society Statement. Diagnosis and treatment of disease caused by nontuberculous mycobacteria. Am J Respir Crit Care Med 1997;156 (Suppl): S1-S25.

Pulmonary Disease Caused by Nontuberculous Mycobacteria in Immunocompetent Patients

Positive sputum cultures for NTM often represent simple colonization but sometimes signify clinically important disease. With the exception of *M. kansasii*, which often responds to standard antituberculous drugs, treatment is likely to be difficult.

Presentation and Progression
Cause

MAC is the most common cause and is widely distributed in the inanimate environment. Person-to-person transmission apparently does not occur. *M. kansasii*, the second most common cause, has a more limited geographic distribution. Unlike MAC, *M. kansasii* is not found in soil or natural water; however, it has been isolated from tap water in certain cities. Rapidly growing mycobacteria such as *M. fortuitum* are the usual cause in persons with aspiration resulting from esophageal disease. *Mycobacterium malmoense* is an important cause of lung disease in northern Europe, and numerous other species occasionally cause human disease.

Presentation

The clinical presentation of nontuberculous mycobacterial infection of the lungs is usually nonspecific and varies to some extent depending on the microorganism and underlying conditions.

With MAC disease about 80% of patients see their physician for a productive cough, and about 20% have hemoptysis. Fever is present in only about one fourth of patients. In the past MAC pulmonary disease was found most commonly in white men with chronic obstructive lung disease. In these patients MAC tends to cause upper lobe cavitary lesions resembling tuberculous cavities, but usually smaller and with thinner walls. The spectrum of illness has shifted, to the extent that a majority of patients are now women, usually nonsmokers. In these patients MAC tends to cause nodular infiltrates, often with bronchiectasis. Older women often have infiltrates in the right middle lobe or lingua. Similar patterns of disease can be seen in younger women, especially those with pectus excavatum, scoliosis, or mitral valve prolapse (the explanation for these associations is unknown). Other patients have worsening of previously diagnosed lung disease such as bronchiectasis, cystic fibrosis, or pneumoconiosis. Others have asymptomatic pulmonary nodules.

M. kansasii also causes cavitary disease resembling tuberculosis but more indolent. This pathogen is relatively common in HIV-infected persons and can also cause serious pulmonary disease in patients with cancer. *M. chelonei* tends to cause pulmonary disease resembling MAC disease in middle-aged and older women.

Rapidly growing mycobacteria such as *M. fortuitum* and various "opportunistic" mycobacteria are frequently associated with indolent pneumonias in patients with esophageal disease and aspiration, which may be occult. Achalasia is a classic underlying disease for this presentation.

When isolated from sputum cultures, *M. gordonae* is usually a nonpathogenic, colonizing organism, even when underlying disease is present.

Diagnosis

Radiographic appearances, as previously noted, are highly variable. Pleural effusions are uncommon. High-resolution CT scan of the chest may show multifocal bronchiectasis and small nodules in certain subsets of patients. Sputum culture is usually the key to diagnosis. A single sputum culture does not suffice to establish the diagnosis, even though the concept of "benign colonization" of the airways by nontuberculous mycobacteria is being increasingly challenged. Current ATS diagnostic criteria can be summarized as follows:

- Clinical criteria include compatible symptoms or documented deterioration of an underlying lung disease (see earlier discussion), with reasonable exclusion of alternative diagnoses that have therapeutic implications, such as cancer, tuberculosis, or histoplasmosis.
- Radiographic criteria include the appearance of new infiltrates with or without nodules (persisting for ≥2 months and progressive), cavitation, multiple nodules, or—by high-resolution CT scan—multiple nodules or multifocal bronchiectasis with or without nodules.
- Bacteriologic criteria include the following: (1) three positive sputum cultures with negative AFB smears *or* two positive sputum cultures with one positive AFB smear; (2) (if the

patient cannot produce sputum and only a single bronchial washing specimen is available), a positive bronchial washing culture with at least 2+ growth or a positive culture with a 2+ positive AFB smear; or (3) if lung biopsy has been performed, any growth from bronchopulmonary sputum, the finding of a granuloma or AFB on histologic examination in combination with at least one positive culture of sputum or bronchial washing, or any growth from a usually sterile extrapulmonary site.

In some patients lung biopsy is necessary to exclude cancer or other disease processes.

Treatment

Methods

M. kansasii is usually treated with a three-drug combination of INH 300 mg/day, rifampin 600 mg/day, and ethambutol 25 mg/kg/day for 2 months and then 15 mg/kg/day. Therapy is continued for 18 months, with a minimum of 12 months after AFB cultures become sterile.

Treatment of MAC pulmonary disease can be extremely difficult and should never be undertaken lightly. Prolonged treatment is necessary, eradication of the infection is difficult to achieve, and resistant strains emerge. Clarithromycin has proved to be an extremely useful addition to the therapeutic armamentarium, but it should never be used alone in this setting because of the emergence of resistance. A currently recommended three-drug regimen consists of clarithromycin 500 mg b.i.d. or azithromycin 250 mg/day, rifampin 600 mg/day or rifabutin 300 mg/day, and ethambutol 25 mg/kg/day for 2 months, then 15 mg/kg/day. Streptomycin should be given two or three times a week if the patient has extensive or cavitary disease or strongly positive sputum smears. Some authorities recommend substituting amikacin for streptomycin. Intermittent dosage (use of four drugs, three times weekly) is being investigated. Surgical resection is useful for selected patients.

Treatment of pulmonary disease caused by rapidly growing mycobacteria is extremely difficult, since these members of the *M. fortuitum* complex tend to be resistant to most antimycobacterial drugs. Clarithromycin, cefoxitin, and amikacin are often helpful, but surgical resection is usually necessary for cure.

Expected Response

M. kansasii pulmonary infection usually responds to therapy if taken with full compliance. Cure rates up to 90% have been reported for treatment of *M. kansasii* infections, but most clinical experience has been disappointing.

Complications

Vision loss from optic neuritis in patients taking ethambutol is likely to occur if renal function is not taken into account in the dosage of this drug, especially in older persons (see later discussion). Use of aminoglycosides carries the risk of ototoxicity and nephrotoxicity (see Chapter 19).

When to Refer

When NTM pulmonary infection is diagnosed, strong consideration should be given to referral to a pulmonary or infectious disease specialist with particular interest in this disease. Treatment is difficult and often complicated. Patients with particularly difficult problems may benefit from referral to the Infectious Diseases Service, National Jewish Medical and Research Center, Denver, Colorado.

Wallace RJ Jr, Cook JL, Glassroth J, et al. Diagnosis and treatment of disease caused by nontuberculous mycobacteria. American Thoracic Society Statement. Am J Respir Crit Care Med 1997; 156 (Suppl): S1-S25.

KEY POINTS

PULMONARY DISEASE CAUSED BY NONTUBERCULOUS MYCOBACTERIA IN IMMUNOCOMPETENT PATIENTS

⊃ Presenting symptoms are usually nonspecific, such as productive cough, fatigue, and weight loss.

⊃ Variable radiographic patterns include upper lobe cavitary lesions suggesting tuberculosis but generally more indolent, especially in male smokers; nodular infiltrates, often with bronchiectasis, especially in older women and sometimes in younger women with pectus excavatum, scoliosis, or mitral valve prolapse; worsening of underlying lung disease such as bronchiectasis, cystic fibrosis, or pneumoconiosis; dense or patchy infiltrates in persons with esophageal disease; and asymptomatic pulmonary nodules. Pleural effusion is uncommon.

⊃ A single positive sputum culture does not establish the diagnosis.

⊃ Diagnosis should be based on ATS criteria, with reasonable exclusion of other diseases such as cancer, tuberculosis, and histoplasmosis.

⊃ M. kansasii infection usually responds to prolonged therapy with INH, rifampin, and ethambutol.

⊃ Treatment of MAC pulmonary disease can be extremely difficult and should never be undertaken lightly. A three-drug regimen is currently recommended, often with the addition of an aminoglycoside. Referral to a physician with special interest in this disease should be strongly considered.

SUGGESTED READING

Bloch KC, Zwerling L, Pletcher MJ, et al. Incidence and clinical implications of isolation of *Mycobacterium kansasii:* results of a 5-year, population-based study. Ann Intern Med 1998; 129: 698-704.

Eckburg PB, Buadu EO, Stark P, et al. Clinical and chest radiographic findings among patients with sputum culture positive for *Mycobacterium gordonae:* a review of 19 cases. Chest 2000; 117: 96-102.

Erasmus JJ, McAdams HP, Farrell MA, et al. Pulmonary nontuberculous mycobacterial infection: radiologic manifestations. Radiographics 1999; 19: 1487-1505.

Griffith DE, Brown BA, Girard WM, et al. Azithromycin-containing regimens for treatment of *Mycobacterium avium* complex lung disease. Clin Infect Dis 2001; 32: 1547-1553.

Hadjiliadis D, Adlakha A, Prakash UB. Rapidly growing mycobacterial lung infection in association with esophageal disorders. Mayo Clin Proc 1999; 74: 45-51.

Hazelton TR, Newell JD Jr, Cook JL, et al. CT findings in 14 patients with *Mycobacterium chelonae* pulmonary infection. AJR 2000; 175: 413-416.

Jacobson KL, Teira R, Libshitz HI, et al. *Mycobacterium kansasii* infections in patients with cancer. Clin Infect Dis 2000; 30: 965-969.

Management of opportunist mycobacterial infections: Joint Tuberculosis Committee Guidelines 1999. Thorax 2000; 55: 210-218.

Lymphadenitis Caused by Nontuberculous Mycobacteria

Cervical lymphadenitis is the usual expression of nontuberculous mycobacterial infection in children, who in contrast to adults seldom have pulmonary infection as a result of nontuberculous mycobacteria. MAC is the most common isolate (80% of cases), followed by *M. scrofulaceum.* Tuberculin skin testing often shows <15 mm of induration, owing to cross-reactivity with *M. tuberculosis.* Fine-needle aspiration can be used to obtain material for cytology and culture, but its use is controversial. Incision and drainage of the involved nodes are discouraged because of the high rate of sinus tracts with drainage. Surgical excision is often recommended as the treatment of choice. Drug therapy as an alternative to excision is being investigated (see Chapter 8 for further discussion and suggested reading).

Skin, Soft Tissue, and Rheumatologic Infections Caused by Nontuberculous Mycobacteria

Nontuberculous mycobacteria occasionally cause localized dermatologic and rheumatologic infections that require a high index of suspicion for correct diagnosis and appropriate therapy.

M. marinum causes a characteristic skin lesion known as "fish tank granuloma" or "swimming pool granuloma." Numerous nontuberculous mycobacteria sometimes cause infections of skin and subcutaneous tissue. These include *M. fortuitum, M. chelonei, Mycobacterium ulcerans,* and *M. abscessus.* *M. marinum* and MAC organisms are frequently associated with tenosynovitis of the hand. *Mycobacterium terrae* complex has also been associated with hand infections.

Some of the prominent syndromes are as follows:

■ "Fish tank granuloma" or "swimming pool granuloma" caused by *M. marinum* generally appears as one or more small, violet papules on an exposed extremity such as the hands, elbows, or knees (Figure 22-4). Suggestive exposure histories include cleaning a fish tank or sustaining a puncture wound from handling a crab or a saltwater fish. The lesions may coalesce, ulcerate, or extend proximally in such a way as to suggest the lymphocutaneous form of sporotrichosis. Opportunistic infections of skin and soft tissue after trauma or surgery are often caused by *M. fortuitum, M. chelonei,* or *M. abscessus.* These microorganisms can also cause opportunistic skin infections in immunocompromised persons (Figure 22-5). They sometimes cause severe subcutaneous disease after plastic surgery procedures (e.g., augmentation mammoplasty or reduction mammoplasty) and in the presence of foreign bodies such as vascular access devices and peritoneal catheters. Outbreaks of nosocomial infection after surgical procedures such as coronary artery bypass have been described.

■ Infections of tendon sheaths, bursae, joints, and bones usually arise after major or minor trauma. Tenosynovitis of the hand is most commonly caused by MAC or *M. marinum,* but numerous mycobacteria occasionally cause this

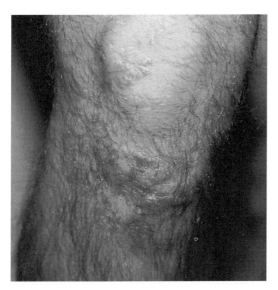

FIG. 22-4 Hyperpigmented nodules over the patella and below the knee in a patient with *Mycobacterium marinum* infection. The patient, a termite inspector, often crawled on his knees in moist soil beneath houses. A specific exposure is often obtained from patients with *M. marinum* infection.

syndrome. An extremely indolent form of tenosynovitis of the hand is caused by *M. terrae* complex (notably *M. nonchromogenicum*). Recent data suggest that *Mycobacterium haemophilum,* which is best known for causing opportunistic infections in immunocompromised patients, also causes skin and soft tissue infections.

■ "Buruli ulcer" (also called Bairnsdale ulcer) is a disease of the tropics caused by *M. ulcerans.*

Diagnosis requires a high index of suspicion. Biopsy typically shows granulomatous inflammation. To reiterate, the microbiology laboratory should be advised to incubate cultures at lower than usual temperatures. The optimal temperature for isolation of *M. marinum,* for example, is 86.8° F (30° C). However, cultures are not infrequently sterile. Attempts have been made to diagnose these infections through PCR of tissue samples, but so far the results are inconclusive.

Appropriate regimens for *M. marinum* infection include clarithromycin 500 mg PO b.i.d., minocycline 100 mg PO b.i.d., or rifampin 600 mg PO b.i.d. plus ethambutol 15 mg/kg/day. Regimens for most of the other pathogens are not standardized. Some patients benefit from consultation with an infectious disease specialist.

 KEY POINTS

SKIN, SOFT TISSUE, AND RHEUMATOLOGIC INFECTIONS CAUSED BY NONTUBERCULOUS MYCOBACTERIA

⊃ *M. marinum* should be suspected with a localized, chronic infection ("fish tank granuloma" or "swimming pool granuloma"). The history often indicates exposure of a wound to water or marine animals. Biopsy usually shows granulomatous histologic features. Treatment is often indicated on clinical grounds because cultures are frequently sterile.

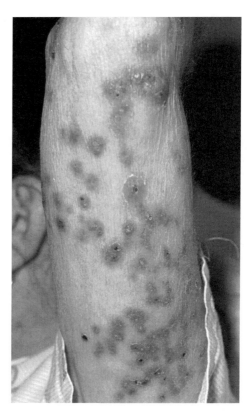

FIG. 22-5 Extensive nodules and plaques caused by *Mycobacterium chelonei* in a patient who had rheumatoid arthritis and was being treated with prednisone.

⊃ When *M. marinum* is suspected, it is important to alert the microbiologist to incubate the specimen at a low temperature (82.4° or 86.8° F [28° or 30° C]) to enhance the yield of culture.

⊃ Nontuberculous mycobacterial skin infections caused by organisms other than *M. marinum* are being recognized with increasing frequency.

⊃ Unusual, indolent cases of tenosynovitis, bursitis, postoperative wound infections, and infections involving foreign bodies should prompt consideration of nontuberculous mycobacterial infection.

SUGGESTED READING

Ang P, Rattana-Apiromyakij N, Goh CL. Retrospective study of *Mycobacterium marinum* skin infections. Int J Dermatol 2000; 39: 343-347.

Bhatty MA, Turner DP, Chamberlain ST. *Mycobacterium marinum* hand infection: case reports and review of literature. Br J Plastic Surg 2000; 53: 161-165.

Busam KJ, Kiehn TE, Salob SP, et al. Histologic reactions to cutaneous infectious by *Mycobacterium haemophilum.* Am J Surg Pathol 1999; 23: 1379-1385.

Ryan JM, Bryant GD. Fish tank granuloma—a frequently misdiagnosed infection of the upper limb. J Accid Emerg Med 1997; 14: 398-400.

Semret M, Koromihis G, MacLean JD, et al. *Mycobacterium ulcerans* infection (Buruli ulcer): first reported case in a traveler. Am J Trop Med Hyg 1999; 61: 689-693.

Smego RA Jr, Castiglia M, Asperilla MO. Lymphocutaneous syndrome: a review of non-*Sporothrix* causes. Medicine (Baltimore) 1999; 78: 38-63.

Smith DS, Lindholm-Levy P, Huitt GA, et al. *Mycobacterium terrae:* case reports, literature review, and in vitro antibiotic susceptibility testing. Clin Infect Dis 2000; 30: 444-453.

Toussirot E, Chevrolet A, Wendling D. Tenosynovitis due to *Mycobacterium avium intracellulare* and *Mycobacterium chelonei:* report of two cases with review of the literature. Clin Rheumatol 1998; 17: 152-156.

Weitzul S, Eichhorn PJ, Pandya AG. Nontuberculous mycobacterial infections of the skin. Dermatol Clin 2000; 18: 359-377.

Leprosy (Hansen's disease)

Leprosy is an ancient disease characterized by a long incubation period and a unique predilection for skin and nerves in the cooler parts of the body. Between 100 and 200 new cases are diagnosed in the United States each year. Most of these patients are immigrants from developing nations, including Mexico and countries in the Caribbean and Southeast Asia. Early diagnosis tremendously improves the prognosis.

Presentation and Progression
Cause

M. leprae is an obligate intracellular parasite infecting humans and nine-banded armadillos. It has never been isolated in cell-free media or tissue cultures. Some data now suggest that it may be transmitted from soil. Human-to-human transmission is thought to be the usual cause, but "prolonged and intimate contact" is required.

Presentation

The wide spectrum of disease is best understood by considering the two polar types: tuberculoid leprosy and lepromatous leprosy. Patients with tuberculoid leprosy have partial T-lymphocyte immunity. The classic early skin lesion is an anesthetic plaque with erythematous borders. In patients with lepromatous leprosy, who have little or no T-lymphocyte immunity to *M. leprae,* symmetric skin nodules, plaques, and dermal thickening develop, eventually leading to "leonine facies" (coarsening of the facial features resulting from massive infiltration of the dermis by *M. leprae*). These patients also manifest hypergammaglobulinemia and are at risk for amyloidosis. Peripheral nerve involvement dominates the clinical features of both types of leprosy. The nerves become enlarged, and the anesthesia results in severe ulcerations and loss of tissue.

Diagnosis

Clinical diagnosis is usually based on the clinical features, such as anesthetic skin plaques (which, however, are not pathognomonic because other skin lesions sometimes cause hypoesthesia), enlargement of peripheral nerves, and demonstration of AFB in tissue biopsy specimens (using a Fite stain rather than the traditional Ziehl-Neelsen stain).

When to Refer

Patients with leprosy should be referred for confirmation of the diagnosis and initiation of appropriate therapy.

 KEY POINTS

LEPROSY

⊃ About 100 to 200 new cases of leprosy occur in the United States each year, mainly in immigrants from developing countries, including Mexico and Southeast Asia.

⊃ Key diagnostic clues include anesthetic skin plaques in tuberculoid leprosy; symmetric nodules, plaques, and dermal thickening in lepromatous leprosy; enlargement of peripheral nerves; and demonstration of AFB in tissue biopsy specimens (preferably using Fite stain).

SUGGESTED READING

Haas CJ, Zink A, Palfi G, et al. Detection of leprosy in ancient human skeletal remains by molecular identification of *Mycobacterium leprae.* Am J Clin Pathol 2000; 114: 428-436.

Haimanot RT, Melaku Z. Leprosy. Curr Opin Neurol 2000; 13: 317-322.

Jacobson RR, Krahenbuhl JL. Leprosy. Lancet 1999; 353: 655-660.

Visschedijk J, van de Broek J, Eggens H, et al. *Mycobacterium leprae—millennium resistant!* Leprosy control on the threshold of a new era. Trop Med Int Health 2000; 5: 388-399.

WHO Expert Committee on Leprosy. 7th Report. World Health Organization Technical Report Series 1998; 874: 1-43.

Antimycobacterial Drugs

Drugs used in the treatment of mycobacterial infections can be grouped into four categories, with some overlap:

- First-line drugs for treatment of tuberculosis: isoniazid (INH), rifampin, pyrazinamide, ethambutol, and streptomycin
- Second-line drugs for treatment of tuberculosis: rifabutin and other rifamycins, quinolones, capreomycin, amikacin, kanamycin, paraaminosalicylic acid, cycloserine, and ethionamide
- Drugs used in the treatment of nontuberculous mycobacterial infections: macrolides (clarithromycin and azithromycin), tetracyclines, sulfonamides, clofazimine, fluoroquinolones, and various drugs in the previous two categories
- Drugs used in the treatment of leprosy: dapsone and other sulfones, rifampin, rifabutin, rifapentine, clofazimine, thiacetazone, and ethionamide

Some of the major toxicities of these drugs are summarized in Table 22-3. Primary care clinicians should be familiar mainly with the first-line antituberculous drugs, which are therefore discussed in more detail.

Isoniazid (INH)

Introduced in 1952, isoniazid (INH) revolutionized the treatment of tuberculosis. However, it soon became apparent that resistant *M. tuberculosis* strains had emerged during therapy when INH was used alone, as had been previously shown to be the case with streptomycin.

Activity, Pharmacokinetics, and Pharmacodynamics

INH is bactericidal against actively multiplying tubercle bacilli in cavities, macrophages (i.e., intracellular bacteria), and necrotic foci, making it useful for all forms of clinical disease. It is bacteriostatic against tubercle bacilli that are not replicating. The mechanism of action involves inhibition of synthesis of mycolic acid in mycobacterial cell walls. About 1 in 10^6 tubercle bacilli are resistant to INH because of mutations.

INH is well absorbed from the gastrointestinal tract and distributed widely throughout the body, with CSF levels about 20% of plasma levels. Initial metabolism of INH involves acetylation of the drug in the liver. Many persons are "slow acetylators," and plasma levels are higher and more sustained in these persons than in "rapid acetylators." However, because peak plasma levels even in rapid acetylators far exceed the minimum inhibitory concentrations of INH against *M. tuberculosis,* acetylator status does not seem to correlate with therapeutic efficacy. After acetylation, INH is excreted in urine, which also contains unmetabolized drug.

Unwanted Effects

The major toxic effect is hepatitis. Hepatitis is rare in persons under 20 years of age, but it occurs in up to 0.3% of persons between 20 and 34 years of age, in up to 1.2% of persons between 35 and 49 years of age, and in up to 2.3% of persons over the age of 50 years. Modest elevation of serum AST and ALT occurs in about 15% of patients but usually resolves during therapy. Hepatitis occurs most commonly during the second month of therapy but can occur at any time. Predisposing factors in addition to age include alcoholism, prior liver damage, pregnancy, and use of acetaminophen. Older African-American women may be at higher risk than other demographic groups.

Peripheral neuropathy is uncommon at today's standard dose of INH but is relatively common at higher doses, especially in persons who are slow acetylators or who have other risk factors for neuropathy such as alcoholism, malnutrition, or diabetes mellitus. Pyridoxine (vitamin B_6) 10 to 50 mg/day is commonly given along with INH to decrease the risk of peripheral neuropathy.

Drug fever from INH occasionally occurs in the absence of hepatitis and can be severe. Other hypersensitivity reactions include rash and hematologic abnormalities. Antinuclear antibodies develop in some patients, but INH-induced lupus erythematosus is rare. Other rare complications are Dupuytren's contracture and shoulder-hand syndrome.

INH inhibits the metabolism of phenytoin (Dilantin) and can thus predispose patients to phenytoin toxicity. INH also predisposes individuals to carbamazepine and theophylline toxicity, and it has been shown to inhibit the metabolism of vitamin D and some of the benzodiazepine tranquilizers. Overdose of INH causes seizures, coma, hyperglycemia, and metabolic acidosis.

Administration

The standard dose of INH is 10 to 20 mg/kg/day for children and 5 mg/kg/day for adults, to whom INH is generally given as a maximum dose of 300 mg/day. Minor dose reduction is sometimes recommended for persons with severe renal disease. The dose should be reduced to 150 to 200 mg/day in patients with severe liver disease who are slow acetylators (measurement of drug levels is necessary to establish slow acetylation). The drug can also be given at a dose of 900 mg two or three times weekly. INH is available as 100- or 200-mg tablets, as a syrup (10 mg/mL), and as capsules or tablets for combination therapy. Combination therapy includes capsules containing 150 mg of INH and 300 mg of rifampin (Rifamate) and tablets containing 50 mg of INH, 120 mg of rifampin, and 300 mg of pyrazinamide (Rifater). Food decreases INH bioavailability.

AST and ALT should be measured before therapy. Whether monitoring of liver function during therapy should be routine remains controversial. Many clinicians monitor the aminotransferases monthly in patients at increased risk of hepatitis, such as those with abnormal baseline liver function tests and elderly persons. Patients should be told to stop the drug and notify their physician in the event of nausea, vomiting, jaundice, or abdominal pain.

 KEY POINTS

ISONIAZID (INH)

⊃ Isoniazid is bactericidal against tubercle bacilli in cavities, macrophages, and necrotic foci.

⊃ Mild elevations of the hepatic AST and ALT levels occur in about 15% of patients but usually resolve with continued therapy.

⊃ Hepatitis, the major side effect, is age related and occurs in up to 2.3% of persons over the age of 50 years. Other risk factors for INH hepatitis include alcoholism, prior liver disease, pregnancy, and use of acetaminophen.

⊃ Peripheral neuropathy is uncommon with the standard doses of INH; the risk can be minimized by coadministration of pyridoxine (vitamin B_6) 10 to 50 mg/day.

⊃ INH increases toxicity from phenytoin and theophylline.

⊃ Aminotransferases (AST, ALT) should be measured before INH therapy. Whether monitoring of liver function during therapy should be routine is controversial. Many clinicians monitor the aminotransferases in patients at increased risk of hepatitis, such as the elderly.

⊃ Patients should be told to stop INH and notify their physician in the event of nausea, vomiting, jaundice, or abdominal pain.

Rifampin

Since its introduction into clinical practice during the late 1960s and early 1970s, rifampin has become standard therapy for all forms of active tuberculosis. Knowledge concerning its adverse effects continues to accumulate.

Activity, Pharmacokinetics, and Pharmacodynamics

Rifampin, like INH, is bactericidal against actively replicating tubercle bacilli in cavities and within macrophages, and it is active to a lesser extent against nonreplicating organisms. The mechanism of action consists of inhibition of DNA-dependent RNA polymerase. Rifampin is well absorbed and widely distributed throughout the body. It is excreted mainly by way of the gastrointestinal tract.

Unwanted Effects

Rifampin causes orange discoloration of urine and various body fluids such as tears, sweat, and saliva. The major adverse reaction is hepatitis. Rifampin, unlike INH, tends to cause elevations of the serum bilirubin and alkaline phosphatase levels, as well as the aminotransferases. Persons with alcoholism or prior liver disease are at increased risk of hepatitis.

Hypersensitivity reactions attributed to rifampin form a diverse spectrum. Drug fever with chills can persist for up to a week after discontinuation of the drug. This "flulike syndrome" is thought to be due to circulating immune complexes. Interstitial nephritis can cause renal failure. Urticaria, vasculitis, eosinophilia, thrombocytopenia, and hemolytic anemia are also seen. Rifampin can also cause IgE-mediated anaphylactic reactions.

Rifampin induces the hepatic cytochrome P450 system and thereby interferes with the metabolism of numerous drugs. Examples of commonly used drugs that are affected by rifampin, resulting in reduced plasma concentrations, include the following:

- Hormones: oral contraceptives, estrogens, prednisone
- Cardiovascular drugs: warfarin (Coumadin), digoxin, propranolol, metoprolol, quinidine, diltiazem, verapamil, and tocainide
- Antiepileptic drugs: phenytoin (Dilantin), barbiturates
- Psychotropic drugs: diazepam, haloperidol, nortriptyline
- Antibacterial drugs: clarithromycin, chloramphenicol
- Antifungal drugs: fluconazole, itraconazole, ketoconazole
- Antiretroviral drugs: indinavir, nelfinavir, retonavir, saquinavir
- Miscellaneous agents: sulfonylureas, cyclosporine, methadone

Rifampin also competes with radiographic contrast agents for biliary excretion and can thereby cause nonvisualization of a normal gallbladder. Recently it has been emphasized that rifampin can cause pseudomembranous colitis with delayed onset. This is important to recognize, especially in patients with advanced HIV disease, whose diarrhea might be attributed to other causes.

Administration

The usual dosage of rifampin is 10 mg/kg/day for adults and 10 to 20 mg/kg/day for children. Rifampin is usually given to adults in the maximum dose of 600 mg/day. Dose reduction is recommended for persons with severe liver disease. When used for intermittent therapy (two to three times per week), rifampin is given at the same dose as is used for daily therapy (maximum dose 600 mg/day). Rifampin is available as 150- or 300-mg capsules and in combination drug preparations (see the preceding section on isoniazid). Rifampin is also available for intravenous infusion.

 KEY POINTS

RIFAMPIN

- ⊃ Rifampin is bactericidal against tubercle bacilli in cavities and macrophages.
- ⊃ Rifampin, like INH, can cause hepatitis, especially in persons with alcoholism or prior liver disease. Rifampin hepatitis tends to cause elevation of the serum bilirubin and alkaline phosphatase levels, as well as aminotransferase (AST, ALT) levels.
- ⊃ Allergic reactions to rifampin include drug fever (which can be severe), a flulike syndrome, interstitial nephritis (which can cause renal failure), and anaphylaxis.

- ⊃ Rifampin occasionally causes pseudomembranous colitis, which should be kept in mind when diarrhea occurs in patients receiving rifampin.
- ⊃ Rifampin induces the cytochrome P450 system and thus increases the metabolism of numerous drugs. The levels of many drugs commonly used in clinical medicine are thus lowered by rifampin.
- ⊃ Patients should be warned of orange discoloration of urine and various body fluids and told to notify their physician in the event of nausea, vomiting, abdominal pain, jaundice, fever, bleeding problems, or rash.

Ethambutol

Ethambutol is used as a companion drug with INH, rifampin, or both to delay the emergence of resistant strains.

Activity, Pharmacokinetics, and Pharmacodynamics

Like INH and rifampin, ethambutol is active against actively replicating tubercle bacilli within cavities or macrophages. Unlike the former agents, however, ethambutol is bacteriostatic rather than bactericidal. The mechanism of action consists of inhibition of enzymes involved in the synthesis of cell wall components. Ethambutol is well absorbed (75% to 80% bioavailability) and widely distributed throughout the body. Most of the drug is eliminated by way of the kidneys.

Unwanted Effects

Ethambutol is generally well tolerated with one important exception: optic nerve damage owing to retrobulbar neuritis. Optic neuropathy is said to occur in 1% of patients given ethambutol 15 mg/kg/day and in 3% of patients given 25 mg/kg/day. It is extremely important to note, however, that high, potentially toxic plasma levels will predictably develop in patients with impaired renal function because of the importance of the kidneys in eliminating the drug (see Chapter 19). Ocular toxicity is manifested as blurred vision that can progress to near-blindness. It is usually slowly reversible. Other unwanted effects are gastrointestinal intolerance, hyperuricemia, and hypersensitivity reaction.

Administration

Ethambutol is available as 100- and 400-mg tablets (Myambutol). In contrast to INH and rifampin (in which a standard dose is often used for adults, irrespective of size), the dose of ethambutol should be calculated on a milligram per kilogram basis and then "rounded off" to determine a practical regimen. The usual dose is 15 to 25 mg/kg/day. As previously noted, optic neuropathy is more common with the higher dose. If the higher dose (25 mg/kg/day) is chosen, the dose should be reduced to 15 mg/kg/day after 60 days of therapy. The dose should also be reduced in patients with impaired renal function (see Table 19-3). Monitoring of plasma levels may be desirable in these patients, but unfortunately, few laboratories are equipped to measure ethambutol levels.

Patients should be warned of the risk of vision loss from optic nerve damage. They should be advised to read newsprint each morning, first with one eye closed and then with the other eye closed, to detect vision impairment in either eye.

Studies suggest that impaired communication between the physician and the patient is a significant risk factor for ethambutol optic neuropathy. Visual acuity and red-green color discrimination should be determined before therapy. Ophthalmology consultation with follow-up should be considered for patients with baseline visual symptoms, for patients given the higher dose (25 mg/kg/day), for patients with renal failure, and for elderly persons.

 KEY POINTS

ETHAMBUTOL

⊃ Ethambutol is bacteriostatic against tubercle bacilli in cavities and macrophages.

⊃ Elimination is mainly by the kidneys.

⊃ Ethambutol dosage should be calculated on a milligram per kilogram basis. For patients with impaired renal function, the dose should be reduced and monitoring of plasma levels may be desirable.

⊃ Patients should be warned of the risk of vision loss from optic neuropathy and should be advised to read newsprint with alternate eyes closed each morning to detect vision problems.

⊃ Visual acuity and red-green color discrimination should ideally be tested before ethambutol use. Patients at increased risk of optic neuropathy because of existing vision disorder, use of the higher dose (25 mg/kg/day), impaired renal function, or advanced age may benefit from consultation and follow-up with an ophthalmologist.

Pyrazinamide

Pyrazinamide (PZA) differs from INH and rifampin in that it is active only in acidic environments. In recent years PZA has become a key part of standard antituberculous regimens.

Activity, Pharmacokinetics, and Pharmacodynamics

PZA is bactericidal against tubercle bacilli within the acid pH environment of macrophages. Like INH, rifampin, and ethambutol, PZA is well absorbed orally and widely distributed throughout the body. Recent data suggest that PZA is highly concentrated within the epithelial lining fluid of the lungs. The drug is metabolized by the liver but excreted mainly by the kidneys.

Unwanted Effects

As with INH and rifampin, liver toxicity is the major unwanted effect. It is less likely to occur at the doses that are now recommended than at the higher doses used in the past. Elevation of the serum uric acid level occurs in about one half of

patients receiving PZA and is usually asymptomatic. The importance of hyperuricemia, however, remains somewhat controversial because occasional cases of severe hyperuricemia and acute arthritis occur. Other unwanted effects are rash, photosensitivity, interstitial nephritis, rhabdomyolysis, and polymyalgia.

Administration

PZA is available as 500-mg tablets or in a combination preparation with INH and rifampin (see earlier discussion). The usual dose is 20 to 35 mg/kg/day, with a maximum dose of 2 g/day for adults. When PZA is used for intermittent therapy, the maximum dose is 4 g when given twice a week and 3 g when given three times a week. Hepatic aminotransferases (ALT, ALT) and uric acid should be measured before therapy and, if abnormal, during therapy. The dose should be reduced in patients with renal failure. Unlike INH, rifampin, and ethambutol, PZA is significantly removed by hemodialysis. Therefore PZA should be given after hemodialysis.

 KEY POINTS

PYRAZINAMIDE

⊃ PZA is bactericidal against tubercle bacilli only in acidic environments, as within the phagolysosomes of macrophages.

⊃ Liver toxicity is the major unwanted effect.

⊃ Hyperuricemia is common (about one half of patients) but usually asymptomatic.

⊃ Hepatic aminotransferases (AST, ALT) and uric acid should be measured before therapy and, if abnormal, during therapy.

⊃ The dose should be reduced in patients with renal failure.

SUGGESTED READING

Byrd RP Jr, Roy TM, Ossorio MA, et al. Delayed onset of pseudomembranous colitis after rifampin therapy. South Med J 1997; 90: 644-646.

Martinez E, Collazos J, Mayo J. Hypersensitivity reactions to rifampin: pathogenetic mechanisms, clinical manifestations, management strategies, and review of the anaphylactic-like reactions. Medicine (Baltimore) 1999; 78: 361-369.

Romero JA, Kuczler FJ Jr. Isoniazid overdose: recognition and management. Am Fam Physician 1998; 57: 749-752.

Self TH, Chrisman CR, Baciewicz AM, et al. Isoniazid drug and food interactions. Am J Med Sci 1999; 317: 304-311.

Van Scoy RE, Wilkowske CJ. Antimycobacterial therapy. Mayo Clin Proc 1999; 74: 1038-1048.

23 Parasitic Infections

DAVID R. HABURCHAK, VALDA CHIJIDE

Primary care physicians in North America and most economically privileged countries rarely encounter or even think about parasitic diseases. Exceptions, of course, include physicians whose practice includes immigrants, travelers, or populations exposed to specific environmental risks. Worldwide, however, parasitic disease is common, and, with the relative ease of travel in the 21st century, more and more physicians have opportunity to care for patients with parasitic infections abroad and at home. In this chapter we emphasize a symptom-based approach to the most common parasitic diseases found in the United States and encountered by American physicians traveling abroad on missionary or humanitarian work. Basic principles of clinical diagnosis, management, and prevention are provided for a limited but representative series of infections, emphasizing cost-effective intervention.

SUGGESTED READING

Cook GC, ed. Manson's Tropical Diseases. 20th ed., London: W.B. Saunders Company; 1996.

DuPont HL, Steffen R. Textbook of Travel Medicine and Health. 2nd ed., Hamilton, Ontario, Canada, BC Decker; 2001.

Goddard J. Infectious Diseases and Arthropods. Totowa, NJ: Humana Press; 2000.

Guerrant RL, Walker DH, Weller PF, ed. Tropical Infectious Diseases: Principles, Pathogens, and Practice. Philadelphia: Churchill Livingstone; 1999.

Gutierrez Y. Diagnostic Pathology of Parasitic Infections with Clinical Correlations. 2nd ed., New York: Oxford University Press; 2000.

Jong EC, McMullen R, eds. The Travel and Tropical Medicine Manual. 2nd ed., St. Louis: W.B. Saunders Company; 1995.

Strickland GT, ed. Hunter's Tropical Medicine and Emerging Infectious Diseases. 8th ed., Philadelphia: W.B. Saunders Company; 2000.

Sun T. Parasitic Disorders: Pathology, Diagnosis, and Management. 2nd ed., Baltimore: Williams & Wilkins; 1999.

Epidemiologic Factors and General Evaluation for Parasitic Disease

Epidemiologic History

The epidemiologic history is crucial to efficient diagnosis and management of parasitic disease because the initial complaints are usually nonspecific. The following are critical questions:

- Travel: Location? Recent or remote? Duration? Activities while traveling? "Off the beaten path"?
- Occupation: Exposure to animals? Exposure to soil? Farming? Military? Child care? Health care?
- Socioeconomic status: Shelter? Crowded conditions? Sanitation? Washing? Homeless, refugee, or immigrant population?
- Recreation: Camping? Adventure sports? Sandy beaches where animals wander?
- Animals: Pets? Hunting? Farm animals? Pests?
- Food and water: Undercooked meat, fish, or game? Raw water? Swimming or diving?

Recent and remote travel, occupation, socioeconomic status, recreation, animal exposure, and living arrangements provide valuable clues. Fever combined with recent travel to tropical or developing countries should prompt consideration of malaria, enteric fever, and arboviral infection. Unusual or imported foodstuffs or consumption of or exposure to untreated water increases the risk of parasites, particularly protozoa. Homeless persons, campers, farm workers, migrants, and refugees are at higher risk of skin and gastrointestinal parasites. Pets associated with parasitic transmission include dogs, cats, mice, rats, hamsters, gerbils, ferrets, snakes, lizards, and primates. Undercooked game meat and fish such as sushi and meat tartare can transmit systemic and gastrointestinal parasitic disease. When was the exposure and how long has it been since the exposure? Most metazoa have relatively long incubation periods (weeks) and duration of parasitosis (months to years), whereas most protozoal infections are more abrupt in onset and of shorter duration.

Further History

Does the patient have chronic underlying disease? Is the patient immunocompromised? Patients with AIDS and patients who are taking immunosuppressive drugs for any reason are subject to reactivation of fungal, mycobacterial, and parasitic infections that would otherwise lie dormant. Most human immunodeficiency virus (HIV)–infected patients with toxoplasmosis, cryptosporidiosis, or other protozoal infections have advanced disease (CD4 count <100/mm³). Patients with lymphoma, leukemia, or advanced HIV disease, and especially patients who have recently started taking immunosuppressive drugs, are vulnerable to dissemination of *Strongyloides* larvae. The resulting hyperinfection syndrome is characterized by massive larval invasion of the lungs and other tissues; complications include ileus, shock, and secondary bacterial infection with sepsis or meningitis caused by gram-negative rods.

What symptoms preceded or accompanied the chief complaint? The symptoms of most parasitic diseases evolve over time as the organisms migrate through tissues or progress through their life cycles. The same disease may cause strikingly different symptoms as the patient goes from one stage to the next. Adding to the confusion, patients—especially those who have lived in underdeveloped countries and those with HIV disease—often have concomitant parasitic and nonparasitic infections. Examples of the latter include tuberculosis, salmonellosis, and sexually transmitted diseases. The clinician should never stop thinking after the first diagnosis. Often valuable clues are elicited only by conducting a thorough review of systems.

The family history can be highly relevant. Are other cases present in the household? Screening of other infected family members and assessment of the household for educational and sanitary deficiencies are often appropriate.

Physical Examination

Vital signs, body mass index, and general appearance give clues to the risk or presence of parasitic disease. Fever, tachycardia, malaise, malnutrition, and pallor suggest severe parasitic disease. Key physical findings include pallor, rashes, lymphadenopathy, muscle wasting, abdominal distention, organomegaly, edema, abnormal heart sounds, and focal neurologic signs. In children, physical and mental or social developmental milestones should be assessed.

Laboratory Assessment

Laboratory assessment for parasitic disease is often expensive and unsatisfactory. Specimen procurement, handling, and interpretation are often less than optimal in practices and communities where the volume of parasitic disease is low. This unfortunate situation prompts many clinicians to treat suspected parasitic disease symptomatically or empirically. Such practice should be avoided. Every effort should be made to secure a laboratory diagnosis before starting therapy. Effective therapy is often quite specific, yet it is expensive, risky, and not always curative. Moreover, family members may need treatment, and a confirmed diagnosis may be necessary for household control.

Patients should be given clear instructions on how to provide stool samples, along with the appropriate kits and directions for prompt laboratory submission. Skin scrapings, tissue biopsy specimens, blood smears, and serologic samples must be obtained and handled properly and interpreted by competent reference laboratories.

Factitious Infection and Pseudoparasitosis

Occasionally patients give a chief complaint of "parasites." The evaluation is not as straightforward as it may sound.

Most parasites are visualized only with the microscope. Exceptions include lice, cutaneous larva migrans, *Ascaris* species, pinworm, and occasionally tapeworm. Immigrants may demonstrate filarial worms in the skin, yet guinea worm is nearly extinct. When a patient describes a real worm in the stool, it usually should either be yellow-white and the size of an earthworm (*Ascaris*) or gray-white and the size of a straight pin (pinworm). Tapeworm proglottids occasionally "swim" or "flip" in the toilet. Cutaneous larva migrans is usually identified easily by inspection and distinguished from more common dermatophyte infections (ringworm, tinea).

Clinicians must be wary of patients who describe or bring in specimens reputed to be parasites. With the aforementioned notable exceptions, most of these patients have delusional or factitious illness. Typically older women, less commonly younger men, often without prior psychiatric history, these patients bring bottles of dirt, lint, dust, mucus, and other objects, claiming they were removed by scratching the skin. More imaginative patients may bring stool, blood, hair, sputum, or other body or toilet samples. We recently encountered a patient who, using a microscope, videotaped his blood to demonstrate his "worms." Most patients are not convinced even if they look at the specimen under the microscope themselves and are shown pictures of real parasites in a textbook. Management has recently been more successful with pimozide (Orap), but unfortunately, the patient may lose the delusion only to develop parkinsonian symptoms and confusion from this drug. Pimozide should be closely supervised and used initially for only a 2-week period.

Occasionally patients bring in insect larvae found in the toilet or in a draining skin lesion. Such maggots are usually identified easily by their segmented bodies when viewed under the microscope. Toilet-trained domestic flies, maggot-infested fruit, or botfly bites during jungle bird watching have been the most common explanations. Most patients with such pseudoparasitosis are easily consoled compared with those who have delusions.

SUGGESTED READING

Goddard J. Imaginary insect or mite infestations. Infect Med 1998; 15:168-170.

Vincent AL, Vincentio RP, Greene JN, et al. Botfly myiasis in a returning traveler. Infect Med 2001; 18: 163-166.

Zanol K, Slaughter J, Hall R. An approach to the treatment of psychogenic parasitosis. Int J Dermatol 1998; 37:56-63.

Parasites Occurring with Skin Manifestations

Ectoparasites

Scabies

Scabies is caused by the "itch mite," *Sarcoptes scabiei* var. *hominis*. Accurate diagnosis is desirable, especially because the disease is highly contagious.

Presentation and Progression

Cause. The adult female mite burrows into the stratum corneum, where it lives and reproduces. Eggs and feces sensitize the skin, causing the characteristic lesions. The disease is usually spread by intimate personal contact, including sexual contact or sharing of bedding. Casual and nosocomial transmission occurs. Epidemics are associated with poverty, war, homelessness, and overcrowding, but casual contact can also transmit the disease. Occasionally, dogs with mange caused by a similar mite, *S. scabiei* var. *canis,* transmit the disease to humans.

Presentation. Scabies usually causes pruritic papules, vesicles, and linear burrows involving interdigital web spaces of the fingers, wrists, ankles, breasts, genitalia, and beltline in older children and adults (Figure 23-1). In infants and children the most likely form of the disease is characterized by pruritic reddish brown nodules, found especially on the penis, scrotum, and axillae. In elderly patients the lesions tend to involve the temples, hairline, forehead, and neck. In some cases the diagnosis is obscured by the development of a secondary eczematous eruption, probably caused by hypersensitivity to the mite, or by secondary bacterial infection, usually caused by *Staphylococcus aureus*. Some patients are seen after treatment with topical corticosteroids, which obscures the nature of the underlying condition (scabies incognito). The most severe form of the disease is known as Norwegian scabies or crusted scabies and is usually encountered in institutionalized and immunosuppressed patients. Patients with Down syndrome or AIDS are especially susceptible. In this form of scabies, hyperkeratotic, crusted nodules and plaques can mimic psoriasis and be complicated by secondary bacterial infection.

Diagnosis

Diagnosis is made by demonstrating the organism or its eggs or feces microscopically in material obtained by scraping or shaving the superficial layers of the skin with a No. 15 scalpel blade to a depth sufficient to cause pinpoint bleeding. Punch biopsy of the skin is sometimes required.

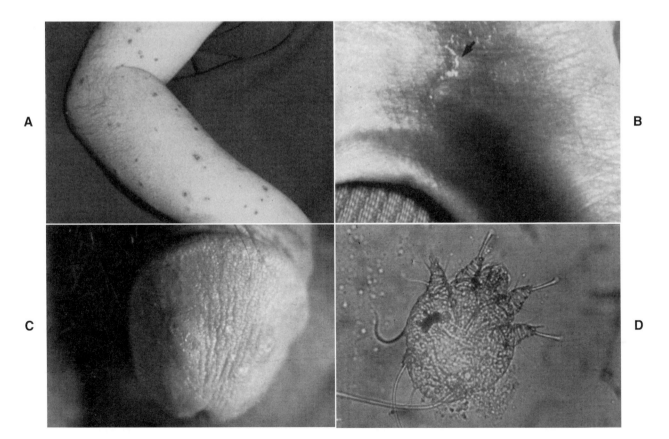

FIG. 23-1 Dermatologic manifestations of scabies and microscopic identification of the causative mite. (Courtesy of The Upjohn Company, Kalamazoo, Michigan.)

Natural History

Expected Outcome. If untreated, scabies tends to persist for long periods, even in immunocompetent individuals.

Treatment

The recommended treatment is permethrin 5% cream (Elimite) applied from the neck down to the toes. This cream is washed off after 8 to 10 hours, and the process is repeated a week later. The safety of permethrin in infants (<2 months) and in pregnant women has not been established; an alternative for these patients is 6% to 10% precipitated sulfur in petrolatum daily for 3 days. Lindane (Kwell, G-well, Scabene) is no longer recommended because of central nervous system toxicity, although such toxicity has been described mainly in infants and very young children and in those who used the drug improperly. Ivermectin (Stromectol) has recently been shown to be effective and has the advantage of single-dose oral administration (200 µg/kg), but it is not yet approved by the Food and Drug Administration (FDA) for this indication and a second course is often necessary. Infants less than 2 months of age and pregnant or lactating women may be treated with precipitated sulfur 6% in petrolatum. Antihistamines and topic antipruritics can be used to control pruritus, which will last weeks after successful therapy to kill the mite. Antibiotics are sometimes necessary for secondary bacterial infection.

Patients should be advised to launder all clothing and bedding in the hot cycle while they are being treated. All family members should be treated simultaneously to prevent recurrence. Patients with Norwegian scabies are highly contagious and should ideally be managed in the hospital setting with careful attention to barrier precautions.

Expected Response. A single application of permethrin cream is usually curative. The nodular form of the disease found in children may persist for months despite adequate therapy, probably reflecting a delayed hypersensitivity reaction to mite products.

When to Refer

Perplexing cases sometimes warrant referral to a dermatologist for confirmation of the diagnosis.

 KEY POINTS

SCABIES

⊃ Scabies, a highly contagious disease caused by the "itch mite," *S. scabiei* var. *hominis,* is usually manifested as pruritic papules, vesicles, and linear burrows. It is often associated with poor hygiene or sexual promiscuity but also affects persons of all ages and social classes.

⊃ In children a nodular form of the disease may develop that can persist for months despite adequate therapy.

⊃ In patients who are institutionalized or severely immunocompromised an extremely contagious form of the disease known as Norwegian scabies and characterized by crusted, hyperkeratotic nodules and plaques can develop.

⊃ Efforts should be made to secure the diagnosis by microscopic demonstration of the mite or its eggs.

⊃ Permethrin 5% cream is now the recommended treatment for most patient groups.

SUGGESTED READING

Chosidow O. Scabies and pediculosis. Lancet 2000; 355: 819-826.
Usha V. A comparative study of oral ivermectin and topical permethrin cream in the treatment of scabies. J Am Acad Dermatol 2000; 42:236-240.

Lice (Pediculosis)

Pediculus humanus capitis (head louse), *Pediculus humanus corporis* (body louse), and *Phthirus pubis* (pubic or crab louse) parasitize humans for blood meals on the skin. Lice can cause pruritus, predispose the skin to bacterial infection, and serve as vectors for epidemic typhus, bartonellosis, and relapsing fever. Adult females produce and glue eggs called nits to body hair and clothing.

Presentation and Progression

Cause. Lice are small (2- to 4-mm), grayish white, wingless insects. The head louse and the body louse have a similar appearance, being elongated with pointed head. The pubic louse resembles a crab (hence its alternative name). The pruritic papules characteristic of lice infestation are attributed to a hypersensitivity reaction to saliva injected into the skin by the lice in the course of obtaining a blood meal.

Lice have a nearly worldwide distribution and cause epidemics during times of war and overcrowding. Persons of all ages and classes are affected. In the United States, lice are especially problematic among schoolchildren, the homeless, and those who are highly sexually active.

Presentation. Pediculosis capitis occurs as severe itching of the scalp. Excoriations from scratching lead to secondary bacterial infection with weeping and crusting of the skin and regional lymphadenopathy. Pediculosis corporis occurs as itching accompanied by erythematous macules, papules, and excoriations, mainly on the trunk. Asymptomatic blue-gray or slate-colored macules (maculae ceruleae) sometimes appear on the trunk, thighs, and buttocks. Secondary impetiginization is common. In persons who have had body lice for a long time, thickened skin with areas of hyperpigmentation (vagabond's disease) can develop. Pubic lice cause severe itching above the genitalia and sometimes affect hairs of the axillae, trunk, and eyelashes as well. Excoriation and secondary bacterial infection, if present at all, are usually less severe than in pediculosis capitis and pediculosis corporis.

Diagnosis

In pediculosis capitis, adult head lice are most commonly found in the temporal and occipital regions, but they can occur in other areas, including the beard. Adult lice may be difficult to find, but the nits can be identified as small globoid protrusions firmly attached to the base of hair shafts. In pediculosis corporis the adult body louse is usually not seen on the skin except in the most severe infestations. Lice can, however, be found in clothing seams.

Natural History

Expected Outcome. Without treatment or improved hygiene, infestation by lice tends to persist and to be complicated by secondary bacterial infection of the skin.

Treatment

Methods. Permethrin 5% cream (Elimite), permethrin 1% (Nix, nonprescription), and piperonyl butoxide (RID) are all effective therapies. Malathion 0.5% lotion (Ovide Lotion) is FDA approved for head lice resistant to standard treatment. Lindane 1% (Kwell) offers no advantage but more toxicity than other agents. However, the toxicity reported from use of lindane for scabies is unlikely to be a problem in treating lice because the application is of short duration.

Nits must be removed from the hair with a fine-toothed comb. One method is to apply a solution of equal parts of vinegar and water; the comb is dipped in the vinegar solution before use. Petrolatum occlusion has been used effectively for treatment of head lice. Eyelid infestations can be treated with petrolatum or 1% yellow oxide of mercury applied to eyelid margins. Ivermectin has been effective for refractory head and eyelid lice in some patients. Insecticides should not be used in the area of the eye.

Body lice do not require treatment. However, the patient's clothes should be discarded or laundered in a hot cycle and dusted with 1% malathion powder or 10% DDT powder.

Expected Response. Response to treatment is usually excellent.

When to Refer

Pediculosis seldom requires referral. When epidemics occur in classrooms, the students' scalps should be examined periodically.

KEY POINTS

LICE (PEDICULOSIS)

⊃ Head lice occurs as itching of the scalp; the nits and occasionally adult lice are found most often attached to the base of hairs in the temporal and occipital areas.

⊃ Body lice occur as itching with small erythematous macules primarily over the trunk; the adult lice can be found in seams of clothing.

⊃ Pubic lice can also affect the hairs of the trunk, axillae, and eyelashes. The nits and occasionally the adult lice are found attached to the base of hairs.

⊃ Infestation with head lice and body lice is often complicated by excoriation and secondary bacterial infection.

SUGGESTED READING

Chosidow O. Scabies and pediculosis. Lancet 2000; 355: 819-826.
Malathion for treatment of head lice. Med Lett 1999; 41: 73-74.
Potts J. Eradication of ectoparasites in children: how to treat infestations of lice, scabies, and chiggers. Postgrad Med 2001: 110, 57-59, 63-64.
Raoult D, Roux V. The body louse as a vector of reemerging human diseases. Clin Infect Dis 1999; 29: 888-911.

Ticks

Ticks, rather than mosquitoes, are now the most important causes of vectorborne disease in the United States (Table 23-1). An alphabetized list of diseases transmitted by ticks includes the following: arbovirus diseases (including yellow fever, dengue, and viral encephalitis), babesiosis, Colorado tick fever, ehrlichiosis, endemic and epidemic relapsing fevers, epidemic typhus, Lyme disease, Q fever, Rocky Mountain spotted fever, tick paralysis, and tularemia.

Despite the impressive list of tickborne diseases, most tick bites are asymptomatic and do not result in disease. Uncomplicated bites can produce pruritic erythematous papules or plaques that may last 1 to 2 weeks. Sometimes a more persistent erythematous nodule develops (tick bite granuloma). Uncomplicated bites can be treated with antipruritics or with topical or intralesional steroids. Rarely, tick bite granuloma requires surgical excision. Patients with systemic infections require specific antibiotics. Tick paralysis can occur after bites with some species, an effect that is believed to be due to a neurotoxin released from the tick salivary gland. Paralysis usually resolves soon after tick removal (see Chapter 6). Answers to frequent questions concerning tick bites are summarized in Table 23-1. The issue frequently arises whether prophylactic antibiotics are useful after a tick bite. The general consensus is no. However, a recent study suggested that doxycycline, given as a single 200-mg dose within 72 hours of *Ixodes scapularis* tick bite, was moderately effective at preventing Lyme disease in a geographic area (Westchester County, New York) where the disease is hyperendemic.

KEY POINTS

MANAGEMENT AND PREVENTION OF TICK EXPOSURES

⊃ When entering tick habitats, individuals should wear protective clothing and insect repellent. Permethrin is more effective and less toxic than DEET (*N,N*-diethylmetatoluamide). Afterward, skin, hair, and pets should be examined for possible infestation.

⊃ Ticks should not be removed with unprotected fingers if possible.

⊃ The best way to remove a tick is to grasp its anterior part with a blunt, rounded forceps (forceps specifically designed for this purpose are available). The tick is then pulled upward, without squeezing but with a slight twisting motion. Occasional ticks (notably the Lone Star tick) are attached more deeply and are difficult to remove, in which case a small excision may be necessary. The tick should be carefully exposed and the hands washed.

⊃ Prophylactic antibiotic administration after tick bites has not been shown to be of value, with the possible exception of exposure in areas where Lyme disease is hyperendemic.

⊃ Medical attention should be sought promptly for the development of fever, rash, or other unusual symptoms.

SUGGESTED READING

Cunha BA, ed. Tickborne Infectious Diseases: Diagnosis and Management. New York: Marcel Dekker; 2000.
Dennis DT, Meltzer MI. Antibiotic prophylaxis after tick bites. Lancet 1997; 350: 1191-1192.
Gayle A, Ringdahl E. Tick-borne diseases. Am Fam Physician 2001; 64: 461-466, 468.

TABLE 23-1
Ticks Commonly Encountered in the United States

Tick	Appearance	Geographic distribution	Characteristics	Diseases
American dog tick (*Dermacentor variabilis*)	Dark brown; rounded mouth parts	Found throughout U.S. except in Rocky Mountains	Favors trails and roadsides near clearings; commonly found on dogs	RMSF (transmission requires ≥24 hours of exposure); tularemia
Rocky Mountain wood tick (*Dermacentor andersoni*)	Dark brown; white markings on scutum*	Rocky Mountains and adjacent areas	Favors brushy vegetation	RMSF; tick paralysis; Colorado tick fever; tularemia
Lone Star tick (*Amblyomma americanum*)	Red-brown; long mouth parts; white spot on the back of females	Central Texas north and east to Iowa and New York	Bites aggressively in southern areas; nicks are common seed ticks	Tularemia; human monocytic ehrlichiosis; possibly Lyme disease or Lyme-like disease in southeastern U.S.
Gulf Coast tick (*Amblyomma maculatum*)	Brown females with mouth parts and metallic markings on scutum	Southeastern Atlantic and Gulf Coast	Bites aggressively	None
Black-legged tick (*Ixodes scapularis*)	Dark brown; long mouth parts	Northern form: eastern and central U.S. to Virginia; southern form: southern U.S. to Mexico	Favors edges of paths and roads; adults active in fall, winter, and spring; immature forms (nymphs), which are important vectors, active in spring and summer	Northern form: Lyme disease (transmission requires >24 hours of exposure for nymphs, 36 hours for adults); human granulocytic ehrlichiosis; babesiosis
Western black-legged tick (*Ixodes pacificus*)	Similar to *Ixodes scapularis*	Canadian Pacific coast south through California	May cause type I hypersensitivity reactions†	Lyme disease (transmission requires 96 hours of exposure for nymphs)
Soft tick (*Ornithodoros hermsi*)	A gray soft tick; mammillated; up to 1 cm in diameter	Western U.S. and Canada	Often found in cabins; bite is painless	
Relapsing fever tick (*Ornithodoros turicata*)	Similar to *Ornithodoros hermsi*	Southwestern and south-central U.S. to northern Florida	Bite is painless, but intense local reaction may occur	Relapsing fever

RMSF, Rocky Mountain spotted fever.
*Scutum: a dorsal plate found on hard ticks.
†Type I hypersensitivity reactions: anaphylaxis, angioedema, urticaria, bronchospasm.

Goddard J. Physician's Guide to Arthropods of Medical Importance. 2nd ed.; Boca Raton, Fla.: CRC Press; 1996.

Nadelman RB, Nowakowski J, Fish D, et al. Prophylaxis with single-dose doxycycline for the prevention of Lyme disease after an *Ixodes scapularis* tick bite. N Engl J Med 2001; 345: 79-84.

Spach DH, Liles WC, Campbell GL, et al. Tick-borne diseases. N Engl J Med 1993; 329: 936-947.

Pinworm (Enterobiasis)

Pinworm is the most prevalent helminthic infection in the United States. Although it affects mainly children in day care centers, institutionalized individuals, and persons liv-ing in crowded positions, it does not make socioeconomic discriminations.

Presentation and Progression
Cause

Enterobius vermicularis is a white worm, about 1 cm in length, that is easily confused with a piece of white thread. After 36 to 53 days of development the adult worms take up residence in the cecum. The mean worm burden is 58 worms in children 4 years to 10 years of age and 16 worms in adolescents. The gravid female contains 11,000 eggs and migrates at night to the perianal and perineal skin, where it lays the eggs. The eggs are infectious for up to 20 days. The adult worms live for 11 to 35 days.

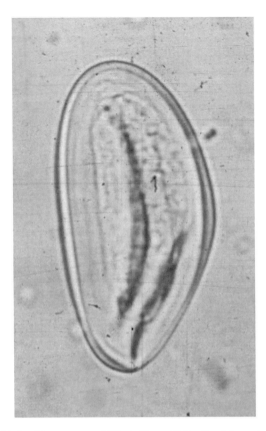

FIG. 23-2 Pinworm egg (100×). (From Walter Reed Army Institute of Research.)

Presentation

The most common complaint prompting evaluation is perianal or perineal itching and insomnia. However, many young patients appear to be asymptomatic. The disease is transmitted most readily by way of the patient's hands. Ova accumulate especially under the fingernails during scratching or handling of linen and undergarments. Multiple family members are commonly affected.

Diagnosis

Diagnosis is easily accomplished by examining for pinworm ova. A piece of cellophane tape is pressed against the perianal skin early in the morning, then placed on a glass slide and examined microscopically. The ovoid egg, flattened on one side, is easily recognized (Figure 23-2). The sensitivity is 50% for a single examination, 90% for three examinations, and 99% for five examinations.

Natural History
Expected Outcome

Pinworm disease is usually benign and eventually self-limited. Appendicitis, salpingitis, and focal ulcerations of the colon have been attributed to migrating worms.

Treatment

Recommend treatment consists of mebendazole (Vermox) as a single oral dose of 100 mg, repeated in 2 weeks. An alternative is albendazole (Albenza) in a 400-mg dose that should

be repeated in 2 weeks. All family members should be treated simultaneously.

Traditionally, patients and their families are given advice about hygiene at the time of treatment. Fingernails should be kept short, hands should be washed before and after meals, shower or stand-up baths (not sit-down baths) should be taken every morning, underwear and bed linen should be changed frequently, toilets should be cleaned regularly, and the house should be vacuumed daily for several days after treatment. With today's effective drug therapy, however, many authorities believe that these exhortations may be excessive, adding unnecessarily to the unfortunate sense of shame over "worms."

Expected Response

Cure rates of 90% to 100% are the rule.

When to Refer

Referral is seldom necessary.

 KEY POINTS

PINWORM

⊃ The most common worm infection in the United States, pinworms most frequently affect children and cause perianal itching and insomnia.
⊃ The "cellophane tape test" for pinworm ova is 50% sensitive for a single specimen and up to 99% sensitive for five examinations.
⊃ Treatment of all family members with mebendazole or albendazole carries a 90% or greater cure rate.
⊃ Although personal and family hygiene should always be encouraged, care must be taken to avoid causing unnecessary psychological trauma.

SUGGESTED READING
Lohiya GS, Tan-Figueroa L, Crinella RM, Lohiya S. Epidemiology and control of enterobiasis in a developmental center. West J Med 2000; 172:305-308.

Cutaneous Larva Migrans (Creeping Eruption)

Cutaneous larva migrans (creeping eruption) is characterized by intensely pruritic, raised, linear or serpiginous skin lesions.

Presentation and Progression
Cause

The usual cause is an infective larva of *Ancylostoma braziliense,* the dog and cat hookworm, but several other animal (e.g., *Ancylostoma caninum, Uncinaria stenocephala, Bunostomum phlebotomum*) and human (e.g., *Strongyloides stercoralis, Gnathostoma spinigerum*) hookworms and, rarely, insect larvae can also cause the disease. The larvae are often acquired by exposure to warm, sandy soils, especially beaches that have been frequented by dogs and cats. In the United States the disease is most prevalent in the southeastern and Gulf Coast states, where seroprevalence up to 50% has been reported. Travelers to tropical and subtropical areas may also become infected.

Presentation

Patients can have intensely pruritic, raised, linear or serpiginous dermatitis (Figure 23-3). The characteristic lesion represents the track taken by the larvae through the skin. Secondary bacterial infection from scratching is sometimes present. The advancing edge of the track is sometimes erythematous and vesicular, whereas older portions fade, becoming dry and encrusted. Eruptions are most often localized to the feet, buttocks, or genitalia, but they can occur anywhere on the skin. Multiple tracks, sometimes hundreds, may be present. Patients often give a history of itching and vesicle formation as the earliest symptoms.

Diagnosis

The diagnosis is made on clinical grounds. Skin biopsies, if performed, show an eosinophilic infiltrate; however, the migrating larvae are seldom identified. The differential diagnosis includes scabies, myiasis, loiasis, *Strongyloides* infection, bacterial or fungal infection, and cercarial or contact dermatitis.

Natural History
Expected Outcome

Without treatment the lesions gradually disappear because the larvae, unable to complete their normal migratory cycle, die within skin or muscle.

Treatment
Methods

Options include topical thiabendazole (Mintezol) applied two to three times daily for 10 days; thiabendazole 25 mg/kg PO b.i.d. for 2 days; albendazole (Albenza) 200 mg b.i.d. for 3 days; or ivermectin (Mectizan, Stromectol) 150 to 200 µg/kg as a single dose. Albendazole and ivermectin are contraindicated during pregnancy. Physicians should not attempt to extract the worm because it has already migrated beyond the visible lesions.

Expected Response

Treatment is usually successful and hastens resolution of the lesions. Most patients treated with albendazole or thiabendazole respond within 1 week.

When to Refer

Referral is seldom necessary.

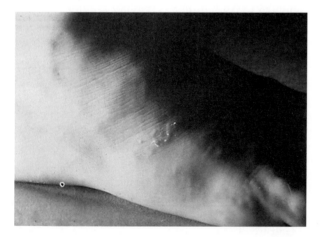

FIG. 23-3 Cutaneous larva migrans. (From Letterman Army Medical Center.)

KEY POINTS

CUTANEOUS LARVA MIGRANS (CREEPING ERUPTION)
⊃ Cutaneous larva migrans is usually caused by the dog and cat hookworm *(A. braziliense)*, acquired from contamination of sandy soil such as beaches.
⊃ Clinical diagnosis is based on the characteristic raised, red, linear, or serpiginous lesions.
⊃ Cutaneous larva migrans is self-limited because the parasite cannot complete its life cycle; however, treatment hastens resolution.

SUGGESTED READING

Caumes E. Treatment of cutaneous larva migrans. Clin Infect Dis 2000; 30: 811-814.

Strongyloidiasis

Strongyloidiasis occurs in the southern United States, where it may affect 0.4% to 4% of the population. Manifestations include skin lesions, abdominal symptoms, and a life-threatening hyperinfection syndrome that can cause shock in immunocompromised persons.

Presentation and Progression
Cause

Strongyloides stercoralis occurs throughout temperate and tropical areas, especially in warm, wet regions. A related nematode, *Strongyloides fulleborni*, is found in Africa and New Guinea. Humans acquire the disease through penetration of the skin by filariform larvae. As in hookworm, the larvae migrate to the lungs and then to the intestines. There females produce eggs, which hatch quickly within the epithelium, releasing first-stage larvae. These larvae, rather than eggs, are usually seen in the stool of infected individuals. Unfortunately, some first-stage larvae can and usually do continue development in the intestinal lumen before exiting the anus, and therefore they can penetrate the intestinal mucosa to establish another round of infection. This allows the parasite to persist with continually renewing infection for many years, despite leaving infected locales. Massive reinfection, termed "hyperinfection," occurs after ileus or immunosuppression and has been reported in former prisoners of war decades after initial exposure.

Presentation

Dermatologic manifestations are usually observed on the lower abdominal wall, buttocks, or thighs with both primary and chronic relapsing infection. Larva currens is an allergic reaction to the migrating larvae manifested as pruritic, urticarial, tortuous tracks. During the intestinal state of the infection, symptoms include abdominal pain, often in the epigastrium, with combinations of nausea, vomiting, diarrhea, and weight loss. In patients with the hyperinfection syndrome, massive larval invasion of the intestines and other tissues develops, causing severe abdominal pain, pulmonary infiltrates, ileus, and shock. Meningitis caused by gram-negative rods such as

Escherichia coli and occasionally by enterococci may occur. In patients with untreated, asymptomatic strongyloidiasis, the hyperinfection syndrome can develop if the patient takes immunosuppressive drugs for any reason.

PATIENT 1

A 50-year-old man who had been a prisoner of war in Vietnam began taking systemic corticosteroids after a lung biopsy demonstrated idiopathic pulmonary fibrosis. Five days later, fever, abdominal pain, and linear erythematous migrating eruptions developed in the skin of his abdomen and trunk (Figure 23-4). The streaks extended at an average rate of 6 mm per 30 minutes. Stool examination disclosed many *Strongyloides* larvae. He responded to thiabendazole therapy.

Diagnosis

Eosinophilia is usually prominent unless the patient is immunosuppressed. The diagnosis is usually made by finding rhabditiform larvae in sputum, stool, or duodenal contents. Serologic tests are highly sensitive in immunocompetent patients.

Natural History
Expected Outcome

About one third of patients with strongyloidiasis are asymptomatic. Persistence of worms in the intestine for up to 35 years after persons left an endemic area has been described.

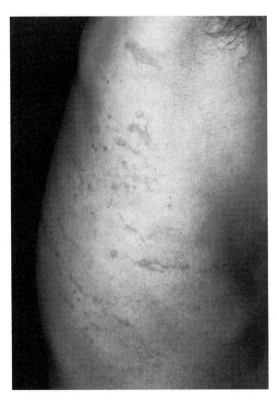

FIG. 23-4   Cutaneous linear eruptions of disseminated strongyloidiasis. (From Eisenhower Army Medical Center.)

Treatment
Methods

Thiabendazole (Mintezol) 25 mg/kg b.i.d. (maximum, 3 g/day) for 2 days is effective therapy. Albendazole and ivermectin are also effective, although not FDA approved.

When to Refer

Patients with the hyperinfection syndrome usually require referral and hospitalization.

 KEY POINTS

STRONGYLOIDIASIS

⊃ Skin manifestations usually occur on the lower abdominal wall, buttocks, or thighs as larva currens, an allergic reaction with pruritic, urticarial, tortuous tracks.

⊃ In immunocompetent patients the main manifestations relate to invasion of the gastrointestinal tract: abdominal pain, nausea, vomiting, and weight loss. Eosinophilia is usually present.

⊃ In immunocompromised patients strongyloidiasis can be a severe, even life-threatening hyperinfection syndrome with abdominal pain, ileus, pulmonary infiltrates, meningitis or sepsis, and shock.

⊃ Strongyloidiasis should be considered before immunosuppressive therapy is initiated in any patient with unexplained eosinophilia.

SUGGESTED READING

Grove DI. Human strongyloidiasis. Adv Parasitol 1996; 38: 251-309.

Heyworth MF. Parasitic diseases in immunocompromised hosts: cryptosporidiosis, isosporiasis and strongyloidiasis. Gastroenterol Clin North Am 1996; 25: 691-707.

Mahmoud AAF. Strongyloidiasis. Clin Infect Dis 1996; 23: 949-952.

Sato Y, Kobayashi J, Toma H, et al. Efficacy of stool examination for detection of *Strongyloides* infection. Am J Trop Med Hyg 1995; 53: 248-250.

Cutaneous Leishmaniasis

Leishmaniasis occurs rarely in the United States, mainly in southern Texas. However, it is endemic in widely scattered parts of the world, including the Middle East, Africa, India, Asia, and Latin America. Interest was renewed recently by its occurrence in veterans of the Persian Gulf War. The three types are cutaneous leishmaniasis, visceral leishmaniasis (kala-azar), and mucosal leishmaniasis (espundia).

Presentation and Progression
Cause

Cutaneous leishmaniasis is produced by protozoal parasites belonging to the genus *Leishmania*. Different species cause the disease in the Eastern Hemisphere (Old World cutaneous leishmaniasis) and Western Hemisphere (New World cutaneous leishmaniasis). The disease is transmitted by *Phlebotomus* sand flies and is prevalent in tropical and subtropical regions.

Presentation

Skin lesions are usually maculopapular before becoming crusted or ulcerated. They heal slowly, usually over several months, and typically leave a flat, atrophic scar. Eczematoid lesions may prompt inappropriate therapy with topical steroids. The lesions of Old World leishmaniasis are commonly called "Oriental sore"; those of New World leishmaniasis, pian bois (bush yaws), uta, or chiclero ulcer. Diffuse or disseminated disease can occur on the face and extremities. Lesions may involve peripheral nerves, producing hypoesthesia and diagnostic confusion with leprosy. Patients may have malaise, lymphadenopathy, and low-grade fever.

Diagnosis

The lesions are diverse, and none are pathognomonic. Diagnosis depends on identification of the organism in Giemsa-stained smears of tissue or aspirates, or of promastigotes in culture (NNN medium or Schneider's *Drosophila* medium supplemented with 30% fetal bovine serum). Punch biopsies should be taken from the border of the lesion and not from an ulcer surface. Serologic diagnosis is unreliable.

Natural History
Expected Outcome

Many lesions gradually heal spontaneously, but others persist and are often unsightly. The visceral form of the disease, which is an important opportunistic infection in HIV-positive persons in some parts of the world, can be life threatening, and the mucosal form of the disease can destroy the nasal septum and other respiratory tissues.

Treatment
Methods

Sodium stibogluconate (antimony sodium gluconate; Pentostam) is effective for treatment of all of the cutaneous leishmanias except the Ethiopian form of diffuse cutaneous disease, which should respond to pentamidine. Meglumine antimoniate (glucantime) can be used in areas where sodium stibogluconate is not available. Other treatments reported to be effective include topical 15% paromomycin and 12% methylbenzethonium chloride in white soft paraffin, intralesional antimony, amphotericin B, and ketoconazole.

Preventive measures include avoiding outdoor activities from dusk to dawn when sand flies are most active, wearing protective clothing, and using DEET on exposed skin and under the edges of clothing. Fine-mesh bed nets impregnated with permethrin may provide additional protection.

Expected Response

Response to treatment is usually slow and often incomplete.

When to Refer

Because cutaneous leishmaniasis is a rare disease in the United States and treatment is difficult, most patients require referral.

 KEY POINTS

CUTANEOUS LEISHMANIASIS

⊃ The diagnosis should be considered when chronic skin lesions develop in tourists, immigrants, and military troops.

⊃ None of the skin lesions are pathognomonic. Diagnosis requires demonstration of the organism or its promastigotes.

⊃ Treatment is sometimes difficult, and most patients require referral.

SUGGESTED READING

Aronson NE, Wortmann GW, Johnson SC, et al. Safety and efficacy of intravenous sodium stibogluconate in the treatment of leishmaniasis: recent U.S. military experience. Clin Infect Dis 1998; 27: 1457-1464.

Norton SA, Frankenburg S, Klaus SN. Cutaneous leishmaniasis acquired during military service in the Middle East. Arch Dermatol 1992; 128: 83-87.

Pearson RD, Sousa AQ. Clinical spectrum of leishmaniasis. Clin Infect Dis 1996; 22: 1-13.

Trichinosis

Consumption of undercooked meat ("jerky," barbecued meat, or microwaved meat) from game animals is increasingly the cause of trichinosis, which is usually asymptomatic but can be life threatening. Fewer than 100 cases occur in the United States each year.

Presentation and Progression
Cause

Trichinella spiralis, a nematode (roundworm), is the usual cause, but other *Trichinella* species have been implicated. These worms are widely distributed in carnivores, including bear, cougar, and wild boar. Herbivores such as horses fed uncooked meat from pigs or other carnivores can also become infectious. Pigs acquire the disease when fed garbage or through ingestion of rats. Common source outbreaks continue to occur in North America and Europe. Dog meat shashliks have caused recent outbreaks in Kazakhstan.

After meat is ingested, larvae are released in the stomach, pass to the small intestine, and molt four times within 30 hours to become adults in the columnar epithelium. The adult worms mate at 30 to 34 hours after ingestion, and 5 days later they begin to release large numbers of larvae. From weeks 2 to 6 the parenteral phase of infection consists of migration of newborn larvae throughout the host via lymphatic and blood vessels to muscle, nervous tissue, and organs throughout the body. Severity and rapidity of onset of symptoms are proportional to numbers of larvae. Patients without enteral symptoms usually have less severe systemic disease.

Presentation

Most infections are subclinical, but symptoms can be severe. The enteral phase of infection is usually asymptomatic, but as many as 20% to 60% of patients have diarrhea, nausea, and upper abdominal pain 3 to 6 days after ingestion. In patients with large worm burdens, myositis develops with weakness, pain, and swelling of muscles that usually begin in the extraocular muscles and later involve other muscles such as the masseters and the muscles of the neck, extremities, and trunk. Other symptoms include headache, dysphagia, rash, and hoarseness. Physical findings often include fever, periorbital or facial edema (15% to 90% of cases), conjunctivitis, and conjunctival hemorrhage.

Diagnosis

The differential diagnosis includes angioneurotic edema, serum sickness, septicemia, polyarteritis nodosa, polymyositis, and allergic reactions to foods and drugs. Useful physical findings include periorbital edema, retinal or subungual splinter hemorrhages, and muscle tenderness. Helpful laboratory findings include eosinophilia, which can be striking after the 10th day of illness, elevation of muscle enzyme levels, and a normal sedimentation rate despite fever. Serologic response is usually delayed until after the second week of infection. Antigen detection tests and the polymerase chain reaction (PCR) are promising but not readily available. Muscle biopsy is specific but insensitive, particularly in mild infection.

Natural History
Expected Outcome

The acute illness wanes by the sixth week, but some patients have chronic myalgia, malaise, fatigue, ocular symptoms, and neuropathic symptoms. Complications of severe infection include abortion, encephalitis, endocarditis, myocarditis, and heart failure. Death may occur from cardiac or neurologic disease during weeks 3 to 5 or, later, from pneumonia.

Treatment
Methods

Therapy consists of observation, supportive fluids, steroids, and albendazole (400 mg/day for 3 days, or 5 mg/kg/day for 4 days in children) or mebendazole (200 mg/day for 3 days). Mebendazole is less expensive, less well absorbed, and more readily available in pharmacies than albendazole. These drugs are in category C and should not be given to pregnant women. Prednisolone is often given at 40 to 60 mg/day in adults for 5 to 7 days.

Expected Response

Treatment is generally considered to be unsatisfactory. Anthelmintic drugs kill the adult worms in the intestines but have little or no effect on the larvae encysted in muscle. Neither anthelmintic drugs nor steroids have been shown convincingly to alter the course of the illness.

When to Refer

Patients with severe trichinosis often require hospitalization for supportive care.

KEY POINTS

TRICHINOSIS
- Trichinosis results from eating undercooked meat.
- Fewer than 100 cases are reported in the United States each year, but outbreaks occur, sometimes attributed to eating unusual meat such as cougar jerky.
- Storage at approximately 59° F (15° C) for 3 weeks usually sterilizes meat, but meat should be cooked until no trace of flesh or pink fluid can be seen (the thermal death point for *Trichina* larvae is 131° F [55° C]).
- Trichinosis should be suspected when patients have any combination of fever, periorbital edema, muscle pain or tenderness, conjunctival or subungual hemorrhage, and eosinophilia.

SUGGESTED READING

Capo V, Despommier DD. Clinical aspects of infection with *Trichinella* spp. Clin Microbiol Rev 1996; 9: 47-54.
Dworkin MS, Gamble HR, Zarlenga DS, et al. Outbreak of trichinellosis associated with eating cougar jerky. J Infect Dis 1996; 174: 663-666.
Greenbloom SL, Martin-Smith P, Isaacs S, et al. Outbreak of trichinosis in Ontario secondary to the ingestion of wild boar meat. Can J Public Health 1997; 88: 52-56.
Wakelin D, Goyal PK. *Trichinella* isolates: parasite variability and host responses. Int J Parasitol 1996; 26: 471-481.

Filariasis

Filariasis is caused by eight insect-transmitted nematodes that parasitize the lymphatic and subcutaneous tissues. Filariasis is a major social and economic burden in tropical and subtropical Asia, Africa, the western Pacific region, and parts of the Americas and is estimated to affect 120 million people in 73 countries (Table 23-2). Most of the morbidity is caused by *Wuchereria bancrofti* (lymphatic filariasis), *Brugia malayi* (lymphatic filariasis), and *Onchocerca volvulus* (river blindness).

Most patients infected with lymphatic filariae are asymptomatic, but nearly two thirds have subclinical renal and lymphatic damage manifested as hematuria, proteinuria, and trace-dependent edema. Nearly one fourth of male patients have hydrocele, and a little over one eighth of infected persons have elephantiasis, lymphedema, or both with accompanying attacks of acute lymphangitis or lymphadenitis. Ultrasonography has been used to detect the twirling motion ("filarial dance sign") of live adult filarial worms and to detect dilated lymphatic channels. Secondary bacterial and fungal infections exacerbate dermal and lymphatic destruction, resulting in elephantiasis of the extremities, scrotum, breasts, and vulva.

O. volvulus causes painless, mobile, subcutaneous nodules, lichenification, depigmentation, atrophy, keratitis, retinitis, and blindness. *Loa loa* causes pruritus, urticaria, and localized angioedema ("Calabar swellings"). The worm may sometimes be seen migrating across the subconjunctiva. Other tropical filariae may cause headache, arthralgias, angioedema, pericarditis, and tropical pulmonary eosinophilia. Demonstration of the causative organism in blood, skin snips, or excised nodules leads to diagnosis. Antigen detection by enzyme-linked immunosorbent assay (ELISA) or PCR has been useful for diagnosis of the nocturnal *W. bancrofti*.

Therapy of filariasis is complex and depends on specific species, presence of eye involvement, and likelihood of

TABLE 23-2
Nematodes Causing Filariasis

Organism	Distribution	Vector	Syndromes
Onchocerca volvulus	Africa, Latin America, Middle East	Blackfly	Skin nodules, blindness
Wuchereria bancrofti	Tropics worldwide	Mosquito	Lymphadenopathy, elephantiasis
Brugia malayi	Asia	Mosquito	Lymphadenopathy, elephantiasis
Mansonella perstans	Africa, South America	Midges	Conjunctival nodules (usually asymptomatic)
Mansonella streptocerca	Africa	Midges	Dermatitis
Mansonella ozzardi	Latin America	Blackfly; midges	Usually asymptomatic
Brugia timori	Indonesia	Mosquito	
Loa loa	Africa	Turbaned fly	Nodules

coinfection. Prevention depends on vector control, hygiene, and mass community therapy to reduce microfilariae.

SUGGESTED READING

Burri H, Loutan L, Kumaraswami V, et al. Skin changes in chronic lymphatic filariasis. Trans R Soc Trop Med Hyg 1996; 90: 671-674.
Michael E, Bundy DA, Grenfell BT. Re-assessing the global prevalence and distribution of lymphatic filariasis. Parasitology 1996; 112: 409-428.
Orihel TC, Eberhard ML. Zoonotic filariasis. Clin Microbiol Rev 1998; 11: 366-381.

Dirofilariasis

Dirofilaria species infect humans as an accidental host, usually causing an asymptomatic pulmonary nodule or a subcutaneous mass. The disease is recognized mainly in the southeastern United States, but the incidence is apparently increasing.

Dirofilaria immitis, the dog heartworm, causes a localized pulmonary vasculitis in humans. Most infections have no symptoms, but some patients have cough, chest pain, or hemoptysis. Eosinophilia is usually absent. A solitary, noncalcified, pleura-based nodule is the most common radiographic finding. Histologic examination usually reveals a dead worm in an infarct with vasculitis and granulomatous or eosinophilic inflammation. Systemic therapy is unnecessary, but the cause of the nodule must be determined to exclude malignancy. Serologic tests lack the sensitivity and specificity to be useful.

Other *Dirofilaria* species include *D. tenuis* (raccoon), *D. ursi* (bear), *D. subdermata* (porcupine), and *D. repens* (dog and cat in Europe and Asia). These latter species cause subcutaneous infections in their respective mammals and also in humans, appearing as skin nodules. Diagnosis is again based on biopsy, which shows an inflammatory mass with eosinophils and a dead worm, although the latter may be difficult to demonstrate.

 KEY POINTS

FILARIASIS AND DIROFILARIASIS

⤳ Filariasis is an important disease worldwide caused by eight mosquito-transmitted nematodes. The most important syndromes include lymphadenopathy, skin nodules, elephantiasis, and blindness.

⤳ Dirofilariasis is encountered in the United States, especially in the Southeast, and is caused by the dog heartworm (*D. immitis*). It occurs most commonly as a pulmonary nodule. Unfortunately, surgical resection is usually necessary to exclude malignancy.

SUGGESTED READING

Nicholson CP, Allen MS, Trastek VF, et al. *Dirofilaria immitis:* a rare, increasing cause of pulmonary nodules. Mayo Clin Proc 1992; 67: 646-650.

Parasites Occurring with Gastrointestinal or Pulmonary Manifestations

Diarrhea is a common, perhaps the most common, manifestation of parasitic infection. Symptoms are usually worst early in the disease process, but they are sometimes the result of coinfecting bacterial or viral pathogens. Abdominal pain with diarrhea, frank dysentery, or skin rash suggests a higher than usual likelihood of protozoal or helminthic disease. Diagnosis usually depends on recovery of eggs, cysts, trophozoites, or larvae from stool or sputa. Stool sample sensitivity depends on the stage, duration, and intensity of infection. Specific

TABLE 23-3
Protozoa Associated with Gastroenteritis

Organism	Epidemiology	Clinical features	Complications	Treatment
Giardia lamblia (giardiasis)	Day care centers; hiking; swimming; camping and foreign travel; men who have sex with men	Asymptomatic in 60% of infections. Early symptoms include bloating, eructation, nausea, and variable fever. Later symptoms include loose, foul-smelling stools, cramps, and flatulence.	Malabsorption; lactase deficiency; weight loss; abdominal pain	Metronidazole (see text)
Entamoeba histolytica (amebiasis)	Developing countries; migrant workers; institutionalized persons; men who have sex with men	Asymptomatic in 90% of infections. Symptoms include dysenteric rectocolitis with ulcers, chronic colitis, and toxic megacolon.	Toxic megacolon; liver abscess; lung abscess; ameboma	Metronidazole; paromomycin (see text)
Cryptosporidium species (cryptosporidiosis)	Surface water; day care centers; swimming; hospitals	Often asymptomatic. Immunocompetent patients tend to have mild diarrhea. Some patients, especially the immunocompromised, including patients with AIDS, have a protracted course with fever, severe cramps, vomiting, and diarrhea.	Weight loss; cholecystitis	Generally unnecessary in immunocompetent persons. Paromomycin plus azithromycin has been used for persons with HIV disease (see Chapter 17).
Cyclospora species (cyclosporiasis)	Developing countries; imported fruits; surface water	Relapsing diarrhea; myalgia; arthralgia.	Severe fatigue	TMP/SMX (one double-strength tablet b.i.d. for 7 days)
Isospora belli (isosporiasis)	Developing countries	Nonbloody diarrhea; fever; headache; abdominal pain.	Dehydration; malabsorption	For patients with HIV disease, TMP/SMX, one double-strength tablet q.i.d. for 10 days, then b.i.d. for 3 weeks or longer.
Microsporidia (microsporidiasis)	Advanced HIV disease	Chronic diarrhea; fever; weight loss.	Disseminated infection	Metronidazole and albendazole have been used with variable success (see Chapter 17).

AIDS, Acquired immunodeficiency syndrome; *HIV,* human immunodeficiency virus; *TMP/SMX,* trimethoprim-sulfamethoxazole.

tests such as the "string test" for *Giardia* species, sigmoidoscopy for amebic dysentery, or future antigen assays for microsporidia may improve diagnosis.

Protozoal Infections: Overview

The major protozoal pathogens causing diarrhea are *Giardia lamblia* (giardiasis); *Entamoeba histolytica* (amebiasis); *Cryptosporidium* species, especially *C. parvum* (cryptosporidiosis); *Cyclospora* species, notably *C. cayetanensis; Isospora belli* (isosporiasis); and a group of parasites collectively known as microsporidia (microsporidiosis). Giardiasis and amebiasis are important pathogens in immunocompetent persons. The other protozoal pathogens can also cause protracted diarrhea, sometimes in the form of outbreaks. *C. parvum* is a major potential threat to water supplies because as few as 30 oocysts can cause disease. Cryptosporidiosis and to a lesser extent microsporidiosis can cause severe disease in persons with advanced HIV disease.

Most patients with diarrhea caused by protozoa contact a physician after days to weeks of protracted watery diarrhea (Table 23-3). Most of these pathogens are resistant to standard chlorination. Many patients give a history of recent travel, cite recreational water exposure, or have children in day care. The symptoms of protozoal diarrhea are usually nonspecific. Symptoms peculiar to specific organisms include eructation of sulfurous gas, bloating, and abdominal cramps (giardiasis); dysentery, abdominal tenderness, and liver abscess

(*E. histolytica*); and relapsing or protracted course (cryptosporidia, *Cyclospora*, microsporidia). The young, the old, and immunocompromised individuals tend to be more severely ill than immunocompetent adults.

Diagnosis requires recovery and identification of the infecting agent from stool or mucosal biopsy in an expert laboratory using special stains. Often two or more specimens are necessary. In some patients with chronic infection and negative stools, *Giardia* species may be diagnosed in the duodenum by the "string test" (Enterotest; Hedeco Corporation, Mountain View, California). Stool antigen detection methods appear promising.

Treatment varies according to the parasite (Table 23-3). Some diseases need therapy directed specifically at cysts as well as trophozoites. Supportive therapy includes avoidance of milk products, gas-forming foods, and caffeine. Patients should be told to abstain from alcohol while taking metronidazole.

SUGGESTED READING

Brown GH, Rotschafer JC. *Cyclospora:* review of an emerging parasite. Pharmacotherapy 1999; 10: 70-75.

Didier ES. Microsporidiosis. Clin Infect Dis 1998; 27: 1-8.

Goodgame RW. Understanding intestinal spore-forming protozoa: cryptosporidia, microsporidia, *Isospora,* and *Cyclospora.* Ann Intern Med 1996; 124: 429-441.

Guerrant RL. Cryptosporidiosis: an emerging highly infectious threat. Emerg Infect Dis 1997; 3: 51-57.

Soave R. *Cyclospora:* an overview. Clin Infect Dis 1996; 23: 429-437.

Giardiasis

G. lamblia is a common cause of diarrhea in both sporadic and epidemic forms. It may be acquired from lake or stream water, contaminated food, and personal contact, particularly in day care centers.

Presentation and Progression

Cause

G. lamblia is a flagellated protozoan found in many mammals, including beavers, dogs, and cats. The organism exists in trophozoite and cyst stages, of which the latter is the environmental and infectious form. Cysts resist chlorination and ultraviolet light, but they may be killed by boiling or removed from water by effective filtration. This organism is the most commonly identified cause of waterborne outbreaks of diarrhea. As few as 10 cysts are capable of producing infection.

Presentation

The incubation period is usually 1 to 2 weeks. Children and previously exposed adults may remain relatively asymptomatic. About 40% of infected individuals have symptoms of bloating, cramping, eructation, and flatulence followed soon by foul-smelling loose stools. Patients often have malaise, weight loss, and anorexia. Diffuse abdominal tenderness may develop with protracted infection. Fever is uncommon after the first few days and should prompt an alternative diagnosis. Many patients have diarrhea for weeks with attendant malabsorption of fats and carbohydrates, especially lactose.

Diagnosis

Diagnosis is usually achieved by examination of multiple stools for cysts. Cysts may be small in number in chronic illness, and new enzyme immunoassay (EIA) antigen tests are highly sensitive and specific. Examination of duodenal or jejunal contents with the string test may be necessary in some cases. Jejunal biopsy may be advantageous in excluding other diseases such as Whipple's disease, lymphoma, or Crohn's disease.

Natural History

About 60% of patients are asymptomatic. Symptomatic patients often have diarrhea for weeks, with resultant malabsorption syndrome. Patients with IgA or other humoral immune deficiency often have a protracted course.

Expected Outcome

Most patients eventually develop immunity, clear the infection, and regain weight.

Treatment

Methods

Metronidazole 250 mg t.i.d. for 5 days and albendazole 400 mg/day for 5 days are considered the drugs of choice at this time. Paromomycin 25 mg/kg/day in three doses for 7 days has been used in the treatment of pregnant women. A lactose-free diet may be helpful.

Expected Response

Most patients respond promptly to treatment. Longer courses or combination regimens may be required for eradication in patients with immunodeficiency.

When to Refer

Recurrent, relapsing, or protracted disease should prompt referral to an infectious disease specialist or gastroenterologist.

 KEY POINTS

GIARDIASIS

⊃ *G. lamblia* resists chlorination. To be safe, campers should boil water from streams or lakes.

⊃ Giardiasis often causes upper abdominal symptoms of belching and cramps before diarrhea.

⊃ Diarrhea, once established, is usually protracted, lasting weeks. It is often associated with abdominal pain, tenderness, weight loss, and signs of fat and carbohydrate malabsorption.

⊃ A diagnosis of giardiasis in the absence of a suggestive travel history should prompt investigation of common sources of infection such as day care centers, water purity, and sexual exposure.

SUGGESTED READING

Gardner TB, Hill DR. Treatment of giardiasis. Clin Microbiol Rev 2001; 14: 114-128.

Ortega YR, Adam RD. *Giardia:* overview and update. Clin Infect Dis 1997; 25:545-550.

Amebiasis

Worldwide, amebiasis is a major threat to the health of millions. Prevalence remains high in many developing countries, in certain institutional and social settings in the United States, and among certain populations, particularly recent immigrants from Mexico.

Presentation and Progression
Cause

E. histolytica exists in trophozoite and cyst forms, and presumably it can be a major contaminant of food and water from cyst carriers. Areas of high endemicity typically have poor sanitation or inadequate access to pure water. More exotic means of infection have been documented, such as cross-contamination of endoscopic equipment, as well as chiropractic (colonic irrigation) and homosexual practices. Unfortunately, a nonpathogenic organism, *Entamoeba dispar,* is morphologically identical to *E. histolytica* and has for years confused epidemiologists and clinicians alike.

Presentation

Up to 90% of patients are asymptomatic and appear only as cyst passers. Other manifestations range from acute nonspecific diarrhea to inflammatory dysentery, colitis with toxic megacolon, and more chronic forms of disease. Liver abscess is the most common of these forms, with complications of rupture or dissemination that include peritonitis, empyema, pericarditis, and lung abscess.

Most patients with acute colitis have pain, urgency, tenesmus, and frequent blood- and mucus-containing stools. Fever and fecal leukocytes are often absent. Left lower quadrant tenderness is common. Children, especially those under the age of 2 years, may have fulminant disease progressing to megacolon and necrosis with fever and right upper quadrant pain.

Patients with liver abscess may have fever and right upper quadrant pain with possible radiation to the right shoulder, back, or epigastrium. Rupture into the pleural space may be associated with dyspnea and cough. Diarrhea is usually not a prominent symptom by the time patients with liver abscess see a physician.

Diagnosis

Identification of trophozoites in stool or involved tissue is diagnostic in symptomatic patients. Ingestion of erythrocytes by trophozoites distinguishes *E. histolytica* from *E. dispar.* Hepatic ultrasound is the diagnostic method of choice for liver abscess, the cause of which may be confirmed by a number of serologic tests. Gel diffusion and counterimmunoelectrophoresis may be more useful in endemic areas because reacting antibodies become negative in 6 to 12 months, but EIA findings may remain positive for years.

Natural History
Expected Outcome

Most patients remain asymptomatic and eventually clear the organism. Metastatic infection to the liver, lungs, and other organs usually requires drainage for cure unless antibiotics are administered.

Treatment
Methods

Treatment of acute or disseminated disease is targeted at the trophozoite with metronidazole 750 mg t.i.d. IV or PO for 10 days. A drug active against cyst forms is required to eradicate the organism, and metronidazole should be followed by a course of paromomycin 500 mg PO t.i.d. for 7 days.

Expected Response

Most patients respond promptly to metronidazole.

When to Refer

Patients often need hospitalization for initiation of therapy.

 KEY POINTS

AMEBIASIS
- Amebiasis should be considered in any patient with dysentery. Before patients are treated with steroids for ulcerative colitis, amebic disease should be excluded.
- Nonpathogenic *E. dispar* may be confused with *E. histolytica* on stool examination.
- Treatment should include therapy for cysts after treatment of invasive disease.

SUGGESTED READING
Petri WA, Singh U. Diagnosis and management of amebiasis. Clin Infect Dis 1999; 29: 1117-1125.
Ravdin JI. Amebiasis. Clin Infect Dis 1995; 20: 1453-1466.

Hookworm

Hookworm, estimated to affect about one fourth of the world's population, still occurs occasionally in the southeastern United States.

Presentation and Progression
Cause

Hookworm is usually caused by either of two small (1 cm in length), grayish white nematodes, *Ancylostoma duodenale* and *Necator americanus.* A canine hookworm, *A. caninum,* usually causes cutaneous larva migrans in humans but was recently shown to cause eosinophilic enteritis.

Infection is acquired by skin exposure to larvae in soil contaminated by human feces. Transmission occurs through 5 minutes or more of skin contact with soil containing viable, third-stage larvae. The larvae pass to venulae, then to the lung, where they break into alveoli. Subsequent to the pulmonary infection, larvae are swallowed and take up residence in the jejunum. Approximately 4 weeks after skin exposure the adult females begin producing oval 40- by 60-μm eggs in large number, allowing diagnosis via stool examination (Figure 23-5).

Presentation

A pruritic rash ("ground itch") may occur at the site of entry, usually bare feet. The pulmonary phase of the infection is

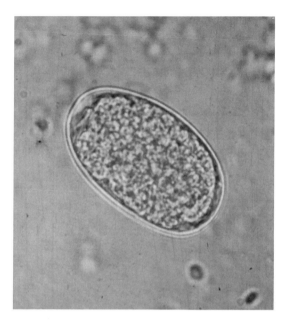

FIG. 23-5 Hookworm egg (100×). (From Walter Reed Army Institute of Research.)

asymptomatic in most cases but can occur with cough, patchy infiltrates, and eosinophilia. Hence hookworm, such as *Ascaris* and *Strongyloides,* may be manifested as the PIE syndrome (pulmonary infiltrates with eosinophilia; also called Löffler syndrome). At this stage it may be possible to find rare larvae in sputum. Early symptoms of intestinal infection are proportional to the intensity of the exposure and may include bloating. Later symptoms usually stem from anemia. Worms consume 0.03 mL (*Necator*) to 0.2 mL (*Ancylostoma*) of blood daily. Anemia is proportional to worm burden, diet, and iron reserves. Populations with low iron consumption tend to have more severe anemia.

Diagnosis

Clinically significant hookworm infections can usually be diagnosed by finding the eggs on direct examination of a fecal smear (Figure 23-5).

Natural History
Expected Outcome

Severe anemia may cause intellectual and physical impairment in children and decreased cardiac performance in adults.

Treatment
Methods

Treatment consists of a single 400-mg dose of albendazole or mebendazole (100 mg b.i.d. for 3 days) plus iron replacement. Mebendazole may be more effective but is more expensive and less convenient. Unfortunately, most treated patients become reinfected within months unless relocated to an area of improved sanitation.

Prevention has been hampered by socioeconomic problems in endemic areas. Successful programs have included economic, sanitary, and mass treatment components but may take years to have an effect. Communitywide single-dose

albendazole chemotherapy at intervals of 18 months is probably the most cost-effective means of control.

Expected Response

Mebendazole, 100 mg b.i.d. for 3 days, results in a 95% cure rate and 99.9% reduction in egg counts. Albendazole is also effective.

When to Refer

Referral is necessary only for the most severe complications.

 KEY POINTS

HOOKWORM
- Hookworm is a common cause of childhood anemia in tropical areas and occasionally occurs in the United States.
- Symptoms and signs include "ground itch" after exposure, pulmonary infiltrates with eosinophilia (PIE syndrome), abdominal pain and nausea, rash, and most commonly anemia.
- Diagnosis is usually made easily by demonstrating eggs in a stool sample.
- Drug therapy is effective, but most infections recur.

SUGGESTED READING

Haburchak DR. Hookworms. EMedicine Textbook of Medicine, Ob-gyn, Psychiatry, and Surgery. www.emedicine.com, April 2000.

Prociv P, Croese J. Human enteric infection with *Ancylostoma caninum:* hookworms reappraised in the light of a "new" zoonosis. Acta Trop 1996; 62: 23-44.

Thompson RCA, Reynoldson JA, Garrow SC, et al. Towards the eradication of hookworm in an isolated Australian community. Lancet 2001; 357: 770-771.

Ascariasis

Ascariasis is the most common helminthic infection, affecting more than 1 billion people worldwide and an estimated 4 million in the United States, mainly in the Southeast. Most patients with these large *Ascaris* nematodes are asymptomatic, but some patients manifest growth retardation, pneumonitis, intestinal obstruction, or hepatobiliary and pancreatic disease.

Presentation and Progression
Cause

Ascaris lumbricoides is a large (15 to 35 cm in length) roundworm. After ingestion of mature eggs from contaminated soil, larvae emerge in the small intestine and migrate to the lung and eventually back to the intestine. Expectorated and swallowed larvae eventually reach the jejunum, where adult females produce prodigious numbers of eggs.

Presentation

Most patients are asymptomatic. With heavy exposure, patients may have early symptoms of cough, dyspnea, asthma, or chest

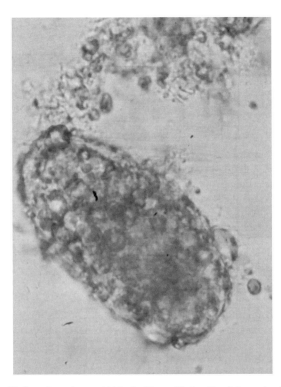

FIG. 23-6 *Ascaris* egg (100×). (From Walter Reed Army Institute of Research.)

pain with eosinophilia (PIE syndrome) as larvae migrate through the lungs. Subsequent symptoms are intraabdominal.

Children in endemic areas, especially between the ages of 3 and 5 years, have the highest prevalence and intensity of infection and are more likely than adults to be symptomatic. Symptoms include abdominal pain, distention, colic, nausea, anorexia, and intermittent diarrhea. These symptoms indicate partial or complete intestinal obstruction by adult worms. Adults are more likely to have biliary or pancreatic complications when worms migrate and obstruct ductal systems. Jaundice, nausea, vomiting, fever, or severe or radiating abdominal pain may suggest cholangitis, pancreatitis, or appendicitis, and worms may be found by serendipity.

Diagnosis

Ascariasis should be suspected in cases of intestinal obstruction. An abdominal x-ray film may show a "whirlpool" pattern of intraluminal worms. Narrow-based air-fluid levels without distended loops of bowel on upright plain films suggest partial obstruction. Wide-based air-fluid levels with distended loops suggest complete obstruction. When the biliary tract is involved, ultrasonography may be extremely useful. Diagnosis is usually based on finding the large (60 by 50 μm), brown, trilayered eggs on direct examination of the stool (Figure 23-6).

Natural History
Expected Outcome

Unless reexposure occurs, the disease resolves within 2 years because the worms do not multiply in the host and by that time have died.

Treatment
Methods

Minimally symptomatic children and adults can be effectively treated with mebendazole 100 mg PO b.i.d. for 3 days. Alternatively, a 400-mg single dose of albendazole is effective. Vitamin A supplementation has helped children with worm-associated growth retardation in Zaire. Unless removed from the contaminating environment, most patients promptly become reinfected.

Surgical care is often needed for complications, which may be life threatening. Conservative management of partial obstruction is usually effective. The patient is kept without oral intake, and partial obstruction usually resolves. Surgical exploration is indicated if the patient exhibits hematochezia, multiple air-fluid levels on abdominal x-ray films, severe abdominal distention with rebound tenderness, unsatisfactory response to conservative therapy, appendicitis and peritonitis, or hepatobiliary or pancreatic disease. The condition of patients with partial obstruction may worsen if they are given paralyzing vermifuges such as pyrantel pamoate or piperazine, so these drugs should be avoided under such circumstances.

Expected Response

Response is usually excellent except in occasional cases of severe intestinal, biliary, or pancreatic obstruction.

When to Refer

Patients with intestinal or hepatobiliary obstruction usually need hospitalization.

 KEY POINTS

ASCARIASIS

- ⊃ Ascariasis affects an estimated 1 billion persons, including up to 4 million persons in the United States, mainly in the Southeast.
- ⊃ Infected individuals are usually asymptomatic, but ascariasis can cause severe intestinal, hepatobiliary, or pancreatic obstruction.
- ⊃ Intestinal obstruction usually develops in children, whereas hepatobiliary obstruction is more common in adults. Plain x-ray films and ultrasound assist in the diagnosis, which is usually made easily by finding the eggs on direct smear of stool specimens.

SUGGESTED READING

Ali M, Khan AN. Sonography of hepatobiliary ascariasis. J Clin Ultrasound 1996; 24: 235-241.
Haburchak D. Ascariasis. EMedicine Textbook of Medicine, Ob-gyn, Psychiatry, and Surgery. www.emedicine.com. February 2000.

Tapeworms

Pork, beef, fish, and dwarf tapeworm infections are uncommon in North America and rarely symptomatic. Outbreaks of fish tapeworm (*Diphyllobothrium latum*) infection have occurred with consumption of raw salmon gefilte fish and other freshwater fish and may appear with acute gastroenteritis. This tapeworm may compete for vitamin B$_{12}$ and thereby produce megaloblastic anemia and neurologic disease after years of infection. *Hymenolepsis nana,* the dwarf tapeworm, is found among institutionalized populations and is acquired by fecal-oral contamination. Children living in substandard housing may acquire *Hymenolepsis diminuta,* a rat tapeworm, by ingesting fleas or beetles that contain its larval elements. These infections are diagnosed by identification of ova in stool and are treated with single-dose praziquantel (25 mg/kg for *Hymenolepsis* species, 5 to 10 mg/kg for others).

Echinococcosis (Hydatid and Alveolar Cyst Disease)

Echinococcus granulosus is a four-segment tapeworm of domestic dogs in many parts of the world where sheep, goats, camels, or horses are raised. The southwestern and mountain states of the United States are areas of relatively high prevalence. *Echinococcus multilocularis* is associated with wolves and other wild canines, primarily in arctic and subarctic regions, but it has also recently been found in red foxes and voles in France and Germany. Human ingestion of eggs from contaminated soil, grass, and foodstuffs produces infection. *E. granulosus* produces so-called hydatid cysts (Figure 23-7) that are self-contained, but they usually grow slowly and may bud off new daughter cysts within the primary lesion. *E. multilocularis* produces expansive, so-called alveolar cystic disease of the liver and lung. Less common sites of infection are brain, heart, bones, and other organs. Many patients with hydatid cysts are asymptomatic and discovered incidentally. Pain associated with an enlarging cyst, obstruction, or rupture is the most common presentation. Cyst rupture may be associated with spillage and dissemination of the daughter cysts or with anaphylaxis. Diagnosis is confirmed by ELISA serologic examination, which has high sensitivity and specificity for liver cysts but less for other organs. The primary therapy for both diseases is surgical, with adjuvant or suppressive therapy with albendazole in 3- to 6-month cycles.

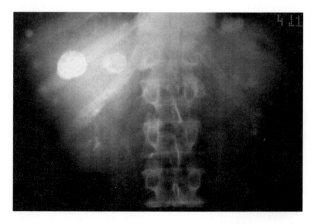

FIG. 23-7 Multiple calcified liver cysts from *Echinococcus granulosus.* (From Letterman Army Center.)

SUGGESTED READING
Franchi C, DiVico B, Teggi A. Long-term evaluation of patients with hydatidosis treated with benzimidazole carbamates. Clin Infect Dis 1999; 29: 304-309.

Romig T, Kratzer W, Kimmig P, et al. An epidemiologic survey of human alveolar echinococcosis in southwestern Germany. Am J Trop Med Hyg 1999; 61: 566-573.

Flukes (Other Than Schistosomiasis)

The liver, lung, and intestine may be parasitized by a variety of flukes that produce infection of specific snail intermediate hosts, mostly in tropical areas, particularly eastern Asia. These include the following:

- *Clonorchis sinensis:* the Chinese liver fluke, endemic in eastern Asia and causing cholangitis and cholangiocarcinoma
- *Opisthorchis felineus* and *Opisthorchis viverrini:* the cat and dog liver flukes, endemic in Southeast Asia, also causing cholangitis or cholangiocarcinoma
- *Fasciola hepatica:* a liver fluke found in sheep-raising areas throughout the world and causing fever, right upper quadrant pain, eosinophilia, and, rarely, biliary obstruction and cirrhosis
- *Fasciola buski:* an intestinal fluke, endemic in eastern Asia and usually asymptomatic
- *Heterophyes heterophyes:* an intestinal fluke found in the Nile Delta, the Far East, and Southeast Asia, causing abdominal pain and mucous diarrhea
- *Paragonimus westermani* and related species: lung flukes occurring with cough, bronchitis, bronchiectasis, lung abscess, lung mass, brain abscess, or a combination of these symptoms

Humans become infected with flukes by eating undercooked fish, crab, crayfish, or aquatic plants such as watercress. Most patients are asymptomatic. Hepatic or pulmonary damage may occur with early migratory stages of infection, usually associated with eosinophilia. Later, patients may have obstructive complications in the biliary or pulmonary system with secondary infection. Most intestinal flukes are carried without symptoms. Diagnosis is usually made by detection of opercular eggs in sputum or stool, although concentration techniques may be required. Praziquantel is the drug of choice for all fluke infections except for fascioliasis.

Parasites Occurring with Fever and Other Systemic Manifestations

Malaria

Malaria continues to be the most important parasitic disease in terms of mortality for both residents of and travelers to tropical climes. Each year it causes an estimated 300 million to 500 million cases, with 2 million to 3 million deaths. The dictum that "any fever in a traveler is malaria until proven otherwise" remains as true today as in the past. Any patient with fever after recent travel should be evaluated first for malaria with a prompt peripheral smear. Parasitemia greater than 5% portends a poor prognosis (Figure 23-8).

Presentation and Progression
Cause

Four *Plasmodium* species cause human malaria: *P. falciparum, P. vivax, P. ovale,* and *P. malariae.* The disease begins when a female anopheline mosquito takes her blood meal. The parasite's life cycle evolves from sporozoites in the bloodstream to schizonts in the liver to merozoites that, released from the liver, invade red blood cells, where they multiply. *P. falciparum* is the most dangerous form of malaria because, unlike the others, it infects red blood cells of all ages, giving rise to massive parasitemia. Also, *P. falciparum* has a unique ability to adhere to endothelial cells, which results in microvascular disease. A current explanation for the unique cytoadherence of *P. falciparum* is the fact that its parasitized red blood cells contain knobs, whereas those of the other species do not.

Presentation

The clinical hallmark of malaria is fever manifested by a three-phase paroxysm: a "cold stage" with chills or shaking lasting 15 minutes to several hours, a "hot stage" of high fever lasting several hours, and drenching sweats. During the period of high fever, the patient may have headache, backache, abdominal pain, nausea, vomiting, cough, hypotension, tachycardia, and altered mental acuity—symptoms that frequently suggest an alternative diagnosis. Cyclic fevers occurring with clockwork regularity characterize malaria that is due to *P. vivax* or *P. ovale* (fever every 48 hours) and *P. malariae* (fever every 72 hours). These fevers correspond to lysis of red blood cells as the schizonts rupture, releasing new merozoites into the bloodstream. In contrast to the regularity of fever in other forms of malaria, nonimmune patients with *P. falciparum* malaria usually have continuous fever with intermittent spikes.

Diagnosis

The broad differential diagnosis includes meningitis, meningococcemia, enteric fever (e.g., typhoid fever), acute rheumatic fever, and commonplace infections such as acute sinusitis, pneumonia, and pyelonephritis. The key to diagnosis is a high index of suspicion and examination of "thick and thin" smears of the peripheral blood. Thick smears have

greater sensitivity, whereas thin smears show better detail. New alternatives to examination of peripheral blood smears, which require some experience, include ELISA kits; these are especially useful for field diagnosis. Other laboratory tests reflect the severity of hemolysis and of complications. These include falling hematocrit percentages and hemoglobin levels with high lactic dehydrogenase and bilirubin levels; thrombocytopenia; and evidence of renal involvement (proteinuria, hemoglobinuria, elevated serum creatinine level).

Natural History
Expected Outcome

P. falciparum malaria is life threatening because of its complications: microvascular obstruction of brain capillaries causing delirium, seizures, and coma (cerebral malaria), or renal failure with hemoglobinuria ("blackwater fever"), pulmonary edema, and hypoglycemia. Another complication is gastroenteritis, especially in young children and anemic individuals. Virtually all of the mortality from malaria is caused by *P. falciparum.* However, in contrast to the other forms, attacks of *P. falciparum* malaria are not complicated by late relapses because the parasite does not establish long-term residence in the liver.

Treatment
Methods

Most travelers should be admitted to the hospital for therapy for *P. falciparum* or if the cause is uncertain (see the Centers for Disease Control and Prevention [CDC] website at www.cdc.gov or call 770-488-7788 for the most recent treatment recommendations) (Table 23-4). Patients with non-*falciparum* malaria and patients with partial immunity may often be treated as outpatients. Intravenous administration of quinidine should be used for patients who are vomiting or severely ill, but always with electrocardiographic monitoring. We prefer quinine plus tetracycline for oral therapy when the cause is not absolutely confirmed as non-*falciparum.* Mild confirmed cases of *P. vivax* and *P. ovale* can usually be treated with chloroquine plus primaquine, except that some chloroquine-resistant *P. vivax* strains have been reported in South America and Oceania. Primaquine resistance has been reported in the Arabian Peninsula and the Horn of Africa. Therapy for *P. malariae* does not require primaquine.

Expected Response

Mortality from severe *P. falciparum* malaria in nonimmune persons remains substantial.

When to Refer

Patients seen in the United States within several weeks of return from a part of the world where malaria is prevalent should usually be hospitalized for management of possible *P. falciparum* malaria unless the diagnosis of a more benign form of the disease (usually *P. vivax*) seems unequivocal on the basis of the peripheral blood smear.

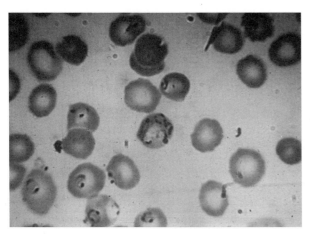

FIG. 23-8 Peripheral blood smear demonstrating high-grade parasitemia with multiple forms of *Plasmodium falciparum.* (From Walter Reed Army Institute of Research.)

 KEY POINTS

MALARIA
⊃ Any fever in a traveler should be considered malaria until proven otherwise.

TABLE 23-4
Suggested Treatment of Malaria in North America

Situation	Regimen
Plasmodium falciparum diagnosed or suspected; oral therapy possible	Quinine sulfate (300 mg) 2 tablets q8h for 7 days, *plus* doxycycline 100 mg q12h for 7 days
P. falciparum diagnosed or suspected, severe disease	Quinidine gluconate 10 mg/kg IV over 1 hour, then 0.02 mg/kg/min for 72 hours, with electrocardiographic monitoring; switch to an oral regimen when possible to complete a 7-day course
Plasmodium vivax or *Plasmodium ovale* confirmed	Chloroquine phosphate 500 mg, 2 tablets (10 mg/kg of the base), then one tablet (5 mg/kg of the base) in 12 hours, 24 hours, and 36 hours (total 2.5 g), *plus* primaquine 26.3 mg (15 mg of the base), one tablet daily for 14 days after screening for severe glucose-6 phosphate dehydrogenase (G6PD) deficiency
P. malariae confirmed	Chloroquine phosphate, as above for *P. vivax* (primaquine is not required)

⊃ Diagnosis is made by examining thick and thin blood smears.
⊃ Malaria is characterized by a three-phase paroxysm (chills, high fever with systemic symptoms, and drenching sweats).
⊃ The broad differential diagnosis of malaria includes both uncommon diseases (e.g., meningococcemia, typhoid fever, acute rheumatic fever) and common diseases (e.g., acute sinusitis, pneumonia, pyelonephritis).
⊃ In the United States, patients with possible *P. falciparum* malaria are nearly always nonimmune and therefore vulnerable to severe complications.

SUGGESTED READING

Baird JK, Hoffman SL. Prevention of malaria in travelers. Med Clin North Am 1999; 83: 923-944.

Kain KC, Keystone JS. Malaria in travelers: epidemiology, disease, and prevention. Infect Dis Clin North Am 1998; 12: 267-284.

Martens P, Hall L. Malaria on the move: human population movement and malaria transmission. Emerg Infect Dis 2000; 6: 103-109.

Newton P, White N. Malaria: new developments in treatment and prevention. Annu Rev Med 1999; 50: 179-192.

Phillips RS. Current status of malaria and potential for control. Clin Microbiol Rev 2001; 14: 208-226.

Babesiosis

Babesiosis is an intraerythrocytic zoonotic infection caused by malaria-like protozoans transmitted by nymph forms of *Ixodes* ticks. Various rodents are the primary hosts. Most of the clinically apparent infections in the United States (<200) have occurred in the northeastern coastal areas. Asymptomatic infection is common; nearly 4% of persons on Cape Cod were found to have antibodies to *Babesia microti*. Moderately severe to severe disease occurs most commonly in older persons and in persons who have undergone splenectomy. The most common reported symptoms are malaise, chills, fever, headache, myalgias, and vomiting. Severe cases

may result in severe hemolytic anemia, shock, and acute respiratory distress syndrome (ARDS). Concomitant infection with the agent of Lyme disease has been reported. Diagnosis is made through identification of ring forms and tetrad merozoites in erythrocytes. PCR and serologic tests are available from the CDC or state health departments. Therapy is unnecessary for mild cases. Severe disease is usually treated with quinine plus clindamycin.

SUGGESTED READING

Boustani MR, Gelfand JA. Babesiosis. Clin Infect Dis 1996; 22: 611-615.

Trypanosomiasis: Chagas' Disease and Sleeping Sickness

Trypanosomes are flagellated protozoa transmitted by insect vectors in tropical Africa and Latin America. *Trypanosoma cruzi* is transmitted by the reduviid bug and causes Chagas' disease in the Americas. *Trypanosoma brucei, Trypanosoma rhodesiense,* and *Trypanosoma gambiense* cause African sleeping sickness after the bite of tsetse flies. Both diseases should be considered in residents or travelers from endemic areas. Blood transfusion has also been responsible for acquisition of Chagas' disease. Expanding outbreaks of sleeping sickness in Africa have recently been attributed to civil strife and subsequent lapse of control programs.

Chagas' disease may occur acutely within a week of exposure. Localized skin induration and edema (a "chagoma") may be followed by regional lymphadenopathy, fever, and malaise. Romaña's sign is painless edema of the eyelid when it is the site of inoculation. Acute encephalitis and myocarditis with congestive failure are rare but often lethal manifestations. Years later, arrhythmias, congestive failure, achalasia, or megacolon may develop. Recent studies indicate that parasite persistence in muscular tissue, rather than autoimmunity, may be the cause of chronic disease. Diagnosis can be confirmed serologically. Nifurtimox (Lampit) therapy should be initiated as early as possible to maximize outcome and should be given for at least 90 days. This drug is available from the CDC, but unfortunately, it has marginal efficacy and significant gastrointestinal and neurologic toxicity.

Sleeping sickness also occurs with a painful chancre a week after infection. Intermittent fevers and generalized lymphadenopathy follow, often associated with facial and periarticular edema and erythematous, pruritic skin rashes. Encephalitis, manifested first as personality change, may occur within weeks of exposure to *T.b. rhodesiense* and months to years after exposure to *T.b. gambiense*. Diagnosis may be made by microscopic examination of wet and stained preparations of chancre, lymph node, or peripheral blood. Serologic tests may assist in diagnosis. Lumbar puncture should be performed to look for elevated pressure, protein levels, and cells. Treatment differs by presence of central nervous system (CNS) involvement: Suramin for non-CNS disease, melarsoprol (Arsobal) for CNS disease. The latter therapy is highly toxic and usually administered in the inpatient setting.

SUGGESTED READING

Kirchhoff LV. American trypanosomiasis (Chagas' disease). Gastroenterol Clin North Am 1996; 25: 517-533.

Mhlanga JD. Sleeping sickness: perspectives in African trypanosomiasis. Sci Prog 1996; 79: 183-214.

Sinha A, Grace C, Alston WK, et al. African trypanosomiasis in two travelers from the United States. Clin Infect Dis 1999; 29: 840-844.

World Health Organization. Control and surveillance of African trypanosomiasis: report of a WHO expert committee. World Health Organ Tech Rep Ser 1998; 881: 1-114.

Zhang L, Tarleton RL. Parasite persistence correlates with disease severity and localization in chronic Chagas' disease. J Infect Dis 1999; 180: 480-486.

Schistosomiasis

Up to 400,000 people in the United States may have schistosomiasis. Most cases are in immigrants from endemic areas, but disease has been reported in tourists and expatriates who have swum in contaminated freshwater. The disease is not transmitted in the United States because of the absence of the specific snails that serve as intermediate hosts for the parasites.

Presentation and Progression
Cause

The disease is caused by five *Schistosoma* species of blood flukes, each with its unique geographic distribution: *S. haematobium* (Africa and the Middle East), *S. japonicum* (China and the Philippines), *S. mansoni* (Africa, Arabia, and South America), *S. mekongi* (Southeast Asia), and *S. intercalatum* (western and central Africa). Human infection with schistosomes follows exposure to water in which snails infected by schistosomal miracidial larvae have liberated cercariae. The cercariae directly penetrate the skin to invade the circulatory system. The immature fluke (schistosomule) remains in the subcutaneous tissue for about 2 days before invading a blood vessel and traveling to the lungs and liver sinusoids. Females deposit eggs in small venulae of the portal and perivesical systems. *S. mansoni* and *S. haematobium* eggs have sharp spines that may aid retention in blood vessels. Two weeks or more after infection, the maturing worms begin migration to their final location in mesenteric or vesicular veins. Schistosomal adults are usually long lived, compared with other parasites, and produce disease by depositing eggs for up to two decades or more.

Presentation

The initial symptom of acute infection may be dermatitis ("swimmer's itch") at the site of skin invasion. Swimmer's itch in North America is likely to come from schistosomal cercariae pathogenic for birds that infect a previously sensitized freshwater swimmer. This dermatitis is relatively common in the Great Lakes region of the United States. Acute systemic disease occurs only with the human-adapted species of schistosomes. In previously uninfected persons fever and malaise may develop 2 to 6 weeks after initial exposure. Heavy exposure to *S. japonicum* and *S. mansoni* produces the syndrome of Katayama fever: high fever, abdominal pain, diarrhea, hematochezia, dry cough, weight loss, myalgia, arthralgia, hepatosplenomegaly, lymphadenopathy, and marked eosinophilia. Early manifestations of *S. haematobium* include terminal hematuria, urinary frequency, dysuria, and eosinophiluria.

Chronic fibrovascular lesions develop in persons exposed to egg deposition for 5 or more years. Organ-specific pathologic changes include stricture and fibrous thickening of the bowel, ureter, or bladder; periportal ("pipestem") fibrosis of the liver; and portal or pulmonary hypertension. Hepatosplenomegaly is common. Neurologic complications include transverse myelitis and granulomas of the conus medullaris or spinal roots. These may occur from several weeks to many years after infection.

Adult flukes can become colonized with salmonellae, subjecting patients to recurrent bacteremia and urinary infection. Concomitant infection with hepatitis B also portends a worse prognosis for liver failure.

Diagnosis

Diagnosis is established in most patients by identification of eggs in concentrated stool or urine. ELISA serologic findings are highly specific and sensitive, but ELISA does not distinguish between remote and current infection. Rectal snip biopsy may be useful if stool examination results are negative. CT scan or ultrasound examination, which is being used increasingly to stage the disease, can detect periportal fibrosis in the liver and document bladder granulomas, polyps, stones, and tumors.

Natural History

Schistosomiasis is often asymptomatic. Chronic disease develops, however, in patients with large worm burdens. Carcinoma of the bladder, liver, and colon may be more frequent in persons with chronic schistosomiasis.

Treatment
Methods

Praziquantel is the drug of choice for all forms of the disease and is given for a single day. The standard dose is

40 mg/kg/day in two divided doses for *S. haematobium* and *S. mansoni* and in three doses for *S. japonicum* and *S. mekongi.* The drug is well tolerated, and when side effects occur, they tend to be mild.

Expected Response

Praziquantel usually eradicates the adult flukes and reduces egg counts, and it has been shown to reverse or reduce mild to moderately severe fibrosis of the liver and urinary tract as demonstrated by ultrasound.

When to Refer

Complications of schistosomiasis usually require referral to a gastroenterologist or urologist.

 KEY POINTS

SCHISTOSOMIASIS

⊃ Schistosomiasis affects more than 200 million people worldwide and up to 200,000 persons in the United States. It is not transmitted in the United States because of absence of the specific snail intermediate hosts.

⊃ The initial symptom is often a dermatitis known as swimmer's itch at the site of skin invasion. Swimmer's itch caused by avian schistosomes is relatively common in the Great Lakes region of the United States.

⊃ Manifestations of chronic schistosomiasis include hepatomegaly and cirrhosis (*S. mansoni, S. japonicum,* and *S. mekongi*), hematuria and dysuria with extensive disease of the liver and bladder (*S. haematobium*), pulmonary hypertension, and, rarely, CNS involvement with space-occupying lesions, encephalopathy, or a transverse myelitis–like syndrome.

⊃ Diagnosis is usually based on identification of eggs in concentrated stool or urine.

⊃ Praziquantel is remarkably effective therapy.

SUGGESTED READING

Lucey DR, Maguire JH. Schistosomiasis. Infect Dis Clin North Am 1993; 7: 635-653.

 ## Parasites Occurring with Neurologic Manifestations

Toxoplasmosis

Acute toxoplasmosis in immunocompetent persons occurs as lymphadenopathy, fever, malaise, sweats, hepatosplenomegaly, macular rash, and chorioretinitis (see also Chapters 5, 8, and 17). Toxoplasmic encephalitis is relatively common in persons with advanced HIV disease, and it occasionally resembles Hodgkin's disease and lymphoma. Serologic testing is the primary means of diagnosis of all forms of toxoplasmosis. Treatment is reserved

---

TABLE 23-5
Treatment of Toxoplasmosis in Immunocompetent Patients

Syndrome	Setting	Treatment
Acute toxoplasmosis	Pregnancy, fetal infection not documented	Spiramycin (available from Food and Drug Administration, telephone 301-827-2335).
	Pregnancy, fetal infection documented	1 to 18 weeks' gestation: sulfadiazine 4 g/day in divided doses; 19 to 40 weeks' gestation: sulfadiazine 4 g/day in divided doses *plus* pyrimethamine 25 mg/day *plus* folinic acid 5 to 15 mg/day.
	Acute severe disease (encephalopathy, ocular)	Sulfadiazine 4-g loading dose, then 1 g q6h; *plus* pyrimethamine 50 mg b.i.d. on day 1, then 25 mg/day; *plus* folinic acid 10 mg/day; *plus* prednisone 1 mg/kg in 2 divided doses daily until ocular inflammation subsides or the cerebrospinal fluid protein content normalizes. Treat for 1 to 2 weeks beyond resolution of symptoms; continue folinic acid 1 week longer.
Ocular toxoplasmosis	Nonpregnant patients, small peripheral reactivation	Observe.
	Pregnancy	Clindamycin 300 mg q6h for minimum of 3 weeks.
Congenital toxoplasmosis		Regimens that have been used include sulfadiazine *plus* pyrimethamine *plus* folinic acid, sometimes alternating with spiramycin. Dr. Rima McLeod at the University of Chicago (773-834-4152) can be contacted for advice about treatment and about the National Collaborative Treatment Trial.

for patients with pregnancy or severe acute disease, ocular manifestations, or congenital infection (Table 23-5).

Visceral Larva Migrans (Toxocariasis)

Visceral larva migrans (VLM) affects mainly children, variably causing fever, eosinophilia, hepatomegaly, and occasionally more severe disease, including myocarditis and CNS infection. The parasite can also affect the eye (ocular larva migrans).

Presentation and Progression
Cause

VLM is usually caused by larvae of *Toxocara canis* acquired from dogs but can also be caused by *T. cati* from cats. Larvae are unable to complete their development in humans and tend to wander in tissues for prolonged periods before encysting as second-stage larvae. Humans acquire infection by ingesting eggs from soil contaminated by dog or cat feces. Eggs may remain viable in soil for months. Rare cases have been attributed to ingestion of raw chicken, rabbit giblets, and lamb liver.

Presentation

VLM primarily affects children. The most severe infections occur in toddlers who have geophagia or exposure to puppies. Patients have abdominal pain, decreased appetite, restlessness, fever, coughing, and wheezing. Hepatomegaly is common, and urticaria and skin nodules may be noted. Laboratory findings include eosinophilia, leukocytosis, hypergammaglobulinemia, and elevated isohemagglutinin titers to A or B blood group antigens. Ocular larva migrans typically occurs unilaterally in children and adults and may be without the systemic signs and symptoms of VLM. Although rare, ocular disease may result in severe inflammation and vision loss. Funduscopic findings include posterior chorioretinitis; a hazy, ill-defined mass lesion; or peripheral granulomas. Serum, vitreous, or aqueous humor titers to *Toxocara* may confirm the diagnosis.

> **PATIENT 2**
> A 24-year-old soldier had painless loss of visual acuity in one eye. Retinal examination revealed necrosis and wormlike tracts in the area of the fovea (Figure 23-9). Serologic findings were positive for *Toxocara* antibodies. The patient had partial recovery with systemic steroids.

Diagnosis

Eosinophilia is usually present in VLM. The differential diagnosis of eosinophilia, which is common, includes allergies, hypersensitivity reactions, parasitic disease, and neoplasia. The diagnosis of VLM is usually made clinically and confirmed by ELISA or histologic examination. Stool examination is of no use. The diagnosis of ocular larva migrans is usually made on clinical grounds because eosinophilia is seldom present and antibodies are present in low titer if at all. The ocular lesions may be mistaken for retinoblastoma.

Natural History

Most cases are asymptomatic. In the southern United States, antibodies to *Toxocara* have been found in 23% of a kindergarten population and in 54% of persons in a rural community.

Moreover, most cases of symptomatic VLM are self-limited. Complications include focal and diffuse CNS disease and myocarditis. Ocular larva migrans can cause loss of vision.

Treatment
Methods

The treatment of choice in adults and children is diethylcarbamazine 6 mg/kg/day in three doses for 7 to 10 days. Acute ocular disease is treated with the addition of prednisone 1 mg/kg/day for 2 to 4 weeks to blunt the intraocular eosinophilic inflammatory response.

Expected Response

The efficacy of treatment has not been established by controlled trials.

 KEY POINTS

VISCERAL LARVA MIGRANS (TOXOCARIASIS) AND OCULAR LARVA MIGRANS

- ⊃ Toxocariasis is mainly a disease of children <6 years of age who often have a history of pica or exposure to puppies.
- ⊃ Most cases are asymptomatic.
- ⊃ Full-blown VLM in children is characterized by fever, eosinophilia, and hepatomegaly. Myocarditis and CNS involvement occasionally occur.
- ⊃ Ocular larva migrans is diagnosed on clinical grounds. It can be mistaken for retinoblastoma, leading to unnecessary enucleation of the eye.

SUGGESTED READING

Elliot DL, Tolle SW, Golberg L, et al. Pet-associated illness. N Engl J Med 1985; 313: 985-995.

Mai EC. Update on therapy of parasitic retinal infection. Ophthalmol Clin North Am 1999; 12:123-144.

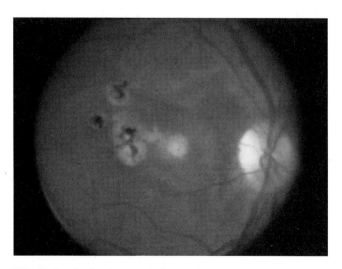

FIG. 23-9 Ocular larva migrans lesions seen on funduscopic examination of a soldier with impaired vision. (From Eisenhower Army Medical Center.)

Cysticercosis

After the ingestion of eggs of the pork tapeworm *Taenia solium,* larval cysts develop in muscle and the CNS ("neurocysticercosis"). This disease is common in many parts of Central America and Southeast Asia, particularly in areas of heavy pork consumption and poor household hygiene. Cities in the United States with many immigrants, such as Los Angeles and Houston, have seen striking numbers of patients recently. Most patients have generalized or focal seizures and less commonly headache, nausea, vomiting, altered mental status, or focal neurologic signs. Diagnosis is usually based on CT scan or magnetic resonance imaging showing single or multiple focal parenchymal, intraventricular, spinal, or subarachnoid lesions that are contrast enhancing, cystic, or calcified. ELISA serologic tests for *T. solium* are highly sensitive and specific for patients with multiple cysts, but less so for single or calcified cysts.

After initial infection and migration to the brain parenchyma, cysts enlarge slowly, usually causing minimum symptoms until they die. Death of the cysts provokes swelling and inflammation that may then lead to the aforementioned symptoms. Cysts in critical areas such as the ventricles, brainstem, intraparenchymal spinal cord, or base of the brain ("racemose cysticercosis") usually cause symptoms as they grow slowly.

Therapy has been controversial. Most authorities no longer recommend routine therapy, but selectively treat those with expanding intraventricular, basilar, and spinal lesions with either albendazole or praziquantel. Symptomatic patients with calcified and apparently dying cysts should receive dexamethasone and, if appropriate, antiepileptic drugs. Patients with ventricular, racemose, or complex neurocysticercosis should be referred to clinics experienced in surgical management of such patients.

SUGGESTED READING

Carpio A, Santillan F, Leon P, et al. Is the course of neurocysticercosis modified by treatment with antihelminthic agents? Arch Intern Med 1995; 155: 1982-1988.

Rosenfeld EA, Byrd SE, Shulman ST. Neurocysticercosis among children in Chicago. Clin Infect Dis 1996; 23: 262-268.

White AC Jr. Neurocysticercosis: a major cause of neurologic disease worldwide. Clin Infect Dis 1997; 24: 101-115.

Naegleria (Amebic Meningoencephalitis)

Naegleria fowleri is an aerobic free-living ameba that feeds primarily on bacteria. It has a worldwide distribution with primary isolation from soil and freshwater sources such as rivers, hot springs, ponds, and lakes. The organism is thermophilic and can survive up to 113° F (45° C).

Primary amebic meningoencephalitis is rare, but it usually occurs in healthy children and young adults who have recently dived into warm freshwater lakes and ponds. The amebae gain access to the CNS by direct invasion through the nasal mucosa and cribriform plate. The incubation period is usually 2 to 5 days. Early disturbances in smell or taste may precede the complaints of headache, stiff neck, and mental status change. The clinical course is usually rapid and dramatic, with coma and death occurring within 1 week of onset.

The diagnosis is based on finding motile trophozoites with blunt pseudopodia on a wet mount of cerebrospinal fluid (CSF). Trophozoites are usually destroyed by the fixation procedure for the Gram stain and therefore may be missed if a wet mount is not performed. The CSF protein level is usually elevated and the glucose level low. The CSF pressure can be elevated, and the fluid is cloudy to frankly purulent. Red blood cells are usually present. Failure to find bacteria on Gram stain of a patient with purulent meningitis should prompt examination for amebae, especially if the patient gives a history of recent swimming.

The mortality rate of this disease is at least 95%. Patients who have survived have been treated with intravenous and intrathecal administration of amphotericin B. A recommended intravenous dose for adults and children is 1 mg/kg/day.

SUGGESTED READING

Barnett ND, Kaplan AM, Hopkin RJ, et al. Primary amoebic meningoencephalitis with *Naegleria fowleri:* clinical review. Pediatr Neurol 1996;15: 230-234.

Kidney DD, Kim SH. CNS infections with free-living amebas: neuroimaging findings. AJR Am J Roentgenol 1998; 171: 809-812.

■ Therapy for Parasitic Infections

Strategic and Cost-Effectiveness Considerations

A decision to treat patients with known or presumed parasitic infection must include analysis of the risks and costs of therapy versus expected short- and long-term benefit. This analysis must take into account specific infections and the health and living circumstances of the patient. Some parasites, particularly helminths, have limited life spans in the host and, in the absence of reinfection, will die within months to weeks. Others, such as falciparum malaria, amebic dysentery, and strongyloidiasis, may be life threatening with primary infection or may produce significant symptoms after years of infestation, as occurs with schistosomiasis. On the other hand, patients who live with poor sanitation and intense vector exposure are likely to be reinfected soon after therapy. Drugs can be relatively expensive and often have mild to major side effects.

Infections discovered in travelers who have recently returned from endemic areas generally require treatment. Symptom resolution may be hastened, complications of chronic infections avoided, psychological distress alleviated, and in some cases transmission to others avoided. Such patients are unlikely to be reinfected at home, and therapy is usually curative.

A strong case has been made for presumptive treatment of all immigrants to the United States from countries where intestinal parasites are endemic. Administration of 400 mg of albendazole daily for 5 days to all 600,000 immigrants per year would prevent 870 patient years of disability, prevent at least 33 deaths and 374 hospitalizations, and save $4.2 million per year. The analysis did not consider the risk of albendazole in unrecognized pregnancy. The primary benefit was in prevention of morbidity and mortality from strongyloidiasis. Two-way sensitivity analysis showed that therapy would benefit populations with a minimum prevalence of 16% infected with *S. stercoralis.* Immigrants from Asia, Latin America, and sub-Saharan Africa might be expected to have this likelihood.

Treatment of patients in endemic areas should be directed to those who are symptomatic and likely to benefit from individual or communitywide therapy as part of an integrated control program. Any intervention should be performed within the context of local health and social programs that ensure community acceptance, surveillance, sanitation, vector control, and health education. Any intervention should be measurable. Sporadic "deworming" by visiting physicians probably does little good. Cost-effectiveness studies have increasingly favored communitywide albendazole treatment of children at 12- to 18-month intervals to limit both the burden of environmental contamination and the prevalence of disease attributable to hookworm until economic conditions permit more comprehensive and expensive control programs. Such modified or "stratified" control programs have been recommended for endemic malaria, leishmaniasis, filariasis, schistosomiasis, onchocerciasis, and African trypanosomiasis, depending on local social and economic circumstances.

Future developments in genomics and other technology may permit new vaccines for the ultimate prevention of parasitic diseases.

SUGGESTED READING

Fradin MS. Mosquitoes and mosquito repellents: a clinician's guide. Ann Intern Med 1998; 128: 931-940.

Mascie-Taylor CG, Alam M, Montanari RM, et al. A study of the cost effectiveness of selective health interventions for the control of intestinal parasites in rural Bangladesh. J Parasitol 1999; 85: 6-11.

Molyneux DH. Control of parasites, parasitic infections and parasitic diseases. In: Cox FEG, Kreier JP, Wakelin D, eds. Parasitology. Vol. 5 in Collier L, Balows A, and Sussman M, eds. Topley & Wilson's Microbiology and Microbial Infections. 9th ed., London; Arnold; 1998.

Muennig P, Pallin D, Sell RL, et al. The cost effectiveness of strategies for the treatment of intestinal parasites in immigrants. N Engl J Med 1999; 340: 773-779.

Drugs Commonly Used to Treat Parasitic Infections

Primary care clinicians in North America and Europe need familiarity with only a short list of antiparasitic agents (Table 23-6), most of which work as invertebrate paralytics. Drug development has been slow because of marginal market incentives. Nevertheless, major advances have occurred with such drugs as ivermectin and praziquantel, both for individual patients and for populations through philanthropy by pharmaceutical firms.

SUGGESTED READING

Rosenblatt JE. Antiparasitic agents. Mayo Clin Proc 1999; 74: 1161-1175.

Acknowledgment

We express our appreciation to Dr. John Fisher for review of the manuscript.

TABLE 23-6
Drugs Used Commonly in the Treatment of Parasitic Infections*

Drug	Indications†	Toxicity

Albendazole (Albenza; Zentel)	Echinococcosis
	   Echinococcus granulosus (hydatid cyst)
	   Echinococcus multilocularis (alveolar)
	Complex neurocysticercosis
	Ascariasis
	   Ascaris lumbricoides (roundworm)
	Hookworm
	   Ancylostoma duodenale
	   Necator americanus
	Trichuriasis
	   Trichuris trichiura (whipworm)
	Trichinosis (trichinellosis)
	   Trichinella spiralis
	Giardiasis
	   Giardia lamblia
		Avoid in pregnancy
		Occasional: abdominal pain, reversible alopecia, abnormal liver function tests (elevated aminotransferase levels)
		Rare: rash, leukopenia

Mebendazole (Vermox)	Ascariasis
	   Ascaris lumbricoides (roundworm)
	Hookworm
	   Ancylostoma duodenale
	   Necator americanus
	Enterobiasis
	   Enterobius vermicularis (pinworm)
	Trichuriasis
	   T. trichiura (whipworm)
		Avoid in pregnancy
		Occasional: diarrhea, abdominal pain
		Rare: leukopenia, hypospermia

Continued

TABLE 23-6—cont'd
Drugs Used Commonly in the Treatment of Parasitic Infections*

Drug	Indications†	Toxicity

Thiabendazole (Mintezol)	Strongyloidiasis
	  S. stercoralis
	Visceral larva migrans
	Cutaneous larva migrans (tropical use)
	  Creeping eruption
		Frequent: nausea, vomiting, vertigo, headache, pruritus, drowsiness
		Occasional: CNS disturbances, rash
		Rare: shock, angioedema

Praziquantel (Biltricide)	Flukes
	  Clonorchis sinensis (Chinese liver fluke)
	  Opisthorchis viverrini (Southeast Asian liver fluke)
	  Heterophyes heterophyes (intestinal fluke)
	  Paragonimus westermani (lung fluke)
	  Fasciolopsis buski (intestinal fluke)
	Schistosomiasis (Bilharziasis)
	Complex neurocysticercosis
	Tapeworms
	  Diphyllobothrium latum (fish)
	  Taenia saginata (beef)
	  Taenia solium (pork)
	  Hymenolepsis nana (dwarf)
	  Dipylidium caninum (dog)
		Frequent: nausea, vomiting, abdominal pain, headache, dizziness, diarrhea
		Occasional: sedation, sweats, fever, eosinophilia
		Rare: pruritus, rash, edema, hiccups

Ivermectin (Stromectol, Mectizan)	Onchocerciasis (river blindness)
	  Onchocerca volvulus
	Strongyloidiasis
	  S. stercoralis
	Lymphatic filariasis (kills only the microfilaria)
	  Wuchereria bancrofti
	  Brugia malayi
		Avoid in pregnancy
		Occasional: pruritus, rash (Mazzotti reaction), fever, lymphadenopathy, headache
		Rare: hypotension

Diethylcarbamazine (Hetrazan, available from CDC‡)	Lymphatic filariasis
	  W. bancrofti
	  B. malayi
	  Loa loa
	Tropical eosinophilia
		Frequent: severe allergic, febrile reactions if patient has microfilaremia; gastric disturbances
		Rare: encephalopathy

Metronidazole (Flagyl)	Amebiasis
	  Entamoeba histolytica
	Giardiasis
	  Giardia lamblia
		Frequent: nausea, headache, anorexia, metallic taste
		Occasional: disulfiram (Antabuse)-like reaction, paresthesias
		Rare: seizures, ataxia, neuropathy

Paromomycin (Humatin)	Amebiasis (cyst form) Giardiasis (in pregnancy)	*Frequent:* nausea, diarrhea *Occasional:* hearing loss, vertigo, pancreatitis

Quinine, quinidine (IV)	Malaria
	  Plasmodium falciparum
	Babesiosis (Nantucket fever)
	  Babesia microti
		Avoid in pregnancy
		Frequent: nausea, abdominal pain
		Occasional: anemia, fevers, arrhythmias, hypotension (IV quinidine should be given with cardiac monitoring)

TABLE 23-6—cont'd
Drugs Used Commonly in the Treatment of Parasitic Infections*

Drug	Indications†	Toxicity
Mefloquine (Lariam)	Malaria prophylaxis	Avoid in pregnancy *Occasional:* insomnia, vertigo, nausea, nightmares, headache, visual disturbance *Rare:* psychosis, seizures, hypotension
Permethrin cream (Nix, Lyclear, Elimite, Rid)	Scabies *Sarcoptes scabiei* (itch mite) Lice *Pediculus humanus* (body lice) *Pediculus capitis* (head lice) *Phthirus pubis* (crab lice)	*Occasional:* burning, rash *Note:* Pruritus may continue weeks after therapy because of retained scabies antigens
Sodium stibogluconate (Pentostam, available from CDC‡)	Cutaneous leishmaniasis (oriental sore, Chiclero's ulcer, espundia) *Leishmania mexicana* *Leishmania braziliensis* Visceral leishmaniasis (kala-azar) *Leishmania donovani*	*Frequent:* muscle pain, nausea, electrocardiographic changes, pancreatitis, hepatitis *Occasional:* weakness, abdominal pain, neutropenia, thrombocytopenia, rash, vomiting *Rare:* diarrhea, shock, death
Nifurtimox (Lampit, available from CDC‡)	Chagas' disease *Trypanosoma cruzi*	*Frequent:* anorexia, vomiting, insomnia, neuropathy *Rare:* seizures, fever, pulmonary infiltrates
Suramin (available from CDC‡)	Trypanosomiasis (non-CNS) *Trypanosoma b. rhodesiense* *Trypanosoma b. gambiense*	*Frequent:* vomiting, pruritus, neuropathy *Occasional:* neuropathy, shock, blood dyscrasia
Melarsoprol (Arosobal, available from CDC‡)	CNS trypanosomiasis (African sleeping sickness)	*Frequent:* encephalopathy, cardiomyopathy, febrile reactions, vomiting, colic, hypertension *Rare:* shock

Data from Drugs for parasitic infections. Med Lett 1998; 40: 1-12; and Gilbert DN, Moellering RC, Sande MA. The Sanford Guide to Antimicrobial Therapy. 30th ed., Hyde Park, Vt.; Antimicrobial Therapy, Inc.; 2000.
CDC, Centers for Disease Control and Prevention; *CNS,* central nervous system.
*See text for dosage, which varies according to the infection. For infrequently used drugs, primary care clinicians are urged to read the package insert before use.
†Indications approved by the Food and Drug Administration may vary from this list.
‡Available from Parasitic Disease Drug Service of Centers for Disease Control and Prevention, telephone 404-639-3670 (or 404-639-3356).

24 Travel and Geographic Medicine

DAVID O. FREEDMAN

Prevention of morbidity in the international traveler should be based on risk-benefit principles. Medical interventions and preventive advice must be highly individualized according to both the travel itinerary and traveler-dependent factors. The primary care clinician should resist the temptation to dispense advice by telephone. A structured pretravel medical interaction is recommended, as follows:

- Step 1. Assess the risk based on itinerary and patient factors.
- Step 2. Provide immunizations, malaria chemoprophylaxis, self-treatment strategies for common problems (such as traveler's diarrhea, jet lag, and motion sickness), and advice to reduce exposure to health risks.

Advice given to individual travelers to a particular country will vary according to the endemic disease zones visited within that country, urban versus rural travel, previous vaccination history, age, deluxe versus basic travel style, duration of stay, and underlying medical history. Aside from vaccination, almost all necessary preventive measures are entirely within the patient's control yet are generally to be initiated only after he or she leaves the physician's office. The volume of information presented to the patient is formidable, and printed instructions are mandatory. Websites maintained by the Centers for Disease Control and Prevention (CDC) and other agencies provide detailed information that can be passed along to the traveler (Table 24-1).

Vaccines and chemoprophylaxis for infectious and exotic diseases constitute only one part of travel medicine practice. Medical care before travel also encompasses the prevention and treatment of travel-related morbidity associated with motor vehicle trauma, swimming, jet lag, altitude sickness, and cross-cultural mental health issues associated with long-term postings in the developing world. The clinician must keep abreast of disease transmission patterns to assess the needs for a given patient. Use of Internet services provided by the World Health Organization (WHO) and CDC, as well as by commercial entities that combine authoritative data, is the best way to accomplish this necessary updating (see Suggested Reading).

PATIENT 1
A 38-year-old man in excellent health is planning a 2-week safari to Kenya and Tanzania. He is not taking any medication at present. His primary care physician has the following plan outlined: (1) vaccinate against hepatitis A, typhoid, yellow fever, and influenza; (2) update, as necessary, tetanus-diphtheria, polio, and measles immunizations; (3) begin 250 mg of mefloquine (Lariam) weekly starting 1 week before the trip and continuing 4 weeks after return; (4) prescribe loperamide and levofloxacin for use as standby therapy for traveler's diarrhea; (5) provide counseling about food and water precautions, sex, jet lag, and freshwater exposure.

Epidemiology of the Most Common Travel-Related Diseases

Every year at least 40 million people, including about 15 million Americans, travel to the developing world from developed countries. Risk for any disease varies by destination. Latin America is the most common destination for U.S. residents,

TABLE 24-1
Some Useful Websites For Travel Medicine

Site	Address
CDC Main Travel Health Information Page	http://www.cdc.gov/travel/index.htm
WHO Yellow Book	http://www.who.int/ith/
WHO Outbreak News	http://www.who.int/emc/outbreak_news/index.html
WHO Weekly Epidemiological Record	http://www.who.int/wer/
EuroSurveillance Weekly	http://www.eurosurv.org
Travel Health On-Line	http://www.tripprep.com
CDC Health Topics A to Z	http://www.cdc.gov/health/diseases.htm
WHO Infectious Disease Health Topics	http://www.who.int/health-topics/idindex.htm

CDC, Centers for Disease Control and Prevention; *WHO*, World Health Organization.

followed closely by Asia. Fewer than 250,000 U.S. citizens travel to Africa each year. Medical problems occur in about 50% of travelers to the developing world, most commonly traveler's diarrhea ("turista"). About 8% of travelers become ill enough to consult a physician during or after travel. Infectious diseases account for significant morbidity among travelers but for only about 1% of deaths.

Classic traveler's diarrhea, as usually defined, consists of three or more unformed stools per day with at least one enteric sign such as abdominal cramps, fever, nausea, or vomiting. Nevertheless, milder diarrheal illnesses can significantly affect the regular activities of travel. The incidence varies from about 7% for travel to developed countries to about 20% in southern Europe, Israel, Japan, South Africa, and some Caribbean islands. In most of Asia, Latin America, Africa, and the Middle East, the risk is 25% to 50% in the first 2 weeks abroad and subsides somewhat thereafter. The most frequent causative agent of diarrhea is enterotoxigenic *Escherichia coli* (6% to 70%). The etiologic agent varies in different parts of the world, but other types of *E. coli, Salmonella, Shigella,* and *Campylobacter* each account for about 5% to 15%. Parasites such as *Entamoeba histolytica, Giardia lamblia, Cryptosporidium,* and *Cyclospora* account for <2% each, and Norwalk virus or rotavirus may rarely be detected in adults. About 30% of diarrheal episodes remain unexplained, but many apparently are of bacterial origin because they resolve with antibiotic therapy. *E. coli* and *Cyclospora* are more common during the summer months and *Campylobacter* during cold months. *Campylobacter* and noncholera *Vibrio* species are more common in Asia. Those at increased risk of traveler's diarrhea include individuals taking proton pump inhibitor drugs (but not those taking H_2 blockers) and persons who are naturally achlorhydric. Presumably because of a propensity to risk-taking behavior, adults between 20 and 29 years of age have a higher incidence of traveler's diarrhea than other age groups do.

Malaria is the most important and potentially life-threatening risk for travelers going to one of the 102 malarious countries (Figure 24-1). Sub-Saharan Africa, India, Brazil, Sri Lanka, Vietnam, the Solomon Islands, and Colombia account for two thirds of all the world's cases. About 90% of all *Plasmodium falciparum* malaria occurs in Africa. The highest risk areas in Central America are Belize, Nicaragua, and Guatemala. During the 1990s malaria caused by *P. falciparum* dramatically increased in the Amazon regions of Peru, Guyana, and Bolivia. Estimates of risk in travelers not taking chemoprophylaxis vary widely by destination but range from 24 per 1000 travelers per month in West Africa to 3.5 per 1000 per month on the Indian subcontinent to 0.5 per 1000 per month in South America. Except in sub-Saharan Africa and India, malaria is a rural disease. Thus persons visiting even highly malarious countries in other parts of the world but traveling only to major urban areas are not at risk of malaria and need not worry about prophylaxis. The majority of cases of imported malaria in the United States and Europe occur in noncitizen immigrants visiting friends and relatives abroad. Malaria chemoprophylactic drugs are underused by these ethnic minority travelers.

For the vaccine-preventable diseases the monthly incidence in developing countries is most significant for symptomatic hepatitis A (3 per 1000 travelers per month). The risk of symptomatic hepatitis B is most significant for long-stay travelers and expatriates (0.25 per 1000 per month). Typhoid fever has a risk of 0.03 per 1000 per month, but the risk on the Indian subcontinent is 10 times higher. Fewer data are available on the risk of yellow fever, meningococcal meningitis, rabies, cholera, polio, measles, and Japanese encephalitis in travelers. Imported measles occurs with regularity in nonimmune individuals and in recent years has accounted for the majority of cases in the United States. The risk of the other aforementioned infections is real but apparently exceedingly

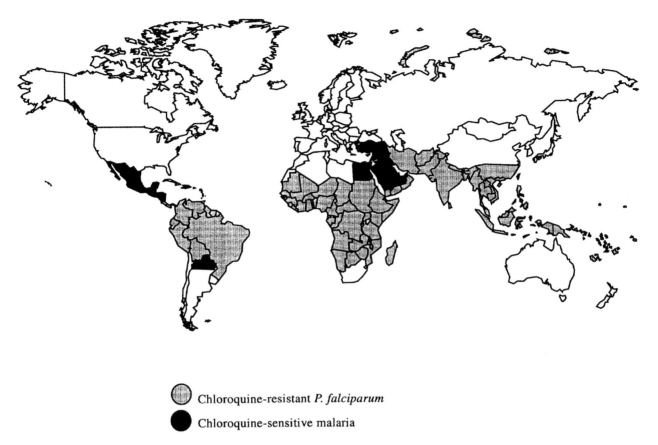

Chloroquine-resistant *P. falciparum*

Chloroquine-sensitive malaria

FIG. 24-1   Distribution of malaria and chloroquine-resistant *Plasmodium falciparum,* 1997. (From the World Health Organization.)

small, even for travel to highly endemic areas. Two fatal cases of yellow fever have occurred in the past 5 years in unvaccinated American travelers visiting Venezuela and Brazil.

Vaccines

Approaches to Vaccination

Prescription of vaccines for travel depends on risk assessment, but travelers differ in their tolerance of risk. Requests for immunization against infectious agents that have bad outcomes if acquired (meningococcal meningitis, Japanese encephalitis) are often difficult for the physician to refuse even if the traveler's risk of acquiring the infection is negligible. Only travel-related vaccine issues are covered here (see Chapter 25 for a general review of vaccines).

Some of the vaccines that are routinely prescribed for certain travel situations have unique factors that must be considered. Vaccines for travelers can be divided into updates of routine immunizations; vaccines indicated for travel to anywhere in the developing world for travelers whose immunization status is not current for that vaccine; and vaccines indicated for specific itineraries. Technical details for all the vaccines discussed are provided in Table 24-2.

Significant reactions to modern vaccines are uncommon, so the indicated immunizations should be given at the same time and can be given in almost any combination. (Immune globulin and cholera vaccine, both of which have interactions with some other vaccines, are now used only in unusual circumstances.) If two live viral antigens are not administered on the same day, they must be spaced by at least a month. Because reactions to modern vaccines are unusual, administration of multiple vaccines at the same sitting is preferable to chancing compliance with a return visit. Contraindications to any vaccine are few. Anaphylactic egg allergy precludes administration of yellow fever, influenza, and measles-mumps-rubella (MMR) vaccines. No current vaccine contains penicillin. Many travel vaccines are available in prefilled syringes at no extra cost.

Update of Routine Immunizations

Because of the greater prevalence of infections in the developing world, routine immunizations need to be current.

Tetanus-Diphtheria (Td) Vaccine

Travelers are at risk for minor or major trauma while far from familiar medical facilities. Adult boosters are normally necessary every 10 years for all adults regardless of travel plans, but boosters at 5-year intervals are suggested for travelers to areas where tetanus immune globulin will be inaccessible. With no proper immunization history, as may occur with immigrants returning home, a complete primary series of three injections is necessary. Diphtheria is prevalent throughout the developing world and in many Eastern European countries.

TABLE 24-2
Synopsis of Vaccines Used by Travelers

Vaccine	Route	Regimen	Duration of protection
Tetanus-diphtheria (toxoid)	IM	Single dose (adult booster)	10 years
Measles (live virus)	SC	Single dose (adult booster)	Lifelong
Poliomyelitis			
Killed virus	IM	Single dose (adult booster)	Lifelong
Live virus	PO*	Single dose (adult booster)	Lifelong
Hepatitis A			
Killed virus	IM	0 and 6 to 12 months	20 years
Immune globulin	IM	Single dose	3 to 5 months
Hepatitis B (killed virus)	IM	0, 1, and 6 months *or 0, 1, 2, and 12 months*	Unknown
Typhoid fever			
Polysaccharide	IM	Single dose	2 to 3 years
Live oral	PO	0, 2, 4, and 6 days	5 years
Whole-cell killed*	IM	0 and 4 weeks	2 to 7 years
Yellow fever (live viral)	SC	Single dose	10 years
Rabies (killed virus)	IM, ID	0, 7, and 21 to 28 days	2 to 3 years
Meningococcal (polysaccharide)	SC	Single dose	2 to 3 years
Japanese encephalitis (killed virus)	IM	0, 7, and 30 days *or 0, 7, 14, and 365 days*	1 to 4 years
Cholera			
Whole-cell killed	ID, SC, IM	0 and 4 weeks	6 months
Live oral*	PO	Single dose	6 months

ID, Intradermally; *IM*, intramuscularly; *PO*, orally; *SC*, subcutaneously.
*Not available in the United States.

Measles Vaccine

In adults measles is a potentially serious disease with a high rate of complications. Intense transmission, which occurs by the respiratory route, is common in developing countries. Persons born in the United States before 1957 or born at any time in the developing world are considered immune to measles. Other travelers over 4 years of age need to have received at least two doses of measles vaccine during their life unless a clinical history of measles infection can be documented. Monovalent measles vaccine should generally be used for adults; MMR should be used for children.

Influenza and Pneumococcal Vaccines

Unvaccinated patients who have the accepted indications for influenza and pneumococcal vaccines should receive them during the pretravel consultation. Influenza is transmitted year round in the tropics, so travelers should be vaccinated with whatever vaccine is available if unvaccinated in the previous 6 months. Vaccine available in the United States differs from that offered in the Southern Hemisphere and may be less efficacious in travelers to those areas. Limited data suggest that

vaccinating all travelers against influenza, regardless of age or health, is beneficial. Travelers have increased risk of upper respiratory infections in general, and influenza vaccine may decrease the risk of all respiratory infections, even those not caused by influenza virus.

Vaccines to Consider for All Travel Destinations in the Developing World
Hepatitis A Vaccine

Hepatitis A is the most common serious infection acquired by travelers, so the hepatitis A vaccine is indicated for every nonimmune traveler visiting a developing country. A single dose of killed hepatitis A vaccine provides high-level protection for ≥1 year. A booster dose administered 6 to 12 months later confers long-term immunity, which has been extrapolated to be at least 20 years but may be lifelong. In almost 100% of individuals seroconversion occurs at 2 weeks (the usual minimum incubation period for hepatitis A infection). Because even postexposure vaccination has been shown to be highly effective in preventing disease, concomitant immune globulin administration for imminent departures is no longer considered necessary. Intramuscular immune globulin, used in the past, provides only short-term (3 to 5 months) passive protection against hepatitis A. It has a long track record of efficacy and low cost, but patients uniformly dislike the intragluteal injection, which is increasingly unavailable in the United States. Individuals born in the developing world should be considered immune to hepatitis A.

Typhoid Fever Vaccine

Typhoid vaccine is indicated for persons traveling to the developing world under all but the most deluxe and protected conditions. Three types of vaccine are licensed in the United States. In distinct contrast to the original whole cell vaccine, which was discontinued in the United States in 2000, the newer preparations (Ty21a, ViCPS) are well tolerated. The Vipolysaccharide vaccine is a single-dose regimen. As with other typhoid vaccines, efficacy is less than 70%, so patients need to be reminded that the vaccine is not a substitute for dietary prudence while traveling. The live attenuated bacterial vaccine (Ty21a) is taken as four capsules, one every other day until finished. Capsules must be refrigerated until used. Ty21a capsules must be taken on an empty stomach (i.e., at least 1 hour before or 3 hours after eating). No antibiotics of any kind can be taken for 2 weeks after beginning the vaccine.

Hepatitis B Vaccine

Because of difficult-to-control transmission-related issues such as sexual contacts, blood transfusions, contaminated medical and dental equipment, sharing of cooking and bathroom facilities, tattooing, and body piercing, hepatitis B vaccine is indicated for all individuals who will be residing for a long time in endemic areas (in addition to individuals with the usual indications for this vaccine). The CDC recommends the vaccine before a stay of at least 6 months in a highly endemic area, and the WHO recommends it for visits of ≥1 month. In practice, the vaccine should be at least discussed with travelers going on all but short vacations or trips. The standard regimen of three vaccinations at day 0, 1 month, and 6 months is generally required for very high seroconversion rates, although two doses offer a 50% chance of protection. Accelerated regimens of vaccinations at day 0, 1 month, and 2 months or alternatively at day 0, 1 week, and 3 weeks (not FDA approved but commonly used in practice) offer good short-term protection. However, both accelerated regimens necessitate a fourth dose at 12 months. This highly effective strategy is suitable for most travelers because it allows rapid onset of protection for a high-risk trip that is beginning in <6 months and most travelers are home in time for the 1-year booster.

Vaccines to Consider Only for Certain Destinations
Yellow Fever Vaccine

Yellow fever is caused by a mosquito-borne arbovirus. The risk for infection is generally not high except in epidemic settings, but the disease has a high case-fatality rate. Certain countries in the yellow fever endemic zone (Amazon basin and sub-Saharan Africa; Figure 24-2) require vaccine certificates from all visitors upon entry. Other infected countries with reasonable risk have no legal requirements, but vaccination of all travelers going to these countries is medically indicated. Still other countries, which have the mosquito vector

but not the infection, particularly countries in Asia and South America, require an official immunization certificate from travelers who have traveled even briefly through any part (not just the infected region) of endemic countries. A special permit is required to administer this vaccine, and these travel medicine clinics are familiar with the complex regulations.

Polio Vaccine

Paralytic poliomyelitis is still present in some developing countries outside the Americas, where the disease has now been eradicated. A single adult booster of injectable polio vaccine before travel to these countries is recommended, even for individuals who had proper immunization against polio as a child. Older adults, generally those ≥60 years of age, with no history of childhood polio immunization should begin a complete series of three primary immunizations of injectable polio vaccine, with at least two doses given before travel. Oral polio vaccine production was discontinued in the United States in 1999.

A global eradication program is decreasing the incidence of polio rapidly in almost all parts of the world outside the Americas. Most remaining cases of polio are in Africa and on the Indian subcontinent. Polio vaccine boosters are now the lowest priority of all the travel vaccines.

Meningococcal Vaccine

Travelers to the "meningitis belt" of sub-Saharan Africa (Figure 24-3) during the dry season from December to June should receive the type A, C, Y, W135 meningococcal vaccine. The incidence of disease in travelers is low, but the effects are devastating. Transmission is respiratory, so all health care workers going to the meningitis belt at any time of year should consider vaccination. In addition, short-term travelers to other areas with current epidemics, as well as Hajj pilgrims to Mecca in Saudi Arabia, require meningococcal vaccine. The vaccine does not protect against serotype B, which is the most common type in the United States.

Japanese Encephalitis Vaccine

Japanese encephalitis is a mosquito-borne arbovirus endemic to certain uncommonly visited rural areas of Southeast Asia and the Indian subcontinent. Very few travelers go to infected areas containing both the pig reservoir and the rice paddies where the vector mosquitoes breed. Transmission is seasonal in most affected areas, peaking during the rainy season. The vaccine is recommended only for those spending a month or more in an infected area or for short-term travelers going into an area known to be having an acute outbreak. A three-dose regimen given at days 0, 7, and 30 provides optimum protection. If insufficient time is available, a days 0, 7, and 14 regimen will give shorter term protection. Some moderate to severe allergic reactions, including facial swelling and laryngeal edema, may occur up to 10 days after vaccine administration. The full duration of protection of the vaccine is unknown at the present time.

Rabies Vaccine

A preexposure rabies series is indicated for long-stay travel to endemic areas of Latin America, Asia, or Africa where the rabies threat is constant and where access to adequate postexposure rabies immune globulin and vaccine is likely to be

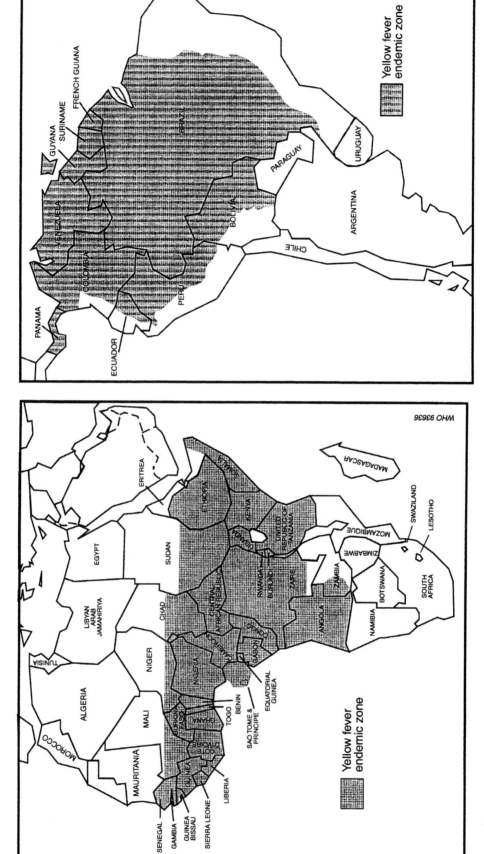

FIG. 24-2 Yellow fever endemic zones of, **A**, Africa and, **B**, South America. (From the World Health Organization.)

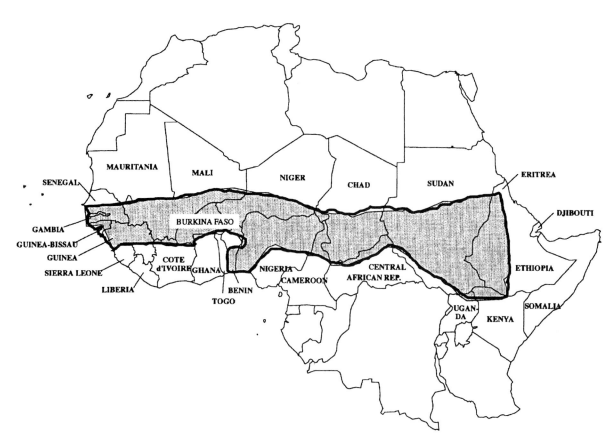

FIG. 24-3 "Meningitis belt" of Africa. (From the World Health Organization.)

limited. Controversy exists over the exact indications for the vaccine. The higher the risk and the more remote the location, the shorter the duration of stay that should be considered as necessitating vaccination. Children are considered to be at high risk for rabies. High-risk situations for adults include adventure travel in rural or remote areas, occupational exposure, or spelunking.

A history of the three-dose preexposure series obviates any need for rabies immune globulin, which is extremely difficult to come by in most developing countries, after a high-risk bite or scratch injury. The regimen for postexposure vaccine (also sometimes difficult to obtain) for vaccinated individuals is two doses at days 0 and 3 instead of the 0-, 3-, 7-, 14-, and 28-day regimen required for unvaccinated individuals.

Cholera Vaccine

Cholera vaccination is no longer required by any country, and the risk to typical travelers is insignificant. Cholera epidemics usually occur in impoverished areas not frequented by travelers. However, aid workers staying for short periods in disaster areas or refugee camps may consider cholera vaccination. The killed whole cell vaccine now available in the United States works poorly and since 1988 has not been recommended by the WHO or the CDC or required for entry into any country. A new oral vaccine that provides reasonable protection for 6 months is currently available only in Canada and Europe. Occasionally travelers encounter a situation in which embassies in the United States working with old documents or forms appear to require

a cholera certificate in order to obtain a visa. A phone call or letter to the embassy in question usually solves the problem.

Plague, Bacille Calmette-Guérin, Anthrax, and European Tickborne Encephalitis Vaccines

Vaccinations with plague, bacille Calmette-Guérin, anthrax, and European tickborne encephalitis vaccines are rarely indicated, and for differing reasons these vaccines are not currently available to clinicians in the United States.

Malaria

Malaria is present in at least some parts of almost every tropical country, 102 in all, and is the most serious risk faced by travelers to these areas (Figure 24-1). Surveillance data indicate that the vast majority of the 2000 or so U.S. residents who contract malaria abroad each year were not taking appropriate medications or precautions to prevent malaria. (For clinical manifestations, diagnosis, and treatment of malaria, see Chapters 6 and 23.)

Although female *Anopheles* mosquitos bite only between dusk and dawn, malaria is highly infectious. A brief exposure—for example, riding in an open train at night or spending a few evening hours visiting a malarious rural area—constitutes a significant enough risk for infection that the institution of full (5 weeks minimum) preventive measures is mandated. Symptoms of malaria are varied and nonspecific at the outset, and most often they start anywhere from 8 to 35 days after an infective bite. Patients should be informed, in writing, of the need to contact a physician and have a malaria smear performed for fever of *any* kind within 2 months of travel to a malarious area.

Principles of Chemoprophylaxis

No single drug will provide optimal protection against malaria in all parts of the world. Chemoprophylactic drug regimens must be tailored to the person's particular itinerary, duration of travel, medical history, access to medical care and curative antimalarial agents abroad, and personal tolerance of risk. Not all regions or cities within a malarious country are malarious. Overall guidelines are shown in Table 24-3, but physicians who prescribe antimalarial drugs must keep up to date on current transmission and drug-resistance patterns. Prudence is always wise, but prescribing long-term medication for a traveler intending to spend months to years in a region of a country where there is no actual risk of malaria is expensive for the patient and has potential for serious drug toxicity. Long-term residents should contact a specialized travel clinic, or physicians may check the CDC website (www.cdc.gov/travel/regionalmalaria/index.htm) or call the CDC physician malaria hotline (1-770-488-7788) for the latest advice. In addition, long-stay travelers must be advised that malaria chemoprophylaxis recommendations are liable to change periodically.

Malaria chemoprophylaxis (except atovaquone-proguanil) must be continued for 4 weeks after the traveler leaves the malarious area because these drugs affect hepatic phase schizonts, which are incubating in the liver (a process that can take 4 weeks or more) and have not yet reached the bloodstream.

Profiles of Drugs in Prophylactic Dosage
Mefloquine (Lariam)

For malaria prevention mefloquine 250 mg once weekly is the drug of choice with two exceptions: in the border areas of Thailand, where, owing to mefloquine resistance, doxycycline or atovaquone-proguanil can be used, and in Central America, Mexico, the Dominican Republic, Haiti, and the Middle East, where chloroquine is still effective. One tablet (250 mg) should be taken once a week, always on the same day and preferably on Sunday, because on that day the daily routine is usually different and the need to take the tablet will be easier to remember. Patients should be told to start taking malaria pills one or two Sundays before entering the malarious area.

The departure date of the traveler does not always correspond with the date of entering the malarious area. On multistop itineraries, one or several intermediate nonmalarious destinations may be included in the trip. If a dose is forgotten, it should be taken later in the week, but the patient should return to the regular day immediately thereafter. However, if a week's dose is forgotten completely, the patient should not double up the following week. Despite considerable anecdotal information to the contrary, side effects are equivalent to those with other antimalarial drugs. In 10% or so of patients, mild stomach upset (the drug may be taken with meals), anxiety, vivid dreams, or insomnia may occur. The real incidence of side effects is difficult to ascertain because most travelers have crossed multiple time zones, are on the move, are in strange surroundings and cultures, and tend to consume more alcohol than at home. If problems arise, it is most often by the second or third dose of mefloquine (hence the advantage of starting at least 2 weeks ahead of time). In general, the benefits of this highly effective drug far outweigh the relatively low rate of side effects. Patients need to be reminded that tolerating mild side effects—such as sleep disturbance one or two nights per week—is far better than stopping the medication and becoming susceptible to a potentially life-threatening disease.

Although still formally advising pregnant women to avoid all travel to chloroquine-resistant areas, the CDC and WHO in carefully worded statements have permitted medical professionals to consider mefloquine usage at all stages of pregnancy when exposure to chloroquine-resistant *P. falciparum* is unavoidable. A wide experience in Europe with mefloquine in infants and toddlers weighing as little as 5 kg has not unearthed any significant adverse effects in this group. Mefloquine is extremely bitter tasting, and the manufacturer has explicitly stated that no liquid formulation of mefloquine is on the horizon. Experienced parents maintain that chocolate syrup is the only vehicle effective in making antimalarial drugs palatable to children.

TABLE 24-3
Recommendations for Malaria Chemoprophylaxis

Drug and dose for adults*	Comments
Mefloquine 250 mg PO weekly	A drug of choice except for countries otherwise noted
Atovaquone-proguanil 250/100 mg daily	A drug of choice for trips <2 weeks or if intolerant of mefloquine
Chloroquine 300 mg PO of base weekly	Drug of choice for Mexico, Central America, Caribbean, and Middle East
Doxycycline 100 mg PO daily	Drug of choice for Thai/Myanmar and Thai/Cambodia border; also indicated for individuals unable to take whichever of the above is otherwise indicated

*Pediatric doses: Mefloquine <20 kg: ¼ tablet; 20-30 kg: ½ tablet; 30-45 kg: ¾ tablet. Atovaquone-proguanil 11-20 kg: 1 pediatric (62.5/25 mg) tablet; 21-30 kg: 2 pediatric tablets; 31-40 kg: 3 pediatric tablets; >40 kg: 1 adult tablet. Chloroquine 5 mg/kg. Doxycycline contraindicated under 8 years of age. Doxycycline and atovaquone-proguanil contraindicated in pregnancy.

Atovaquone-Proguanil (Malarone)

Atovaquone-proguanil combination tablets (250 mg atovaquone and 100 mg proguanil) have recently become available in the United States. Studies in several different regions of the world suggest that this combination is as effective as mefloquine or doxycycline for malaria prevention. In addition, it appears to be extremely well tolerated in the relatively small populations in which it has been tested. The drug is effective against incubating hepatic phase parasites. One tablet per day starting 2 days before entering the malarious area and continuing for just 7 days after the last possible exposure make this drug more convenient than doxycycline but still less convenient than weekly mefloquine. The cost of the daily drug will make it expensive for most patients needing long-term coverage but competitive with mefloquine for a typical 1- to 2-week vacation stay.

Chloroquine

Chloroquine is indicated and preferable for all malarious areas within Central America, Mexico, the Dominican Republic, Haiti, and the Middle East, where chloroquine is still effective. The dosage schedule (one 500-mg tablet once a week) is the same as for mefloquine. A pediatric liquid preparation is available in many malarious countries overseas but not in the United States, so crushed tablets in chocolate syrup must again be used. Aside from mild gastrointestinal upset, chloroquine is one of the safest and best tolerated of all drugs. At present chloroquine-resistant *Plasmodium vivax* occurs only in areas where mefloquine and atovaquone-proguanil are already indicated for prophylaxis because of the concomitant presence of resistant *P. falciparum*.

Doxycycline

If contraindications or intolerance to mefloquine exists, daily doxycycline can be used, but atovaquone-proguanil is preferable if cost is not a concern. One doxycycline tablet (100 mg) once a day should be taken starting 1 to 2 days before entering the malarious area and continuing for 4 weeks afterward. Esophageal ulceration and gastric irritation, photosensitivity skin rash, candidal vaginitis, and jock itch occur. Women taking doxycycline should always carry single-dose fluconazole for self-treatment of candidal vaginitis. Topical anticandidal agents are difficult to use in tropical climates.

Other Drugs

The preceding agents constitute a complete armamentarium for malaria chemoprophylaxis. Nevertheless, a large number of antimalarial drugs not licensed in the United States are in use overseas, and patients may have questions about them. A travel medicine specialist should be consulted for information about proguanil (Paludrine), halofantrine (Halfan), pyrimethamine-dapsone (Maloprim or Deltaprim), and artesunate, to name a few.

Personal Protection Measures

Antimalarial chemoprophylactic drugs are significantly less than 100% effective in many parts of the world, and resistance is increasing. Minimizing mosquito bites means minimizing incidence of malaria and is more important than ever. Antimosquito measures during feeding hours (dusk to dawn) should be emphasized to every patient:

- After dark, cover up exposed skin, use repellent containing ≥30% DEET (*N,N*-diethylmetatoluamide) liberally on remaining exposed skin, and stay indoors in well-screened areas if possible.
- Impregnate clothing with permethrin.
- Use knockdown insect sprays or mosquito coils in sleeping areas before bed, and sleep under permethrin-impregnated mosquito netting.

Personal protection to minimize mosquito bites will protect travelers not only against malaria but also against dengue, filariasis, and a number of important arboviral diseases. *Aedes* species and culicine mosquitoes are usually daytime biters, so vigilance at all hours of the day will best protect individuals against a full spectrum of arthropod-borne infectious agents.

Self-Treatment of Malaria

For travel to areas with very low transmission rates of malaria, some authorities (notably in Europe) advise that only a standby drug be carried, which is to be taken in the event that symptoms suggestive of malaria occur and the patient has no access to a physician or facility that can competently perform a malaria smear within 6 to 12 hours. In areas with chloroquine-resistant *P. falciparum,* the drug of choice for this purpose is atovaquone-proguanil in treatment doses. In areas without chloroquine-resistant *P. falciparum,* chloroquine is the drug of choice. Owing to the uniform development of side effects, self-treatment with quinine is no longer advocated because atovaquone-proguanil is now available. Even after a good clinical response, the patient should be instructed to consult a physician as soon as possible.

Traveler's Diarrhea

Traveler's diarrhea is generally mild. Only 25% of those affected have more than six bowel movements per day. One half of patients suffer abdominal cramps, and roughly 15% have nausea, vomiting, fever, or blood admixed in the stools. None of the clinical symptoms are pathognomonic for a specific agent. Untreated, the syndrome is self-limited, with an average duration of 4 to 7 days. Persistent diarrhea, defined as diarrhea lasting >14 days, occurs in 1% to 2% of travelers and has a different spectrum of causes.

Prevention Strategies

The incidence of traveler's diarrhea can be reduced but not eliminated by educating the traveler to avoid dietary indiscretions. Unfortunately, data show that despite the considerable time spent by most travel clinics in such education, <3% of travelers avoid all potentially risky food and drink items. Even in the most expensive and luxurious hotels, the water and many of the foods are simply not safe. Street vendors should be avoided at all costs; as few as 10 *Shigella* organisms can cause full-blown dysentery. The safest foods are those served steaming hot, fruits that can be peeled, and bread. Hot soup, coffee, or tea, as well as bottled carbonated beverages (preferably multinational brands), beer, and wine, are generally safe. Clearly high-risk items include undercooked shellfish and meats, salads, creamy desserts, sauces sitting for long periods at room temperatures, and ice cubes, which may be made from contaminated water. Dairy products should in general be avoided unless pasteurization can be ascertained.

If available, commercial bottled water (carbonated or uncarbonated) that has a tamper-proof top and is opened personally by the traveler (or is opened in front of him or her) is almost always safe. Where boiled, bottled, or other safe sources of drinking water are not likely to be available, travelers should carry either halogen-based water purification tablets or an iodine resin–based filtration device.

Routine antibiotic prophylaxis for diarrhea is not recommended for the typical traveler because of the potential for adverse drug effects, rashes, or allergies while away from medical care. The most important reason to avoid routine antibiotics is that an effective rapid-onset therapy is available for traveler's diarrhea should it occur (see Tables 12-3 and 12-4). However, chemoprophylaxis can be considered for travelers with HIV infection, individuals with an underlying chronic medical problem that makes them more prone to adverse consequences from diarrhea, and those on a vital mission for a short period (<1 week) who cannot afford to lose a working day because of disability. Bismuth subsalicylate (two tablets four times per day) during travel and for 1 to 2 days after returning may reduce the incidence of diarrhea by up to 60% but is inconvenient to take. Antimicrobial agents are more effective, but their use may complicate therapy if breakthrough illness occurs. Quinolone antibiotics are recommended. These include norfloxacin 400 mg, ciprofloxacin 500 mg, ofloxacin 300 mg, or levofloxacin 500 mg once daily during travel and for 1 to 3 days after returning home. Antibiotic prophylaxis should be used only for trips of ≤2 weeks. For longer trips chemoprophylaxis is not advised.

Self-Treatment of Traveler's Diarrhea

Because even travelers in developed countries may have diarrhea while away from easily accessible medical care, all travelers should be instructed in self-therapy for diarrheal disease. The traveler's medical kit should include loperamide and a quinolone antibiotic. In contrast to the case with diphenoxylate-atropine (Lomotil), in which antimotility therapy was shown to be harmful to some patients with diarrhea, loperamide has now been shown to provide an actual therapeutic advantage in cases of bacillary dysentery caused by *Shigella* or enteroinvasive *E. coli*. It can now be cautiously recommended even for travelers with dysentery.

Diarrhea that does not respond to loperamide within a few hours can be treated with a 3-day course of a quinolone (see "Prevention Strategies" for drugs and dosages) during loperamide therapy. About 80% of patients respond to this regimen within 24 hours. The other 20% of patients, who may have more invasive bacterial disease and take 2 to 3 days to respond, should continue therapy for up to 5 days. Those who have dysentery or do not respond to 5 days of antibacterial medication should seek medical attention as soon as possible.

Some authorities endorse a single 750-mg dose of ciprofloxacin for mild traveler's diarrhea. Data also now indicate that azithromycin is effective against most of the causes of traveler's diarrhea, including quinolone-resistant *Campylobacter* strains now emerging in Southeast Asia. Azithromycin (e.g., 500 mg/day for 3 days) can therefore be recommended for patients unable to take a quinolone, such as those with known hypersensitivity. However, the demonstrated superior efficacy of quinolones makes them the drug of choice in difficult situations, including serious febrile diarrheal illness in children when medical care is unavailable.

Bismuth subsalicylate by itself is often curative but is clearly slower and less effective than the loperamide-antibiotic combination. Traveler's diarrhea is not dehydrating, and salty crackers and oral fluids suffice in almost all cases. Persons going to remote regions where a dehydrating illness might be devastating and persons with significant underlying medical problems should carry packets of oral rehydration salts (ORS). Both the standard WHO formulation and rice-based ORS (better flavor) are available in the United States from a number of catalog and Internet vendors. Pedialyte should always be carried when traveling with infants and toddlers, who are prone to dehydrating illness. Patients should be instructed to avoid antidiarrhea drugs sold over the counter in pharmacies overseas—some of them are very dangerous.

Other Preventive and Self-Treatment Strategies
General Considerations

A predeparture dental checkup will lessen the risk of oral infections during travel. A baseline tuberculin skin test with annual retesting is indicated before long-stay travel to developing countries. Aggressive treatment of skin test converters will prevent cases of active tuberculosis later.

Travelers should carry a compact medical kit (Table 24-4). Simple first-aid supplies such as bandages, gauze, antiseptic, antibiotic ointment, and splinter forceps will allow early self-treatment of minor wounds before infection ensues. Commercially available kits contain compact combination needles, syringes, suture material, and intravenous tubing. The kit may include an extended spectrum quinolone such as levofloxacin or a macrolide such as azithromycin, which will permit early self-treatment of respiratory or soft tissue infections. Antifungal creams or powders will alleviate mycotic infections prevalent in humid tropical environments. Travelers to high-risk areas should have a thermometer to document elevations in temperature so that they can determine early the need to take antimalarial or antimicrobial drugs or seek medical attention.

Walking barefoot in tropical areas predisposes travelers to hookworm, *Strongyloides* infection, cutaneous larva migrans, and tungiasis. Scabies and lice are prevented by close attention to personal hygiene and careful laundering of clothes. In Africa all clothes dried outdoors should be ironed to avoid cutaneous myiasis caused by the tumbu fly.

Long-stay travelers should seek out the local expatriate medical infrastructure immediately after arrival so they can rapidly seek competent care for any ensuing infectious disease early in its course.

Sex

Freed from the normal social constraints of everyday life and often with an overlay of alcohol consumption, a remarkable number of travelers (4% to 25%, depending on the population studied) engage in casual travel sex (CTS). Most of these contacts are with fellow travelers, but this is still risky sex. More pernicious is sex tourism, travel specifically arranged for encounters with male or female professional sex workers. Risk factors for CTS include traveling alone, traveling on business, making more than two trips to the same destination, and having had a sexually transmitted disease in the previous 5 years. Alarmingly, of 273 Swedish women having CTS, only 15% regularly used condoms.

TABLE 24-4
Travel Medical Kit

Essential	Necessary if applicable	Of practical importance
Travel-related medications prescribed by physician Acetaminophen or similar antiinflammatory drug Disinfectant for skin cuts and wounds Bandages, gauze, Band-Aids, tweezers Neosporin (or similar) antibiotic ointment Sun block Sun hat DEET-based insect repellent (minimum 30%) (may damage plastic watch crystals, contact lenses, etc.) Cold and flu medication (to contain pseudoephedrine as one ingredient) Antihistamine (i.e., Chlor-Trimeton, Benadryl) Plastic water bottle or flask All of the above items to be carried in hand luggage	Oversupply of regular prescription drugs Copy of important prescriptions using generic names Nasal decongestant spray Oil of wintergreen (for toothache) and emergency dental kit Antifungal skin cream (Lotrimin) and foot powder (e.g. Tinactin) Heating coil (to boil water) Iodine tablets or hand-filter (to treat water if no electricity) Oral rehydration packets (for travel to remote areas) Motion sickness pills (e.g., Bonine) or Scopolamine patches Cough syrup or tablets Thermometer Sunburn cream Insect sting kit (Epi-Pen) Ipecac (if traveling with small children)	Mosquito bed net Permethrin insect spray or liquid to impregnate clothes AIDS-free certificate (for long-term visitors, students, or workers) Swiss Army Knife Sunglasses, spare eyeglasses, copy of eye prescription Sewing kit Small flashlight Knockdown insect spray Facial tissues and toilet paper Commercial AIDS prevention kit (needles, syringes, intravenous infusion tubing) Photocopy of passport front page, airline ticket, important phone numbers (i.e., U.S. embassy, personal physician), credit card data Supplementary health insurance information

Human nature is not to be denied: 15 years into the HIV epidemic, large numbers of individuals still travel to such places as Nairobi and Bangkok and avail themselves of local sex workers. Verbal and written education at the time of the pretravel visit is important, and some travel clinics make free condoms discreetly available to clients on their way out the door. Education on the incidence of HIV and sexually transmitted diseases among professional sex workers abroad, on the use of condoms, and on the failure rate of condoms (3% to 5% breakage or slippage) should be given to every traveler regardless of apparent circumstances.

Motor Vehicle Trauma

Traffic accidents are the most common cause of death in travelers. Many multinational corporations prohibit their employees from driving in much of the developing world. Vacationers should be advised similarly and particularly advised against renting mopeds and motorbikes.

Motion Illness

With the exception of scopolamine patches, all drugs used for motion sickness are essentially antihistamines and work to some extent by their sedative effect. Meclizine, cyclizine, dimenhydrinate, and ginger root are effective over-the-counter preparations available in the United States, and no statistically significant difference in efficacy exists among these medications. No treatment is truly satisfactory. In practice, a balance between efficacy and oversedation needs to be achieved if the traveler's goal of seeing and doing as much as possible is to be met. All preparations are more effective if predisposed persons begin using them before the potentially offending activity.

Jet Lag

Patients can be prescribed short-acting sedatives such as zolpidem (Ambien) and instructed to take one tablet at bedtime for 2 or 3 days after arrival to allow them to fall asleep at the appropriate time for their current location. The temptation to nap at other times of day should be fought. Melatonin is a natural substance and variably effective in different studies, but patients have trouble either understanding or adhering to the somewhat complicated and lengthy regimens that have been proposed.

Altitude

For patients not allergic to sulfa, acetazolamide 250 mg PO b.i.d. for 24 hours before and 48 hours after ascending rapidly to 11,000 feet or more can prevent altitude sickness. If altitude symptoms persist beyond the day after ascent, travelers can continue to take one tablet each evening. This diuretic quickly alters acid-base balance to shift the oxyhemoglobin curve and improve oxygen-carrying capacity. Patients need to be educated about the necessity for an experienced professional to accompany any group ascending to an altitude >15,000 feet. Individuals in whom high-altitude pulmonary edema or cerebral edema develops are in no position to treat themselves.

Swimming

Clean water in the developing world is rare. Swimming, rafting, or wading in freshwater should be actively discouraged, especially in Africa, where schistosomiasis-free lakes or rivers are few and far between. A significant risk of leptospirosis exists in freshwater throughout the developing world owing to excretion of the spirochetes (which can penetrate intact skin) in the urine of rodents and other animals.

Treatment After Return

The most common syndromes encountered in returning travelers are fever, diarrhea, and skin problems. The most perplexing problem is eosinophilia. Diagnosis of medical problems in travelers requires knowledge of world geography, the epidemiology of disease patterns in some 250 countries, and the clinical presentation of a wide spectrum of disorders. The history is vital:

- Where exactly did the traveler go? At what altitudes? During what season?
- When did the symptoms occur? Was there periodicity? Were the symptoms multiphasic?
- What exposures took place? Occupation? Accommodation? Eating habits? Sex? Swimming? Contact with sick persons?
- What vector contact occurred? Mosquitos? Flies? Arthropods? Snails? Animals?
- What immunizations were received, and when? What antimalarial prophylaxis was taken, and when? What medications were taken, including drugs with unfamiliar names?

The meticulousness with which the exact itinerary within each country visited and the chronology of travel must be dissected cannot be overemphasized. Many clinics employ waiting-room questionnaires for this purpose. A key consideration is that common causes *are common,* and clinicians are frequently so excited about the potential for an exotic diagnosis that they fail to consider the everyday concerns in their differential diagnosis. Generating two mental lists for the differential diagnosis is frequently helpful. The second list would include all the possibilities for a patient appearing with the same clinical syndrome who had never left his or her current hometown.

Fever

The instinctive performance of serial malaria smears for all appropriate febrile travelers could prevent the unnecessary deaths caused by *P. falciparum* malaria that still occur each year in the United States. Fever in a traveler returning from a malarious area should be considered an emergency, and all diagnostic tests should be obtained and performed on an urgent basis. Overt hemorrhagic manifestations in patients should likewise be treated as emergencies because of the possibility of hemorrhagic fever or meningococcemia. The most common tropical causes of undifferentiated fever without localizing signs in the returned traveler are malaria, typhoid fever, hepatitis, and dengue. Other frequent causes include amebic disease, typhus, arboviral disease, leptospirosis, brucellosis, acute schistosomiasis, rickettsial disease, and acute fungal infection.

At present malaria is overwhelmingly an African disease. About 90% of the world's cases of *P. falciparum* malaria, the life-threatening form of the disease, occur in Africa. Of the remaining cases, approximately one half occur in Brazil and India and another one quarter in the countries of Southeast Asia. The nonuse or improper use of malaria prophylactic medication by the majority of individuals with imported malaria has been noted repeatedly. However, a history of adequate prophylaxis properly taken greatly lessens but does not eliminate the possibility of malaria. The initial signs and symptoms of imported malaria remain protean enough to mimic a number of common nontropical conditions. These include gastroenteritis, pyelonephritis, pharyngitis, upper respiratory tract infection, and undifferentiated viral syndromes. Classic periodic malarial fever, as is described in medical school curricula and textbooks, is not a usual manifestation of imported malaria.

Every fever in an individual who has been present, no matter how briefly, in a malaria-endemic area during the preceding 3 months requires an urgent malaria smear. Non-*falciparum* malaria is rarely life threatening and can appear much later after arrival in the United States. A single negative malaria smear, even one properly prepared and read by an expert, does not rule out malaria. Smears must be repeated at least every 12 to 24 hours for a minimum of 3 days to rule out malaria. Deterioration can occur over a period of hours. Smear-negative patients whose illness suggests malaria should be admitted to the hospital for inpatient observation.

Many other serious infections are present in malarious areas. The search for malaria should not hamper the simultaneous workup for other pathogens in smear-negative patients. Similarly, partially immune residents of endemic areas may be mildly parasitemic on a chronic basis with little ill effect, so a positive malaria smear in these patients should not hamper a workup for any other clinically suspected infections. Other mandatory diagnostic tests in the workup of every tropical fever are blood cultures (typhoid), complete blood cell count (CBC) with differential and platelet counts, liver function tests, urinalysis, and at the slightest clinical indication a chest x-ray examination. If the patient's condition is stable, no laboratory abnormalities or clinical evidence of end-organ damage is found, and the patient has a reliable companion, follow-up on an outpatient basis is appropriate during the clinical evolution. The workup can be pursued according to the clinical findings. At least one fourth of febrile illnesses are viral and self-limiting.

Ciprofloxacin is sometimes given orally as empiric therapy for typhoid fever because of the ease of treatment and difficulty in making the diagnosis. Empiric therapy for malaria without a positive blood smear is appropriate only if clinical evidence of cerebral dysfunction or other end-organ damage consistent with malaria is present. Otherwise, examination of these patients and of serial blood smears over several days by someone with appropriate experience will lead to the parasitologic diagnosis of malaria if it is present, and such expertise is rarely so far away as to compromise patient care. In addition to exposing the patient to possible drug toxicities, empiric treatment will eliminate any possibility of determining the species if the patient does in fact have malaria. After empiric treatment the clinician is probably obligated to a course of primaquine, a potentially toxic drug, to cover the possibility that the antecedent infection was due to relapsing *P. vivax* or *Plasmodium ovale* malaria. (For the clinical approach to proven malaria, see Chapters 6 and 23.)

Diarrhea

Most traveler's diarrhea is bacterial or viral and is self-limited, with a duration of about 5 to 7 days. As previously described, many patients self-treat with quinolone antibiotics and are told to seek medical assistance if diarrhea does not resolve after a 3-to 5-day course of antibiotics. Returned travelers with diarrhea who have not yet had a course of quinolone antibiotic can be prescribed an empiric course without any workup or stool culture. Antibiotic nonresponders should then have stool tests, including bacterial cultures, examination for ova and parasites (O&P), acid-fast bacillus staining to detect *Cryptosporidium* and *Cyclospora* species, enzyme-linked immunosorbent assay (ELISA) to detect *Giardia* and *Entamoeba,* and toxin assay on stool specimen to detect *Clostridium difficile.* Quinolone-resistant *Campylobacter* is increasing, so an empiric course of azithromycin can be given while culture results are awaited if the patient is still acutely ill.

In a small proportion of travelers without immediate diagnosis, chronic diarrhea develops and lasts a month or more. The diagnosis is often elusive despite extensive diagnostic testing. Appropriate studies include serologic tests for HIV, testing for malabsorption, and upper and lower endoscopy with all aspirates sent for parasitologic examination. Biopsy almost always yields nonspecific findings, although cases of tropical sprue are occasionally discovered. In many of these individuals the cause of the nonspecific villus blunting that is often found is unclear. This syndrome has often been called tropical enteropathy or postinfective tropical malabsorption, and it is thought to be the residual damage from an initial bacterial or other insult. Diarrhea may persist for months before resolving. Lactose-free, high-fiber diets are sometimes beneficial.

Skin Diseases

Common eruptions include pyodermas, arthropod bites (infected or not), cutaneous larva migrans, furuncular myiasis, dermatophytosis, and drug eruptions. Ulcerative lesions include leishmaniasis, mycobacterial disease, and deep mycoses. Rickettsial diseases frequently include black eschars at the site of the arthropod bite.

Eosinophilia

Peripheral blood eosinophilia may be associated with a wide spectrum of immunologic, inflammatory, dermatologic, neoplastic, and idiopathic etiologies, as well as parasitic causes. Returning travelers and natives of tropical countries are as prone to nonparasitic causes of eosinophilia as is the general population, and all of these must be considered when taking the clinical history and initiating the workup in a patient with a travel history. Generally eosinophilia is a reaction to a tissue-invasive helminth. Its intensity is proportional to the degree of tissue invasion.

Although most laboratory reports express the eosinophil count solely as a percentage of the total white blood cell count, this practice can make serial determinations difficult to follow in an individual patient. The absolute eosinophil count can be calculated by simple arithmetic and ranges from 0 to $350/mm^3$ (mean, $120/mm^3$) in normal patients. During the progressive course of a new infection with a specific parasite, such as hookworm, in an individual patient, intense eosinophilia (up to $5000/mm^3$) may occur during the migration of the infective larvae through the lungs. The most frequent parasitic causes of massive eosinophilia are lymphatic filariasis and toxocariasis. Because the list of helminths causing eosinophilia is extensive, and because many of the parasitologic and serologic techniques required for specific diagnosis are laborious and expensive, an epidemiologic history carefully obtained by a physician knowledgeable about current epidemiology is vital to narrow the differential diagnosis to a manageable size.

Clearly the cornerstone of any workup for eosinophilia is the examination of stools for O&P. Unfortunately, this crucial diagnostic procedure is totally dependent on the expertise of the laboratory. A concentration technique should be used and at least three separate stools examined. The following ancillary procedures are indicated when epidemiologically appropriate or when dictated by specific symptoms: day and night blood concentrations (filariasis); skin snips (onchocerciasis); rectal snips (schistosomiasis); urine concentration (schistosomiasis); string test (strongyloidiasis); sputum for O&P (migrating larvae, paragonimiasis); and biopsy of any abnormal lesions. Serologic tests are available for many of the common helminthic infections, but such testing is hampered by lack of standardization and broad cross-reactivity among many helminth species. Nevertheless, serologic tests can be extremely helpful when the results are positive for an expatriate individual with a history of exposure to only one or a few specific parasites. Lifelong residents of tropical areas with constant and intense exposure to a wide variety of pathogens may be seropositive to many parasites without actually harboring current infection.

The detection of one parasitic infection does not preclude the presence of another. Patients should complete the diagnostic workup that is clinically and epidemiologically indicated. Similarly, follow-up is necessary for treated patients to be certain that both infection and eosinophilia have resolved.

When to Refer

The special medical needs of some travelers, such as those with HIV infection, immunocompromising conditions, pregnancy, or chronic disease, are dealt with elsewhere in the text. These patients are best referred to a specialized travel medicine clinic.

SUGGESTED READING

American Academy of Pediatrics. 2000 Red Book. Report of the Committee on Infectious Diseases. Elk Grove, Ill.: American Academy of Pediatrics; 2000. http://www.aap.org/aapstore/default.htm.

Auerbach PS, Donner HJ, Weiss EA. Field Guide to Wilderness Medicine. St. Louis: Mosby; 1999.

Centers for Disease Control. Health information for international travel. 1999-2000 Edition. US Department of Health and Human Services, Centers for Disease Control and Prevention (Order from the Catalogue #017-023 00202-3 of the US Government Printing Office).

Chin J. Control of Communicable Diseases Manual. 17th ed. Washington, DC: American Public Health Association; 2000.

Freedman DO, ed. Travel medicine. Infect Dis Clin North Am 1998; 12: 249-554.

Guerrant RL, Walker DH, Weller PF, eds. Essentials of Tropical Infectious Diseases. New York: Churchill Livingstone; 2001.

Hertzstein JA. International Occupational and Environmental Medicine. St. Louis: Mosby; 1998.

Jong EC, McMullen R. The Travel and Tropical Medicine Manual. 3rd ed. Philadelphia: W.B. Saunders Company; 2001.

Juckett G. Malaria prevention in travelers. Am Fam Physician 1999; 59: 2523-2530, 2535-2536.

Keystone JS, Kozarsky PE, Freedman DO. Internet and computer-based resources for travel medicine practitioners. Clin Infect Dis 2001; 32: 757-765.

Matteelli A, Carosi G. Sexually transmitted diseases in travelers. Clin Infect Dis 2001; 32: 1063-1067.

Monooee A, Rickman LS. Infectious diseases on cruise ships. Clin Infect Dis 1999; 29: 737-744.

Partiff K. Martindale, the Complete Drug Reference. 32nd ed. London: PhP Pharmaceutical Press; 2000.

Strickland GT, ed. Hunter's Tropical Medicine and Emerging Infectious Diseases. 8th ed., Philadelphia: W.B. Saunders Company; 1999.

Thompson RF. Travel and Routine Immunizations 2000, a Practical Guide for the Medical Office. Milwaukee, Wisc.: Shoreland, Inc.; 2000. http://www.shoreland.com.

Wilson ME. A World Guide to Infections. New York: Oxford University Press; 1991.

25 Immunization

WILLIAM H. BARKER

With the exception of environmental hygiene directed at waterborne, foodborne, and airborne transmission of disease, no general strategy can compare with immunization for protecting against infectious diseases and their complications. The impact of immunization, although dramatized by the 20th-century eradication of smallpox and the imminent global eradication of polio, is perhaps most immediately apparent to clinicians in the remarkable record of decline in the annually reported cases of once common vaccine-preventable diseases of childhood in the United States:

- Measles has been reduced from a maximum of nearly 900,000 cases in 1921 to only 86 cases in 1999.
- Mumps has been reduced from a maximum of >152,000 cases in 1968 to only 352 cases in 1999.
- Rubella has been reduced from nearly 58,000 cases in 1969 to 128 cases in 1995.
- Diphtheria has been reduced from >200,000 cases in 1921 to no cases in 1995.
- Pertussis has been reduced from >265,000 cases in 1934 to just over 1000 cases in 1976.
- Invasive infections caused by *Haemophilus influenzae* type b in children <5 years of age have been reduced from an estimated 20,000 cases per year before 1985 to 230 cases in 1999.

However, the unrealized potential for immunization, particularly among adults, is manifest by the estimated 50,000 to 60,000 influenza- or pneumococcal-related deaths and the 5000 to 6000 hepatitis B–related deaths annually in the United States, many of which could be averted by more effective use of available vaccines.

The task of effectively using vaccines is preeminently that of primary care practitioners and their colleagues in community-based services, such as local health departments, home care agencies, and student health programs. This chapter first covers general knowledge and principles applicable to vaccines and their successful delivery. The major content of the chapter comprises succinct reviews of knowledge regarding selected vaccine-preventable diseases and the composition, effectiveness, side effects, and current recommended use of licensed vaccines for their prevention. These begin with brief sections on standard combined childhood vaccinations (diphtheria-pertussis-tetanus and measles-mumps-rubella) followed by sections on individual vaccines currently used in the United States, which are covered in alphabetical order. Updated recommendations and further information are available from the National Immunization Program at the Centers for Disease Control and Prevention (CDC) website at www.cdc.gov.

SUGGESTED WEBSITES

Immunization Action Coalition, a public-private-funded clearinghouse for a wide variety of current immunization information for health care professionals and consumers: www.immunize.org.

Periodic Reports of the Advisory Committee on Immunization Practices (ACIP), which include current recommendations for specific vaccine-preventable diseases and for selected population subgroups, including children, adolescents, adults, pregnant women, immunocompromised persons, and health care workers: www.cdc.gov/nip/publications/ACIP.

Red Book 2000: Report of the Committee on Infectious Diseases, American Academy of Pediatrics: www.aap.org.

SUGGESTED READING

American Academy of Pediatrics, Committee on Infectious Diseases. Report of the Committee on Infectious Diseases. 25th ed., Elk Grove Village, Ill.: American Academy of Pediatrics; 2000.

American College of Physicians Task Force on Adult Immunization and Infectious Diseases Society of America. Guide for Adult Immunization. 4th ed., Philadelphia: American College of Physicians; 2001.

Centers for Disease Control and Prevention. National Childhood Vaccine Act: Requirements for permanent vaccination records and for reporting selected events after vaccination. MMWR 1988; 37: 97-100.

Dennehy PH. Active immunization in the United States: developments over the past decade. Clin Microbiol Rev 2001; 14: 872-908.

Gardner P, Peters G. Vaccine recommendations: challenges and controversies. Infect Dis Clin North Am 2001; 15: 1-333.

Humiston SG, Good C. Vaccinating Your Child: Questions and Answers for the Concerned Parent. Atlanta: Peachtree Publishers; 2000.

Jenson HB. Pocket Guide to Vaccination and Prophylaxis. Philadelphia: W.B. Saunders Company; 1999.

Plotskin SA, Orenstein WA, eds. Vaccines. 3rd ed., Philadelphia: W.B. Saunders Company; 1999.

Yu VL, Merigan TC, Barriere SL, eds. Antimicrobial therapy and vaccines. Baltimore: Williams & Wilkins; 1999.

Principles of Immunization

The primary care clinician should be familiar with the basic types of vaccines and also with systems or strategies that have been shown to be useful for enhancing the effective use of vaccines in office settings.

Vaccine Classification: Live Attenuated and Inactivated

Vaccines are broadly divided into two basic types, which determine how they are used.

Live attenuated vaccines are produced by modifying the disease-causing "wild" form of a virus or bacterium to an innocuous form, which will multiply and induce an immune response in the recipient without causing the disease. Such vaccines tend to confer long-lasting immunity after a single parenteral inoculation, except for orally administered agents (e.g., live polio vaccine), which require a series of doses to immunize. A protective immune response, identical to that with natural infection, occurs within 2 to 3 weeks. Live vaccines are labile and must be handled properly to avoid damage by heat and light. The most common side effects include soreness and redness at the administration site and an occasional mild transient form of the primary disease occurring within a typical incubation period of 7 to 21 days (e.g., a mild rash following measles or rubella vaccine.) These attenuated vaccines may grow out of control and cause serious illness in immunodeficient persons (e.g., patients with leukemia or receiving immunosuppressive drugs), and hence they should not be given to such persons. Commonly used live attenuated vaccines include those for measles, mumps, rubella, polio, yellow fever, varicella, and (formerly) vaccinia for smallpox.

Inactivated vaccines are derived from killed viruses or bacteria and may comprise the whole organism or fractional components such as toxoids, subunits, or polysaccharide surface antigen. An immune response often requires multiple doses spaced over time, as well as periodic booster inoculations, to attain and maintain protective antibody levels. Because they do not replicate in the recipient, inactivated vaccines cannot cause the disease against which they immunize and can safely be given to immunocompromised persons. Principal adverse reactions or side effects occurring within 1 to 3 days and of brief duration consist of local soreness; redness and swelling at the inoculation site, which is quite common; and systematic malaise or mild fever, which is less common.

Inactivated vaccines in current use include inactivated whole viruses and bacteria (polio, influenza, rabies, and hepatitis A; pertussis and cholera); viral or bacterial subunits (influenza and hepatitis B; acellular pertussis, typhoid Vi, and Lyme disease); pure polysaccharides (pneumococcal, *Haemophilus influenzae* type b, meningococcal); conjugated polysaccharides (*H. influenzae* type b and pneumococcal); and toxoids (diphtheria, tetanus, botulinum).

Allergic reactions may be caused by attenuated or inactivated vaccines related to the vaccine antigen proper or to material used in vaccine production or preservation. Such reactions, which may be life threatening, are fortunately exceedingly rare.

Vaccine Delivery

Successful delivery of vaccines to those for whom they are intended is greatly enhanced when practitioners make optimal use of opportunities to vaccinate individuals and employ simple systems to reach all eligible persons in their practices and communities.

(Missed) Opportunities

At the heart of making optimal use of opportunities to vaccinate is a sound understanding of valid and invalid contraindications to administering vaccines to specific individuals. Contraindications and precautions for administering live attenuated and inactivated vaccines are relatively few (Table 25-1). Pregnancy is a true contraindication to receiving live attenuated vaccines, on the hypothetical chance that such vaccines might infect and harm the fetus. Pregnancy is not, however, a contraindication to administering live vaccine to children with whom a pregnant woman (e.g., a mother or a classroom teacher) will come in contact. Immunocompromised individuals, as previously noted, should not receive live vaccines. Persons who have received antibody-containing blood products will respond well to killed vaccine but may not respond to live attenuated vaccines, which should accordingly be deferred for 5 to 6 months.

Mistaken perceptions by practitioners and the public regarding invalid contraindications account for costly and frequent missed opportunities to vaccinate children and adults. These include the following:

- Mild illness
- Antibiotic therapy
- Disease exposure or convalescence
- Pregnancy in the household
- Breast-feeding

TABLE 25-1

General Contraindications and Precautions for Administering Attenuated Live Vaccines and Inactivated Vaccines

Medical circumstances	Live attenuated vaccines	Inactivated vaccines
Allergy to component	Contraindicated	Contraindicated
Encephalopathy	—	Contraindicated
Pregnancy	Contraindicated	Vaccinate if indicated
Immunosuppression	Contraindicated	Vaccinate if indicated
Severe illness	Precaution	Precaution
Recent blood products	Precaution	Vaccinate if indicated

- Premature birth
- Allergies to products that are not in the vaccine
- Family history unrelated to immunosuppression
- Need for tuberculin skin testing
- Need for multiple vaccines

Certain of the preceding mistaken perceptions merit special emphasis. First and foremost, minor illness with low-grade fever such as upper respiratory infection, otitis media, or mild diarrhea does not reduce the immune response and should not be invoked as a reason to defer indicated immunizations. Simultaneous administration of attenuated as well as inactivated childhood and adult vaccinations does not result in decreased immune response to individual antigens; therefore multiple vaccines may be given simultaneously, with certain qualifications, as follow. The vaccines should not be combined in one syringe but should be administered separately and at separate sites. If two indicated live attenuated vaccines are not given the same day, the second should be administered after 30 days.

The common failure of adults to receive indicated vaccination is illustrated in the following typical vignettes, all of which represent mistaken reasons for not receiving annual influenza vaccination.

- A 27-year-old medical resident has had a runny nose for 10 days. She considers this not severe enough to keep her from working 10 to 12 hours a day on the medical wards, but good reason to put off receiving a flu shot because her immune system is "too taxed to respond to vaccine."
- An 81-year-old widow who has chronic bronchitis and adult-onset diabetes mellitus, controlled by daily insulin injections, lives in an apartment with her sister. She refuses to go to the public clinic with her sister for a free flu shot because last year she developed a bad cold and cough 4 days after "that no-good flu shot that just made me sick with the flu!"
- A 20-year-old clerk in a clothing store, who is infected with human immunodeficiency virus (HIV), is advised by a medical student friend not to get a flu shot because of his HIV status.
- A 68-year-old college professor has a history of hypertension with enlarged heart and onset of congestive heart failure 2 years ago, now well managed with medication. He received a flu shot a little over a year ago and sees no reason to get a flu shot again this year, even though his physician has recommended it. "After all, I only get a tetanus shot once every 10 to 15 years."

Practice-Based Systems

Numerous studies have demonstrated a significant increase in the percentage of patients receiving indicated vaccinations when simple office-based management strategies are used to remind the clinician and the patients in his or her practice population when vaccinations are due. Such strategies are of two basic types.

The first type of strategy targets the individual patient during an office visit scheduled for any reason. Such approaches include displaying health maintenance schedules prominently in the front of patients' medical records and designating an office staff member to check routinely on patients' current vaccination status and offer the vaccinations that are currently indicated.

The second type of strategy targets the entire population of patients in the clinician's practice. This has the obvious advantage of reaching patients who have no other reason to schedule an office visit. Such approaches include using chart audits or registries to identify patients who are due for routine vaccinations and sending postcards or making telephone calls to remind such patients of their needed vaccinations. A particularly innovative denominator-driven technique, which has been used successfully to enhance provision of annual influenza vaccination to older patients, is shown in Fig. 25-1. The practice first enumerates its census of Medicare patients, easily done from computerized billing systems, and then charts on a weekly basis the number and percentage of Medicare patients who receive flu shots during the fall months. The patients who are not seen are then contacted by telephone or other means.

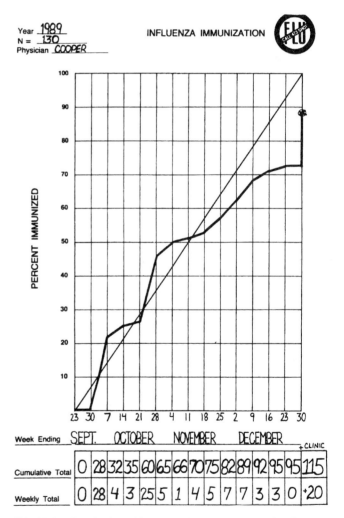

FIG. 25-1 Practice-based immunization strategy: completed poster from a physician. N is the target population of patients ≥65 years of age. The weekly and cumulative numbers of immunizations are tallied below the graph, and the percentage of the target population immunized is plotted weekly. "Clinic" refers to patients in the practice who were immunized in public health clinics. (From Buffington J, Bell KM, LaForce FM, et al. A target-based model for increasing influenza immunizations in private practice. J Gen Intern Med 1991; 6: 204-209.)

KEY POINTS

PRINCIPLES OF IMMUNIZATION

- ➲ Live attenuated vaccines currently in use include those for measles, mumps, rubella, polio, yellow fever, and varicella-zoster viruses. Except for orally administered agents (e.g., live polio vaccine), these vaccines tend to confer long-lasting immunity after a single inoculation. In immunocompetent persons these vaccines are extremely safe, although occasionally a mild, transient form of the primary disease develops. Live attenuated vaccines may, however, cause serious diseases in persons who are immunocompromised because of diseases (e.g., leukemia) or immunosuppressive drugs.

- ➲ Inactivated vaccines, derived from killed viruses, bacteria, or their products, often require multiple doses and periodic booster inoculations to ensure protective antibody levels. Because these vaccines do not replicate in the recipient, they can be given safely to immunocompromised persons. Allergic reactions can be life threatening but are exceedingly rare.

- ➲ Unfortunately, there are widespread misconceptions concerning contraindications to vaccination. Factors mistakenly believed to contraindicate vaccination include mild illnesses, antibiotic therapy, disease exposure, pregnancy in the household, breast-feeding, premature birth, allergies to products that are not in the vaccine, the need for tuberculin skin testing, and the need for multiple vaccines.

- ➲ Primary care clinicians should develop and maintain strategies for efficient use of vaccines.

- ➲ One strategy consists of keeping a health maintenance schedule at the front of patients' records and designating an office staff member to check routinely on each patient's vaccination status before or during an office visit.

- ➲ A second and complementary strategy consists of chart audits or registries to identify persons due for routine vaccinations, with postcards or telephone calls to remind such patients of needed vaccinations. Innovative ways to reach target populations continue to be developed.

SUGGESTED READING

Association of Teachers of Preventive Medicine. What works: computer assisted instruction on strategies to improve adult vaccination rates. For information visit the website www.atpm.org.

Briss PA, Rodewald LE, Hinman AR, et al. Reviews of evidence regarding interventions to improve vaccination coverage in children, adolescents, and adults. Am J Prev Med 2000; 18(1S): 97-140.

Combination vaccines for childhood immunization: recommendations of the Advisory Committee on Immunization Practices (ACIP), the American Academy of Pediatrics (AAP), and the American Academy of Family Physicians (AAFP). Pediatrics 1999; 103: 1064-1077.

Gellin BG, Curlin GT, Raginovich NR, et al. Adult immunization: principles and practice. Adv Intern Med 1999; 44: 327-352.

Handal GA. Adolescent immunization. Adolesc Med 2000; 11: 439-452.

Hensrud DD. Clinical preventive medicine in primary care: background and practice. II. Delivering primary preventive services. Mayo Clin Proc 2000; 75: 255-264.

Muñoz FM, Englund JA. A step ahead: infant protection through maternal immunization. Pediatr Clin North Am 2000; 47: 449-463.

Plotkin SA. Immunologic correlates of protection induced by vaccination. Pediatr Infect Dis J 2001; 20: 63-75.

Szilagyi PG, Bordley C, Vann JC, et al. Effect of patient reminder/recall interventions on immunization rates: a review. JAMA 2000; 284: 1820-1827.

Vaccine-Preventable Diseases: Overview

The list of diseases that are amenable to prevention by vaccines continues to expand. In this section are reviewed the major vaccines in general use in the United States, beginning with the long-standing combined childhood vaccinations. Recommended childhood immunizations are summarized in Chapter 4. Recommended adult immunizations are summarized in this chapter. Vaccines recommended for travel to other parts of the world are discussed in Chapter 24.

Diphtheria, Pertussis, and Tetanus

Diphtheria, pertussis, and tetanus, caused respectively by bacterial pathogens *Corynebacterium diphtheriae* and its toxin, *Bordetella pertussis,* and *Clostridium tetani* and its toxin, were among the first serious infectious diseases to be dramatically reduced in the United States and elsewhere by universal childhood vaccination (Table 25-1). Noteworthy current epidemiologic observations remind us of the continuing potential threats posed by these vaccine-preventable diseases. Serosurveys in the United States since the late 1970s indicate that a substantial proportion of adults may lack protective levels of circulatory antitoxin against both diphtheria and tetanus, presumably in most instances because of waning vaccine-induced immunity from childhood. Pertussis, a traditionally highly communicable disease of childhood, with particularly severe complications among the very young, has in recent years been increasingly diagnosed and reported among adults, who may in turn become a source of transmission to unvaccinated or incompletely vaccinated young children.

Since the late 1940s a series of inoculations with inactivated vaccine combining diphtheria and tetanus toxoid with pertussis bacterial antigen has been a mainstay of well-child care. Diphtheria and tetanus toxoids are produced by formaldehyde treatment of the respective toxins, with the amount incorporated in vaccine varying according to the age of the vaccine recipients (Box 25-1). Pertussis vaccine, originally comprising inactivated whole cell *B. pertussis,* administered in combination with the diphtheria and tetanus toxoids as DTP, was in the 1990s largely supplanted by the equally effective and much safer acellular pertussis antigen. This antigen, first licensed in 1991, is given with the diphtheria and tetanus toxoids in combined form as DTaP vaccine. The original whole cell pertussis vaccine often causes pain at the inoculation site and high fever, as well as infrequent but distressing hypotonic episodes, seizures, and inconsolable crying. All of these adverse effects are markedly reduced with the acellular vaccine. Side effects of tetanus and diphtheria toxoids are limited to mild soreness at the inoculation site. Current recommendations of the CDC's Advisory Committee on Immunization Practices (ACIP) are summarized in Box 25-1.

SUGGESTED READING

Conrad DA, Jenson HB. Using acellular pertussis vaccines for childhood immunization: potential benefits far outweigh potential risks. Postgrad Med 1999; 105: 165-168, 171-173, 177-178.

Eskola J, Ward J, Dagan R, et al. Combined vaccination of *Haemophilus influenzae* type b conjugate and diphtheria-tetanus-pertussis containing acellular pertussis. Lancet 1999; 354: 2063-2068.

Matheson AJ, Goa KL. Diphtheria-tetanus-acellular pertussis vaccine adsorbed (Triacelluvax; DTaP3-CB): a review of its use in the prevention of *Bordetella pertussis* infection. Paediatr Drugs 2000; 2: 139-159.

Measles, Mumps, and Rubella

Measles, mumps, and rubella, once a group of extremely common communicable diseases of childhood, have been all but eliminated in the United States through the widespread use of live attenuated vaccines developed in the latter part of the 20th century. All three diseases are caused by viruses for which humans serve as the reservoir. The viruses infect the respiratory tract initially, spread readily from person to person, and confer lifelong immunity after natural infection.

Measles has an incubation period of 10 to 14 days, with characteristic widespread rash, coryza, and fever developing in virtually all infected persons. Diarrhea, otitis media, and pneumonia are common complications, and encephalitis or death occurs in approximately 1 in 1000 cases. Mumps occurs after an incubation period of 16 to 18 days, with classic clinical manifestations of parotitis often accompanied by low-grade fever or upper respiratory tract symptoms; complications, which occur most often in adults, include aseptic meningitis and orchitis. The incubation period for rubella is 12 to 24 days, with illness consisting of a relatively mild rash, often accompanied by transient low-grade fever, lymphadenopathy, or arthralgia. The arthralgia occurs more commonly among adults. Rubella infection during pregnancy can severely affect the fetus (see Chapter 5).

Although individual live attenuated vaccines were originally developed for the respective diseases, the preferred product for current use is the combined measles-mumps-rubella (MMR) vaccine (Box 25-2). Each of the components produces protective antibodies in 90% to 95% of recipients following a single dose offered after 1 year of age, and with a second dose some 99% are protected. Vaccine-induced immunity appears to be lifelong. Side effects of MMR vaccine, seen in approximately 5% of vaccine recipients, include temperature $\geq 103°$ F ($39.4°$ C), mild rash, and lymphadenopathy, all of which occur 7 to 12 days after vaccination and are of short duration. More severe adverse events have been postulated, and evidence supports a causal relation between MMR and thrombocytopenia, febrile seizures, and acute arthritis.

Postexposure prophylaxis with immune globulin (IG) administered within 6 days of exposure may prevent or reduce severity of measles infection in persons lacking natural or vaccine-induced immunity. Postexposure IG does not protect against rubella or mumps infection.

SUGGESTED READING

Afzal MA, Minor PD, Schild GC. Clinical safety issues of measles, mumps and rubella vaccines. Bull World Health Organ 2000; 78: 199-204.

Robertson SE, Cutts FT, Samuel R, et al. Control of rubella and congenital rubella syndrome (CRS) in developing countries. Part 2: Vaccination against rubella. Bull World Health Organ 1997; 75: 69-80.

Wild TF. Measles vaccines, new developments and immunization strategies. Vaccine 1999; 17: 1726-1729.

BOX 25-1
Diphtheria-Tetanus-Pertussis (DTP) Vaccine (2000)

- All children should receive a full course of primary vaccination with combined vaccine, preferably DTaP, at standard recommended intervals of 2 months, 4 months, 6 months, 15 to 18 months, and 4 to 6 years of age. If encephalopathy develops within 7 days of vaccination, it is presumed to be caused by central nervous system sensitivity to pertussis antigen, and the vaccination schedule should be completed with diphtheria-tetanus (DT) vaccine only.
- Adults with uncertain history of completion of a primary DTaP vaccination series should receive a primary series using the combined Td toxoid, which contains a smaller quantity of diphtheria toxoid than that contained in TD.
- All persons who have completed primary DTP immunization should receive a booster inoculation with Td at approximately 10-year intervals.
- Postexposure prophylaxis in persons with severe unclean wounds, and therefore risk of exposure to tetanus spores, may be provided with tetanus immune globulin given simultaneously with Td booster. Passive immunization is of no proven benefit for susceptible persons exposed to pertussis, and use of diphtheria antitoxin, a highly allergenic and questionably protective product prepared from equine sera, is not generally recommended for susceptible persons exposed to diphtheria.

Practices recommended by the Advisory Committee on Immunization Practices of the Centers for Disease Control and Prevention.

BOX 25-2
Measles-Mumps-Rubella (MMR) Vaccine (1998)

- All children should receive a two-dose regimen of MMR, with the initial dose administered at 12 to 15 months of age and second dose at 4 to 6 years of age, before entrance into kindergarten or first grade.
- Adults born before 1957, with the exception of women who could become pregnant, can be considered immune to measles, mumps, and rubella by virtue of natural infection. Those born since 1957 who lack history of vaccination or natural disease or lack serologic evidence of immunity should be considered susceptible and should receive a two-dose course of MMR vaccine. This recommendation is particularly important for health care workers.
- Women of childbearing age who lack evidence of rubella immunity should be vaccinated with MMR, but not during pregnancy. As a rule, MMR should not be administered to immunocompromised persons, including those with congenital or acquired immunodeficiency disorders or those receiving immunosuppressive treatment, including high-dose corticosteroids. MMR is, however, recommended for human immunodeficiency virus–infected persons who are not severely immunocompromised as reflected in their CD4 and T-lymphocyte counts.

Practices recommended by the Advisory Committee on Immunization Practices of the Centers for Disease Control and Prevention.

Haemophilus Influenzae Type B

Before the development of the *H. influenzae* type b (Hib) vaccine, invasive Hib disease occurred in 1 in 200 children before 5 years of age. Meningitis developed in 60% of these cases, and 20% to 30% of survivors had permanent sequelae ranging from hearing loss to mental retardation. Humans are the reservoir for Hib, and asymptomatic carriage is relatively common. Airborne droplets or discharges from infected or colonized persons spread this pathogen; the portal of entry is the nasopharynx, and the incubation period is usually 2 to 4 days. Pathogenicity is conferred by the polyribosylribitol phosphate (PRP) capsule of Hib, and antibody to PRP is the primary basis for protection.

A pure polysaccharide Hib vaccine, licensed in the United States in 1985, was displaced after 1988 by polysaccharide-protein conjugated vaccines. The former, like other T-cell–independent polysaccharide antigens, is poorly immunogenic in children under 2 years of age (those at greatest risk from invasive Hib disease). By contrast, the T-cell–dependent protein antigen in the latter product confers highly immunogenic properties. In multiple field trials the several variant conjugate vaccines were shown to confer efficacy levels exceeding 90% against invasive Hib disease. Since their widespread use among infants in the United States and other developed countries, these diseases have been mostly eliminated. Adverse effects of Hib conjugated vaccines are largely limited to short-lived local swelling, redness, or pain at the inoculation site and occasional fever. ACIP recommendations for Hib conjugated vaccine administration, which varies slightly in frequency depending on product, are shown in Box 25-3.

SUGGESTED READING

Galil K, Singleton R, Levine OS, et al. Reemergence of invasive *Haemophilus influenzae* type b disease in a well-vaccinated population in remote Alaska. J Infect Dis 1999; 179: 101-106.
Peltola H. Prophylaxis of bacterial meningitis. Infect Dis Clin North Am 1999; 13: 685-710.
Peltola H. Worldwide *Haemophilus influenzae* type b disease at the beginning of the 21st century: global analysis of the disease burden

---

BOX 25-3
Haemophilus Influenzae Serotype B (Hib) Vaccine (1991)

- A multiple-dose schedule of vaccine should be given universally to children beginning at 6 to 8 weeks of age, but no sooner, and ending with the final dose at 12 to 15 months of age.
- Children less than 2 years of age who have had invasive Hib disease should be vaccinated because many young children fail to develop immunity after natural Hib disease.
- Previously unvaccinated children 15 to 59 months of age should receive a single dose of vaccine.
- In general, unvaccinated children ≥5 years of age do not require Hib vaccine. However, unvaccinated older children and adults with high risk for invasive Hib disease, including those with functional asplenia, immunodeficiency, immunosuppression from cancer chemotherapy, or HIV infection, should receive at least one dose of conjugate vaccine.

Practices recommended by the Advisory Committee on Immunization Practices of the Centers for Disease Control and Prevention.

---

25 years after the use of the polysaccharide vaccine and a decade after the advent of conjugates. Clin Microbiol Rev 2000; 13: 302-317.

Hepatitis A

Hepatitis A virus (HAV; see Chapter 13) is associated with low mortality but substantial morbidity. Inactivated and attenuated HAV vaccines have been developed, but only the former—Havrix and Vaqta—have been licensed for use in the United States. Both are administered in a two-dose schedule intramuscularly in the deltoid muscle and have been shown to elicit protective antibody levels in over 95% of children and adults within 1 month of the first dose. Double-blind randomized clinical trials have documented 95% to 100% efficacy in preventing clinical hepatitis A. Side effects are largely limited to short-lived soreness at the injection site, headache, or malaise, and to date, after millions of vaccinations of adults and children, virtually no serious adverse events have been attributed to hepatitis A vaccine. As shown in Box 25-4, the ACIP (1999) recommends hepatitis A vaccination for two broad groups.

Postexposure prophylactic administration of pooled immune globulin, once the mainstay of clinical prevention of hepatitis A, is currently recommended only for persons with known exposure to hepatitis A (e.g., at home, at work, or at a restaurant) who had not been vaccinated against hepatitis A at least 1 month earlier. IG should be administered within 2 weeks of exposure.

SUGGESTED READING

Marcus EL, Tur-Kaspa R. Viral hepatitis in older adults. J Am Geriatr Soc 1997; 45: 755-763.

Hepatitis B

Hepatitis B virus (HBV; see Chapter 13) causes chronic liver disease and continues to be a major public health problem. Inactivated vaccines, first licensed in the United States in the 1980s, consist of HBsAg produced by recombinant DNA technology. Immunization involves a series of injections in the deltoid muscle, which induces a readily detectable antibody response in over 90% of children and adults, with 80% to 95% protective efficacy against infection, as demonstrated in field trials. Immunologic memory has been found to persist for at least 15 years; therefore to date there is no apparent need for booster vaccination. Mirroring hepatitis A vaccine, side effects

---

BOX 25-4
Hepatitis A Virus (HAV) Vaccine (1999)

- HAV vaccine is appropriate for children living in states, counties, or defined areas (e.g., Native American communities) with average annual hepatitis A rates during the past decade of ≥20 cases per 100,000 population (approximately twice the national average). The ultimate goal is to reduce high rates of transmission while protecting individuals.
- Vaccination is recommended for individuals in subgroups at increased risk of exposure or serious complications, including travelers to countries with high endemic occurrence of hepatitis A, injecting drug users, men who have sex with men, and persons with chronic liver disease.

Practices recommended by the Advisory Committee on Immunization Practices of the Centers for Disease Control and Prevention.

have been mild and self-limited and serious adverse events exceedingly rare. For long-term reduction of hepatitis B infections in the general population and to protect individuals currently at high risk of exposure, the ACIP recommends a multifaceted strategy for hepatitis B vaccine (Box 25-5).

Vaccination is recommended for selected high-risk groups, including persons with occupational risk of exposure to blood products; all persons involved in personal health care, who should preferably be vaccinated during training in professional school; clients, and staff who work closely with clients, in institutions for the developmentally disabled; hemodialysis patients; household contacts and sex partners of HBV carriers; men who have sex with men; injecting drug users; and inmates of correctional facilities with histories of aforementioned high-risk behaviors.

Postexposure prophylaxis with HBIG is indicated for any person in the preceding categories and others who have known percutaneous, sexual, or mucosal exposure to HBV and who have not been fully vaccinated against the disease.

SUGGESTED READING

Mast EE, Mahoney FJ, Alter MJ, et al. Progress toward elimination of hepatitis B virus transmission in the United States. Vaccine 1998; 16 (Suppl): S48-S51.
Scheifele D. Universal childhood hepatitis B vaccination: infants vs. preadolescents, the Canadian perspective. Pediatr Infect Dis J 1998; 17 (Suppl 7): S35-S37.

Influenza

Types A and B influenza virus (see Chapter 11) are responsible for mild to severe epidemics virtually every year in the winter months and infrequent pandemics (1889, 1918, 1957, 1968), which are caused, respectively, by a minor "drift" or a major "shift" in the virus's hemagglutinin (H) or neuraminidase (N) glycoprotein surface antigens. Annual epidemic influenza is caused most often by influenza A strains (H3N2 and H1N1 have been predominant since the 1970s) owing to greater mutability of their surface glycoproteins, although epidemics caused by type B or involving both type A and B occur every several years. Transmission is predominantly by airborne droplets. After an incubation period of 1 to 4 days, illness often commences with abrupt onset of fever, myalgia, headache, dry cough, and sore throat. Clinical attack rates during annual epidemics range from 10% to 30% in the general population, with the highest rates in

children. Secondary bacterial pneumonia or complications of underlying chronic cardiopulmonary disease, occurring primarily among frail older persons, cause high rates of excess mortality and morbidity ranging from 10,000 to 40,000 deaths and 150,000 to 200,000 hospitalizations annually.

Inactivated vaccine, derived from virus grown in embryonated hens' eggs, is produced annually and consists of a combination of antigens from each of the wild strains of influenza predicted to cause epidemic illness in humans during the coming year. In recent years these have been trivalent vaccines, containing H1N1, H3N2, and B antigen. Vaccine, injected in the deltoid muscle, is given during the autumn months: a single dose of whole virus vaccine is given to adults, and two doses of less pyrogenic split or purified vaccine is given to young children. Protective antibodies are present within 2 to 3 weeks. Efficacy in preventing clinical influenza caused by strains matched to those in the vaccine is 70% to 90% among healthy persons <65 years of age. The major benefit conferred among older persons, including those residing in nursing homes, and among persons of all ages with high-risk chronic disease (see later discussion), is protection against influenza-related hospitalization and deaths, with observed levels of effectiveness ranging from 30% to 70%.

Soreness at the injection site is a relatively common side effect, and systemic symptoms (fever, malaise) may occur less often, beginning within 6 to 12 hours and lasting 1 to 2 days. It is important to recognize that the vaccine contains noninfectious killed virus and cannot cause influenza. During 1976 some influenza vaccine was associated with the occurrence of Guillain-Barré syndrome at a rate of 10 excess cases per million vaccine recipients. However, close surveillance in subsequent years reveals an exceedingly small risk, if any, of Guillain-Barré syndrome, which is far outweighed by the excess morbidity prevented by vaccination against influenza. Current ACIP recommendations are shown in Box 25-6. Persons who provide essential community services (e.g., firefighters, police officers) should also be considered for annual influenza vaccination.

BOX 25-5
Hepatitis B Virus (HBV) Vaccine (1991)

- Universal vaccination of newborns should preferably begin before the infant is discharged from the hospital. If the mother is HBsAg positive, hepatitis B immune globulin (HBIG) should be administered to the newborn within 12 hours for immediate immunoprophylaxis as well as to initiate the routine schedule of hepatitis B vaccination.
- All children through age 18 years, if not vaccinated earlier as part of universal newborn vaccination, should be vaccinated.

Practices recommended by the Advisory Committee on Immunization Practices of the Centers for Disease Control and Prevention.

BOX 25-6
Influenza Vaccine (2000)

- Influenza vaccine is recommended for those at increased risk for complications, including all persons aged ≥50 years (revised in 2000 from previous recommendation to vaccinate all persons aged ≥65 years); residents of nursing homes and other chronic care facilities; adults and children of any age who have chronic cardiovascular or pulmonary conditions, including asthma, or who require regular medical follow-up for chronic metabolic disease (e.g., diabetes mellitus), renal dysfunction, hemoglobinopathies, or drug- or disease-induced immunosuppression, including human immunodeficiency virus infection; children receiving chronic aspirin therapy who might be at risk for Reye's syndrome if infected by influenza; and women who will be in the second or third trimester of pregnancy during the influenza season.
- Persons with increased potential to transmit influenza to high-risk individuals—including health care workers, employees of nursing homes and residential facilities for older persons, and members of households where high-risk persons live—should also be vaccinated.

Practices recommended by the Advisory Committee on Immunization Practices of the Centers for Disease Control and Prevention.

SUGGESTED READING

Bradley SF. Long-Term-Care Committee of the Society for Healthcare Epidemiology of America. Prevention of influenza in long-term-care facilities. Infect Control Hosp Epidemiol 1999; 20: 629-637.

Centers for Disease Control and Prevention. Prevention and control of influenza: recommendations of the Advisory Committee on Immunization Practices (ACIP). MMWR 2001; 50 (RR-4): 1-44.

Cox NJ, Subbarao K. Influenza. Lancet 1999; 354: 1277-1282.

Maassab HF, Bryant ML. The development of live attenuated cold-adapted influenza virus vaccine for humans. Rev Med Virol 1999; 9: 237-244.

Nichol KL. Cost-benefit analysis of a strategy to vaccinate healthy working adults against influenza. Arch Intern Med 2001; 161: 749-759.

Nguyen-Van-Tam JS, Keal KR. Clinical effectiveness, policies, and practices for influenza and pneumococcal vaccines. Semin Respir Infect 1999; 14: 184-195.

Zimmerman RK. Lowering the age for routine influenza vaccination to 50 years: AAFP leads the nation in influenza vaccine policy. Am Fam Physician 1999; 60: 2061-2066, 2069-2070.

Lyme Disease

Lyme disease (see Chapter 7), caused by the spirochete *Borrelia burgdorferi,* is a tickborne zoonosis transmitted to humans by the bite of infected ticks of the genus *Ixodes.* Over 60,000 clinical cases were reported in the United States between 1993 and 1997, with the highest risk among persons who live in regions of high endemicity and engage in extensive occupational, residential, horticultural, recreational, or leisure activities in wooded or overgrown brush settings likely to serve as tick habitats. Incubation period from tick bite to appearance of characteristic bull's eye erythema migrans rash is typically 1 to 2 weeks, but it may range from 3 to 30 days.

Lyme disease vaccine, first licensed for use in the United States in 1998, is a recombinant-derived vaccine composed of the *B. burgdorferi* outer surface protein OspA. The vaccine is administered intramuscularly in the deltoid muscle as a three-dose regimen, with second and third doses given at 1 and 12 months after the initial dose. In randomized clinical trials involving subjects between 15 and 70 years of age living in Lyme disease–endemic areas, individuals taking two doses of vaccine attained 49% protective efficacy, and those

taking three doses attained 76% protective efficacy against occurrence of laboratory-confirmed clinical Lyme disease. Vaccine side effects consist of soreness at the injection site and, in a small percentage, short-lived fever and myalgia. Late-onset musculoskeletal adverse effects have not been observed. The ACIP recommendations for use of Lyme disease vaccine are shown in Box 25-7. The duration of protection and need for booster inoculation of this recently released vaccine remain to be determined. Vaccination appears to be cost effective only when the seasonal probability of *B. burgdorferi* infection is greater than 1%.

SUGGESTED READING

Gerber MA. Lyme disease vaccine. Pediatr Infect Dis J 1999; 18: 825-826.

Hayney MS, Grunske MM, Boh LE. Lyme disease prevention and vaccine prophylaxis. Ann Pharmacother 1999; 33: 723-729.

Lyme disease vaccine. Med Lett 1999; 41: 29-30.

Morey SS. Advisory Committee on Immunization Practices. ACIP issues recommendations for Lyme disease vaccine. Am Fam Physician 1999; 60: 2171-2172.

Orloski KA, Hayes EB, Campbell GL, et al. Surveillance for Lyme disease—United States, 1992-1998. MMWR 2000; 49: 1-11.

Shadick NA, Liang MH, Phillips CB, et al. The cost-effectiveness of vaccination against Lyme disease. Arch Intern Med 2001; 161: 554-561.

Thanassi WT, Schoen RT. The Lyme disease vaccine: conception, development, and implementation. Ann Intern Med 2000; 132: 661-668.

Meningococcal Disease

Neisseria meningitidis is a leading cause of meningitis and sepsis in older children and young adults in the United States (see Chapter 6). Although serogroup A organisms were the major causes of epidemics earlier in the century, since the 1990s most cases in the United States have been caused by groups B, C, and Y. Some 3000 cases occur in the United States annually, for a rate approaching 1 per 100,000. More than 95% of cases occur sporadically. Somewhat increased rates have been well documented in healthy young adults residing in congregated circumstances, particularly new military recruits living in barracks and college freshmen living in dormitories.

Quadrivalent polysaccharide vaccine for meningococcal serogroups A, C, Y, and W-135 is licensed for use in the United States. Administered as a single subcutaneous dose to children and adults, the vaccine elicits protective levels of antibody within 2 weeks, which wane over time but are still detectable for up to 10 years. Side effects are generally mild, consisting of transient pain and redness at the injection site, as well as low-grade fever in a small percentage of young children. Clinical protective effectiveness rates of >85% have been well documented in children and young adults. The meningococcal vaccine is not recommended for universal use. Current ACIP recommendations for its use or consideration are shown in Box 25-8.

BOX 25-7
Lyme Disease Vaccine (1999)

- Vaccination is recommended for persons aged 15 to 70 years who live in regions of high Lyme disease endemicity and engage in frequent occupational, property maintenance, recreational, or leisure activities in tick-infested habitats.
- Vaccination is not recommended for persons living, working, or taking part in recreation in areas of low Lyme disease endemicity.
- Vaccination should be considered for persons with a history of previously uncomplicated Lyme disease who are at continued high risk of exposure; however, such persons with treatment-resistant Lyme arthritis should not be vaccinated because of the association between this condition and immune reactivity to OspA antigen.

Practices recommended by the Advisory Committee on Immunization Practices of the Centers for Disease Control and Prevention.

SUGGESTED READING

Harrison LH. Preventing meningococcal infection in college students. Clin Infect Dis 2000; 30: 648-651.

Harrison LH, Dwyer DM, Maples CT, et al. Risk of meningococcal infection in college students. JAMA 1999; 281: 1906-1910.

MacLennan JM, Shackley F, Heath PT, et al. Safety, immunogenicity, and induction of immunologic memory by a serogroup C meningococcal conjugate vaccine in infants: a randomized controlled trial. JAMA 2000; 283: 2795-2801.

Peltola H. Meningococcal vaccines: current status and future possibilities. Drugs 1998; 55: 347-366.

Prevention and control of meningococcal disease: recommendations of the Advisory Committee on Immunization Practices (ACIP). MMWR 2000; 49 (RR-7): 1-10.

Pneumococcal Disease

Streptococcus pneumoniae is a ubiquitous bacterial pathogen for which the upper respiratory tract of healthy humans serves as reservoir, and transmission occurs primarily person-to-person via airborne droplet spread. *S. pneumoniae* is a leading cause of preventable illness among children, particularly the very young, and adults, particularly the very old. It accounts for an estimated 3000 cases of meningitis, 50,000 cases of bacteremia, 500,000 cases of pneumonia, 7 million cases of otitis media, and 40,000 deaths annually in the United States. Mortality is highest among individuals contracting meningitis and bacteremia, with case-fatality rates ranging from 15% to 20% among all adult patients to 30% to 40% among elderly patients. These high fatality rates occur despite treatment with appropriate antibiotics and intensive medical care and may be expected to be exacerbated with the increasing emergence of antibiotic-resistant strains of pneumococcus (see Chapters 1 and 11). Invasive pneumococcal disease is especially common among African-American adults, Alaska natives, and Native Americans (American Indians).

Two forms of inactivated pneumococcal vaccine are now available for use in the United States. A 23-valent polysaccharide pneumococcal vaccine (PPV) was licensed in 1983, and a heptavalent pneumococcal conjugate vaccine was licensed in 2000. Characteristics of these two classes of pneumococcal vaccine and recommendations for their use are covered separately.

23-Valent Polysaccharide Pneumococcal Vaccine

The 23-valent PPV (Pneumovax-23; Pnu-Imune-23) is composed of capsular polysaccharide antigen from pathogenic strains that account for more than 80% of bacteremic pneumococcal infections in adults in the United States. Administered as a single dose by either subcutaneous or intramuscular injection, PPV elicits type-specific opsonizing antibody within 2 to 3 weeks in >80% of healthy young adults. Antibody responses are variable among the 23 antigens, are lower among persons with chronic disease and older persons, and are poor to nonexistent among children <2 years of age, whose maturing immune systems are relatively unresponsive to polysaccharide antigen. In numerous observational and experimental evaluations among adults with and without chronic disease, under and over 65 years of age, PPV has been shown to confer high levels of protection, ranging from 50% to 81%, against bacteremic disease caused by strains included in the vaccine. By contrast, these studies have found little evidence of PPV protection against nonbacteremic pneumonia or common upper respiratory disease (sinusitis, otitis media). In approximately one third of vaccine recipients, self-limited local side effects develop at the site of injection, and these effects have been found to be somewhat more likely among persons who are revaccinated 5 years or more after primary vaccination. Serious or life-threatening adverse reactions are virtually nonexistent. ACIP recommendations for the 23-valent PPV target the groups shown in Box 25-9, with the principal goal of preventing invasive, potentially fatal pneumococcal disease. Fig. 25-2 provides a helpful algorithm.

BOX 25-8
Meningococcal Vaccine (2000)

- Vaccine is used to control serogroup C meningococcal disease outbreaks, defined as occurrences of three or more confirmed cases within ≤3 months, with a resulting community attack rate of at least 10 cases per 100,000 population.
- Certain high-risk individuals, including persons with terminal complement component deficiency or functional asplenia, and laboratory workers or others at risk of aerosolized exposure to *Neisseria meningitidis* organisms, should have the vaccine.
- College freshmen (and their parents), particularly students planning to live in residence halls, should be made aware of the modest but real increased risk of meningococcal disease and of the availability of a safe and effective vaccine. Those who provide routine medical care to such students, either family physicians or college health services, should make the vaccine easily available to persons who wish to receive it. (These guidelines have been developed and disseminated in cooperation with the American College Health Association.)
- Persons planning extended residence in hyperendemic areas, particularly sub-Saharan Africa (see Chapter 24) should receive the vaccine.

BOX 25-9
23-Valent Polysaccharide Pneumococcal Vaccine (Pneumovax-23; Pnu-Imune-23) (1997)

- Vaccination is recommended for all persons >65 years of age, including revaccination of such persons who have not received PPV for at least 5 years and were <65 years of age when previously vaccinated.
- Immunocompetent persons between 2 and 64 years of age should be vaccinated if they have chronic cardiovascular, pulmonary, liver, or renal disease; have anatomic asplenia (e.g., sickle cell disease or splenectomy); or reside in a nursing home.
- Vaccination is recommended for immunocompromised persons >2 years of age, including those with leukemia, lymphoma, Hodgkin's disease, or human immunodeficiency virus infection, all of whom may or may not respond well to vaccine but are at risk for severe life-threatening pneumococcal infections. Persons scheduled to receive immunosuppressant chemotherapy or radiation therapy should be vaccinated at least 2 weeks before therapy is initiated.
- Native Americans (Alaskans and Indians) and others residing in communities with documented high endemic rates of invasive pneumococcal disease should receive the vaccine.

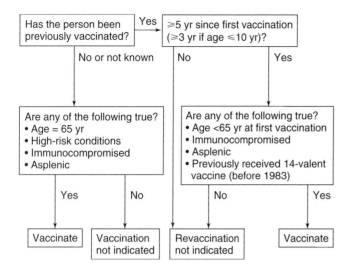

FIG. 25-2 Algorithm for using the 23-valent pneumococcal polysaccharide vaccine. The optimum frequency of revaccination for persons who have received two doses is unknown, but revaccination every 5 to 7 years for patients belonging to high-risk groups is a growing trend.

Pneumococcal Conjugate Vaccine

The newly licensed pneumococcal conjugate vaccine (PCV7; Prevnar) contains seven capsular antigens from strains that account for >80% of pneumococcal meningitis and bacteremia in very young children and that have been rendered highly immunogenic in this target population by conjugation with a protein carrier. Large randomized, controlled field trials have demonstrated >90% protection against invasive disease among vaccinees, as well as modest but significant reduction in otitis media–related morbidity. The vaccine is given intramuscularly in one of several schedules, according to the age of recipients, as follows:

- Age 2 to 6 months: three doses, 6 to 8 weeks apart, followed by a booster dose at 12 to 15 months of age
- Age 7 to 11 months: two doses, 6 to 8 weeks apart, followed by a booster dose at 12 to 15 months of age
- Age 12 to 23 months: two doses, 6 to 8 weeks apart
- Age ≥24 months: one dose

Observed side effects are limited to mild fever or soreness and redness at the site of injection. Recommendations of the American Academy of Pediatrics (AAP) Committee on Infectious Disease and ACIP for PCV7 are shown in Box 25-10.

SUGGESTED READING

Butler JC, Cetron MS. Pneumococcal drug resistance: the new "special enemy of old age." Clin Infect Dis 1999; 28: 730-735.

Butler JC, Shapiro ED, Carlone GM. Pneumococcal vaccines: history, current status, and future directions. Am J Med 1999; 107 (1A): 69S-76S.

Dagan R, Fraser D. Conjugate pneumococcal vaccine and antibiotic-resistant *Streptococcus pneumoniae:* herd immunity and reduction of otitis morbidity. Pediatr Infect Dis J 2000 ; 19 (Suppl 5): S79-S87.

Eskola J. Immunogenicity of pneumococcal conjugate vaccines. Pediatr Infect Dis J 2000; 19: 388-393.

BOX 25-10
Pneumococcal Conjugate Vaccine (Prevnar)

- Universal vaccination of children ≤23 months of age is recommended. The vaccination should be given concurrently with other recommended childhood vaccinations, with a reduced number of doses for those initiating vaccination between 7 and 23 months of age (see also Table 25-2).
- A two-dose regimen should be provided for children 24 to 59 months of age; persons at high risk for invasive pneumococcal disease, including those with any form of asplenia, human immunodeficiency virus infection, and any major predisposing congenital or chronic medical condition; and children of Native American or African-American descent.

Practices recommended by the American Academy of Pediatrics Committee on Infectious Disease and the Advisory Committee on Immunization Practices of the Centers for Disease Control and Prevention.

Pneumococcal vaccine. Med Lett 1999; 41: 84.

Rubin LG. Pneumococcal vaccine. Pediatr Clin North Am 2000; 47: 269-285.

Poliomyelitis

The three serotypes of poliovirus, as well as enterovirus, are highly contagious. Most infections are asymptomatic, but 1 in 100 to 1 in 1000 infected persons contract paralytic poliomyelitis. Symptomatic cases typically begin with nonspecific febrile illness, followed in a small percentage of cases by aseptic meningitis or rapidly progressing paralysis, classified according to locus of involvement as spinal, bulbar, or spinobulbar. Humans represent the sole reservoir for poliovirus, which is spread either directly by fecal-oral contact or indirectly by contaminated sewage or water. The incubation period for symptomatic disease is 7 to 21 days, and the period of communicability may range from 4 to 6 weeks, beginning in the presymptomatic stage of infection.

Following widespread use of polio vaccines, cases of paralytic polio in the United States declined from an epidemic high of 20,000 in 1952 to an average of 8 to 9 cases annually between 1980 and 1994. With the exception of a few imported cases, virtually all cases in the United States during the 1990s represent vaccine-associated paralytic polio (VAPP), an adverse outcome that occurs at a rate of 1 case per 2.4 million doses of live polio vaccine. Global polio eradication was initiated by the World Health Organization (WHO) in 1988. As of 2000 the disease had been eradicated from the Western Hemisphere (since 1994) and was rapidly succumbing to organized public health efforts in the remaining endemic areas of the developing world.

Trivalent inactivated polio vaccine (IPV) was introduced in the United States and other countries in the mid-1950s and was replaced by live attenuated oral polio vaccine (OPV) in the early 1960s. Both vaccines, given in multidose schedules as part of well-child care, attain 90% to 100% immunity. During the late 1990s, to eliminate VAPP, which was accounting for all new indigenous polio in the United States, the ACIP and other advisory groups recommended a transition first in 1997 to a sequential IPV-OPV vaccination schedule (two doses of IPV followed by two doses of OPV) and then, effective in

TABLE 25-2
Adult and Adolescent Immunization Schedule

Vaccine	Timing of immunization
Hepatitis A	First dose (for international travelers, at least 4 weeks before departure) Second dose: 6 to 12 months after first dose
Hepatitis B	First dose Second dose: at least 1 month after first dose Third dose: at least 5 months after first dose
Influenza	One dose annually, usually between September and December, to adults ≥50 years of age and also to younger persons with chronic illness or other risk factors*
Measles-mumps-rubella (MMR)†	First dose Second dose: 28 days or more after first dose
Pneumococcal vaccine	One dose given to persons ≥65 years of age First dose for persons 2 to 64 years of age with chronic illness and at high risk One "booster" dose given 5 years after the first dose (applies only to persons who were 2 to 64 years of age at the time of the first dose)
Tetanus-diphtheria (Td)	Three-dose initial series (if not given in childhood): First dose Second dose: 1 to 2 months after first dose Third dose: 6 to 12 months after second dose Booster series: Every 10 years thereafter
Varicella‡ for susceptible individuals§	First dose Second dose: 28 days or more after first dose

Based on recommendations of the Advisory Committee on Immunization Practices of the Centers for Disease Control and Prevention.
*Patients should consult their physicians to determine their level of risk.
†Should not be given to a pregnant woman. Pregnancy should be avoided for 3 months after receipt of the MMR vaccine.
‡Should not be given to a pregnant woman. Pregnancy should be avoided for 1 month after receipt of the varicella vaccine.
§Susceptible individuals include those who have not been immunized previously and who do not have a reliable history of chickenpox.

2000, to an all-IPV schedule. Current ACIP recommendations, in concert with those of the American Association of Family Physicians and the AAP, are shown in Box 25-11.

SUGGESTED READING

Dowdle WR, Featherstone DA, Birmingham ME, et al. Poliomyelitis eradication. Virus Res 1999; 62: 185-192.
Fine PE, Carneiro IA. Transmissibility and persistence of oral polio vaccine viruses: implications for the global poliomyelitis eradication initiative. Am J Epidemiol 1999; 150: 1001-1021.
Prevots DR, Strebel PM. Poliomyelitis prevention in the United States: new recommendations for routine childhood vaccination place greater reliance on inactivated poliovirus vaccine. Pediatr Ann 1997; 26: 378-383.

Rabies

Rabies is an almost invariably fatal encephalomyelitis caused by various rabies virus strains belonging to the lyssaviruses. The disease, which is restricted to warm-blooded mammals, is found worldwide except in a few rabies-free areas, most of which are islands, including Hawaii. An estimated 30,000 to 100,000 rabies deaths occur annually, almost all of them in developing countries as a result of bites from infected dogs. In the United States 36 human cases were reported between 1980 and 1997, of which 58% were caused by domestic exposure to the bat variant of rabies virus and 33% by exposure to the dog variant of rabies virus outside of the country.

Rabies is transmitted by direct exposure to saliva of an infected animal via bite or scratch wounds. Person-to-person spread, although theoretically possible, has not been documented. Airborne transmission in bat-infected caves and in laboratory settings has occurred, but this is extremely rare. Infected mammals may spread the virus in their saliva for up to 2 weeks before the onset of clinical evidence of rabies. The incubation period in humans is usually 2 to 8 weeks, but it may be as long as a year.

Rabies immunoprophylactic products licensed for use in the United States include three inactivated vaccines (human diploid cell vaccine [HDCV]; purified chick embryo cell vaccine [PCEC]; and rabies vaccine adsorbed [RVA]) and two rabies immune globulin (RIG) products prepared from plasma of hyperimmunized human donors (Bay Rab and Imogam Rabies-HT). The vaccines induce a protective immune response in 7 to 10 days, with approximately 2 years' duration. RIG provides immediate passive immunity with a short duration of several weeks. Side effects from vaccine, which are far less common or serious than those of past rabies vaccines, include pain and erythema at the inoculation site and occasional transient headache, nausea, muscle ache, and dizziness. RIG is associated with occasional inoculation site pain and transient fever and has not been associated with transmission of any pathogenic virus from donors.

Immunization against rabies in humans takes two distinct forms: preexposure vaccination of persons at increased risk of exposure to rabies and postexposure prophylaxis of persons following proven or presumed exposure to rabies. ACIP (1999) recommendations for these respective indications follow.

Preexposure vaccination is recommended for veterinarians, animal handlers, laboratory workers likely to be exposed to rabies, persons whose activities bring them in frequent contact with potentially rabid animals (e.g., spelunkers visiting bat caves), and international travelers to areas where dog rabies is enzootic (see Chapter 24). Primary vaccination comprises three intramuscular injections, with second and third injections at 7 days and 21 to 28 days after the initial injection. HDCV vaccine may also be administered intradermally according to the same timetable. Vaccinated laboratory workers, veterinarians, and others with either continuous or highly likely occupational exposure to rabies (e.g., individuals working in areas where rabies is highly endemic) should have regular serologic testing and receive booster vaccination if antibody titers are below levels established as protective against rabies.

BOX 25-11

Polio Vaccines: Use of Trivalent Inactivated Polio Vaccine (IPV) and Oral Polio Vaccine (OPV) (2000)

- Routine childhood vaccination should comprise four doses of IPV, given at ages 2 months, 4 months, 6 to 18 months, and 4 to 6 years.
- Children whose vaccination was initiated with OPV should complete their series with IPV.
- Adults in the following categories of increased risk of exposure to poliovirus should receive a three-dose schedule of IPV, with two doses administered at 4-week to 8-week intervals and a third dose 6 to 12 months later: travelers to polio endemic areas, laboratory workers handling specimens potentially contaminated with polio, health care workers in close contact with patients who may be excreting poliovirus, and unvaccinated adults whose children will be receiving OPV.
- Neither IPV or OPV should be administered to pregnant women or to persons allergic to streptomycin, polymyxin B, or neomycin, trace amounts of which are contained in media for producing vaccine.

Practices recommended by the American Academy of Pediatrics Committee on Infectious Disease, the American Academy of Family Physicians, and the Advisory Committee on Immunization Practices of the Centers for Disease Control and Prevention. OPV can now be used, after thorough counseling, in only five circumstances: (1) mass vaccination campaigns during outbreaks of paralytic polio; (2) unvaccinated children who will be traveling in <4 weeks to areas where polio is endemic; (3) persons with life-threatening allergic reaction to a dose of IPV; (4) persons with life-threatening allergy to neomycin, streptomycin, or polymyxin B; and (5) children of parents who do not accept the recommended number of vaccine injections.

PEP comprises immediate local protection at the bite wound site, as well as passive and active immunoprophylaxis for persons with proven or presumed exposure to rabies. Exposures consist most commonly of a direct bite that penetrates the skin or less commonly of nonbite contamination of open wounds or mucous membranes with saliva or other potentially infectious material from a rabid animal. The essential PEP regimen for previously unvaccinated persons is thorough washing of a bite wound with soap and water; administration of one course of RIG to provide immediate passive immunization; and a five-dose course of vaccination to begin immediately, with follow-up doses administered 3 days, 7 days, 14 days, and 28 days after the first dose. Previously vaccinated persons should receive two booster doses of vaccine, one immediately and one 3 days later, but need not receive RIG.

Assessment of whether an individual has experienced definite or likely rabies exposure—and hence is a candidate for PEP—first requires careful review of the nature (bite or nonbite) and circumstances (provoked or unprovoked bite) of the exposure and second requires review of whether the animal responsible for the exposure is likely or unlikely to be carrying rabies in the particular geographic area in which the exposure occurs. Rabies in bats is endemic throughout the United States, making bat exposure always suspect, but local health authorities must be consulted to determine the likelihood of exposure to rabies from other animal species (e.g., foxes, raccoons, skunks) in the area. Small rodents (e.g., squirrels, rats, mice, and hamsters), although far and away the most frequently reported biting animals, are almost never infected with rabies and have not been known to transmit rabies to humans. Experience suggests that PEP for rabies is frequently inappropriate.

 KEY POINTS

RABIES

- Preexposure use of rabies vaccine is recommended for veterinarians, animal handlers, certain laboratory workers, persons whose activities bring them in frequent contact with potentially rabid animals (e.g., spelunkers visiting bat caves), and international travelers to areas where dog bites are enzootic.
- Postexposure prophylaxis against rabies involves immediate local protection at the bite wound site, passive immunization with rabies immune globulin, and active immunization with the rabies vaccine.
- Assessment of whether a person has had a definite or likely rabies exposure and should therefore receive postexposure prophylaxis involves review of the nature of the exposure (bite or nonbite), the circumstances (provoked or unprovoked), and the likelihood that the animal responsible for the exposure might be carrying the rabies virus.
- Currently in the United States, 58% of rabies cases are caused by bat exposures and 33% are caused by dog bites sustained in other countries.
- Bats, dogs, foxes, raccoons, and skunks are among the animals that sometimes cause rabies in humans.
- Small rodents such as squirrels, rats, mice, and hamsters frequently cause bites but have not been shown to transmit rabies to humans.

⊃ Postexposure prophylaxis for rabies is frequently inappropriate.

⊃ Specific advice concerning possible rabies exposures is nearly always available from local and state health departments.

SUGGESTED READING

Mackowiak M, Maki J, Motes-Kreimeyer L, et al. Vaccination of wildlife against rabies: successful use of a vectored vaccine obtained by recombinant technology. Adv Vet Med 1999; 41: 571-583.

Moran GJ, Talan DA, Mower W, et al. Appropriateness of rabies postexposure prophylaxis treatment of animal exposures. JAMA 2000; 284: 1001-1007.

Plotkin SA. Rabies. Clin Infect Dis 2000; 30: 4-12.

Rose VL. CDC issues revised guidelines for the prevention of human rabies. Am Fam Physician 1999; 59: 2007-2008, 2013-2014.

Wilde H, Tipkong P, Khawplod P. Economic issues in postexposure rabies treatment. J Travel Med 1999; 6: 238-242.

Wilkerson JA. Rabies update. Wilderness Environ Med 2000; 11: 31-39.

Wyatt JD, Barker WH, Bennett NM, et al. Human rabies postexposure prophylaxis during rabies epizootic in New York, 1993 and 1994. Emerg Infect Dis 1999; 5: 415-423.

Varicella-Zoster Virus

The varicella-zoster virus (VZV) is highly contagious and causes varicella (chickenpox) and herpes zoster (shingles).

BOX 25-12
Varicella-Zoster Virus Vaccine (1999)

- A single dose of the vaccine is recommended for all susceptible children before their 13th birthday. Preferably this vaccination will be administered routinely between 12 and 18 months of age at the same time that measles-mumps-rubella vaccination occurs. Children between 19 months and 12 years of age who do not have a reliable history of clinical chickenpox should be considered susceptible and be vaccinated.

- Persons ≥13 years of age without reliable history of chickenpox should be considered susceptible and should receive two doses of vaccine at 4- to 8-week intervals. Because most adults without reliable history are actually immune from past infection, serologic testing before vaccination is likely to be cost effective.

- High priority should be given to vaccinating the following high-risk susceptible adults:
  - Health care workers and family members of immunocompromised persons who are at high risk for severe complications from varicella
  - Persons who live or work in environments where varicella is likely to occur, including teachers of young children, day care staff, and individuals in other group settings
  - Nonpregnant women of childbearing age
  - Selected subsets of human immunodeficiency virus–infected persons (consult the Centers for Disease Control and Prevention for current guidelines)
  - Persons requiring postexposure prophylaxis, if given within 3 days of exposure to an infected individual, and susceptible persons exposed to a varicella outbreak that may persist for several months in such settings as schools, day care centers, and institutions

Practices recommended by the Advisory Committee on Immunization Practices of the Centers for Disease Control and Prevention.

Live attenuated varicella-zoster vaccine (Varivax), originally developed in Japan, was licensed for use in the United States in 1995. Administered subcutaneously as a single dose to children 12 months to 12 years of age and as a two-dose regimen to persons ≥13 years old, the vaccine elicits readily detectable antibody in 97% to 99% of healthy recipients. In field trials involving children, VZV vaccine has been shown to provide >90% protection against clinical chickenpox and significantly less severity in those clinical cases that do occur in vaccinees. Detectable antibody and protective effectiveness have been shown to persist for at least 10 years after vaccination. The vaccine has also been shown to provide >90% postexposure protection against infection in persons vaccinated within 3 days of exposure. Pain and redness at the vaccination site and transient varicella-like rash are seen in a small percentage of vaccinees, whereas postvaccination zoster is exceedingly rare. ACIP recommendations for varicella vaccination are shown in Box 25-12.

Postexposure prophylaxis with varicella-zoster immune globulin (VZIG), if administered within 3 to 4 days of exposure to varicella, is effective in preventing infection in susceptible healthy individuals and in preventing or modifying clinical illness in susceptible immunocompromised persons.

SUGGESTED READING

Freeman VA, Freed GL. Parental knowledge, attitudes, and demand regarding a vaccine to prevent varicella. Am J Prev Med 1999; 17: 153-155.

Meyer PA, Seward JF, Jumaan AO, et al. Varicella mortality: trends before vaccine licensure in the United States, 1970-1994. J Infect Dis 2000; 182: 383-390.

Taylor JA, Newman RD. The Puget Sound Pediatric Research Network. Parental attitudes toward varicella vaccination. Arch Pediatr Adolesc Med 2000; 154: 302-306.

Vazquez M, LaRussa PS, Gershon AA, et al. The effectiveness of the varicella vaccine in clinical practice. N Engl J Med 2001; 344: 955-960.

Watson B, Seward J, Yang A, et al. Postexposure effectiveness of varicella vaccine. Pediatrics 2000; 105: 84-88.

Future Directions

In the wake of prolific expansion of available vaccines and vaccine technology in the last quarter of the 20th century, a number of promising new developments in vaccines and biologic vaccine delivery systems are on the horizon in the early years of the 21st century.

Among vaccines, intranasally administered inactivated and live attenuated influenza vaccines that stimulate respiratory mucosal immunity have proved efficacious in clinical trials in children and adults and are likely to be licensed soon for use in the United States. Live attenuated varicella vaccine has been shown to be well tolerated and to produce a significant booster response to varicella-zoster virus in older adults, giving rise to the potential for preventing shingles in this age group, a possibility currently being studied in a large, multicenter, placebo-controlled trial. Vaccines against respiratory syncytial virus, *Pseudomonas,* and HIV infection, among others, are in varying stages of development and field testing.

A number of expanded combination vaccines, including DTP combined with Hib, inactivated polio, or hepatitis vaccine and MMR combined with varicella vaccine, which could reduce the number of separate childhood inoculations, have been developed but had not yet been licensed for use in the United States as of early 2001.

With regard to novel biologic vaccine delivery modalities, which may enhance or simplify immunization in the near future, two are especially noteworthy: vector vaccines and microencapsulation vaccines. Vector vaccines, building on genetic engineering technology, are produced by inserting or cloning genes that code for a pathogen's immunizing antigen into attenuated bacterial or viral vectors through genetic recombinant techniques. The recipient host is inoculated with the genetically engineered vector, which expresses the desired antigen, which in turn elicits an immune response. Candidate vectors include attenuated *Salmonella* and *E. coli* bacteria for oral administration and adenovirus and canarypox viruses for inducing respiratory tract and systemic immunity. Microen-capsulation vaccines under development incorporate multiple immunizing antigens into a biodegradable material that allows pulsed release of antigens at intervals of weeks or months, comparable with the timetable for vaccines given in multidose immunization schedules. Such vaccines could significantly reduce the need for frequent medical visits to complete a series of immunizations.

SUGGESTED READING

Cleland JL. Single-administration vaccines: controlled-release technology to mimic repeated immunizations. Trends Biotechnol 1999; 17: 25-29.

Kurstak E. Towards new vaccines and modern vaccinology: introductory remarks. Vaccine 1999; 17: 1583-1586.

Letvin NL, Bloom BR, Hoffman SL. Prospects for vaccines to protect against AIDS, tuberculosis, and malaria. JAMA 2001; 285: 606-611.

Plotkin SA. Vaccination in the 21st century. J Infect Dis 1993; 168: 29-37.

26 Preexposure and Postexposure Prophylaxis

CHARLES S. BRYAN, ROBERT T. BALL

Postexposure Management and Prophylaxis After
    Occupational Blood and Body Fluid Exposure:
    Overview
Postexposure Prophylaxis for Human Immunodeficiency
    Virus
Postexposure Prophylaxis for Viral Hepatitis
Postexposure Prophylaxis After Sexual Assault
Postexposure Prophylaxis After Bite Wounds
Postexposure Prophylaxis After Other Forms of Trauma
Preexposure Prophylaxis for Endocarditis
Preexposure Prophylaxis for Surgical Procedures

Antimicrobial prophylaxis (from the Greek *pro,* "before," and *phylassein,* "to preserve") works best when therapeutic drug levels are present in serum and tissues *before* the exposure. Strictly speaking, drug administration *after* an exposure is therapeutic rather than prophylactic, because unless the drug is given immediately, the invading microorganisms are able to multiply. Postexposure prophylaxis (PEP) is discussed first in this chapter because the clinical scenarios usually involve both management and therapeutic urgency, especially for health care workers potentially exposed to one or more of the three major bloodborne pathogens (hepatitis B virus, hepatitis C virus, and human immunodeficiency virus [HIV]). Postexposure prophylaxis is discussed elsewhere for meningococcal disease (Chapter 6), influenza (Chapter 10), tuberculosis (Chapter 22), tick bites (Chapter 23), tetanus (Chapter 25), rabies (Chapter 25), and varicella-zoster virus (Chapter 25).

Postexposure Management and Prophylaxis After Occupational Blood and Body Fluid Exposure: Overview

Occupational exposures and postexposure prophylaxis are frequent issues for health care workers (HCWs). Up to one half of HCWs report at least one percutaneous exposure to blood during their careers, and up to one quarter sustain an exposure within a given 12-month period. However, for various reasons, up to one third of HCW exposures go unreported. Exposures are also an issue in the wider community, as illustrated by the recent case of a police officer, who, while making an arrest, sustained a clenched fist injury that resulted in his infection by both the hepatitis C virus and HIV. The optimum strategy is prevention, using standard (previously,

"universal") precautions (gloves, gowns, masks, and goggles, depending on the circumstances) before anticipated blood and body fluid exposures. Because accidental exposures inevitably occur, all primary care clinicians need general familiarity with management and PEP measures. The basic principles are as follows:

- First, immediately irrigate the exposed areas. Mucous membranes, puncture wounds, or lacerations should be irrigated with copious amounts of water or sterile saline solution. Basic wound care is appropriate, but no data are available for or against the common use of topical antiseptics or attempts to squeeze fluid out of the wound.

- Expedite triage. Exposure to infected or potentially infected body fluids commonly generates acute anxiety, and the exposed person should be evaluated as quickly as possible. Primary care clinicians who are not equipped to manage exposures in their offices should have an established system of expedited referral to an infectious disease specialist or other specialist in the community.

- Document the time, date, and precise nature of the exposure. When, where, and how did it occur? If an instrument was involved, was it a hollow needle (highest risk), a nonhollow needle (such as a suture needle), or a sharp instrument? Did the instrument contain visible blood? If so, was the blood fresh (highest risk) or dried? Did it contain other materials, such as cerebrospinal fluid (CSF), saliva, or stool? Did the instrument penetrate the skin, and if so, how far? Was there evidence that blood was injected into the exposed person's tissues? If the exposure involved a splash, did it involve mucous membranes, intact skin, or nonintact skin (e.g., an open wound or weeping dermatitis)?

- Obtain information about the source person or patient, if identified. Obtain the source person's name and, if possible, the name of the source person's physician (or medical record number). If the source person is known to be HIV positive, what antiretroviral drugs has he or she taken, and what is the current viral load? Is the source person known to have had hepatitis B or hepatitis C? Is the source person an injecting drug user, or does the person have other risk factors for bloodborne diseases? *Most important, obtain serum from the source or patient for testing for bloodborne pathogens; this is allowed in most states even without expressed consent.*

- Obtain information about the exposed person. Has a course of vaccination against hepatitis B been completed? If the exposed person has been shown to have had a positive serologic test for hepatitis B (anti-HBs), that person is considered to have protective immunity and no further

597

management for hepatitis B is needed. What underlying diseases may be present, and what are the person's current medications?

■ Obtain baseline laboratory studies from the exposed person when indicated (i.e., when the source person is known to be infected with a bloodborne pathogen or when the source is unknown). These include an HIV antibody test, hepatitis B serologic tests (HBsAg, anti-HBs, anti-HBc), and hepatitis C serologic tests (anti-HCV) (see Chapter 13). Baseline laboratory studies are not indicated if the source is confirmed to be uninfected, and further testing or follow-up of the exposed person is unnecessary except in cases of inordinate anxiety.

■ Make decisions. Is PEP for HIV indicated (see "Postexposure Prophylaxis for Human Immunodeficiency Virus")? Is PEP for hepatitis B indicated (see "Postexposure Prophylaxis for Hepatitis B")?

■ Provide or arrange for adequate counseling and follow-up.

Management of blood and body fluid exposures can be time consuming. It is important to act promptly, to evaluate the injury in a systematic fashion as previously outlined, to provide accurate information, and to make PEP available if indicated.

In 1991 OSHA published its Bloodborne Pathogen Standards, a set of federal regulatory requirements that health care employers must meet to protect their workers. These include a requirement to have a written detailed exposure control plan (including the management of exposures) and to provide hepatitis B vaccination. In November 1999 OSHA updated its enforcement directive, requiring adherence to the latest Centers for Disease Control and Prevention (CDC) guidelines, which had been previously published in separate issues of *Morbidity Mortality Weekly Report* but were at that time combined into a single update. OSHA also mandated evaluation and implementation of needle safety devices, which have

been shown to reduce the incidence of needlestick injuries by up to 76%. In November 2000 the federal Needlestick Safety and Prevention Act became law, requiring updated Bloodborne Pathogen Standards, which were published in January 2001. These and other mandates *require* health care workers to use safety devices with "built-in safety features" and to observe the CDC guidelines, including use of PEP.

 KEY POINTS

POSTEXPOSURE MANAGEMENT AND PROPHYLAXIS AFTER BLOOD AND BODY FLUID EXPOSURE: OVERVIEW

⊃ Exposures to blood and body fluids usually engender acute anxiety. Management must be prompt and thorough.

⊃ The time and nature of the exposure should be documented, and information should be obtained about the source person and the exposed person.

⊃ It is essential to test both the source person and the exposed person for HIV, hepatitis C, and possibly hepatitis B (HBsAg).

⊃ Immediate decisions must be made about the need for antiretroviral PEP for HIV exposure and (rarely) PEP for hepatitis B.

SUGGESTED READING

Abel S, Césaire R, Cales-Quist D, et al. Occupational transmission of human immunodeficiency virus and hepatitis C virus after a punch. Clin Infect Dis 2000; 31: 1494-1495.

Beltrami EM, Williams IT, Shapiro CN, et al. Risk and management of blood-borne infections in healthcare workers. Clin Microbiol Rev 2000; 13: 385-407.

Centers for Disease Control and Prevention. Updated Public Health Service (PHS) guidelines for the management of occupational

TABLE 26-1
Some Resources and Registries Concerning Postexposure Prophylaxis for Human Immunodeficiency Virus

Resource	Comments
National Clinician's Postexposure Hotline (PEPline) (1-888-448-4911)	Information and 24-hour consultations are available through San Francisco General Hospital, supported by the Public Health Service website: http://pepline.ucsf.edu/pepline
Hepatitis Hotline of Centers for Disease Control and Prevention (1-888-443-7232)	Website: http://www.cdc.gov/hepatitis
HIV Postexposure Prophylaxis Registry (1-888-737-4448)	Address: 1410 Commonwealth Drive, Suite 215, Wilmington NC 28405
Antiretroviral Pregnancy Registry (1-800-258-4263; Fax 1-800-800-1052)	Address: 1410 Commonwealth Drive, Suite 215, Wilmington NC 28405
Food and Drug Administration (1-800-332-1088)	For reporting unusual or severe toxicity or side effects from antiretroviral drugs; website: http://www.fda.gov/medwatch
Centers for Disease Control and Prevention (1-404-639-6425)	For reporting seroconversions in health care workers who received postexposure prophylaxis against human immunodeficiency virus

exposures to HBV, HCV, and HIV and recommendations for post-exposure prophylaxis (PEP). MMWR 2001; 50 (RR11); 1-42.

Hersey JC, Martin LS. Use of infection control guidelines by workers in healthcare facilities to prevent occupational transmission of HBV and HIV: results from a national survey. Infect Control Hosp Epidemiol 1994; 15: 243-252.

Moran GJ. Emergency department management of blood and body fluid exposures. Ann Emerg Med 2000; 35: 47-62.

Postexposure Prophylaxis for Human Immunodeficiency Virus

In recent years few if any issues in clinical medicine have engendered more controversy and anxiety than occupational exposure to the human immunodeficiency virus. Management of potential exposures, like management of HIV disease (see "Antiretroviral Drug Therapy" in Chapter 17), is fraught with a great deal of complexity. Primary care clinicians should understand the basis for management and PEP, have a framework for getting the source person tested immediately, have a system in place for helping exposed persons to make the initial decision whether to take postexposure drugs, and know where to find assistance.

Basis for Postexposure Prophylaxis Against Human Immunodeficiency Virus

It is highly unlikely that PEP will ever be supported by a randomized, prospective, controlled trial in humans. The manufacturer of zidovudine (AZT), to its credit, attempted such a trial, but enrollment proved insufficient. Several lines of evidence support the concept of postexposure prophylaxis:

- In a case-control study of health care workers, the risk of HIV infection was reduced by about 81% for those who took AZT after the exposure (95% confidence interval for 43% to 94%).
- In a randomized, prospective, controlled trial it was shown that AZT reduces the risk of perinatal transmission of HIV from infected mothers to their infants by about 67%.
- In several animal models PEP prevented HIV infection or attenuated its severity.

Data from animal models suggest that PEP is most effective when begun early and continued for a substantial duration (i.e., several weeks).

The use of AZT as monotherapy after potential HIV exposure is now inappropriate because potent combination regimens are now available and today's source patients have usually received antiretroviral drugs and may therefore have drug-resistant strains. Exposed persons must therefore take at least two and sometimes three drugs that may have significant side effects. Currently available antiretroviral drugs do not prevent HIV from entering target cells. The rationale behind PEP is to suppress viral activity until no cells contain viral particles capable of infecting other cells. Stated differently, the rationale is to "hit early, hit hard, and hit often." Much depends on the first clinical contact. A decision must be made whether to give the initial doses of PEP. *The exposed person's life may literally depend on this decision.* Thereafter both the clinician and the patient can consult with a specialist or obtain information through one of many available sources (Table 26-1).

Decision to Begin Postexposure Prophylaxis Against Human Immunodeficiency Virus

The decision to begin PEP, which should be made jointly by the exposed person and the treating clinician, is based on the nature of the exposure and the extent to which the source person is thought to be infectious.

Percutaneous exposures carry the greatest risk, now estimated at about 1 in 300 (Table 26-2). Factors associated with increased risk from percutaneous exposure include hollow needles (as opposed to solid needles, including suture needles), deep injury, visible blood on the device (fresh blood probably carries a greater risk than dried blood), and the previous presence of a needle in the source person's vein or artery. Mucosal exposures, such as splashes into the eye, carry a lesser risk, currently estimated at about 1 in 1000. Infection by HIV after exposure to skin that is completely intact is rare, if it occurs at all. However, HIV seroconversion has been reported in instances in which the exposed skin was severely chapped, abraded, or inflamed as by dermatitis. Documented transmission has also occurred after various wounds, including bite wounds.

Knowing that the source person is HIV positive facilitates the initial decision. The HIV status of the source person is usually unknown at the time of the injury. The introduction in 1998 of rapid HIV antibody tests (turnaround time of an hour or less) led to wide reliance on such tests in hospital settings.

TABLE 26-2
Some Risks of Blood and Body Fluid Exposures and Potential Prophylaxis

Disease	Risk to health care workers after percutaneous exposure	Risk after mucosal exposure	Effective prophylaxis available?
Human immunodeficiency virus infection	0.3% (95% C.I., 0.2% to 0.5%*)	0.09% (95% C.I., 0.006% to 0.5%*)	Yes; antiretroviral drug therapy
Hepatitis B (carriers; positive for HBsAg)	2% (HBeAg absent) to 40% (HBeAg present); averages about 1 in 3 to 1 in 4	Estimated to be about 1 in 10	Yes; hepatitis B immune globulin (HBIG) and vaccine
Hepatitis C	Average 1.8% (range 0% to 7%)	Undetermined (apparently low)	No; theoretically, interferon and other antiviral agents may help

*Range values for the estimated true risk, based on data in the literature and expressed as a 95% confidence interval (95% C.I.).

At the time of this writing the continued availability of these tests is uncertain. However, several rapid HIV antibody tests may soon become available, and many laboratories can now perform the HIV enzyme immunoassay (EIA) antibody screen on a same- or next-day basis.

The window of opportunity for beginning PEP in humans is unknown. On the basis of animal experiments, most authorities believe that PEP should be given as soon as possible, preferably within hours, although it may be useful if begun up to 3 days after the exposure. When a significant exposure has occurred and doubt exists about whether the source is HIV positive, our preference is to recommend the first doses of PEP while awaiting HIV test results on the source patient.

The complexities of PEP against HIV are such that the concept is difficult to capture with a single algorithm (for a simplification, see Figure 26-1). The 2001 CDC guidelines are summarized in Tables 26-3 to 26-5. The three steps are as follows:

- Classify the exposure (Tables 26-3 and 26-4). If it is bona fide, is it trivial, less severe, or more severe?
- Classify the source (Tables 26-3 and 26-4). Is the source person HIV negative or HIV positive? If the person is HIV positive, is the viral titer known or likely to be at lower levels (HIV Class 1) or higher levels (HIV Class 2)? Or is the HIV status of the source person unknown (HIV Class Unknown)?

- Recommend whether to begin PEP on the basis of the exposure category and the source category (Tables 26-3 to 26-5). The clinician should explain in lay terms (even when the exposed person is medically sophisticated, which is often the case) the likelihood of HIV infection based on the exposure category and the source category. When doubt exists in the exposed person's mind, it is usually best to offer PEP because the drugs can always be discontinued later. Pregnancy is not considered a contraindication to

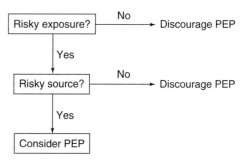

FIG. 26-1 Overview of postexposure prophylaxis for human immunodeficiency virus (see Tables 26-3 to 26-5).

TABLE 26-3

Recommendations of Centers for Disease Control and Prevention for Postexposure Prophylaxis for Human Immunodeficiency Virus After Percutaneous Exposures (2001)

Exposure type	HIV-positive, Class 1: asymptomatic HIV infection or known low viral load (e.g., <1500/mm³)*	HIV-positive, Class 2: symptomatic HIV infection, AIDS, acute seroconversion, or known high viral load*	HIV status unknown or source unknown	HIV-negative or trivial exposure, or no contamination with blood or body fluids†
Less severe (e.g., solid needle; superficial injury)	Recommend basic two-drug PEP regimen (see Table 26-5)	Recommend expanded three-drug PEP regimen (see Table 26-5)	Generally, no PEP warranted; however, basic PEP regimen‡ might be considered for a source with HIV risk factors§	No PEP warranted
More severe (e.g., large-bore hollow needle, deep puncture, visible blood on device, or needle used in patient's artery or vein)	Recommend expanded three-drug PEP regimen (see Table 26-5)	Recommend expanded three-drug PEP regimen (see Table 26-5)	Generally, no PEP warranted; however, basic PEP regimen‡ might be considered for a source with HIV risk factors§	No PEP warranted

Modified from Centers for Disease Control and Prevention. Updated Public Health Service (PHS) guidelines for the management of occupational exposures to HBV, HCV, and HIV and recommendations for post-exposure prophylaxis (PEP). MMWR 2001; 50 (RR-11).
AIDS, Acquired immunodeficiency syndrome; *HIV,* human immunodeficiency virus; *PEP,* postexposure prophylaxis.
*If drug resistance is a concern, obtain expert consultation. Initiation of PEP should not be delayed pending expert consultation, and because expert consultation alone cannot substitute for face-to-face counseling, resources should be available to provide immediate evaluation and follow-up care for all exposures.
†Semen or vaginal secretions; cerebrospinal fluid; synovial, pleural, peritoneal, pericardial, or amniotic fluid; or tissue. The nature of the exposure or incident should be documented carefully in the patient's record.
‡Consideration of PEP indicates that PEP is optional and should be based on an individualized decision between the exposed person and the treating clinician.
§If PEP is offered and taken and the source is later determined to be HIV negative, PEP should be discontinued.

using a reverse transcriptase inhibitor (such as those recommended in the basic PEP regimen, Table 26-5). Most authorities, however, advise against the use of protease inhibitors during pregnancy.

The following cases illustrate how these three steps can be applied to different scenarios.

PATIENT 1

A 36-year-old nurse sustained a splash in the face while giving medication by nasogastric tube to a patient with end-stage HIV disease. The medication had consisted of a crushed tablet, and the splash occurred when high pressure in the nasogastric tube caused the plunger to become disconnected from the syringe. No blood was visible. The extent, if any, to which the material splashed in the face came from the patient was unclear. Although the source category was high risk, the exposure category was judged to have been trivial because gastric juice is not on the list of potentially infected body fluids (see footnote to Table 26-3). The nurse decided not to continue PEP because the risk of transmission was estimated to be extremely low.

PATIENT 2

A 46-year-old nurse's aide sustained a prick on the finger, drawing "a drop or two" of blood, from a lancet that had been used for blood glucose determination in a patient recently determined to be HIV positive. The lancet, which had been left on a countertop, did not contain visible blood. The patient, who was asymptomatic from HIV disease, had recently started highly active antiretroviral therapy (HAART) with an excellent response (reduction in viral load from 122,000 to 600 copies/mm³ within 6 weeks). Both the exposure category and the source category were considered to be of low to moderate risk. The aide was offered a basic two-drug regimen (AZT plus 3TC [Combivir]) for 4 weeks but discontinued the regimen within 7 days because of side effects.

Continued PEP therapy should ideally be supervised by a physician knowledgeable about the complexities of antiretroviral therapy (see Chapter 17). A review of the source person's medical record is often useful. What is the current viral load? What antiretroviral drugs are currently being

TABLE 26-4

Recommendations of Centers for Disease Control and Prevention for Postexposure Prophylaxis for Human Immunodeficiency Virus After Mucous Membrane Exposures and Nonintact Skin Exposures (2001)

Exposure type	HIV-positive, Class 1: asymptomatic HIV infection or known low viral load (e.g., <1500/mm³)*	HIV-positive, Class 2: symptomatic HIV infection, AIDS, acute seroconversion, or known high viral load*	HIV status unknown or source unknown	HIV-negative or trivial exposure, or no contamination with blood or body fluids†
Small volume (e.g., a few drops)	Recommend basic two-drug PEP regimen (see Table 26-5)	Recommend basic two-drug PEP regimen (see Table 26-5)	Generally, no PEP warranted; however, basic PEP regimen‡ might be considered for a source with HIV risk factors§	No PEP warranted
Large volume (e.g., a major blood splash)	Recommend basic two-drug PEP regimen (see Table 26-5)	Recommend expanded three-drug PEP regimen (see Table 26-5)	Generally, no PEP warranted; however, basic PEP regimen‡ might be considered for a source with HIV risk factors§	No PEP warranted

Modified from Centers for Disease Control and Prevention. Updated Public Health Service (PHS) guidelines for the management of occupational exposures to HBV, HCV, and HIV and recommendations for post-exposure prophylaxis (PEP). MMWR 2001; 50 (RR #), (in press).
AIDS, Acquired immunodeficiency syndrome; *HIV*, human immunodeficiency virus; *PEP*, postexposure prophylaxis.
*If drug resistance is a concern, obtain expert consultation. Initiation of PEP should not be delayed pending expert consultation, and because expert consultation alone cannot substitute for face-to-face counseling, resources should be available to provide immediate evaluation and follow-up care for all exposures.
†Semen or vaginal secretions; cerebrospinal fluid; synovial, pleural, peritoneal, pericardial, or amniotic fluid; or tissue. The nature of the exposure or incident should be documented carefully in the patient's record. Contact of blood or other body fluids with intact skin is usually not considered a risk factor for HIV transmission. However, because transmission has been reported in cases involving *prolonged* contact of blood with skin that was abraded or inflamed, PEP might be considered in instances that involve (1) large volumes of blood or certain other body fluids as defined above, and (2) prolonged contact. Examples of nonintact skin are open wounds, abrasions, dermatitis, and chapped skin.
‡Consideration of PEP indicates that PEP is optional and should be based on an individualized decision between the exposed person and the treating clinician.
§If PEP is offered and taken and the source is later determined to be HIV negative, PEP should be discontinued.

TABLE 26-5
Postexposure Prophylaxis for HIV: Drug Regimens (2001)

Type of regimen	Appropriateness	Drugs*
Basic (two-drug) regimen for 4 weeks	Situations in which the estimated risk of HIV transmission is considered to be low (see Tables 26-4 and 26-5)	Basic PEP: AZT plus 3TC; or 3TC plus d4T; or DDI plus D4T. The first regimen is most conveniently given as Combivir (300 mg of AZT *plus* 150 mg of 3TC), twice daily. The other regimens are 3TC 150 mg b.i.d. *plus* d4T 40 mg b.i.d., or didanosine EC 400 mg daily *plus* d4T 40 mg b.i.d.
Expanded (three-drug) regimen for 4 weeks	Situation in which the estimated risk of HIV is considered to be significant (see Tables 26-4 and 26-5)	Basic PEP (i.e., one of the above basic regimens) *plus* a protease inhibitor or efavirenz or abacavir. Protease inhibitors include nelfinavir (750 mg t.i.d., with meals) or indinavir (800 mg q8h, on an empty stomach and with ample fluid intake). Efavirenz is given 600 mg daily at bedtime. The dose of abacavir is 300 mg b.i.d.
Individualized regimen for 4 weeks (expert referral advised)	Situations in which the source person has received antiretroviral drugs, including HAART	Therapy must be individualized. Ideally the exposed person takes two or three drugs that have not been previously taken by the source person (and to which cross-resistance would therefore not be expected to occur).

Modified from Centers for Disease Control and Prevention. Updated Public Health Service (PHS) guidelines for the management of occupational exposures to HBV, HCV, and HIV and recommendations for post-exposure prophylaxis (PEP). MMWR 2001; 50 (RR-11).
HAART, Highly active antiretroviral therapy; *HIV,* human immunodeficiency virus; *PEP,* postexposure prophylaxis.
*Drug abbreviations: *AZT,* zidovudine (also abbreviated ZDV); *3TC,* lamivudine; *d4T,* stavudine; *ddI,* didanosine. See Chapter 17 for further discussion of individual drugs and toxicities.

PATIENT 3
A 24-year-old phlebotomist sustained a needlestick injury after drawing blood from a patient with end-stage HIV disease. He had removed the needle used for the phlebotomy and had attached a new needle to the blood-filled syringe in order to inoculate a blood culture bottle. The injury occurred to the hand containing the blood culture bottle as he prepared for the inoculation. Since he had placed no pressure on the plunger, he believed that injection of blood had not occurred. However, because he could not be certain about the latter point, the exposure category was judged to be high risk. Because the source was also high risk, he was encouraged to take an expanded three-drug regimen (Combivir [AZT and 3TC] plus a protease inhibitor) for 4 weeks.

used, and what drugs have been used in the past? The exposed person may need an antiretroviral regimen against drug-resistant strains of HIV. Many exposed persons who begin PEP regimens later discontinue them. A follow-up of 449 health care workers who began PEP regimens indicated that only 43% completed the PEP regimen as initially prescribed and that 44% of the exposed persons discontinued all of the PEP drugs. Side effects become a significant issue for many exposed persons. Life-threatening toxicity has also occurred, especially in persons given nevirapine for prophylaxis. With the complexities of PEP, more recent CDC guidelines take into account the frequent need to obtain consultation and follow-up from a physician with special interest in this area.

 KEY POINTS

POSTEXPOSURE PROPHYLAXIS FOR HUMAN IMMUNODEFICIENCY VIRUS

⊃ Risk is about 1 in 300 after a percutaneous injury and 1 in 1000 after a mucosal exposure. Risk factors are vascular access device, fresh visible blood, or a source person with active disease or high viral load. No cases have been documented after exposure of blood to intact skin.

⊃ The decision to begin PEP for HIV should be reached between the exposed person and the clinician and is based on the nature of the exposure and the likelihood that the source is high risk.

⊃ In the acute situation, when the best course of action is unclear in the mind of the exposed person or the clinician, it is often best to give the first dose of PEP (or a 3-day supply) provided early pregnancy can be reasonably excluded. The decision whether to continue PEP can be made after the acute anxiety has subsided.

⊃ Because most of today's source patients have received antiretroviral drugs, PEP regimens often must be individualized. Ideally the physician supervising continued PEP therapy is thoroughly steeped in the complexities of antiretroviral therapy.

SUGGESTED READING

Cardo DM, Culver DH, Ciesielski CA, et al. A case-control study of HIV seroconversion in health care workers after percutaneous exposure. N Engl J Med 1997; 337: 1485-1490.

Centers for Disease Control and Prevention. Updated Public Health Service (PHS) guidelines for the management of occupational exposures to HBV, HCV, and HIV, and recommendations for post-exposure prophylaxis (PEP). MMWR 2001; 50 (RR-11).

Centers for Disease Control and Prevention. Serious adverse effects attributed to nevirapine regimens for postexposure prophylaxis after HIV exposures—worldwide, 1997-2000. MMWR 2001; 49: 1153-1156.

Connor EM, Sperling RS, Gelber R, et al. Reduction of maternal-infant transmission of human immunodeficiency virus type 1 with zidovudine treatment. N Engl J Med 1994; 331: 1173-1180.

Henderson DK. Postexposure chemoprophylaxis for occupational exposures to the human immunodeficiency virus. JAMA 1999; 281: 931-936.

Postexposure Prophylaxis for Viral Hepatitis

Clinicians should be familiar with indications for PEP for hepatitis B. Although transmission of hepatitis C by percutaneous exposure is a major issue, recommendations for PEP are unavailable at the time of this writing. A recent study suggests that treatment of acute hepatitis C with interferon-α prevents chronic infection (see "Hepatitis C" in Chapter 13). It may therefore be appropriate to follow persons exposed to hepatitis C by monitoring alanine aminotransferase (ALT) levels, keeping in mind that the incubation period for acute hepatitis C ranges from 2 weeks to 6 months with an average of 6 to 7 weeks. Percutaneous or mucous membrane exposures are not risk factors for hepatitis A transmission.

Hepatitis B

Hepatitis B (see Chapter 13) continues to be an important disease despite the availability of a vaccine. For postexposure prophylaxis the vaccine is sometimes used in combination with hepatitis B immune globulin (HBIG), depending on the status of the source patient and the exposed person.

Household Exposure

In cases of household exposure to acute hepatitis B, indications for prophylaxis include an exposed person who is an infant <12 months of age and has not been previously vaccinated against hepatitis B, and a person who has had an identifiable blood exposure—for example, by sharing a razor or toothbrush. These persons should receive HBIG 0.06 mL/kg IM and begin hepatitis B immunization (first dose immediately, then complete the series). When household contact with a person who has chronic hepatitis B (i.e., a chronic HBsAg carrier) has occurred, all previously unvaccinated household members should begin the vaccine.

Percutaneous or Permucosal Exposure

The issue of percutaneous or permucosal exposure arises most frequently after accidental injury to health care workers but also arises after sexual exposures (see "Postexposure Prophylaxis after Sexual Assault" later in the chapter), perinatal exposures, and instances of trauma. HBsAg carriers who are also HbeAg positive are extremely infectious. However, the HBeAg status is usually unknown at the time decisions must be made and is not taken into account in the standard CDC recommendations (Table 26-6).

Hepatitis C

The risk of hepatitis C virus (HCV) infection after an accidental needlestick injury is about 1.8% (range 0% to 7% in reported studies). Immune globulin has been tried in the past

but is not currently recommended. Current recommendations for postexposure management are as follows:

- Obtain a baseline serologic test for anti-HCV antibodies from the exposed persons.
- Repeat anti-HCV testing at 6 weeks, 3 months, and 6 months. Many authorities also recommend obtaining an HCV polymerase chain reaction (PCR) test 2 to 3 weeks after the exposure in order to make an early diagnosis of HCV infection. Exposed persons who demonstrate seroconversion or a positive HCV PCR test result should be referred to a physician (such as a hepatologist) with experience in α-interferon therapy for hepatitis C.

 KEY POINTS

POSTEXPOSURE PROPHYLAXIS FOR VIRAL HEPATITIS

⊃ Hepatitis B. Prophylaxis includes hepatitis B immune globulin (HBIG) or the hepatitis B vaccine, depending on the circumstances.

⊃ Hepatitis C. There is no effective postexposure prophylaxis. Exposed persons should be tested for HCV antibodies, and the test should be repeated at 6 weeks, 3 months, and 6 months. Persons who seroconvert may be candidates for α-interferon therapy.

SUGGESTED READING

AIDS/TB Committee of the Society for Healthcare Epidemiology of America. Management of healthcare workers infected with hepatitis B virus, hepatitis C virus, human immunodeficiency virus, or other bloodborne pathogens. Infect Control Hosp Epidemiol 1997; 18: 349-363.

Centers for Disease Control and Prevention. Updated Public Health Service (PHS) guidelines for the management of occupational exposures to HBV, HCV, and HIV and recommendations for post-exposure prophylaxis (PEP). MMWR 2001; 50 (RR-11).

Eddleston AL. Hepatitis B and health-care workers. Lancet 1997; 349: 1339-1340.

Henderson DK. Occupational infection with hepatitis B virus—waging war against an insidious, intractable, intolerable foe. Clin Infect Dis 1998; 26: 572-574.

Mast EE, Alter MJ, Margolis HJ. Strategies to prevent and control hepatitis B and C virus infections: a global perspective. Vaccine 1999; 17; 1730-1733.

Postexposure Prophylaxis After Sexual Assault

The estimated lifetime risk of attempted or completed rape in the United States is about 1 in 6 (or even higher) for women and 1 in 33 for men. Most instances are never reported. The risk of contracting a sexually transmitted disease (STD), including HIV, can be substantial. Studies suggest that up to 5% of women who are raped have gonorrhea or chlamydial infection as a result and up to 20% have trichomoniasis as a result. The risk of HIV transmission, although not precisely defined, is probably higher than with voluntary sexual activity (estimated to be three to nine HIV transmissions per 10,000 exposures for insertive vaginal sex) because of the physical trauma that is usually involved.

Most hospitals have sexual assault nurse examiner (SANE) programs designed to address the needs of the rape victim. According to a recent survey, nearly all of these programs provide

TABLE 26-6
Postexposure Prophylaxis for Hepatitis B After Percutaneous or Permucosal Exposure

Vaccination status of exposed person	Anti-HBs titer status of exposed person	HBsAg status of source person	Recommendations
Unvaccinated	Not applicable*	Positive Negative Unknown	HBIG† as soon as possible; begin hepatitis B vaccine series Begin hepatitis B vaccine series Begin hepatitis B vaccine series
Previously vaccinated	Protective (i.e., responder)†	Positive, negative, or unknown	No treatment
	Nonprotective (i.e., nonresponder)‡	Positive Negative Unknown	HBIG at time of exposure and repeat in 1 month; *or* HBIG at time of exposure and hepatitis B vaccine booster dose No treatment If the source is thought to be high risk (e.g., an injecting drug user), treat as though the source were HBsAg positive
	Unknown (i.e., titer result unavailable)	Positive Negative Unknown	Test the exposed person for anti-HBs; if the titer is protective, no treatment; if the titer is nonprotective, give HBIG and a hepatitis B vaccine booster dose. No treatment Test the exposed person for anti-HBs; if the titer is protective, no treatment; if the titer is nonprotective, give a hepatitis B vaccine booster dose

Modified from Centers for Disease Control and Prevention. Protection against viral hepatitis: recommendations of the Immunization Advisory Practices Committee (ACIP). MMWR 1990; 39 (RR-2): 15-16.
*It is presumed that an unvaccinated person lacks protective antibodies. An occasional person will have developed protective anti-HBs antibodies as a result of previous, subclinical hepatitis B. No clinical evidence has shown that giving hepatitis B vaccine to such persons is harmful (remotely and theoretically, hepatitis B vaccine could trigger immune complex disease in persons with antibodies to the virus).
†HBIG (hepatitis B immune globulin), 0.06 mL/kg body weight, should be given intramuscularly as soon as possible, preferably within 24 hours of the exposure and in all cases within 7 days.
‡Responders and nonresponders to hepatitis B vaccination are defined on the basis of anti-HBs titers as determined by radioimmunoassay or enzyme immunoassay (responders, ≥10 mIU/mL; nonresponders, <10 mIU/mL).

pregnancy testing, pregnancy prophylaxis, and STD prophylaxis. However, less than one half of the programs offer HIV testing. A growing body of literature indicates that HIV testing and PEP should be an integral part of the care of the rape victim. Unfortunately, and in contrast to most percutaneous exposures in the hospital setting, the identity of the assailant is often unknown and even more frequently the assailant is unavailable for testing. The basic rape protocol for women includes the following:

- Appropriate documentation for legal purposes and chain of custody assurances for forensic medical evidence collected during the extensive postrape examination
- Blood tests: complete blood cell count (CBC), liver enzyme levels, HIV antibody test, hepatitis B antibody test (anti-HBs), and rapid plasma reagin (RPR) and Venereal Disease Research Laboratory (VDRL) tests for syphilis
- Pelvic examination: culture for *Neisseria gonorrhoeae* and *Chlamydia trachomatis;* vaginal secretion specimen to be saved for legal purposes
- Pregnancy test
- Empiric treatment for syphilis, gonorrhea, and chlamydial infection
- Immunization for hepatitis B if the victim was not previously vaccinated

- Emergency contraception measures
- Consideration of postexposure prophylaxis for HIV

If the HIV status of the assailant is known, the previously outlined PEP protocol for HIV can be followed. When this information is unavailable (as is usually the case), it is best to begin the basic PEP protocol, using a two- or three-drug regimen depending on the estimated likelihood that the source person may be HIV positive. Expert consultation is recommended, and close follow-up is required. Experience indicates that follow-up with PEP regimens is often suboptimal.

 KEY POINTS

POSTEXPOSURE PROPHYLAXIS AFTER SEXUAL ASSAULT
- ⊃ The lifetime risk of sexual assault in the United States is about 1 in 4 to 6 women and 1 in 33 men.
- ⊃ Rape victims should be tested for STDs, including serologic testing for hepatitis B and HIV.
- ⊃ Treatment should be given for syphilis, gonorrhea, and chlamydial infection, and vaccination against hepatitis B should be started if the person has not been previously immunized.

⊃ PEP for HIV should be considered because the HIV status of the assailant is usually unknown.

⊃ Close medical follow-up (as well as psychological counseling) should be arranged.

SUGGESTED READING

Babl FE, Cooper ER, Damon B, et al. HIV postexposure prophylaxis for children and adolescents. Am J Emerg Med 2000; 18: 282-287.

Bamberger JD, Waldo CR, Gerberding JL, et al. Postexposure prophylaxis for human immunodeficiency virus (HIV) infection following sexual assault. Am J Med 1999; 106: 323-326.

Ciancone AC, Wilson C, Collette R, et al. Sexual assault nurse examiner programs in the United States. Ann Emerg Med 2000; 35: 353-357.

Hampton HL. Care of the woman who has been raped. N Engl J Med 1995; 332: 234-237.

Jenny C, Hooton TM, Bowers A, et al. Sexually transmitted diseases in victims of rape. N Engl J Med 1990; 322: 713-716.

Linden JA. Sexual assault. Emerg Med Clin North Am 1999; 17: 685-697.

Wiebe ER, Comay SE, McGregor M, et al. Offering HIV prophylaxis to people who have been sexually assaulted: 16 months' experience in a sexual assault service. CMAJ 2000; 162: 641-645.

Postexposure Prophylaxis After Bite Wounds

Bites are extremely common in primary care. They account for an estimated 1% of all emergency room visits and about 800,000 medical visits in the United States. The lifetime prevalence of bite wounds in the United States is about 50%, and the cost of managing these lesions exceeds $100 million. Most bite wounds appear to be of trivial extent when first seen, and indeed only about 20% of patients seek medical attention. Serious complications are necrotizing soft tissue infection, osteomyelitis, and systemic infection, including endocarditis and overwhelming sepsis. Complications are more common after human bites than after animal bites, and bite wounds following clenched-fist injuries (from striking a person in the mouth) are especially likely to be serious.

Dog and Cat Bites

Animal bites occur more frequently in children than adults, especially in boys between the ages of 5 and 9 years. Dog bites occur more often in men than in women, but the opposite is true of cat bites. Bites that come to medical attention are likely to involve the dominant hand or, in children, the face. About 85% of dog bites, and probably most cat bites, are caused by the victim's own pet or by an animal known to the victim. *Pasteurella multocida* is the major pathogen associated with cat bites and is also relatively common in dog bite wounds (up to 50%), along with other *Pasteurella* species such as *Pasteurella canis*. *Capnocytophaga canimorsus* (formerly known as DF-2) is another important pathogen associated with dog bites, and it causes fatal sepsis in asplenic persons (see Chapter 6). However, recent studies confirm that the contaminating flora in dog and cat bites is nearly always

polymicrobial, with a mixture of aerobic and anaerobic pathogens in more than one half of all contaminated wounds. Aerobic pathogens include *Staphylococcus aureus* and various streptococci. Anaerobic pathogens include *Bacteroides, Fusobacterium, Prevotella,* and *Porphyromonas* species. Rarely, *Francisella tularensis* (the cause of tularemia) and *Erysipelothrix rhusiopathiae* (the cause of fish handler's disease) have been transmitted by cat bites. Although optimum management of dog and cat bites remains somewhat controversial, some general principles are as follows:

- Routine culture of the fresh bite wound is not recommended. Results of such cultures correlate poorly with pathogens later isolated from infections.

- The wound should be irrigated copiously with saline solution and débrided, and a decision then made about closure. Facial wounds are usually closed if possible. Most authorities advise against routine closure of puncture wounds (which are usually caused by cat bites) and dog bite wounds of the hand.

- Prophylactic antibiotics (for options, see "Postexposure Prophylaxis After Other Forms of Trauma" later in the chapter) should be given after dog bites in the following circumstances: hand wound, deep puncture wound (especially if tendons, joints, or bone is involved), wound requiring surgical débridement, wound located near a prosthetic joint, wound in an extremity with compromised venous or lymphatic drainage, or wound in an older or immunocompromised person. Whether prophylactic antibiotics should be given routinely is somewhat controversial. According to one analysis, 14 patients would need to be given antibiotics after dog bites to prevent a single infection.

- The need for rabies prophylaxis should be addressed if the biting animal was a mammal (see Chapter 25). The local health department should be informed even if the victim was the animal's owner.

- The need for tetanus immunization should be addressed (see Chapter 25).

- Close follow-up should be arranged. Indications for hospitalization include rapidly progressive cellulitis; suspicion of deep infection involving tendons, joints, or bones; and failure of oral therapy. Joint pain, swelling, or limitation of motion should raise the possibility of septic arthritis.

Human Bites

Human bites are more dangerous than dog and cat bites and often carry legal implications. Some are self-inflicted, some are "love nips," often associated with alcohol or drug use, and some result from altercations. A notorious example of the latter is the clenched-fist injury sustained by striking someone in the mouth. The "knuckle sandwich" with its short (<2 cm) lacerations may appear unimpressive when first seen, but infection can easily spread to key structures of the hand such as joint capsules, tendons, fascial planes, and web spaces. At least 42 bacterial species have been isolated from the human mouth (see Chapter 1 for a brief overview). *Eikenella corrodens,* a microaerophilic gram-negative rod, has been associated with about 25% of infections caused by clenched-fist injuries and is frequently associated with deep infections such as osteomyelitis. *S. aureus* is sometimes associated with human bite wounds, and infections by methicillin-resistant strains have now been reported. Important anaerobic bacteria include *Fusobacterium nucleatum, Bacteroides* and *Prevotella* species, and peptostreptococci. Necrotizing fasciitis caused by group A streptococci, HIV infection, and hepatitis C transmission has rarely been reported. HIV transmission from the biter is a matter of great concern to the bite victim, although saliva without blood contains negligible amounts of HIV and has not been proved to transmit HIV. More realistically, blood from the victim may expose the oral mucosa of the biter (for an excellent discussion see the *2000 Red Book* by the American Academy of Pediatrics, cited in "Suggested Reading"). Management of human bites involves the following principles:

- Careful documentation by diagram, photograph, or both is essential.
- A swab specimen of the wound for PCR-based testing of DNA in saliva can be useful for forensic purposes when the criminal intent seems possible or likely.
- Wounds should be copiously irrigated with saline solution and débrided. Most authorities advise against routine closure, but this should be determined on an individual basis.
- Prophylactic antibiotics (for options, see "Postexposure Prophylaxis After Other Forms of Trauma" later in the chapter) are indicated for patients who are seen relatively early after the bite.
- The need for tetanus immunization should be addressed.
- Evaluation for the possibility of HIV, hepatitis B, and hepatitis C transmission should proceed along the lines outlined in previous sections of this chapter (with evaluation of the source person if possible). Rarely, human bites transmit syphilis (mainly in the event that the source person had a mucous patch lesion of secondary syphilis; see Chapter 7).
- Close follow-up should be arranged as outlined for dog and cat bites.
- Consideration may be needed for postexposure prophylaxis for hepatitis B, but not for hepatitis C or HIV.

Other Types of Bites

Rat bites can transmit *Streptobacillus moniliformis* and *Spirillum minus,* which cause two different types of rat-bite fever. Bites by reptiles of all types may transmit *Salmonella* species. Snake bites are associated with a wide variety of aerobic and anaerobic bacteria, reflecting the fecal flora of their prey, but the need for prophylactic antibiotic therapy is not well defined. Bite wounds inflicted by large cats (lions, tigers, and cougars) typically contain *P. multocida,* thus resembling those of their smaller domestic cousins.

Choice of Antimicrobials for Postexposure Prophylaxis After Bites

Analysis of the relative activity of various antimicrobials against pathogens isolated from bite wounds (Table 26-7) makes it clear that the optimum drug of choice is usually a β-lactam–β-lactamase inhibitor combination. Thus amoxicillin-clavulanate (Augmentin) is a near-ideal agent for oral therapy, and ampicillin-clavulanate (Unasyn) is appropriate when intravenous therapy is warranted. Reliance should not be placed on first-generation cephalosporins because of the likelihood that anaerobic pathogens and *E. corrodens* may be resistant. The optimum duration of prophylactic, or expectant, therapy for bite wounds is not well established, but most authorities advise a 3- to 5-day course.

 KEY POINTS

POSTEXPOSURE PROPHYLAXIS AFTER BITE WOUNDS

- ⊃ Bacteria notoriously associated with bite wounds include *P. multocida* after cat bites, *Pasteurella* species and *C. canimorsus* after dog bites, and *E. corrodens* after human bites. However, most infections after bite wounds are polymicrobial.
- ⊃ Expectant antimicrobial therapy should be considered for patients seen within 8 hours of a bite wound. Patients seen more than 8 hours after the wound generally have established infection, and definitive therapy should be based—ideally—on the results of Gram stains and cultures.
- ⊃ Antibiotics are unnecessary for most open, uncomplicated bite wounds.
- ⊃ Antibiotics are indicated for high-risk bite wounds from dogs, cats, and other animals if the bites involve the hands, feet, joints, tendons, or bones, if thorough irrigation and débridement are not possible, or if the patient is immunocompromised or asplenic.
- ⊃ Antibiotics are indicated for human bites, especially for clenched-fist injuries.
- ⊃ Amoxicillin-clavulanate (Augmentin) is the most useful antibiotic for expectant therapy of bite wounds on the basis of currently available data.
- ⊃ Asplenic patients who have been bitten by dogs should be considered for hospitalization and intravenous antibiotics because of the risk of overwhelming *C. canimorsus* sepsis.
- ⊃ The optimum duration of expectant antibiotic therapy after bite wounds is not well established, but most authorities recommend a 3- to 5-day course.

SUGGESTED READING

American Academy of Pediatrics, Committee on Infectious Diseases. 2000 Red Book: Report of the Committee on Infectious Diseases. 25th ed., Elk Grove, Ill.: American Academy of Pediatrics; 2000.

Eron LJ. Targeting lurking pathogens in acute traumatic and chronic wounds. J Emerg Med 1999; 17: 189-195.

Fleisher GR. The management of bite wounds. N Engl J Med 1999; 340: 138-140.

Goldstein EJ. Current concepts on animal bites: bacteriology and therapy. Curr Clin Top Infect Dis 1999; 19: 99-111.

Hoff GL, Brawley J, Johnson K. Companion animal issues and the physician. South Med J 1999; 92: 651-659.

Oral and dental aspects of child abuse and neglect. American Academy of Pediatrics. Committee on Child Abuse and Neglect. American Academy of Pediatric Dentistry. Ad Hoc Work Group on Child Abuse and Neglect. Pediatrics 1999; 104: 348-350.

Pretty IA, Anderson GS, Sweet DJ. Human bites and the risk of human immunodeficiency virus transmission. Am J Forensic Med Pathol 1999; 20: 232-239.

Smith PF, Meadowcroft AM, May DB. Treating mammalian bite wounds. J Clin Pharm Ther 2000; 25: 85-99.

Sweet D, Lorente JA, Valenzuela A, et al. PCR-based DNA typing of saliva strains recovered from human skin. J Forensic Sci 1997; 42: 447-451.

Talan DA, Citron DM, Abrahamian FM, et al. Bacteriologic analysis of infected dog and cat bites. N Engl J Med 1999; 340: 85-92.

TABLE 26-7
Relative Activity of Various Antibiotics Against Bacteria Commonly Found in Bite Wounds

Agent	*Pasteurella multocida**	Anaerobes	*Eikenella corrodens*	*Capnocytophaga canimorsus*	*Staphylococcus aureus*	*Staphylococcus intermedius*	Comments
Amoxicillin-clavulanate	++++	++++	++++	+++	++++	++++	Overall, the most useful agent for prophylaxis of bite wounds.
Penicillin	++	++	+++	+++	+	++	Some oral anaerobes such as fusobacteria are resistant.
Dicloxacillin	++	++	–	NA	++++	++++	Activity against *P. multocida* and oral anaerobes can be marginal.
Cephalexin	+	++	+	NA	+++	+++	Activity against *P. multocida* and oral anaerobes can be marginal.
Cefuroxime	+++	++	++	NA	+++	+++	Offers reasonably good coverage against the common pathogens.
Erythromycin	+	++	+	+++	++	++	Activity against *P. multocida* and oral anaerobes can be marginal.
Azithromycin	++++	++	+++	+++	+++	NA	Limited clinical experience in this setting.
Clindamycin	0	++++	0	+++	+++	+++	Limited activity against *P. multocida* and *E. corrodens* is a major limitation.
Tetracycline	+++	++	+++	+++	++	++	An acceptable alternative in patients with history of penicillin allergy.
Trimethoprim-sulfamethoxazole	+++	0	+++	+ to ++	+++	NA	Lack of anaerobic coverage is a limitation; could be combined with metronidazole if necessary.
Levofloxacin	++++	++	++++	++++	+++	+++	Quinolones are potentially useful in this setting; major limitations are limited anaerobic coverage and limited experience.

Data from multiple sources, especially Goldstein EJC. Bites. In: Mandell GL, Bennett JE, Dolin R, ed. Mandell, Douglas, and Bennett's Principles and Practice of Infectious Diseases. 5th ed., Philadelphia: Churchill Livingstone; 2000: 3202-3206.
Scale: 0, inactive; ++++, highly active; NA, data unavailable.

Postexposure Prophylaxis After Other Forms of Trauma

Minor trauma is a common event in primary care, and the inevitable contamination of traumatic wounds by bacteria and other microorganisms tempts clinicians to prescribe prophylactic, or—more properly—expectant, antimicrobial therapy.

- For simple lacerations, including lacerations involving the hand, numerous randomized, placebo-controlled trials have failed to demonstrate a benefit of antibiotic therapy for uncomplicated lacerations. Cleaning of the wound such as irrigation with povidone-iodine reduces potential contamination to a low level.
- For open (compound) fractures involving an extremity, the efficacy of prophylactic therapy with antistaphylocccal antibiotics has been clearly established by randomized trials. A short course (24 hours) of antistaphylococcal therapy was shown to be as efficacious as the traditional 3- to 5-day regimen. Antibiotics are sometimes given after facial fractures and basilar skull fractures as well, but the evidence for efficacy is much less convincing.
- For puncture wounds involving the foot, prophylactic therapy with an antipseudomonal drug (such as ciprofloxacin) is sometimes recommended because of the risk of osteomyelitis caused by *Pseudomonas aeruginosa* (see Chapter 15). Unfortunately, quinolones are contraindicated in children and adolescents, and no convenient alternatives are available.
- Wounds that have been exposed to water are vulnerable to infection caused by a wide variety of pathogens, including *Aeromonas hydrophila* (freshwater), *Vibrio vulnificus* (saltwater or brackish water), *E. rhusiopathiae, Edwardsiella tarda,* and *Mycobacterium marinum.* These same bacteria are sometimes transmitted by wounds sustained from handling fish or other marine animals. Recently, *Streptococcus iniae* (not previously known to be a human pathogen) was found to cause severe cellulitis in persons who had handled fish, especially tilapia, which are used in Asian cooking. Again, there may be a theoretical rationale for short-course prophylaxis, but properly designed studies have not established this point.

 KEY POINTS

POSTEXPOSURE PROPHYLAXIS AFTER OTHER FORMS OF TRAUMA

- ⊃ Antibiotics are not indicated after simple lacerations.
- ⊃ Antibiotics are indicated after open fractures.
- ⊃ On theoretical grounds, prophylactic antibiotics might be useful for nail puncture wounds of the plantar surfaces of the feet and for fresh wounds that have been exposed to water. However, comparative trials are lacking.
- ⊃ By no means should antimicrobial therapy be viewed as a substitute for aggressive wound care, which remains the most important measure for prevention of infection after trauma of any kind.

SUGGESTED READING

Dellinger EP, Caplan ES, Weaver LD, et al. Duration of preventive antibiotic administration for open extremity fractures. Arch Surg 1988; 123: 333-339.

Hoffman RD, Adams BD. The role of antibiotics in the management of elective and post-traumatic hand surgery. Hand Clin 1998; 14: 657-666.

Talan DA. Infectious disease issues in the emergency department. Clin Infect Dis 1996; 23: 1-14.

Tsai E, Failla JM. Hand infections in the trauma patient. Hand Clin 1999; 15: 373-386.

Weinstein MR, Litt M, Kertesz DA, et al. S. iniae Study Group. Invasive infections due to a fish pathogen, *Streptococcus iniae*. N Engl J Med 1997; 337: 589-594.

Preexposure Prophylaxis for Endocarditis

Prophylaxis of infective endocarditis before dental and other procedures in patients with certain preexisting heart conditions is well established in clinical practice. Endocarditis is difficult to diagnose and uniformly fatal if untreated, and even when successfully treated it often results in long-term morbidity and reduced life expectancy.

Unfortunately, no data convincingly demonstrate that endocarditis can be prevented in humans. The obstacles to such a demonstration are formidable. A leading researcher in this area points out that, assuming that the risk of endocarditis after dental extraction is 1 in 500, that an antibiotic is 100% effective for prophylaxis, and that a hospital ethics committee would approve the protocol, a randomized study involving 6000 patients would be necessary to obtain a marginally significant result ($\chi^2 = 4.2, p < .05$). The benefit of prophylactic antibiotics has been challenged by several studies in recent years, prompting the suggestion that prophylaxis might be reserved for patients with significant predisposing lesions who are undergoing dental extraction or gingival surgery, for patients with prosthetic heart valves, and for patients with previous episodes of endocarditis.

Given the above, what is the standard of care? Four issues should be addressed for each patient:

- What risk is imposed by the patient's heart condition? The patient's risk should be classified as "relatively high," "intermediate," or "very low or negligible" on the basis of the nature of the lesion and the consequences of endocarditis, should it occur (Table 26-8). Endocarditis is especially likely when a lesion causes blood to flow abnormally and across a narrow orifice from a high-pressure vessel or chamber to a low-pressure vessel or chamber. Examples include aortic regurgitation, mitral regurgitation, ventricular septal defect, and coarctation of the aorta. The consequences of endocarditis are usually serious in patients with prosthetic valves and in patients with significant hemodynamic abnormalities.
- What risk is imposed by the procedure? Procedures can be classified as "relatively high risk" or "lower risk" on the basis of the likelihood that bacteremia will occur (Table 26-9). Estimates of the risk of bacteremia associated with various procedures were derived from numerous studies in which frequent blood cultures were obtained during and just after the procedure. Highest risks of bacteremia have been associated with periodontal surgery (up to 90%), dental extraction (about 60%),

TABLE 26-8
Stratification of Heart Conditions According to Risk of Endocarditis

Risk category	Examples	Comments
Relatively high risk	Prosthetic heart valves Aortic regurgitation Mitral regurgitation Ventricular septal defect Patent ductus arteriosus Coarctation of the aorta Aortic stenosis with hemodynamic abnormality Cyanotic congenital heart disease Previous endocarditis Residual hemodynamic abnormality after surgical repair of a cardiac lesion	Patients with prosthetic heart valves are at high risk (in one study, odds ratio 75:1 compared with persons with normal heart valves) and also have high morbidity because replacement of the prosthetic valve is often necessary for cure. Aortic regurgitation, mitral regurgitation, ventricular septal defect, patent ductus arteriosus, and coarctation of the aorta have in common the abnormal flow of blood from a high- to a low-pressure chamber across a narrow orifice, which promotes the formation of vegetations and deposition of bacteria in the low-pressure chamber, just distal to the orifice (Rodbard's rules).
Intermediate risk	Mitral valve prolapse with regurgitant murmur or valve thickening or redundancy by echocardiogram Aortic stenosis (bicuspid valve or calcific aortic sclerosis) with minimal hemodynamic abnormality Degenerative valvular disease (such as calcification of the mitral valve annulus) Asymmetric septal hypertrophy Tricuspid valve disease Pulmonary stenosis Mitral stenosis without regurgitation (pure mitral stenosis) Surgical repair of a cardiac lesion within the past 6 months, no significant hemodynamic abnormality	The extent to which patients with mitral valve prolapse should receive prophylaxis against endocarditis is controversial. Mitral valve prolapse is extremely common in the general population, and routine use of antibiotics for all persons with this diagnosis is undesirable (see text). Similarly, degenerative lesions such as calcific aortic sclerosis and calcification of the mitral valve annulus are common in older persons, yet endocarditis in this setting is uncommon. Although the need for prophylaxis may be arguable, the diagnosis of endocarditis should nevertheless be obtained when patients with the cardiac conditions here have unexplained fever or signs and symptoms suggesting embolic phenomena or immune complex disease.
Low or negligible risk	Mitral valve prolapse without regurgitant murmur and without valvular thickening or redundancy by echocardiography Isolated atrial septal defect Tricuspid regurgitation by echocardiogram with otherwise-normal tricuspid valve Coronary artery disease Arteriosclerotic plaques Cardiac pacemaker	None of these settings features abnormal flow of blood from a high- to a low-pressure chamber across a narrow orifice, and therefore "Rodbard's rules" (see above) are not met. Endocarditis occasionally occurs in these settings, but the number of patients who would need to receive prophylaxis to prevent a single case of endocarditis is currently believed to be prohibitive.

Modified from Durack DT. Prevention of infective endocarditis. N Engl J Med 1995; 332: 38-44.

and prostatectomy in patients with infected urine (about 60%). Transient bacteremia is a frequent event of everyday life—for example, during vigorous brushing of the teeth—and occurs occasionally after such routine medical events as normal delivery, barium enema, or proctoscopy.
- Are antibiotics indicated? Depending on the answers to the previous questions, the practitioner determines whether

antibiotics are indicated based on the underlying heart condition and the risk of the procedure (Table 26-10). The answer is sometimes black or white, but there are also many shades of gray. Erring toward the side of prophylaxis is often best when the complications of endocarditis could be disastrous, as in patients with prosthetic heart valves or patients with significant cardiac lesions such as aortic regurgitation with heart failure.

TABLE 26-9
Risk of Bacteremia with Various Procedures

Risk category	Examples	Comments
Relatively high-risk procedures	Dental procedures that induce gingival or mucosal bleeding, including professional cleaning and scaling Tonsillectomy or adenoidectomy Surgery involving the gastrointestinal or upper respiratory mucosa Bronchoscopy with a rigid bronchoscope Sclerotherapy for esophageal varices Esophageal dilatation Gallbladder surgery Cystoscopy for urethral dilatation Urinary catheterization in the presence of urinary tract infection Surgery on the urinary tract, including the prostate Incision and drainage of any infected tissue Vaginal hysterectomy Vaginal delivery complicated by infection	These procedures are associated with relatively high rates of bacteremia. Compilation of data from various studies indicates the following risks of bacteremia: periodontal surgery, 88%; dental extraction, 60%; prostatectomy in the presence of infected urine, 60%; esophageal dilatation, 45%; rigorous tooth brushing or irrigation, 40%; tonsillectomy, 35%; dilatation of genitourinary strictures, 28%; bronchoscopy with a rigid bronchoscope, 15%.
Lower risk procedures	Dental procedures that are unlikely to cause bleeding, such as simple fillings above the gum line or adjustment of orthodontic appliances Intraoral injection of local anesthetic Tympanostomy tube insertion Endotracheal tube insertion Bronchoscopy with a flexible bronchoscope, with or without biopsy Cardiac catheterization Gastrointestinal endoscopy, with or without biopsy Cesarean section Urethral catheterization, uncomplicated vaginal delivery, dilatation and curettage, therapeutic abortion, insertion or removal of an intrauterine device, or laparoscopy in the absence of infection	These procedures are associated with relatively low rates of bacteremia. Compilation of data from various studies indicates the following risks of bacteremia: insertion and removal of a urinary catheter, 13%; barium enema, 10%; hemorrhoidectomy, 8%; endoscopic retrograde cholangiopancreatography, 5%; colonoscopy 5%; sigmoidoscopy with a rigid sigmoidoscope, 5%; normal delivery, 3%; proctoscopy, 2%; cardiac catheterization, 2%; bronchoscopy with a flexible bronchoscope, 0%; insertion or removal of an intrauterine device, 0%.

Modified from Durack DT. Prevention of infective endocarditis. N Engl J Med 1995; 332: 38-44.

Withholding of prophylaxis when the cardiac lesions are relatively trivial is often preferable. When, for example, should antibiotics be given to patients with mitral valve prolapse who are scheduled for dental procedures? Two researchers calculated the outcome for 10 million patients with mitral valve prolapse undergoing dental procedures: (1) With no prophylaxis, two fatal and 47 nonfatal cases of endocarditis would occur; (2) with penicillin, five cases of endocarditis and 175 deaths from drug reaction would occur; and (3) with erythromycin,

TABLE 26-10
Recommendations for Use of Prophylactic Antibiotics for Prevention of Endocarditis

Underlying heart condition*	High-risk procedures†	Low-risk procedures†
Relatively high risk	Prophylaxis recommended	Prophylaxis optional‡
Intermediate risk	Prophylaxis recommended	Prophylaxis not recommended
Low or negligible risk	Prophylaxis not recommended	Prophylaxis not recommended

Modified from Durack DT, Prophylaxis of infective endocarditis. In: Mandell GL, Bennett JE, Dolin R. Mandell, Douglas, and Bennett's Principles and Practice of Infectious Diseases. 5th ed., Philadelphia: Churchill Livingstone; 2000: 917-925.
*See Table 26-8.
†See Table 26-9.
‡Whether to give prophylaxis becomes a judgment decision between the physician and the patient.

one fatal and 12 nonfatal cases of endocarditis would occur. A reasonable strategy is to give antibiotics only to patients with mitral valve prolapse who have a significant murmur or thickening of the valve as shown by echocardiography.

■ What should be the recommended therapy? The recommendations issued from time to time by expert committees assembled by the American Heart Association take into account the preceding issues (Table 26-11). Prophylaxis before dental and upper respiratory procedures is targeted against viridans streptococci. Prophylaxis before gastrointestinal and genitourinary procedures is targeted against enterococci. Patients with prosthetic heart valves who are undergoing gastrointestinal and genitourinary procedures are given gentamicin in addition to ampicillin or vancomycin in the attempt to obtain maximum protection against enterococcal endocarditis. The continued emergence of drug resistance among enterococci, however, makes optimum prophylaxis increasingly problematic.

The primary care clinician should determine the need for prophylaxis for each patient with a significant heart lesion (Figure 26-2). The patient should be educated about any such need and be able to convey recommendations to dentists and other health care professionals.

TABLE 26-11
American Heart Association Recommendations for Prophylaxis of Endocarditis

Setting	Regimen	Dose for adults	Dose for children
DENTAL AND UPPER RESPIRATORY PROCEDURES			
Oral regimen, no penicillin allergy	Amoxicillin	2 g 1 hour before the procedure	50 mg/kg 1 hour before the procedure
Alternative oral regimens, penicillin allergy	Clindamycin Cephalexin or cefadroxil Azithromycin or clarithromycin	600 mg 1 hour before the procedure 2 g 1 hour before the procedure 500 mg 1 hour before the procedure	20 mg/kg 1 hour before the procedure 50 mg/kg 1 hour before the procedure 15 mg/kg 1 hour before the procedure
Parenteral regimen, no penicillin allergy	Ampicillin	2 g IM or IV 30 minutes before the procedure	50 mg/kg IM or IV 30 minutes before the procedure
Alternative parenteral regimens, penicillin allergy	Clindamycin Cefazolin	600 mg IV within 30 minutes before the procedure 1 g IM or IV within 30 minutes before the procedure	20 mg/kg IM or IV 30 minutes before the procedure 25 mg/kg IM or IV within 30 minutes before the procedure
GASTROINTESTINAL OR GENITOURINARY PROCEDURES			
Oral, no penicillin allergy	Amoxicillin	2 g 1 hour before the procedure	50 mg/kg 1 hour before the procedure
Parenteral, no penicillin allergy	Ampicillin, with or without gentamicin Gentamicin*	2 g IM or IV within 30 minutes before the procedure 2.5 mg/kg (120 mg, maximum) IM or IV 30 minutes before the procedure	50 mg/kg IM or IV 30 minutes before the procedure 2 mg/kg IM or IV 30 minutes before the procedure

Continued

TABLE 26-11—cont'd
American Heart Association Recommendations for Prophylaxis of Endocarditis

Setting	Regimen	Dose for adults	Dose for children
Penicillin allergy	Vancomycin, with or without gentamicin	1 g IV infused slowly over 1 hour beginning 1 hour before the procedure	20 mg/kg IV infused slowly over 1 hour beginning 1 hour before the procedure
	Gentamicin*	1.5 mg/kg (120 mg, maximum) IM or IV 30 minutes before the procedure	2 mg/kg IM or IV 30 minutes before the procedure

From Dejani AS, Taubert KA, Wilson W, et al. Prevention of bacterial endocarditis: recommendations by the American Heart Association. JAMA 1997; 27: 1794-1801.

*Parenteral regimens that include gentamicin are recommended for patients with prosthetic heart valves and for those with advanced underlying heart disease who would tolerate cardiac surgery poorly. These combination regimens (ampicillin or vancomycin, plus gentamicin) are designed to give optimum coverage against enterococci.

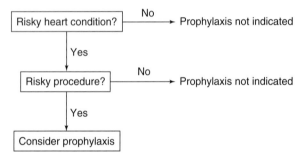

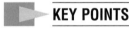

FIG. 26-2   Overview of prophylaxis for endocarditis (see Tables 26-8 to 26-11).

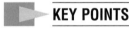   **KEY POINTS**

PREEXPOSURE PROPHYLAXIS FOR ENDOCARDITIS
⊃ The ability of prophylactic antibiotics to prevent infective endocarditis has not been established by rigorous controlled trials.
⊃ In practice, however, antibiotics are commonly given to patients with significant underlying heart conditions who are scheduled for procedures that carry a high risk for bacteremia.
⊃ When to give prophylactic antibiotics to patients with mitral valve prolapse, which is an extremely common lesion, is controversial. Antibiotics should probably be reserved for patients with a significant murmur or with significant valvular thickening shown by echocardiography.

SUGGESTED READING
Bor DH, Himmelstein DU. Endocarditis prophylaxis for patients with mitral valve prolapse: a quantitative analysis. Am J Med 1984; 76: 711-717.

Dajani AS, Taubert KA, Wilson W, et al. Prevention of bacterial endocarditis: recommendations by the American Heart Association. JAMA 1997; 277: 1794-1801.

Durack DT. Antibiotics for prevention of endocarditis during dentistry: time to scale back? Ann Intern Med 1998; 129: 829-831.

Durack DT. Prophylaxis of infective endocarditis. In: Mandell GL, Bennett JE, Dolin R, et al. Mandell, Douglas, and Bennett's Principles and Practice of Infectious Diseases. 5th ed., Philadelphia: Churchill-Livingstone; 2000: 917-925.

Kantoch MJ, Collins-Nakai RL, Medwid S, et al. Adult patients' knowledge about their congenital heart disease. Can J Cardiol 1997; 13: 641-645.

Osmon DR. Antimicrobial prophylaxis in adults. Mayo Clin Proc 2000; 75: 98-109.

Seto TB, Kwiat D, Taira DA, et al. Physicians' recommendations to patients for use of antibiotic prophylaxis to prevent endocarditis. JAMA 2000; 284: 68-71.

Taubert KA, Dajani AS. Preventing bacterial endocarditis: American Heart Association guidelines. Am Fam Physician 1998; 57: 457-468.

Preexposure Prophylaxis for Surgical Procedures

Controlled therapeutic trials and clinical experience have led to general consensus in most areas of prophylaxis of surgical wound infection. Prophylaxis is indicated when the likelihood of postoperative infection is high or when the consequences of postoperative infection are grave. Antimicrobial prophylaxis is given before prosthetic heart valve or joint replacement, for example, because infection in these circumstances can be disastrous to the patient. Most surgeons have in place set protocols for administration of prophylactic antimicrobials. For the past quarter century cephalosporins, and especially cefazolin, have been the most popular drugs for this purpose. A concern that heavy use of cefazolin may promote the emergence of methicillin-resistant *S. aureus* and the vancomycin-resistant enterococcus *Streptococcus faecium* has yet to be resolved.

Some current recommendations are summarized in Table 26-12, but these recommendations engender a number of controversies and are subject to change from time to time. The duration of prophylaxis should be brief—in most instances no longer than 24 hours—and in some instances

TABLE 26-12
Prophylaxis Before Surgical Procedures: Summary of Current Recommendations

Procedure	Likely organisms	Drugs of choice	Alternative drugs
CARDIAC SURGERY			
Prosthetic valve, coronary artery bypass, pacemaker, or defibrillator implant	*Staphylococcus epidermidis, Staphylococcus aureus, Corynebacterium,* enteric gram-negative bacilli	Cefazolin or cefuroxime	Vancomycin*
GASTROINTESTINAL SURGERY			
Esophageal or gastroduodenal surgery, *high-risk*	Enteric gram-negative bacilli; gram-positive cocci	Cefazolin	
Biliary tract surgery, *high-risk*	Enteric gram-negative bacilli, gram-positive cocci, clostridia	Cefazolin	
Colorectal surgery	Enteric gram-negative bacilli, anaerobes, enterococci	Oral: neomycin *plus* erythromycin base IV: cefoxitin, cefotetan, or cefoxitin-metronidazole	
Appendectomy, nonperforated	Enteric gram-negative bacilli, anaerobes, enterococci	Cefoxitin or cefotetan	
GENITOURINARY TRACT SURGERY			
Prostatectomy, *high-risk*	Enteric gram-negative bacilli, enterococci	Ciprofloxacin	
GYNECOLOGIC AND OBSTETRIC SURGERY			
Vaginal or abdominal hysterectomy	Enteric gram-negative bacilli, enterococci, group B streptococci, anaerobes	Cefazolin or cefotetan or cefoxitin	
Cesarean section, *high-risk*	Enteric gram-negative bacilli, enterococci, group B streptococci, anaerobes	Cefazolin	
Abortion, first trimester, *high-risk*	Enteric gram-negative bacilli, enterococci, group B streptococci, anaerobes	Aqueous penicillin G or doxycycline	
Abortion, second semester, *high-risk*	Enteric gram-negative bacilli, enterococci, group B streptococci, anaerobes	Cefazolin	
HEAD AND NECK SURGERY			
Incisions through oral or pharyngeal mucosa	Anaerobes, enteric gram-negative bacilli, *S. aureus*	Clindamycin *plus* gentamicin	
NEUROSURGERY			
Craniotomy	*S. aureus, S. epidermidis*	Cefazolin	Vancomycin*
OPHTHALMIC SURGERY			
Various procedures	*S. epidermidis, S. aureus,* streptococci, enteric gram-negative bacilli, *Pseudomonas* species	Gentamicin, tobramycin, ciprofloxacin, ofloxacin, or neomycin–gramicidin–polymyxin B or cefazolin	

Continued

TABLE 26-12—cont'd
Prophylaxis Before Surgical Procedures: Summary of Current Recommendations

Procedure	Likely organisms	Drugs of choice	Alternative drugs
ORTHOPEDIC SURGERY			
Total joint replacement, internal fixation of fractures	*S. aureus, S. epidermidis*	Cefazolin	Vancomycin*
THORACIC (NONCARDIAC) SURGERY			
Lobectomy, pneumonectomy	*S. aureus, S. epidermidis,* streptococci, enteric gram-negative bacilli	Cefazolin or cefuroxime	Vancomycin
VASCULAR SURGERY			
Arterial surgery involving a prosthesis, the abdominal aorta, or a groin incision	*S. aureus, S. epidermidis,* enteric gram-negative bacilli	Cefazolin	Vancomycin
Lower extremity amputation for ischemia	*S. aureus, S. epidermidis,* enteric gram-negative bacilli, clostridia	Cefazolin	Vancomycin

*Vancomycin is often preferred for implant surgery such as prosthetic heart valve implantation.

limited to a single dose. Primary care clinicians should have a general familiarity with these recommendations so that they can counsel patients before surgery and coordinate care when patients are admitted for "same-day" surgery or undergo surgery in the outpatient setting. Intravenous antibiotics should in most instances be given 30 minutes before the anticipated skin incision.

SUGGESTED READING

Antimicrobial prophylaxis in surgery. Med Lett 1999; 41: 75-80.
Barie PS. Antibiotic-resistant gram-positive cocci: implications for surgical practice. World J Surg 1998; 22: 118-126.
Fry DE, ed. Surgical Infections. Boston: Little, Brown; 1995.
Gyssens IC. Preventing postoperative infections: current treatment recommendations. Drugs 1999; 57: 175-185.
Polk HC Jr, Christmas AB. Prophylactic antibiotics in surgery and surgical wound infections. Am Surg 2000; 66: 105-111.
Schentag JJ, Hyatt JM, Carr JR, et al. Genesis of methicillin-resistant *Staphylococcus aureus* (MRSA), how treatment of MRSA infections has selected for vancomycin-resistant *Enterococcus faecium,* and the importance of antibiotic management and infection control. Clin Infect Dis 1998; 26: 1204-1214.

27 Parenteral Antimicrobial Therapy in the Ambulatory Setting

R. BROOKS GAINER II

Outpatient parenteral antimicrobial therapy (OPAT) was one of the major developments in medicine during the last quarter of the 20th century. Previously patients requiring prolonged intravenous therapy for such diseases as endocarditis, staphylococcal sepsis, osteomyelitis, systemic fungal infections, and viral infections remained in the hospital for 4 to 6 weeks or longer just to receive their medication. Many of these patients can now be treated successfully as outpatients.

The purpose of this chapter is to outline the historical aspects of OPAT development, the various models available, patient selection, choice of therapy and methods of delivery, monitoring, medicolegal issues, reimbursement, and what the future may portend for this form of treatment.

Historical Perspectives

Intravenous administration of antibiotics outside the hospital was first described in 1974 for children with cystic fibrosis. Soon thereafter, OPAT was used to treat adults with osteomyelitis. As interest grew, numerous studies documented the safety, efficacy, and cost savings of OPAT for a wide variety of serious infections. Interested physicians, home health agencies, and visiting nurse agencies began to collaborate to improve the mechanics of OPAT. During the early 1980s entrepreneurs formed infusion companies of various types. These included joint ventures among physicians, hospitals, and home health agencies. Unfortunately, some of these relationships were used by partners in these ventures to gain referrals to their agencies (Table 27-1).

The introduction of OPAT stimulated tremendous growth in related technologies. The introduction of plastic bags overcame the problem of glass container breakage. The need for superb venous access prompted the development of the intravenous devices we now enjoy. New mechanical and electrical pumps provided safe volume- and time-controlled administration of drugs in the outpatient setting. Meanwhile, researchers addressed the frequency with which intravenous catheters needed to be changed both inside and outside the hospital. Studies were also designed to address how long intravenous solutions remain safe at room temperature.

New antimicrobial agents with longer serum half-lives and broader spectrums of activity simplified treatment. The introduction of ceftriaxone (Rocephin) in 1985 revolutionized OPAT for many gram-positive and gram-negative bacterial infections. Researchers were then stimulated to determine how frequent the doses of other agents really needed to be in order to provide adequate bactericidal and bacteriostatic activity (see Chapter 19). Pharmaceutical firms were encouraged to develop new drugs with prolonged serum half-lives.

The availability of OPAT shortens hospitalization and in some cases makes it unnecessary. Patients benefit from the psychological support of family, friends, and caregivers in their homes. Often patients can return to work while receiving treatment, which reduces the economic impact of serious infections on patients and their employers. The risk of iatrogenic infection (now called "nosohusial" when acquired in the home or outpatient setting, as opposed to "nosocomial" in

TABLE 27-1

Essentials of an Outpatient Parenteral Antimicrobial Therapy (OPAT) Program

Aspect	Essential components
Stringent patient selection	Appropriate therapy for an identified infection; clinically stable patient; well-tolerated antimicrobial agent; adequate home environment; "teachable" patient and caregiver; patient confidence and proficiency in home care; financial feasibility
Adequate support personnel	Nursing staff and pharmacy (maintain vascular access; prepare, deliver, and oversee administration of drugs; monitor patients for problems related to drug toxicity or to vascular access)
Physician	Availability of 24-hour on-call emergency care; provision of regular follow-up; monitoring of therapeutic efficacy; monitoring for drug toxicity (based on clinical reports and selected laboratory tests)
Laboratory	Expeditious determination and reporting of serum drug levels and other laboratory tests
Oversight entity (physician, practice, or firm providing OPAT)	Collection of data from each patient pertaining to efficacy, safety, and cost of OPAT; tabulation and analysis of data; ideally, comparison of data with those of other practices using the OPAT registry of the Outpatient Infusion Therapy Association (see text)

the inpatient setting) is lower outside the hospital. Properly carried out, OPAT results in enormous cost savings.

OPAT also carries risk. Patients give up the safety net of having nurses and other health care workers a "call light away" in the event of emergency or change in clinical condition. Patients have to learn about maintaining sterility, flushing lines, changing intravenous bags or antibiotic-filled syringes, and setting electrical pumps. They need to know about the potential adverse reactions to their intravenous devices, mechanical devices, and drugs. Despite these risks the growth of OPAT and its enthusiastic endorsement by patients have been phenomenal; indeed, the effect on the treatment of infectious diseases in the United States has been revolutionary.

During the mid-1980s physicians had to convince third party payers of the efficacy and safety of OPAT. Conversely, by the mid-1990s physicians faced the need to convince patients and caregivers that OPAT carries risks and that a team approach is important to prevent serious complications. In recent years payers have seemed to be concerned primarily with the costs of OPAT rather than its quality. The 1997 guidelines of the Infectious Diseases Society of America (IDSA) emphasize the importance of having a knowledgeable physician oversee any OPAT program.

Various Models of Outpatient Parenteral Antimicrobial Therapy

No single model of OPAT fits the needs of all patients. The models used are influenced by many factors, such as geography, weather, and philosophy of payers in the particular location. Also, with a few exceptions, Medicare does not cover self-administered infusion therapy or infusion therapy administered by home health agencies.

Infusion Center Model

Infusion centers may be created in a variety of medical settings, including a hospital clinic or outpatient area, an urgent

care center, an emergency department, a physician's office, or an independent facility. The infusion center model is ideal for the Medicare patient. The patient can be discharged from the hospital and treated in the infusion center with appropriate reimbursement from Medicare. The infusion center has a physician on site, as well as nursing personnel and often laboratory facilities.

Major disadvantages of the infusion center model are the need for patients to leave home and travel to the center during the recuperative phase of their illnesses and the need to make multiple visits each day if the antimicrobial agent must be given more frequently than every 24 hours. The physician office–based infusion center is usually the most efficient and cost-effective model. The patients are not encumbered by the administrative restrictions of the hospital-based center, and they have immediate access to the prescribing physician. The disadvantage of the physician office–based infusion center is that the physician or nurse practitioner or physician's assistant must be present in the facility while Medicare patients receive therapy. A tertiary care facility or a multispecialty clinic facility can be as efficient as the physician office–based infusion center if properly organized. The size of such facilities, however, is intimidating to some patients.

Self-Infusion Model

The ideal method of OPAT is for the patient to prepare, administer, and monitor therapy at home. Patients must become familiar with the antimicrobial agent and with the management of the intravenous device, including how to obtain access, how to flush the device, and how to minimize the risk of infection. Printed educational materials covering the properties and common side effects of the drug and maintenance of intravenous access must be provided. Ongoing support systems must be available 24 hours a day to address questions pertaining to drugs, intravenous devices, and other equipment. Antimicrobial agents and other supplies can be delivered to homes by appropriate support agencies if a commercial firm or visiting nurse agency is involved. Patients can also return to their physician's office facilities to be evaluated, to have appropriate laboratory work performed, and to pick up their drugs and supplies.

In this model the team approach is essential. The prescribing physician must be confident that the patient has access to the support system vital to overcoming the trade-offs between in-hospital therapy (continuous monitoring by trained health care workers) and OPAT (convenience and cost savings).

Visiting Nurse Model

A third model for OPAT uses a visiting nurse, who is usually an employee of a home health agency or a nursing association. This model is useful for situations in which the patient is unable to travel to an infusion center because of physical or psychological factors and cannot self-administer the drug. The visiting nurse model offers the advantage of having a professional in the home every day to assess the patient, evaluate venous access, and watch for adverse reactions. The major disadvantage is the increased cost of having a trained nurse visit the patient's home daily. The health care professional also faces risk, in some situations, from entering dangerous neighborhoods.

Extended Care–Nursing Home Model

The extended care–nursing home model is applicable for Medicare patients who are not covered for self-administration and cannot come to an infusion center for one reason or another. In this model the staff members of an extended care facility administer the drug, monitor the patient for adverse effects, and obtain the requisite laboratory studies. The attending physician periodically visits the patient at the facility, or the patient returns to the physician's office for evaluation of the infection being treated, vascular access, and evidence of drug toxicity. This model is usually the most expensive method of OPAT because of the cost associated with an extended care facility. Unfortunately, Congress has yet to modify the Medicare law to allow for self-administration.

Hospital Multispecialty Model

In some areas the patient has no choice but to return to the emergency room or to the outpatient facility of a local hospital to receive OPAT. This may be necessary if self-administered therapy is not covered by the patient's insurance plan or if the physician lacks facilities for office-based infusion therapy. In this model OPAT is typically given in the emergency room. Long waits are frequently necessary while legitimate emergencies are handled in the treating facility. Ideally, hospitals should develop outpatient infusion suites to accommodate both Medicare patients and patients whose only alternatives are to remain in the hospital or in an extended care facility. In some situations the hospital multispecialty model might even be less expensive than the visiting nurse model for OPAT.

Patient Selection for Outpatient Parenteral Antimicrobial Therapy

Patient selection for OPAT is based on the medical condition, the home situation, and, last but not least, the payer. The patient's insurance program, whether an indemnity plan or a health maintenance organization (HMO), must be contacted to clarify the terms of coverage.

Patient's Medical Condition

OPAT, if it is to be used, must clearly be in the patient's best interest. The patient must receive the best care, not just the least expensive care. A physician or anyone else would find it difficult to acknowledge before a jury that well-established criteria for use of OPAT were violated for social or economic reasons. Rarely a patient refuses prolonged parenteral therapy. When this happens, the clinician must document in great detail that the risks of cessation of treatment have been explained in depth.

To use OPAT, the patient must be clinically stable. Removing the safety net of the hospital environment increases the risk of treatment and places greater responsibility on the patient and caregivers. The feasibility of OPAT often becomes clear during the initial discussion with the patient and his or her caregivers. Caregivers may be reluctant to assume the responsibilities of assisting the patient in self-administration of drugs. Transportation to and from an infusion center may impose a physical and an economic hardship. In addition, underlying medical problems may render OPAT inappropriate even when the clinical condition is stable. Examples include poor manual dexterity because of arthritis, poor vision, dementia, or a history of injecting drug use (substance abuse). The clinician must ascertain that the patient has the mental and physical dexterity to handle self-administered therapy.

Oral therapy may be an option. Antimicrobial agents with excellent oral bioavailability are now available (see Chapter 19). Oral therapy becomes ideal when the patient's infection has been stabilized and when adequate serum levels can be attained through this route of administration.

Patient's Home Situation and Social Environment

The Americans with Disabilities Act places significant emphasis on assessing the home situation:

- Is the home environment sufficiently sanitary for safe administration of intravenous drugs?
- Does the home refrigerator or freezer have sufficient capacity for a week's supply of drugs, either in a frozen form or in bags to be maintained by refrigeration?
- Is electricity available for infusion pumps?
- Is a knowledgeable, trainable, and reliable caregiver available? (Ideally, the clinician and the infusion therapy team should evaluate the caregiver before the patient's discharge from the hospital.)
- Is a telephone adjacent to the patient's bed to allow communication with the infusion therapy team and to arrange for transportation to the hospital if necessary?

Serious adverse reactions such as anaphylaxis are rare, but they must be considered as a possibility.

The clinician should never bow to the pressures of a payer or of hospital administration (e.g., utilization review staff) to discharge a patient to an unsafe situation. Whether the patient, a visiting nurse, or an infusion center administers OPAT, the physician is ultimately responsible for the patient's protection.

Timely communication is essential to success with OPAT. The clinician must respond to situations that arise with OPAT in a prompt and appropriate manner. The patient, the infusion team (i.e., the extended care facility, the nurse, or the proprietary agency), and the pharmacy must have 24-hour access to the on-call physician. Adverse drug reactions and complications with equipment often occur after the usual office hours. The entire OPAT team must be well informed from the beginning, with a protocol for reaching appropriate personnel when urgent situations arise. If the physician, as captain of the team, is uncomfortable with this communication network, OPAT may need to be deferred.

Patient's Insurance Program

In the past, physicians have not dealt well with discussing the financial aspects of health care. OPAT, when self-administered, may cost several hundred dollars per day, depending on the drug and frequency of administration. The financial issues must be addressed and clarified. Sadly, patients sometimes receive promises from payers that OPAT will be covered, only to have reimbursement for OPAT challenged after therapy has been completed. Reimbursement issues are discussed in more detail later in the chapter.

 KEY POINTS

PATIENT SELECTION FOR OUTPATIENT PARENTERAL ANTIMICROBIAL THERAPY

⊃ OPAT must always be in the patient's best interest. The clinician is ultimately responsible for the patient's care and should never bow to pressures from payers or hospital administration (utilization review) to discharge a patient into an unsafe situation.

⊃ Oral therapy may be an option. The excellent oral bioavailability of newer antimicrobial agents (see Chapter 19) enables oral therapy for many patients whose conditions are stabilized.

⊃ The patient's medical condition, home environment, and insurance coverage must be carefully evaluated.

Antimicrobial Selection and Methods of Delivery

Nearly any infectious disease can now be treated in the outpatient setting if stringent criteria are met. In 1997 IDSA published a major set of guidelines for OPAT.

Antimicrobial Selection

During the early years of OPAT the pharmacokinetics and serum half-lives of available agents made drug selection difficult. Administering drugs intravenously every 4 to 6 hours was emotionally stressful and time consuming for the patient. The development of newer agents with longer serum half-lives allowed administration every 12 to 24 hours, making OPAT easier for all concerned. Ceftriaxone was the first agent shown to be effective when given once every 24 hours. Recently introduced drugs such as levofloxacin, azithromycin, and linezolid broaden the therapeutic options for once-daily therapy. Other drugs with long serum half-lives, such as MK-0826 (ertapenem) and daptomycin, are now being investigated.

Complementing the development of new drugs were advances in technology, such as the programmable infusion pump. Continuous infusion of older antimicrobial agents was shown to be reliable and cost effective in maintaining a favorable ratio of the peak serum level to the minimum inhibitory concentration (C_{max}/MIC), or a favorable ratio of the magnitude

and duration of serum levels (area under the curve [AUC]) to the MIC (AUC/MIC ratio) (see Chapter 19). This proved to be the case because some drugs are sufficiently stable at room temperature for continuous intravenous infusion over prolonged periods. Continuous infusion is an especially cost-effective means of treatment with time-dependent antimicrobial agents (see Chapter 19) because the serum level can usually be kept well above the MIC for the infecting microorganism, even with drugs that have short serum half-lives. For example, penicillin G can be given continuously at room temperature for 3 days for treatment of serious pneumococcal infections or neurosyphilis. Oxacillin is sufficiently stable at room temperature that it can be given over 7 days. When oxacillin is given for a staphylococcal infection, rather than administering 2 g of oxacillin every 6 hours, the OPAT provider can place 56 g of the drug into an infusion bag and give the medication continuously for the entire week. Cephalosporins such as cefazolin are stable in normal saline solution for 96 hours at room temperature and for 7 days when refrigerated. On the other hand, some agents, such as ampicillin, are difficult to administer in the outpatient setting because of their poor stability at room temperature. The main disadvantage of continuous infusion is that the patient must be continuously connected to the intravenous line and the infusion device.

Clinical studies established that some of the older agents could be given by intermittent infusion less frequently than was previously deemed necessary. For example, vancomycin can usually be given every 24 hours to elderly patients who have impaired renal function even when the serum creatinine level is normal (see Chapters 3 and 19) without compromising therapeutic efficacy. A once-daily aminoglycoside dose is now considered by many authorities to be the appropriate way to give these potentially toxic drugs. Pharmacodynamic studies also indicate that metronidazole can be given every 24 hours with favorable outcomes.

In selecting an appropriate antimicrobial regimen for OPAT, the clinician must address several additional points:

■ Is oral therapy a reasonable option? It should again be stressed that oral administration of certain drugs provides serum levels comparable to those achieved with intravenous administration. With rare exceptions, such as linezolid (Zyvox), oral therapy is not only more convenient but also much less expensive.

■ What other drugs is the patient taking? The clinician should evaluate not only prescription medications but also over-the-counter or self-administered drugs and should review the potential interactions.

■ Is combination antimicrobial therapy necessary? For a few infections, such as enterococcal endocarditis, combination therapy is nearly always required for cure. However, most infections caused by a single pathogen can be cured with one antimicrobial agent. For example, adding an aminoglycoside increases the risk of toxicity and should therefore not be done merely "to achieve synergy," but only when a clear rationale exists.

Methods of Delivery

When delivery methods are being considered, the first issue to address is venous access. The intravenous catheters and heparin locks that were available during the 1980s required changing every 24 to 48 hours. Newer devices need less frequent changes. Midline catheters can be left in place for up to 90 days, and peripherally inserted central catheters (PICC lines) can be left in place for up to 6 months. Tunneled catheters and implantable ports can be used for patients with difficult venous access. A surprising observation is that heparin locks often function for 5 to 7 days in the outpatient setting without phlebitis or infiltration, perhaps because the catheter is less frequently manipulated than in the hospital setting. Many new products have been designed to reduce the risk of catheter-associated infections. These include catheters impregnated with silver or coated with vancomycin and minocycline.

A second issue is the method of administration. Some patients choose to have OPAT administered by the older gravity method because they do not want the expense or trouble of mechanical or electronic infusion devices. Gravity infusion usually takes longer but avoids the cost of mechanical or programmable pumps. Slow intravenous injection (as opposed to infusion) has gained popularity both in the hospital and in the OPAT setting because this method reduces the cost of supplies and administration. However, this "slow IV push" method is currently suitable only for the penicillins and cephalosporins. The aminoglycosides, vancomycin, and the available antifungal drugs should not be given by "slow IV push." The clinician and the caregivers need to know the appropriate dilution of the drug and the risks, if any, of infusion.

Electronic syringe pumps offer a controlled way to administer medications and are generally less expensive than gravity systems because of the elimination of the minibag. The medication is appropriately diluted and drawn into a syringe to a maximum of 100 mL. The syringe pump can then be programmed to infuse the drug over varying intervals or by continuous infusion. Ambulatory infusion pumps are extremely versatile. Current models include single- and multiple-chamber devices. These pumps are convenient not only for the patient who needs intermittent doses of antimicrobial drugs but also for the patient who needs other forms of intravenous therapy, such as nutritional support. Disposable programmable pumps can be cost effective because they eliminate the need to retrieve, clean, and test the device when therapy has been discontinued. Pumps are also available that allow support personnel to address programming and access problems by telephone.

In summary, a combination of antimicrobial agents, intravenous catheters, and infusion devices permits the clinician to customize OPAT therapy to suit each patient's needs. Financial issues must also be addressed, because more technology usually implies greater cost. If patients must assume a significant portion of the expense, they may be willing to sacrifice convenience for cost savings (e.g., by using the gravity method rather than the newest programmable pump). Financial considerations are especially important for elderly patients, for whom OPAT is often the most appropriate form of therapy.

KEY POINTS

ANTIMICROBIAL SELECTION AND METHODS OF DELIVERY

- Patients selected for OPAT should meet stringent criteria such as those enumerated in 1997 by the IDSA.
- Newer drugs with long serum half-lives (such as ceftriaxone, levofloxacin, azithromycin, and linezolid) can be given every 24 hours by intermittent infusion.
- Older drugs with short serum half-lives (such as penicillin G and oxacillin) can be given by continuous intravenous infusion, often for a period of several days to as much as a week (with oxacillin).
- Studies have shown that some drugs (e.g., vancomycin, the aminoglycosides, and metronidazole) require less frequent administration by intermittent intravenous infusion than was formerly thought to be the case.
- Newer catheters can be left in place longer than the older models can.
- Some patients prefer gravity infusion of antimicrobial agents because of its simplicity and low cost.
- Slow intravenous injection ("slow IV push") can be cost effective for penicillins and cephalosporins but is inappropriate for most other antimicrobial agents.
- Newer programmable pumps offer enormous flexibility.

Monitoring of Outpatient Parenteral Antimicrobial Therapy and the Outpatient Parenteral Antimicrobial Therapy Program

In addition to monitoring the clinical response to therapy, clinicians overseeing OPAT must monitor drug toxicity, complications related to venous access, and the efficacy of the overall program (outcomes monitoring).

Monitoring for Drug Toxicity

Monitoring for drug toxicity requires clinical evaluation supplemented by appropriate laboratory tests. The prescribing clinician should make sure that a system and schedule for monitoring are in place, based on the known adverse effect of the drugs being given and the patient's clinical stability. Although the optimum frequency of laboratory monitoring has not been established by controlled trials, reasonable schedules (as set forth in the 1997 IDSA practice guidelines) include the following:

- Penicillins and cephalosporins. Evaluate the complete blood cell count (CBC) and serum creatinine level weekly (for children monitoring can be less frequent, such as every 2 weeks). Liver function tests may also be appropriate for patients receiving nafcillin, oxacillin, or ceftriaxone. Measurement of serum potassium levels may be appropriate for patients receiving antipseudomonal penicillins such as ticarcillin.
- Vancomycin. Evaluate CBC weekly, serum creatinine level twice weekly, and serum levels as clinically indicated (e.g., trough serum level once or twice weekly).
- Aminoglycosides. Check CBC weekly, serum creatinine level twice weekly, and serum levels as clinically indicated (e.g., trough serum level once or twice weekly). Also, consider a baseline audiogram and repetition of the audiogram every 2 weeks during therapy.
- Clindamycin. Evaluate CBC and serum creatinine level weekly.
- Trimethoprim-sulfamethoxazole. Evaluate CBC, serum creatinine, and serum potassium level weekly.
- Amphotericin B. Check CBC weekly; evaluate serum creatinine, potassium, and magnesium levels twice weekly.
- Pentamidine. Check CBC and serum creatinine, potassium, and magnesium levels twice weekly, and examine blood glucose level (by finger stick) daily.

- Acyclovir. Check CBC and serum creatinine and magnesium levels weekly.
- Ganciclovir. Check CBC twice weekly and serum creatinine weekly.
- Foscarnet. Evaluate CBC weekly and serum creatinine, potassium, and magnesium levels twice weekly; also, run a weekly chemistry profile, including serum calcium level.
- Cidofovir. CBC and serum creatinine level should be evaluated weekly.

In younger patients who are clinically stable, less frequent monitoring may be appropriate. However, it is best to err toward more frequent monitoring in older patients and those who are clinically unstable.

In a recent study of adverse drug reactions during OPAT, it was determined that hematologic toxicity such as leukopenia (16% of all study patients), thrombocytopenia (4%), and eosinophilia (12%) was most common during therapy with β-lactam agents. Nephrotoxicity occurred in 8% of patients, most frequently with amphotericin B. Diarrhea, which can be caused by *C. difficile*, occurred in 7% of patients. Cephalosporins, currently the most commonly used drugs for OPAT, are consi-

dered by many physicians to be almost without adverse effects. However, in patients on long-term cephalosporin therapy, for example, Coombs-positive hemolytic anemia, leukopenia, thrombocytopenia, azotemia, and abnormal liver function tests can develop. The aminoglycosides not infrequently cause ototoxicity in older patients, many of whom have subclinical hearing impairment. Fluoroquinolones have been associated with transient, usually reversible abnormalities of hematologic, renal, and liver function, and prolonged use can cause rupture of the Achilles tendon. Amphotericin B nearly always causes impairment of renal function and also causes anemia and hypokalemia. Patients should be forewarned of the potential toxicities of the drugs being used, especially when therapy is prolonged.

Monitoring for Complications Related to Venous Access

Complications related to vascular access devices are a major cause of morbidity and even mortality among hospitalized patients. Acute complications such as pneumothorax and hemothorax are unlikely to occur during OPAT because venous devices of the types associated with these complications are usually inserted in the hospital or in an ambulatory

TABLE 27-2
Essentials of Guidelines for Care of Vascular Access Devices from the Centers for Disease Control and Prevention

Component	Aspect	Recommendations (quality of supporting data)*
Catheter insertion	Preparation of site	The skin should be cleaned with 70% alcohol, 10% povidone-iodine, or 2% tincture of iodine (1A).
	Dressing	Sterile gauze or a transparent dressing should be used to cover the site (1A). The dressing can be left in place until the catheter is removed (1B) unless the site becomes moist or tender (1A).
	Documentation	The date and time of catheter insertion should be documented (1B).
Peripheral IV catheters	Type of needle	Teflon, polyurethane, or steel needles are preferred (1B); do not use steel needle, however, if extravasation of the drug will cause tissue necrosis (1A).
	Insertion site	Upper extremities should be used for insertion if possible for adults (1A); scalp, hand, or foot for children (II).
	Topical antimicrobials	Value of topical antimicrobial agents is unclear (NR).
	Flush solutions	Normal saline solution should be used routinely for flushing (1B). Heparin (10 μg/mL) should be used after blood sampling (1B).
	Frequency of catheter changes	Remove catheter if there is any sign of phlebitis (1A). In adults, rotation every 48 to 72 hours reduces the risk of phlebitis (1B). In children, and also for midline catheters, the ideal frequency of changing catheters is unknown (NR).
Central venous catheters	Number of lumens	Single-lumen CVC devices are preferred unless multiple lumens are essential (1B).
	Insertion method	For adults and for children >4 years of age, tunneled CVC devices or implantable ports should be used if the catheter is needed for >30 days (1A). For children <4 years of age, a totally implanted port should be used (1A).
	Insertion site	Subclavian site is preferred over jugular or femoral site (1B).
	Precautions during insertion	Sterile gown, gloves, mask, and large sterile drape should be used during CVC insertions even if performed in the operating room (IIB).

surgery center. Patients receiving OPAT are vulnerable to bloodstream infection or "line sepsis." For surveillance purposes, to be considered a laboratory-confirmed primary bloodstream infection (i.e., a bloodstream infection presumed to result from a vascular access device), the infection must meet one of the following criteria:

- It is caused by a recognized pathogen isolated from blood culture, *and* the pathogen is not clearly related to an infection at another site.
- The patient has fever, chills, or hypotension, *and* either of the following applies: (1) a common skin contaminant (such as coagulase-negative staphylococci) is isolated from two blood cultures drawn on separate occasions *and* the organism is not related to infection at another site, *or* (2) a common skin contaminant is isolated from a blood culture from a patient with a vascular access device *and* the physician institutes appropriate antimicrobial therapy.

Line sepsis caused by virulent microorganisms such as *Staphylococcus aureus* usually attracts attention because of acute clinical phenomena such as fever, chills, and hypotension. However, many instances of line sepsis involve opportunistic microorganisms such as coagulase-negative staphylococci and *Candida* species. Line sepsis caused by relatively avirulent pathogens can be extremely indolent; however, these infections can result in serious complications such as endocarditis or vertebral osteomyelitis.

Blood cultures obtained with scrupulous attention to skin preparation for the venipuncture are crucial to the diagnosis of line sepsis. When a central line is removed from the patient because of suspected sepsis, two segments (each 2 to 3 cm in length) of the catheter—the catheter tip and the intracutaneous portion of the catheter—can be submitted to the microbiology laboratory for culture. Semiquantitative culture using the "roll-plate" method is much more useful than broth culture, which frequently reflects contamination rather than true infection of the line. The clinician, the home health nurse or agency, and the patient should be familiar with the general principles of the Centers for Disease Control (CDC) guidelines for care of vascular access devices (Table 27-2). Sometimes what appears to be a minor infection at the site of vascular access results in serious, even life-threatening sepsis (Figure 27-1).

TABLE 27-2—cont'd
Essentials of Guidelines for Care of Vascular Access Devices from the Centers for Disease Control and Prevention

Component	Aspect	Recommendations (quality of supporting data)*
	Topical antimicrobials	Topical antimicrobial agents should *not* be applied on a routine basis to a CVC insertion site (1B).
	Flush solutions	Heparin (10 µg/mL) should be used to flush Broviac and Hickman catheters but is not required for Groshong catheters (IB)
	Blood sampling through the catheter	The risk to the patient of obtaining blood through a CVC is unclear. When sepsis is suspected, obtaining blood by peripheral venipuncture is preferable (the test should not rely only on a "through the catheter" specimen) (NR).
	Dressing changes	Dressings should be changed if they become damp, soiled, or loose or if inspection of the insertion site is necessary. The optimal timing for dressing change is unknown (NR).
	Frequency of catheter changes	PICC lines should be changed at least every 6 weeks (1B), although they may be safe for >6 weeks in some cases (NR). However, frequent or routine changing of PICC lines should not be done strictly to prevent catheter-related infections (1A). The need for routine change of ports and access needles is unclear (NR). Changing a CVC over a guidewire is safe provided no evidence of infection is present (1B).
Surveillance for phlebitis and infection	Evaluation of the site	Sites should be palpated daily for evidence of tenderness (1B). The dressing should be removed so that the site can be inspected if signs or symptoms of infection are present (1B).
	Blood cultures	The unexpected occurrence of fever, chills, or hypotension should prompt evaluation of the site and also blood cultures [author's addition].

Data from Occupational Safety and Health Administration: Occupational exposure to bloodborne pathogens; final rule. Federal Register 1991; 56 (235): 64004-64182. 29 CFR Part 1910.1030; and Wade BH, Rush SE. Infection control and outpatient parenteral antibiotic therapy. Infect Dis Clin North Am 1998; 12: 979-994.
CVC, Central venous catheter; *PICC,* peripherally inserted central catheter.
*Quality of evidence: *1A,* strongly recommended on the basis of excellent data; *1B,* strongly recommended on the basis of experience and the opinion of authorities in this area; *II,* suggested, and supported by suggestive clinical or epidemiologic studies; *NR,* no recommendation because the issue is unresolved or because there is insufficient evidence or consensus among experts.

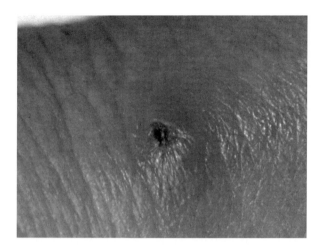

FIG. 27-1 Localized area of inflammation caused by a peripheral intravenous device was associated with life-threatening sepsis from *Staphylococcus aureus.* (Courtesy of Dr. Charles S. Bryan.)

Monitoring of the Efficacy of the Outpatient Parenteral Antimicrobial Therapy Program (Outcomes Monitoring)

Outcomes monitoring is becoming an important issue to both patients and payers in the rapidly evolving U.S. health care system. Unfortunately, data obtained through such monitoring can be disadvantageous to the physician who attempts to manage complicated problems in which the clinical outcome of OPAT is unpredictable.

Physicians using OPAT should expect, in the near future, a requirement to supply data demonstrating the efficacy (clinical success) and safety (complication rate) of the OPAT program. Recognizing the importance of such data, the Outpatient Infusion Therapy Association designed in 1993 a comprehensive questionnaire that includes multiple variables for each course of therapy. This questionnaire established the basis for a national OPAT registry. By completing the questionnaire for each patient, the physician can identify a problem or potential problem in his or her practice, including problems related to a particular antimicrobial agent, intravenous solution, catheter, or infusion pump. The physician can also compare the data from his or her practice with comparable practices throughout the United States. Individual practices are also encouraged to develop monitoring systems specific to their needs.

 KEY POINTS

MONITORING OF OUTPATIENT PARENTERAL ANTIMICROBIAL THERAPY AND THE OUTPATIENT PARENTERAL ANTIMICROBIAL THERAPY PROGRAM

⊃ The physician prescribing OPAT should ensure that a system and schedule for monitoring for drug toxicity are in place, based on the known adverse effect of the drugs being given and the patient's clinical stability.
⊃ The CDC guidelines for care of vascular access devices should be observed.

⊃ Primary bloodstream infection ("line sepsis") caused by vascular access devices can be an acute illness with fever, chills, hypotension, or a combination of these, or, when caused by relatively avirulent microorganisms such as coagulase-negative staphylococci or *Candida* species, can be a smoldering process that can nevertheless cause serious complications.
⊃ Diagnosis of line sepsis is established by blood cultures. When central catheters are removed because of suspected sepsis, both the catheter tip and the intracutaneous portion of the catheter, in separate sterile containers, should be submitted for semiquantitative cultures by the "roll-plate" method.
⊃ Outcomes monitoring for OPAT programs will assume increasing importance. The Outpatient Infusion Therapy Association has established a national OPAT registry for this purpose.

Legal Considerations

Physicians desiring to develop a program for OPAT must address a series of local, state, and federal regulations and laws. Initially the physician must contact the state medical association, the medical licensing board, and the board of pharmacy to determine what limitations or restrictions apply to OPAT in the office setting. Existing regulations and laws may determine the structure and scope of the OPAT program. For example, the laws governing in-office infusion may differ distinctly from those governing a program in which the physician's office dispenses drugs for self-administration at home. There may be state requirements or limitations pertaining to physician ownership of a licensed retail pharmacy, compounding or dispensing of parenteral medications in the physician's office, the physician's employment of a pharmacist or use of a consulting pharmacist, or the physician's ability to purchase drugs. In many states the board of pharmacy is the best place to look for information concerning issues related to medication compounding, administration, and dispensing.

Issues pertaining to the nursing services required for OPAT must also be investigated. The nurse practice act of each state must be reviewed to determine whether it requires a registered nurse (RN) to compound the drug or whether a licensed practical nurse (LPN) may do so. Who can and who cannot insert intravenous devices? What are the community standards? Even if it is legal for a person with certain levels of skill to insert devices such as PICC or midline catheters, the prevailing community standard may restrict these procedures to RNs. If a problem occurs, the question may arise as to which standard the physician and practice will be held in court. If the OPAT program plans to use an RN or LPN to monitor patients in the home environment, is the practice required by state law to obtain additional licensure for a home health agency? What, exactly, can the RN or LPN do in the home setting? Activities may be restricted to one skilled service such as overseeing infusion therapy, or a range of services (e.g., wound care, education about diabetes, and monitoring of blood pressure) may be permitted.

Federal regulations must also be addressed. Medicare, when enacted in the 1960s, provided no coverage for self-administered therapy in the home. It did, however, provide coverage for durable medical equipment such as infusion pumps. In the early 1990s the Health Care Financing Administration (HCFA) determined that because the cost of an infusion pump was covered, the cost of the materials administered by the pump should also be covered. In 1992 a limited formulary of parenteral medications was approved that included vancomycin, amphotericin B, acyclovir, ganciclovir, and foscarnet. Because vancomycin was the only parenteral antibiotic covered, many physicians overused this drug to allow patients to receive treatment for gram-positive bacterial infections at home. In 1993 HCFA removed vancomycin from the Medicare formulary. Several bills have been introduced in Congress to expand parenteral antimicrobial therapy for Medicare patients. At this writing, none of these bills have survived committee hearings. Also, regulations pertaining to a specific geographic area must be investigated; for example, many Medicaid programs do not cover self-administered antimicrobial agents.

Federal Medicare and Medicaid Anti-Kickback Statutes

In 1972 criminal statutes were enacted prohibiting intentional payments of anything of value to a physician for referral of a patient or for any business associated with a federal program. The Medicare-Medicaid Protection Act of 1987 expanded this prohibition to joint ventures and to other financial arrangements between physicians and home infusion companies to whom they refer patients. Numerous situations arose that, while technically violating this law, were not necessarily abusive. The Department of Justice therefore published a list of "safe harbors" that could protect nonabusive arrangements from enforcement. In 1991 Congress gave the Office of the Inspector General of Health and Human Services (OIG) civil sanction authority on the topic of kickback violations, but it did not require OIG to publish safe harbor regulations that could allow practitioners to understand more clearly the Inspector General's thinking or intent. In 1993 a new set of safe harbor regulations was published that expanded the protection in certain defined situations. In 1999 the Inspector General again expanded the list of safe harbors to eight new areas, including OPAT.

Stark I and Stark II

The Ethics and Patient Referral Acts of 1989 became law as part of the Omnibus Budget Reconciliation Act. This act was called the Stark Act because of the strong support of Rep. Fortney "Pete" Stark (D-California). The Stark Act made it unlawful for a physician to refer a Medicare patient to a clinical laboratory for tests in which the physician or a member of his or her immediate family held any ownership or other financial interests. The act did not apply, however, to the in office laboratory of a physician or a multispecialty group practice. These clinical laboratory facilities were free-standing in the proprietary market.

In 1993 the Omnibus Budget Reconciliation Act contained a provision commonly known as Stark II that expanded the self-referral prohibition to include Medicaid patients. The list of designated health services included home health services, outpatient prescription drugs, parenteral and enteral nutrients, equipment and supplies, and durable medical equipment. Included in this act were penalties for violations including fines of up to $15,000 for each Medicare claim covering services as the result of a prohibitive referral. Each violation of

the requirements of this law about which the physician knew or should have known carries a fine of up to $100,000. The Stark II Act also includes a $10,000 per day fine, as well as exclusion from Medicare and Medicaid programs, for failure to report information concerning the physician's ownership, investment, and compensation arrangements.

Through the extensive efforts of infectious disease specialists and oncologists to educate members of Congress, infusion pumps were specifically omitted from the prohibitions for durable medical equipment provided under the Medicare and Medicaid programs. The Stark prohibitions do not apply to services that are not covered by Medicare or Medicaid. Also, the restrictions do not apply to patients who receive neither Medicare nor Medicaid. Some individual states have passed self-referral laws dealing with all patients in that particular state. Services provided by an individual physician or by a group practice, as part of a professional organization, are exempt from the self-referral prohibition.

Interpretation of the Stark II legislation is ongoing. It remains unclear whether a physician may submit a claim for dispensing covered infusion drugs for home use to Medicare and Medicaid patients, or even to a private insurer that may be a primary payer for Medicare and Medicaid patients. If the physician's Medicare carrier has a written policy that it will not cover the services, the physician is not in violation of the Stark restrictions. Even the bill's primary author, Pete Stark, has reportedly expressed concern about how HCFA has interpreted various provisions of the 1993 act. Apparently there was no intent to restrict direct care by infectious disease specialists or oncologists in treating complex problems as an extension of their office practices. The main concern was to restrict entrepreneurial activities that might not be in the patient's or the public's best interest. Unfortunately, the complexity of the published rules interpreting the intent of Stark II has made it extremely difficult for many physicians to know whether they are in compliance. The latest version of the proposed rules fills approximately 450 pages of text.

Safe Harbors

What constitutes a "safe harbor" merits further comment. The 13 safe harbors designated in 1991 by the OIG covered various investment ventures and compensation arrangements. These included investments in publicly traded companies, small entity joint ventures, patient equipment rentals, personal service arrangements, sale of practices, and discounts. Certain types of activities were identified that, although technically covered by the statute, would not be subject to criminal or civil prosecution provided certain conditions were met.

Failure to qualify for safe harbor protection does not mean that the activity violates the anti-kickback statute. Instead, it means that a transaction will not automatically be protected from prosecution. Whether or not an activity violates the law depends on the facts and circumstances. The eight additional areas designated as safe harbors by the OIG in 1999 are as follows: (1) investment interest in underserved areas; (2) investment in ambulatory surgical centers; (3) investment in group medical practices; (4) practitioner recruitment in underserved areas; (5) obstetric malpractice insurance subsidies in primary health care professional shortage areas; (6) referral agreements for specialty services; (7) cooperative hospital service organizations; and (8) sale of practices in underserved areas. Clarifications of existing safe harbors address such issues as (1) investment interests; (2) space and equipment for personnel, parenteral services, and management contracts; (3) referral services; (4) discounts; and (5) sham transactions and devices.

The OIG recognizes that many physicians who have structured their business arrangements under the good faith of interpretation of older safe harbors may need time to arrange their affairs to comply with revisions and with new safe harbors. The OIG indicates its intent to "exercise discretion to be fair to the parties" when providers work diligently and in good faith to restructure their arrangements in order to comply with the most recent determinations.

The safe harbor terminology related to ambulatory surgical centers allows for investment by individuals in entities that are not in a position to refer patients. The terminology also allows for hospital-physician relationships. The regulations for ambulatory surgical centers permit the leasing of space, equipment, or personnel from a hospital investor if the existing safe harbor criteria are met. The safe harbor criteria related to ambulatory surgery centers are quite similar to the criteria that could be used for infusion centers. Clarification of this issue by the OIG would allow joint venture activities between physicians, hospitals, and private investors. At present, expansion of Medicare to cover self-administered outpatient therapy is considered unlikely. However, the expansion of infusion centers would allow many Medicare patients to be treated outside of the hospital environment in a way that is both cost effective and psychologically beneficial.

 KEY POINTS

LEGAL CONSIDERATIONS

➲ Before starting an OPAT program, the practitioner must carefully review the relevant local, state, and federal laws and regulations.

➲ The Ethics and Patient Referrals Act of 1989 (commonly known as the Stark Act and later modified as Stark II) was designed to curb conflicts of interest arising from self-referral.

➲ Beginning in 1991 the Office of the Inspector General of Health and Human Services has outlined a number of "safe harbors."

➲ Financial arrangements for OPAT must be structured in such a way as to comply with the Stark acts and the safe harbor provisions, and legal advice should be obtained.

Reimbursement

Physicians considering the development of an OPAT program must pay close attention to the economic aspects. In the early 1980s, when OPAT was in its infancy, the problem was reimbursement. Many payers, including HCFA, considered OPAT experimental. Reimbursement became easier when payers recognized the potential savings. By 1985 it was recognized that the average cost of OPAT was about $250 per day compared with a hospital per diem cost of about $1000. The rapid proliferation of local, regional, and national infusion companies

attested to the enormous growth potential of OPAT. Today, as physicians are confronted with issues pertaining to cost containment from multiple directions, public and private policies have a significant impact on reimbursement for OPAT.

Medicare, Part B

Antimicrobial agents given in the office-based infusion center are reimbursed at 80% of reasonable cost, with the patient providing a 20% copayment. In the past, the physician was required to be present or immediately available during treatment. Decisions made by several Medicare intermediaries now allow the supervisory role to be filled by an RN, LPN, or physician's assistant if reimbursement is based on the estimated acquisition cost (EAC) or average wholesale price (AWP) of the drug. The infusion center needs to use a J-code for billing the number of units administered. Medicare stipulates that the drug be used only for FDA-approved indications (i.e., on-label use). Reimbursement for intravenous infusion is based on CPT-Code 907.80. A different code (907.88) is used for antimicrobial agents given intramuscularly. At times, additional supplies are reimbursed using HCFA Common Procedure Coding (HCPC) codes. The patient visit to the physician is billed using the appropriate evaluation and management (E & M) codes. When the physician does not physically see the patient, nursing fees can be billed at a level of service with the appropriate coding. The physician or the billing staff must be thoroughly familiar with the appropriate coding policies. To avoid suspicion of fraudulent billing, the staff must be continually updated because the codes change from year to year.

Medicaid

Federal and state governments jointly fund the Medicaid program to provide medical care to certain populations, primarily the indigent. Reimbursement for OPAT varies from state to state. Most Medicaid programs are currently underfunded. However, many Medicaid programs offer options not available to Medicare recipients, including self-administered home infusion of antimicrobial agents. Physicians must, however, be familiar with the local reimbursement rates. At times, reimbursements fail to cover the costs inherent in OPAT. Some statues mandate that if a physician treats a public employee, the physician is thenceforth obligated to treat patients covered only by Medicaid or Workers' Compensation at risk of exclusion from all three programs.

Third Party Payers

Most third party payers have adopted procedures for reimbursement of antimicrobial infusion in the office setting. Many commercial insurers and Blue Cross/Blue Shield plans have established limits based on the prevailing usual and customary charges. Drug costs are usually based on AWP. During the 1990s many insurers negotiated a per diem rate for OPAT separate from drug acquisition costs. The per diem fee covers administration, supplies, nursing care, pharmaceutical services, and fixed overhead costs when treatment is given in the infusion center. If the treatment is self-administered at home, allowance is also made for the provider who is on call to deal with oversight issues. The per diem fee gives the provider and the payer a better understanding of the expenses involved in OPAT. For severely ill patients, additional allowance is often made for the expenses incurred through frequent nursing visits or office visits. However, in these situations providers should contact their major carriers before they initiate OPAT. There should be clarification of the services covered, the projected reimbursement, and the services (e.g., which nursing services) to be used. Many Blue Cross/Blue Shield plans and other national carriers have developed preferred provider arrangements for home infusion. Often, prearrangement for antimicrobial therapy excludes the physician from providing OPAT even if the physician's charges are lower than those of the preferred provider. Some physicians have been able to negotiate disease-related reimbursements (e.g., for acquired immunodeficiency syndrome) whereby insurers provide coverage for OPAT, laboratory tests, home and office visits, and nursing visits.

Capitation agreements should be reviewed carefully. Providers need to have data pertaining to the patients they serve and the cost of providing OPAT in order to decide whether this form of risk sharing is appropriate.

Billing

The physician and billing staff must understand the policies and procedures of each carrier. Failure to review these policies and procedures carefully can inflate administrative costs to the extent that reimbursement for OPAT fails to cover the expense. Some carriers require itemized bills. If bills are not properly submitted with appropriate documentation, the carriers will uniformly reject the claims. The billing staff must know which carriers, including Medicaid, require prior approval. When therapy is begun in the hospital, the institution's discharge planners must be familiar with the requirements of each program. Companies employ case managers who can provide the information and policies needed to decide whether OPAT is feasible. Preauthorization should be obtained by facsimile or by e-mail and should include the name of the carrier's employee who is issuing the preauthorization. More than one provider has been unable to collect its charges, after giving OPAT for many weeks, because of lack of documented preauthorization.

A Cautionary Note

It should be clear that thorough review of the marketplace and its restrictions is necessary to determine the economic feasibility of starting an OPAT program. However, the prescribing physician is ultimately liable for injuries that occur to the patient irrespective of who is administering OPAT. In situations where a question exists about the quality of services given by a contracted agency, the physician, as the patient's advocate, may have to refuse to continue services in an oversight capacity. In these situations the physician must keep the patient in the hospital or arrange for someone else to provide coverage. If the patient suffered harm, the practitioner would have difficulty defending in court his or her reservations about an agency providing OPAT.

The Future

The number of courses of OPAT given in the United States each year is now estimated to be more than 250,000, which represents a 100% increase since the mid-1990s. The maximum growth of OPAT has yet to be realized, at least in some geographic areas. Increasingly, data support the use of OPAT for infections that previously mandated hospitalization, such as fever in a neutropenic cancer patient, bacterial meningitis, endocarditis, and disseminated fungal infection. All primary care clinicians will need to become familiar with OPAT as more patients are discharged from the hospital to receive this form of therapy. Many primary care clinicians will find the office-based infusion center to be a convenient, cost-effective way to treat serious infections when appropriate therapy includes a drug with favorable pharmacokinetics, such as ceftriaxone. Some primary care clinicians will want to explore more elaborate models of OPAT, perhaps in collaboration with infectious disease specialists.

Still, OPAT will probably be subject to increasing scrutiny by government, by third party payers, and by the public. The OPAT registry established by the Outpatient Infusion Therapy Association is an important step toward self-regulation. Perhaps the major threat to the future of OPAT, as a cost-effective form of treatment that is also in the patient's best interests, is the tendency of payers to view OPAT in mainly economic terms. Because OPAT eliminates the safety net of the hospital environment, each practice must establish and maintain rigorous internal policies and procedures. Data derived from the growing experience with OPAT will continue to be used as a way to evaluate dosage schedules, intravenous devices, management of vascular access sites, and the potential adverse effects of long-term use of antimicrobial agents. Already, in its brief existence over the past quarter century, OPAT has been a tremendous stimulus to the development of new drugs and new infusion technologies. No doubt this is only the beginning. Advances in methods of drug administration, combined with advances in diagnostic methods, will increasingly move the management of serious infectious diseases out of the hospital and into the ambulatory care setting.

SUGGESTED READING

Anthony TU, Rubin LG. Stability of antibiotics used for antibiotic-lock treatment of infections of implantable venous devices (ports). Antimicrob Agents Chemother 1999; 43: 2074-2076.

Embry FC, Chinnes LF. Draft definitions for surveillance of infections in home health care. Am J Infect Control 2000; 28: 449-453.

Gilbert DN, Dworkin RJ, Raber SR, et al. Outpatient parenteral antimicrobial-drug therapy. N Engl J Med 1997; 337: 829-838.

Hoffman-Terry ML, Fraimow HS, Fox TR, et al. Adverse effects of outpatient parenteral antibiotic therapy. Am J Med 1999; 106: 44-49.

Leggett JE. Ambulatory use of parenteral antibacterials: contemporary perspectives. Drugs 2000; 59 (Suppl 3): 1-8.

Mermel LA, Farr BM, Sheretz RJ, et al. Guidelines for the management of intravascular catheter-related infections. Clin Infect Dis 2001; 32: 1249-1272.

Tice AD. Handbook of Outpatient Parenteral Therapy for Infectious Diseases. New York: Scientific American, Inc.; 1997.

Tice AD. Pharmacoeconomic considerations in the ambulatory use of parenteral cephalosporins. Drugs 2000; 59 (Suppl 3): 29-35.

Tice AD, ed. Outpatient parenteral antimicrobial therapy. Infect Dis Clin North Am 1998; 12: 827-1050.

Williams DN, Rehm SJ, Tice AD, et al. Practice guidelines for community-based parenteral anti-infective therapy. Clin Infect Dis 1997; 25: 787-801.

Empiric Antibiotic Therapy for Syndromes That Can Often Be Treated on an Outpatient Basis

CHARLES S. BRYAN

Syndrome	Diagnosis	First-line therapy	Alternative therapy	Comments
PHARYNGITIS (see Chapter 10)				
Acute pharyngitis with exudate or diffuse erythema, gonococcal pharyngitis unlikely	The rapid streptococcal antigen test is highly specific (>95%), but the sensitivity varies (60% to 100%). Throat cultures may be performed if the antigen test is negative and the clinical picture strongly suggests a streptococcal etiology.	Penicillin V PO for 10 days. Benzathine penicillin G IM if compliance is unlikely. (For dosages, see Table 10-11.)	Erythromycin, azithromycin, clarithromycin, or oral cephalosporin (For dosages, see Table 10-11.)	The major goal of treatment is prevention of acute rheumatic fever caused by group A streptococci. The other etiologies (see Table 10-9) are not associated with risk of acute rheumatic fever. The optical immunoassay test may not need throat culture backup.
Acute pharyngitis, gonococcal pharyngitis proven or likely (see Chapters 10 and 16)	Throat culture using modified Thayer-Martin media. The usual indication for treatment is a positive culture for *Neisseria gonorrhoeae*.	Ceftriaxone 125 mg IM (1 dose) plus azithromycin or doxycycline (see "Comments")	Ciprofloxacin 500 mg PO (1 dose), ofloxacin 400 mg PO (1 dose), or gatifloxacin 400 mg (1 dose), plus azithromycin or doxycycline (see "Comments")	Azithromycin 1 g PO (1 dose) or doxycycline 100 mg PO b.i.d. for 7 days is used for possible coinfection with *Chlamydia trachomatis*.
Asymptomatic group A streptococcal carrier state following treatment	Routine follow-up culture after treatment of streptococcal pharyngitis is not recommended.	None		Treatment of the asymptomatic carrier state is not advised.
Recurrent symptomatic pharyngitis with frequent positive cultures for group A streptococci	Rapid streptococcal antigen test or throat culture. (See "Comments.")	Clindamycin or amoxicillin-clavulanate. Rifampin is also used with penicillin V or benzathine penicillin G.	Benzathine penicillin G IM. Tonsillectomy is sometimes considered.	In this situation it is difficult to be sure whether the symptoms are caused by group A streptococci or by recurrent viral pharyngitis, the streptococcal carrier state being coincidental.
Vesicular or ulcerative pharyngitis	Viral culture for herpes simplex in severe cases. Etiologies include herpes simplex (types 1 and 2), coxsackieviruses A9 and B 1 through 5, echoviruses (multiple types), and enterovirus type 71.	Acyclovir for proven or strongly suspected herpes simplex infection (For dosages and alternative drugs in this class, see Table 20-3.)		Aphthous stomatitis should be considered in the differential diagnosis (see Chapter 10).

Continued

Syndrome	Diagnosis	First-line therapy	Alternative therapy	Comments
LARYNGITIS (see Chapter 10)				
Acute laryngitis	Studies are not indicated except in cases of persistent hoarseness.	Symptomatic therapy only	See "Croup" in Chapter 4.	Laryngoscopy should be carried out for persistent hoarseness.
SINUSITIS (see Chapter 10)				
Acute uncomplicated sinusitis in an afebrile patient, symptoms less than 7 to 14 days' duration	Clinical diagnosis. Imaging studies and cultures are not indicated (see Table 10-2).	Symptomatic therapy only (see Table 10-2)		Mild sinusitis is a typical feature of the common cold (hence the term "rhinosinusitis"). Therapeutic restraint and patient education are usually advisable.
Acute sinusitis with fever or with symptoms of greater than 14 days' duration, frontal or sphenoid sinusitis unlikely (see Chapter 10)	Clinical diagnosis. Imaging studies are not indicated except in unusually severe cases (see Chapter 10).	Amoxicillin and TMP/SMX are the most cost-effective regimens. Other regimens include amoxicillin-clavulanate, cefuroxime axetil, and fluoro-quinolones (for dosages see Table 10-6).	Cefdinir, cefprozil, cefpodoxime, or clarithromycin	For a detailed discussion of when and how to treat acute bacterial sinusitis, see Chapter 10. Agents other than amoxicillin and TMP/SMX may be appropriate if the patient has received antibiotics within the previous 2 weeks.
Acute sinusitis with systemic toxicity, severe generalized headache, or severe localized headache over frontal bone or orbit	Imaging studies (CT scan preferred)	Parenteral antibiotics may be indicated depending on CT scan findings (see Chapter 10).		Severe frontal, ethmoid, or sphenoid sinusitis can be life threatening (see Chapters 6 and 10).
Acute sinusitis in a patient who has recently been treated for diabetic ketoacidosis (see Chapter 3)	Consider rhinocerebral mucormycosis; studies include CT scanning and careful examination of the palate and nasal mucosa for black eschars.	If mucormycosis is not present, treatment is the same as for acute sinusitis in a nondiabetic patient.		A high index of suspicion of mucormycosis mandates hospitalization or referral.
Chronic sinusitis in the adult patient	Imaging (CT scan preferred) is useful to confirm the diagnosis. Various bacteria, including anaerobes, are often isolated, but their significance is unclear.	Antibiotics tend to be ineffective except during acute exacerbations.	Endoscopic sinus surgery, treatment of allergic disorders, and treatment of periodontitis of the maxillary teeth may be useful in selected patients.	For discussion, see Table 10-2.
EAR INFECTIONS (see Chapter 10)				
Acute diffuse otitis externa ("swimmer's ear")	*Pseudomonas aeruginosa* is the usual cause; other etiologies include Enterobacteriaceae, acute infection caused by *S. aureus,* and (rarely) fungi.	Topical therapy: polymyxin *B plus* neomycin *plus* hydrocortisone ear drops q.i.d. *or* ofloxacin 0.3% solution b.i.d. (see Table 10-7)		Gentle cleaning of the ear should be carried out. Ointments should not be used in the ear.
Acute external otitis	Look for pustule or furuncle suggesting *S. aureus.*	Dicloxacillin 500 mg PO q.i.d. (for administration of dicloxacillin, see Chapter 19)	Amoxicillin-clavulanate or cephalexin (in children)	Ointments should not be used in the ear.

Syndrome	Diagnosis	First-line therapy	Alternative therapy	Comments
Chronic otitis externa	Look for evidence of seborrheic dermatitis, the usual cause	Ear drops (polymyxin B+ neomycin + hydrocortisone) q.i.d. + selenium sulfide	See Table 10-9	Dandruff control with a shampoo containing selenium sulfide (Selsun) or ketoconazole shampoo + a medium-potency steroid solution such as triamcinolone 0.1%
Acute otitis media	Pneumatic otoscopy showing lack of mobility of the tympanic membrane with inflammation; tympanocentesis is useful for etiologic diagnosis.	High-dose amoxicillin (80 to 90 mg/kg/day in children) or amoxicillin-clavulanate or TMP/SMX (in adults, not children) or oral second- or third-generation cephalosporin (see text, Chapter 10; not all second-generation cephalosporins are appropriate)	Erythromycin-sulfisoxazole or clarithromycin or azithromycin (adults, not children)	In children, about 80% of earaches resolve without antimicrobial therapy.
Persistent, prolonged, suppurative, or recurrent episodes of acute otitis media	As above, plus clinical history	Amoxicillin-clavulanate, cefuroxime axetil, or ceftriaxone (IM)	Oral second- or third-generation cephalosporin (not all second-generation cephalosporins are appropriate)	Suspect a drug-resistant microorganism. Tympanocentesis for culture and sensitivity may be indicated to guide therapy. Clindamycin may be useful but lacks activity against *Haemophilus influenzae* and *Moraxella catarrhalis.*
Acute mastoiditis	Evidence of acute otitis media with pain and tenderness over mastoid process	Same as for acute otitis media. Dicloxacillin or IV antistaphylococcal antibiotics if *S. aureus* is present.		Acute mastoiditis is now rare. Referral to an otolaryngologist is indicated, since intracranial extension can have serious consequences.
Chronic mastoiditis	Evidence of chronic otitis media with pain or tenderness over mastoid process	Parenteral antibiotics should be given in conjunction with surgery.		

EYE INFECTIONS (see Chapter 9)

Syndrome	Diagnosis	First-line therapy	Alternative therapy	Comments
Blepharitis	Clinical appearance. Culture is sometimes indicated.	Topical therapy with bacitracin or erythromycin ointment after washing off debris with baby shampoo and warm compresses.		The actual value of topical antibiotics is unclear. Artificial tears should be prescribed if dry eye is present.
Internal hordeolum (acute meibomianitis)	Clinical appearance. *S. aureus* is the usual cause.	Dicloxacillin plus hot packs		The internal hordeolum seldom drains spontaneously.
External hordeolum	Clinical appearance. *S. aureus* is the usual cause.	Hot packs. Systemic antibiotic therapy is unnecessary.		The external hordeolum usually drains spontaneously.

Continued

Syndrome	Diagnosis	First-line therapy	Alternative therapy	Comments
Conjunctivitis with painless suffusion (pink eye)	Clinical appearance	No treatment is necessary. Topical antibiotics are often used.		In an adult, presence of ocular pain and photophobia suggests associated keratitis (rare). Etiology is often viral in children.
Inclusion conjunctivitis	Demonstration of *Chlamydia trachomatis* by culture, antigen detection system, or PCR	Doxycycline 10 mg b.i.d. for 1 to 3 weeks; erythromycin in children	Erythromycin 250 mg q.i.d. for 1 to 3 weeks	Usually unilateral; an oculogenital disease
Trachoma		Azithromycin 20 mg/kg as a single dose	Doxycycline 100 mg b.i.d. (or tetracycline 250 mg q.i.d.) for 14 days	Topical therapy is of little help.
Suppurative conjunctivitis	Distinguish between gonococcal and nongonococcal disease.	For gonococcal disease, ceftriaxone 125 mg IV or IM; for nongonococcal disease, ophthalmic erythromycin, gentamicin, or bacitracin–polymyxin B	Ophthalmic tobramycin, ciprofloxacin, ofloxacin, or polymyxin B–trimethoprim	Nongonococcal suppurative conjunctivitis is often self-limited. Avoid use of topical neomycin and other aminoglycosides (can cause punctate staining of cornea) and chloramphenicol.
Canaliculitis (infection of lacrimal apparatus)	Exudate appears at the lacrimal punctum with digital pressure; Gram stain reveals bacteria, usually *Actinomyces*	Irrigation with 10% sulfacetamide drops after removal of granules; for children, amoxicillin-clavulanate or an oral second-generation cephalosporin	Irrigation with penicillin G (100,000 units/mL) or clindamycin	Some authors suggest that penicillin G is the drug of first choice.
Dacryocystitis (infection of lacrimal sac)	Exudate appears at the lacrimal punctum with little or no digital pressure; culture and sensitivity should be requested	Oral first-generation cephalosporin or dicloxacillin	Erythromycin	Ophthalmology consultation is indicated. Usual etiologic agents are *S. pneumoniae*, *S. aureus*, *H. influenzae*, and group A streptococci. In young infants rule out dacryostenosis.
Herpes simplex keratitis	Clinical diagnosis. Dendritic ulcers are demonstrated with fluorescein staining of the cornea.	Trifluridine, one drop per hour 9 times a day for up to 21 days	Vidarabine ointment	Acyclovir, 400 mg PO b.i.d. has been shown to reduce the frequency of recurrences.
Keratitis in contact lens users	Clinical diagnosis. Alginate swab for culture and sensitivity testing, looking especially for *P. aeruginosa*	Tobramycin (14 mg/mL) plus piperacillin or ticarcillin (6 to 12 mg/mL) eye drops q15-60 min for 24 to 72 hours, then slow tapering	Ciprofloxacin or ofloxacin, 0.3% drops q15-60 min round the clock for 24 to 72 hours, then slow tapering	Pain, photophobia, and impaired vision suggest the diagnosis. *P. aeruginosa* is the most common pathogen. *Ophthalmology referral is advised.*
LOWER RESPIRATORY INFECTIONS (see Chapter 11)				
Bronchiolitis in infant or child ≤3 years of age manifested by expiratory wheezing ("wheezy bronchitis") (see Chapter 4)	Rapid diagnosis of RSV (50% of cases) can be made with antigen detection systems. Parainfluenza viruses cause 25% and other viruses about 20% of cases.	Supportive care with oxygen	Preventive treatment with monthly palivizumab in high-risk infants.	Aerosolized ribavirin is not beneficial. IV ribavirin has not been well studied, but there is currently little enthusiasm for its use.

Syndrome	Diagnosis	First-line therapy	Alternative therapy	Comments
Bronchitis in child ≥5 years of age (see Chapter 4)	Clinical diagnosis. Adenovirus causes most cases in children; other causes are RSV and parainfluenza 3 virus.	Symptomatic therapy unless complications are present (see "Comments")	Palivizumab injections for high-risk infants	Indications for antibiotic therapy include associated sinusitis; heavy growth of *S. pneumoniae, H. influenzae,* or group A streptococci on throat culture; or no improvement in 1 week.
Acute bronchitis in adolescent or healthy adult (acute tracheobronchitis; "chest cold") (see Chapter 11)	Clinical diagnosis, but chest x-ray examination is indicated to exclude pneumonia in patients with respiratory symptoms, abnormal chest examination, fever, or tachycardia. Usual etiologies are viruses, *Mycobacterium pneumoniae,* and *Chlamydia pneumoniae.*	Symptomatic therapy		Antibiotic therapy is indicated only if pneumonia is present. Purulent sputum is not an indication for antibiotic therapy. Persistent cough should raise the possibility of pertussis (see below).
Cough lasting >14 days in infant or adult; pertussis (whooping cough) (see Chapters 4 and 11)	Consider postnasal drip, gastroesophageal reflux, and asthma, especially in adults. In both children and adults, consider whooping cough *(Bordetella pertussis;* sometimes *Bordetella parapertussis).*	Erythromycin, azithromycin, clarithromycin, or (in adults) TMP/SMX (see Chapter 11)		Whooping cough is now being recognized as a cause of bronchitis in adults.
Acute exacerbations of chronic bronchitis in patients with underlying chronic lung disease (see Chapter 11)	Clinical diagnosis; chest x-ray examination is indicated in presence of fever or marked respiratory distress.	TMP/SMX, doxycycline, or newer antibiotics (see Table 11-1)	See Table 11-1.	The role of antibiotics in COPD exacerbations is debatable. All patients should receive pneumococcal vaccine and yearly influenza vaccination.
Pneumonitis syndrome and pneumonia, birth to 5 years of age (see Chapter 4)	Chest x-ray examination; hospitalization is often indicated; etiologies include RSV and other respiratory viruses, *B. pertussis, S. pneumoniae, H. influenzae, M. pneumoniae, C. pneumoniae,* and *S. aureus* (rare)	For older infants (3 months to 5 years) with mild to moderate disease to be treated as outpatients, erythromycin or clarithromycin (see Chapter 4)		Neonates and most infants <24 months of age with significant pneumonia should be treated in the hospital (see Chapter 4).
Pneumonia in patient 5 to 18 years of age, mild to moderately severe (see Chapters 4 and 11)	Chest x-ray examination; sputum culture in patients with sudden onset and copious, purulent sputum. Etiologic agents include *M. pneumoniae, C. pneumoniae,* respiratory viruses, and *S. pneumoniae.*	Clarithromycin or azithromycin if *M. pneumoniae* or *C. pneumoniae* is suspected; amoxicillin if *S. pneumoniae* is suspected.	Doxycycline in children >8 years; erythromycin; ceftriaxone IM by daily injection	Pneumococcal pneumonia should be suspected in patients with sudden onset and copious, purulent sputum. Prolonged treatment (2 or 3 weeks) is indicated for *M. pneumoniae* or *C. pneumoniae.*

Syndrome	Diagnosis	First-line therapy	Alternative therapy	Comments
Pneumonia in adult, mild to moderately severe, not presumed to be of viral etiology, with no clues as to a specific etiology by history, physical examination, or initial laboratory studies (see Chapter 11)	Chest x-ray examination; sputum culture in patients with sudden onset and copious, purulent sputum. In patients without comorbidity, "atypical agents" (*M. pneumoniae, C. pneumoniae,* and viruses) are relatively common. Bacteria (*S. pneumoniae, H. influenzae,* and *M. catarrhalis*) are relatively more common in cigarette smokers. There are numerous potential causative agents, including *M. tuberculosis* (see Chapters 11, 20, 21, and 22).	Azithromycin or clarithromycin (see Table 11-6)*	Fluoroquinolone (levofloxacin, moxifloxacin, or gatifloxacin); oral cephalosporin; amoxicillin-clavulanate	Hospitalization should be strongly considered in elderly patients, in patients with severe underlying diseases, and in patients with severe pneumonia (see Chapters 3 and 11).
Pneumonia in adult, presumed to be viral (see Chapter 11)	Influenza is the most likely etiology between December and March. Other causes include parainfluenza viruses, adenoviruses, RSV, and the Hantavirus pulmonary syndrome (see Chapter 6).	For influenza A or B, PO oseltamivir or inhaled zanamivir (see Table 11-10 and Chapter 20)	For influenza A, rimantadine or amantadine	Hospitalization is indicated for severe pneumonia. Consider possibility of *Pneumocystis carinii* pneumonia in a patient with HIV disease previously undiagnosed.
Pneumonia in HIV-positive patient (see Chapter 17)	In patients with acute onset, pleuritic pain, discrete infiltrates, or purulent sputum, consider bacteria (*S. pneumoniae, H. influenzae,* and gram-negative rods); in patients with subacute onset, dry cough, progressive dyspnea, or diffuse infiltrates consider *P. carinii* pneumonia; in all patients, consider *M. tuberculosis.*	For suspected *P. carinii* pneumonia, TMP/SMX or (in mild cases) dapsone plus trimethoprim.	Since up to 20% of *S. pneumoniae* strains are resistant to TMP/SMX, it is often appropriate to add a more effective drug for pneumococcal pneumonia (e.g., ceftriaxone) when this possibility cannot be excluded.	Hospitalization is usually indicated.

GASTROINTESTINAL INFECTIONS (see Chapter 12)

Syndrome	Diagnosis	First-line therapy	Alternative therapy	Comments
Gastroenteritis in an infant (see Chapter 4)	Stool culture looking especially for enteropathogenic strains of *E. coli* if dysentery or bloody diarrhea is present	Symptomatic therapy unless dysentery is present.		Adequate hydration must be maintained. Most cases are of viral etiology. Dysentery syndrome requires stool culture.
Gastroenteritis in adult	Stool for fecal leukocytes and culture, since therapy will usually depend on the specific organism (see Figure 12-1).	Ciprofloxacin while awaiting results of culture	TMP/SMX	See Table 12-4 for therapy for specific pathogens.
Traveler's diarrhea (see Chapters 12 and 24)	Obtain stool culture if patient has significant systemic symptoms, tenesmus, bloody diarrhea, or presence of fecal leukocytes.	Oral quinolone (ciprofloxacin 500 mg, norfloxacin 400 mg, or ofloxacin 300 mg) b.i.d. for 3 days. For mild cases, a single dose of ciprofloxacin (750 mg) may suffice. TMP/SMX in children.	TMP/SMX, one double-strength tablet b.i.d. for 3 days	For symptomatic therapy, loperamide (Imodium), 4 mg and then 2 mg after each loose stool. When significant systemic symptoms are present, consider diverse etiologies: *Salmonella, Shigella, Entamoeba histolytica, Escherichia coli* O157:H7; *Clostridium difficile, Cryptosporidium, Cyclospora.*

Syndrome	Diagnosis	First-line therapy	Alternative therapy	Comments
Diverticulitis (see Chapter 12)	Patients with marked systemic symptoms should be given parenteral therapy	TMP/SMX (one double-strength tablet b.i.d.) or ciprofloxacin 500 mg b.i.d. *plus* metronidazole 500 mg PO q6h	Amoxicillin-clavulanate 500 mg/125 mg PO t.i.d.	Close outpatient follow-up is warranted for potential complications.

URINARY TRACT INFECTIONS (see Chapter 14)

Syndrome	Diagnosis	First-line therapy	Alternative therapy	Comments
Asymptomatic bacteriuria in pregnancy (see Chapters 5 and 14)	Screening urine culture during the first trimester	Amoxicillin if the organism is sensitive	Nitrofurantoin; oral cephalosporin; TMP/SMX; trimethoprim alone	Repeat urine culture monthly to screen for recurrence.
Asymptomatic bacteriuria, preschool child (see Chapters 4 and 14)	Urine culture; if positive, repeat in 3 to 7 days for confirmation.	Amoxicillin if the organism is sensitive	TMP/SMX	See Chapters 4 and 14. In most other situations asymptomatic bacteriuria does not require treatment (see Table 14-4).
Acute uncomplicated cystitis, young woman	Leukocyte esterase test (dipstick urinalysis); consider sexually transmitted disease as an alternative diagnosis.	Three-day regimen with fluoroquinolone (ciprofloxacin 250 mg b.i.d. or norfloxacin 500 mg b.i.d. or ofloxacin 200 mg b.i.d. or enoxacin 200 mg b.i.d. or levofloxacin 250 mg b.i.d.) or TMP/SMX (1 double-strength tablet b.i.d.) (see Table 14-7)	Three-day regimen: oral cephalosporin; nitrofurantoin; doxycycline; amoxicillin-clavulanate (see Table 14-7)	Fluoroquinolones have replaced TMP/SMX as drugs of choice whenever primary resistance of *E. coli* to TMP/SMX is expected to exceed 20% (see Chapter 14). Three-day regimens are more effective than single-dose regimens. Nitrofurantoin is not effective against *Staphylococcus saprophyticus,* which causes some episodes. Single-dose therapy with fosfomycin (3 g) has been used but is less effective than 3-day regimen with TMP/SMX or a fluoroquinolone.
Recurrent cystitis (three or more episodes per year), uncomplicated, young woman	As above; consider culture and sensitivity to confirm *E. coli* or *S. saprophyticus* as pathogen.	Treat acute infection as above, then consider strategy for prevention (see Table 14-8).		Most patients do not require urologic evaluation.
Recurrent cystitis (three or more episodes per year), postmenopausal woman	As above, but also evaluate for potentially correctable problems such as cystocele, urinary incontinence, and urinary retention (residual volume >50 mL).	As above		
Acute uncomplicated pyelonephritis without nausea and vomiting	Urine culture and sensitivity; Gram stain on uncentrifuged urine may help guide initial therapy.	Oral fluoroquinolone (ciprofloxacin 500 mg b.i.d. or norfloxacin 400 mg b.i.d. or ofloxacin 400 mg b.i.d. or levofloxacin 250 mg daily or enoxacin 400 mg b.i.d.) (see Table 14-9)	TMP/SMX if organism is sensitive; amoxicillin-clavulanate; oral cephalosporin (see Table 14-9)	Treatment for 14 days is generally recommended, although some data indicate that 7 days may be sufficient with quinolones. Nausea or vomiting calls for parenteral therapy.
Acute prostatitis, younger man (<35 years)	Urethral culture (alginate swab) for gonococci and *Chlamydia*	Ofloxacin 400 mg, then 300 mg q12h for at least 7 days	Ceftriaxone (250 mg IM, one dose), then doxycycline (100 mg PO b.i.d. for 10 days)	Evaluation of partners is indicated when sexually transmitted pathogens are demonstrated.

Continued

Syndrome	Diagnosis	First-line therapy	Alternative therapy	Comments
Acute prostatitis, older man (>35 years)	Urine culture	Oral fluoroquinolone (ciprofloxacin 500 mg b.i.d. or norfloxacin 400 mg b.i.d. or ofloxacin 200 mg b.i.d.) for 10 to 14 days	TMP/SMX; specific therapy based on Gram stain and culture	Optimum duration of therapy is unclear, and some authorities would treat for a much longer duration (3 to 4 weeks)
Chronic bacterial prostatitis	Four-cup test (see Chapter 14)	Oral fluoroquinolone (ciprofloxacin 500 mg b.i.d. or ofloxacin 300 mg b.i.d.) for 4 to 6 weeks	TMP/SMX	Consider prostatic calculi in patients who fail to respond to treatment.
Nonbacterial prostatosis	Four-cup test (see Chapter 14) to exclude other diagnoses	Doxycycline 100 mg PO b.i.d. for 14 days	Erythromycin 500 mg PO q.i.d. for 14 days	This entity remains highly controversial (see Chapter 14).

SKIN AND SKIN STRUCTURE INFECTIONS (see Chapter 15)

Syndrome	Diagnosis	First-line therapy	Alternative therapy	Comments
Impetigo, nonbullous	Clinical diagnosis, with typical "stuck-on," honey-colored crust; may be caused by group A streptococci or *S. aureus*	First-generation oral cephalosporin (see Chapter 15)	Mupirocin (Bactroban) ointment t.i.d. or oral erythromycin, azithromycin, clarithromycin; or oral second-generation cephalosporin; or dicloxacillin	Some data suggest that cure rates are higher with oral cephalosporins than with oral penicillins. Some authors suggest that oral dicloxacillin (or cloxacillin) is now the drug of choice.
Bullous impetigo	Presence of bullae or, if the bullae are ruptured, a thin, "varnishlike" crust	Oral dicloxacillin, oxacillin, or a first-generation cephalosporin other than cefixime	Mupirocin (Bactroban) ointment or amoxicillin-clavulanate or azithromycin or clarithromycin	Bullous impetigo is usually caused by *S. aureus.*
Furuncle (boil)	Clinical diagnosis; Gram stain and culture of pus are usually confirmatory of *S. aureus* but unnecessary in most cases.	Hot packs and drainage. Antistaphylococcal antibiotics (dicloxacillin PO or nafcillin or oxacillin IV) are indicated if there is evidence of cellulitis or sepsis.		Systemic antibiotics do not shorten the duration of the lesion; for prevention of recurrences, see Table 15-2.
Hidradenitis suppurativa	Clinical diagnosis; Gram stain and culture of an aspirate of the lesion or drainage from pus should be used to guide therapy.	Based on results of culture and sensitivity studies of pus from the lesion. Topical clindamycin may be useful.		Antibiotics are used to treat secondary pathogens such as *S. aureus,* aerobic gram-negative rods, including *P. aeruginosa,* and anaerobes. Overall utility of antibiotics, however, is unclear.
Facial cellulitis, mild	Clinical diagnosis; Gram stain and culture of any primary lesions may be helpful	Dicloxacillin 500 mg PO q6h	First- or second-generation cephalosporin	*S. aureus* and group A streptococci are important pathogens.
Infected wound, extremity, without fever or systemic toxicity	Clinical findings (look for history of freshwater or saltwater exposure); Gram stain may be useful	Amoxicillin-clavulanate (875/125 mg or 500/125 mg) PO b.i.d. or an oral cephalosporin	Erythromycin, azithromycin, clarithromycin, or clindamycin.	Aggressive wound care and débridement are indicated. Unusual etiologies are often suggested by the exposure history (see below).

Syndrome	Diagnosis	First-line therapy	Alternative therapy	Comments
Cellulitis of the extremities or trunk, mild, patient without diabetes mellitus	Clinical diagnosis; Gram stain and culture of any primary lesions may be helpful; consider unusual etiologies based on exposure history (see Table 15-3). When cellulitis complicates varicella, consider virulent group A streptococci; consider hospitalization and treatment with penicillin G, ampicillin, or a third-generation cephalosporin plus clindamycin.	Dicloxacillin 500 mg PO q6h	Amoxicillin-clavulanate, first-generation cephalosporin, erythromycin, azithromycin, or clarithromycin	Streptococci (group A and occasionally others such as groups B, C, or G) are the usual cause; *S. aureus* is sometimes present; consider unusual causes such as *Aeromonas hydrophila* (freshwater exposure), *Vibrio vulnificus* (saltwater exposure), and *Erysipelothrix rhusiopathiae* (fish handling) based on history, or *Cryptococcus neoformans* in an immunocompromised patient.

BONE, JOINT, AND BURSA INFECTIONS (see Chapter 15)

Syndrome	Diagnosis	First-line therapy	Alternative therapy	Comments
Septic arthritis, sexually active young adult (arthritis-dermatitis syndrome or Gram stain of aspirate is negative) (see Chapters 7, 15, and 16)	Tenosynovitis with a few hemorrhagic bullae is virtually diagnostic of *N. gonorrhoeae*; other bacteria should be excluded by Gram stain and culture when a joint effusion is present	Ceftriaxone 1 g IV or IM daily	Cefotaxime or ceftizoxime	In all other settings acute septic arthritis is best managed in the hospital.
Septic bursitis	Gram stain and culture on pus aspirated from bursa	Dicloxacillin 500 mg PO q.i.d.	Based on results of aspirate	*S. aureus* is the usual pathogen. Consider *M. tuberculosis* and *M. marinum* if Gram stain and culture are unrevealing. Daily aspiration should be carried out initially, and the duration of antibiotic therapy should be at least 14 to 21 days (and often longer). Aggressive initial treatment may prevent recurrence and the need to excise the bursa.

SEXUALLY TRANSMITTED DISEASES (see Chapter 16)

Syndrome	Diagnosis	First-line therapy	Alternative therapy	Comments
Urethritis, cervicitis, or proctitis suspected to be due to *Chlamydia trachomatis*, non-pregnant patient	Clinical examination, Gram stain of discharge (urethritis or cervicitis), culture or nonculture test (antigen detection, amplification) for *Chlamydia*	Azithromycin 1 g PO (one dose, on an empty stomach); or doxycycline 100 mg PO b.i.d. for 10 days	Ofloxacin, erythromycin	A 7-day course of generic doxycycline is less expensive than a single dose of azithromycin, but compliance must be addressed.
Urethritis or cervicitis, suspected to be due to *C. trachomatis*, pregnant patient	Same as above	Amoxicillin 500 mg PO t.i.d. for 10 days; or erythromycin base 500 mg PO q.i.d. for 7 days	Azithromycin 1 g PO as a single dose; erythromycin ethylsuccinate 800 mg PO q.i.d. for 7 days.	The safety of azithromycin in pregnancy has not been established. Erythromycin estolate should not be used in pregnancy.

Continued

Syndrome	Diagnosis	First-line therapy	Alternative therapy	Comments
Urethritis, cervicitis, or proctitis suspected to be due to *Neisseria gonorrhoeae*	Gram stain (for urethritis in male patients); culture; nonculture tests (antigen detection and amplification)	Cefixime 400 mg PO (one dose); ciprofloxacin 500 mg PO (one dose); ofloxacin 400 mg PO (one dose); or ceftriaxone 125 mg IM (one dose)	Spectinomycin, 2 g IM (one dose)	Ciprofloxacin and ofloxacin should not be used during pregnancy. Spectinomycin is reserved for pregnant patients with history of severe allergy (especially type I) to β-lactam antibiotics. Patients should also be treated for *Chlamydia trachomatis* because of possible coinfection.
Epididymitis caused by *N. gonorrhoeae*	Physical examination plus (ideally) demonstration of *N. gonorrhoeae* in urethral discharge	Ofloxacin 300 mg PO b.i.d. for 10 days	Ceftriaxone 250 mg IM (one dose), then doxycycline 100 mg PO b.i.d. for 10 days	Acute epididymitis in men <35 years old is more commonly due to *C. trachomatis* than to *N. gonorrhoeae*; ofloxacin covers both possibilities.
Genital herpes simplex virus infection, first episode	Physical examination plus culture or nonculture test (antigen detection test or amplification)	Acyclovir 400 mg PO t.i.d. for 7 to 10 days; famciclovir 250 mg PO t.i.d. for 7 to 10 days; or valacyclovir 1 g PO b.i.d. for 7 to 10 days.	Acyclovir 200 mg PO 5 times daily for 7 to 10 days	Unusually severe episodes can be treated in the hospital with IV acyclovir (5 to 10 mg/kg q8h for 5 to 7 days); first episodes of proctitis caused by herpes simplex virus should be treated with higher doses, e.g., acyclovir 800 mg PO t.i.d. or 400 mg PO 5 times daily.
Genital herpes simplex virus infection, recurrent episode	Same as above; symptoms and signs suffice if there is previous adequate documentation of the virus	Acyclovir 400 mg PO t.i.d. for 5 days or famciclovir 125 mg PO b.i.d. for 5 days or valacyclovir 500 mg PO b.i.d. for 5 days		Treatment is likely to be effective only if started early. Long-term suppressive therapy can be attempted (see Chapters 5, 16, and 20).
Vaginitis, suspected to be due to *Trichomonas vaginalis*	Physical examination plus wet mount preparation	Metronidazole 2 g PO (one dose)	Metronidazole 375 mg or 500 mg PO b.i.d. for 7 days	Metronidazole is now considered safe during pregnancy. Male sexual partners should also be treated. Higher doses of metronidazole (e.g., 2 to 4 g/day for 7 to 10 days) can be used for metronidazole-resistant strains.
Bacterial vaginosis	Physical examination; wet mount and KOH preparation	Metronidazole 500 mg PO b.i.d. for 7 days; or metronidazole gel, 0.75%, 5 g intravaginally qhs for 7 days; or clindamycin, 2% cream, 5 g intravaginally qhs for 7 days	Metronidazole 2 g PO (one dose); or metronidazole 750 mg PO daily for 7 days; or clindamycin 300 mg PO b.i.d. for 7 days	Single-dose therapy is less effective and is recommended mainly for patients in whom compliance is likely to be poor.

Syndrome	Diagnosis	First-line therapy	Alternative therapy	Comments
Vulvovaginal candidiasis	Physical examination; wet mount and KOH preparation	Fluconazole, 150 mg PO (one dose); or intra-vaginal butoconazole, clotrimazole, miconazole, terconazole, or tioconazole	Nystatin 100,000-unit vaginal tablet once daily for 14 days; itraconazole 200 mg PO b.i.d. for 1 day	Single-dose fluconazole therapy is convenient and preferred by many patients. All regimens are associated with a high rate of recurrence. Treatment failures may be due to azole-resistant *Candida glabrata*.
Pelvic inflammatory disease, mild to moderate extent	Pelvic examination; cultures or nonculture tests of cervical specimens for *N. gonorrhoeae* and *C. trachomatis*	Ofloxacin 400 mg PO b.i.d. for 14 days plus metronidazole 500 mg PO b.i.d. for 14 days; ceftriaxone 250 mg IM (one dose) plus metronidazole 500 mg PO b.i.d. for 14 days plus doxycycline 100 mg PO b.i.d. for 14 days; or cefoxitin 2 g IM (one dose, with 1 g probenecid PO) plus metronidazole 500 mg PO b.i.d. for 14 days plus doxycycline 100 mg PO b.i.d. for 14 days		More seriously ill patients should be hospitalized. Treatment must provide coverage not only against *N. gonorrhoeae* and *C. trachomatis* but also against the broad range of aerobic and anaerobic pathogens that may be involved, plus *Mycoplasma hominis*.
Syphilis, early (primary, secondary, or latent for less than 1 year)	Clinical findings (chancre; rash of secondary syphilis) plus serologic tests (RPR)	Benzathine penicillin G 2.4 million units IM (one dose)	Doxycyline 100 mg PO b.i.d. for 14 days; ceftriaxone (125 mg daily, or 250 mg every other day, for 10 days) has also been used.	Some authorities advise a second dose of benzathine penicillin after 7 days, especially in HIV-positive patients. Doxycycline is contraindicated during pregnancy. Efforts should be made to document penicillin allergy before turning to alternatives.
Syphilis, late (>1 year's duration, cardiovascular, late-latent, or gumma)	Serologic tests (late-latent syphilis) plus clinical findings (for cardiovascular syphilis and gumma). Lumbar puncture is recommended if serum RPR (VDRL) is 1:32 or greater, if the patient is HIV positive, if neurologic symptoms or signs are present, if evidence of aortitis (e.g., diastolic murmur at right sternal border) is present, or if treatment has failed.	Benzathine penicillin G, 2.4 million units IM weekly for 3 weeks	Doxycycline 100 mg PO b.i.d. for 14 days	Optimally, lumbar puncture should be performed to exclude neurosyphilis. The value of routine lumbar puncture in patients without risk factors for neurosyphilis (see "Diagnosis" column at left) is being debated. Doxycycline is contraindicated during pregnancy.
Neurosyphilis	Clinical findings plus serologic tests plus analysis of CSF (cell count, glucose, protein, RPR)	Aqueous (crystalline) penicillin G, 18 to 24 million units IV for 10 to 14 days	Procaine penicillin G, 2.4 million units IM daily plus probenecid 500 mg PO q.i.d., both for 10 to 14 days	Crystalline penicillin G can be given by continuous IV infusion (my preference) or by intermittent infusion (q3h or q4h). Probenecid should not be used with IV penicillin. Patients allergic to penicillin should be desensitized.

Continued

Syndrome	Diagnosis	First-line therapy	Alternative therapy	Comments
Lymphogranuloma venereum	Clinical findings (inguinal lymphadenopathy plus often inconspicuous primary lesion)	Doxycycline 100 mg PO b.i.d. for 21 days	Erythromycin 500 mg PO q.i.d. for 21 days	
Chancroid	Clinical findings (painful soft chancre as opposed to the painless hard chancre of syphilis)	Azithromycin 1 g PO (one dose, on empty stomach); or ceftriaxone, 250 mg IM (one dose)	Ciprofloxacin 500 mg PO b.i.d. for 3 days; or erythromycin 500 mg PO q.i.d. for 7 days	All regimens are less effective in HIV-infected patients
Genital warts (human papillomavirus [HPV] infection)	Clinical findings. Papanicolaou smear should be performed in women because of high incidence of cervical dysplasia and neoplasia. Detection of HPV DNA has been recently introduced as a specific test (see Chapter 2).	Topical tricholoroacetic acid or podophyllin in the office setting; imiquimod 5% cream or podofilox 0.5% solution or gel for self-treatment at home; cryotherapy with liquid nitrogen or a cryoprobe	Laser therapy; surgery	No regimen has been shown to be uniformly effective in removing warts, preventing recurrence, eradicating the virus, or modifying the risk of cervical dysplasia or neoplasia

Data from various sources, including Gilbert DN, Moellering RC Jr, Sande MA. The Sanford Guide to Antimicrobial Therapy. 31st ed., Hyde Park, Vt.: Antimicrobial Therapy, Inc.; 2001; The Medical Letter on Drugs and Therapeutics (especially 1999; 41: 85-90 [Drugs for sexually transmitted infections] and 2001; 43: 69-78 [The choice of antibacterial drugs]); Bartlett JG. Pocket Book of Infectious Disease Therapy. 10th ed., Philadelphia: Williams & Wilkins; 2000; Mandell GL, Bennett JE, Dolin R, eds. Mandell, Douglas, and Bennett's Principles and Practice of Infectious Diseases. 5th ed., Philadelphia: Churchill Livingstone; 2000.

COPD, Chronic obstructive pulmonary disease; CSF, cerebrospinal fluid; CT, computed tomography; HIV, human immunodeficiency virus; HPV, human papillomavirus; KOH, potassium hydroxide; PCR, polymerase chain reaction; RPR, rapid plasma reagin; RSV, respiratory syncytial virus; TMP/SMX, trimethoprim-sulfamethoxazole; VDRL, Venereal Disease Research Laboratory.

*The preference for a macrolide or a fluoroquinolone in the treatment of mild to moderately severe community-acquired pneumonia is controversial, and the literature should be watched.

2

Empiric Therapy for Syndromes That Usually Require Admission to the Hospital

CHARLES S. BRYAN

Syndrome	Diagnosis	First-line therapy	Alternative therapy	Comments
EYE INFECTIONS (see Chapter 9)				
Orbital cellulitis (see Chapter 9)	Clinical diagnosis; *Streptococcus pneumoniae, Staphylococcus aureus, Moraxella catarrhalis,* anaerobic bacteria, *Streptococcus pyogenes,* and *Haemophilus influenzae* are potential pathogens.	IV second- or third-generation cephalosporin or ampicillin-sulbactam	IV ticarcillin-clavulanate or piperacillin-tazobactam	Consider mucormycosis especially for patients recently recovered from diabetic ketoacidosis.
UPPER RESPIRATORY INFECTIONS (see Chapters 4 and 11)				
Acute malignant otitis externa (see Chapter 3)	External otitis in a patient with diabetes mellitus, complicated by fever, headache, or cranial nerve palsies	IV imipenem or meropenem or ceftazidime or antipseudomonal penicillin plus an aminoglycoside	IV ciprofloxacin	Often a medical emergency. Hospitalization or referral is usually indicated. Mild cases are sometimes treated on an outpatient basis with ciprofloxacin.
Membranous pharyngitis caused by diphtheria (see Chapter 10)	Diphtheria is suggested by a membrane that often extends to the uvula and soft palate; other signs include systemic toxicity, hoarseness, stridor, palatal paralysis, and nasal discharge.	Diphtheria antitoxin plus penicillin or erythromycin		Suspicion of diphtheria should usually prompt referral or admission to the hospital. Definitive diagnosis is made by isolation of *Corynebacterium diphtheriae* on Löffler's medium or tellurite selective media such as Tindale's agar.
Membranous pharyngitis caused by Vincent's angina	The membrane is coated with a purulent exudate, and the breath often has a purulent odor reflecting the anaerobic component.	High-dose IV penicillin G	IV clindamycin	This now uncommon disease is caused by anaerobic bacteria and spirochetes; *S. pyogenes* and *S. aureus* are important in some cases.
Septic thrombophlebitis of the internal jugular vein (Lemierre syndrome) (see Chapter 6)	Tenderness along the sternocleidomastold muscle (carotid sheath) with systemic toxicity and often septic emboli to the lungs	High-dose IV penicillin G	IV clindamycin	*Fusobacterium* species, especially *Fusobacterium necrophorum,* are the usual pathogens in this syndrome, which arises from head and neck infection.

Continued

Syndrome	Diagnosis	First-line therapy	Alternative therapy	Comments
Acute epiglottitis (see Chapter 6)	Sore throat with respiratory distress; when the diagnosis is strongly suspected in a child, immediate attention should be given to maintaining the airway.	Newer cephalosporin IV (cefuroxime or cefotaxime or ceftriaxone)	IV ampicillin-sulbactam or TMP/SMX	Maintaining airway patency takes first priority. Intubation should be considered. Although the diagnosis is easily confirmed radiologically, patients (and especially children) should not be sent unattended to the x-ray department.
Necrotizing soft tissue infections of the fascial spaces of the head and neck (see Chapter 6)	Clinical or radiologic evidence of inflammation involving the submandibular, lateral pharyngeal, retropharyngeal, or pretracheal soft tissues	High-dose IV penicillin G plus IV metronidazole or cefoxitin	IV clindamycin, ampicillin-sulbactam, ticarcillin-clavulanate, or piperacillin-tazobactam	These infections typically involve both aerobic and anaerobic bacteria. *Eikenella corrodens,* a potential pathogen, is resistant to cephalosporins.
PNEUMONIA (SEVERE) (see Chapter 11)				
Community-acquired pneumonia, severe but not requiring admission to an intensive care unit	Blood cultures; sputum Gram stain and culture; consider serologic tests, urine test for *Legionella* antigen	IV ceftriaxone or cefotaxime plus azithromycin or erythromycin	IV cefuroxime plus erythromycin, or a "respiratory quinolone" (levofloxacin, moxifloxacin, or gatifloxacin)	If high-level resistance to penicillin is suspected, add vancomycin.
Community-acquired pneumonia, severe and requiring admission to an intensive care unit	Same as above	IV ceftriaxone or cefotaxime plus a "respiratory quinolone" or azithromycin ± vancomycin	IV "respiratory quinolone" (levofloxacin, moxifloxacin, or gatifloxacin)	If high-level resistance to penicillin is suspected, add vancomycin.
Aspiration pneumonia with lung abscess, caused by "mouth flora"	Suspect the diagnosis if breath has a foul odor, oral hygiene is poor, and clinical setting is appropriate.	IV clindamycin	IV cefoxitin or ticarcillin-clavulanate or piperacillin-tazobactam	Consider bronchoscopy. Occasionally, aerobic bacteria such as *S. aureus, Klebsiella pneumoniae,* and type 3 *S. pneumoniae* cause lung abscess.
INFECTIONS OF THE CENTRAL NERVOUS SYSTEM (see Chapter 6)				
Acute bacterial meningitis, age 1 to 3 months	Blood cultures; CSF cultures	IV ampicillin plus ceftriaxone or cefotaxime	IV vancomycin plus ceftriaxone or cefotaxime	Corticosteroids are now recommended: dexamethasone, 0.4 mg/kg IV q12h for 2 days or 0.15 mg/kg IV q6h for 4 days, with the first dose given 15 to 20 minutes before the first dose of antibiotics.
Acute bacterial meningitis, age 3 months to 50 years	Blood cultures; CSF cultures; test any *S. pneumoniae* isolate for penicillin susceptibility	IV ceftriaxone or cefotaxime plus vancomycin	IV meropenem plus vancomycin	Vancomycin is recommended for additional coverage against penicillin-resistant *S. pneumoniae;* meropenem is less prone to cause seizures than imipenem.

Syndrome	Diagnosis	First-line therapy	Alternative therapy	Comments
Acute bacterial meningitis, age >50, years of alcoholism	Blood cultures; CSF cultures	Same as above plus IV ampicillin	Same as above	Ampicillin is added to cover *Listeria monocytogenes.* Consider corticosteroids (dexamethasone 0.4 mg/kg IV q12h for 2 days, with the first dose before the first dose of antibiotics).
Encephalitis	Herpes simplex encephalitis, the currently "treatable" cause, is suggested by clinical, CT or MRI, and CSF findings.	IV acyclovir		If herpes simplex virus encephalitis is suspected, antiviral therapy is recommended while awaiting the results of PCR on CSF for herpes simplex virus.
Brain abscess	CT or MRI scan of brain; aspiration or open surgical drainage	High-dose IV penicillin G or third-generation cephalosporin (cefotaxime or ceftriaxone) plus IV metronidazole		Patients in the early stages ("cerebritis") are sometimes treated empirically with close observation. Common pathogens include *Streptococcus intermedius* group and anaerobic bacteria.
Subdural empyema	CT or MRI scan of brain	Same as above		Urgent surgical drainage is recommended.
Cavernous sinus thrombosis	CT or MRI scan of brain with clinical findings such as proptosis and third nerve involvement	IV nafcillin or oxacillin plus third-generation cephalosporin or imipenem	IV vancomycin or meropenem	Heparin is indicated as adjunctive therapy. Fungal pathogens including mucormycosis should be considered, especially in patients with diabetes mellitus or malignant disease.
Spinal epidural abscess	Clinical findings of fever, back pain, or spinal cord compression with confirmation by MRI scan	IV nafcillin or oxacillin	IV vancomycin	*S. aureus* is the usual pathogen. Surgical exploration and drainage with bacteriologic confirmation are urgent.
SEPSIS SYNDROME, SOURCE UNDETERMINED (see Chapter 6)				
Child, not immunocompromised	Blood cultures	IV ceftriaxone or cefotaxime or cefuroxime	IV nafcillin or oxacillin plus cefuroxime	Ampicillin-sulbactam and ticarcillin-clavulanate are not FDA approved for children.
Adult, not immunocompromised	Blood cultures	IV third- or fourth-generation cephalosporin (ceftriaxone, cefotaxime, ceftazidime, or cefepime), ticarcillin-clavulanate or piperacillin-tazobactam or imipenem or meropenem plus aminoglycoside	IV third or fourth-generation cephalosporin (ceftriaxone, cefotaxime, ceftazidime, or cefepime) plus clindamycin or metronidazole; or fluoroquinolone plus clindamycin	Add vancomycin if there is strong reason to suspect methicillin-resistant *S. aureus.* Anaerobic coverage, desirable to cover the possibility of occult intraabdominal sepsis, is provided in these regimens by ticarcillin-clavulanate, piperacillin-tazobactam, imipenem, meropenem, clindamycin, or metronidazole.

Continued

Syndrome	Diagnosis	First-line therapy	Alternative therapy	Comments
Adult, asplenic (see Chapter 6)	Blood cultures	IV ceftriaxone or cefotaxime		Hospitalization is usually indicated.
Adult, injecting drug user	Blood cultures	IV nafcillin or oxacillin plus aminoglycoside (gentamicin)	IV vancomycin plus aminoglycoside	These regimens are for *S. aureus*. Keep in mind other possibilities such as intraabdominal sepsis and septic arthritis or osteomyelitis caused by *Pseudomonas aeruginosa.*
Adult, decubitus ulcers	Blood cultures	IV imipenem, meropenem, ticarcillin-clavulanate, or piperacillin-tazobactam	IV ciprofloxacin or levo-floxacin plus clindamycin or metronidazole	Sepsis is usually polymi-crobial; anaerobic bacteria including *Bacteroides fragilis* are usually present; consider the possibility of methicillin-resistant *S. aureus,* which requires vancomycin.
Staphylococcal toxic shock syndrome	Clinical diagnosis (see Chapter 6)	IV nafcillin or oxacillin	IV cefazolin	Use vancomycin if a methicillin-resistant strain is likely
Streptococcal toxic shock syndrome	Clinical diagnosis (see Chapter 6)	High-dose IV penicillin G plus clindamycin	IV erythromycin or IV ceftriaxone plus clindamycin	Clindamycin is used to inhibit toxin production.

ENDOCARDITIS (see Chapter 6)

Syndrome	Diagnosis	First-line therapy	Alternative therapy	Comments
Injecting drug user or other reason to suspect *S. aureus*	Blood cultures (three sets)	High-dose IV nafcillin or oxacillin plus gentamicin	Vancomycin plus gentamicin	Nafcillin and oxacillin are more effective than cefa-zolin and vancomycin against mutually suscep-tible strains. Vancomycin should be used in initial regimen if there is a high index of suspicion of methicillin-resistant *S. aureus.*
Endocarditis, other settings, acutely ill patient	Blood cultures (three sets)	High-dose IV penicillin G or ampicillin plus nafcillin or oxacillin plus gentamicin	Vancomycin plus gentamicin	Isolation of the infecting microorganism by blood culture is extremely desir-able (see comment below).
Endocarditis, suspected, patient not acutely ill	Blood cultures (three sets on each of 2 consecutive days)	See comment	See comment	For patients with sub-acute illness, most authorities prefer to await the results of blood cul-tures while observing the patient closely for complications.

SKIN AND SOFT TISSUE INFECTIONS (see Chapter 15)

Syndrome	Diagnosis	First-line therapy	Alternative therapy	Comments
Facial cellulitis (erysipelas), adult	Clinical diagnosis; *S. aureus* is a potential pathogen	IV nafcillin or oxacillin	IV cefazolin or vancomycin	Ampicillin-sulbactam is appropriate therapy in mild to moderately severe cases
Breast abscess or severe mastitis, postpartum	Aspiration or surgical drainage	IV nafcillin, oxacillin, or cefazolin	IV vancomycin or clindamycin	*S. aureus* is the usual pathogen.

Syndrome	Diagnosis	First-line therapy	Alternative therapy	Comments
Breast abscess or severe mastitis, nonpuerperal	Aspiration or surgical drainage	IV nafcillin, oxacillin, or cefazolin plus metronidazole	IV ampicillin-sulbactam or vancomycin plus metronidazole	Subareolar abscesses commonly involve anaerobic bacteria in addition to *S. aureus;* peripherally located abscesses are usually due to *S. aureus.*
Cellulitis, extremities	Clinical diagnosis; group A streptococci the usual cause of erysipelas; *S. aureus* sometimes present as sole pathogen or copathogen; exposure history may suggest unusual etiology such as *Aeromonas hydrophila* or *Vibrio vulnificus* (see Chapter 15).	IV nafcillin or oxacillin	IV cefazolin or ampicillin-sulbactam	Culture of any primary lesion may be worthwhile; cultures of "tissue aspirates" are sometimes helpful in immunocompromised persons.
Infected wound, extremity, with systemic toxicity	Clinical findings including any history of freshwater or saltwater exposure, bite, or osteomyelitis; Gram stain of material may be useful.	IV nafcillin or oxacillin plus clindamycin plus aminoglycoside	IV ampicillin-sulbactam or ticarcillin-clavulanate plus aminoglycoside	Consider gas gangrene (anaerobic myonecrosis) and necrotizing fasciitis; unusual etiologies of cellulitis calling for specific therapy (e.g., *Vibrio vulnificus),* and, if there is a history of osteomyelitis treated with multiple antibiotics, drug-resistant gram-negative bacilli or *S. aureus.*
Infected foot, patient with diabetes mellitus, acute with toxicity	Clinical findings; radiologic imaging (looking for gas and evidence of osteomyelitis); "probe-to-bone" test	IV cefoxitin; or a quinolone (e.g., ciprofloxacin) plus metronidazole or clindamycin	IV imipenem or meropenem or ticarcillin-clavulanate or ampicillin-sulbactam or piperacillin-tazobactam or nafcillin (or oxacillin) plus an aminoglycoside (or aztreonam) plus metronidazole or clindamycin	For milder infections, treatment as an outpatient with oral antibiotics (e.g., amoxicillin-clavulanate or a quinolone or TMP/SMX plus metronidazole is often effective (see Chapter 15).
Necrotizing fasciitis (see Chapter 6)	Clinical findings (pain disproportionate to inflammation; crepitance; systemic toxicity); radiologic imaging can be confirmatory but should not be performed if it will delay surgical exploration in urgent cases.	High-dose IV penicillin G plus clindamycin	IV third-generation cephalosporin (cefotaxime or ceftriaxone) or erythromycin plus clindamycin	Clindamycin is used to reduce toxin production. Surgical exploration is indicated on an urgent basis.

INTRAABDOMINAL INFECTIONS (see Chapter 12)

Syndrome	Diagnosis	First-line therapy	Alternative therapy	Comments
Acute cholecystitis or cholangitis	Imaging studies; surgical consultation	Piperacillin-tazobactam or ticarcillin-clavulanate or ampicillin-sulbactam or ampicillin plus gentamicin ± metronidazole; piperacillin ± metronidazole	Ceftriaxone or cefotaxime plus metronidazole or clindamycin; aztreonam plus clindamycin	Close surgical follow-up is highly desirable.

Continued

Syndrome	Diagnosis	First-line therapy	Alternative therapy	Comments
Spontaneous bacterial peritonitis (see Chapter 3)	Paracentesis; blood and ascitic fluid cultures	Cefotaxime	Ceftriaxone, β-lactam/β-lactamase inhibitor combination; or a fluoroquinolone	Suspect in a febrile patient with cirrhosis and ascites. High mortality resulting in part from severity of underlying disease.
Secondary bacterial peritonitis caused by ruptured viscus, including acute appendicitis and acute diverticulitis	Imaging studies; CT- or ultrasound-guided aspiration; surgical exploration	Gentamicin plus clindamycin is the historical "gold standard," but numerous regimens are effective (e.g., ticarcillin-clavulanate, piperacillin-tazobactam; ceftriaxone or cefotaxime plus metronidazole).	Many alternative regimens continue to be evaluated; the principle is that therapy must cover aerobic gram-negative bacteria and also anaerobic bacteria, including *Bacteroides fragilis*.	Close surgical follow-up is mandatory.
OBSTETRIC AND GYNECOLOGIC INFECTIONS (see Chapters 5 and 16)				
Pelvic inflammatory disease, severe (see Chapter 16)	Pelvic examination; ultrasound examination	IV cefoxitin or cefotetan plus doxycycline	IV clindamycin plus gentamicin; ciprofloxacin or ofloxacin plus metronidazole; ampicillin-sulbactam plus doxycycline	Treatment should include coverage against *Chlamydia trachomatis*; sex partners should also be evaluated and treated.
Septic abortion	Pelvic examination; history; presence of marked systemic toxicity	IV ticarcillin-clavulanate, piperacillin-tazobactam, ampicillin-sulbactam, or cefoxitin	IV clindamycin plus ceftriaxone or cefotaxime plus gentamicin or tobramycin	Coverage should include aerobic gram-negative rods and anaerobic pathogens, including *Bacteroides* species and *Clostridium perfringens* (which can cause gas gangrene of the uterus).
BONE AND JOINT INFECTIONS (see Chapter 15)				
Septic arthritis, child	Blood cultures; Gram stain and culture of synovial fluid	IV nafcillin or oxacillin plus ceftriaxone or cefotaxime	Vancomycin plus ceftriaxone or cefotaxime	Coverage should be effective against *S. aureus*, gram-negative bacilli, *H. influenzae*, and *Neisseria* species
Septic arthritis, sexually active adult	Same as above	IV ceftriaxone; consider adding nafcillin or oxacillin	Severe β-lactam allergy: IM spectinomycin or IV ciprofloxacin; consider adding nafcillin or oxacillin	Ceftriaxone is reasonable therapy if clinical presentation strongly suggests *N. gonorrhoeae* (see Chapters 7, 15, and 16). Add antistaphylococcal coverage if there is strong reason to suspect *S. aureus*.

Syndrome	Diagnosis	First-line therapy	Alternative therapy	Comments
Septic arthritis, older adult	Same as above; look for uric acid (gout) and calcium pyrophosphate (pseudogout) crystals in synovial fluid.	IV nafcillin or oxacillin plus ceftriaxone	Severe β-lactam allergy: IV vancomycin plus ciprofloxacin	Coverage should include *S. aureus*, gram-negative bacilli, and *N. gonorrhoeae*. Consider *S. aureus* especially in patients with severe rheumatoid arthritis.
Hematogenous osteomyelitis, child	Bone aspirate; blood culture	Nafcillin or oxacillin	Vancomycin or clindamycin	*S. aureus* or GABHS most commonly; occasionally gram-negative rods, in which case ceftriaxone is appropriate.
Hematogenous osteomyelitis, adult	Bone aspirate; blood culture	Nafcillin or oxacillin; cefazolin	Vancomycin	*S. aureus* is the most common agent, but etiologic diagnosis is highly desirable. Consider *Salmonella* in patients with sickle cell disease; consider *P. aeruginosa* in injecting drug users or patients receiving hemodialysis.
Osteomyelitis after nail puncture wound of foot through tennis shoe	Bone aspirate	Ceftazidime or (except in children) ciprofloxacin	Ciprofloxacin (except in children)	*P. aeruginosa* is the usual pathogen (93% of cases).
Osteomyelitis, chronic	Bone aspirate or biopsy, or (ideally) culture of material obtained at sequestrectomy			Empiric therapy is not appropriate unless patient has sepsis, in which case management is the same as for acute hematogenous osteomyelitis (but taking into account any previous bacteriologic findings).

Data from various sources, including Gilbert DN, Moellering RC Jr, Sande MA. The Sanford Guide to Antimicrobial Therapy. 31st ed., Hyde Park, Vt.: Antimicrobial Therapy, Inc.; 2001; The Medical Letter on Drugs and Therapeutics (especially 1999; 41: 85-90 [Drugs for sexually transmitted infections] and 2001; 43: 69-78 [The choice of antibacterial drugs]); Bartlett JG. Pocket Book of Infectious Disease Therapy. 10th ed., Philadelphia: Williams & Wilkins; 2000; Mandell GL, Bennett JE, Dolin R, eds. Mandell, Douglas, and Bennett's Principles and Practice of Infectious Diseases. 5th ed., Philadelphia: Churchill Livingstone; 2000.
CSF, Cerebrospinal fluid; *CT*, computed tomography; *FDA*, Food and Drug Administration; *MRI*, magnetic resonance imaging; *PCR*, polymerase chain reaction; *TMP/SMX*, trimethoprim-sulfamethoxazole.

3 For Patients: Acute Infection and You— The "Buddy Check"

CHARLES S. BRYAN

Acute Infection and You—The "Buddy Check"

Your doctor may have determined that you have symptoms and signs consistent with an acute viral illness, or "viral syndrome." Symptoms of acute viral illness may include fever, chilliness, muscle aches, headache, dizziness, photophobia (pain on looking into light), nausea, and diarrhea. Physical examination usually shows only mild abnormalities, if any. The problem that your doctor faces is as follows.

- Most of the time, patients with acute "viral syndrome" recover within several days without treatment. The disease is self-limited.
- Rarely, previously healthy persons come to their doctors with symptoms and signs consistent with an acute "viral syndrome" that turn out to be caused instead by life-threatening acute infectious disease.
- Unfortunately, there is sometimes no practical way to distinguish between "viral syndrome" and the initial manifestations of acute life-threatening illness.

The more important life-threatening infections that can occur in this way in the United States include meningococcal (pronounced "men-IN-go-COCK-al") sepsis, acute bacterial meningitis, Rocky Mountain spotted fever, staphylococcal sepsis, and (in travelers) falciparum malaria.

The following recommendations are intended to help you through this period of uncertainty:

1. *Be on the lookout for symptoms and signs that are out of the ordinary for an acute viral illness.* If you have headache, is it the worst you've ever had? Infectious causes of extremely severe headache include meningitis, brain abscess (which usually presents with gradual onset), Rocky Mountain spotted fever (a consideration especially during the summer months in much of the United States), and acute sphenoid sinusitis (which is rare). Does your neck hurt? If so, are you able to put your chin between your knees without severe pain? Inability to do so suggests meningitis. Unusually forceful vomiting, sometimes called "projectile vomiting," is another symptom of meningitis. If you have aches and pains, are they localized in any one place? Severe localized pain is sometimes caused by acute staphylococcal ("staph") infection, which can be life threatening. Inspect your skin closely for little red spots. Called "petechiae" (pronounced "pit-TEAK-e-EYE"), little red spots on the skin can be an extremely important clue to meningococcal sepsis, Rocky Mountain spotted fever, and other serious illnesses. Look for them especially on the chest, near the armpits, and on the extremities. Are your symptoms and signs different in any way from whatever illness seems to be "making the rounds" in your community?
2. *Do not take medications or other substances such as alcohol that might mask the severity of your symptoms.* Be careful about taking sleeping pills, muscle relaxants, and other drugs that cause drowsiness. Also, be careful about taking large doses of aspirin or any of the newer, potent antiinflammatory drugs. Fever can cause seizures in children but is seldom harmful to adults, who usually tolerate temperatures of 105° F with little or no difficulty. In fever, the body's thermostat remains intact; it has simply been "reset" upward (in contrast to heatstroke, in which the body's thermostat is broken and which must therefore be treated differently). Many authorities advise taking analgesics only for comfort.
3. *Do not hesitate to report back to your doctor if your symptoms do not get better, or if new symptoms and signs develop.* You may wish to ask your doctor or his or her assistant to have your "CBC and differential" checked. Even if the white blood cell count is normal, the differential cell count sometimes shows more "bands and polys" than should be present in acute viral illness. A low platelet count can also be important. If you have severe headache or neck stiffness or both, and especially if you have severe nausea or vomiting, you may need a spinal tap (lumbar puncture) to exclude meningitis. If you have a history of heart murmur, you may need blood cultures to exclude endocarditis (infection of the heart valves). If you do not have a spleen, you may need to be admitted to the hospital because sepsis can be extremely severe in this instance.

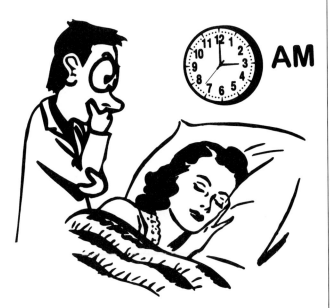

The buddy check. At 3 AM, or about 4 hours after you retire, your "buddy" (spouse, parent, roommate, or significant other) should awaken you, ask about your symptoms, and help you look for little red spots on your skin, especially on the chest.

4. *Arrange for a "buddy check" at 3 AM, or about 4 hours after you go to sleep.* Each year, occasional persons go to sleep only to be found moribund the next morning because of an acute infectious disease such as meningitis or meningococcemia. Do you remember the "buddy check" from the lake or swimming pool at summer camp? When the lifeguard blew a whistle, every camper found his or her "buddy" and the pair raised their joined hands. Have someone in your household— parent, spouse, roommate, or significant other—set an alarm clock for 3 AM, or about 4 hours after you retire. Your buddy should speak to you or shake you gently and then, when you awake, ask you about your symptoms and look for little red spots. If you have no new symptoms and no little red spots, both of you can go back to sleep. If things have changed, you should strongly consider calling your doctor or reporting to the nearest emergency room.

Special instructions for _____

4 For Patients: Antibiotics and You— Why Less Is Sometimes More

CHARLES S. BRYAN

Antibiotics and You—Why Less Is Sometimes More

An old truism holds that "if something seems too good to be true, it probably is." Penicillin, introduced in the 1940s, indeed seemed too good to be true. It cured certain infections that were previously incurable, and it lowered the death rates from diseases caused by such common bacteria as "group A strep," "staph," and the pneumococcus (the common cause of acute bacterial pneumonia). It attacked a piece of bacterial machinery that had no counterpart in humans, and therefore it was a "magic bullet." The result: everyone wanted penicillin, and its use was often inappropriate.

Bacteria did not take long to figure out ways to dodge the bullet. Some bacteria manufactured enzymes that destroy penicillin. Others made it more difficult for penicillin to pierce their armor. New drugs were needed to kill some organisms, such as the staphylococcus. The story of penicillin and resistant bacteria has been repeated with almost every new class of antibiotics. A "wonder drug" is discovered and found to be effective. It is used inappropriately. Bacteria (and other germs that cause infections, including viruses and fungi) become resistant. Pharmaceutical manufacturers retrench to their research laboratories. Another new drug is introduced. And the cycle continues.

The problem of overuse of antibiotics and the development of drug-resistant microbes is receiving national and international attention from government agencies and health care organizations. The following are of particular concern:

- The growing resistance of the pneumococcus to penicillin and many other antibiotics
- The growing resistance of staphylococci to methicillin and most other antibiotics
- The growing resistance of enterococci (a common bacterium found in the intestines) to vancomycin, which has been the "drug of last resort"
- The recognition that staphylococci can also become resistant to vancomycin

Physicians are now beginning to see bacterial infections for which no effective drug treatment is available. What can and should be done? This is a case in which we must "think globally and act locally." Will you be part of the problem, or part of the solution?

Nobody, and especially not your doctor, would want to deny you antibiotics for a serious or life-threatening infection. Problems enter when evidence of serious infection is equivocal or even absent, yet patients want "something to be done." Physicians, who are often pressed for time, find it much easier to prescribe than to educate. As one doctor put it, "It takes me 5 seconds to write a prescription for antibiotics and 5 minutes to explain why it isn't indicated." Many physicians have found that some patients accept such explanations begrudgingly if at all.

They may even change doctors! This pressure to prescribe explains, at least in part, why nearly one half of the antibiotic prescriptions written in primary care settings may be inappropriate.

Fortunately, the public is becoming aware that we *must* use antibiotics more judiciously if our children and grandchildren are to benefit from these lifesaving drugs. Two points need emphasis. First, many infections, especially infections involving the upper respiratory tract, are caused by viruses rather than by bacteria. These infections are usually self-limited, and antibiotics are irrelevant. Second, use of antibiotics promotes the development of resistance in bacteria that normally colonize body surfaces, including "staph" and the pneumococcus.

The following recommendations, adapted in part from *Consumer Reports* (January 2001), reflect commonsense advice concerning antibiotics:

1. Do not insist on antibiotics for symptoms of upper respiratory infection such as "sinus trouble," sore throat, or acute bronchitis with cough. More often than not, viruses rather than bacteria cause these infections.
2. Ask your doctor whether, in his or her opinion, your problem is likely to be a bacterial infection.
3. Ask whether it's appropriate to obtain a culture. Treatment for "strep throat," for example, is usually inappropriate unless supported by a positive culture or other test for the group A streptococcus.
4. Ask whether it's appropriate to use "tincture of time" rather than drugs. Most community-acquired infections are self-limited. All too often, antibiotics receive the credit for an infection that would have resolved within 48 to 72 hours anyway.
5. If your doctor believes that an antibiotic is indicated, ask whether it's a relatively narrow-spectrum drug designed to cover the most likely bacteria or a broad-spectrum drug. Broad-spectrum drugs are sometimes used inappropriately and are more likely to cause problems such as overgrowth of harmful bacteria and fungi. Also, ask about the optimum duration of antibiotics.
6. Discard any unused antibiotics, or donate them to a health clinic. Do not keep antibiotics around the house unless you have a specific indication for doing so that you have discussed with your doctor. Do not share your antibiotics with others.

Wise use of antibiotics is the key to curbing the alarming spread of drug-resistant bacteria and other microbes. In this instance the saying that "less is more" may indeed hold true.

For further information you may wish to consult a website maintained by the Centers for Disease Control and Prevention: http://www.cdc.gov/ncidod/dbmd/antibioticresistance/. Drug-resistant bacteria are becoming everyone's problem. Pitch in!

APPENDIX

5 Useful Websites for Information About Infectious Diseases

ERIC R. BRENNER, DAVID GREENHOUSE

Only 10 years ago few physicians had ever used the Internet. Recent surveys, however, show that 70% of practitioners today have access to the Internet in their office and that they use it not only as a communication tool (e-mail), but also as a professional tool to access medical news and information. This trend has been made possible by the availability of increasingly powerful yet relatively inexpensive personal computers (PCs), by new communication technologies that have literally "wired" the world, and most of all by the startlingly rapid development of the World Wide Web (usually simply referred to as "the Web"). Thanks to the Web (and related technologies such as compact disks), physicians who in the past might have felt isolated in suburban or rural practice now enjoy rapid and convenient access to current information previously available only to those who practiced in proximity to large medical libraries. However, the amount of information on the Web can, at times, appear overwhelming and unstructured. Furthermore, it is said to increase by more than 1 million pages per day! The challenge for the practicing physician thus lies in being able to extract truly useful information from the Web in a reasonable amount of time. This appendix presents examples of useful websites pertaining to infectious diseases and also provides tips and suggestions for optimal Web use.

Websites with Infectious Disease Content

Because the Web is so vast and dynamic, no list of sites, however long, can be complete or even meet all the needs of any individual Web user. The sites presented here have been chosen either because of their recognized excellence and utility or because they are good examples of the sites available in a subject area. While some sites are useful for their content, others are useful because of their well-organized lists of links to other sites.

As the nation's premier agency for communicable disease control, the Centers for Disease Control and Prevention (CDC) has resources extraordinary in their scope and quality. Their

TABLE 1
General Infectious Diseases Websites

www.cdc.gov	U.S. Centers for Disease Control and Prevention (see further details in Table 2)
www.niaid.nih.gov	National Institute of Allergy and Infectious Diseases (at National Institutes of Health)
www.who.ch	World Health Organization, Geneva, Switzerland
www.who.int/infectious-disease-report/index.htm	Two major WHO reports about infectious diseases: the global perspective
www.paho.org	Pan American Health Organization (Washington, D.C.)
www.fda.gov	U.S. Food and Drug Administration
www.sermed.com/infect.htm	Links to a variety of infectious disease resources
www.medscape.com	An "infectious disease" portal with news, reviewed articles, and more
www.icanprevent.com	An excellent site for information on communicable disease and infection control. Paid membership required (but can be tried free for 30 days)
home.idac.org/idac/idlinks.html	Numerous useful infectious disease links provided by the Infectious Disease Association of California

Web offerings are so extensive that even skilled "Web browsing and searching" starting from the CDC "home page" (www.cdc.gov) can fail to lead efficiently to useful resources. Table 2 therefore offers a more detailed guide to the CDC's Web resources.

Whereas the listings in Table 1 are institutions or other sites that focus on many different infectious diseases, some websites are devoted exclusively to specific individual infections. Examples of these are presented in Table 3. (Yahoo's health page http://dir.yahoo.com/Health/ can be used as a portal to many hundreds of other sites devoted to specific infectious and noninfectious conditions.)

Accessing Major Medical Journals Via the Web

Most major medical journals now maintain Web pages. However, their policies concerning the content they make available to Web users and the terms of use vary widely. A few, such as the *British Medical Journal*, make full text of all content freely available. More commonly, however,

TABLE 2
A More Detailed Guide to the Website of the Centers for Disease Control and Prevention

www.cdc.gov/	CDC's home page
www.cdc.gov/travel/index.htm	Health recommendations for international travelers
www.cdc.gov/nip/	National Immunization Program (outstanding resources on vaccines)
www.cdc.gov/nchstp/tb/	Tuberculosis news and recommendations
www.cdc.gov/nchstp/dstd/dstdp.html	Sexually transmitted diseases
www.cdc.gov/hiv/dhap.htm	HIV/AIDS
www.cdc.gov/ncidod/diseases/index.htm	Authoritative patient fact sheets for dozens of different infectious diseases
www.cdc.gov/ncidod/dvrd/disinfo/disease.htm	Information about numerous viral diseases
www.cdc.gov/ncidod/dbmd/diseaseinfo/default.htm	Patient and professional information about numerous bacterial and mycotic infections
www.cdc.gov/ncidod/diseases/hepatitis	Viral hepatitis A to E
www.cdc.gov/ncidod/dpd/default.htm	Parasitic diseases
www.cdc.gov/ncidod/dvrd/rabies	Rabies
www.cdc.gov/ncidod/dvrd/default.htm	Viral and rickettsial diseases
www.cdc.gov/ncidod/hip/abc/abc.htm	ABCs of Safe and Healthy Child Care (guidelines and fact sheets for day care staff and parents)
www.cdc.gov/ncidod/diseases/flu/fluvirus.htm	Influenza—in-depth general information
www.cdc.gov/ncidod/diseases/flu/weekly.htm	Influenza—weekly surveillance information from around the country. Interesting to follow during the "flu season."
www.cdc.gov/ncidod/dbmd/antibioticresistance	Information and resources regarding antibiotic resistance in clinical practice (see Appendix 4)
www.cdc.gov/od/oc/media/archives.htm	Press releases from the past several years. Often helpful to answer patient questions.
www2.cdc.gov/mmwr	Access to current and past issues of the famed CDC *Morbidity and Mortality Weekly Report* (includes weekly issues as well as official "Recommendations and Reports" and "Surveillance Series".)
aepo-xdv-www.epo.cdc.gov/wonder/PrevGuid/PrevGuid.htm	Links to numerous official prevention guidelines

journal sites make abstracts available to all but require a subscription for full-text access. Rather than presenting a list of journal websites, Table 4 presents sites that in turn offer links to hundreds of medical journals. Physicians need only follow these links to the journals most important to their practice and then add the URLs (Uniform Resource Locators or Web addresses) to their catalog of favorite Web bookmarks.

Searching MEDLINE Through the National Library of Medicine

At one time, physicians could perform MEDLINE searches only with the assistance of a medical librarian or through a service that required a subscription or other form of payment. However, since 1996 the U.S. National Library of Medicine (NLM), has made MEDLINE, a searchable database of the world's medical periodical literature published since 1966, free and universally available via the Web (Table 5). Two interfaces can be used for performing these Web-based MEDLINE searches: PubMed and Internet Grateful Med (IGM). The PubMed interface is particularly simple: author names, title words, or NLM Medical Subject Headings (MESH) can be entered in any order on a single line, and a single click then initiates the search, which can also be refined by clicking on a button marked "Limits." The IGM interface is slightly more complex but is more flexible. Separate lines can be used to enter search criteria for authors, title words, and MESH headings, and options for using Boolean operators (AND, OR) are particularly convenient. The options for further refining searches go beyond those of PubMed. The user can, for example, easily specify just which journal(s) should be searched, a convenient option for a physician who has local access to just a particular group of journals. Both PubMed and IGM permit the user not only to view and print citations and abstracts, but also to save search results to disk in a variety of formats, some of which can then be saved directly to commercial bibliographic software packages such as Reference Manager and End Notes. In this manner a physician can gradually develop a database of references most relevant to his or her practice. The database will consist of articles initially iden-

TABLE 3
Examples of Websites Devoted to Individual Infections

www.hivatis.org	The HIV/AIDS Treatment Information Service, a central resource for federally approved treatment guidelines for HIV and AIDS
www.ama-assn.org/special/hiv	*JAMA*'s excellent site for AIDS clinicians and researchers
www.aap.org/new/immpublic.htm	American Academy of Pediatrics' excellent information and links for professionals and parents with questions about immunizations
www.hepnet.com	Canada's Hepatitis Information Network
www.ntca-tb.org/tbWeb.htm	Useful links relating to tuberculosis
www.headlice.org	The Web page of the National Pediculosis Association
www.hsph.harvard.edu/headlice.htm	A Harvard School of Public Health entomologist's page on head lice
www.lymenet.org	A patient-oriented site devoted to Lyme disease

TABLE 4
Medical Journals on the Web

www.cdc.gov/ncidod/EID/index.htm	CDC's acclaimed journal on emerging infectious diseases (full text)
www.sciencekomm.at/journals/medicine/med-bio.html	Links to websites of hundreds of medical journals. Follow the links, and save your favorites.
www.coreynahman.com/medical_journals.html	More links to medical journals

TABLE 5
Searching MEDLINE on the Web

www.nlm.nih.gov	Home page of the National Library of Medicine Can then access MEDLINE by following links.
www.ncbi.nlm.nih.gov/ entrez/query.fcgi	PubMed system for searching MEDLINE. Straightforward and easy to use.
igm.nlm.nih.gov	Grateful Med system for searching MEDLINE. Slightly more complex than the PubMed but offers more flexibility and options.

TABLE 6
Illustration: Searching the Web for Information About Malaria Prophylaxis for Travelers

Terms of Altavista search	Yield
+malaria	78,000 hits
+malaria +travel	32,000 hits
+malaria +travel +precautions	7000 hits
+title:malaria +text:travel +url:cdc.gov*	47 hits—a number with titles that could easily be scanned, and one containing a brochure the patient could download

*This search used more advanced options, which indicates that the physician was looking for a site having the word "malaria" in the title, containing the word "travel" somewhere in the body of the site's text pages, and located on any of the pages maintained at the giant website of the Centers for Disease Control and Prevention, www.cdc.gov.

tified via on-line MEDLINE searches but will then be maintained and managed by use of bibliographic software on the physician's PC.

Using Web Search Engines

Most Web users are familiar with sites that can be used to "search the Web." These come in two main types, directories and search engines. The former is exemplified by Yahoo (www.yahoo.com), which maintains a list of thousands of websites organized by a professional staff into hierarchies of lists. Thus from the Yahoo main page a physician can click on "Health," then on the next page, click on a variety of subheadings such as "Children's Services" and "Diseases and Conditions," which lead, respectively, to approximately 150 or 7500 additional subsubheadings or sites. Eventually, by drilling down in this manner through the hierarchy of links, the user can identify specific sites within the catalog containing content of interest. The search engine approach is quite different and is perhaps best exemplified by Altavista (www.altavista.com). There the user enters search terms of interest and clicks to launch a search that finds sites indexed by Altavista's computers as containing terms of interest. Unless the user is careful, this approach can yield thousands (or tens or hundreds of thousands) of hits, often far too many to be useful. Altavista, like other search engines, offers various approaches to refine searches. A click on "HELP" (at Altavista or other search engine sites) will bring up explanations that are usually quite clear. In the case of Altavista, taking the time to learn how to perform a more refined search can yield enormous rewards. For example, a physician might be seeking to advise a patient about prophylaxis for malaria before travel in the tropics. Table 6 illustrates the results of using Altavista and a variety of different search strategies.

Of course, the physician might have located the same information more quickly had he or she previously bookmarked the CDC site with recommendations for travelers shown in Table 2. This simple example thus illustrates that a variety of paths can be used to access information on the Web.

Although Yahoo and Altavista have been mentioned here, numerous other excellent Web directories and search engines have been developed. The site www.lib.auburn.edu/madd/

docs/searchengine contains explanations about and links to many of the top Web search engines. Most busy physicians will find it more useful to become proficient in both basic and advanced search techniques using just one or two search engines that fit their style.

Other Medical Resources on the Web

Although the focus in this appendix is on websites related to infectious disease, sites of major medical organizations and of commercial and nonprofit organizations devoted to medicine in general can serve as portals to Web resources that include sections devoted to infectious diseases or provide links to other sites that do. Some of these are presented in Table 7. The last two sites in Table 7, one official and one private, are devoted to debunking medical rumors, hoaxes, and quackery.

Web Resources for Patients

The focus in this appendix is on Web resources for physicians. However, patients also surf the Web seeking information about their medical problems and now commonly arrive at their physician's office armed with printouts of their latest Web research. Information gleaned by nonprofessionals can range from excellent to poor and from the innocuous to the potentially harmful. Physicians have found it helpful to become familiar with some of these sites and to tell their patients the ones with which they feel comfortable. Some reputable sites for the general public to which interested patients can be referred are shown in Table 8.

The CDC recently published its Web page tips to help the general public evaluate information on the Internet. These are presented in Box 1.

TABLE 7
Websites of Selected Professional Organizations and Other Web Resources of General Medical Interest

www.ama-assn.org	American Medical Association
www.aap.org	American Academy of Pediatrics
www.aafp.org	American Academy of Family Physicians
www.acponline.org	American College of Physicians–American Society of Internal Medicine
www.uwo.ca/fammed/clfm/sites.html	Outstanding links of interest to family physicians (from the Canadian Library of Family Medicine staff)
www.medinfo.ufl.edu/cme/inet/inetres.html	Internet resources for family physicians (compiled by an individual)
www.ohsu.edu/cliniWeb	Oregon Health Sciences University's portal for links to medical sites, which have been screened for content
www.gimg.com/LINKS.HTM	A general internal medicine group's links to the Web
www.slackinc.com/child/pednet-x.htm	Web links for pediatricians
www.cmecourses.com	Gateway to on-line continuing medical education courses
www.quackwatch.com	Site offering a guide to health fraud and quackery
www.cdc.gov/hoax_rumors.htm	Site of the Centers for Disease Control and Prevention, devoted to debunking Internet rumors and urban legends often relating to infectious disease

TABLE 8
Some Websites to Which Patients Can Be Referred

www.nlm.nih.gov/ medlineplus	NIH maintained repository of information for the general public. Outstanding quality.
www.drkoop.com	A commercial popular site for the public
www.healthfinder.gov	A U.S. government site with links and resources for the general public (many links useful to physicians as well; e.g., see journals listings)
www.healthgate.com	An all-purpose medical site for the general public
www.cdc.gov	The CDC home page is user friendly and especially useful for questions about international travel.

BOX 1
Ten Tips for Evaluating Medical Information on the Internet

1. The ownership of the site should be clear.
2. The information provided should be based on sound scientific study.
3. The site should carefully weigh the evidence and acknowledge the limitations of the work.
4. The user should beware of "junk science" and suggestions of "conspiracies."
5. The individuals or group providing the information should be qualified to address the subject matter.
6. Arguments should be based on facts, not conjecture.
7. The motives of the site should be clear.
8. The information provided should make sense.
9. One sign of a scientifically sound Internet site is that it contains references from and to peer-reviewed publications.
10. The user should be able to obtain additional information if needed.

Miscellaneous Tips and Tricks
Hardware and Connectivity Issues

As anyone who has leafed through a computer magazine knows, the personal computer industry is in perpetual motion. Yesterday's "hottest PC" is today's relic. However, most PCs manufactured in the last several years can be used for efficient Web access. This is because the factor limiting efficient Web use is generally the speed of the PC's connection to the Internet, not the speed of the PC's microprocessor. Through the late 1990s most users accessed the Internet from home or office using dial-up modems, which provided connection speeds of 14.4, 28.8, 33.6, and then 56 kilobits (Kbps) per second. Only physicians based in hospitals or in other large institutions enjoyed special "hard-wired" rapid connections. However, a new generation of high-speed Internet services is becoming available to homes and offices in most communities. One type of service uses so-called digital subscriber lines (DSL). DSL offers connection speeds of the order of 1.0 or 1.5 megabits (Mbps) per second, 20 to 40 times as fast as that of the common dial-up modem. DSL services are attractive because they use existing phone lines and thus can be set up in most offices and homes. Furthermore, the connection does not tie up the phone line, so users can simultaneously carry on normal voice communications and browse the Web. Cable TV companies provide another type of high-speed Internet connection with speeds similar to those of DSL. Homes equipped with cable service are already "wired" for this service and require only installation of a special cable modem. Although the respective merits of DSL and cable can be debated, from a practical viewpoint both technologies offer tremendous improvement in Web access, can end the frustrating wait times while Web pages with extensive graphics load, cost about the same (about $50 per month at this writing), and for most physicians upgrade performance to transform the Web into a truly useful professional tool.

Web Browsers

The most commonly used Web browsers (the software packages that let PC users access the Web) are Microsoft Internet Explorer (IE) and Netscape Navigator (NN). Again, although each has its partisans, recent versions of either browser provide similar features and functionality. Both of these browsers allow users not only to create and maintain a list of sites to which they can later return with a single click of the mouse, but also to organize these sites logically into "folders." Although using a browser to follow hyperlinks on the Web is an intuitive process requiring essentially no training, many physicians fail to take advantage of the numerous features offered by current versions of browser software. A modest investment in a half-day course or in one of the excellent introductory books dealing with browsers and the Web (see "Suggested Reading") can pay for itself many times over in pleasure and convenience.

Saving Favorite Bookmarks to a Website

As mentioned previously, current Web browsers allow users to save their favorite websites as bookmarks or favorites to which they can return at the click of a mouse. However, having a good set of Web bookmarks at home or at the office is useless to a physician seated at a PC in a hospital unit or a medical library. A number of websites now give users the option of saving their private bookmarks to a password-protected Web page, allowing them to add to, manage, and access these bookmarks from any PC in the world that is connected to the Web. Some sites that provide this service are www.yahoo.com; www.visto.com; and www.oneview.com, although many others are available, each with slightly different features. Physicians whose information needs are met in part by rapid access to their favorite websites will benefit from taking the time to select and use one of these services, most of which are free.

Portable Document Format Files

Over the past several years portable document format (PDF) files have become a common format for distribution of documents over the Internet or between computers of different types (e.g., from an IBM-compatible PC to an Apple Macintosh). For example, all the back issues of CDC's *Morbidity and Mortality Weekly Report* (MMWR), including those with new U.S. Public Health Service guidelines for use of vaccines, are available as PDF files from the CDC's Web page. Many journals that allow users to download full-text versions of their articles make these available as PDF files. Reading PDF files on-line can be awkward and slow because a PDF file reader must be opened within the browser window. A cleaner approach is to download the PDF file from the posting website (where it will always be clearly labeled as a PDF file) to the browsing PC. On a PC this is done by right-clicking on the file's icon, then using "Save As" to save the file as a PDF file on the PC's hard drive. Downloaded PDF files can be conveniently saved in a separate folder that is created for that purpose and is commonly called C:\PDF. Once downloaded, the PDF files can be read off-line using the PDF file reader Acrobat Reader, which can be downloaded from www.adobe.com at no cost.

Getting Help

In the interest of saving valuable time, most physicians will benefit from having professional assistance in configuring their office and home PCs for most efficient Web use. Exceptions might be physicians who are computer hobbyists or have an interested teen-age or college-age child in the home.

Conclusion

A commitment to lifelong learning has always been necessary for practicing physicians, and the need to maintain this commitment has never been more pressing than it is today. Fortunately, the Internet, which is in part responsible for the increased volume and flow of information, now offers physicians convenient tools to keep up with official recommendations and reports, consensus guidelines, journal articles, and much more. Regular, skillful use of the World Wide Web is increasingly an integral part of becoming and remaining a well-educated and well-informed physician.

SUGGESTED READING

Bryson DM, Ingebretson M. The Physician's Guide to Internet Explorer: A Quick-Start Tutorial. Chicago, Ill.: American Medical Association; 1999.

Graber MA, Bergus GR, York CAD. Using the World Wide Web to answer clinical questions: how efficient are different methods of information retrieval? J Fam Pract 1999; 48: 520-524.

Kim P, Eng TR, Deering MJ, et al. Published criteria for evaluating health related web sites: review. BMJ 1999; 318: 647-649.

Pandolfini C, Impicciatore P, Bonati M. Parents on the web: risks for quality management of cough in children. Pediatrics 2000; 105: e1.

Shortliffe EH, Fagan LM, Yu V. The infectious diseases physician and the Internet. In: Mandell GL, Bennett JE, Dolin R, eds. Mandell, Douglas, and Bennett's Principles and Practice of Infectious Diseases. 5th ed., Philadelphia: Churchill Livingstone; 2000: 3258-3263.

6 Temperature Equivalents

Degrees Fahrenheit	Degrees Centigrade
95.0	35.0
96.0	35.5
96.8	36.0
97.0	36.1
98.0	36.6
98.6	37.0
99.0	37.2
100.0	37.7
100.4	38.0
101.0	38.3
102.0	38.8
102.2	39.0
103.0	39.4
104.0	40.0
105.0	40.5
105.8	41.0
106.0	41.1
107.0	41.6
107.6	42.0
108.0	42.2

$^\circ F = (^\circ C \times \frac{9}{5}) + 32$
$^\circ C = (^\circ F - 32) \times \frac{5}{9}$

APPENDIX

7 Abbreviations

AAFP American Academy of Family Physicians
AAP American Academy of Pediatrics
ABW Actual body weight
ACE Angiotensin-converting enzyme
ACIP Advisory Committee on Immunization Practices of the Centers for Disease Control and Prevention
ACOG American College of Obstetricians and Gynecologists
AFB Acid-fast bacillus
AIDS Acquired immunodeficiency syndrome
ALPS Alcoholism, leukopenia, and pneumococcal sepsis
ALT Alanine aminotransferase (also known as SGPT)
AOM Acute otitis media
AP Alkaline phosphatase
APHA American Public Health Association
ARDS Acute (also, adult) respiratory distress syndrome
ASCUS Atypical squamous cells of uncertain significance
ASD Adult Still's disease
ASO Antistreptolysin O
AST Aspartate aminotransferase (also known as SGOT)
ATLL Acute (also, adult) T-cell leukemia lymphoma
ATP Adenosine triphosphate
ATS American Thoracic Society
AUC Area under the curve (serum level of a drug plotted against time after a dose)
AWP Average wholesale price
AZT* Zidovudine (azidothymidine; Retrovir) (also abbreviated ZDV)
BCG Bacille Calmette-Guérin
bDNA Branched DNA
BUN Blood urea nitrogen
BV Bacterial vaginosis
CBC Complete blood count
CDC Centers for Disease Control and Prevention (Atlanta, Georgia)
CF Complement fixation
CFS Chronic fatigue syndrome
CFU Colony-forming unit
CLIA Clinical Laboratories Improvement Act (Public Law 100-578)
C$_{max}$ Peak serum concentration after a dose of a drug

CMV Cytomegalovirus
CNS Central nervous system
COPD Chronic obstructive pulmonary disease (also abbreviated COLD)
CPK Creatinine phosphokinase
CRP C-reactive protein
CSF Cerebrospinal fluid
CT Computed tomography
CTS Casual travel sex
CVA Costovertebral angle
CVC Central venous catheter
DAEC Diffusely adherent *Escherichia coli*
ddI Didanosine
DEET *N,N*-Diethylmetatoluimide
DFA Direct fluorescent antibody
DGI Disseminated gonococcal infection
DHHS Department of Health and Human Services
DMSA Dimercaptosuccinic acid
DNA Deoxyribonucleic acid
DNSSP Drug-nonsusceptible *Streptococcus pneumoniae* strains (also abbreviated DRSP)
DOT Directly observed therapy (for tuberculosis)
DRSP Drug-resistant *Streptococcus pneumoniae* (also abbreviated DNSSP)
DT Diphtheria-tetanus
DtaP Diphtheria and tetanus toxoids and acellular pertussis vaccine
DTC Division of tuberculosis control
DTP Diphtheria-tetanus-pertussis
DWCF Dose weight correction factor
E & M Evaluation and management
EAC Estimated acquisition cost
EAEC Enteroaggregative *Escherichia coli*
EBNA Epstein-Barr virus nuclear antigen
EBV Epstein-Barr virus
ECFV Extracellular fluid volume
EEG Electroencephalography
EHEC Enterohemorrhagic *Escherichia coli*
EIA Enzyme immunoassay
EIEC Enteroinvasive *Escherichia coli*
ELISA Enzyme-linked immunosorbent assay
EM Erythema multiforme
EMB Ethambutol
EPA Environmental Protection Agency
EPEC Enteropathogenic *Escherichia coli*
ESBL Extended-spectrum β-lactamase
ESR Erythrocyte sedimentation rate

---

*Many authorities now prefer "ZDV" over "AZT" because (1) the preferred generic name has been changed from azidothymidine to zidovudine and (2) "AZT" might be confused with the immunosuppressive drug azathioprine (Imuran). Because "AZT" sems to be the preferred abbreviation among most practicing clinicians, at least in our experience, "AZT" has been generally used throughout this text.

ETEC Enterotoxigenic *Escherichia coli*
FA Fluorescent antibody
FDA Food and Drug Administration
FESS Functional endoscopic sinus surgery
FTA-ABS Fluorescent treponemal antibody absorption
FUO Fever of undetermined origin
G6PD Glucose-6 phosphate dehydrogenase
GABHS Group A β-hemolytic streptococcus (*Streptococcus pyogenes*)
GAS Group A streptococcus (GABHS)
GBS Group B streptococcus (*Streptococcus agalactiae*)
GERD Gastroesophageal reflux disease
GGT Gamma-glutamyl transferase
GI Gastrointestinal
GUD Genital ulcer disease
HAART Highly active antiretroviral therapy
HACEK *Haemophilus* species, *Actinobacillus actinomycetemcomitans, Cardiobacterium hominis, Eikenella corrodens,* and *Kingella* species
HAV Hepatitis A virus
HBc Hepatitis B core antigen
Hbe Hepatitis B "e" antigen
HBeAg Hepatitis B early antigen
HBIG Hepatitis B immune globulin
HBsAg Hepatitis B surface antigen
HBV Hepatitis B virus
HCC Hepatocellular carcinoma
HCFA Health Care Financing Administration
HCPC Common Procedure Coding of the Health Care Financing Administration
HCV Hepatitis C virus
HCW Health care worker
HDCV Human diploid cell vaccine
HDV Hepatitis D virus
HEV Hepatitis E virus
HGV Hepatitis G virus
HHV Human herpesvirus
Hib *Haemophilus influenzae* type b
HIV Human immunodeficiency virus
HMO Health maintenance organization
HPF High-power field (on microscopic examination)
HPV Human papillomavirus
HSV Herpes simplex virus
HTLV Human T-cell leukemia virus; human T-cell lymphotropic virus
HUS Hemolytic-uremic syndrome
IBW Ideal body weight
IC Inhibitory concentration
ICD Implantable cardioverter-defibrillator
ICU Intensive care unit
IDSA Infectious Diseases Society of America
IFA Indirect fluorescent antibody
IG Immune globulin
IgA Immunoglobulin A
IgE Immunoglobulin E
IgG Immunoglobulin G
IgM Immunoglobulin M
IM Intramuscular; intramuscularly
INH Isoniazid
IPV Inactivated polio vaccine
IUD Intrauterine contraceptive device

IV Intravenous; intravenously
IVP Intravenous pyelography
KOH Potassium hydroxide
KUB Kidney-ureter-bladder
LCM Lymphocytic choriomeningitis
LCR Ligase chain reaction
LDH Lactate dehydrogenase
LGV Lymphogranuloma venereum
LP Lumbar puncture
LPN Licensed practical nurse
LRI Lower respiratory infection
MAC *Mycobacterium avium-intracellulare* complex
MALT Mucosa-associated lymphoid tissue
MBC Minimum bactericidal concentration
MHA-TP *Treponema pallidum* microhemagglutination assay for antibodies to *Treponema pallidum*
MIC Minimum inhibitory concentration
MLC Minimum lethal concentration
MMPI Minnesota Multiphasic Personality Inventory
MMR Measles-mumps-rubella
MMWR *Morbidity and Mortality Weekly Report,* CDC Surveillance Summaries (Atlanta, Georgia)
MPC Mucopurulent cervicitis
MRI Magnetic resonance imaging
MRSA Methicillin-resistant *Staphylococcus aureus*
MTT Methylthiotetrazole
NA Nuclear antigen
NADH Nicotinamide adenine dinucleotide
NASBA Nucleic acid sequence–based amplification
NGU Nongonococcal urethritis
NIH National Institutes of Health, U.S. Public Health Service
NNRTI Nonnucleoside reverse transcriptase inhibitor
NNT Number needed to treat (or number needed to test)
NRTI Nucleoside reverse transcriptase inhibitor
NSAID Nonsteroidal antiinflammatory drug
NTB Nontuberculous mycobacteria
O&P Ova and parasites
OIG Office of the Inspector General of the U.S. Department of Health and Human Services
OPAT Outpatient parenteral antimicrobial therapy
OPV Oral polio vaccine
ORS Oral rehydration salts
ORT Oral rehydration therapy
OSHA Occupational Safety and Health Administration, U.S. Department of Health and Human Services
PABA Paraaminobenzoic acid
PAE Postantibiotic effect
Pap Papanicolaou
PCEC Purified chick embryo cell
PCP *Pneumocystis carinii* pneumonia
PCR Polymerase chain reaction
PCV Pneumococcal conjugate vaccine
PEP Postexposure prophylaxis
PFADA Periodic fever, aphthous stomatitis, pharyngitis, and cervical adenitis; Marshall's syndrome
PI Protease inhibitor
PICC Peripherally inserted central catheter
PID Pelvic inflammatory disease
PIE Primary infiltrates with eosinophilia
PMN Polymorphonuclear neutrophil

PO Oral; orally
PPD Purified protein derivative
PPI Proton pump inhibitor
PPM Provider-performed microscopy
PPV Polysaccharide pneumococcal vaccine
PRP Polyribosylribitol phosphate
PRSP Penicillin-resistant *Streptococcus pneumoniae*
PSA Prostate specific antigen
PSI Pneumonia severity index
PZA Pyrazinamide
RBC Red blood cell
RIBA Recombinant immunoblot assay
RIG Rabies immune globulin
RN Registered nurse
RPR Rapid plasma reagin (nontreponemal test for syphilis)
RST Rapid streptococcal test
RSV Respiratory syncytial virus
RT-PCR Reverse transcription polymerase chain reaction
RVA Rabies vaccine adsorbed
SANE Sexual assault nurse examiner
SBT Serum bactericidal titer
SDA Strand-displacement amplification
SJS Stevens-Johnson syndrome
SLE Systemic lupus erythematosus
SMAC Sorbitol-MacConkey
SPECT Single photon emission computed tomography
STARI Southern tick-associated rash illness
STD Sexually transmitted disease
STEC Shiga toxin–producing *Escherichia coli* (also known as EHEC)
TB Tuberculosis
TCA Trichloroacetic acid
TCBS Thiosulfate–citrate–bile salts–sucrose
Td Tetanus-diphtheria
TEE Transesophageal echocardiography

TEN Toxic epidermal necrolysis
TK Thymidine kinase
TMA Transcription-mediated amplification
TMP/SMX Trimethoprim-sulfamethoxazole (Bactrim, Septra, and others)
TNF Tumor necrosis factor
TORCHES Toxoplasmosis, rubella, cytomegalovirus, herpes, and syphilis
TP Tube precipitin
TP-PA *Treponema pallidum* particle agglutination
TRUST Toluidine red unheated serum test (test for syphilis)
TSH Thyroid-stimulating hormone
TST Tuberculin skin test
TTV Transfusion-transmitted virus
T½ Serum half-life
URI Upper respiratory infection
USR Unheated serum reagin (test for syphilis)
UTI Urinary tract infection
VAPP Vaccine-associated paralytic polio
VCA Viral capsid antigen
VCUG Voiding cystourethrogram
V$_d$ Volume of distribution
VDRL Venereal Disease Research Laboratory (nontreponemal test for syphilis)
VISA Vancomycin-intermediate *Staphylococcus aureus*
VLM Visceral larval migrans
VRE Vancomycin-resistant enterococci
VRSA Vancomycin-resistant *Staphylococcus aureus*
VVC Vulvovaginal candidiasis
VZIG Varicella-zoster immune globulin
WBC White blood cell; white blood cell count
WHO World Health Organization
ZDV Zidovudine (Retrovir; also commonly known as AZT)

Index